HAGAN AND BRUNER'S INFECTIOUS DISEASES OF DOMESTIC ANIMALS

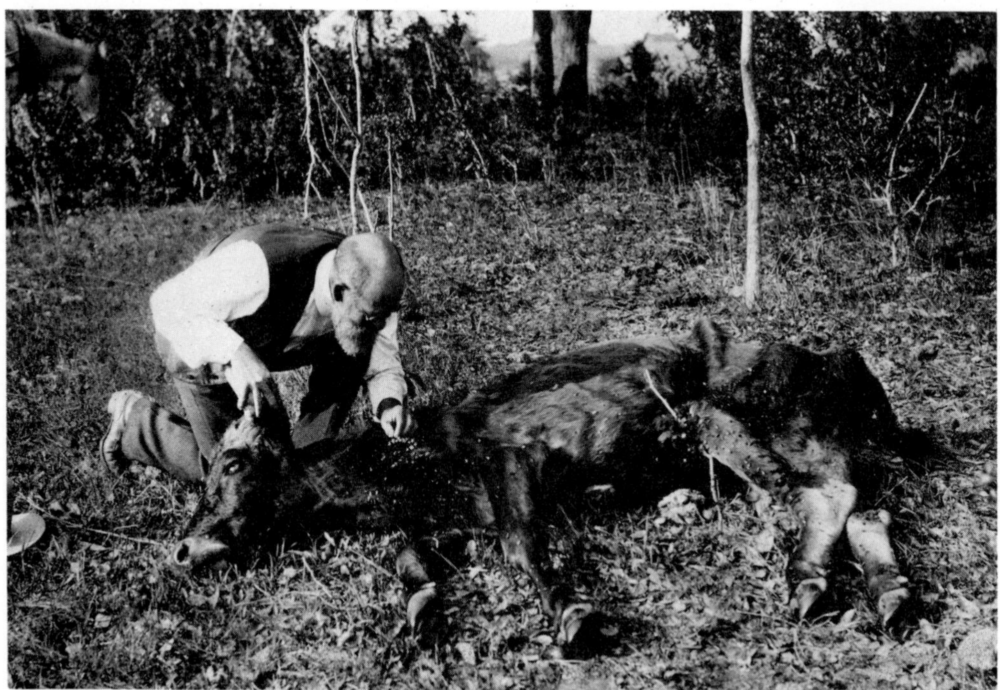

Dr. Cooper Curtice examining ticks on a cow dead of Texas fever. The work of Salmon, Smith, Kilborne, and Curtice (1889–1893) on the causation and mode of transmission of Texas fever is one of the epochal accomplishments in the field of medical history because it was the first to show that arthropods were capable of acting as carriers of agents of diseases of mammals. Curtice championed the "tick theory" of the transmission of this disease, and he was responsible in greater degree than any other person in proving that the southern cattle tick (*Boophilus annulatus*) was the sole carrier of the agent of this disease. (Courtesy *The Nation's Business*.)

HAGAN AND BRUNER'S INFECTIOUS DISEASES OF DOMESTIC ANIMALS

WITH REFERENCE TO ETIOLOGY, PATHOGENICITY, IMMUNITY, EPIDEMIOLOGY, DIAGNOSIS, AND BIOLOGIC THERAPY

JAMES HOWARD GILLESPIE, V.M.D.

Professor of Veterinary Microbiology
Chairman, Department of Veterinary Microbiology
New York State College of Veterinary Medicine
Cornell University

JOHN FRANCIS TIMONEY, B.S., M.V.B., M.S., Ph.D.

Associate Professor of Veterinary Bacteriology
Department of Veterinary Microbiology
New York State College of Veterinary Medicine
Cornell University

SEVENTH EDITION

COMSTOCK PUBLISHING ASSOCIATES *a division of*
CORNELL UNIVERSITY PRESS *Ithaca and London*

First edition, 1943, entitled THE INFECTIOUS DISEASES OF DOMESTIC ANIMALS, by W. A. Hagan. Second edition, 1951, by W. A. Hagan and D. W. Bruner. Third edition, 1957. Fourth edition, 1961.

Fifth edition, 1966, entitled HAGAN'S INFECTIOUS DISEASES OF DOMESTIC ANIMALS, by D. W. Bruner and J. H. Gillespie. Sixth edition, 1973.

Seventh edition, 1981, published by Cornell University Press.
Published in the United Kingdom by Cornell University Press, Ltd., 2–4 Brook Street, London W1Y 1AA.

International Standard Book Number 0-8014-1333-8
Library of Congress Catalog Card Number 80-15937

Printed in the United States of America

Librarians: Library of Congress cataloging information appears on the last page of the book.

For
Bea C. Bruner, Virginia A. Gillespie,
and M. Enid Timoney

In memory of
Esther L. Hagan

Preface to the Seventh Edition

In recognition of Dorsey William Bruner's contributions as coauthor of five earlier editions, the authors of this edition are pleased to add his name to its title. The expertise and devotion he brought to this book are beyond comprehension or appreciation except to those who know Dorsey as a colleague and a close friend. Although he is not listed as an author of this edition, he served as an adviser and editor. Without this assistance, its preparation would have been difficult.

The original objective in writing this book was the creation of a satisfactory textbook for veterinary students in their courses dealing with pathogenic microbiology, immunology, virology, and infectious diseases of domestic animals. The textbook should continue to be valuable to practitioners as well because it covers all aspects of a disease—properties and cultivation of the pathogenic organism, disease characteristics, immunity, epidemiology, diagnostic considerations, prophylaxis, treatment, and the disease in man. Research scientists with an interest in animal disease or comparative microbiology will also find the book useful because it contains many references that provide more detail about a disease. To assure reasonable documentation of the literature, the authors drew heavily upon the computerized system of MEDLARS (Medical Literature Analysis and Retrieval System), which provides abstracts of approximately 2,200 of the world's biomedical journals.

This is an extensive revision of the sixth edition. All chapters of the book covering the pathogenic bacteria, the mycoplasma, and the pathogenic fungi were almost completely rewritten. The chapters on the virales and on the mechanisms of infection and the causes of disease underwent major revisions in this edition. The virology chapters have been reorganized to conform with the latest information on viral taxonomy, which has made great strides since 1971 and now approaches the taxonomical sophistication achieved by bacteriologists and presented in the eighth edition of *Bergey's Manual of Determinative Bacteriology*.

Because it has proved successful in past editions, the format for covering the diseases has not been changed. We have reluctantly dropped the section on pathogenic protozoology so that we could produce a textbook of more manageable size. That decision was aided by the recent appearance of several excellent textbooks that cover pathogenic protozoa of domestic animals. The section on chemotherapy has also been deleted, but the information it contained has been moved to the appropriate sections on individual diseases.

With each new edition the mass of literature covering the various disciplines of pathogenic microbiology, immunology, virology, and epidemiology that contributes to our knowledge of the infectious diseases of domestic animals continues to increase at an incredible rate. It was a humbling experience to review the literature and screen the material for a student textbook.

The listing of only two authors for this edition is misleading because so many fine people contributed to its completion. Dr. Dorsey Bruner assembled the index and aided the authors in reading the proof. Dr. S. Gordon Campbell wrote the chapters on *Brucella, Mycobacterium,* and *Corynebacterium*—a major contribution to the book. Dr. Fernando Noronha assisted the senior author in preparing the section on feline leukemia. Dr. Bruce Calnek, Dr. Neil Norcross, Dr. Leroy Coggins, Dr. Alexander Winter, Dr. Peter Timoney, and other Cornell colleagues provided valuable input and advice. Many professional colleagues, particularly Dr. Frederick Murphy, Dr. Douglas Gregg, and Dr. Jerry Callis, supplied illustrations and suggestions, and to them we are grateful. The efforts of those who assisted the authors in their literature search—Susan Markowitz, Donald McArthur, Antonio Cusano, Deborah Cogan, Christine Pinello, and Janet Gillespie—must be acknowledged. The authors are grateful to those who typed the manuscript—Virginia Gillespie, Angela Jackmin, Polly Marion, and Patricia Mahoney. The staff at Cornell University Press was extremely helpful and supported our task in an efficient, professional, and dedicated manner, particularly Allison Dodge and Daniel Snodderly. We needed all the encouragement and assistance we could obtain, and the Press staff cheerfully obliged us.

In everyone's life there are individuals who greatly influence his or her career. Without the support, sacrifice, and encouragement of his parents, sisters, and brother, the senior author would never have had the opportunity to obtain his professional degree during the Great Depression. Dr. John F. Timoney, Sr., provided the stimulus and inspiration that led to the junior author's chosen career. We humbly pay tribute to these wonderful people.

James H. Gillespie
John F. Timoney

Ithaca, New York

Preface to the First Edition

This book is an outgrowth of a lecture course on pathogenic bacteriology and immunology which the author has given during the last twenty years to students of veterinary medicine. The work is less than a textbook of bacteriology in that a knowledge of the general principles of the subject is taken for granted and this part of the usual text is omitted. It is somewhat more, on the other hand, in that the fungi, protozoa, and viruses that are pathogenic for the domestic animals are included in addition to the bacteria. Also, somewhat greater consideration is given to the nature of the diseases produced by the various agents and to the biological products which are available for their diagnosis, prevention, and cure than is found in most texts of this type.

Since students of animal diseases are interested in microorganisms more because of what they do than for what they are, the work is not a systematic discussion of disease-producing organisms but rather a discussion of the infectious diseases of animals with special reference to their etiological factors.

With regard to the difficult matter of nomenclature of bacteria, *Bergey's Manual* has been followed in general except in the case of the Gram-negative enteric organisms for which the old name *Bacterium* is retained. This is done because it is felt that the numerous divisions which have been made in this group on the basis of cultural features are highly artificial. The newer methods of antigenic analysis do not support these divisions but rather suggest that we have a large group in which there are minor gradations from the colon bacillus at one end to the dysentery organisms at the other without sharp divisions anywhere. Until lines can be drawn more sharply it is felt that there is no justification for the creation of numerous genera within this group.

In instances in which the animal pathogens are transmissible to man, this fact is pointed out and brief discussions of the nature of the human diseases are given, together with what is known of the manner in which the transmission to man occurs. It is felt that veterinarians should be informed on these matters both for their own protection and for the assistance which they often can give to physicians in such cases.

The text will be used by the author in connection with his course in Infectious Diseases of Animals. It is hoped that it will prove suitable for such courses in other schools. In addition it is hoped also that the compilation of brief accounts of the biological characteristics of the etiological agents of all of the more important infectious diseases of animals in a single volume will make it useful to veterinary practitioners, laboratory workers who are called upon to make diagnoses of these conditions, and research workers who utilize animals in their daily work. Because of the wide scope of the field covered and the necessary limitations in a book designed for student use, the discussions are not exhaustive. Diseases which are known to occur in North America are treated more exhaustively than those which do not occur here. Since experience shows, however, that diseases which are thought to occur only in remote parts of the world often exist here in an unrecognized form, and that it is always possible that remote diseases may be imported, an effort has been made to include brief descriptions of all of the more important of such diseases and their causative agents. A few references are given at the end of each subject so those who wish to read more exhaustively may find the more important papers in the literature. Since most students and practitioners do not have a working knowledge of foreign languages, the greater part of the references are to papers published in English. By consulting the bibliographies given in most of these papers one can obtain leads which will open the entire literature to him.

The author is indebted to many friends for various kinds of assistance. The illustrations, in particular, have been borrowed from many sources, acknowledgment being made in each case. The author is especially grateful to Dr. William H. Feldman, of the Mayo Foundation, for reading and making numerous criticisms of the copy, criticisms which undoubtedly have contributed to greater clarity and greater accuracy in the volume. To all of those who have helped he wishes to extend his hearty thanks.

In a first edition of this kind many errors undoubtedly have been included. The author will appreciate having these called to his attention in order that they may be eliminated from future editions if the reception of the work warrants future revisions. In many instances it is realized that subjects are still in the stage of controversy. An attempt has been made not to be too didactic in the treating of such matters; however, in the interest of good pedagogical practice some sort of a stand usually is taken in such matters after it has been indicated that uncertainty exists.

W. A. HAGAN

New York State Veterinary College
Cornell University, Ithaca, New York
June 1942

Contents

PART III
THE MYCOPLASMAS

PART IV
THE RICKETTSIAE

PART V

THE PATHOGENIC FUNGI

PART VI

THE VIRALES

SECTION I GENERAL VIROLOGY

HAGAN AND BRUNER'S INFECTIOUS DISEASES OF DOMESTIC ANIMALS

PART I

THE MECHANISMS OF INFECTION AND RESISTANCE

1 The Mechanisms of Infection and the Causes of Infectious Disease

Disease may be defined as an alteration of the state of the body, or of some of its organs, which interrupts or disturbs the proper performance of the bodily functions. Functional disturbance soon is manifested by physical signs which the patient detects by his sensations and which usually can be detected by others.

Disease may be of external or of internal origin. Little is known about the fundamental causes of the intrinsic diseases. These include metabolic and endocrine disturbances, degeneration of organs from age, neoplasms, and possibly autoimmunity. It is probable that many of these disorders are initiated by extrinsic causes as yet unrecognized. The external causes of disease may be living agents such as bacteria, protozoa, or viruses, or they may be nonliving agents such as traumatism, heat, cold, chemical poisons, or food deficiencies.

When living agents enter an animal body and set up a disturbance of function in any part, *infection* is said to have occurred. The word *infection* is derived from the Latin *inficere,* meaning "to put into." An *infectious disease* is one caused by the presence in or on an animal body of a foreign living organism, which creates a disturbance leading to the development of signs of illness.

Most infections are caused by living organisms that have escaped from another individual of the same species, but sometimes they come from another species. This occurs when man develops rabies from a dog bite, or when a lap dog contracts tuberculosis from its consumptive master. Sometimes the infection is obtained indirectly, as when typhoid fever is contracted by a man from infected drinking water, or anthrax by a stable-fed horse in midwinter from hay that had been grown the previous summer on anthrax-infected soil. Some infections originate from organisms that normally live a free existence in nature, as, for example, the bacillus of tetanus. Presumably at some remote periods in evolutionary history, all the disease-producing organisms lived a free existence, becoming parasitic and pathogenic through gradual adaptation.

The Fates of Infecting Organisms

Several possible fates await organisms that cause infections. This is a matter of considerable practical interest, because the transmission of the disease to other individuals occurs by vertical or horizontal means, usually by the latter mechanism.

1. Some organisms are destroyed by the host tissue. Infections are not accomplished without resistance on the part of the host, because the host-parasite relationship is not a natural one. The capacity of the host to destroy invading agents is so great that a large majority of the foreign living agents that manage to reach living tissues and fluids of the body are rapidly and completely destroyed. This is a continual process. Sometimes the resistance is not sufficient to prevent growth and multiplication in the tissues, but the infection does not become extensive, and after a brief time the invading organisms are destroyed. Sometimes the agent persists and makes slow headway against the resistance of the host, in which case the infection is called *chronic*. In a few infections such an anthrax in the herbivorous animals, the resis-

tance of the host is overwhelmed so quickly that the organism multiplies in all parts and early death of the hosts ensues. These cases are known as *acute*, or *peracute*.

2. Some organisms usually are eliminated in the secretions or excretions of the host. Except in the peracute cases, when possibly no infecting organisms escape from the host, the diseased animal usually eliminates, in a manner that varies with the disease, the organism that causes it. In chronic infections the host usually eliminates large numbers of the infecting agent. Sometimes this agent is removed through pus, as when an abscess bursts or is lanced; sometimes through droplets that are discharged when the individual is suffering from one of the respiratory infections, as canine distemper, bovine tuberculosis, avian coryza, or human diphtheria; sometimes in the intestinal discharges (feces), as in the various forms of intestinal coccidiosis of animals and in the enteric infections of man; sometimes in the urine, as in cholera of swine and in typhoid fever of man. In some diseases that become extensive and even fatal, the causative organism may be eliminated in small numbers or not at all, as in some cases of tuberculosis. The more chronic the disease becomes, the less likelihood there is that the host will continue to retain all the infecting organisms. In some diseases the mechanism by which the infection escapes from one animal to another is peculiar, as, for example, in rabies, in which the seat of the infection is the central nervous system and the means of escape is through the salivary glands.

3. If the disease proves fatal to the host, many of the infecting organisms are destroyed with the carcass. Death of the host from infection always traps in the carcass a large number of the involved organisms. If the carcass is disposed of properly by incineration or deep burial, these organisms perish. Improper disposal of the dead bodies of animals may result in serious outbreaks of disease.

4. In some instances the organism and host reach an impasse. The organism is unable to cause serious damage to the host, and yet the host is unable to eliminate the organism. This situation may continue throughout the lifetime of the animal, or it may be terminated either by the final elimination of the infection or by a change in which the infection becomes more active and signs of disease are manifested by the host. In tuberculosis of both man and animals, the tubercle bacilli may become walled off by dense tissue in some of the organs and the case is said to be *arrested*. Such cases are not entirely cured because living tubercle organisms may continue to exist in the tissues and sometimes they break forth and cause a flare-up of the disease. In man, recovery from typhoid fever usually leaves the individual with many typhoid bacilli in his urine and stools, and these may persist for weeks, months, and years. Individuals who discharge virulent organisms with their excretions, although apparently normal otherwise, are said to be *carriers*. One who has had a recognized disease and who has not rid himself of the infecting agent is said to be a *convalescent carrier*. Sometimes individuals eliminate virulent infection although they have no history of ever having suffered from the disease themselves. These individuals are immune but are a source of great danger to others who lack the same amount of resistance. They are known as *immune carriers* or sometimes as *asymptomatic carriers*. At times individuals harbor and eliminate a dangerous organism that they have picked up from close contact with another individual. These are known as *contact carriers*.

The carrier is one of the great problems in the control of many infectious diseases. Animals that are obviously diseased may be recognized, but there is no simple way of recognizing the carrier.

Sources of Infection

The courses by which infections reach new hosts often are indirect and complicated. Some of the more common ways by which infections are contracted by new hosts are as follows.

1. Direct or immediate contact with a diseased individual. This involves actual contact between a diseased and a normal surface, such as when a cow licks the external genitals of another animal and thus picks up the organism of Bang's disease or brucellosis, or when ringworm is contracted by an animal's rubbing against the affected skin of another, or when venereal infections are transferred through sexual contact, or when an infection is transmitted by an animal's bite.

2. Contact through fomites. *Fomites* (fomes) are inanimate objects that may serve to carry infections from one animal to another, such as a bran sack that may convey dried discharge of an aborting cow to another cow, perhaps in a different herd, or a railroad stock car or a motor truck that has not been properly cleaned and disinfected after carrying diseased stock.

3. Contact with disease carriers. A disease carrier may infect others either directly or indirectly just as is done by a frankly diseased individual.

4. Infection from soil. Certain spore-bearing or-

ganisms that live in soil are able to produce disease in animals if chance carries them into the tissues, usually through wounds in the skin. Tetanus and gas gangrene infections are of this type.

5. Infections from food and water. Serious infections derived from food and water are more common in man than in animals, because animals do not suffer from the typhoid and dysentery organisms that are the principal menaces to man. Water often is suspected of spreading animal diseases from one pasture to another when small streams flow between them, and occasionally the suspicion has been confirmed. Leptospirosis often is transmitted in this way. Anthrax is conveyed to animals through hay and straw raised on lowlands infected with anthrax spores. There have been a considerable number of reports of deaths of horses from eating ensilage which proved innocuous to cattle, and the organism of botulism has been incriminated in some of these cases.

6. Air-borne infections. Disease organisms do not spread very far through the air, though it was formerly believed they did. When individuals are close together and especially indoors, droplets of moisture sneezed and coughed from the upper air passages often convey the organisms of respiratory disease from diseased to well individuals. The common cold of man, influenzal infections of man and animals, and glanders are good examples of diseases transmitted in this way. Tuberculosis of the lungs is usually transmitted in this fashion. Dust particles less often convey viable disease-producing organisms, but there are some examples such as the anthrax spore (in woolsorter's disease), *Escherichia coli* (in hospital outbreaks of infant diarrhea), and spores of the higher fungi (in coccidioidomycosis and histoplasmosis).

7. Infections from bloodsucking arthropods. Some diseases of man and animals are normally transmitted through the bites of flies, fleas, mosquitoes, lice, or ticks. Malaria and yellow fever are good examples of such diseases of man, and Texas fever, anaplasmosis, anthrax, and the trypanosome diseases are examples in animals. In some instances, the infecting organism must pass a part of its life cycle in the invertebrate host, as, for example, the malaria and yellow fever parasites in the mosquito, in which case the arthropod is known as a *biological vector*. In other instances, such as anthrax, the black horsefly merely carries the bacillus mechanically, not being affected by it in any way. In these cases, the arthropod carrier is known as a *mechanical vector*.

8. Infections from organisms normally carried. Pathogenic streptococci, pneumococci, *Pasteurella*, and some other organisms can often be found on the mucous membranes of the head of apparently normal individuals. It is believed that infections sometimes occur from such organisms when the normal defensive forces of the body are weakened in any way.

9. Infections acquired in the laboratory. These usually appear in those who work with highly virulent and infectious microorganisms such as *Brucella melitensis, Pasteurella tularensis, Coxiella burneti,* and *Coccidioides immitis*.

Infection and Contagion

A contagious disease is one that may be transmitted from one individual to another by direct or indirect contact. All contagious diseases are also infectious, but it does not follow that all infectious diseases are contagious. Tetanus and gas gangrene infections, caused by organisms that live in the soil, are infectious but not contagious, because they are not transmitted from one animal to another. The contagiousness of infectious diseases depends on the way the parasites are eliminated from the body of the diseased animal and the opportunity they have of reaching others. Some infectious diseases are highly contagious, some are slightly contagious, and a few are not contagious at all.

Superinfection, Mixed Infection, and Synergistic Relationships

Superinfection refers to a fresh invasion or reinfection added to an already existing infection. Some definitions limit the use of the term to organisms of the same species that caused the initial infection. A *mixed infection* is one in which more than one species of organism is present. This same phenomenon has been referred to as a *secondary infection* when it is established that the primary infection presents conditions favorable for invasion by another organism.

Superinfection has been reported *in vitro* in a study of Daudi cells (human Burkitt's lymphoma) that are superinfected with the P3HR-1 strain of Epstein-Barr virus (20), and recently in an *in vivo* study in which it became evident that a polyoma-virus-induced tumor became infected with an endogenous mouse virus when passaged through nude mice (15).

The bovine mammary gland is often the residence of mixed infections of *Corynebacterium pyogenes* and various species of streptococci and staphylococci (21).

Canine distemper is caused by a paramyxovirus that often gives rise to very few pathological changes. The typical clinical and necropsy picture associated with canine distemper is attributable to the mixed secondary invasion that almost invariably occurs. The commonest secondary invader is *Bordetella bronchiseptica* but *Mycoplasma, Toxoplasma,* and coccidia species may also be present (6).

There are many examples of *synergism* in animal diseases. The term *synergism* refers to the action of two or more agents to produce a result (clinical state) that neither could effect alone. Suppurative infections of the liver in cattle fall into this descriptive category. *Fusobacterium necrophorum* and *Corynebacterium pyogenes* are frequently found in combination, the former being established in the anaerobic conditions of the necrotic damaged liver tissue (4). *Treponema hyodysenteriae* has been established as the primary causal agent in swine dysentery; however, the fibrinonecrotic colitis seen in the disease is thought to be caused by the synergistic effect of this spirochete and normal gut flora such as *Campylobacter* species. This conclusion is based in part on studies using gnotobiotic pigs, in which the intestinal anaerobes are lacking and consequently the clinical disease is not manifest (4, 14).

Properties of Pathogenic Organisms

Virulence. *Virulence* is an attribute of all pathogenic or disease-producing organisms. The word has reference to their disease-producing power or malignancy. A highly virulent organism has great malignancy, a slightly virulent one has little, and a nonvirulent one has none. The property of virulence varies greatly, both among different species of parasitic forms and among different strains of the same species. In some parts of the world smallpox was a highly malignant disease; in others it was very mild. In some years influenzal infections are mild; in others, severe. In the laboratory one may sometimes cause the death of a white mouse by inoculating it with as little as 0.001 ml of a strain of *Streptococcus,* whereas another strain of the same species of *Streptococcus* may not kill a mouse when 0.1 ml is inoculated. The one strain in this case may be said to be at least 100 times as virulent as the other.

Alteration of Virulence. The pathogenic power, or virulence, of many disease-producing organisms can be altered readily in the laboratory; others resist such alteration. It has been suggested that possibly the ability to change virulence is evidence that the organism has only recently acquired this property, and thus it is not a firmly fixed characteristic.

The process of diminishing the virulence of an organism is known as *attenuation.* Attenuated organisms often are used as vaccines. Attenuation of virulence is readily accomplished in most instances; in fact the mere procedure of artificial cultivation is enough to attenuate most organisms to some extent. Many methods are available for reducing the disease-producing power of organisms. Some of the more common for bacteria are as follows.

1. Cultivating the organism at an unfavorable temperature. Pasteur found that anthrax bacilli quickly lost virulence when they were incubated at 42 to 43 C, a temperature about 5 degrees above their optimum.
2. Heating cultures or infective material for a short time to a point a little below the thermal death point of the organism.
3. Cultivating the organism on a medium rendered unfavorable by the presence of small amounts of acids, alkalies, metallic salts, dyes, or other substances. On such media many organisms may grow well if the concentration of the attenuating agent is gradually increased from day to day.
4. Plating the organism on a suitable medium and selecting a nonvirulent colony. Usually this is accomplished by picking the more granular-appearing type of colony. (See the next section, "Microbic Dissociation and Change of Virulence.")
5. Injecting the organism into a species of animal that is quite resistant naturally, or whose resistance has been increased by partial immunization, and recovering it after a sojourn there.
6. Injecting the organism into an animal and, after permitting its multiplication in this host for a time, passing it to a second individual of the same species. From the second animal it is carried in the same way to a third, and so on in a series of individuals. However, by such process some disease organisms may be *adapted* to a certain animal species and become highly virulent for it. Frequently in the process of adaptation to the one species of animal, it loses much or all of its virulence for others.

When an increase in the virulence of an organism is desired, all methods often fail, particularly if the organism has become highly attenuated. The procedure usually followed is to inoculate heavily an animal known to be highly susceptible, with the hope of overwhelming it with the infection. If this succeeds, another animal is immediately inoculated from the first, and so on. The virulence of some disease-producing agents may be enormously increased in this way. As a rule, the practice of growing avirulent bacteria in fresh animal serum, or in immune serum, fails to enhance virulence.

Burnet (5) in 1925 indicated that the cultivation of one species of microorganism in the presence of another enabled the first to acquire properties of the second. He called this phenomenon *entraînement*. In 1927 Frobisher and Brown (13) were able to cause a harmless *Streptococcus* from cheese to acquire the property of forming erythrogenic toxin (scarlet fever toxin) by growing it in contact with scarlet fever streptococci. In 1932 Alloway (1) found that extracts of dead, smooth Type 3 pneumococci would induce live, rough non-type-specific forms of Type 2 pneumococci to change into smooth Type 3 pneumococci. The new Type 3, like other Type 3 pneumococci, was highly virulent.

In 1951 Freeman (12) reported that it was possible to isolate virulent strains of *Corynebacterium diphtheriae* from avirulent cultures by exposing them to diphtheria bacteriophage. His studies indicated an association between lysogenicity and virulence (toxigenicity) in diphtheria bacilli. Later studies have confirmed that toxigenicity in *Corynebacterium diphtheriae* is the result of the action of phage genes which direct the synthesis of toxin in the host cell.

Bacteriophage can also transfer genes from one bacterium to another. These phenomena are discussed more fully in Chapter 3.

Microbic Dissociation and Change of Virulence. Certain growth phenomena that may be observed both macroscopically and microscopically are associated with change in virulence in many bacterial cultures. These were first described by Arkwright (2) in England in 1920 and by De Kruif (9) in the United States in 1921. Many of these phenomena had been seen earlier, but their significance had not been fully appreciated. The changes of the type of which we speak may easily be observed on ordinary culture media, especially of the solid type. When cells of a single bacterial culture are streaked on the surface of a solid medium, the colonies that develop are often not alike but may be differentiated into several types. The extremes of these are the so-called S-type (smooth type) and the R-type (rough type). Between these two there may be several intergrading forms. These types may be seen even when the culture is the progeny of a single bacterial cell; thus it is not a matter of a cultural mixture of types, except insofar as the progeny of single cells may vary from one another. In most cases certain other characteristics are associated with each of the colony types. The more important of these characteristics are described below.

S-type colonies are recognized by a smooth, glistening surface and rather regular margins. In consistency such colonies usually are soft and buttery. When grown in broth, these organisms usually produce uniform clouding of the medium, and, when suspended in physiological salt solution, uniform and stable suspensions are formed. Organisms of the smooth type usually are good antigens. They are excellent immunizing agents and, when agglutinated with specific antisera, produce large flocculi. If the organism is pathogenic, this form usually is highly virulent. Such organisms frequently produce capsules and are relatively resistant to phagocytosis.

R-type colonies differ from the preceding in that they have a rough or uneven contour, or at least show a granular structure under magnification and proper illumination that is not seen in the S-types. In consistency such colonies are friable or granular. When grown in a fluid medium, the growth usually is in the form of a pellicle and sediment, and when attempts are made to suspend such cells in salt solution, they usually fail because the cells form into flakes and clumps which settle out. While, in general, changed colony formation, stability in broth, and changed serological characteristics go hand in hand, many cultures produce colonies that are quite rough in appearance; yet their broth cultures are stable and they retain most of their normal antigenic complex. In *Salmonella* studies the Pampana (18) trypaflavin test for the deduction of roughness follows the serological behavior of S and R antigens more closely than does any other test (11). If the parent culture was pathogenic, the R-type variant usually is not. Capsules are not produced, and such cells usually are easily phagocytosed. Such strains usually are poor antigens, that is, they immunize poorly.

Intermediate types usually have some of the characteristics of both R- and S-types. In some cultures several intermediate types may be recognized; in others they are not seen.

Dissociation of most bacterial cultures into S- and R-forms occurs naturally when the cultures are growing in culture media, and in many cases also when growing in tissues. Various ways have been found to force dissociation to occur in culture media when it does not occur readily otherwise. Many smooth strains, for example, can be made to develop the rough form by cultivating them in culture media to which immune serum has been added. In general, S-R dissociation takes place more rapidly in fluid than on solid culture media. Spontaneous dissociation from the S- to the R-form occurs readily in most cultures, sometimes to the extent that the S-form disappears entirely. The R- to S-form of dissociation, however, is not often seen spontaneously and is not easily forced.

The significance of dissociation in relation to virulence is clear. It affords a possible clue to the reason why pathogenic bacteria in artificial culture tend to become less virulent, why such organisms in chronic infections often are attenuated in virulence, why vaccines sometimes are efficacious and sometimes not, and why some strains of organisms make satisfactory antigens for agglutination tests and others do not. If virulence is to be retained, if vaccines are to be effective, and if cultures are to make good agglutination antigens, means of keeping the strain in the S-form must be found. In many cases this is not difficult, it being necessary only to make frequent plate cultures and to select S-type colonies for propagating the strain. Inoculation of susceptible animals is another way to eliminate rough and intermediate variants from a culture. If the culture has not lost all virulence, the animal will act selectively, destroying the nonvirulent types and yielding finally only the smooth type.

Evolution of Pathogenicity. Many diseases apparently are not so destructive today as they once were. The reasons for this obviously are not simple, and probably they have to do with changes in both host and parasite. Mass immunization or "herd immunity," which gradually raises the resistance of populations, probably is a factor. It will be discussed later. Better nutrition and better hygienic conditions of many kinds probably have played a part. Genetic factors evidently are at work because destructive disease tends to eliminate the more susceptible and leave the resistant strains. Years ago Theobald Smith (22) suggested that it should be expected that infectious diseases would evolve into more chronic, less virulent forms in the course of time, even if the host resistance did not change in the meantime. The reasoning behind this conclusion was that in acute disease the parasite quickly destroys its host and thus quickly terminates its own chances of escaping to new hosts, whereas in chronic disease the opportunity for escape is much better because of the prolonged course of the disease. Under such conditions, Smith concluded that the chronic form had a better chance of propagating itself and would, in time, become the predominating form.

The Mechanism of Disease Production by Pathogenic Organisms

The possession of the property of virulence distinguishes pathogenic organisms from the nonpathogenic. In the final analysis virulence depends on two properties of the organism:

(*a*) The ability to propagate in the tissues or on the surface of the body.

(*b*) The ability to form chemical substances that injure or destroy body cells, organs, or tissues.

Ability to Propagate in Tissues. The ability to grow in an animal body is something that an organism acquires in its evolution toward a parasitic existence. Obviously the organism has to "learn" how to protect itself against forces in the body that are antagonistic to it. Virulent organisms usually, but not invariably, are of the S-type, which means that they are more or less resistant to phagocytosis and often possess capsular or surface substances that serve to protect them from harmful influences in the tissue fluids.

The ability to invade and multiply in living tissues varies a great deal among disease-producing organisms. Some organisms that are malignant-disease producers have little invasive ability and do most of their damage while growing in restricted parts of the body, in which they generate powerful poisons, or toxins, that are absorbed and circulated throughout the body. The tetanus organism, for example, usually remains localized in a wound which may be very insignificant in size, but in this wound the tetanus toxin is generated, which is carried to the nervous system, where the damage is done. The organism of human diphtheria is rarely found in the internal organs but is usually restricted to the membranes of the throat, where the diphtheria toxin is generated. These bacteria produce systemic diseases only because of the absorption of their toxins.

The organisms that lack soluble toxins must have considerable powers of invasiveness if they are to produce systemic disease, or disease of any of the vital organs. Such organisms produce their principal damage at the points where they are multiplying. Sometimes they localize near the point where they enter the body and do not extend far from this site. These are known as *local infections*. Most wound infections are of this type. Others characteristically invade lymph and blood vessels, whence they are carried to many other parts of the body, a process known as *metastasis,* where secondary localizations occur. These are the *systemic* or *general infections*.

In speaking of invasiveness we should not develop the idea that organisms actively drive or bore their way into tissues. Many actively invading organisms are nonmotile. In most instances, bacteria probably enter the tissues in the same way that inanimate particles do. Organisms on mucous membranes are often picked up by wandering phagocytic cells which find their way back into the tissues carrying their bacterial load with them. These cells often destroy their bacterial meal, in which case nothing happens; but in other cases the bacterial load survives, destroys the cell that harbors it, and then proceeds to initiate an infection of the tissues where it finds itself. Other organisms colonize on surfaces and reach the subepithelial tissues by direct extension of growth through glands and hair follicles. Certain bacteria produce the enzyme hyaluronidase. This enzyme may aid in the spread of these bacteria throughout the tissues by hydrolyzing hyaluronic acid, a viscous mucopolysaccharide that binds water in the interstitial tissues, thereby holding cells together in a jellylike matrix and acting ordinarily as a physical barrier to invasion by foreign substances (17). This acid also is present in synovial fluid, and its destruction in joint cavities appears to be related to certain rheumatic diseases. If the organism possesses the property of virulence, it will go on from this point to produce an infection; if it does not, it will be picked up by the fixed or wandering phagocytic cells of the tissue and destroyed.

As a general rule, bacteria do not multiply in the circulating fluids of the body. When many bacteria are found in the blood, a condition we call *bacteremia,* it means that there are foci in the tissues from which the organisms are being poured forth in such large numbers that the blood-clearing mechanism is temporarily overwhelmed.

At one time it was seriously believed that microorganisms might produce disease in a purely mechanical way, that is, by blocking capillaries or tissue spaces. This idea is untenable because it is known that the body has mechanisms for dealing with rather large amounts of foreign solids, more than the total bulk of bacteria present even in overwhelming infections. The damage caused by infecting organisms is clearly due to their metabolic activities.

Ability to Form Toxins. Toxins are divided into three groups according to the type of organism that produces them:

1. The phytotoxins, such as *ricin* of the castor bean plant, and the *amanita toxin* of the poisonous fungi of that name (toadstools).
2. The zootoxins, such as the venoms of certain snakes, spiders, and fish.
3. The bacterial toxins, such as those of the organisms causing diphtheria, tetanus, and botulism.

Toxins usually exhibit specific affinities for certain cells or tissues; thus we have *neurotoxins,* such as those of tetanus and botulism, *hemolytic toxins,* such as those of many streptococci and the organism of tetanus, and leukotoxins or *leukocidins,* such as those of the pyogenic staphylococci. The first type combines with and injures or destroys nerve cells, the second destroys erythrocytes, and the third destroys leukocytes. When toxins are injected into the blood of susceptible animals, they quickly disappear from it; furthermore, in diseases in which toxins play a predominating role, seldom can more than traces be found in the circulating blood. Toxins are quickly absorbed by the cells or tissues for which they have affinities. This can easily be demonstrated *in vitro;* suspensions of nerve cells will combine with and inactivate the neurotoxins, and erythrocytes will do likewise with the hemolytic toxins. Suspensions of other types of cells will not do this. It is interesting to note also that tetanus toxin will circulate for days in the blood of some cold-blooded animals, and diphtheria toxin disappears very slowly from the blood of rats. These animals are not susceptible to these toxins, and their tissues have little affinity for them.

Endotoxins. It is clear that substances mildly toxic to animal tissues are contained in most bacteria. Extracts of many purely saprophytic organisms often are distinctly poisonous when injected into animals. These substances apparently occur intracellularly as lipid-polysaccharide-polypeptide complexes and are structural components of the bacterial cell that represent O antigen and occur, for the most part, in the cell wall. Endotoxins may be extracted or they may be released by the mechanical disruption of bacterial cells. They are heat-stable and resistant to proteolytic enzymes, but are destroyed by mild acid hydrolysis. Systemic injection of endotoxins produces a variety of effects including fever, thrombosis (resulting in the Shwartzman phenomenon), abortion, and vascular shock. Endotoxins are excellent antigens in stimulating the formation of agglutinins, but these antibodies fail to neutralize the toxic effects of the endotoxin, although they combine with it.

It is possible that the difference between a pathogenic and a nonpathogenic organism, if pathogenicity depends upon endotoxins, is that the former has the ability to penetrate into the body in the face of the resistance offered by the body's protective mechanism, to multiply and colonize in various tissues and organs, and there to release its poisons, while the latter lacks this ability. Pathogenic bacteria that do not form any recognizable poisons, other than endotoxins, must have the property of invasiveness.

Exotoxins. Certain plants and animals and a few bacteria secrete or excrete substances that are highly toxic to animals. These products have a number of properties in common, yet each toxin is highly distinctive or specific. The cardinal characteristic of exotoxins is that they are *antigenic,* that is, that they will stimulate in animals *antibodies* which will neutralize them *in vivo* or *in vitro.*

Physical Properties of Toxins. 1. Most toxins are comparatively thermolabile. Heating to 58 to 60 C for 10 minutes will inactivate most toxins. A few are more resistant.

2. All toxins deteriorate with age. Some lose their potency very rapidly, while others deteriorate rather slowly. The speed of deterioration depends on the conditions under which they are held. They usually keep best when stored in darkness and at a low temperature. If carefully dried and stored in a dry atmosphere, many toxins can be maintained with little change for long periods.

When toxins deteriorate, it is the poisonous portion that disappears first. Antigenicity is retained long after all traces of toxicity have been lost. Toxins that have lost their poisonous properties but have retained antigenicity are known as *toxoids.*

3. Toxins are composed of relatively large molecules. They will diffuse through parchment but not through the thicker collodion membranes. Their molecular size evidently is less than that of albumins and globulins but larger than that of the amino acids.

4. Most toxins require a "period of incubation" before showing their poisonous effects. Many of the bacterial toxins, and some of the others, do not cause signs of illness immediately after injection. Even when enormous doses are given to experimental animals, there usually is a delay of several hours before signs appear. This is quite different from the action of other highly active poisons such as prussic acid and strychnine, in which the signs of intoxication are immediate. Most poisons have small molecules and are readily diffusible; the toxins have large molecules and do not readily diffuse through membranes. Because poisoning does not occur until the poison has diffused into the susceptible cells, the lag period shown by toxins can be explained on this basis. It is possible, too, that toxins have to be activated in some way before they become poisonous.

Chemical Properties of Toxins. 1. All toxins are antigenic poisons. It has already been stated that this is the prime, or cardinal, characteristic that separates these poisons from all others. The antibodies stimulated by the presence of toxin in the tissues of animals are always highly specific, that is, they will neutralize only the type of toxin that caused their production.

2. Toxins can be precipitated from solution by concentrated alcohol, metallic salts, and ammonium sulfate. In these respects their reactions are like those of proteins.

3. Toxins can be concentrated and purified by adsorption on aluminum hydroxide gels and elution from them. In this respect they resemble enzymes.

4. Toxins can be crystallized. This is the highest degree of purification yet attained. Crystalline botulism toxin may be prepared by initial acid precipitation of the poison from solution, followed by shaking with chloroform, and salting out with ammonium sulfate (16). The crystals are in the form of needles and are pure protein, having the properties of globulin. Accordingly, certain toxins are protein in nature, but whether this applies to all toxins, or whether some of them are merely adsorbed to proteins, remains to be answered.

5. Most toxins are readily destroyed by proteolytic enzymes. Peptic or tryptic digestion quickly destroys the majority of toxins. The toxin of *Clostridium botulinum,* which causes botulism because of its absorption through the digestive tract, is quite resistant.

6. Toxins can be changed to toxoids by chemical treatment. It has already been stated that toxins tend to deteriorate naturally into nonpoisonous substances called *toxoids.* The importance of toxoids lies in the fact that they retain the immunizing properties of toxins while losing their poisonous properties. Toxins can quickly be converted into toxoids by treatment with certain chemicals, notably formaldehyde. Formaldehyde-treated toxins are used for immunization against human diphtheria and against tetanus. Ramon (19), who developed the method, calls these products *anatoxins,* and they are so designated in the French literature. The term is used in English, but the word *toxoid* is more common.

Other Active Constituents Produced by Pathogenic Bacteria. Many years ago (1900), Bail (3) and his coworkers in Germany showed that sterile filtrates of the exudate which collect under the skin of animals after the injection of any of a number of pathogenic organisms had remarkable properties. The phenomena are highly specific for the organism used for injection. Several of the more important of these observations are as follows.

1. When the filtrate alone is injected into normal animals, no reactions are observed at the time, but later it can be shown that the animals have developed antibodies specific for the organism.

2. When the filtrate is injected with sublethal doses of the organism, the combination becomes lethal.

3. When the filtrate is injected with a dose of the bacterial culture that would have caused a chronic disease, the disease produced is acute.

4. When the filtrate is injected with a strain of the organism that has been attenuated so it no longer will produce infection when injected alone, the mixture will cause infection.

The agent in the exudate that apparently increases the virulence of the specific organism was called *aggressin*. Others called it *virulin*. It is now apparent that the word *aggressin* does not refer to a single substance secreted by bacteria, as Bail supposed, but to a property dependent on the release from bacteria, in or out of the body, of substances such as capsular material, bacterial protein, secretions, excretions, enzymes, and toxins that have a deleterious effect on the tissues of the host, thereby interfering with the host's defensive mechanism and permitting multiplication of the organism in the tissues.

Thus certain pathogenic *Staphylococcus aureus* strains were shown to produce a coagulase that accelerated the clotting of human and rabbit plasma (8), and Tillet and Garner (23) demonstrated an antigenic substance in hemolytic streptococci that dissolved human fibrin. This fibrinolysin behaves in many ways like an enzyme and is produced by most Group A, C, and G streptococci associated with suppurative and invasive types of human infection. For the most part these activities are broadly related to virulence.

Among the more important bacterial products can be listed the "spreading" or "diffusing" factors (10). These substances are elaborated by certain strains of staphylococci, streptococci, pneumococci, diphtheria bacilli, and clostridia. The identity of these bacteria-spreading factors with the enzyme hyaluronidase was suggested by Chaine and Duthie (7). This enzyme hydrolyzes hyaluronic acid, an ingredient of the intercellular ground substance of mesodermal tissue, and by so doing permits the ready diffusion of fluid and bacteria through the intercellular spaces. In certain experimental infections it appears that the addition of hyaluronidase to the inoculum enhances the virulence of the organisms. However, the role of hyaluronidase in infections by organisms that produce this substance themselves is not entirely clear because there is no complete correlation between invasiveness and hyaluronidase production. In fact, this enzyme may even interfere with the virulence of certain encapsulated microorganisms by digesting their mucoid capsules.

Other enzymes besides those mentioned above also influence infection by alteration of the metabolism of the tissues.

REFERENCES

1. Alloway. Jour. Exp. Med., 1932, *55*, 91.
2. Arkwright. Jour. Path. and Bact., 1920, *23*, 358.
3. Bail. Zentrbl. f. Bakt., I Abt., 1900, *27*, 10 and 517; 1902, *33*, 343.
4. Blood, D. C., J. A. Henderson, and O. M. Radostits. Veterinary medicine, 5th ed. Lea and Febiger, Philadelphia, 1979.
5. Burnet. Comp. rend. Soc. Biol. (Paris), 1925, *93*, 1422.
6. Catcott, E. J. (ed.). Canine Medicine, 4th ed. American Veterinary Publications, Inc., Wheaton, Ill., 1979.
7. Chain and Duthie. Brit. Jour. Exp. Path., 1940, *21*, 324.
8. Chapman, Berens, Peters, and Curcio. Jour. Bact., 1934, *28*, 343.
9. De Kruif. Jour. Exp. Med., 1921, *33*, 773.
10. Duran-Reynals. Bact. Rev., 1942, *6*, 197.
11. Edwards and Bruner. Ky. Agr. Exp. Sta. Cir. 54, 1942.
12. Freeman. Jour. Bact., 1952, *63*, 407.
13. Frobisher and Brown. Johns Hopkins Hosp. Bull., 1927, *41*, 167.
14. Hughes, Olander, and Williams. Am. Jour. Vet. Res., 1975, *36*, 971.
15. Kuzumaki, Fenyo, Giovanella, and Klein. Int. Jour. Cancer, 1978, *21*, 62.
16. Lamanna, McElroy, and Eklund. Science, 1946, *103*, 613.
17. Meyer. Physiol. Rev., 1947, *27*, 335.
18. Pampana. Jour. Hyg. (London), 1933, *33*, 402.
19. Ramon. Comp. rend. Soc. Biol. (Paris), 1922, *86*, 661.
20. Sairenjl, Hinuma, Sekizawa, and Yoshida. Jour. Gen. Virol., 1978, *38*, 111.
21. Schalm, O. W., E. J. Carroll, and N. C. Jain. Bovine mastitis. Lea and Febiger, Philadelphia, 1971.
22. Smith. Jour. Am. Med. Assoc., 1913, *60*, 1591.
23. Tillet and Garner. Jour. Exp. Med., 1933, *58*, 485.

2 The Host's Response to Infection

When microorganisms penetrate into or through the primary epithelial barriers, they are usually quickly recognized as foreign by the host, which then mounts a sequence of responses that may be local and/or systemic. The nature and extent of these responses vary according to the site of invasion, the pathogenicity of the invading microorganisms, and the immunologic status of the host. In the case of microorganisms such as *Bordetella bronchiseptica* or enterotoxigenic *Escherichia coli* there may be no actual penetration of epithelium by the organism itself, but rather the organism's toxins or other products are absorbed and cause various ill effects. Some infections may be superficial and clinically inapparent, as is the case with colonization of the tonsil of the pig by *Erysipelothrix rhusiopathiae* or *Mycoplasma hyosynoviae*. However, although the infections may be clinically inapparent, the host animal often detects their presence and produces antibody.

In this chapter we will describe the salient features of the host's response to infection beginning with inflammation and fever and progressing to the humoral and cellular phases of the immune response as they relate to infection at both the systemic and local levels. The reader's knowledge of the general principles of pathology and immunology is assumed, and the reader is referred to other excellent sources on these subjects (16, 31, 37, 42).

INFLAMMATION AND MICROBIAL CLEARANCE

After penetrating the epithelial barrier, microorganisms are physically hindered from spreading more deeply by the interlacing meshwork of connective-tissue fibers in the subepithelial or submucosal tissues. Within a few minutes, the invader's presence is detected and causes rapid changes in the caliber and flow of the local vasculature. These are followed by vasodilation, plasma leakage into the surrounding areas, and movement of cells from the bloodstream through the walls of the blood vessels into the extravascular tissue. Initially these cells are predominantly neutrophils, which, before moving through the walls of the blood vessels, have become adherent to the vascular endothelium.

The migrating neutrophils soon make contact with the invading microorganisms and, in many cases, become adherent to them. This permits the neutrophil to engulf the microorganism within newly formed projections of its cytoplasm. These projections wrap around the organism and form a phagosome. Subsequently, the phagosome fuses with a lysosomal granule to form a phagolysosome which has a high concentration of a variety of lytic enzymes that are lethal to many microorganisms. In the case of capsulated bacteria and fungi such as *Klebsiella pneumoniae, Bacillus anthracis,* and *Cryptococcus neoformans,* phagocytosis is greatly hindered. *Bacillus anthracis* and some other bacteria also produce substances that are lethal to neutrophils and other phagocytic cells.

Some bacteria such as *Brucella abortus, Listeria monocytogenes,* and *Erysipelothrix rhusiopathiae* exhibit a high rate of survival in the phagolysosome and are known as *facultative intracellular parasites*. Infections caused by these organisms tend to be persistent, and their eventual control and elimination require the production of cell-mediated immunity in the host animal.

The presence of specific antibody greatly enhances phagocytosis because it coats or "opsonizes" the microorganism thus facilitating adhesion to the phagocytic cells and thereby stimulating phagocytosis. Complement present in the extravascular transudate is also bound and activated by the reaction of antibody with its antigen on the surface of the microorganism. This improves immune adherence as well as producing lysis of Gram-negative bacterial cells by damaging the membrane surface and allowing lysozyme to hydrolyse the mucopeptide layer beneath. In addition, activation of complement results in formation of (*a*) anaphylatoxin (C3a, C5a), which causes release of histamine from mast cells and results in further increase in vascular permeability at the invasion site and (*b*) chemotactic factors (C5a, C5b, C6, C7), which attract even more neutrophils to the area.

Complement may also be activated by interaction with bacterial endotoxin in the absence of antibody, and so the beneficial effects of complement activation may still be available in part during invasions of nonimmune hosts by endotoxin containing Gram-negative bacteria.

Antibodies to invading bacteria also inhibit their metabolism and multiplication (*Mycoplasma hyopneumoniae, Leptospira pomona, Erysipelothrix rhusiopathiae*). Antibody to viruses may prevent their adherence to specific receptors on target cells, thus limiting their spread from the focus of invasion.

In the peritoneum, neutrophils are suspended in a transudate of plasma and are the dominant cells for the first day of the infection. They are then replaced by eosinophils and mononuclear cells. In immune animals the mononuclear response is much greater than in the nonimmune. The mononuclear cells include many macrophages which, after they ingest bacteria or other foreign material, tend to clump together by intertwining their cytoplasmic processes (38). These clumps also include lymphocytes and neutrophils and in a few days become attached to the omentum where they become vascularized and organize into granulomas. Fibroblasts become prominent and synthesize collagenic fibers. Histologically, the granuloma consists of a central area composed of necrotic cells, bacteria, or other foreign material, and scattered macrophages and neutrophils. The outer layer consists of macrophages, plasma cells, lymphocytes, eosinophils, fibroblasts, epithelioid, and giant cells. The latter two cell types are derivatives of macrophages and are actively pinocytotic rather than phagocytic. Giant cells are formed when epithelioid cells fuse together. Bacteria and fungi such as *Mycobacterium bovis* or *Histoplasma capsulatum* may survive indefinitely in macrophages in chronic granulomata.

Microorganisms that enter the blood stream are filtered out by fixed macrophages in the blood sinusoids of the liver, lymph nodes, bone marrow, and spleen. This is known as the reticuloendothelial system. In bacteremic or septicemic infections these organs remove great numbers of bacteria. Virulent bacteria such as *B. anthracis, Salmonella typhimurium,* and *E. rhusiopathiae* and virulent pneumococci eventually overcome the ability of the reticuloendothelial system to remove them and their numbers then increase progressively in the blood (Table 2.1). Immune animals, particularly those that have developed a cell-mediated response, exhibit very rapid and permanent clearance.

Table 2.1. Numbers of pneumococci in the peripheral blood of normal rabbits after single intravenous doses

Time after injection	Avirulent	Slightly virulent	Highly virulent
Immediately	8,900,000	1,030,000	1,070,000
2 hours	206	20,800	137,000
5 hours	2	340	25,000
24 hours	0	1,300	1,510,000
48 hours	—	134	Animal dead
96 hours	—	0	—

From N. D. Wright, *Jour. Path. Bact.*, 1927, *30*, 189.

FEVER

Elevation of body temperature is frequently the earliest and most readily recognized host response to infection since most infectious processes follow a febrile course of varying degree and duration. There are two mechanisms by which infectious processes produce fever. First, the lipid A component of bacterial endotoxin or intact bacteria stimulates release of a polypeptide (M.W. 13,000) after ingestion by neutrophils, macrophages, Kupffer cells, and blood monocytes. The function of this polypeptide, known as endogenous pyrogen (EP), is to inhibit thermosensitive neurons in the anterior hypothalamus. These neurons in turn inhibit the "thermal blind" neurons of the posterior hypothalamus. When the latter are no longer inhibited, peripheral vasoconstriction occurs and heat loss is reduced.

The second mechanism by which infection produces fever involves exposure to and activation of lymphocytes of previously sensitized individuals by antigens derived from the infectious agent. Antigen-antibody complexes are also effective in this respect. Lymphocytes so activated produce lymphokine, which acts on neutrophils causing them to release EP.

The effect of increased body temperature on the infectious process is as yet unknown.

THE IMMUNE RESPONSE TO INFECTION

Exposure to a microorganism or its products during infection usually results in synthesis of immunoglobulins with specific antibody activity by the host animal. Macrophages that have ingested and digested the infectious agent process its antigens and present them to B (bursa-derived) lymphocytes. The exact manner by which this occurs is unknown. There is evidence that macrophages can pass on a modified form of the antigen and information concerning the antigen in the form of soluble factors, one form of which is a small molecular weight RNA fraction known as "immune RNA." B lymphocytes carry surface markers that act as antigen-specific receptor molecules.

These surface markers can be IgG, IgM, or IgD, and reflect the synthetic capacity of the cells. They also carry receptors for antigen-antibody complexes (Fc receptor) and for antigen-antibody-complement complexes (C3 receptor).

T (thymus-derived) lymphocytes can also bind antigen, but do so by a different receptor. There is evidence that this receptor is an immunoglobulinlike protein akin to the H2 histocompatibility antigen. B lymphocytes that receive this information are activated and, with the aid of T lymphocyte helper cells, become differentiated into plasma cells which synthesize immunoglobulin with specific antibody activity.

The Humoral (Immunoglobulin) Response

Antibody activity has long been known to be associated with the gamma globulin fraction of serum. This fraction contains five major structural classes that have been designated Immunoglobulins G, M, A, D, and E. (IgG, IgM, IgA, IgD, and IgE). Their main properties and functions in defense against infection are summarized in Table 2.2.

Following its first exposure to a particular infectious agent, the infected animal produces a primary antibody response, which is slow to develop and of low intensity. It is characterized by a relatively high proportion of IgM-type antibodies.

If the infection persists or if there is a second exposure to the infectious agent or its antigen, the host produces antibody that belongs principally to the IgG class at a more rapid rate and at a higher level. This is known as the anamnestic or secondary response. The small lymphocyte is essential for both primary and secondary responses and carries the memory of the original exposure to the infectious agent that is activated during the secondary response. The plasma cells that synthesize antibodies in these responses are derived from these small lymphocytes.

IgA. IgA antibodies are the dominant defensive antibody on mucosal surfaces of the eye, nasopharynx, and lower respiratory, intestinal, and vaginal tracts. Their importance in local protection can be gauged from the fact that their concentration in intestinal juice of swine is 13 times higher than that of IgG (4). In sow's milk the level of IgA is twice as high as that of IgG whereas levels of the latter are 10 times higher in serum. IgA antibodies have been shown to block adherence of *E. coli* that have the K88 adhesive antigen (23). There is also evidence that they inhibit or otherwise change bacterial growth (5). In the bovine vagina, they have been shown to have an immobilizing effect on *Campylobacter fetus* (9). In the canine trachea and bronchi they may prevent adhesion of *Bordetella bronchiseptica* to cilia of the tracheobronchial epithelium. It is known that plasma cells producing IgA are much more numerous than IgG- or IgM-producing cells in the lamina propria of the respiratory mucosa (6). In respiratory virus infections IgA plays an important part in the host response (43).

IgA is present in serum mainly as a 7S monomer but occurs as a dimer in secretions. The latter is composed of two 7S molecules joined by a polypeptide chain (J chain) and also containing a secretory component (T piece). The dimer with secretory component is resistant to digestive enzymes.

The IgA antibody response is short-lived; it lasts but a few months at the longest. There is no memory established, and a second response is no greater than the first. Thus continuous or intermittent exposure to the infectious agent is necessary to maintain local immunity to it.

IgG. Antibodies of this immunoglobulin class are important in neutralization of bacterial toxins and viruses, in opsonization and complement-mediated lysis of Gram-negative bacteria, and in inhibition of bacterial

Table 2.2. Properties and defensive functions of the immunoglobulins

Immunoglobulin class	Molecular weight	Sedimentation constant	Serum concentration	Complement fixing	Defensive function
IgA	160,000 (serum) 380,000 (colostrum and secretions)	7S 11S	1-4 mg/ml	No	Protects mucosal surfaces by: 1. Blocking microbial adherence 2. Inhibiting bacterial growth 3. Immobilizing motile bacteria 4. Neutralizing viruses 5. Limiting entry of nonviable antigens
IgG	150,000	7S	8-16 mg/ml	Yes	Combats microbial infections in blood, tissues, and extravascular spaces by: 1. Neutralizing bacterial toxins 2. Neutralizing viruses 3. Opsonizing bacteria 4. Lysing bacteria (bacteriolysis) in presence of complement 5. Inhibiting bacterial metabolism and multiplication
IgM	900,000	19S	0.5-2.0 mg/ml	Yes	Combats microbial infections in their early stages by: 1. Opsonizing bacteria 2. Lysing bacteria in presence of complement
IgD	185,000	7S	3-40 μg/ml	—	Unknown
IgE	200,000	8S	0-1.0 μg/ml	—	Functions in defense against parasites

growth. IgG immunoglobulins are further divided into subclasses, IgG_1, IgG_2, etc.

In cattle, only IgG_1 is found in the normal fetus. It differs in biological properties from IgG_2 in being unable to bind complement or to participate in an Arthus reaction.

IgG is the dominant immunoglobulin in the secondary response to an infectious agent. There is evidence (36) that IgG antibodies are more effective in opsonizing Gram-negative bacteria in man than IgM. The reverse is true in swine and cattle.

IgM. IgM molecules are pentamers that have either 5 or 10 combining sites arranged in a circle. They are therefore much more efficient than dimeric IgG molecules in agglutinating particulate antigens, in opsonization, and in binding complement. This is so because only one molecule of IgM is required to initiate complement fixation whereas two closely spaced IgG molecules are needed for this. Most IgM synthesis occurs in the spleen.

There is growing evidence that IgM have a much more potent antibacterial action than IgG antibodies (8, 31), especially in newborn piglets, calves, and other species in which prevention of Gram-negative bacteremia is critical. They also neutralize some of the effects of endotoxin (20). Another valuable characteristic of IgM antibodies received in the colostrum by the newborn is that they do not suppress the individual's own active immune responses when infectious agents are encountered against which the individual already has IgM antibodies.

The sera of animals with chronic bacterial infections such as those of *Brucella abortus* frequently have significant titers of antibodies of the IgM class which are useful diagnostically and can be detected by their sensitivity to mercaptoethanol. The microscopic agglutination test for leptospiral antibody is a test based on IgM antibody (15). However, in leptospirosis, these antibodies are not important in protection.

IgD. This immunoglobulin class is present in only trace amounts in serum. It is found on the surface of large numbers of lymphocytes and is apparently an immunoglobulin receptor for antigen.

IgE. IgE, also a minor immunoglobulin with respect to concentration in serum, is the immunoglobulin class that contains the reaginic antibodies. These are antibodies produced by the host against allergens and are responsible for immediate hypersensitivity or allergy. The role of IgE in the host's response to an infectious agent is presently unknown.

Cell-Mediated Immunity

The host's immune response to facultative or obligate intracellular parasites includes not only an antibody response but also, and of much greater importance in protection, a heightened microbicidal activity of (activated) macrophages.

This enhanced cell-mediated immunity is transferable with the T lymphocytes of an immune animal. T lymphocytes belong to different subpopulations, each of which has a particular role in cell-mediated immune responses. For instance, the subpopulation of T lymphocytes known as Ly 1 behaves as affector cells in delayed hypersensitivity reactions, and T lymphocytes with helper cell activity in this reaction belong to other subpopulations.

T lymphocytes sensitized to antigens of the infectious agent begin to appear about 6 to 10 days after a primary infection begins.

Their induction is highly specific—animals previously sensitized to mycobacterial antigens have an immunological memory of the sensitization that can be recalled only by the same antigen. However, the enhanced microbicidal activity of macrophages produced as a result of the sensitization is not so specific and can be expressed against unrelated bacteria. After activation, macrophages are more actively mobile, phagocytic, and microbicidal (Figure 2.1).

Activation of macrophages is effected by means of soluble substances (lymphokines) produced by the immune T lymphocytes that have interacted with the antigen. One of these substances is transfer factor, a dialyzable low molecular weight compound that is effective in immune reconstitution of individuals lacking normal cell-mediated responses. Migratory inhibitory factor (MIF) is another lymphokine and inhibits migration of macrophages.

Cell-mediated responses involving activated macrophages have been described in infections caused by *Brucella abortus, Mycobacterium tuberculosis, Listeria monocytogenes, Salmonella enteritidis, Francisella tularensis,* and *Erysipelothrix rhusiopathiae* (2, 39). They are also produced in response to living vaccines of these organisms, and activation persists as long as the vaccine strain survives in the tissues (21).

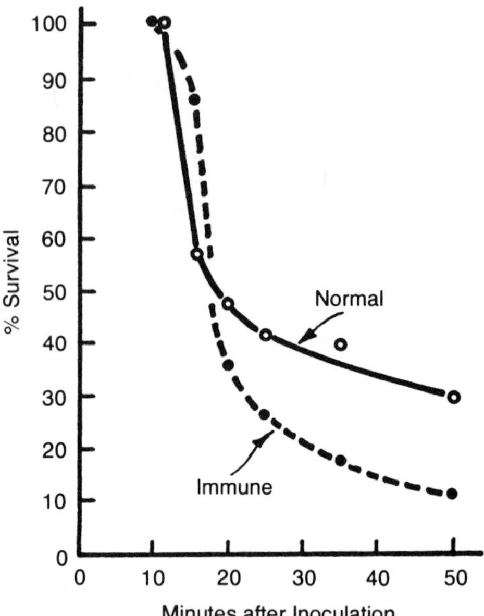

Figure 2.1. Curves showing the intracellular inactivation of *Erysipelothrix rhusiopathiae* in macrophages from normal mice and immune erysipelothrix-infected mice. (From John F. Timoney, *Res. Vet. Sci.*, 1969, *10*, 301.)

Cell-mediated immunity may also be expressed as a delayed hypersensitivity (DS) reaction or by a cytotoxic effect of the sensitized lymphocytes on target cells. The DS reaction is characterized by swelling of the skin of a sensitized individual about 24 to 48 hours after the intradermal inoculation of the antigen (bacterial, fungal) to which it is hypersensitive. The area is edematous and contains infiltrates of lymphocytes and macrophages. A different subpopulation of T lymphocytes is responsible for this reaction than is involved in the development of cellular immunity as described above.

The DS reaction is of great diagnostic importance in veterinary medicine. It is used in detection of infection with *Mycobacterium bovis, M. avium, M. paratuberculosis,* and *M. tuberculosis; Pseudomonas mallei; Mycoplasma mycoides* var. *mycoides; Histoplasma capsulatum;* and *Coccidioides immitis.* Its protective value in the host response, however, is doubtful. It may in fact be harmful because it can cause quiescent lesions to become hyperactive resulting in necrosis, liquefaction, and release of bacteria from their intracellular nidi. Vascularization of the area may lead to possible systemic dissemination of the bacteria via the bloodstream following their entry into blood vessels near the lesion (24).

The cytotoxic manifestation of cell-mediated immunity is a direct effect of mediators released by immune T lymphocytes onto other nearby cells that contain antigen to which the lymphocytes are sensitized. This arm of the cell-mediated response is probably particularly important in viral infections in which a viral antigen is associated with or inserted in a cell membrane.

It may also be important in acquired resistance to ringworm in which infections of *Microsporum* and *Trichophyton* sp. affect the nonliving stratum corneum and are remote from the direct effect of macrophages and other phagocytic cells. The cell-mediated response in this situation must be mediated via soluble factors that diffuse outwards from lymphocytes in the dermis to the stratum corneum.

There is indirect evidence that cell-mediated immune responses tend to be inversely related to antibody response. Individuals with progressive fungal infections, for instance, often have high antibody titers but a diminished cell-mediated response. A similar observation has been made about Johne's disease in cattle in which animals with the highest titers of antibody are more severely affected, shed greater numbers of *Mycobacterium paratuberculosis*, and have a poor prognosis (11). This phenomenon has been termed the "immunoprotective niche."

Local Immune Responses

Respiratory Tract. Evidence for a local immune response in the nasal cavity was first obtained by Walsh and Cannon in the 1930s (44). Fazekas de St. Groth and Donnelley (12) later showed that antibody to influenza virus in mice is stimulated most effectively when the antigen is applied intranasally and that the resulting antibody is produced locally.

The tonsils are an important site of local antibody production for the nasopharynx. This has been shown in studies of immunity to poliomyelitis virus in children. Tonsillectomized children had much lower titers of antibody to the virus in their nasopharyngeal secretions (43). Furthermore, paralytic polio has long been known to be less common in children who have not been tonsillectomized.

In the lower respiratory tract, the lamina propria of the trachea and bronchi contains many macrophages, neutrophils, lymphocytes, eosinophils, and plasma cells. The majority of these plasma cells produce IgA; the remainder produce IgG and IgM (6). Some IgE plasma cells may also be present.

Antibodies against a number of important virus infections in animals are produced locally in the trachea and bronchi (42).

As the local infectious process develops, the inflammatory response in the respiratory mucosa increases the permeability of the area to immunoglobulins in the plasma which then pass into the secretions, and so local concentrations of IgG and IgM increase. Neutrophils may also migrate into the mucosa and are actively phagocytic and microbicidal. They are especially effective in killing *Bordetella bronchiseptica* in the canine respiratory tract (1).

The duration of the local response is believed to be short, and there is no memory. Persisting antigenic stimulation is necessary for continuing specific IgA synthesis.

The alveolar macrophage is a vital component of the defense of the lung parenchyma. Microorganisms that penetrate this far are phagocytosed and destroyed. Viruses such as parainfluenza III in cattle, however, can depress the antibacterial abilities of these macrophages and so make the lung more susceptible to secondary bacterial invasion (18, 22). When experimental mice were previously immunized to the bacteria, virus-induced suppression of the alveolar macrophages was less effective (17). As well as the cellular immunity expressed by the alveolar macrophages, locally sensitized lymphocytes have also been demonstrated in the lower respiratory tract (45). Their significance in the local host response to infection is unknown.

Intestine. Acquired resistance to infection in the intestine is mediated locally by means of IgA antibody synthesized by plasma cells in the lamina propria. This antibody is in the form of secretory dimeric IgA (SIgA) consisting of two 7S monomers joined by a J chain and containing secretory component. SIgA is thereby protected from enzymatic digestion.

Antigens of the infectious agent are presented to immunocompetent cells in the lamina propria by epithelial cells known as M cells (46). There is evidence that the IgA-producing plasma cells in the lamina propria originate as lymphoid precursor cells in Peyer's patches or other lymphoid areas on the intestinal mucosa. These cells are originally transformed by exposure to locally available antigen and then migrate via the mesenteric and ileocecal lymph nodes, thoracic duct, and blood stream in which they travel back, or "home," to the lamina propria of the intestine. Some of these cells also home to the mammary gland and the spleen. In the neonate, these plasma cells synthesize IgM immunoglobulin for the first week before they mature and make IgA.

Locally synthesized IgA prevents microbial adhesion, inhibits bacterial growth, neutralizes enterotoxin activity (14, 35), and limits viral replication. An example of the latter is resistance of piglets to transmissible gastroenteritis (TGE) virus which is mediated by colostrum-derived IgA (3).

There is no memory in the local intestinal immune responses tend to be inversely related to antibody response. tion requires persisting antigenic stimulation (4).

Evidence of local cell-mediated immunity in the intestine that is independent of systemic cell-mediated responsiveness is available for TGE and polio virus infections (13, 27).

Substantial macrophage and neutrophil populations occur in the lamina propria and great numbers of neutrophils may pass through the mucosa in enteric salmonellosis and can be recognized in the stool.

The local immune response also undoubtedly plays an important role in control of regional colonization of the intestine by the normal flora. The manner by which this control is achieved is not yet understood.

Female Genital Tract. The local immune response of the cow to infection by *Brucella abortus, Campylobacter fetus venerealis* and the protozoon parasite *Trichomonas fetus* has been recognized for many years and has been used in diagnosis of infection by these organisms (30).

The local immune response to *C. fetus venerealis* has been studied extensively (9, 10). Neutrophils are present in the early stages and are later replaced by foci of mononuclear cells including plasma cells. The plasma cells in the vagina and cervix produce IgA antibodies that have an immobilizing effect on the flagella of the organism and thereby inhibit its spread in the tract. In the uterus, antibodies are predominantly of the IgG class and are very effective in clearance of infection.

Infection in the cervicovaginal area tends, however, to be persistent. This is probably due to the organism's ability to change its surface antigens, allowing survival of variants that have antigenic configurations that do not react with the IgA antibody being synthesized at the time (9).

Urinary Tract. Infection of the urinary tract by *Corynebacterium renale* in the cow causes a purulent urethritis and cystitis that later may extend via the ureter to the kidney and cause pyelonephritis. At this stage of the disease, agglutinating antibodies appear in the serum and antibody-coated bacteria appear in the urine (25). These antibodies are mostly IgG, but some IgA are present also. The latter are probably of local origin; the former are derived from transudates of plasma that have leaked out of the inflammatory focus in the kidney.

The host immune response in the urinary tract is generally inhibited by the high urea content, poor phagocytic activity of neutrophils, and diminished effect of complement.

Eye. IgA containing plasma cells are numerous in the interstitial region of lacrimal glands, and IgA is the only immunoglobulin found in human tears (43). It is also the predominant immunoglobulin in bovine tears (28). In cattle, a local resistance has been observed following infection of the eye by *Moraxella bovis.* This resistance correlated with the presence of specific precipitins in the lacrimal secretions (26).

During acute inflammation, IgG is selectively transferred from the blood to the tears (29) and may be responsible for the precipitin activity present. This is suggested because the highest and most persistent antibody titers are associated with IgG and not IgA (19).

In dogs, the ocular disorder known as *blue eye,* associated with infectious canine hepatitis virus infection, is due to infiltration of the posterior surface of the cornea by neutrophils. This infiltration is believed to be a host response to the presence of virus-antibody complexes in the region (7).

Joints. Synovial tissue has the capacity to develop immunocompetence and mount a local immune response. Infection of pig joints by *Erysipelothrix rhusiopathiae* (40) and by *Mycoplasma hyorhinis* (32) result in accumulations of plasma cells. In the case of *E. rhusiopathiae* arthritis these plasma cells contain antibody to the causative bacterium and this antibody is predominantly of the IgG class (41) (Figure 2.2).

The type A synoviocytes of the synovial lining are phagocytic cells but, being fixed, are unable to escape from the joint with their burden of ingested microorganisms. Antigens of infectious agents therefore tend to be held in the synovial tissue and so are a continuing local source of immune stimulus. This may explain the chronicity of some forms of infectious arthritis in animals and man.

Mammary Gland. Neutrophils are probably the most important component of the host defense mechanism in the bovine mammary gland. They rapidly increase in number in the milk following bacterial invasion of the quarter and phagocytose and kill large numbers of bac-

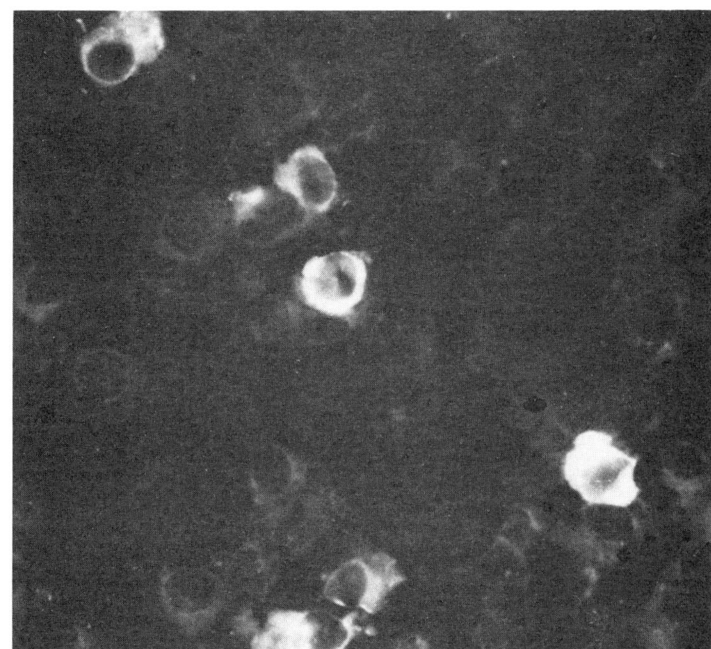

Figure 2.2. Plasma cells containing antibody to *Erysipelothrix rhusiopathiae* (ER) in the synovial tissue of a pig affected with arthritis caused by ER. The tissue section was treated with a soluble extract of ER followed by a fluorescent antiserum to ER.

teria. Endotoxin from Gram-negative bacteria is a very effective chemotactic stimulus for neutrophils within the udder and can be used in treatment of persisting infections when the udder's response by itself appears to be insufficient.

There is also a local antibody response to the antigens of *Staphylococcus aureus* (47) and of *Streptococcus agalactiae* (see Chapter 17). The presence of antibodies to the alpha toxin of *Staphylococcus aureus* is important in resistance of the gland to gangrenous mastitis.

Antibodies of the IgM and IgA classes confer protection against *Streptococcus agalactiae,* and IgA antibody levels can be increased by intramammary vaccination. Local antibody synthesis occurs in the supramammary lymph node (47) and in plasma cells scattered through the secretory parenchyma.

The great dilution effect of the milk flow probably results in inadequate amounts of antibody for effective protection of the secretory parenchyma. As well, complement activity is negligible in milk, and so there is no complement-enhanced opsonization and bacteriolysis.

The delayed hypersensitivity reaction is involved in the pathogenesis of chronic staphylococcal and possibly other forms of mastitis as well.

INTERFERON

Interferons are a family of soluble glycoproteins produced by virus-infected cells, which, when released, are capable of protecting other cells from virus infection. Interferons are host-cell-specific but not virus-specific. They mediate protection by inducing cells to produce a protein that increases the cells' resistance to infection by blocking virus takeover of ribosomes for viral protein synthesis. Their role is a primary defensive one in restricting spread of virus infection (see Chapter 36).

RESPONSE OF THE FETUS TO INFECTIOUS AGENTS

The immune system of the fetus develops some time before birth (Figure 2.3). The calf is capable of responding to infectious agents about halfway through gestation (33, 34, 42), while the piglet develops immunocompetence about 3 months after conception. Puppies, perhaps because of their relatively short gestation period, develop humeral immune responsiveness only within a week or two of birth.

Of all the domestic animals, the ruminants are most prone to fetal invasions by infectious agents. Examples of these are *Brucella abortus, Leptospira pomona, Campylobacter fetus (venerealis* and *intestinalis*), *Aspergillus fumigatus,* infectious bovine rhinotracheitis (IBR) virus, and bovine virus diarrhea (BVD). If virus infection of the fetus occurs before it is immunocompetent, the outcome is usually fetal death and subsequent abortion. Virus infections occurring late in gestation are often limited in part by the fetal immune response and

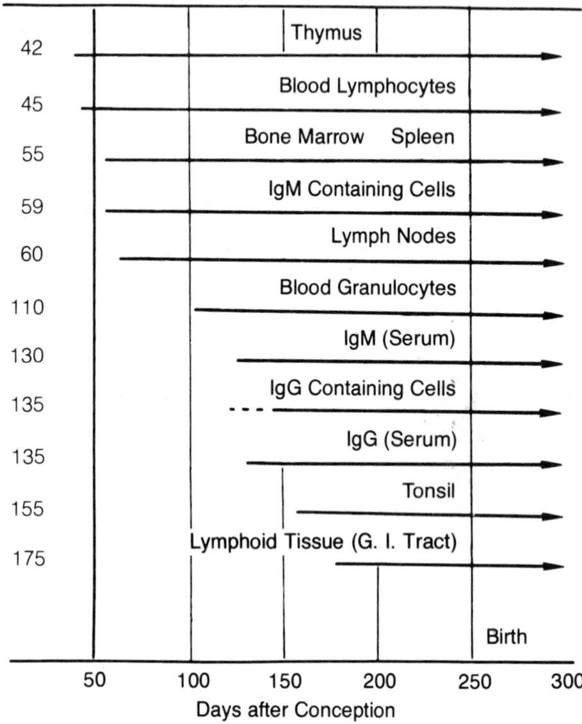

Figure 2.3. The development of the immune system in the bovine. (From R. D. Schultz, *Cornell Vet.*, 1973, *63*, 513.)

have less severe effects. Most bacterial infections result in fetal death irrespective of the stage of fetal development.

The immune response of the fetus to infection consists of lymphoreticular hyperplasia and significant levels of immunoglobulins in the serum at birth. Normally, only trace amounts of immunoglobulins are present at this time. IgM levels are raised in most species. In the calf, IgG_1 and IgG_2 are present to a significant degree. IgG_2 is normally absent from calf serum at birth. Thus the presence in serum of this immunoglobulin subclass at birth is good evidence of fetal infection *in utero*.

Calves infected *in utero* with *Mycobacterium bovis*, although sensitized to tuberculin, may be unable to mount a delayed hypersensitivity response because of fetal glucocorticoid synthesis just before parturition.

EFFECT OF CORTICOSTEROIDS ON THE HOST'S RESPONSE TO INFECTION

Corticosteroids have marked anti-inflammatory and immunosuppressive activity in relation to host resistance to infectious agents. They delay attachment of leukocytes to the endothelium and so reduce and delay migration through blood vessels into inflammatory foci. Corticosteroids also reduce chemotaxis and are antiphagocytic. They stabilize lysosomes and so prolong intracellular survival of phagocytosed infectious agents as well as delaying antigen processing.

Furthermore, they suppress the activity of T lymphocytes and cause macrophages to be less responsive to lymphokines. Activation of latent microbial infections is a well-known effect of corticosteroid administration and can be used to detect animals carrying virus such as that of bovine rhinotracheitis.

REFERENCES

1. Bemis, Greisen, and Appel. Jour. Inf. Dis., 1977, *135*, 753.
2. Blanden, Mackaness, and Collins. Jour. Exp. Med., 1966, *124*, 585.
3. Bohl, Gupta, and Olquin. Inf. and Immun., 1972, *6*, 289.
4. Bourne. Vet. Rec., 1976, *98*, 499.
5. Brandtzaeg, Fjellanger, and Gjeruldsen. Science, 1968, *160*, 789.
6. Breeze, Wheeldon, and Pirie. Vet. Bull., 1976, *46*, 319.
7. Carmichael. Pathol. Vet., 1964, *1*, 73.
8. Chidlow and Porter. Res. Vet. Sci., 1978, *24*, 245.
9. Corbeil, Schurig, Bier, and Winter. Inf. and Immun., 1975, *11*, 240.
10. Corbeil, Schurig, Duncan, Corbeil, and Winter. Inf. and Immun., 1974, *10*, 422.
11. de Lisle, Geoffrey. Ph.D. thesis, Cornell University, Ithaca, N.Y., 1979.
12. Fazekas de St. Groth and Donnelley. Austral. Jour. Exp. Biol. Med. Sci., 1950, *28*, 61.
13. Frederick and Bohl. Jour. Immunol., 1976, *116*, 1000.
14. Gibbons. Adv. Exp. Med. Biol., 1974, *45*, 315.
15. Hanson. Jour. Dairy Sci., 1974, *59*, 1166.
16. Herbert, N. J. Veterinary immunology, Revised ed. Blackwell Scientific Publications, Oxford, 1974.
17. Jakab and Green. Jour. Clin. Invest., 1973, *52*, 2878.
18. Jericho and Langford. Can. Jour. Comp. Med., 1978, *42*, 269.
19. Killinger, Weisiger, Helper, and Mansfield. Am. Jour. Vet. Res., 1978, *39*, 931.
20. Kim and Watson. Jour. Exp. Med., 1965, *121*, 751.
21. Kuramasu, Imamura, Sameshima, and Tajima. Zentrbl. f. Vet.-Med., 1963, *9B*, 362.
22. Lopez, Thomson, and Savan. Can. Jour. Comp. Med., 1976, *40*, 385.
23. Miler, Corma, Trovnicek, Rejnek, and Krumel. Folia Mikrobiologica, 1975, *20*, 433.
24. Myrvik, Kohlweiss, and Harpold. *In* Microbiology 1975, ed. David Schlessinger. Am. Soc. of Microbiology, Washington, D.C., 1975, pp. 227–35.
25. Nicolet and Fey. Vet. Rec., 1979, *105*, 301.
26. Noyar and Saunders. Can. Jour. Comp. Med., 1975, *39*, 22.
27. Ogra, Wallace, and Umana. Adv. Exp. Med. Biol., 1974, *45*, 271.

28. Pedersen, Neils. Infectious Keratoconjunctivitis in Cattle. Thesis, Royal Vet. and Ag. Univ., Copenhagen, Denmark, 1973.
29. Pedersen. Acta Path. et Microbiol. Scand., 1973, *81B,* Fasc. 2, 245.
30. Pierce. Vet. Rev. Annot., 1939, *5,* 17.
31. Roitt, Ivan. Essential immunology, 2nd ed. Blackwell Scientific Publications, Oxford, 1975.
32. Ross. Ann. N.Y. Acad. Sci., 1973, *225,* 359.
33. Schultz. Cornell Vet., 1973, *63,* 507.
34. Schultz, Wang, and Dunne. Am. Jour. Vet. Res., 1974, *32,* 1331.
35. Sock, Johnsen, and Pierce. Jour. Inf. Dis., 1976, *134,* 15.
36. Smith, Barnett, May, and Sanford. Jour. Immunol., 1967, *98,* 336.
37. Smith, Hilton A., Thomas C. Jones, and Ronald D. Hunt. Veterinary pathology, 4th ed. Lea and Febiger, Philadelphia, 1972.
38. Spiers and Spiers. *In* White cells in inflammation, ed. Gordon Van Arman. Thomas, Springfield, Ill., 1974, pp. 54–92.
39. Timoney. Res. Vet. Sci., 1970, *11,* 189.
40. Timoney and Berman. Am. Jour. Vet. Res., 1970, *31,* 1405.
41. Timoney and Yarkoni. Vet. Microbiol., 1976, *1,* 467.
42. Tizard, Ian R. An introduction to veterinary immunology. Saunders, Philadelphia, 1977, pp. 156–57.
43. Tomasi, Thomas B. The Immune system of secretions. Prentice-Hall, Englewood Cliffs, N.J., 1976.
44. Walsh and Cannon. Jour. Immunol., 1938, *35,* 31.
45. Weldman and Henney. Jour. Exp. Med., 1971, *134,* 482.
46. Welliver and Ogra. Jour. Am. Vet. Med. Assoc., 1978, *173,* 560.
47. Willoughby. Am. Jour. Vet. Res., 1966, *27,* 522.

PART II

THE PATHOGENIC BACTERIA

3 The Genetics of Virulence and Antibiotic Resistance

Genetic information in bacteria is mainly contained in the chromosomal deoxyribonucleic acid (DNA), where specific sequences of nucleotides form genes which code for specific polypeptide chains. Large numbers of genes are usually carried on DNA molecules whose size is measured in megadaltons (1 megadalton = 10^6 daltons). The DNA of the bacterial chromosome is in the form of a circle, and it has been estimated that in *Escherichia coli* it weighs about 2.5×10^3 megadaltons. Each 3 to 5 megadaltons of DNA can potentially code for up to 5 proteins.

The complement of genes representing the genetic potential of the cell is referred to as its genotype. The bacterial genotype may be changed or added to by (*a*) mutations, (*b*) sexual conjugation, (*c*) phage transduction and phage conversion, (*d*) transformation by foreign DNA, and (*e*) loss or acquisition of plasmids.

Mutations

Alterations in nucleotide sequence occasionally occur, and these may be recognized by changes in the phenotype of the cells such as loss of a biochemical function, change in morphology, or acquisition of antibiotic resistance. Mutations may also lead to increased or decreased virulence, or to the appearance of colonial roughness. They may occur spontaneously, usually at a frequency of less than 10^{-6} but often much less frequently. However, in the presence of a selection pressure such as that of an antibiotic, the occurrence of even a very low-frequency event can be of importance, because only the antibiotic-resistant mutant can survive, and it soon becomes the dominant clone. Within the animal, mutants that enhance the virulence of the organism tend to be selected, because these mutant clones are better able to survive the antibacterial defenses of the host. When pathogenic bacteria are cultivated on artificial media and without the selection pressure of the host defenses, reversion mutants that have lost their virulence tend to be selected. This is so because synthesis of virulence factors imposes a metabolic demand on these clones; thus they tend to be crowded out in competition with less virulent clones that are in position to devote all their metabolic energy toward multiplication.

Mutational resistance to penicillin, the tetracyclines, kanamycin, and some other antibiotics arises by a stepwise process whereby clones with low-level resistance appear first, and then mutants with a higher level of resistance are selected from among these clones. Resistance to streptomycin, however, can be found at a high level in the first generation of mutants, and these are described as "one-step" mutants.

Sexual Conjugation

A process resembling mating has been described in the genera *Salmonella, Shigella, Vibrio, Escherichia, Pseudomonas,* and the fecal streptococci. In the case of members of the Enterobacteriaceae, donor cells, which are known as F^+ cells (male), possess a sex factor (F) which codes for synthesis of a tubelike connection between the donor cell and the recipient, F^- (female), cell.

The F factor and chromosomal DNA pass through this tube into the recipient cell. In the recipient cell the F factor may integrate into the host chromosome and cause the new host bacterium to exhibit a high frequency of recombination (Hfr). This means that Hfr donors rarely transfer the F factor to recipients but instead transfer their own chromosomal genes at a high frequency.

Sexual conjugation among pathogenic bacteria of veterinary interest does not at present appear to be of great importance. However, *Salmonella* strains have occasionally been isolated that were lactose-positive because of the presence of F-like factors which carried a lac^{+} gene (8).

Phage Transduction and Conversion

Phage transduction is the process by which bacteriophage transfers bacterial genes from one cell to another. The process is described as *general transduction* when the bacteriophage can transfer any bacterial gene and as *restricted transduction* when the phage can transfer only the bacterial genes adjoining the prophage position on the bacterial chromosome.

The plasmid containing the gene for beta lactamase (penicillinase) in *Staphylococcus aureus* may be transferred in this way, and this transfer can occur within the body of the animal. Production of botulinum toxin by *Clostridium botulinum* types C and D is also phage-transduced, although the exact source or location of the gene in donor cells has not yet been determined.

In phage conversion, phage genes direct the synthesis of bacterial antigens or toxins in the host cell. The phage-coded toxins or antigens are synthesized independently of the progeny phage. Examples of phage conversion important in infectious disease include the synthesis of diphtheria toxin by *Corynebacterium diphtheriae,* the synthesis of the O antigens 15 and 36 in *Salmonella,* the synthesis of hyaluronidase by *Streptococcus pyogenes* and *equi,* and the production of alpha hemolysin and enterotoxin by *Staphylococcus aureus.*

Transformation

When free DNA released by one bacterium is taken in through the cell wall of another and the new gene(s) are expressed in the host bacterium, the latter is described as having undergone transformation. Transformation is important in conversion of rough, avirulent pneumococci to the smooth, virulent form. It is also involved in genetic changes in *Hemophilus* sp., *Streptococcus* sp., and *Bacillus* sp. Its full significance in veterinary bacteriology has still to be discovered.

Plasmids (Episomes)

Plasmids are composed of covalently closed circular molecules of DNA which replicate somewhat independently of the bacterial chromosome. They are found in the cytoplasm and can be transferred between bacteria via contact (conjugation) or by transduction. One means of contact is the pilus, a hollow tube which extends between the donor and recipient cells. The genes for pilus synthesis and for transfer function may be carried on the plasmid, which is then described as conjugative. However, many nonconjugative plasmids exist which lack genes for transfer. The transfer gene complex is called the transfer factor which can sometimes exist by itself as a separate plasmid. Nonconjugative plasmids which lack transfer factors can sometimes be mobilized by other coexisting conjugative plasmids. In this situation they apparently slip through the pilus close behind the conjugative plasmid.

Plasmids range in size from about 0.6 to 200 megadaltons. They are usually isolated from bacteria by detergent lysis followed by selective precipitation of membrane-associated chromosomal DNA. They can then be separated and measured by electrophoresis in agarose gels (Figure 3.1). Purified plasmid DNA can be photographed in the electron microscope and the contour length of the molecule measured to estimate its molecular weight (Figures 3.2 and 3.3).

Another method of separating plasmid from chromosomal DNA is by dye-bouyant density centrifugation in cesium chloride. In this procedure, the dye (ethidium bromide) is taken up to a much greater extent by the linear fragments of chromosomal DNA than by the closed circular, supercoiled plasmid molecules and bands at a different level in a cesium chloride gradient during ultracentrifugation.

Genes carried on plasmids can mediate a wide variety of important functions that include antibiotic and heavy metal resistance, virulence, and metabolic characteristics such as sucrose and lactose fermentation. In the case of *E. coli,* enterotoxin production, adhesion and colonization factors (such as K88 and K99 antigens), colicin and hemolysin production, and other factors involved in lethality are plasmid-mediated.

Plasmids Mediating Antibiotic Resistance. Plasmids coding for antibiotic resistance in the Enterobacteriaceae

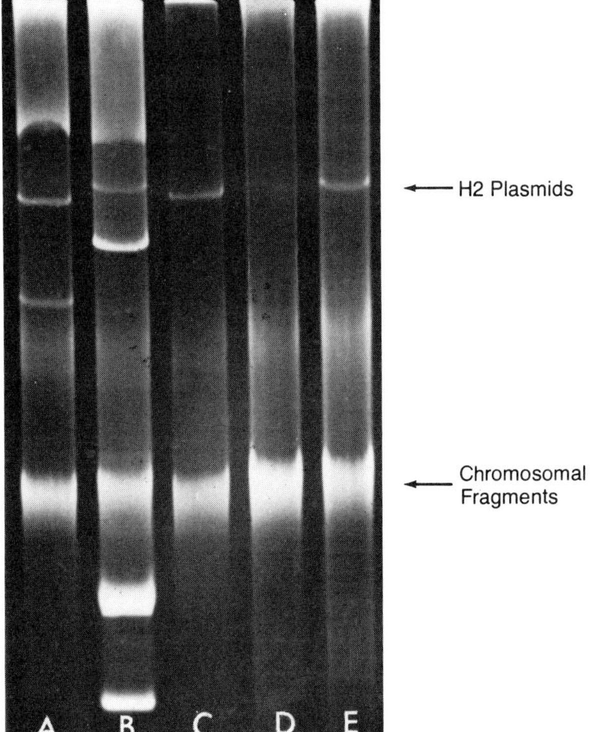

Figure 3.1. Agarose gel electrophoresis of plasmid DNA's from a series of *Salmonella typhimurium* strains with multiple antibiotic resistance and an antibiotic-sensitive strain (Track D). The narrow bands at the top of the picture are H2 incompatibility group plasmids of molecular weight greater than 140 megadaltons. The wide bands at the same level on all the tracks in the lower half of the picture are produced by chromosomal fragments (10 megadaltons). The two bands toward the lower end of track B are small plasmids of less than 6 megadaltons. The logarithm_{10} of the distance of plasmid migration is proportional to the logarithm_{10} of its molecular weight.

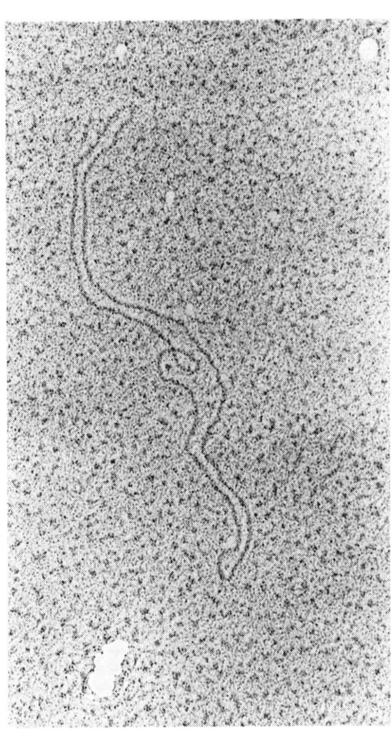

Figure 3.2. Electron micrograph of a small plasmid (6.1 megadaltons). × 60,000.

Figure 3.3. Electron micrograph of a large plasmid (110 megadaltons) of the H1 incompatibility group. × 21,000.

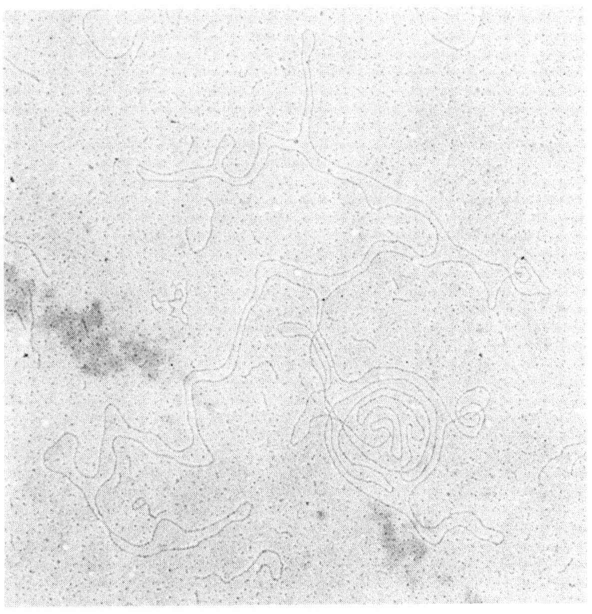

are termed R (resistance) factors (7). R factors were first found in the genus *Shigella* in 1959 in Japan and since then have been found in all the other genera of the Enterobacteriaceae and in the genera *Pasteurella, Vibrio,* and *Pseudomonas*. Resistance to a number of different antibiotics can be mediated by the same R factor, and these resistances can transfer readily by conjugation to other bacteria of the same or different genera of the Enterobacteriaceae.

Classification of R factor plasmids is based mainly on compatibility grouping, DNA homology, and endonuclease digest pattern (Figure 3.4) studies, but other characteristics can be helpful in classification—such as thermosensitivity of transfer, phage restriction, fertility inhibition, the level of resistance mediated, the resistance determinants carried, and the type of pilus produced (3, 4). Incompatibility (Inc) grouping is based

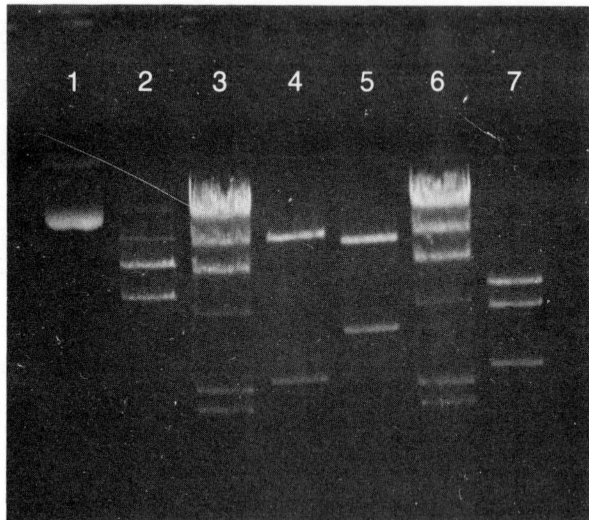

Figure 3.4. Patterns of endonuclease digests of plasmid pUB1661 following electrophoresis on agarose gel. Track 1 contains the undigested plasmid. Tracks 2, 4, 5, and 7 contain digests of pUB1661 produced by endonucleases Bgl II, Hind III, Bam H1 and EcoR1 respectively. Tracks 3 and 6 contain λ bacteriophage DNA digested with Hind III endonuclease. The λ fragments are of known size and are used as a standard against which the pUB1661 fragments can be measured. Each endonuclease cleaves at specific sites, and the resulting digest patterns can be used to "fingerprint" an unknown plasmid and to identify it by comparing it with digests of known plasmids. (Courtesy Andrew Docherty.)

on the fact that similar plasmids cannot coexist in the same cell: one will kick the other out. Unlike plasmids, however, can coexist. Inc groups are designated by letters, for example, FI, FII, H1, H2, I, N, etc.

Inc H plasmids are of especial interest because they are thermosensitive for transfer and are very common in *Salmonella typhimurium* from animals (26). These plasmids do not transfer at temperatures above 34 C, and so they are unlikely to transfer in the intestine unless mobilized by another plasmid whose transfer is not thermosensitive. Resistance to tetracycline, chloramphenicol, kanamycin, and streptomycin in *S. typhimurium* is commonly carried on these plasmids. Ampicillin resistance is usually carried on nonthermosensitive plasmids—a potential disadvantage of oral ampicillin therapy because it will exert a selection pressure for these kinds of plasmids in the intestine and so promote rapid transfer of resistance among the gut flora. Inc H plasmids are uncommon in enteropathogenic *E. coli* from calves, although they are common in *S. typhimurium* strains from this source (Table 3.1). Thus R factor plasmids are not shared equally among the pathogenic members of the Enterobacteriaceae, and the host bacterium is an important factor in the kinds of plamids hosted.

R factors from human and animal sources appear to be similar, and it has been suggested that they share a common reservoir (2, 18). Resistance genes such as those for ampicillin, tetracycline, and streptomycin have also been found to be similar among a wide range of pathogenic bacteria. This is so apparently because these genes are transposable from one location on a plasmid to another, from one plasmid to another, and even from a plasmid to a chromosomal location (10). The ampicillin resistance gene is known to reside on a transposon of about 3.0 megadaltons and this transposon is widespread among plasmids of the Enterobacteriaceae and in *Hemophilus* and *Neisseria* sp.

The Public Health Significance of Antibiotic Resistance in Animals

The feeding of low levels of antibiotics such as tetracycline and penicillin to poultry, swine, and calves in order to promote growth has resulted in a great increase in the reservoir of bacteria that are resistant to antibiotics. This increase has been such that resistant bacteria from animals may be contributing to the reservoir of

Table 3.1. The occurrence of H incompatibility group plasmids in multiresistant *Salmonella typhimurium* and enteropathogenic *Escherichia coli* from calves in New York State (1974–78)

	Percentages of strains with			
Host organism	H only	H and non H*	Non H* only	No transfer
S. typhimurium (134)†	37	37	16	10
E. coli (115)†	1	0	69	30

*Plasmids of incompatibility groups other than H.
†The numbers in parentheses are the number of strains studied.

antibiotic resistance in man's bacterial flora, and this may be compromising the efficacy of antimicrobial therapy in man. Although there is considerable evidence that antibiotic-resistant *E. coli* can colonize man's intestine long enough for transfer of antibiotic resistance to occur (5, 27), there is as yet no direct evidence—with the exception of two epidemics of *S. typhimurium* infection in man in England (1, 25)—that the problem of antibiotic resistance in animals is adversely affecting therapy of bacterial disease in man. However, antibiotic resistance in *E. coli*, *Salmonella typhimurium*, and *Staphylococcus aureus* has made therapy of diseases caused by these organisms in animals very difficult. The extent to which feed and therapeutic use of antibiotics has contributed to this situation is unknown. It is known, however, that the therapeutic use of antibiotics by itself can exert a selection pressure for resistant clones of *S. typhimurium* (26) and that this was probably important in the emergence of resistant clones of *S. typhimurium* in intensively raised calves in England.

Although antibiotic resistance is common among the Enterobacteriaceae, *Staphylococcus aureus*, *Pasteurella multocida*, and *Pseudomonas aeruginosa*, other pathogenic bacterial populations of veterinary importance appear to have been unaffected by antibiotic usage and are still sensitive to antibiotics.

Genetics of Virulence in Enteropathogenic *E. Coli*

Enterotoxins. Toxigenic strains of *E. coli* elaborate two types of toxins, one of which is heat-stable (ST), the other heat-labile (LT). The genetic determinants for these toxins can occur together on the same or on separate plasmids (9). Sherman *et al.* (15) found that ST-LT plasmids from humans and swine had approximately the same molecular weight (55 to 60 megadaltons) but that the molecular weight of ST plasmids was highly variable. Later, So *et al.* (21) showed that ST plasmids from swine strains had no homology with ST-LT plasmids from either swine or humans but that there was considerable homology between ST-LT plasmids from each of these sources. However, they found that these plasmids belonged to different incompatibility groups—the porcine ST-LT plasmid was an FI and the human plasmid was an FII. This difference in incompatibility group did not involve a substantial amount of DNA because, as So *et al.* (22) were able to show by DNA hybridization studies, ST-LT plasmids have a majority of nucleotides in common regardless of origin. Thus there is good evidence that a substantial part of the ST-LT plasmid is common to both swine and human strains of enterotoxigenic *E. coli*. The DNA fragment in this plasmid which encodes for LT toxin is no greater than 3.0 kilobases (23).

The ST determinant from a plasmid containing ST alone has been cloned in a DNA fragment of 3.4 kilobases and has been shown to be a transposon flanked by inverted repeats of IS 1 (24). This transposability probably accounts for the differing molecular weight of ST plasmids.

These findings suggest that the ST genes in *E. coli* from a variety of hosts could be the same because they have the potential for transfer from one plasmid to another. Furthermore, there are indications that the genes for ST-LT are also on a transposon. Inverted repeat sequences are known to bound the area containing the genes on a plasmid with ST-LT function (17).

Colonizing Antigens. A number of pilus- and capsule-associated antigens are known to be important in the colonization of the small intestine of pigs, calves, lambs, and humans by enteropathogenic *E. coli*. These include the K88 and K99 antigens, the pilus antigen of porcine *E. coli* 987P (11), and the colonization factor associated with the human *E. coli* strain H-10407 (6). Only the genetic basis of the K88 antigen has been well studied. Shipley *et al.* (16) have shown that the genes for the K88 antigen are located on 50 and 90 megadalton plasmids. The larger plasmid is autotransmissible, but the smaller is not. More recently it has been shown that the genes for $K88^{ab}$ synthesis lie on a DNA sequence of 4.3 megadaltons or less (12). Studies to compare DNA sequences for K88 synthesis with DNA sequences from human *E. coli* strains that possessed colonization factors have not yet been reported. Because the K88 antigens have been found only on *E. coli* strains specific for swine (13), it is likely that the genes for factors with similar function in human *E. coli* strains will prove different.

The K99 antigen is found in enteropathogenic *E. coli* from calves and lambs (14) and on porcine *E. coli* of O groups 101 and 64 (13). No studies on the characteristics of the K99 genes have yet been reported.

Other Virulence Plasmids in *E. coli*. Smith (19, 20) has described two plasmids that increase the lethality of *E. coli* for experimental animals. The first of these, the Vir plasmid, was found in about 2 percent of *E. coli* from cases of *E. coli* septicemia in lambs and calves. This plasmid mediates the production of a toxin which causes extravasation of fluid into the pericardial and abdominal cavities and leads to death of the animal because of circulatory failure.

The second plasmid involved in virulence is the Col V plasmid, which, besides coding for colicin V production, also codes for increased resistance of the host organism to serum bactericidal action. This plasmid was found in 0.5 percent of *E. coli* from cases of bacteremia in humans and chickens.

REFERENCES

1. Anderson. Ann. Rev. Microbiol., 1968, *22,* 131.
2. Anderson and Threlfall. Jour. Hyg. (London), 1974, *72,* 471.
3. Anderson, Humphreys, and Willshaw. Jour. Gen. Microbiol., 1975, *91,* 376.
4. Datta. Microbiology—1974, ed. David Schlessinger. Am. Soc. Microbiol., Washington, D.C., 1974, p. 9.
5. Dorn, Trutakawa, Fein, Burton, and Blender. Am. Jour. Epidemiol., 1975, *102,* 319.
6. Evans, Silver, Evans, Chase, and Gorbach. Inf. and Immun., 1975, *12,* 656.
7. Falkow, Stanley. Infectious multiple drug resistance. Pion Ltd., London, 1975.
8. Falkow and Baron, Jour. Bact., 1962, *84,* 581.
9. Gyles, So, and Falkow. Jour. Inf. Dis., 1974, *130,* 40.
10. Hedges and Jacob. Mol. Gen. Genet., 1974, *132,* 31.
11. Isaacson, Nagy, and Moon. Jour. Inf. Dis., 1977, *135,* 531.
12. Mooi, de Graaf, and Van Embden. Nucleic Acid Res., 1978, *6,* 849.
13. Moon, Nagy, Isaacson, and Orskov. Inf. and Immun., 1977, *15,* 614.
14. Orskov, Orskov, Smith, and Sojka. Acta. Path. et Microbiol., Scand., Sect. B, 1975, *83,* 31.
15. Sherman, Formal, and Falkow. Inf. and Immun., 1972, *5,* 622.
16. Shipley, Gyles, and Falkow. Inf. and Immun., 1978, *20,* 559.
17. Silva, Maas, and Gyles. Proc. Natl. Acad. Sci., 1978, *75,* 1384.
18. Silver and Mercer. *In* Nutrition and drug interrelations, ed. Hathcock and Coon. Academic Press, New York, 1978, pp. 649–64.
19. Smith. Jour. Gen. Microbiol., 1974, *83,* 95.
20. Smith and Higgins. Jour. Gen. Microbiol., 1976, *92,* 335.
21. So, Crosa, and Falkow. Jour. Bact., 1975, *121,* 234.
22. So, Boyer, Betlach, and Falkow. Jour. Bact., 1976, *128,* 463.
23. So, Dallas, and Falkow. Inf. and Immun., 1978, *21,* 405.
24. So, Heffron, and McCarthy. Nature, 1979, *277,* 453.
25. Threlfall, Ward, and Rowe. Vet. Rec., 1978, *103,* 438.
26. Timoney. Jour. Inf. Dis., 1978, *137,* 67.
27. Wells and James. Jour. Hyg. (London), 1973, *71,* 209.

4 The Genus *Pseudomonas*

Members of this genus are commonly found in aquatic habitats and in soil. One species (*P. mallei*) is a specialized mammalian parasite. Two other species (*P. pseudomallei* and *P. aeruginosa*) are occasional parasites of animals. All are motile by means of polar flagella and are rod-shaped and oxidase-positive.

Pseudomonas aeruginosa

SYNONYMS: *Pseudomonas pyocyaneus*, bacillus of green pus

This is an organism of comparatively low virulence found frequently in suppurative processes in domestic animals. It causes severe epidemics of respiratory disease in mink and chinchillas. Many infections are opportunistic and are commonly associated with immunosuppressive therapy, prolonged broad-spectrum antibiotic administration, burns, or debilitating operations. The organism is especially common in chicken intestinal contents and may lead to early spoilage of chicken meat. It has also caused a "green wool" condition in sheep (16, 24).

Morphology and Staining Reactions. *P. aeruginosa* is a straight, slender rod, 2.5 by 0.4 μm. Young cultures are rapidly motile by means of one to three polar flagella. Spores are not formed and a capsule is sometimes present. The organism is Gram-negative and stains readily with the ordinary dyes (Figure 4.1).

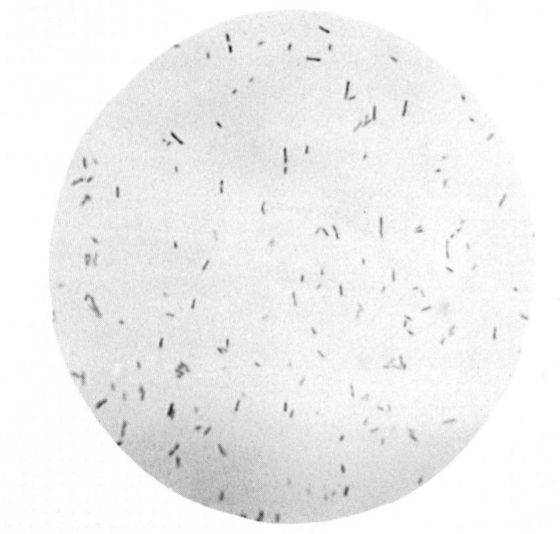

Figure 4.1. *Pseudomonas aeruginosa*, from a culture on a slant agar incubated for 18 hours at 37 C. × 1,150.

Cultural Features. This organism is readily recognized by the bright green pigment and characteristic odor that it produces. There are really two pigments. One of these, known as fluorescein, is yellowish green when fresh and oxidizes to yellow. Fluorescein is produced by a number of organisms other than *P. aeruginosa* which have their habitat in water. The second pigment is a bluish green that oxidizes to brown. It is known as pyocyanin, and is produced only by *P. aeruginosa*. Both fluorescein and pyocyanin are water-soluble; hence in culture the green pigment diffuses throughout the medium. This is best seen when the organism is growing on a solid medium. Pyocyanin is soluble in chloroform to a greater degree than in water, whereas fluorescein is insoluble in chloroform. If a few drops of chloroform are added to a culture and thoroughly shaken through it, the chloroform, when it settles out, will be colored a deep blue. This is a rapid and reliable test for the presence of pyocyanin.

Both of the pigments of this organism are products of oxidation and do not appear unless the organism is growing under aerobic conditions. If the organism is cultivated under anaerobic conditions in a fluid medium and then exposed to oxygen by shaking the culture or blowing air through it, the colorless medium will assume the characteristic deep green color within a few seconds. Some strains lose their ability to produce pigment upon prolonged culture. Apyocyanogenic strains are fairly common and must be identified by their mucoid growth on potassium gluconate medium.

P. aeruginosa may be cultivated upon the simplest of media. Most strains produce smooth, shiny, moist, fimbriate and spreading colonies. Colonies have thin, irregular margins, and the translucent centers are cream-colored, although this color often is disguised by the green pigment that stains the surroundings. An opalescent sheen characteristically appears on the surface of growths on solid media.

It is nonfermentative of carbohydrates, but some strains have been shown to produce acid from D-arabinose, L-arabinose, D-glucose, D-mannose, and D-xylose. It is indol-, methyl-red-, and Voges-Proskauer-negative and is catalase- and oxidase-positive. Most strains liquefy gelatin and are urease-positive and hemolytic. The organism grows well at a wide range of incubation temperatures (4 to 42 C).

P. aeruginosa produces bacteriocins known as pyocins which act on other *P. aeruginosa* strains and therefore have been used for typing. Holloway (10) has written a good review of pyocins. Other, less specific bactericidal substances may also be produced. These include alpha-oxyphenarine and a lipoidal fraction (pyocyanase), both of which are effective against various Gram-positive organisms.

By using precipitation tests in which trichloracetic acid extracts were used as antigen, Van den Ende (23) classified strains of *P. aeruginosa* into six serological groups. Verder and Evans (25) studied 326 cultures and by means of agglutination tests divided them into 10 O groups and 13 O types. Ten H factors were found to occur in eight distinct combinations. On the basis of these O and H antigens, 29 serotypes were established. Besides serological methods, *P. aeruginosa* may be typed by bacteriophage (21) and pyocin (9). In North America, strains from animals seem to belong mainly to pyocin types 1 and 3 (14). Type 1 strains are most important also in Israel, where 80 percent of strains from mastitis cases were of this type (17).

Pathogenesis. The organism produces lecithinase and protease, which appear to be responsible for edema and induration of the skin and for the hemorrhagic and necrotic skin lesions (13). Elastase activity is associated with the proteases of most strains. Toxin production *in vivo* is apparently enhanced by the ready availability of the amino acids, aspartic acid, glutamic acid, and alpha-alanine in animal tissue. The extracellular slime produced by the organism is antiphagocytic and aids penetration of tissue. However, the organism is not very pathogenic in normal animals and requires circumstances such as immunosuppression or tissue debilitation to enter and multiply. Protease production is greater in tissue with an elevated lactic acid concentration; thus the organism would have greater penetration ability in injured tissue.

Pathogenicity for experimental animals. Intraperitoneal injection of freshly isolated cultures into guinea pigs usually produces death within 24 hours. Rabbits are not so susceptible as guinea pigs; mice and pigeons are even less susceptible. According to Gorrill (8), the intravenous injection of *P. aeruginosa* in mice is followed either by (*a*) septicemic death within 24 to 48 hours, (*b*) renal-abscess formation and death in 3 to 14 days, or (*c*) survival. The results depend on the virulence and number of organisms injected.

Pathogenicity for domestic animals. This organism is often found in necrotic pneumonias of swine. Frequently it reaches these organs by aspiration of pus from necrotic rhinitis, a disease in which it is believed to be a secondary invader. The organism also appears in the intestinal lumen of swine in cases of necrotic enteritis. It often is found in foul-smelling abscesses of the spleen and liver of both swine and cattle. In traumatic pericarditis of cattle, this organism commonly accompanies the foreign body. In most abscesses other bacteria are present, and the role of each of the organisms present is uncertain. Poels (18) has described a form of scours in calves in which *P. aeruginosa* was thought to be the causative agent. It was found in almost pure culture in the watery stools. Occasionally cases of septicemia are observed, the organism being found in pure culture in the blood and all organs shortly after death. It has been recognized in outbreaks of bovine mastitis and has been known to erupt from this gland into systemic infection (7). Tucker (22) has stated that some outbreaks of *Pseudomonas* mastitis have been caused by the introduction of the organism into the udder during administration of penicillin for infusion therapy.

Water used for udder washing or rinsing of milking machines has also been noted as a source of infection for the bovine mammary gland (15). In this outbreak, carrier cows were later responsible for secondary cases. In England, *Pseudomonas* mastitis appears to have an increased incidence in August, September, and October (1)—the reason for this is unclear. The disease may be characterized by chronic inflammation with periodic flare-ups, and the organism may be difficult to culture from affected animals. Infusion of endotoxin is sometimes effective in removal of infection because of the leukocytosis which is thereby induced.

P. aeruginosa has been implicated as a cause of bovine infertility (3). Heifers inseminated with semen containing this pathogen developed varying degrees of uteritis, cervicitis, and vaginitis. It has also been reported as the cause of sporadic abortions in cattle. The organism has been shown to be spermicidal (19) and has caused balanoposthitis in bulls (4). It is also transmitted by the stallion and may cause infertility in the mare (12). Older mares are more susceptible. Abortion caused by *P. aeruginosa* has also been described in this host.

In dogs, the organism causes a suppurative otitis externa as a complication of injury, mange, and other bacterial and fungal infections. Postoperative septicemia caused by *P. aeruginosa* has been described in dogs following experimental cardiovascular surgery (5).

Blue *et al.* (2) recommend lavage of affected ears with ethylene diamine-tetraacetic acid (EDTA)-trimethamine-lysozyme solution. Over 80 percent of cases respond well according to these authors.

P. aeruginosa infection is perhaps most devastating in mink (6) and chinchillas, where it causes hemorrhagic pneumonia (Figure 4.2). Infection apparently enters when the animal sniffs its food. Vaccination of mink is highly successful, but vaccines must contain the common protective antigen endotoxin and toxoids of the proteases and elastases produced by the organism (11). A nasal vaccine consisting of the protein moiety of the *Pseudomonas* endotoxin has recently been shown to protect mice against homologous and heterologous strains (20).

"Green wool" in sheep in Australia is believed to be a result of overgrowth of *P. aeruginosa* in fleeces subjected to prolonged wetting (16). The bacterial overgrowth is caused by protein which leaks out of the macerated skin. Oviposition by flies is stimulated by odors

Figure 4.2. A colony of *Pseudomonas aeruginosa* in a section of lung of mink with hemorrhagic pneumonia. × 700. (Courtesy Farrell, Leader, and Gorham, *Cornell Vet.*)

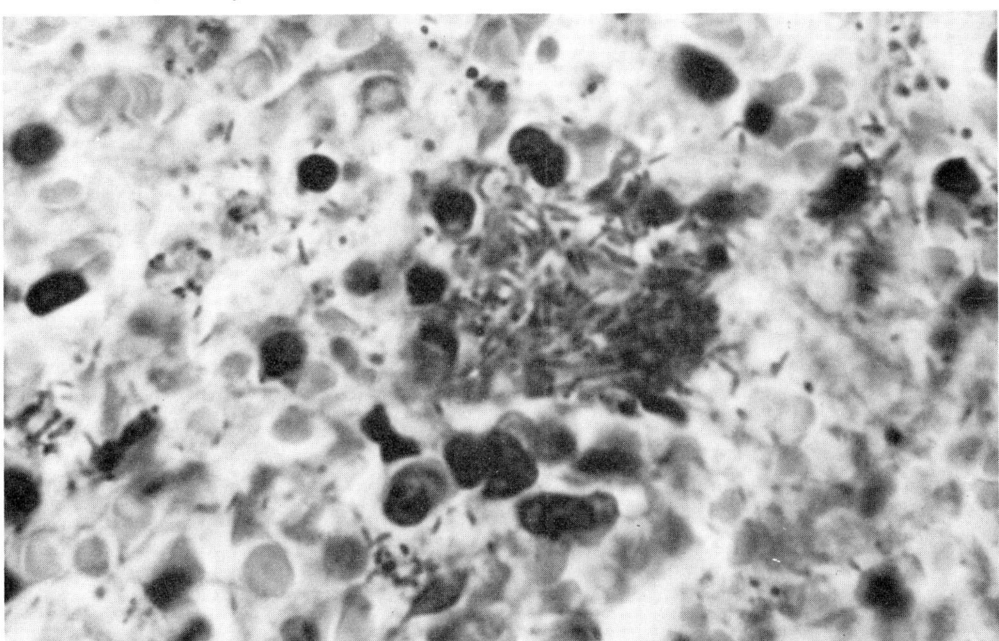

from the protein breakdown, and so affected sheep are predisposed to *strike*.

Treatment. The majority of strains of *P. aeruginosa* from lesions in animals have multiple antibiotic resistance. These resistances are mediated by R factors. Antibiotics to which strains are likely to be sensitive include polymixin B, carbenicillin, and gentamicin. One percent acetic acid has been used in treating otorrhea in dogs.

REFERENCES

1. Anonymous. Vet Rec., 1977, *100*, 441.
2. Blue, Wooley, and Eagon. Am. Jour. Vet. Res., 1974, *35*, 1221.
3. Corradini and Binato. Vet. Ital., 1961, *12*, 320.
4. Corrias and Mollinari. Atti Soc. Ital. Sci. Vet., 1958, *12*, 243.
5. Cross, Cooper, and Needham. Jour. Comp. Path., 1975, *85*, 445.
6. Farrell, Leader, and Gorham. Cornell Vet., 1958, *48*, 378.
7. Gardiner and Craig. Vet. Rec., 1961, *73*, 372.
8. Gorrill. Jour. Path. and Bact., 1952, *64*, 857.
9. Govan and Gillies. Jour. Med. Microbiol., 1969, *2*, 17.
10. Holloway. Bact. Rev., 1969, *33*, 419.
11. Honda, Homma, Abe, Tanomota, Noda, and Yanagowa. Zentrbl. f. Bakt., 1977, *237A*, 297.
12. Hughes, Ashury, Loy, and Burd. Cornell Vet., 1966, *57*, 53.
13. Liu. Jour. Inf. Dis., 1966, *116*, 112.
14. Lusis and Soltys. Vet. Bull., 1971, *41*, 169.
15. Malmo, Robinson, and Morris. Austral. Vet. Jour., 1972, *48*, 137.
16. Merritt and Watts. Austral. Vet. Jour., 1978, *54*, 517.
17. Murkin and Ziv. Jour. Hyg. (London), 1972, *71*, 113.
18. Poels. Berl. Tierärztl. Wchnschr., 1901, *17*, 290.
19. Schwerdtner. Zuchthyg. Forpl. Stor. Besam. Haustiere, 1961, *5*, 260.
20. Shinizu, Homma, Abe, Tansmoto, Aoyoma, Okada, Yanagwa, Fujimoto, Noda, Takaschima, Honda, and Minamide. Am. Jour. Vet. Res., 1976, *37*, 1441.
21. Sutter, Hurst, and Fennell. Health Lab. Sci., 1965, *2*, 7.
22. Tucker. Cornell Vet., 1950, *40*, 95.
23. Van den Ende. Jour. Hyg. (London), 1952, *50*, 405.
24. Van Tonder, Kellerman, and Bolton. Jour. S. Afr. Vet. Assoc., 1976, *47*, 223.
25. Verder and Evans. Jour. Inf. Dis., 1961, *109*, 183.

Pseudomonas (Malleomyces) pseudomallei

SYNONYMS: Bacillus of Whitmore, *Malleomyces whitmori*

In vitro DNA hybridization experiments suggest a close relationship of *P. pseudomallei* to *P. mallei*.

P. pseudomallei produces melioidosis, a glanderslike disease originally described by Whitmore and Krishnaswami (14) in Rangoon. For many years it was thought to be primarily a disease of rodents, occasionally communicable to man, and limited in occurrence to southeast Asia. It is now known to occur in man in the Western Hemisphere and in wild and domestic animals in France, Australia, and the Caribbean. It has been found in soil and water in southeast Asia and is probably an accidental pathogen (11).

Morphology and Staining Reactions. It is a Gram-negative bacillus with a single polar flagellum and closely resembles *P. aeruginosa*. It may show bipolar staining.

Cultural Features. Colonies are readily formed on simple media and range from rough to mucoid and from cream to orange in color. Acid is usually produced from glucose, maltose, sucrose, and mannitol.

Pathogenicity. The organism is pathogenic for rodents, cats, dogs, pigs, goats, sheep, horses, and man. The characteristic lesion produced is a small caseous nodule. These nodules may coalesce to form large areas of caseation or break down into abscesses. They may be found in lymph nodes, in the spleen, lungs, liver, joints, nasal cavity, and tonsils, and in fact in almost any tissue, including the brain (9). Guinea pigs and rabbits are highly susceptible to infection, and inoculated male guinea pigs may produce the Strauss reaction. *P. pseudomallei* has been isolated from an aborted goat fetus (12). It has been reported as the cause of vertebral abscesses on the spinal cord of lambs resulting in posterior flaccid paralysis (3). In cattle, acute fatal infection is characterized by pneumonia, placentitis, and endometritis (4). In the same report a chronic form characterized by encapsulated caseous lesions in the lung and arthritis is also described.

Infection was common in military dogs in Vietnam. Dogs affected with melioidosis exhibit fever, myalgia, dermal abscesses, and epididymitis (6). Many infections are inapparent.

Diagnosis. Diagnosis of the disease depends on the isolation and identification of the organism rather than on clinical findings or serologic tests, although Olds and Lewis (8) reported some success with the melioidin test, and Nigg and Johnston (7) and Omar (10) have employed complement-fixation and agglutination tests with apparent success. A complement fixation test (CFT) titer of 1:20 indicates active or recent infection. Moe *et al.* (6) diagnosed canine melioidosis by culture of blood and lesions and by means of a hemagglutination (HA) test on serum.

Transmission. The disease occurs naturally in rodents, and transmission among these animals by biting insects such as mosquitoes and fleas has been reported (5). Studies by Strauss *et al.* (13) revealed no evidence to suggest that this microorganism requires the rat or any other animal as a maintenance host. They concluded that, in Malaysia, *P. pseudomallei* is a normal inhabitant of the soil and water. In man there is evidence that melioidosis often follows trauma.

Treatment. The organism is sensitive to trimethoprim-sulfamethoxazole (1) and to a combination of novobiocin and tetracyline (2). Sulfamylan is effective for topical application.

REFERENCES

1. Bassett. Jour. Clin. Path., 1971, *24,* 798.
2. Calabi. Jour. Med. Microbiol., 1973, *6,* 293.
3. Ketterer and Bomford. Austral. Vet. Jour., 1967, *43,* 79.
4. Ketterer, Donald, and Rogers. Austral. Vet. Jour., 1975, *51,* 395.
5. Mirick, Zimmerman, Maner, and Humphrey. Jour. Am. Med. Assoc., 1946, *130,* 1063.
6. Moe, Stedham, and Jennings. Am. Jour. Trop. Med. and Hyg., 1972, *21,* 351.
7. Nigg and Johnston. Jour. Bact., 1961, *82,* 159.
8. Olds and Lewis. Austral. Vet. Jour., 1954, *30,* 253.
9. Omar. Jour. Comp. Path. and Therap., 1963, *73,* 359.
10. Omar. Brit. Vet. Jour., 1962, *118,* 421.
11. Redfearn, Palleroni, and Stainer. Jour. Gen. Microbiol., 1966, *43,* 293.
12. Retnasabapathy. Vet. Rec., 1966, *79,* 166.
13. Strauss, Grones, Mariappan, and Ellison. Am. Jour. Trop. Med. and Hyg., 1969, *18,* 698.
14. Whitmore and Krishnaswami. Indian Med. Gaz., 1912, *47,* 262.

Pseudomonas (Malleomyces) mallei

SYNONYMS: *Actinobacillus mallei, Bacterium mallei, Bacillus mallei, Pfeifferella mallei, Loefflerella mallei, Corynebacterium mallei, Mycobacterium mallei*

P. mallei is the cause of *glanders,* a disease primarily of solipeds (horses and the horse family). It also affects man, and cases have been described in lions that have fed on infected horse meat. The disease is one of the oldest known and was described by the ancient Greeks and Romans. As early as the seventeenth century it was recognized as contagious, but the organism was not isolated and shown to be the etiological agent by Loeffler and Schultz (9) until 1882.

Morphology and Staining Reactions. In young cultures the cells are long, slender rods. Older cultures often are quite pleomorphic, the bacilli varying in size and shape from coccoid elements to long, slender filaments. The longer rods usually are distinctively beaded because of accumulated granules of poly B-hydroxybutyrate; the shorter may be bipolar because of granules lying in each end of the cell. The width is 0.3 to 0.5 μm and the length 0.7 to 5.0 μm. The cells are always Gram-negative. With the weaker dyes the organism stains rather poorly. Spores are not formed; there are no capsules and no flagella.

Cultural Features. *P. mallei* grows well but rather slowly upon ordinary laboratory media. Growth on such media generally is enhanced by the addition of glycerol. The organism is rather insensitive to acidity and will grow well on media that are too acid for most pathogenic bacteria.

After a few days' incubation at 37 C, the surface of glycerol agar slants becomes covered with a confluent growth, slightly cream-colored, smooth, moist, and viscid. Continued incubation causes the blanket of growth to increase in thickness and the color to darken until it is dark brown. It is now so viscid as to make it difficult to remove bits of growth with the inoculating loop. Upon plain agar the growth is much less luxuriant.

Very characteristic is the growth upon glycerol potato. Old potato cultures generally become exceedingly luxuriant, the blanket of growth being slimy and then viscid, light tan in the beginning and a mahogany brown finally.

In glycerol broth a viscid sediment forms, and if the cultures are not disturbed a heavy, slimy pellicle forms from which stalactites stretch in the medium toward the bottom of the tube or flask. The broth gradually darkens. Cultures several weeks old become coffee-colored.

The growth on gelatin usually is poor, and ordinarily there is no liquefaction. Litmus milk is slightly acidified, and coagulation may occur after long incubation. Carbohydrates usually are not fermented, but glucose media may be slightly acidified.

Indol is not produced, nitrates are not reduced, and blood is not hemolyzed.

According to Cravitz and Miller (2), strains of *P. mallei* can be separated into at least three serologic groups. Furthermore, a strong relationship exists between the serotypes in one of their groups and *P. pseudomallei.* In fact they were unsuccessful in preparing a complement-fixation antigen that would differentiate between the two species. This is not surprising because DNA hybridization indicates a close relationship of *P. mallei* and *P. pseudomallei.*

Resistance. The organism possesses only slight powers of resistance to drying, heat, and chemicals. Outside the body it probably cannot, under the most favorable of conditions, exist longer than 2 or 3 months.

Pathogenicity. The organism is highly pathogenic for horses, mules, and asses. It is less so for cats (wild and tame), dogs, goats, and man. Sheep, swine, and cattle are highly resistant. Guinea pigs are easily infected artificially, rabbits less easily. The disease occurs almost entirely in the horse species and in carnivora that have consumed infected meat. Man is infected only occasionally when handling animals.

The infection in horses may be either acute or chronic. The latter is by far the more common form. In mules and asses the acute form is more frequent than it is in horses.

The mode of infection is a disputed question; however, it appears probable that ingestion is more important than inhalation. Infection of wounds of the skin occurs, though probably rather rarely. According to the work of Nocard (13) and of McFadyean (10), infection can easily be produced by feeding infected materials. In some cases lesions occur in the mesenteric lymph glands, but many times the lesions appear in the lungs and the mucosa of the upper air passages without evidence of disease processes in the intestine where the infection took place. The intestinal tract therefore probably has a considerable degree of organ immunity. The lungs appear very susceptible, because they are nearly always involved irrespective of the portal of entry.

The organisms are initially spread via the lymph system, but eventually bacteremia occurs with dissemination to the lungs and nasal mucosa.

The lung lesions may take the form of nodules or of a diffuse, pneumonic process (Figure 4.3). The nodules have a characteristic histologic structure by which they may be recognized (3, 10). This structure is not unlike that of a tubercle. Through the rupture of lung nodules into bronchi and the carrying of infective material upward, the upper air passages frequently become the seat of characteristic lesions. Apparently, these lesions can

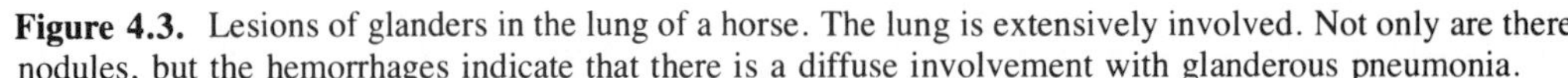

Figure 4.3. Lesions of glanders in the lung of a horse. The lung is extensively involved. Not only are there nodules, but the hemorrhages indicate that there is a diffuse involvement with glanderous pneumonia.

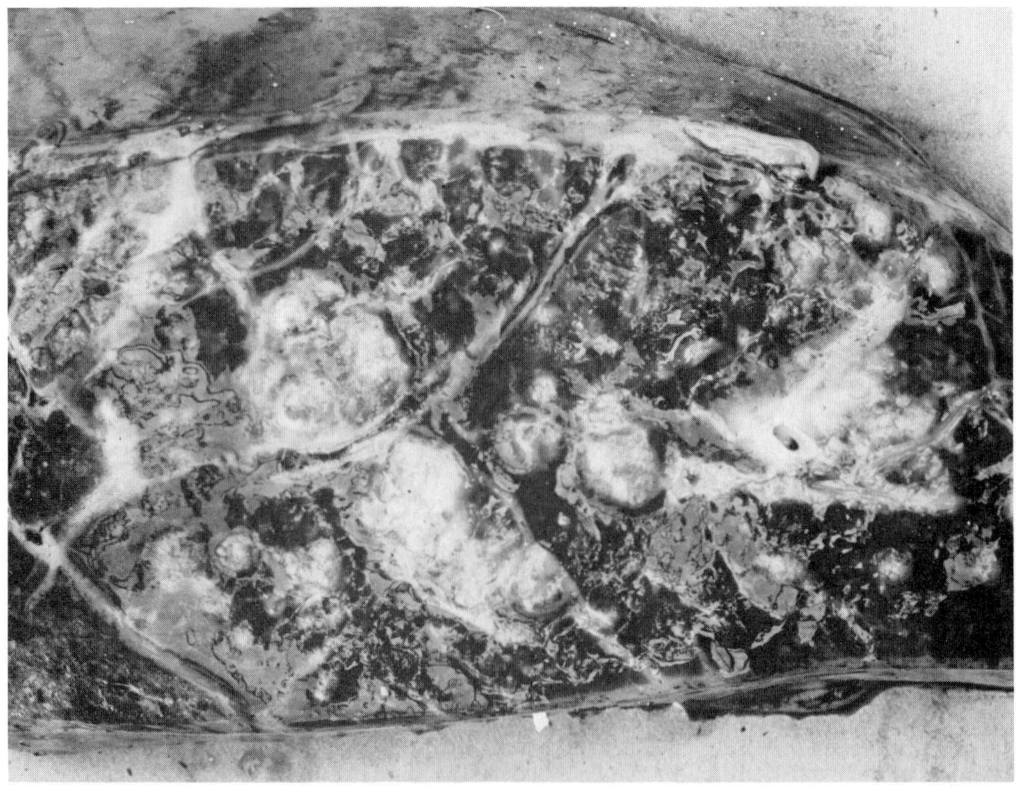

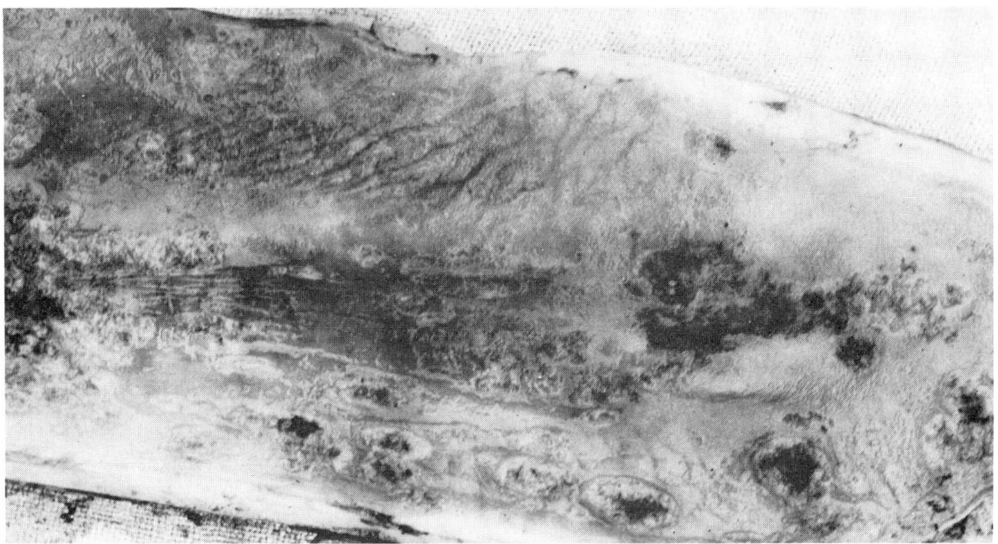

Figure 4.4. Lesions of glanders in the nasal septum of a horse. Shown are ecchymotic hemorrhages and the superficial ulcers from which a sticky discharge exudes.

also occur in animals by direct metastasis from the portal of entry, for sometimes well-marked lesions are found in the upper air passages when few or none exist in the lungs. The lesions in the nasal passages begin as submucosal nodules (Figure 4.4), which quickly rupture forming shallow, craterlike ulcers that exude a thick, sticky purulent material. This is discharged from the nostrils, constituting a highly dangerous exudate.

Glanders nodules may be found in other organs, especially in the liver and spleen. Frequently nodules form under the skin, particularly of the legs (Figure 4.5). These occur in the lymph channels, the infection localizing here and there and forming chains of nodules connected by indurated cords. The nodules usually break down, forming craterlike ulcers that discharge a sticky, honeylike exudate containing the glanders bacillus. This form of glanders is known as *farcy*. Farcy can be a manifestation of local wound infection, but usually it is accompanied by lesions in the internal organs. McFayden (10), who had much experience with glanders in London, stated, "No case of glanders with lesions elsewhere than in the lungs and with those organs healthy, has ever been recorded."

Distribution and Mode of Infection. Infection is contracted in most instances through ingestion, according to McFadyean (10), although it probably can occur through inhalation and through wound infection. Glanders has always, until recently, been the scourge of army horses. From ancient to modern times, wars have always caused the disease to flourish, and the distribution of army animals in civilian service afterward had served to spread the disease far and wide. The American Civil War caused the disease to extend over the eastern parts of the United States. It flourished mostly in the cities, where there were great concentrations of horses in the days of the horsecar and the great livery and delivery stables, but it was by no means unknown in rural districts. During the early part of the present century, after excellent diagnostic tests had been developed, the disease was rapidly brought under control, and the advent of the motor car

Figure 4.5. Skin glanders or farcy of the horse.

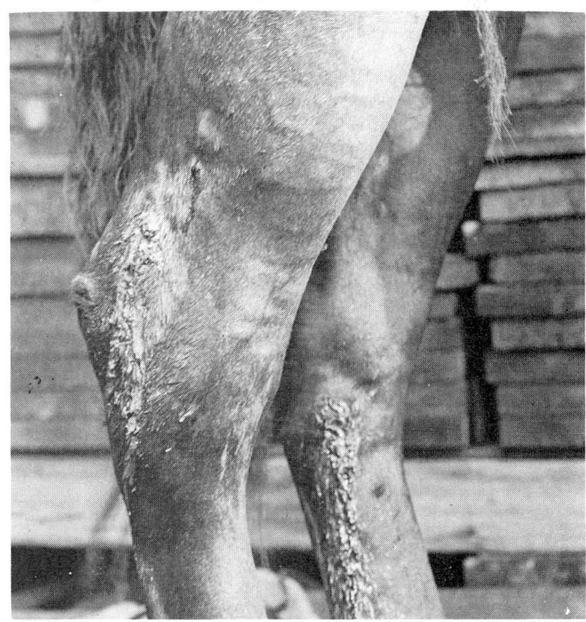

and the motor truck, which diminished the horse populations of all cities, helped greatly in stamping out the disease. It has been eliminated from the United States and the countries of western Europe. It continued to exist in the Balkan states and in Russia, however, until recent years.

Infections are contracted mostly from the highly infectious nasal discharges which contaminate the surroundings, especially harnesses and feeding and watering troughs. Carnivorous animals usually are infected by the eating of meat of glanderous horses. A number of serious outbreaks have occurred in zoological parks from the practice of feeding horse meat to members of the cat family (7). Human infections occur principally among persons whose work brings them into close association with diseased horses. Infections may also occur through wounds while conducting autopsies or while handling meat from glanderous animals. A large number of laboratory infections have been reported, a rather surprising fact in view of the comparatively slight infectivity of glanderous carcasses for man (11).

Diagnosis of Glanders. There are a number of ways by which this disease can be definitely diagnosed. The most important of these are:

1. Physical examination and postmortem lesions. Well-developed clinical cases of glanders are generally easily diagnosed by the symptoms, and the lesions are easily recognized by endoscopy and at necropsy in the majority of cases. Unfortunately such diagnoses can be made only after the animals are well advanced in the disease and have become dangerous spreaders of the infection.

2. Detection of the organism. *P. mallei* may be readily cultivated from closed lesions on plain or glycerol potato, or upon glycerol agar (preferably acid in reaction). When the lesion is open and other organisms are present, it is surer to inoculate several guinea pigs rather than to depend on cultures. If male guinea pigs are inoculated intraperitoneally with not too great a number of *P. mallei* organisms, a localized peritonitis involving the scrotal sac usually develops. As a result the scrotal sac becomes enlarged and painful. Usually the process requires several days to reach its height. The testicle itself becomes involved in a short time, and the whole organ is reduced to a mass of caseous pus which will break through the skin and discharge to the surface. This is known as the *Strauss reaction* (4). A similar reaction sometimes occurs owing to other organisms, for example, *Pseudomonas aeruginosa, Corynebacterium, Brucella,* and *Actinobacillus* species; thus it is not diagnostic of glanders. If too many glanders organisms are injected, the guinea pig will develop a generalized peritonitis and die in a day or two without showing the scrotal changes. If the injection is made subcutaneously instead of intraperitoneally, an ulcer usually forms at the site of injection and the animal will die after 4 or 5 weeks with nodules in many of the internal organs.

3. Serological tests. (*a*) *Complement fixation.* This test has proved to be the most accurate of the serological methods of diagnosing glanders. It was first applied to the disease in Germany about 1909 and soon afterward was introduced into the United States as a diagnostic procedure.

(*b*) *Agglutination.* This is generally admitted to be not so accurate as the previous test. Failures occur in chronic cases. Normal agglutinins exist in a concentration as high as 1:500 in many horses, whereas infected animals usually react in dilutions of 1:1,000 and higher (12).

(*c*) *Hemagglutination.* The use of the hemagglutination test has been proposed for the diagnosis of glanders (6). An HA titer above 1:640 is considered to be positive and it was claimed that this test was more sensitive than the mallein test.

4. Mallein tests. Mallein is a glycoprotein, somewhat analogous to tuberculin, produced by *P. mallei* in glycerol broth and can be extracted by alcohol precipitation. It is nontoxic for normal animals. Animals infected with *P. mallei* become allergic to mallein and exhibit local and systemic hypersensitivity following its inoculation.

Mallein is used in three ways: (*a*) subcutaneous test, (*b*) ophthalmic test, (*c*) intrapalpebral test. When injected subcutaneously it gives rise to fever, which appears and subsides again within 24 hours after the injection. There is usually a marked swelling at the point of injection. Normal horses may show some swelling at this point, but the temperature curve is absent. The ophthalmic test consists of instilling some concentrated mallein into the eye (conjunctival sac). A pus-forming inflammation of the eye occurs within a few hours when the animal is glanderous. The intrapalpebral test consists of injecting a small amount of concentrated mallein into the skin of the lower eyelid (Figure 4.6). A local swelling and a pus-forming inflammation of the eye occur. The intrapalpebral test is more accurate than the ophthalmic and accordingly is more often used.

Shumilov (14) has reported that a double intradermal mallein test detected twice as many infected horses in Mongolia as a double ophthalmic test. Both tests were

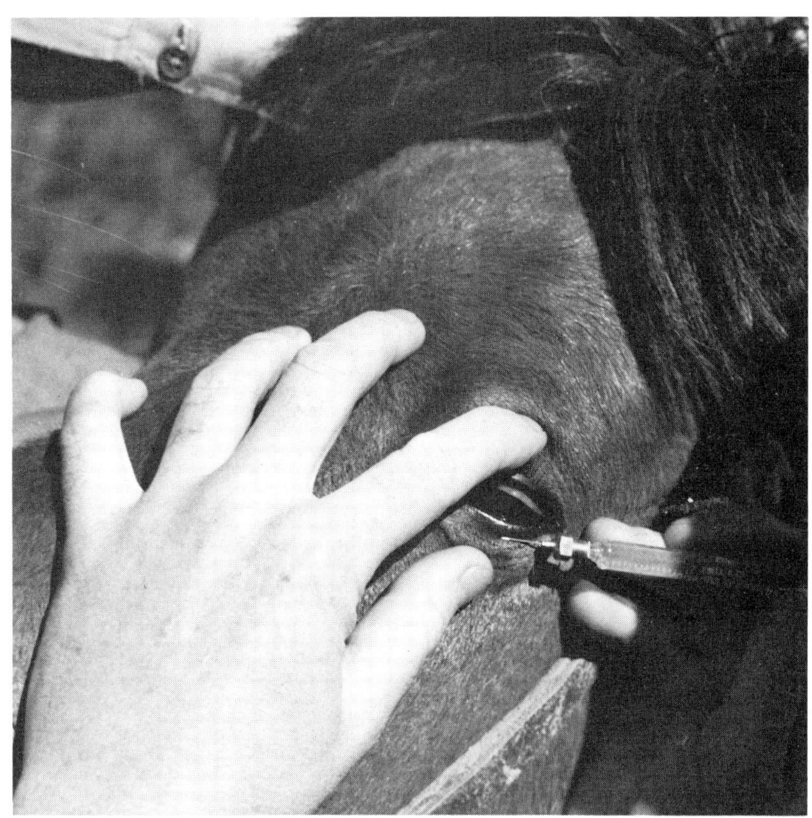

Figure 4.6. Injection of mallein in the intrapalpebral test for the detection of glanders. (Courtesy Col. W. E. Jennings, Veterinary Corps, U.S. Army.)

more reliable when double rather than single inoculations were used. The inoculations of mallein did not induce complement-fixing antibody.

A useful diagnostic feature of mallein tests is that partially healed lesions on the nasal mucosa are activated and become easy to see some 12 to 36 hours after inoculation.

Control Measures. Since spontaneous recovery is rare in this disease and since no efficacious vaccines have been developed, control of the disease has been accomplished wholly by methods which involve early diagnosis and elimination of the reacting animals. Clinical examinations at frequent intervals, the use of mallein and the serological tests, and the destruction of animals that give evidence of infection by any of these tests have proved adequate. These methods have practically eliminated the disease from many European countries. It should be noted that serologic tests are not entirely reliable in diagnosing glanders in areas where melioidosis also exists because of the common somatic antigens possessed by the causative organism (2). The organism is sensitive to sulfonamides and tetracyclines (8).

Glanders in Man. Man is not highly susceptible to glanders; yet numerous infections have occurred in persons caring for glanderous animals, especially stablemen and veterinarians (1). The disease is characterized by swelling and pain at the point of infection (usually the hand, the lip, or the eye), which comes on in 3 to 5 days, swelling of the neighboring lymph glands, development of nasal and mouth ulcers (in about half the cases), development of abscesses and pustules in the skin, joint inflammations, and general symptoms accompanied by fever. The cases usually end fatally in from 2 to 4 weeks. A few cases of glanders in man occurred in Russia during World War I. Chronic glanders in man has been vividly described by Gaiger (5), a British veterinarian who contracted the disease in India.

REFERENCES

1. Coleman and Ewing. Jour. Med. Res., 1903, *4*, 223.
2. Cravitz and Miller. Jour. Inf. Dis., 1950, *86*, 46 and 52.
3. Duval and White. Jour. Exp. Med., 1907, *9*, 352.
4. Frothingham. Jour. Med. Res., 1901, *1*, 331.
5. Gaiger. Jour. Comp. Path. and Therap., 1913, *26*, 233; 1916, *29*, 26.
6. Gangulee, Sen, and Sharma. Indian Vet. Jour., 1966, *43*, 386.
7. Hart. Jour. Am. Vet. Med. Assoc., 1916, *49*, 659.
8. Ipatenko. Trudy Moskow Veter. Akad., 1972, *61*, 142.

9. Loeffler and Schutz. Deut. med. Wchnschr., 1882, *8,* 707.
10. McFadyean. Jour. Comp. Path. and Therap., 1904, *17,* 295.
11. McFadyean. Jour. Comp. Path. and Therap., 1905, *18,* 23.
12. Moore and Taylor. Jour. Inf. Dis., 1907, Supp. 3, 85.
13. Nocard. Bull. Soc. Cent. Med. Vet., 1894, *48,* 225 and 367.
14. Shumilov. Trudy Vsesoyuz Inst. Eksper. Veter., 1974, *42,* 274.

5 The Spirochetes

GENERAL CHARACTERISTICS

The spirochetes are slender, flexuous, helically coiled, unicellular bacteria that range from 3 to 500 μm in length. They are motile through rapid rotation along the axis of the helix, flexion of the cells, and by movement along a corkscrew or serpentine path.

Morphology. The form is spiral. In some species the spirals are tight, in others quite open and variable. Terminal filaments are seen in some types, but these do not behave like flagella. Some forms may show an axial filament, a lateral crista or ridge, or transverse striations.

Staining Properties. Most of the spirochetes are difficult to stain. Few of the pathogenic species may be stained with methylene blue. All are Gram-negative. The Giemsa stain is useful, some staining red, others blue. Those that stain blue generally are saprophytes that can be stained with methylene blue. For demonstration in tissues, Levaditi's stain is most useful. This stain contains silver nitrate. After the tissue block has been saturated with the silver compound, it is treated with a reducing agent that removes the silver from the tissues and other bacteria but not from the spirochetes. These are then seen as intensely black organisms. The dark-field method of examination often is used when these organisms are sought, because it is practically impossible to see them unstained in ordinary light due to their extreme tenuousness. India ink, nigrosin, and similar background-filling agents also are useful in making organisms visible in film preparations.

Resistance. In general, the resistance of spirochetes is very low. Drying is rapidly fatal. Temperatures of 50 to 60 C generally kill within a short time. Resistance to chemical disinfectants is not great.

Cultivation. The spirochetes generally are less easily cultivated than other bacteria. Some, especially the *Leptospira,* can be grown without great difficulty, but others require elaborate media and the results are uncertain at best. The majority are strict anaerobes. Even the aerobic forms thrive best when the oxygen tension is lowered.

Classification. The family Spirochaetaceae contains three genera which include species that cause disease in domestic animals. These genera are *Borrelia, Leptospira,* and *Treponema.*

THE GENUS *BORRELIA*

In this genus are found a number of parasitic forms. They are pathogenic for man, other mammals, and birds. Some are transmitted by the bites of arthropods.

Morphology and Staining Reactions. These organisms are loosely spiraled and irregular. They generally taper terminally into fine filaments. They stain easily with ordinary aniline dyes and are Gram-negative. Their refractive indices are approximately the same as those of other bacteria. However, they can be demonstrated best by dark-field illumination, the India ink method, or the Levaditi stain.

Cultural Features. Noguchi (15) cultivated a number of species in a medium consisting of a tall column of ascitic fluid that contained a bit of sterile rabbit kidney overlaid with paraffin oil. A few drops of infected blood were used as the inoculum, and the tubes were incubated at body temperature. In such tubes the spirochetes grew rather rapidly for 4 or 5 days, then appeared to disintegrate into granules. The report of Bohls *et al.* (2) indicates that the spirochete of relapsing fever can be cultivated in the developing chick embryo. Krizanova *et al.* (10) found that the best method of cultivation of *Borrelia*like organisms was on BHI agar with 20 percent fresh defibrinated ram's blood. Incubation should be carried out in a atmosphere of 10 percent CO_2.

Relapsing Fever Spirochetes (*Borrelia*)

Relapsing fever is a disease of man that occurs throughout the world. In the febrile paroxysms of this disease, members of *Borrelia* can be demonstrated in the blood, and these organisms undoubtedly are the cause of the disease. The organisms differ in various localities, although all forms of relapsing fever are clinically identical. Two epidemiological types of the disease are distinguished, the one tick-borne and representing transmission from an animal reservoir of infection to man, and the other louse-borne and spread from man to man (4). The organisms undergo a developmental cycle in these insects; the tick can transmit the infection by biting, but the louse transmits infection by its feces or by being crushed on the skin. The tick-borne disease appears to be the only one that occurs in the United States, and endemic foci of infection exist in Arizona, California, Colorado, Idaho, Kansas, New Mexico, Nevada, Oklahoma, Oregon, and Texas. According to Francis (8), the infection may survive in ticks for as long as 6.5 years and be transmitted to offspring of the third generation. In 1969 an outbreak occurred on Brown mountain near Spokane, Washington, in boy scouts and scoutmasters who camped there. *Ornithodoros hermsi* ticks were shown to be infected with spirochetes and it was suggested that chipmunks and pine squirrels were the reservoir for the disease (21).

Mice, rats, and hamsters can be infected by inoculation of relapsing fever spirochetes, but guinea pigs are more resistant. Natural infection of lower animals occurs with some frequency in endemic areas, and it is quite possible that small mammals, especially rodents, constitute a natural reservoir of the tick-borne infection.

Practical laboratory diagnosis is based on mouse inoculation and blood-smear demonstrations of the *Borrelia* organism (7).

Borrelia theileri

SYNONYMS: *Treponema theileri, Spirocheta theileri*

This organism was found by Theiler (20) in the blood of South African cattle in 1902. It is a large, loosely twisted spiral, measuring 20 to 30 μm in length. The organism can be easily demonstrated in the blood during the febrile stage of the infection, but it disappears later. It is actively motile. Artificial cultivation of this organism has not been reported.

The disease apparently is fairly benign. The symptoms resemble those of anaplasmosis but are less severe. One or more febrile attacks are followed by recovery. Transmission is by the ticks *Margaropus decoloratus* and *Rhipicephalus evertsi*.

It has been shown that *Boophilus annulatus,* usually thought to be harmless, can be an efficient vector for *B. theileri* (22).

An organism similar to *B. theileri* has been found associated with febrile attacks in sheep and horses. These diseases are not serious.

Borrelia anserina

SYNONYMS: *Spirocheta anserina, Spirocheta gallinarum, Borrelia gallinarum, Spironema gallinarum*

This organism was first described by Sakharoff (18), in Russia, as the cause of "goose septicemia" in 1891. It is probable that it is the same as the cause of "fowl spirochetosis" or "fowl spirillosis," which was recognized in Brazil by Marchoux and Salimbeni in 1903. The disease was found a little later in the Sudan. The spirochete of the chicken disease is regarded as a separate species by some and given the name *Borrelia gallinarum*. A similar disease has been reported in ducks and turkeys. It seems likely that geese, chickens, ducks, and turkeys are affected by the same species. If this is the case, the correct name of the organism, inappropriate as it may seem, is that first applied to the goose infection.

In California, outbreaks of avian spirochetosis have been reported in turkeys (11) and in Mongolian pheasants. It was readily transmitted from the pheasants to Muscovy ducklings and to chickens (13). The avian spirochete was believed to be the cause of epizootics in Arizona poultry (17). The infection occurs in Australia (9).

The disease is manifested by signs of acute septicemia. The affected birds develop fever, they are depressed, a profuse diarrhea occurs, and they soon die. The mortality rate is very high. Autopsy examination reveals a swollen spleen, a pale and swollen liver, and a serofibrinous exudate in the pericardial sac. During the early stages of the febrile reaction the spiral organisms can readily be found in the blood. At the time of death they usually are absent, or abnormal or clumped forms may be found.

A *B. anserina* antigen is normally demonstrable in the liver of infected birds by agar gel immunodiffusion. However, Al-Attar and Johanly (1) have shown that extracts of other organs also become positive for antigen when treated with bile salts to dissolve the spirochetes. Fluorescent-antibody techniques provide a rapid method of detecting *Borrelia* in blood films as well as serving as a basis for serotyping strains of *B. anserina*.

The disease is generally believed to be transmitted by argasid ticks; transovarial transmission has been demonstrated in *Argas persicus* and *Argas arboreus*. However, California workers suggested (11, 13) that infected droppings represented the most probable means of transmission in the outbreaks that they studied. The fowl mite, *Dermanyssus gallinae,* has been suspected of being a transmitting agent. There is some evidence that mosquitoes that have fed recently on infected birds can transmit the disease to other birds.

The disease is easily transmitted to a variety of birds such as sparrows, canaries, and guinea fowl. Pigeons are relatively resistant. Ten or fewer spirochetes constitute an infective dose for susceptible chickens. A specific protein in serum of infected fowls may represent catabolic products of the spirochete (19). With homologous antisera, spirochetes exhibit bright yellow-green fluorescence, and often large, intensely fluorescing granules are present as well; in heterologous reactions, there is dull blue-green fluorescence and no granules. It is suggested that granules represent some type-specific antigen located in cell membranes (5). In argasid ticks, the spiral forms disappear in 3 to 4 months but the ticks remain infected. The infective form in this situation is probably the granule, since these persist in infected ticks.

Immunity. Recovery from the disease leaves the bird refractory to further infection for a considerable period of time. The fresh serum of recovered geese causes disintegration and destruction of the spirochetes in a short time when incubated at 37 C. This is similar to the action that goes on in the blood of the recovering bird. Immune horse serum has been found effective as a prophylactic agent but ineffective when administered to birds in which the organism had begun to multiply.

Marchoux and Salimbeni (12) prepared an effective vaccine by heating the fresh blood of affected birds to 55 C for 5 minues. They also found that the organism loses its virulence when stored in blood for 48 hours, and that such blood may be used as a vaccine. Rao *et al.* (16), Uppal and Rao (23), and Gorrie (9) have developed embryonated egg vaccines that promise durable immunity in vaccinated birds.

Antibodies have been demonstrated in eggs of vaccinated hens 8 weeks after vaccination, and these antibodies possibly protected chicks for the first 2 weeks of life (6).

Chemotherapy. Arsphenamine and its derivatives have been used successfully in treating some of the relapsing fever infections of man. Morcos *et al.* (14) reported that Arrhenal, sulfonamides, and penicillin had no curative effect in avian spirochetosis. On the other hand, Myosalvarsan, Atoxyl, and Spirocide were almost specific as curatives and had the further advantage of serving as tonics. Rao *et al.* (16) reported that penicillin administered as a therapeutic agent at 4,000 units per pound of body weight is fully effective in curing avian spirochetosis at the height of infection.

Injection of a single subcutaneous dose of benzathine chlortetracycline (a long-acting drug) or administration of tetracycline hydrochloride in the drinking water have proved effective in the treatment of infected birds. Infected goslings respond well to tylosin, erythromycin, and spectinomycin (3).

REFERENCES

1. Al-Attar and Johanly. Avian Dis., 1974, *18,* 463.
2. Bohls, Irons, and De Shazo. Proc. Soc. Exp. Biol. and Med., 1940, *45,* 375.
3. Bok, Somberg, Rubina, and Hadoni. Refuah Veter., 1975, *32,* 147.
4. Burrows, William. Textbook of microbiology. 20th ed. W. B. Saunders, Philadelphia and London, 1973.
5. Djankov, Sumrov, and Lozeva. Vet. Nauki. Sofia, 1975, *12,* 29.
6. Dutta, Mehta, and Muley. Indian Jour. An. Sci., 1977, *47,* 554.
7. Felsenfeld. Bact. Rev., 1965, *29,* 46.
8. Francis. Pub. Health Rpts. (U.S.), 1938, *53,* 2220.
9. Gorrie. Austral. Vet. Jour., 1950, *26,* 308.
10. Krizanova, Beseda, Koppel, Halosa, and Horvath. Vet. Med., 1972, *17,* 527.
11. Loomis. Am. Jour. Vet. Res., 1953, *14,* 612.

12. Marchoux and Salimbeni. Ann. Inst. Pasteur, 1903, *17,* 569.
13. Mathey and Siddle. Jour. Am. Vet. Med. Assoc., 1955, *126,* 123.
14. Morcos, Zaki, and Zaki. Jour. Am. Vet. Med. Assoc., 1946, *109,* 112.
15. Noguchi. Jour. Exp. Med., 1912, *16,* 620.
16. Rao, Thakral, and Dhanda. Indian Vet. Jour., 1954, *31,* 1.
17. Rokey and Snell. Jour. Am. Vet. Med. Assoc., 1961, *138,* 648.
18. Sakharoff. Ann. Inst. Pasteur, 1891, *5,* 564.
19. Simionescu and Chisui. Recueil de Med. Vet., 1972, *148,* 349.
20. Theiler. Jour. Comp. Path. and Therap., 1904, *17,* 47.
21. Thompson, Burgdorfer, Russell, and Francis. Jour. Am. Med. Assoc., 1969, *210,* 1045.
22. Trees. Trop. An. Health and Product., 1978, *10,* 93.
23. Uppal and Rao. Indian Vet. Jour., 1966, *43,* 191.

THE GENUS *LEPTOSPIRA*

Leptospirae are chiefly saprophytic aquatic organisms which are found in river and lake waters, in sewage, and in the sea. Some species are pathogenic for man and animals. The pathogenic types are not known to multiply outside infected animal tissues.

Morphology and Staining Reactions. Leptospirae are the smallest of the spirochetes. Individual cells are not more than 0.3 μm in breadth, but vary from 6 to 30 μm in length. Frequently their spirals are so fine and so closely wound that, when observed in the dark field, only the outer curves are seen. They are further characterized by being bent into a hook at one or both ends (Figure 5.1). Their motion consists of a writhing and flexing movement and a rapid rotation around the long axis. They stain with difficulty except with Giemsa's stain and silver impregnation. They are readily filterable through Berkefeld V and N candles—a means of separating them from bacteria and treponemas.

Cultural Features. The leptospirae are readily cultivated. They may be grown on serum diluted with 5 to 10 parts of Ringer or Locke solution. A medium devised by Noguchi which contains a mixture of one part of 2 percent nutrient agar, one part of rabbit serum, and eight parts of physiological salt solution may be used. Semisolid meat infusion agar containing 10 percent serum makes a very good medium (42). Semisynthetic media has also been recommended (15, 26, 50). Incubation at 30 C or slightly below usually produces the best

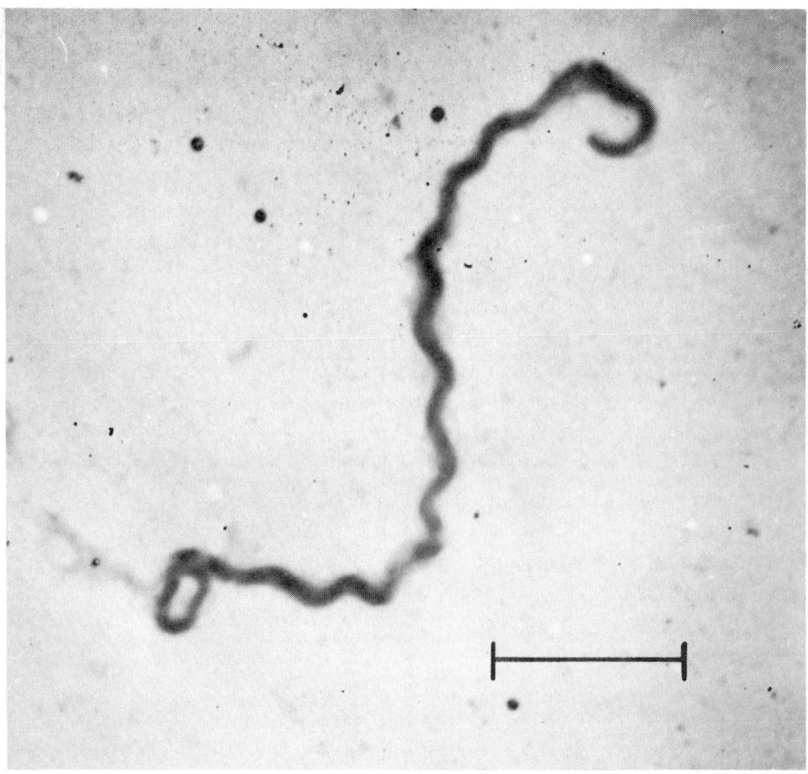

Figure 5.1. Electron micrograph of bovine *Leptospira*. Scale = 1 micron. × 26,500 approximately. (Courtesy J. A. Baker.)

growth. The organisms can be cultivated in embryonated chicken eggs. They will grow in bovine fetal kidney cell tissue cultures (31).

The respiratory mechanism of leptospirae is peculiar in that they require gaseous oxygen, and to this extent are strict aerobes, but in a limited sense they are microaerophilic. In a solid or semisolid media they grow a few mm below the surface, they are cyanide-sensitive, lack catalase, have slight reducing activity, and fail to produce recognizable traces of hydrogen peroxide (12). Apparently they do not ferment sugars. It appears that virulence can be maintained by serial cultivation in animals or embryos but not in artificial media. Some strains such as *L. hardjo* are difficult to maintain in artificial media.

Serotypes. The eighth edition of *Bergey's Manual* lists *Leptospira interrogans* as the only species in the genus. The seventh edition listed two—the parasitic (pathogenic) *L. icterohemorrhagiae* and the saprophytic *L. biflexa*. It is at present uncertain which of the classifications will prevail. In any event, the pathogenic strains are identified in the veterinary and medical literature by the name of the serotype which is the basic taxon. The serotype is determined on the basis of agglutination tests with specific typing antisera. Pathogenic serotypes are similar to one another with respect to morphological, cultural, and biochemical characteristics. There are approximately 150 serotypes divided among 18 serogroups. These groups have been designated Icterohemorrhagiae, Javanica, Celledoni, Canicola, Ballum, Pyrogenes, Cynopteri, Autumnalis, Australis, Pomona, Grippotyphosa, Hebdomadis, Bataviae, Tarassovi, Panama, Shermani, Semaranga, and Andamana.

Epidemiology. In general, the leptospiral serotypes are associated with one or more mammalian species. The principal reservoirs are rodents, especially rats, mice, and voles, and domestic animals such as dogs, cattle, and pigs. For many years, rats and dogs were considered to be the primary animal carriers. Although leptospirosis is still prevalent in dogs and infection in rats ranges from 30 to 60 percent, the disease in now a major problem in cattle and swine, and in some areas sheep, goats, and horses become infected. There is evidence of a wide distribution of leptospirae in a variety of wild animals throughout the world.

Besides the rat other rodent carriers are mice and voles, and the wild animal reservoirs include bats, mongooses, shrews, bandicoots, jackals, and hedgehogs. In the United States deer, opossums, raccoons, skunks, foxes, wildcats, beaver, nutria, armadillos, woodchucks, and rabbits have been infected.

Survival of *Leptospira* sp. in the environment is usually brief and requires suitable conditions of moisture, pH, and temperature. Slightly alkaline conditions favor survival (67). The natural reservoir of *Leptospira* sp. is the lumen of nephritic tubules, from which the organism is shed in the urine and spreads to other hosts. The production of urease by pathogenic *Leptospira* sp. may be significant in renal colonization (38). Shedding in the urine takes place during the later clinical phase and during the convalescent and recovery phases and persists for a variable period. In dogs, cattle, and swine, shedding is usually heavy for the first few months after infection and then becomes lighter or may cease altogether. Rodents are persistent heavy shedders. Although urine is the most important vehicle of infection, milk, placental material, and aborted fetuses have also been sources of the organism for other animals.

Leptospirae easily penetrate the mucosae of the digestive tract, the conjunctiva and the genitalia (56). They also penetrate skin that has been abraded or softened by exposure to moisture.

Serotypes such as *L. icterohemorrhagiae, L. canicola, L. grippotyphosa, L. bataviae, L. hebdomadis, L. australis, L. pyrogenes, L. pomona, L. ballum,* and *L. tarassovi* show widespread global distribution. Other serotypes (*L. autumnalis, L. sejroe,* and *L. andamana*) appear to be restricted to particular areas of the world. Primary problems in the United States usually are associated with the more common types, *L. icterohemorrhagiae, L. canicola,* and *L. pomona,* in domestic animals and man (21). Numerous other serotypes have been isolated, and the findings suggest the presence of many more. *L. autumnalis* has been identified in man and in wild animals. *L. ballum* has appeared in mice, opossums, rats, an eastern hog-nosed snake, and man. *L. grippotyphosa* was obtained from wild animals in Florida, along with *L. pomona, L. australis,* and *L. autumnalis*. Other serotypes belonging to the Tarassovi serogroup have been isolated from wild animals in the southeastern United States and have been designated *L. bakeri* and *L. atlantae*. A new subserotype of the Hebdomadis serogroup was named *L. mimi georgia*. This type has now been derived also from human infection. Serologic evidence suggests the presence of *L. bataviae* infection in man and in cattle. *L. sejroe* occurs in cattle and man and a closely related serotype, *L. hardjo,* has been obtained in Louisiana, Nebraska, and Pennsylvania from animals both with and without signs of disease. A member of the Bataviae serogroup (*L. paidjan*) has been found in Louisiana in nutria (52), and *L. manilae,* a new serotype in the Pyrogenes group, was derived from rats (20).

L. icterohemorrhagiae is carried by rats, dogs, and occasionally cattle and swine; *L. canicola* is primarily an infection of dogs but also is seen in swine and cattle; and *L. pomona* is the organism most frequently incriminated as the cause of bovine, equine, and porcine leptospirosis. Although it seems that certain leptospiral serotypes have a primary host, none are completely host-adapted. It is not unusual for a so-called *primary host* to become infected with other serotypes. *L. canicola* is found principally in dogs, but has been isolated from cattle, swine, jackals, hedgehogs, and skunks. Serologic evidence suggests that it may infect raccoons. In addition to *L. canicola* dogs have been found to harbor at least nine serotypes, including *L. pomona.*

Bovine Leptospirosis

Leptospirosis in cattle is a cause of serious economic loss throughout the world. In the United States, six serotypes have been isolated from disease in the bovine: *L. canicola, L. icterohemorrhagiae, L. hardjo, L. pomona, L. szwajizak,* and *L. grippotyphosa.*

Although *L. icterohemorrhagiae* and *L. canicola* occur in cattle, the predominant serotypes in the bovine species appear to be *L. hardjo* and *L. pomona* in the United States and Australia, *L. australis* and *L. hebdomadis* in Japan, and *L. grippotyphosa* in Russia and Israel. Many of the recognized serotypes have been isolated from cattle in widely scattered parts of the world.

The Natural Disease. The incubation period varies from 4 to 10 days and is followed by a leptospiremia which lasts for 1 to 5 days. This phase is terminated by the appearance of antibody in the animal's blood. The organism is now rapidly cleared from the bloodstream but localizes and remains in the kidneys (8). The site of localization is the lumen of the convoluted tubule where the organism multiplies and is shed in the urine. Leptospiruria lasts for 1 to 3 months, but the organism may persist in the kidney for longer periods.

Animals with acute leptospirosis may show a transient fever and loss of appetite. Lactating cows exhibit agalactia and a mild secretion that is yellow, clotted, and often blood-stained. Severely affected animals develop anemia, jaundice, hemoglobinuria, and pneumonia. These effects may be fatal in calves.

In pregnant cows, the leptospirae may invade the fetus, which dies and is aborted 1 to 4 weeks after the leptospiremic phase. The organism is usually difficult to culture from aborted fetuses because of autolytic changes in the tissues after death and before abortion occurs (58).

Infertility in cattle has been associated with enzootic infections by *L. hardjo* and *L. szwajizak* (2, 17, 23). The immunosuppressive effects of concurrent infection by infectious bovine rhinotracheitis virus have been suggested as important in the pathogenesis of *L. hardjo* abortion in heifers (37).

The local immune response of the animal's endometrium appears to play a role in infertility problems associated with *L. hardjo* and *L. szwajizak* (2), although vaccination with specific bacterins has improved fertility in infected herds (23).

Stoenner *et al.* (62) have reported neurologic manifestations of leptospirosis in a dairy cow and have observed survival of the organism in the cerebrospinal fluid despite intensive antibiotic therapy.

Immunity. Antibodies of the IgM class are detectable a few days after the febrile and leptospiremic phases. These antibodies are agglutinins and are probably responsible for initial clearance of the organism from the bloodstream. Agglutinin titers rise to a peak for a month and persist at high level in most animals for up to 2 years (30). Antibodies of the IgG class appear a few days after the IgM (45). These antibodies have neutralizing activity and are detectable by the hamster passive-protection test (45). They persist for several years.

Persistence of antibody in cattle may be promoted by further field exposure to *Leptospira* sp. similar to or related to the serotype involved in the primary infection (64).

Vaccination with killed bacterins protects against clinical leptospirosis for up to a year, but the bacterin must contain the antigens of the strain to which the cattle are subsequently exposed. Both IgM and IgG antibodies are produced. The former are present in low titer and fall below diagnostic levels in a few weeks (66). The protective antibodies, which are not agglutinating and belong to the IgG class, persist for 6 months to a year. Most herds are vaccinated at intervals of 6 months to a year depending on the expected level of field exposure (29).

Calves born of immunized dams are protected by colostral antibodies for the first few months of life. Passively immune calves should not be vaccinated before 3 months because the vaccine response will be of short duration (22).

Swine Leptospirosis

At least twelve different serotypes of *Leptospira* are known to infect swine, the most important of which are *L. pomona, L. canicola, L. hyos,* and *L. icterohemorrhagiae*. Swine infected with *L. pomona* have been a source of infection for their caretakers—the resultant disease in whom has been appropriately named *swineherd's disease* (19, 27).

The Natural Disease. Transmission of *L. pomona* from pig to pig occurs readily by contact via urine, and the pig is widely believed to be the primary reservoir of this serotype. *L. canicola* and *L. icterohemorrhagiae* are also spread from pig to pig in the urine, but rodents and dogs are probably important as primary sources of these serotypes for swine. *L. pomona* can be transmitted from swine to calves (8).

The symptoms in swine vary widely. Many infections are subclinical and only recognizable by seroconversion, by isolation of the organism from the kidneys of normal swine at slaughter, or by cases of leptospirosis in swineherds.

Acute or subacute infections are observed in young pigs infected by *L. icterohemorrhagiae* or *L. canicola* (3, 46). There is fever, anorexia, icterus, hemoglobinuria, and a heavy mortality. Petechial hemorrhages occur in the lungs, kidneys, and other abdominal visera. Diarrhea, irritability, conjunctivitis, tremors of the legs, weakness of the hind limbs, stiffness of the neck, and encephalitic symptoms have also been described (55).

Infertility, abortions, and stillbirths associated with *L. canicola, L. pomona, L. hyos,* and *L. icterohemorrhagiae* are also widely observed (43). Aborted fetuses are jaundiced, and piglets born alive are weak and die soon after birth.

Immunity. A mixed *L. pomona*-*L. hyos* bacterin has been shown to protect sows and gilts against abortions (9). However, the immunity stimulated by *L. pomona* bacterin in swine does not protect against renal colonization (61). Interestingly, attenuated *L. pomona* vaccine does protect against the renal carrier state (60).

Canine Leptospirosis

L. canicola and *L. icterohemorrhagiae* are very frequent canine infections throughout the world. Antibodies to serotypes such as *L. pomona* and *L. sejroe* have also been found in dog sera and indicate that other serotypes cause canine infections as well. In the United States,

canine leptospirosis is uncommon in the northeast but more common in other regions.

Leptospirosis is more common in male than in female dogs (53), and *L. canicola* infection is more often found in city dogs than in dogs from sporting kennels, where *L. icterohemorrhagiae* infection is more frequent.

The Natural Disease. Three types of leptospirosis in dogs are recognized: (*a*) the acute hemorrhagic type; (*b*) the icteric, less acute type; and (*c*) the uremic type, commonly known as *Stuttgart disease*.

L. icterohemorrhagiae has been associated with the first two syndromes, whereas *L. canicola* has been most often implicated in renal disease (Figures 5.2 and 5.3). However, there is evidence that *L. icterohemorrhagiae* also causes a substantial proportion of renal lesions in dogs (63). Meningeal involvement results occasionally from infection by either serotype.

The acute hemorrhagic disease is characterized by high fever, prostration, and early death. Hemorrhages occur throughout the organs, especially in the lungs and alimentary tract. The second type is less acute and is characterized by intense icterus, hemorrhages with blood-stained feces, and pigmented urine. The third type is characterized by uremia because of extensive kidney damage; by a foul odor from the mouth because of ulcerative stomatitis; and by hemorrhagic enteritis, coma, and death in a high percentage of cases.

The kidneys of dogs with acute interstitial nephritis

Figure 5.2. Normal kidney (259D) and a kidney from a dog with chronic interstitial nephritis caused by *Leptospira icterohemorrhagiae*.

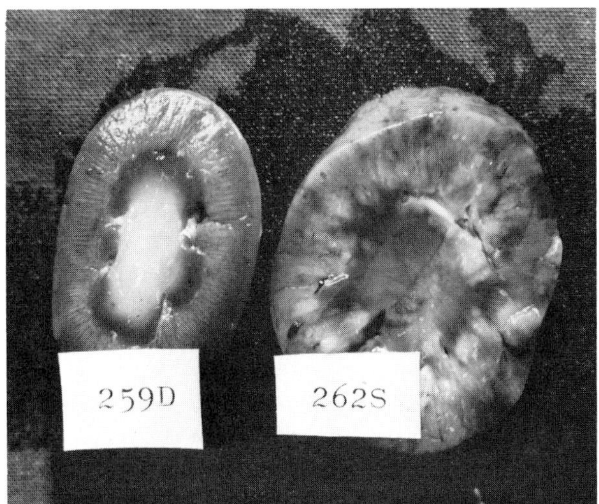

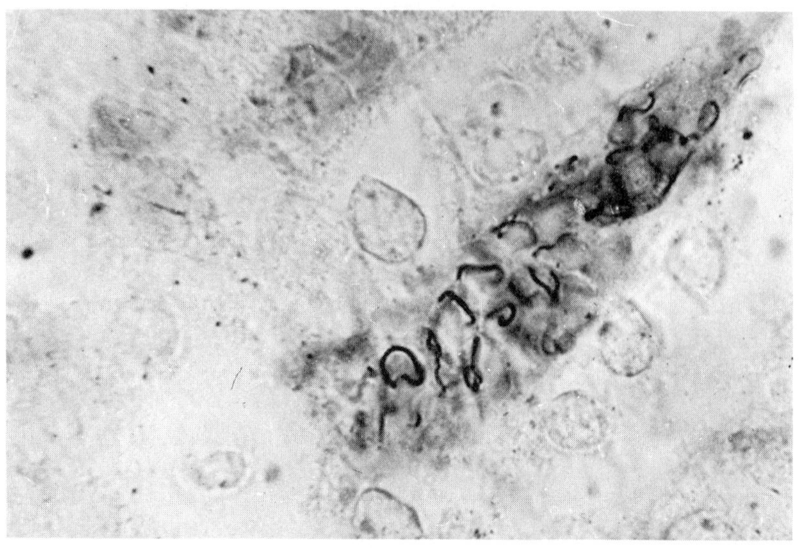

Figure 5.3. *Leptospira canicola* in the kidney of an artificially infected guinea pig. Warthin-Starry stain. × 2,300. (Courtesy John T. Bryans and Peter C. Kennedy.)

caused by *L. canicola* exhibit extensive accumulations of plasma cells which have been shown to contain IgG antibodies to leptospira antigens (44). These antibodies appear to be ineffective in clearing renal infection since many dogs continue to shed the organism in the urine. It is probable, however, that these organisms are less virulent than organisms shed during the phase before antibody is produced. This phenomenon is already known to occur in the mouse (18, 34).

Immunity. Dogs are successfully vaccinated against clinical leptospirosis with formalin or phenol-killed vaccines that contain the antigens of *L. canicola* and *L. icterohemorrhagiae*. Hyperimmune serum has also been used for passive protection and for treatment of early cases (43, 47). A vaccine against *L. canicola* and *L. icterohemorrhagiae* which protects against the renal carrier state has recently been described (39).

Ovine and Caprine Leptospirosis

L. pomona has been shown to be responsible for clinical leptospirosis in sheep and lambs (35). The disease resembles that described for cattle (4, 32). Antibodies to a variety of leptospira serotypes have been found in various countries (43).

Equine Leptospirosis

In 1948, Heusser (33) suggested that equine periodic ophthalmia of horses in Switzerland might be caused by infection with leptospirae. He did not succeed in isolating any leptospirae but based his conclusions on the results of serological tests. Noting that most cases of this disease in Switzerland occurred in areas where swineherd's disease prevailed, he tested 291 affected horses and as many controls. Nine types of leptospirae were used. Positive reactions were obtained with only three—*L. pomona, L. australis,* and *L. grippotyphosa*. The titers varied among these species, but most diseased animals agglutinated one or more of the cultures in dilutions varying from 1:4 to 1:25,000. The titers of normal horses did not exceed 1:400. Tests made with the aqueous humor of acute cases showed much higher titers than the blood of the same individuals.

On the basis of serological tests Yager *et al.* (69) indicated that *L. pomona* is the cause of recurrent iridocyclitis of horses in the United States, but Bryans (7) in his studies on equine leptospirosis concludes that the disease in horses, as caused by *L. pomona,* does not present pathognomic symptoms. Because of the mild nature of the disease in horses and the failure to demonstrate a carrier state in experimental animals, it appears that leptospirosis is of little importance to the light horse industry of the United States. However, serological evidence does indicate that a relatively high percentage of horses possess antibodies against leptospirae, and a few naturally occurring cases of *L. pomona* infection have been described with symptoms of fever, anorexia, depression, and icterus (28, 51). Abortion in mares has been reported to be caused by *Leptospira* sp. (36). Abortion caused by a mixed infection of equine herpes virus and *Leptospira* sp. has also been reported in a group of mares (16). Vaccination of horses has been shown to be protective (5).

Feline Leptospirosis

The sera of cats has been shown to contain antibodies to a variety of leptospira serotypes (43). The disease appears to be unimportant in cats (68).

Leptospirosis in Man

The epidemiology of leptospirosis in man is not related to age or sex, but to occupation. *L. icterohemorrhagiae* infections (Weil's disease) are frequently observed in miners and in sewer and abattoir workers, whereas *L. canicola* infections (canicola fever) are found predominantly in veterinarians and in breeders and owners of dogs. In Europe *L. grippotyphosa* infection attacks farmers and agricultural and flax workers. *L. pomona* infection occurs in swineherders, creamery workers, cheese makers, and swine slaughterers. *L. australis* infection is found in sugarcane plantation workers, and *L. bataviae* infection attacks rice-field workers.

Infection of man occurs either directly from urine or tissues of a diseased animal or indirectly through contact with water or soil contaminated by animals; and in the United States the animals most likely to be involved are dogs, rats, cattle, swine, and certain wild animals that may contaminate streams. The portals of entry are most likely to be the mucous membranes of the eyes, nose, and mouth or the broken skin.

Symptoms of leptospirosis in man vary. Although they are frequently severe, the mortality rate is low. The disease is manifested by fever, headache, conjunctivitis, muscle pains, and encephalitic symptoms. There may be muscular tenderness, pharyngeal inflammation, skin rash, and minor hemorrhagic episodes. In some cases meningitis is a conspicuous symptom. Orchitis has been reported. The urine frequently contains albumin, a few erythrocytes, and casts. Jaundice frequently does not occur. Agglutinins and lytic antibodies for *Leptospira* sp. appear in the 2nd week of the disease and reach maximum titers several weeks later. The specific organism has often been isolated from the blood during the febrile period and from the urine later.

Although Weil's disease and canicola fever have been known to exist in the United States for some time, information with regard to the presence of other types is more recent. In 1951, Schaeffer (54) reported a water-borne outbreak of *L. pomona* in Alabama that attacked 50 out of 80 adolescents and young adults. In 1952, Gochenour *et al.* (25) clearly established that the so-called Fort Bragg fever was a leptospiral infection caused by *L. autumnalis*. Since then *L. ballum*, *L. grippotyphosa*, *L. mimi georgia*, and *L. hardjo* have been implicated in human infection.

In Israel, where about 30 percent of the cases of leptospirosis appearing annually are canicola fever (48), it seems that jackals are the main reservoir of the spirochete and are responsible for its transmission to pigs and cattle. The source of infection for man is most likely to be swine or rats.

Laboratory Diagnosis of Leptospirosis

Direct Examination. Direct dark-field examination of body or tissue fluids from acutely affected clinical cases may result in detection of the organism. Blood (heparinized) should be centrifuged at low speed to deposit cellular elements and the plasma then examined. These techniques are of value only when large numbers of leptospirae are present.

The fluorescent-antibody technique is more sensitive and is of particular value for examination of urinary sediments. It can be used also on tissue sections or impressions (41) and to identify serotypes (13, 14). The microscopic-agglutination test is the most reliable and widely used of the serologic diagnostic methods. A titer of 1:100 or greater is evidence of past exposure to *Leptospira* antigen. Titers may reach enormous levels in some animals (10). This test detects IgM agglutinins about 7 to 9 days after the onset of the clinical disease.

The agglutination test with killed antigen is less reliable and is more difficult to read.

The hamster passive-protection test and the growth-inhibition tests detect IgG neutralizing antibodies and become positive about 2 to 3 weeks after signs of clinical disease. These antibodies are protective and persist much longer than the IgM (30).

Animal Inoculation. Guinea pigs and hamsters are susceptible to *Leptospira* infection and may be used for detection of the organism in tissue or urinary specimens.

Cultural Examination. During the acute phase of the disease, blood culture in Fletcher's, Stuart's, or Ellinghausen's medium is the most reliable method of detecting the organism. In the later phases of the disease, when leptospiruria has commenced, urine samples collected aseptically may be inoculated into these media. Both undiluted and 10-fold dilutions of urine should be inoculated. The undiluted urine may contain growth-inhibitory substances. To inhibit other contaminating bacteria 5-fluorouracil (200 μg per ml) may also be added. Cultures should be examined at weekly intervals for 5 weeks before discarding.

Detection of Antibodies. Serologic examination is of immense value for retrospective diagnosis. Acute and convalescent sera should be examined. A positive diagnosis requires a 4-fold or greater increase in titer. A high titer that remains stationary indicates past infection.

Tests for antibody commonly used are (*a*) the microscopic-agglutination test using live or killed leptospirae, (*b*) the plate and tube agglutination test using formalin-treated leptospirae, (*c*) a hemolytic test involving absorbtion of antigen onto erythrocytes (11), (*d*) the hamster passive-protection test, and (*e*) the growth-inhibition test (65).

Chemotherapy of Leptospirosis

Smadel (57) concludes from studies on infected animals that penicillin, streptomycin, Aureomycin, and Terramycin are effective prophylactic agents but relatively ineffective therapeutic agents. These four antibiotics show appreciable activity against leptospirae in the laboratory but do not produce dramatic results in treating a patient unless given within the first day or two of the disease. On the other hand, Brunner (6) used streptomycin to treat six dogs that had survived experimental infection (five with *L. canicola* and one with *L. icterohemorrhagiae*) and were shedding large numbers of the organisms in the urine. He found the antibiotic to be fully effective in eliminating these organisms. Lococo *et al.* (40) used dihydrostreptomycin and Baker *et al.* (1) employed Terramycin in effectively eradicating leptospiruria in swine. Terramycin was used at levels of 500 and 1,000 g per ton of feed. Ringen and Bracken (49) reported no evidence of leptospiruria in cattle treated with high levels of tetracycline. Quinapyramine sulfate given subcutaneously in doses of 10 μg per kg of body weight has been shown to be effective in calves infected by *L. pomona* (24). During an active infection in cattle herds, *Leptospira* bacterins can be administered together with dihydrostreptomycin—the idea being that the antibiotic will control the infection until antibody appears (59).

REFERENCES

1. Baker, Gallian, Price, and White. Vet. Med., 1957, *52,* 103.
2. Belloni and Ruggers. Clin. Vet. Milani., 1969, *91,* 237.
3. Bezdenieznykh and Kaszanova. Jour. Microbiol. Epid. Immunol., Moscow, 1956, *4,* 101.
4. Bokori, Kemenes, Szemeredi, Gy, and Szeky. Acta Vet. Acad. Sci. Hung., 1969, *10,* 2.
5. Brown, Creamer, and Scheidy. Vet. Med., 1956, *51,* 556.
6. Brunner. North Am. Vet., 1949, *30,* 517.
7. Bryans. Cornell Vet., 1955, *45,* 16.
8. Burnstein and Baker. Jour. Inf. Dis., 1954, *94,* 53.
9. Caleffi. Clin. Vet. Milani, 1966, *89,* 215.
10. Coffin and Stubbs. Jour. Am. Vet. Med. Assoc., 1944, *104,* 152.
11. Cox, Alexander, and Murphy. Jour. Inf. Dis., 1957, *101,* 210.
12. Czekalowski, McLeod, and Rodican. Brit. Jour. Exp. Path., 1953, *34,* 588.
13. Dacres. Am. Jour. Vet. Res., 1961, *22,* 570.
14. Dacres. Am. Jour. Vet. Res., 1963, *24,* 1321.
15. Ellinghausen and McCullough. Am. Jour. Vet. Res., 1965, *26,* 39.
16. Ellis, Bryson, and McFerran. Vet. Rec., 1976, *98,* 218.
17. Ellis and Michna. Vet. Rec., 1976, *99,* 409.
18. Faine. Jour. Hyg. (London), 1962, *60,* 435.
19. Frey. Schweiz. med. Wchnschr., 1948, *78,* 531.
20. Galton, Aragon, Jacalne, Shotts, and Sulzer. Jour. Inf. Dis., 1963, *112,* 164.
21. Galton, Menges, Shotts, Nahmias, and Heath. Leptospirosis: Epidemiology, clinical manifestations in man and animals, and methods in laboratory diagnosis. U.S. Public Health Service, Center for Disease Control, Atlanta, Ga., 1962.
22. Gillespie and Kerzy. Vet. Med., 1958, *53,* 401.
23. Glosser, Sulzer, Reynolds, and Whitsett. Proc. 78th Ann. Meeting, U.S. Animal Health Assoc., Roanoke, Va., 1974, p. 119.
24. Gloukovschi, Topciu, Levin, Glavan, Stan, and Nistort. Rev. Zootech. Med. Vet. Bucuresti, 1964, *4,* 52.
25. Gochenour, Smadel, Jackson, Evans, and Yager. Pub. Health Rpts. (U.S.), 1953, *67,* 811.
26. Greene, Camien, and Dunn. Proc. Soc. Exp. Biol. and Med., 1950, *75,* 208.
27. Gsell. Presse Med., 1954 (Sept.), 525.
28. Hall and Bryans. Cornell Vet., 1954, *44,* 345.
29. Hanson, Tripathy, and Killinger. Jour. Am. Vet. Med. Assoc., 1972, *161,* 1235.
30. Hanson. Jour. Dairy Sci., 1974, *59,* 1166.
31. Harrington and Sleight. Am. Jour. Vet. Res., 1966, *27,* 249.
32. Hartley. Austral. Vet. Jour., 1952, *28,* 169.
33. Heusser. Schweiz. Arch. f. Tierheilk., 1948, *90,* 287.
34. Hirschberg and Vaughn. Vet. Med./Small An. Clin., 1973, *68,* 67.
35. Hodges. New Zeal. Vet. Jour., 1974, *22,* 151.
36. Jackson, Jones, and Clark. Jour. Am. Vet. Med. Assoc., 1957, *131,* 564.
37. Johnson, Allan, and Bennett. Austral. Vet. Jour., 1974, *50,* 325.
38. Kadis and Pugh. Inf. and Immun., 1974, *10,* 793.
39. Kerr and Marshall. Vet. Med./Small An. Clin., 1974, *69,* 1157.

40. Lococo, Bohl, and Smith. Jour. Am. Vet. Med. Assoc., 1958, *132,* 251.
41. Maestrone. Can. Jour. Comp. Med. and Vet. Sci., 1963, *27,* 109.
42. Menges and Galton. Am. Jour. Vet. Res., 1961, *22,* 1085.
43. Michna. Vet. Rec., 1970, *86,* 484.
44. Morrison and Wright. Jour. Path., 1975, *120,* 83.
45. Negi, Meyers, and Segre. Am. Jour. Vet. Res., 1971, *32,* 1915.
46. Nisbet. Jour. Comp. Path. and Therap., 1951, *61,* 155.
47. Nowakowski. Medycyna Wet., 1977, *32,* 611.
48. Pertzelan and Pruzanski. Am. Jour. Trop. Med. and Hyg., 1963, *12,* 75.
49. Ringen and Bracken. Jour. Am. Vet. Med. Assoc., 1956, *129,* 266.
50. Ringen and Gillespie. Jour. Bact., 1954, *67,* 252.
51. Roberts, York, and Robinson. Jour. Am. Vet. Med. Assoc., 1952, *121,* 237.
52. Roth, Adams, Sanford, Greer, and Mayeux. Pub. Health Rpts. (U.S.), 1962, *77,* 583.
53. Ryu. Int. Jour. Zoonoses, 1975, *2,* 16.
54. Schaeffer. Jour. Clin. Invest., 1951, *30,* 670.
55. Sippel. North Am. Vet., 1953, *34,* 111.
56. Sleight and Williams. Jour. Am. Vet. Med. Assoc., 1961, *138,* 151.
57. Smadel. *In* Symposium on the leptospiroses. Army Medical Service Graduate School, Washington, D.C., Med. Sci. Pub. No. 1, 1953.
58. Smith, Reynolds, and Clark. Cornell Vet., 1970, *60,* 40.
59. South and Stoenner. Proc. 78th Ann. Meeting, U.S. Animal Health Assoc., Roanoke, Va., 1974, p. 126.
60. Stalheim. Am. Jour. Vet. Res., 1968, *29,* 1463.
61. Stalheim. Proc. 69th Ann. Meeting, U.S. Livestock Sanit. Assoc., 1966, p. 170.
62. Stoenner, Hadlow, and Ward. Jour. Am. Vet. Med. Assoc., 1963, *142,* 491.
63. Timoney, Sheehan, and Timoney. Vet. Rec., 1974, *94,* 316.
64. Tripathy and Hanson. Am. Jour. Vet. Res., 1973, *34,* 503.
65. Tripathy, Hanson, and Mansfield. Proc. 77th Ann. Meeting, U.S. Animal Health Assoc., St. Louis, 1974, p. 113.
66. Tripathy, Smith, and Hanson. Am. Jour. Vet. Res., 1975, *36,* 1735.
67. Twigg and McDiarmid. Vet. Rec., 1972, *90,* 598.
68. White, Stoliker, and Galton. Am. Jour. Vet. Res., 1961, *22,* 650.
69. Yager, Gochenour, and Wetmore. Jour. Am. Vet. Med. Assoc., 1950, *117,* 207.

THE GENUS *TREPONEMA*

Members of the genus *Treponema* are found in the oral cavity, intestinal tract, and genital regions of man and animals. They are unicellular, helical rods, 5 to 20 μm long, with tight regular or irregular spirals. The cells have one or more axial fibrils inserted at each end of the protoplasmic cylinder. Those that have been cultivated are anaerobic.

Only two species are of known significance in veterinary bacteriology—*T. hyodysenteriae* and *T. cuniculi.* These organisms cause dysentery and vent disease in swine and rabbits, respectively.

Treponema hyodysenteriae

Swine dysentery (*bloody scours*) was first described in 1921 by Whiting *et al.* (17) but definitive characterization and confirmation of the primary infectious agent was not accomplished until the early 1970s (4, 14).

Although *T. hyodysenteriae* is the primary inciting agent in swine dysentery, the disease process requires the interaction of other components of the normal colonic flora (1, 5, 9). It appears (5) that *Bacteroides vulgatus* and *Fusobacterium necrophorum* are two such organisms. In gnotobiotic pigs, swine dysentery could only

Figure 5.4. A carbol fuchsin stain of *Treponema hyodysenteriae* demonstrating the spiral shape of the organism. × 1,400. (From Harris, Glock, Christensen, and Kinyon. *Vet. Med./Small An. Clin.,* 1972, *67,* 62.)

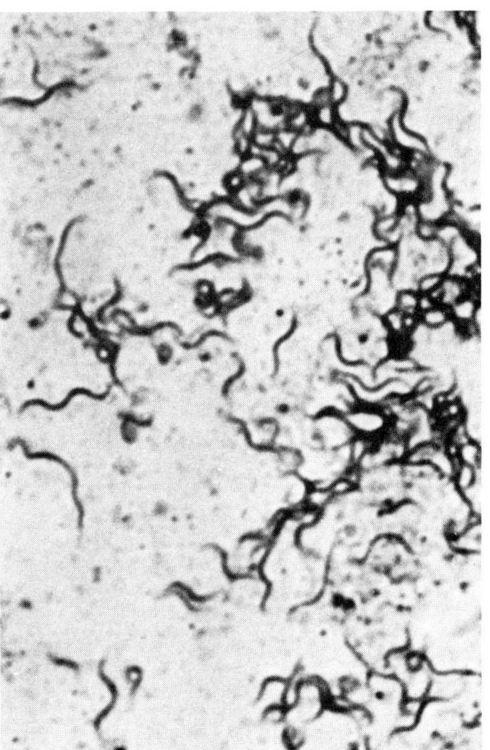

be produced when *T. hyodysenteriae* and these organisms were administered together.

Morphology and Staining Reactions. *T. hyodysenteriae* is 6 to 9 μm in length and 0.3 μm in diameter (Figure 5.4). It is loosely coiled, tapered at the ends, and possesses 7 to 9 axial fibrils inserted at each end which overlap near the middle of the cell. The organism may be stained with crystal violet or dilute carbol fuchsin. In sections of mucosa, the organism may be stained by the Goodpasture or Warthin-Starry procedures. It is Gram-negative.

Cultivation. Although *T. hyodysenteriae* is an anaerobe, it is tolerant of oxygen. It grows readily under anaerobiasis on freshly poured trypticase soy agar containing 5 percent bovine or equine blood. The plates should be examined for hemolysis every 2 days. The organism produces small, gray, hazy colonies within the hemolytic zones and can be transferred by taking a piece of agar from the edge of the zone and using it as inoculum for a new culture. Prereduced trypticase soy broth containing 10 percent fetal calf serum can also be used for propagation (8). A selective medium that contains spectinomycin for isolation has been described (12).

It is oxidase- and catalase-negative and produces acid from glucose.

The organism is readily separated from other intestinal bacteria by passing it through cellulose acetate filters of porosity 0.8, 0.65, and 0.45 μm and culturing the filtrate on blood agar.

Epidemiology and Pathogenesis. Swine dysentery is most common in feeder swine that weigh between 30 and 140 pounds. The pig is the only known reservoir of pathogenic strains, and transmission is by means of ingestion of feces from clinically affected or carrier animals. The organism can survive in feces for not more than 24 hours at 37 C but survives for up to 48 days at temperatures between 0 and 10 C (2).

The incubation period is variable but averages about 10 to 14 days. After infection, the spirochetes are first observed in the crypts of Lieberkühn (Figures 5.5 and 5.6), where they proliferate onto the luminal surface (7) and cause a mucohemorrhagic colitis. Blood and mucus or mucus alone is passed in the feces, which is thin and watery. Some pigs have elevated temperatures. Fibronecrotic membranous material is formed on the colonic mucosa, and large numbers of *Treponema hyodysen-*

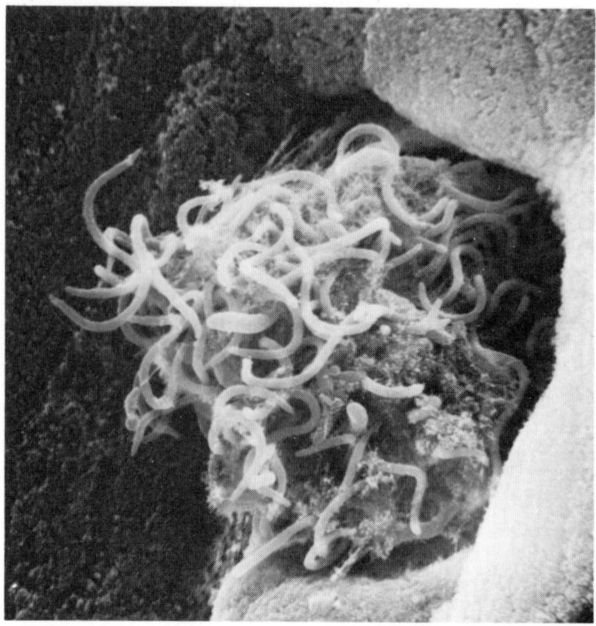

Figure 5.5. *Treponema hyodysenteriae* in a colonic crypt of a pig affected with swine dysentery. P.W. = 20.5 μm. (Courtesy George A. Kennedy. From *Scanning Electron Microscopy,* vol. 2, ed. Om Johari and Robert Becker, Chicago, 1977, p. 287.)

Figure 5.6. Scanning electron micrograph of spirochetes and associated *Vibrio*like organisms (V) in the colon of a pig affected with dysentery. × 9,300. (From George A. Kennedy, *Jour. Am. Vet. Med. Assoc.*, 1973, *163,* 54.)

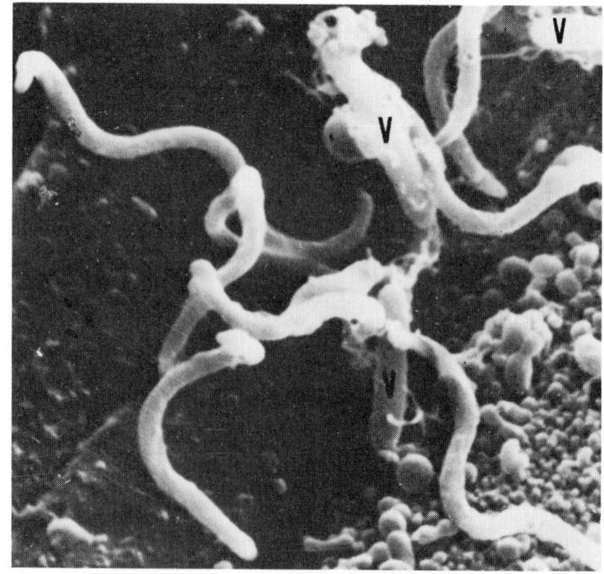

teriae and of other *Vibrio*like organisms are present in this material. The walls and mesentery of the large intestine are hyperemic and edematous, and the rugose texture of the mucosal surface is lost.

Up to 50 percent of untreated swine die of the disease. Death is caused by dehydration and acidosis. Recovered animals may continue to shed the organism and infect other in-contact animals for up to 90 days (13).

Immunity. Resistance to reinfection has been demonstrated in convalescent pigs (10), and antibodies have been found in sera of convalescent animals (16). Intravenous hyperimmunization with formalin-killed antigen has been shown to increase serum antibody titers and to protect against challenge with a homologous strain (3). Passively immunized pigs are not protected against infection, but the onset of the disease is delayed (11).

Fluorescent-antibody (16), passive hemolysis (6), and microtiter agglutination tests (7) have been described for the assay of antibodies. The reliability of these techniques for detection of carrier animals is as yet unclear.

Diagnosis. Confirmation of clinical diagnosis must be made in the laboratory. The presence of numerous large, loosely coiled spirochetelike organisms in mucosal scrapings, as detected by phase or dark-field microscopy, the fluorescent antibody test, or in stained preparations, is tentative evidence for a diagnosis of swine dysentery. Attempts to culture the organism from filtrates of mucosal scrapings should also be made.

Campylobacter sp. and closely coiled spirochetes may also be present in swine dysentery and in other enteric conditions of swine and may complicate interpretation of microscopic preparations.

Chemotherapy. Ronidazole has been shown to be effective in the treatment and prophylaxis of experimentally induced swine dysentery (15). Organic arsenicals are also useful in areas where strains of the organism have not become resistant to the compounds. Tiamutilin, tylosin, neomycin, furazolidone, and other antimicrobials have been successfully used, but strains of *T. hyodysenteriae* resistant to some of these drugs have been found.

Depopulation is an effective measure to eliminate infection in a herd but must be done in association with sanitation measures and a rest period of 30 to 60 days.

REFERENCES

1. Brandenburg, Miniats, Geissinger, and Ewert. Can. Jour. Comp. Med., 1977, *41,* 294.
2. Chia and Taylor. Vet. Rec., 1978, *103,* 68.
3. Glock, Schwartz, and Harris. Proc. Int. Pig Vet. Soc., Ames, Iowa, 1976.
4. Harris, Glock, Christensen, and Kinyon. Vet. Med./Small .An. Clin., 1972, *67,* 61.
5. Harris, Alexander, Shipp, Robinson, Glock, and Matthews. Jour. Am. Vet. Med. Assoc., 1978, *172,* 468.
6. Jenkins, Sinba, Varice, and Reese. Inf. and Immun., 1976, *14,* 1106.
7. Joens, Harris, Kinyon, and Kaeperle. Jour. Clin. Microbiol., 1978, *8,* 293.
8. Kinyon and Harris. Vet. Rec., 1974, *95,* 219.
9. Meyer, Simon, and Byerly. Vet. Path., 1974, *11,* 515.
10. Olsen. Can. Jour. Comp. Med., 1974, *38,* 7.
11. Schwartz and Glock. Proc. Int. Pig Vet. Soc., Ames, Iowa, 1976.
12. Songer, Kinyon, and Harris. Jour. Clin. Microbiol., 1976, *4,* 57.
13. Soyer. Diss. Abstr. Int., 1977, *37B,* 5553.
14. Taylor. Vet. Rec., 1970, *86,* 416.
15. Taylor. Vet. Rec., 1976, *99,* 453.
16. Terpstra, Akkermans, and Oninerkerk. Neth. Jour. Vet. Sci., 1968, *1,* 5.
17. Whiting, Doyle, and Spray. Swine dysentery. Purdue Univ. Agr. Exp. Sta. Bull., 1921, *257,* 3.

Treponema cuniculi

This organism is the cause of *rabbit syphilis* (*vent disease*) and is spread during sexual activity. The lesions are superficial ulcerated areas on the genital and perineael areas. The organism is very slender, 6 to 14 μm in length, and has not been cultured.

Organic arsenicals and penicillin are effective in therapy. Small and Newman give a good description of the disease (1).

REFERENCE

1. Small and Newman. Lab. An. Sci., 1972, *22,* 77.

6 The Enterobacteriaceae—The Lactose Fermenters

Members of the family Enterobacteriaceae are straight Gram-negative rods. They may be motile or nonmotile. The motile strains have peritrichous flagella. All species grow well on artificial media and attack glucose, with the formation of acid, or acid and gas. With some exceptions in the genus *Erwinia* they reduce nitrates to nitrites. Their antigenic composition constitutes a mosaic of interlocking serological relationships among the several genera. The family contains many animal parasites and some plant parasites. Frequently many of these bacteria occur as saprophytes in nature.

For the purpose of orientation the classification of the Enterobacteriaceae given by the eighth edition of *Bergey's Manual of Determinative Bacteriology* is presented.

Tribe I. Escherichiae
- Genus 1. *Escherichia*—Intestinal inhabitant of animals.
- Genus 2. *Edwardsiella*—Intestinal inhabitant of snakes, also found in water.
- Genus 3. *Citrobacter*—Found in water, feces, and urine.
- Genus 4. *Salmonella*—Pathogen of man and animals.
- Genus 5. *Shigella*—Enteric pathogen of primates.

Tribe II. Klebsielliae
- Genus 1. *Klebsiella*—Widely distributed, intestines, environment, etc.
- Genus 2. *Enterobacter*—Found in feces, water, etc.
- Genus 3. *Hafnia*—Found in feces, water, etc.
- Genus 4. *Serratia*—Found widely in soil, water, etc. Opportunistic pathogen of man and animals.

Tribe III. Proteeae
- Genus 1. *Proteus*—Intestinal inhabitants.

Tribe IV. Yersineae
- Genus 1. *Yersinia*—Pathogens of man and animals.

Tribe V. Erwinieae
- Genus 1. *Erwinia*—Pathogens of plants.

For years the species and genera of the Enterobacteriaceae were characterized according to source of isolation and biochemical behavior. However, physiological characteristics proved to be variable even among members of the same species, and accurate identifications were impossible. Finally, recognition of the antigens possessed by the bacteria became the basis of identification, and serological methods have largely replaced the biochemical tests.

The isolation of enteric bacteria is accomplished by means of various selective and enrichment mediums (21). Before attempting serological classification, a preliminary grouping based on certain physiological characteristics of the enteric isolate is often made. These groups are presented in Table 6.1. It must be understood that the differences listed for each group are not fixed but tend to vary according to the species examined. At best, Table

Table 6.1. Some differential characteristics of enteric groups concerned in animal diseases

	Cultural features													
Enteric groups	Semisolid motility medium	Gelatin	Hydrogen sulfide	Indol	Urea	Methyl red	Voges-Proskauer	Citrate medium	Glucose	Lactose	Sucrose	Salicin	KCN medium
Escherichia coli	v	−	−	+	−	+	−	−	ag	ag	v	v	−
Klebsiella-Enterobacter	(−)	(−)	−	−	s	v	v	+	ag	ag	ag	ag	+
Citrobacter	+	−	+	v	s−	+	−	+	ag	v	v	v	+
Proteus	+	+	+	+	+	−	−	−	av	−	av	−	+
Salmonella	+	−	+	−	−	+	−	+	ag	−	−	−	−
Salmonella arizona	+	s	+	−	−	+	−	+	ag	s	−	−	−
Shigella	−	−	−	(−)	−	+	−	−	a−	(−)	(−)	−	−

v = variable; − = negative; (−) = usually negative, but important exceptions occur; + = positive; s = slow utilization; s− = slow utilization or negative; ag = acid and gas; av = acid with or without gas; a− = acid without gas.

6.1 presents only a very general biochemical classification of each group.

Polyvalent antiserums (8, 21) and bacteriophage (11) are useful tools in grouping members of the Enterobacteriaceae. The fluorescent antibody (FA) technique is occasionally helpful in detecting *Salmonella* types, but has proved quite useful in detecting enteropathogenic *Escherichia coli* types (17, 44). Wide-spectrum bacteriophages can be used to separate salmonellae from other enteric bacteria, but not to differentiate the serotypes (51).

For purposes of presentation the Enterobacteriaceae are divided into lactose-fermenting and non-lactose-fermenting groups. This chapter will deal with the lactose-fermenters; Chapter 7 will examine the genera that do not ferment lactose.

Among the organisms that ferment lactose are the members of the genera *Escherichia, Enterobacter, Klebsiella, Citrobacter, Erwinia,* and *Serratia.* Because *Citrobacter* and *Erwinia* are not animal pathogens, they are not discussed. Chromogenic *Serratia* have been reported in bovine mastitis and in septicemias in man and are assuming an increasing importance as opportunistic pathogens. In the genus *Escherichia* the type species is *E. coli.* It is quite strictly parasitic in its habits and is not found abundantly anywhere in nature except in intestinal tracts, in feces, and in materials that have been subjected to fecal pollution. Kauffmann (32) claims that the members of the genus listed in *Bergey's Manual* as *Klebsiella* are serologically identical with members of the *Enterobacter* genus. Accordingly, we will consider them in the *Klebsiella-Enterobacter* group. These species may be found in the alimentary tract of animals. Some members of the *Klebsiella-Enterobacter* group grow freely in nature on grains and plants, and others are found in the respiratory, intestinal, and genitourinary tracts of man and animals. The members of the Escherichiae are frequently referred to as the *colon-aerogenes,* or the *coliform* group of bacteria. Strains of this group are sought in bacteriological examination of water, and their presence is interpreted as evidence of fecal pollution.

THE GENUS *ESCHERICHIA*

Escherichia coli

This organism is a normal inhabitant of the lower bowel of all warm-blooded animals. It usually is absent from the intestines of fish and other cold-blooded animals. Few or none are found in the stomach and anterior portions of the bowel. Carnivora and omnivora usually harbor the organism in greater abundance than the herbivora. The feces of cows and horses frequently show very few.

Morphology and Staining Reactions. *E. coli* is a small rod-shaped organism that varies widely in morphology under varying conditions. Usually it is a short, plump rod; sometimes rather long filaments are seen. It may be motile or nonmotile. Spores are never formed, and capsular material is absent from most but not all strains. It stains readily and evenly with ordinary stains and is Gram-negative.

Cultural Features. *E. coli* grows readily on all ordinary media. Its optimum temperature is about that of the body, but it will grow through a wide range. It is aerobic and facultatively anaerobic. Most strains show motility of a sluggish type.

In broth there is uniform clouding within 12 to 18

hours. On old cultures friable pellicles form, and very old cultures show considerable viscid sediment. Agar surface colonies are slightly raised, smooth, glistening, unpigmented, and circular in outline. Deep colonies usually are lenticular in shape and brownish. On slants the growth becomes confluent, and the water of syneresis, turbid. Gelatin colonies are thin, bluish-white, translucent, and glistening. The surface usually shows radial ridges, and the margins are somewhat irregular, giving the colonies the shape of a grape leaf. The gelatin is not liquefied. Growth on potato is less abundant than on agar, brownish and rather dry. Some strains are strongly hemolytic, producing wide zones of beta-type hemolysis around colonies on blood agar plates. Others have no hemolytic action. According to Smith (52), the hemolytic stains produce at least two hemolysins which he designates *alpha* and *beta*. The alpha-hemolysin is filterable and the beta-hemolysin is not. Litmus milk is acidified and coagulated within 24 hours at 37 C. The litmus is reduced except near the surface. Glucose and lactose are attacked by all strains, both acid and gas being formed. On other carbohydrate media, acid and gas are formed from some and not from others, depending upon the strain.

Indol is formed, usually in abundance; nitrates are vigorously reduced; and the Voges-Proskauer reaction is negative. This last reaction is considered valuable in distinguishing *E. coli* types from *Enterobacter aerogenes*, which give a positive reaction.

Resistance. *E. coli* is fairly resistant to drying and to the action of many chemical disinfectants. Usually it is destroyed by pasteurization, but certain heat-resistant strains may withstand this exposure (56).

Antigens. The surface structures of *E. coli* are expressed as O (somatic), K (capsular), and H (flagellar) antigens (31). There are at least 150 recognized O antigens, 90 K, and 50 H. Each serotype is designated by the numbers of the antigens it carries, e.g., O139: K82: H2. The O antigen determinant is located on the polysaccharide part of the lipopolysaccharide molecule. K antigens are polysaccharide and/or protein. The H antigens are proteinaceous and are found in the flagella. Most isolates of *E. coli* from humans can be serotyped with available grouping antisera, but a large proportion of isolates from animals cannot be grouped. Only the enteropathogenic *E. coli* from animals have been well categorized serotypically.

Epidemiology and Pathogenesis. Enteropathogenic *E. coli* are defined as strains with the potential of causing disease in the gastrointestinal tract (40). Most of these strains are host-specific, and a limited number of well-defined serotypes are closely associated with specific disease entities in each animal host. These diseases are characteristically found in the newborn or young animal.

***E. coli* Infections in Swine.** There are three distinct manifestations of enteric colibacillosis in swine (45): (*a*) neonatal *E. coli* diarrhea—enteritis of piglets 1 to 4 days old; (*b*) weanling enteritis—enteritis at the time of weaning; (*c*) edema disease—edema in various body tissues of pigs soon after weaning.

Neonatal enteritis. Neonatal *E. coli* enteritis occurs during the first 4 days of life in piglets raised under intensive conditions of husbandry. The piglets appear normal for the first 12 hours of life and then develop a profuse pale-yellow watery diarrhea, which frequently leads to fatal dehydration within 18 hours. Most of the litter is usually affected and the mortality may be as high as 90 percent. Predisposing factors include poor sanitation and ventilation, high humidity, and stress caused by cold. The disease is especially a problem in farrowing units with a large proportion of young sows farrowing for the first time. The litters of older sows are less likely to be severely affected.

The serotypes involved mainly belong to groups O8, O101, O138, O141, O147, O149, and O157. Closed herds are affected by only one or two serotypes, open herds by up to 7. The pathogenesis of the diarrhea centers on the effect of the enterotoxin(s) produced by the *E. coli* serotype. After infection of the baby piglet, the *E. coli* strain colonizes the epithelium of the small intestine. This phase is favored by the possession of colonizing antigens such as the K88 pilus protein, which mediates adhesion to the microvilli of the intestinal epithelial cells (Figure 6.1). Enterotoxin production and release then follows. About 50 percent of *E. coli* isolates from piglet enteritis are enterotoxigenic by the available assays. Both heat-labile (LT) and heat-stable (ST) forms may be found in the same strains. All strains produce ST and some also produce LT toxin (53). The properties and effects of ST and LT toxins are listed in Table 6.2. The effects of LT toxin are ameliorated by high intraluminal glucose (9) and by chlorpromazine (36). LT toxin is neutralized by specific antiserum and by antiserum to cholera toxin, which is similar biochemically and in its mode of action.

Vaccination of gilts and sows with vaccines prepared from the fimbrial K88 antigen or other pilus-associated antigens has been shown to reduce morbidity and mortality caused by *E. coli* neonatal enteritis (41, 43,

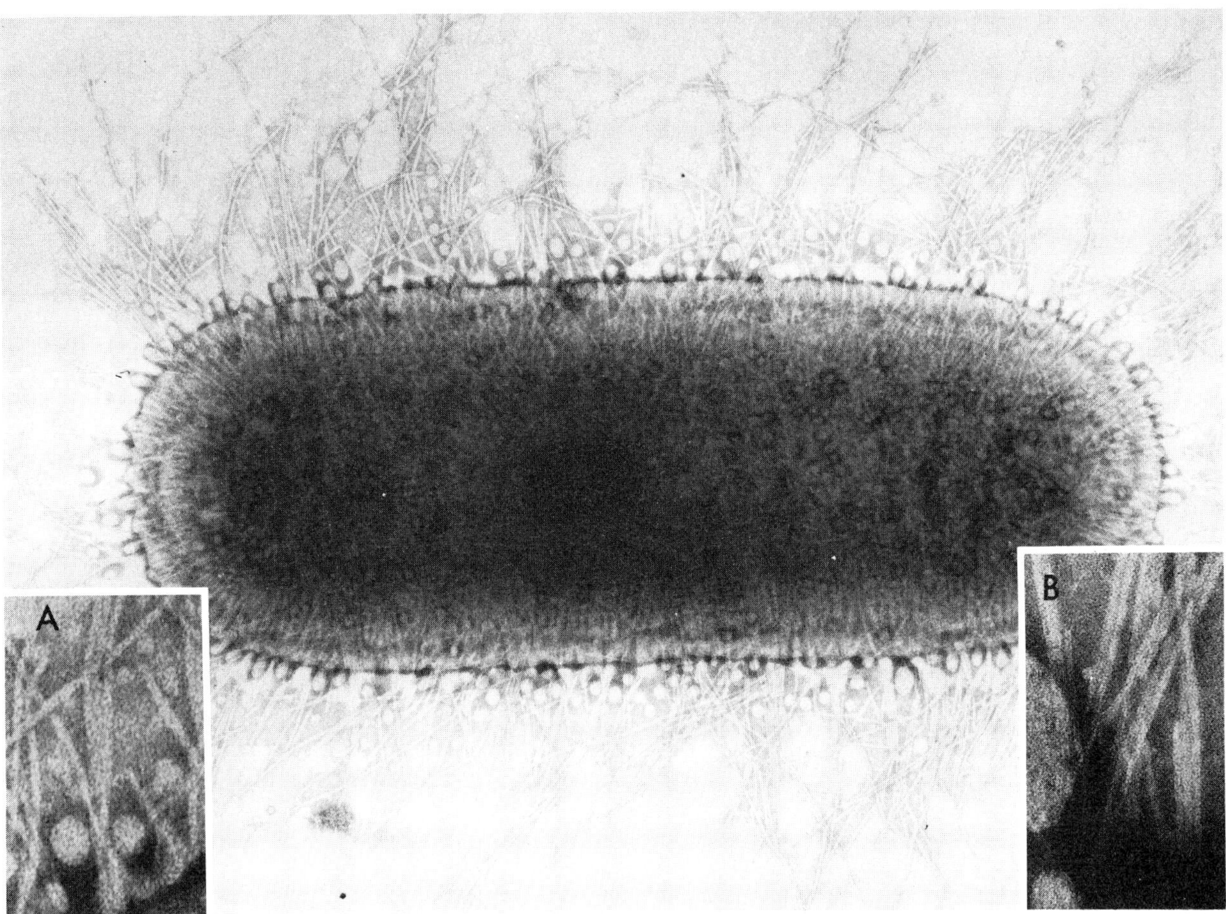

Figure 6.1. Electron micrograph of a negatively stained *Escherichia coli*. Numerous pili can be seen. Inserts *A* and *B* show pili of bacteria grown *in vitro* and *in vivo* respectively. The pili are identical under both sets of growth conditions. × 35,343. (Reprinted from R. E. Isaacson, B. Nagy, and H. W. Moon, "Colonization of Porcine Small Intestine *Escherichia coli:* Colonization and Adhesion Factors of Pig Enteropathogens That Lack K88," *Journal of Infectious Diseases,* 1977, *135,* 534 by permission of the University of Chicago Press. Copyright © 1977 by the University of Chicago. All rights reserved.)

Table 6.2. Properties and effects of *E. coli* enterotoxins

Property	Heat stable toxin (ST)	Heat labile toxin (LT)
Mol. wt.	5,000 (1)	100,000? (14)
Antigenic	No	Yes
Mode of action	Stimulates guanylate cyclase activity of ileal epithelial cells (23).	Stimulates adenyl cyclase activity of intestinal and capillary epithelium
Onset and duration of action	Rapid and short-lived	Slower and more prolonged
Effect	Cyclic GMP levels elevated Net Cl^- absorption abolished Efflux of Na^+, H_2O and HCO_3^- into intestinal lumen	Cyclic AMP levels elevated Net Cl^- absorption abolished Efflux of Na^+, H_2O and HCO_3^- into intestinal lumen

50). Oil adjuvants have been shown to increase the antibody response (49). Antibody reduces bacterial colonization in and shedding from the intestine and thus reduces the mass of infection in a population of piglets.

Vaccination of sows 3 weeks before farrowing with live organisms has also been shown to protect piglets (33) but is perhaps judiciously used only on a limited basis in herds from which the strain used for vaccine production was derived. Chidlow and Porter (13) used a combination of orally and intramuscularly administered vaccine in sows to obtain optimum levels of specific IgM antibodies in the colostrum.

Weanling enteritis (post-weaning diarrhea). Enteritis caused by hemolytic *E. coli* of O groups O8, O138, O139, and O141 (45) in feeder pigs is a very common complication of weaning. The disease is usually seen in pigs that are thriving on a heavy grain diet a short time after weaning. Change of diet apparently leads to massive colonization of the anterior small intestine by an enteropathogenic clone. Affected pigs exhibit diarrhea, depression, anorexia, and fever which may persist for 2 to 3 days. Although large thriving pigs often collapse and die after a short period of diarrhea, the overall mortality from weanling diarrhea is much lower than that in neonatal *E. coli* diarrhea. The pathogenesis of the diseases appears to be similar. Oral vaccination of young pigs with multivalent *E. coli* heat-inactivated vaccine resulted in better weight gains post weaning (48).

Edema disease (enterotoxemia, bowel edema). This disease was first described in Ireland in 1938 and has since been reported from swine-raising areas throughout the world. According to Timoney (59) and Lamont *et al.* (35), four fairly constant conditions are associated with the occurrence of edema disease: (*a*) age—weanlings, are most commonly involved, but occasionally pigs of any age may be affected; (*b*) change of feed—frequently a change either in feed or methods of feeding has been made; this is a natural occurrence at weaning time; (*c*) rapid growth—the disease is seen most frequently in thriving animals; (*d*) diarrhea—mild diarrhea often occurs a day or two before the attack. The disease is associated with proliferation of *E. coli* that belong principally to the somatic O groups O8, O45, O138, O141.

The disease occurs suddenly, has a short course, and usually ends in death of the pig. Affected animals exhibit a staggering gait, which may be slight at first but becomes more severe, and the animal is eventually unable to rise. Muscular tremors and spasms may also be present. The squeal is hoarse, and edema of the eyelids and face may be present. Body temperature is usually normal or subnormal, and the animal is often constipated. However, some cases exhibit diarrhea, which is a reflection of simultaneous enterotoxin production by the causative *E. coli* strain.

The first experimental production of the disease was achieved by Timoney in 1949 (58). He injected experimental swine intravenously with supernatants of intestinal contents from naturally occurring cases of the disease and produced the typical disease. He suggested that edema disease was an enterotoxemia. Later, he showed that a heat-labile toxin was present in the small intestine but is not found in the stomach of affected pigs and that alum-precipitated material derived from formalinized intestinal supernatant fluid could be used to hyperimmunize swine whose serum would then passively protect other swine against the experimentally induced disease. Both he (60) and others (22, 25) later showed that extracts of strains of hemolytic *E. coli* from cases could be used to produce the disease experimentally. It was also shown that a procedure effective for the extraction of the neurotoxin of *Shigella shigae* was effective for the extraction of the edema-disease-producing toxin from an *E. coli* strain (O139: K82(B): H1 (26, 62).

Clugston and Nielsen (15) showed that the toxin was precipitated by ammonium sulfate, was thermolabile, was insoluble at acidic pH but readily soluble at alkaline pH, and had a molecular weight of between 50,000 and 100,000.

Edema is the characteristic lesion of the disease and is found in the eyelids, the facial area, the cardiac zone of the stomach between the mucosa and the muscle layers, the mesentery and the mesenteric lymph nodes, the gall bladder, the larynx, and other tissues (Figure 6.2). The extent of the edema is variable, and some cases may show very little.

Clugston *et al.* (16) have described the microscopic features of the disease. They observed accumulations of noninflammatory edema and arterial changes in the cardiac submucosa, the large intestinal mucosa, lymph nodes, spinal cord, cerebral cortex, and brain stem. The arterial changes consisted of mural edema and hyaline degeneration. In cases that recovered, medial necrosis was evident. Clugston *et al.* concluded that the changes in the small arteries were responsible for the outward movement of fluid resulting in the edema and were similar to those seen in cases of human hypertension.

Kurtz and Quast (34) found areas of malacia in the brain stem that they felt were the result of ischemia. They characterized the lesions of edema disease as a

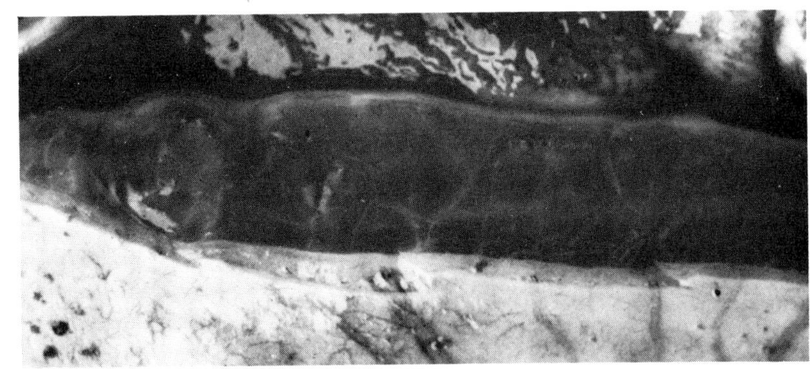

Figure 6.2. Edema disease of swine. Section of stomach wall showing thick layer of edema.

vascular myolysis and panarteritis of the central nervous system.

Clugston and Nielsen (15) have proposed that the toxin in edema disease be termed a vasotoxin because of its effect on arteries and its hypertensive effect. Interestingly enough, the hypertension they observed coincided with the development of the characteristic nervous signs of edema disease.

There is no effective treatment for edema disease. Preventive measures have included the use of a saline cathartic and reduction in amount of feed during the critical period after weaning. Both of these procedures apparently reduce the population of strains of *E. coli* that produce edema disease.

***E. coli* Infections in Calves.** Enteric disease (*white scour*) caused by specific serotypes of *E. coli* is a very frequent and serious disorder of calves during the first week of life (5). It occurs in all breeds of beef and dairy calves, and outbreaks of the disease occur constantly on premises where large numbers of calves are raised in confinement. In small herds the disease will be seen only sporadically during the calving season. Calves left with their dams on pasture rarely develop white scour.

The strains involved belong principally to O groups O8, O9, O20, and O101 (24, 42). Specific serotypes may predominate on certain farms.

An important distinction must be made between the serotypes found in enteritis and those found in cases of septicemia where the *E. coli* invades and multiplies in the bloodstream and tissues of the calf. Serotypes belonging to O groups O15, O26, O35, O78, O86, O115, O117, and O137 (24, 55) commonly are involved in the invasive form of colibacillosis in the calf.

About 12 percent of *E. coli* isolates from calves with diarrhea are enterotoxin-producing by the available methods of assay (38). This enterotoxin is usually the ST form and is nearly always associated with the K99 antigen.

There are three distinct *E. coli* syndromes in calves: (*a*) the enteric, (*b*) the enterotoxemic, and (*c*) the septicemic (24). The pathogenesis of the enteric form is in dispute (54) because there is as yet no clear-cut evidence of the role of *E. coli* in the disease in colostrum-fed calves. It is likely that factors other than *E. coli* contribute to the pathogenesis of enteritis in these calves. However, the limited range of non-enterotoxin-producing serotypes found in the enteric syndrome and the protective effect of K25 and K30 antibodies against challenge by serotypes containing these antigens suggests that these serotypes do have an important role in calf enteritis (38).

The enterotoxemic syndrome is produced by strains of O8, O9, O20, and O101 groups. After infection by these strains, there is rapid multiplication of the strain in the anterior small intestine. Colonization of this area is promoted by the adhesive abilities of the K99 antigen. ST enterotoxin is then released and mediates net outward flow of water and electrolytes as in piglet diarrhea.

The septicemic form of colibacillosis in calves is a common sequel of colostrum deprivation and is often preceded or accompanied by diarrhea (55). The serotypes involved belong to a limited range of O groups; a common one being O78. The important colostral immunoglobulin class in prevention of *E. coli* septicemia is IgM (46).

Calves with the enteric and enterotoxemic forms develop a severe diarrhea, the feces being full of gas bubbles and whitish. The animal may die in a few days from dehydration and acidosis. Septicemic calves become weak and sleepy, and soon die. Some cases survive longer but exhibit polyarthritis and meningitis, which is frequently fatal.

The success of vaccination of cows with *E. coli* to prevent diarrheal disease in calves appears to depend on formation of the appropriate K antibodies (42). Antibodies to O antigens are not significant in protection.

The fact that ST enterotoxin is not antigenic precludes the use of immunologic methods for prevention or neutralization of the toxic phase of the enterotoxemic syndrome. Vaccines must be multivalent in respect of K antigen content so that calves exposed under field conditions to a variety of enteropathogenic serotypes may be protected.

Vaccine failures are attributable to poor immune response of dams, involvement of other etiologic agents, and exposure to such vast numbers of *E. coli* under conditions of poor hygiene that antibody protection is overwhelmed.

***E. coli* Infections in Lambs.** Sojka (55) classified *E. coli* infections in lambs as being of two kinds, enteric and bacteremic. The enteric form occurs in lambs 2 to 8 days old and is caused by the proliferation of enteropathogenic, noninvasive strains in the upper small intestine. The serotypes studied have been similar to those producing enterotoxemia in the calf and have K99 antigen. These strains produce ST enterotoxin. However, Ansari *et al.* (4) found that only a proportion of diarrhea-producing strains in lambs have produced enterotoxin in a ligated loop test in the lamb, suggesting that another category of enteropathogenic *E. coli* exists in lambs.

Strains that produce bacteremia are different serotypically from the strains producing enteric disease, the most frequent serotype being O78: K80 (57).

Lambs with enteric colibacillosis exhibit diarrhea, depression, and some mortality. The bacteremic form often results in sudden death. Less severe manifestations include meningitis and/or arthritis. Ansari *et al.* (4) found that in an intensive shed lambing operation, colibacillosis appeared sooner in lambs born during inclement weather than in those born during good weather.

***E. coli* Infections in Horses and Dogs.** In a 26-year study of infections in fetuses and foals, Dimock, Edwards, and Bruner (20) found that *E. coli* accounted for approximately 1 percent of the abortions observed in mares and for about 5 percent of the deaths of foals. Foals that succumbed to *E. coli* infection usually were ill at birth (29). They presented symptoms of increased temperature and pulse rate and were dull and weak. Death frequently occurred within 24 hours after the onset of the disease. In foals examined before postmortem decomposition the microorganisms were isolated from the internal organs and from synovial fluids. Congenitally defective foals are more prone to the disease (47).

In mares, *E. coli* (groups O2, O4, O6, O75) often are initial invaders of the genital tract after dystocia but usually are rapidly cleared from the tract. Occasionally, they cause acute metritis.

In puppies, bacteremias caused by *E. coli* (group O42) have been implicated in the "fading-puppy syndrome" in which affected puppies become weak and anorectic, and die. This syndrome is also associated with herpesvirus infection, however, and the etiology may be multifactorial.

E. coli are present in about 70 percent of cases of pyometra in the bitch but are not believed to have primary etiologic significance. Serotypes of groups O4, O6, and O22 predominate (10, 27).

***E. coli* Infections in Poultry.** *E. coli* are rarely implicated in avian diarrheal disease: the diarrhea seen in avian colibacillosis is a result of urinary water loss and is not a sequel to enteritis. Typical colibacillosis in older chickens and turkeys involves primarily the respiratory tract as a result of inhalation of feces-contaminated litter dust. The organism then spreads into the bloodstream and causes either (*a*) acute colisepticemia with high mortality, (*b*) fibrinopurulent serositis, or (*c*) coligranuloma (Hjàrre's disease). Hjàrre's disease is usually chronic in course and is characterized by granulomatous lesions in the wall of the intestinal tract, the liver, and the lungs.

Colibacillosis in newly hatched chickens usually results from *E. coli* contamination of eggs, either from feces or from infection in the ovary of the hen. The chicks exhibit omphalitis and mushy-yolk disease.

The serotypes involved in avian colibacillosis belong predominantly to groups O1, O2, O36, and O78 (12).

Vaccines consisting of inactivated O78: K80 strains have been shown to be protective (12).

***E. coli* Mastitis (Bovine).** *E. coli* is by far the most important of the Gram-negative environmental organisms that cause mastitis in dairy cattle (3). The incidence can be very high on certain farms and usually peaks during the winter months. There is good evidence that *E. coli* mastitis is more frequent in herds where dry cow therapy and teat dipping is practiced (37). These procedures reduce the population of commensal organisms such as *Corynebacterium bovis* and nonpathogenic staphylococci on and in the udder. These organisms normally promote a low-level cellular response in the secretion which helps protect against other infections.

There is also a positive correlation between contamination of the environment by *E. coli* and the occurrence of *E. coli* mastitis (6). Furthermore, the wide range of serotypes involved suggests that environmental rather than cow-to-cow transfer occurs.

Irregular vacuum fluctuations and inadequate machine sanitation contribute to the incidence of the disease (7). Entry of the organism occurs through the meatus. Adherence of some strains of fimbriate *E. coli* to epithelial cells in the mammary gland may be important in pathogenesis of the disease (2, 30). In some cases, colonization may be limited to the streak canal and the lower teat cistern. These organisms release endotoxin, which incites an inflammatory response in more remote parts of the gland. In most cases of *E. coli* mastitis, however, there is true intramammary infection by the organism. Endotoxin released during bacteriolysis causes a great increase in mammary bloodflow (19). There is marked swelling of the gland, and a serous fluid replaces the milk. Absorption of endotoxin into the animal's bloodstream leads to high fever, depression, a leukopenia followed by a leukocytosis, prolonged hypoglycemia, and, in severe cases, irreversible shock and death of the animal. Because recovery of damaged mammary tissue is slow, losses in milk production may be substantial.

Diagnosis of *E. coli* Infections. Enteric colibacillosis is characteristically associated with abnormally large numbers of a single clone of *E. coli* (usually beta-hemolytic and mucoid) in the anterior and distal segments of the small intestine. Culture of fresh intestinal contents or even of freshly voided stool will frequently yield almost pure cultures of *E. coli.*

The fluorescent-antibody test, using conjugates prepared against the K99 colonizing antigens, has been employed to diagnose enteric colibacillosis in calves (39). In this procedure, sections of ileum from fresh carcasses are stained with the conjugate. After isolation, serotyping may be performed and representative isolates checked for production of enterotoxins by the suckling mouse and hamster ovary cell assays (18, 28).

Septicemic and avian colibacilloses are diagnosed by demonstrating pure cultures of *E. coli* in the blood, parenchymatous organs, and lesions.

In cases of mastitis, the organism may be difficult to culture. In these cases, endotoxin may be detected by the limulus amoebocyte lysate test.

REFERENCES

1. Alderete and Robertson. Inf. and Immun., 1978, *19,* 1021.
2. Anderson, Burrows, and Bramley. Vet. Path., 1977, *14,* 618.
3. Anon. Vet. Rec., 1977. *100,* 441.

4. Ansari, Renshaw, and Gates. Am. Jour. Vet. Res., 1978, *39,* 11.
5. Barnum, Glantz, and Moon. Colibacillosis. CIBA Veterinary Monograph Series No. 2, 1967.
6. Bramley. Ph.D. thesis, University of Reading, England, 1974.
7. Bramley and Neave. Brit. Vet. Jour., 1975, *131,* 160.
8. Bruner. Cornell Vet., 1957, *47,* 491.
9. Bywater, Jour. Comp. Pathol., 1970, *80,* 565.
10. Chaffaux, Person, and Renault. Recueil de Med. Vet., 1978, *154,* 465.
11. Cherry, Davis, Edwards, and Hogan. Jour. Lab. and Clin. Med., 1954, *44,* 51.
12. Cheville and Arp. Jour. Am. Vet. Med. Assoc., 1978, *173,* 584.
13. Chidlow and Porter. Vet. Rec., 1979, *104,* 496.
14. Clements and Finkelstein. Inf. and Immun., 1979, *24,* 760.
15. Clugston and Nielsen. Can. Jour. Comp. Med., 1974, *38,* 22.
16. Clugston, Nielsen, and Smith. Can. Jour. Comp. Med., 1974, *38,* 34.
17. Davis and Ewing. Am. Jour. Clin. Path., 1963, *39,* 198.
18. Dean, Ching, Williams, and Handen. Jour. Inf. Dis., 1972, *125,* 407.
19. Dhondt, Burnemich, and Peeters. Jour. Dairy Res., 1977, *44,* 433.
20. Dimock, Edwards, and Bruner. Cornell Vet., 1947, *37,* 89.
21. Edwards, Philip R. and William H. Ewing. Identification of enterobacteriaceae, 3rd ed. Burgess, Minneapolis, Minn., 1972.
22. Erskine, Sojka, and Lloyd. Vet. Rec., 1957, *69,* 301.
23. Field, Graf, Laird, and Smith. Proc. Natl. Acad. Sci., 1978, *75,* 2800.
24. Gay. Bact. Rev., 1965, *29,* 75.
25. Gregory. Vet. Med., 1958, *53,* 77.
26. Gregory. Vet. Rec., 1960, *72,* 1208.
27. Grindley, Renton, and Ramsay. Res. Vet. Sci., 1973, *14,* 75.
28. Guerrant, Brunton, Schnaitman, Rebhun, and Gilman. Inf. and Immun., 1974, *10,* 320.
29. Gunning. Vet. Jour., 1947, *103,* 47.
30. Harper, Turvey, and Bramley. Jour. Med. Microbiol., 1978, *11,* 117.
31. Kauffmann. Jour. Immunol., 1946, *57,* 71.
32. Kauffmann. Acta Path. et Microbiol. Scand., 1949, *26,* 381.
33. Kohler, Cross, and Bohl. Am. Jour. Vet. Res., 1975, *36,* 757.
34. Kurtz and Quast. Proc. Int. Pig. Vet. Soc., Ames, Iowa, June 1976.
35. Lamont, Luke, and Gordon. Vet. Rec., 1950, *62,* 737.
36. Lonnroth, Andren, Lange, Martinsson, and Holmgren. Inf. and Immun., 1979, *24,* 900.
37. Marr. Vet. Rec., 1978, *102,* 132.
38. Meyers and Guinee. Inf. and Immun., 1976, *13,* 117.

39. Moon, McClurkin, Isaacson, Poblenz, Skartvedt, Gillette, and Baetz. Jour. Am. Vet. Med. Assoc., 1978, *173,* 577.
40. Moon. Adv. Vet. Sci., 1974, *18,* 179.
41. Morgan, Isaacson, and Brinton. Proc. Ann. Conf. Res. Workers in Animal Disease, Chicago, 1977.
42. Myers. Am. Jour. Vet. Res., 1978, *39,* 761.
43. Nagy, Moon, Isaacson, To, and Brinton. Inf. and Immun., 1978, *21,* 269.
44. Nelson, Whitaker, Hempstead, and Harris. Jour. Am. Med. Assoc., 1961, *176,* 26.
45. Nielsen, Moon, and Roe. Jour. Am. Vet. Med. Assoc., 1968, *153,* 1590.
46. Penhale, Christie, McEwan, Fisher, and Selman. Brit. Vet. Jour., 1970, *126,* 30.
47. Platt. Brit. Vet. Jour., 1973, *129,* 221.
48. Porter, Kenworthy, Holme, and Horsfield. Vet. Rec., 1973, *92,* 630.
49. Rutter. Vet. Rec., 1975, *96,* 171.
50. Rutter, Jones, and Brown. Inf. and Immun., 1976, *13,* 667.
51. Silliker and Taylor. Jour. Lab. and Clin. Med., 1957, *49,* 460.
52. Smith. Jour. Path. and Bact., 1963, *85,* 197.
53. Smith and Gyles. Jour. Med. Microbiol., 1970, *3,* 387.
54. Sojka. Vet. Bull., 1971, *41,* 509.
55. Sojka. Can. Inst. Food Sci. Technol., 1973, *6,* 52.
56. Stark and Patterson. Jour. Dairy Sci., 1936, *19,* 495.
57. Teklecki and Sojka. Brit. Vet. Jour., 1965, *121,* 462.
58. Timoney. Vet. Rec., 1949, *61,* 710.
59. Timoney. Vet. Rec., 1950, *62,* 748.
60. Timoney. Vet. Rec., 1956, *68,* 849.
61. Timoney. Vet. Rec., 1957, *69,* 1160.
62. Timoney. Vet. Rec., 1960, *72,* 1252.

THE *KLEBSIELLA-ENTEROBACTER* GROUP

Although certain members of this group are lacking in pathogenicity, some of the types are associated with bovine mastitis (1), with respiratory and urogenital infections in man, with genital infections of animals, and possibly with endotoxemia in horses (5). The mucoid (encapsulated) types within the group, known as *klebsiellas,* are of most importance. In man, *Klebsiella pneumoniae* (Friedlander's bacillus) has been recognized in respiratory, urogenital, and intestinal (severe diarrheal) diseases.

Strains of *Klebsiella* have been classified serologically by Kauffman (9). Among these encapsulated types is the organism *Klebsiella pneumoniae* var. *genitalium* described in 1927 by Dimock and Edwards (6) as the cause of a particular type of urogenital infection of mares.

Klebsiella pneumoniae var. *genitalium*

Morphology and Staining Reactions. This microorganism is a Gram-negative, nonmotile, non-spore-bearing, encapsulated rod. The capsules are readily demonstrable and are responsible for an excessively mucoid form of growth on culture media.

Cultural Features. The organism grows readily on ordinary laboratory media. On agar slants there occurs an excessively dirty-white to slightly yellow growth that is moist, spreading, glistening, and very viscid. Agar colonies are large, raised, round, and entire. Broth becomes turbid, with a ropy sediment. A typical nailhead growth appears in gelatin; no liquefaction occurs. Acid and coagulation are produced in litmus milk. Nitrates are reduced to nitrites and ammonia. Indol is not formed. Most strains are methyl-red-negative and Voges-Proskauer-positive.

K. pneumoniae may be differentiated from *Enterobacter aerogenes* by the urease and ornithine decarboxylase tests. The former is positive in the first, and negative in the second of these tests. Also, *K. pneumoniae* is not motile.

Antigens. Cultures are classified on the basis of their K (capsular) and O (somatic) antigens. There are at least 80 capsular types (designated 1, 2, 3, etc.) and 11 different O types.

Epidemiology and Pathogenesis. *K. pneumoniae* is commonly found as a saprophyte in nature and as a commensal in the intestinal tract of healthy animals. It is also found on wood shavings.

Mares have been shown to carry strains of *K. pneumoniae* in the vestibule, urethra, or clitoris as normal flora. These infections do not usually involve the cervix or uterus (8). In some mares, opportunistic invasion of these sites does occur and results in metritis and infertility. Strains isolated from cases of metritis predominantly belong to capsular types 1, 5, and 7 (10). The stallion may transmit infection from mare to mare but is not believed to be important as a reservoir of infection. Stallions clear infections within 10 to 12 days of ceasing service (4). Contaminated instruments and hands may also serve as vehicles of transmission.

K. pneumoniae is also a cause of environmentally derived bovine mastitis. The organism has been shown to be present on wood shavings used for bedding and to infect cows from this source. A variety of capsular types has been found among isolates from individual herds (3)—further proof of the environmental origin of the infection. The form of the mastitis is acute or peracute (3).

Mastitis caused by this organism also occurs in sows (7, 11) and produces a severe leukopenia (2).

Chemotherapy. Most strains appear to be sensitive to kanamycin, neomycin, gentamicin, polymixin B, and furazolidone.

REFERENCES

1. Adler, North Am. Vet., 1951, *32,* 96.
2. Bertschinger, Pohlenz, Middleton, and Williams. Schweiz. Arch. f. Tierheilk., 1977, *119,* 265.
3. Braman, Eberhart, Asbury, and Hermann. Jour. Am. Vet. Med. Assoc., 1973, *162,* 109.
4. Cadazza and Sampien. Folia Vet. Latina, 1973, *3,* 424.
5. Carroll, Schalm, and Wheat. Jour. Am. Vet. Med. Assoc., 1965, *146,* 1300.
6. Dimock and Edwards. Jour. Am. Vet. Med. Assoc., 1927, *70,* 469.
7. Done. Acta Vet. Acad. Sci. Hung., 1975, *25,* 211.
8. Greenwood and Ellis. Vet. Rec., 1976, *99,* 439.
9. Kauffmann. Acta Path. et Microbiol. Scand., 1949, *26,* 381.
10. Platt, Atherton, and Orskov. Jour. Hyg. (London), 1977, *77,* 401.
11. Ross, Zimmerman, Wagner, and Cox. Jour. Am. Vet. Med. Assoc., 1975, *167,* 231.

7 The Enterobacteriaceae—The Non-Lactose-Fermenters

The important non-lactose-fermenting genera of the Enterobacteriaceae with respect to animal disease are *Salmonella, Proteus,* and *Yersinia.* The genus *Salmonella* belongs to the tribe Escherichiae, while *Proteus* and *Yersinia* belong to the tribes Proteeae and Yersinieae, respectively.

The eighth edition of *Bergey's Manual* includes *Arizona* as subgenus III of the genus *Salmonella* because members of the groups are biochemically and antigenically very similar. However, many strains of *S. arizona* are delayed lactose fermenters. Notwithstanding this incongruity, we feel that they are best discussed with the other salmonellas and have placed them accordingly.

THE GENUS *SALMONELLA*

Soon after the isolation of the "hog cholera bacillus" by Salmon and Smith (27) in 1885, paratyphoid bacteria were found by numerous workers in a variety of diseases of animals and in enteric fever and gastroenteritis of man. Smith and Stewart (31) in 1897 stated that these microorganisms "belong to one great group (or species) in virtue of the identity of their morphological and biological characters." However, the identity of the individual members was not clearly established until White (36) recognized the importance of antigenic analysis of paratyphoid strains. The pioneer work of White, confirmed and greatly extended by Kauffmann (18), resulted in the Kauffmann-White schema for the rapid and exact identification of paratyphoid bacteria. Because Salmon and Smith (27) had isolated and described the first member of the group, the generic name of *Salmonella* was chosen, and *Salmonella choleraesuis* became the type species.

Morphology and Staining Reactions. The cells are Gram-negative, short rods (2 to 4 by 0.5 μm) that have peritrichous flagella and frequently also carry fimbriae (Figure 7.1). *S. pullorum* and *S. gallinarum* do not have flagella.

Cultural and Biochemical Characteristics. Salmonellas are aerobic and facultatively anaerobic and will grow on defined media without special growth factors. (The

Figure 7.1. *Salmonella typhimurium* showing flagella and many short fimbriae. Negative stain. × 25,300. (From Tanaka and Katsube, *Jap. Jour. Vet. Sci.*, 1978, *40,* 681.)

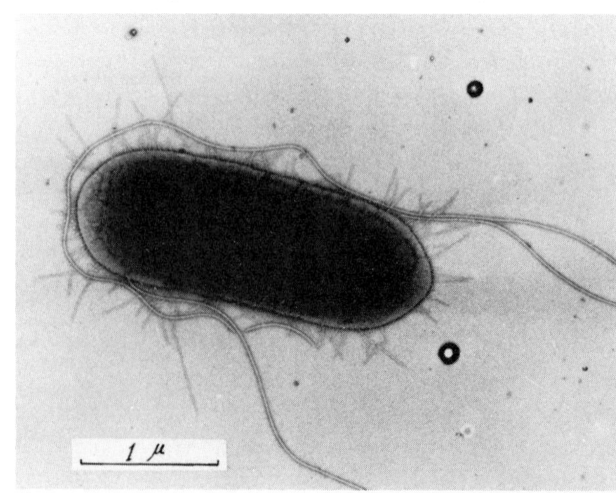

common biochemical characteristics are listed in Table 6.1.) They can use citrate as a carbon source and are usually aerogenic, producing gas from glucose. They can selectively utilize tetrathionate or sodium selenite; thus very small numbers can be detected in highly contaminated specimens using these substrates as enrichment media. Many specially formulated differential and selective media for the isolation of salmonellas have been devised. The most useful of these in veterinary bacteriology are brilliant green, McConkey, and bismuth sulfite agars.

The optimum growth temperature is 37 C, but good growth also occurs at 43 C—a characteristic often used to reduce the growth of other bacteria in highly contaminated specimens.

Antigens. Three kinds of antigens are used for the identification of salmonellas: the O (somatic), the H (flagellar), and the Vi (virulence) antigens. The O antigenic specificity is determined by the structure and composition of the lipopolysaccharide of the cell wall, and the different O antigens are designated by Arabic figures, for example, 4,12. The H antigens, unlike the O, are heat-labile and composed of protein. They can exist in either a single (monophasic) or in two separate forms (diphasic), only one of which is expressed at a given time. This phenomenon is known as the phase variation of Andrewes (2). Antigens of phase 1 are assigned small letters, for example, a,b and those of phase 2 are given Arabic numbers or small letters.

The antigens of phase 1 and phase 2 flagella are determined by two genes, H1 and H2, which code for the flagellar protein, flagellin. H2 flagellin synthesis is controlled by a recombinational event which inverts the section of the chromosome containing the H2 gene. When the H2 gene is activated, another gene close by is also active and synthesizes a repressor substance which inhibits expression of the H1 gene (29). The "switch" mechanism controlling the recombinational event on the chromosome which turns on phase 2 is as yet unknown.

The Vi antigen is found on *S. typhi* and is of no importance with regard to the salmonellas that cause disease in animals.

The antigenic formulas (serotypes) of some common salmonellas are given in Table 7.1. There are more than 1,300 known salmonella serotypes.

Form Variation in *S. pullorum*. Younie (41) called attention to the occurrence of *S. pullorum* infection in the progeny of flocks that contained no reactors to the standard agglutination test. Cultures of *S. pullorum* recovered from the chicks of such flocks differed serologically from standard antigen strains of *S. pullorum*. Sera of chicks infected with these variant cultures failed to agglutinate the standard antigen strains but did agglutinate the infecting cultures in high dilution.

Table 7.1. Antigenic formulas of some common *Salmonella* serotypes

Serotype	Antigenic formula
S. choleraesuis	6,7: c-1,5 (diphasic)
S. dublin	9,12: g,p-(monophasic)
S. pullorum	9,12:-(nonmotile)
S. typhimurium	1,4,5,12: i-1,2 (diphasic)

Edwards and Bruner (4) studied the "standard" and "variant" strains of *S. pullorum* and noted that the antigenic formula of *S. pullorum* is $9,12_1$ (12_2), 12_3. In normal cultures the 12_2 factor is variable, and forms containing a large amount or a negligible amount of 12_2 can be isolated from the same strain. It is possible for cultures to become fairly well stabilized in either form, thus giving rise to the so-called *standard* strains and *variant* or X strains. The standard strains contain only a small amount of 12_2, but the X strains contain a large amount of the antigen. Although the strains lacking 12_2 and the strains containing 12_2 cross-agglutinate to a certain titer, each strain agglutinates to a much higher titer when exposed to its homologous serum. Therefore, the presence of the variant type of infection in a flock of birds necessitates the use of the variant antigen if the disease is to be eradicated by removing the agglutination reactors.

Another variation in the O antigen can result in a change in the colonial appearance of the strain from smooth (S) to rough (R). This change is accompanied by loss of the O antigen and sometimes of virulence.

Bacteriophage Typing. Phage typing is based on the sensitivity of cultures to a series of bacteriophage at appropriate dilutions. The technique was first used on *S. typhi* and has since been applied to *S. typhimurium* and to other salmonellas (1). It is of great value for source tracing in epidemiologic studies. Typing schemes for *S. typhimurium* strains from one country, however, are not necessarily applicable in another, and the schemes devised for use in the United States are different from those used in Britain (9, 38). The presence of certain R-factor plasmids complicates the interpretation of phage typing results because of plasmid-mediated effects such as altered receptor sites on the cell surface or synthesis of endonucleases which destroy the phage after it enters the cell.

Epidemiology. The feco-oral route is the most important mode of transmission of salmonellas in animals. However, the cycle of infection may be more complex in some animal populations; in poultry, for example, the primary source of infection may be contaminated feed, and subsequent spread may occur via the feco-oral route or from egg to chick in the hatchery. A variable percentage of animals, once infected, remain carriers and shed the organism intermittently.

The salmonellas are classified as either host-adapted or non-host-adapted depending on their host range (Table 7.2). The host-adapted serotypes rarely cause disease in hosts other than the one to which they are adapted. *S. dublin* is traditionally host-adapted to cattle but in some areas is showing a tendency to spread into swine (20, 34).

Young animals are more susceptible to salmonellosis than older ones. Poor sanitation, overcrowding, inclement weather, stress of hospitalization and surgery, parturition, parasitism, transportation, overtraining, and concurrent viral infections are all factors which predispose animals to clinical salmonellosis. Many animals suffer inapparent infections during their lifetimes. This is especially true of swine and poultry fed rations that contain salmonellas.

Animal feeds are frequently contaminated by a variety of serotypes (23), which usually enter the feed mixture in the protein supplement. Meat and bone meal, fish meal, and soybean meal have all been shown to be frequently and heavily contaminated. The salmonellas enter these materials during or after processing. In the case of meat and bone meal, the percolator phase that removes fat after cooking is an important contaminative stage: the organisms are maintained and multiply in the material as it cools (33).

Table 7.2. Some host-adapted and non-host-adapted *Salmonella* serotypes

Host-adapted	Non-host-adapted
S. abortusequi	*S. anatum*
S. abortusovis	*S. derby*
S. choleraesuis	*S. newport*
S. dublin	*S. tennessee*
S. gallinarum	*S. typhimurium*
S. paratyphi (A, C)	
S. pullorum	
S. typhi	

Salmonellas are killed at 56 C in about 10 to 20 minutes, although more heat-resistant strains of *S. senftenburg* have occasionally been found. They survive for months or longer in manure, feces (17), and the sediments of streams and ponds (12).

Wild birds and rodents such as rats and mice may also be a source of infection for livestock via feces contamination of feed or buildings.

Pathogenesis. Salmonellosis is usually an enteric disease but sometimes becomes generalized with bacteremia or septicemia and involvement of other organ systems. Abortion and meningitis are two other less common manifestations of salmonella infection.

The pathogenesis of *Salmonella* enteritis occurs in three stages: (*a*) colonization of the intestine, (*b*) invasion of the intestinal epithelium, and (*c*) stimulation of fluid exsorption.

(*a*) *Colonization of the intestine.* Colonization of the distal small intestine and the colon is a necessary first step in the pathogenesis of enteric salmonellosis. Indigenous fusiform bacteria that lie in the mucous layer investing the epithelium of the large intestine normally inhibit growth of salmonellas by producing volatile organic acids (14). The normal flora also block access to attachment sites needed by the salmonellas. Factors which disrupt the normal colonic flora, such as antibiotic therapy, diet, and water deprivation, greatly increase the host's susceptibility to enteric and septicemic salmonellosis (22, 32, 35). Reduced peristalsis also enhances colonization by salmonellas because it allows temporary overgrowth to occur, especially in the small intestine. Peristalsis is stimulated by an active indigenous microflora, suppression of which increases the host's susceptibility to colonization. Swine that are stressed by transportation exhibit greatly increased rates of colonization by a variety of salmonellas (37). The physiological basis of this phenomenon is poorly understood.

(*b*) *Invasion of the intestinal epithelium.* The invasion phase involves the villous tips of the ileum and colon. The brush border is penetrated, and the salmonellas enter the cell, apparently without killing it, as there is no morphologic change until later in the disease process. The organisms may multiply and infect other adjoining cells or pass into the lamina propria, where they continue to multiply and are phagocytosed and trapped in the regional lymph nodes. After invasion, the villous tips contract and are invaded by neutrophils.

(*c*) *Stimulation of fluid exsorption.* There is evidence that this is a result of activation of adenylcyclase with net secretion of water, HCO_3^-, and Cl^- (10). The activation of adenylcyclase may be due to the effects of prostaglandins induced by the inflammatory response to the invading salmonellas. However, some strains of *S. typhimurium* are known to produce enterotoxinlike substances (28). An inflammatory enteritis quickly develops and is characterized by extensive neutrophil invasion of villous cores with acute ileitis and colitis. Neutrophils are also shed in the stool, and their presence has diagnostic value.

Salmonella *septicemia*. The pathogenesis of the septicemic phase of salmonellosis appears to be related to the effects of endotoxin released from bacterial cells. In salmonellas, endotoxic activity resides in the lipopolysaccharide of the cell wall. The lipopolysaccharide is composed of an O-specific chain, a core oligosaccharide common to all salmonellas, and a lipid A component. The latter is the part of the lipopolysaccharide molecule that contains endotoxin activity (8).

The effects of endotoxin on the host include fever, mucosal hemorrhages, a leukopenia followed by a leukocytosis, thrombocytopenia, and depletion of liver glycogen with prolonged hypoglycemia and shock. The shock effect may be severe and irreversible and lead to the death of the animal.

Immunity to Salmonellas. There is widespread agreement that cell-mediated immunity is more important than humoral antibodies in resistance to salmonellosis. Woolcock (39) provides an excellent review of the issues involved in this question. Cell-mediated immunity has its basis in enhanced microbicidal activity of the host's macrophages for the organism and is not serotype-specific. Humoral immunity contributes to bacterial clearance, and is serotype-specific.

Local mucosal immunity in the intestine to salmonellas is poorly understood, but the cell-mediated response appears to be less important in intestinal protection.

Antibodies to lipid A do not appear to protect against the effects of endotoxin (21) unless certain complement factors are present in excess (8).

Bovine Salmonellosis

The two serotypes of greatest important in bovine salmonellosis are *S. dublin* and *S. typhimurium*. Occasional outbreaks are caused by other, mostly feed-derived, serotypes. *S. dublin* is host adapted to the bovine and occurs throughout Europe, in the United States west of the Rocky Mountains, and in South Africa.

Carrier animals are the main reservoir of *S. dublin*

infection between outbreaks, although the organism can survive in feces for up to 4 months and elsewhere in the environment for over a year (11).

Carriers are less important in the epidemiology of salmonellosis caused by *S. typhimurium*, the reservoir of which includes a wide range of species and sources, including feed.

Calves are more susceptible to salmonellosis than adult animals, and losses are frequently severe in intensive rearing units. A number of factors may be involved in outbreaks of salmonellosis in calves, including the manner in which the calves were purchased and transported, housing, penning, and standards of husbandry.

Calves purchased in sales yards by dealers often have not received colostrum and are derived from a variety of sources. The stress of transportation before and after marketing under poor hygienic and crowded conditions favors rapid transfer of the organism. Cases of salmonellosis usually appear within a few days, and the number of cases peaks at about 3 weeks. The spread of infection is greater among calves penned loosely and able to contact each other than in groups penned separately (19); one reason for this is that calves with salmonellosis secrete the organism in the saliva and thus may pass the infection to others by licking or by means of contaminated buckets. However, feco-oral transfer among calves is the single most important mode of transfer.

On farms which do not bring in calves from outside sources, *S. dublin* infection is often derived from adult carriers (6). Carrier cows shed the organism at parturition, and the newborn calves are thereby exposed to infection.

The disease in young calves is characterized by foul-smelling diarrhea, depression, anorexia, fever, weakness, and death in a day or two. The stool may be blood-stained and contain mucus and shreds of mucosa (Figure 7.2). Postmortem examination reveals petechial hemorrhages in the peritoneum and areas of hemorrhagic inflammation on the colon and distal small intestine. The mesenteric lymph nodes are also hemorrhagic and edematous. There may be areas of necrosis in the liver.

In calves that do not die in the acute phase there may be later signs of joint involvement and, rarely, ischemic necrosis of the tips of the ears, tail, and feet.

The mortality in calf salmonellosis may be as high as 75 percent, but losses are usually of the order of 5 to 10 percent. Losses are generally much higher among purchased than among home-bred calves (16).

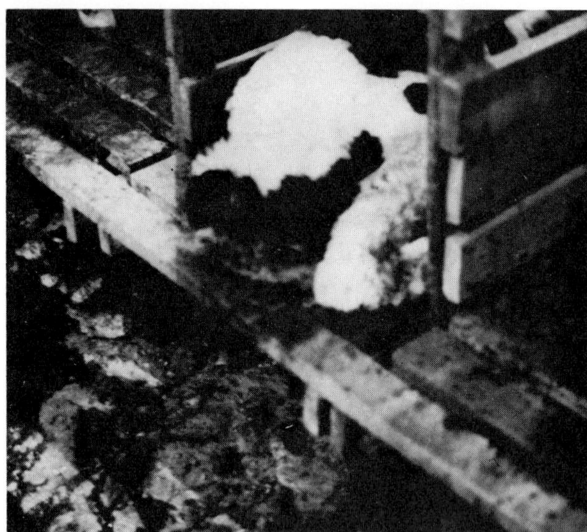

Figure 7.2. Dysentery in a veal calf caused by *Salmonella typhimurium*. Note the dark blood-stained area in the center of the pool of diarrheic feces.

Salmonellosis among adult cattle is much less common and more sporadic than among calves. Predisposing factors include parturition, parasitism, inclement weather, poor nutrition, and stress of transportation. The disease is similar to that in calves. Animals in the later stages often lapse into irreversible endotoxic shock. The organism may be shed in the milk and urine of bacteremic/septicemic cows.

S. dublin and to a lesser extent, a variety of other serotypes are well established as causes of abortion in the bovine in Northern Europe and the United States. Abortion may occur in association with the enteric and septicemic forms of the disease but often occurs by itself (15). *S. dublin* abortions are more common from August to November in Europe (7). The organism apparently enters the fetus from the maternal circulation via the placenta and causes septicemia and death of the fetus. There is no evidence of venereal transmission. The aborted fetus exhibits edema of the subcutis and serosanguineous fluid in the peritoneal cavity. Abortion due to salmonellas occurs on average about 200 days after conception (7).

Serologic Response. The available serologic tests (agglutination, antiglobulin) are not reliable for the detection of individual infected bovines but are of value in detection of infected herds (40). Both O and H titers can be measured. O titers of at least 1:80 and H titers of at least 1:320 are diagnostic (3). However, many infected animals do not have positive titers either because the serum was collected too early or because the infection was not severe enough to stimulate an immune response. Also, animals may passively transfer the organism through their intestines without developing an immune response. The antigenic stimulus associated with clinical salmonellosis is much more effective in eliciting an antibody response (24) and so recovered animals or animals that have aborted due to *Salmonella* sp. usually have positive titers (7).

Calves respond much more to the H antigens than to the O antigens of salmonellas, so H titers must be measured in these animals (5). Ideally, paired serum samples should be tested.

Vaccination. Salmonella bacterins, although capable of stimulating an antibody response, are less effective in promoting a solid immunity than live vaccines (25). Vaccination of pregnant cattle with *S. dublin* to protect calves for the first few weeks of life has been shown to be effective (13), and this procedure also reduces fecal excretion in exposed calves (26). Attenuated live vaccines prepared from rough strains of *S. gallinarum*, *S. dublin*, and *S. choleraesuis* have been shown to be protective in poultry, calves, and swine in Britain (30). The calf and swine vaccines are commercially available in Britain but not in the United States. They appear to be most effective when field exposure is kept to a minimum and the use of antibiotics is avoided.

REFERENCES

1. Anderson. *In* The world problem of salmonellosis, ed. E. Van Oye. Junk, the Hague, 1974, pp. 84–110.
2. Andrewes. Jour. Path. and Bact., 1922, *25*, 505.
3. Clarenburg and Vink. Rep. XIV Int. Vet. Congr., London, 1949, *2*, 262.
4. Edwards and Bruner. Cornell Vet., 1946, *36*, 318.
5. Field. *In* Diseases due to bacteria, Vol. 2, ed. Arthur Stableforth and Ian Galloway. London, Butterworth, 1959.
6. Field. Vet. Jour., 1968, *104*, 251, 294.
7. Frik. Profschrift Fac. Diergeneesk., Rijksuniv., Utrecht, 1969.
8. Galanos, Freudenburg, Hose, Joy, and Ruschman. Microbiology 1977, 269.
9. Gershman. Jour. Clin. Microbiol., 1976, *3*, 214.
10. Grainello, Gots, and Charney. Gastroenterology, 1975, *69*, 1238.
11. Gibson. Vet. Rec., 1961, *73*, 1284.
12. Hendricks. Appl. Microbiol., 1971, *21*, 378.
13. Henning. Onderstepoort Jour. Vet. Res., 1953, *26*, 45.
14. Hentges and Maier. Inf. and Immun., 1970, *2*, 364.
15. Hinton. Vet. Bull., 1971, *41*, 973.
16. Hughes. Bull. Off. Int. Epiz., 1964, *62*, 525.

17. Joselord. Austral. Vet. Jour., 1951, *27,* 264.
18. Kauffmann, Fritz. Die Bakteriologie der Salmonellagruppe. Enjnar Munksgaard, Copenhagen, 1941.
19. Linton, Howe, Pethiyagoda, and Osborne. Vet. Rec., 1974, *94,* 581.
20. McErlean. Vet. Rec., 1968, *82,* 257.
21. Mullan, Newsome, Cunnington, Palmer, and Wilson. Inf. and Immun., 1974, *10,* 1195.
22. Nelson, Pediatrics, 1971, *48,* 248.
23. Pomeroy and Grady. Proc. U.S. Livestock Sanit. Assoc., 1961, *65,* 449.
24. Richardson. Vet. Rec., 1975, *96,* 329.
25. Roantree. Ann. Rev. Microbiol., 1967, *21,* 443.
26. Royal, Robinson, and Loken. Vet. Rec., 1969, *86,* 67.
27. Salmon and Smith. Report on swine plague. U.S. Bur. Anim. Indus., 2nd Ann. Rpt., 1885.
28. Sedlock, Koupal, and Deibel. Inf. and Immun., 1978, *20,* 375.
29. Silverman, Zieg, and Simon. Jour. Bact., 1979, *137,* 517.
30. Smith. Jour. Hyg. (London), 1965, *63,* 117.
31. Smith and Stewart. Boston Soc. Med. Sci. Jour., 1897, *16,* 12.
32. Tamnock and Smith. Jour. Med. Microbiol., 1972, *5,* 283.
33. Timoney. Vet. Rec., 1968, *83,* 541.
34. Timoney. Irish Vet. Jour., 1970, *24,* 141.
35. Timoney, Niebert, and Scott. Cornell Vet., 1978, *68,* 211.
36. White. Med. Res. Council (Brit.), Spec. Rpt. Ser. 103, 1926.
37. Williams and Newell. Jour. Hyg. (London), 1968, *66,* 281.
38. Wilson, Hierman, and Balows. Appl. Microbiol., 1971, *21,* 774.
39. Woolcock. Austral. Vet. Jour., 1973, *49,* 307.
40. Wray, Sojka, and Callow. Brit. Vet. Jour., 1977, *133,* 25.
41. Younie. Can. Jour. Comp. Med., 1941, *5,* 164.

Equine Salmonellosis

It has been estimated that 5 to 10 percent of the equine population in the United States becomes infected with salmonellas during its lifetime (18). *S. typhimurium* is by far the most common serotype isolated but *S. enteritis, S. newport,* and *S. heidelberg* are also occasionally found. *S. absortusequi,* a once common cause of abortion in horses in the United States, appears to have been eradicated. The infection is still present in parts of Europe, South Africa, and South America.

Various stresses including overtraining, hospitalization, worming, transportation, early weaning, and hot weather have been observed to be predisposing factors for equine salmonellosis (18). The disease may be devastating in foals under 6 months of age. A peracute, septicemic, and fatal infection frequently occurs in this age group.

Morse *et al.* (18) also describe an acute form with fever, weakness, and diarrhea and a chronic form characterized by intransigent diarrhea persisting for weeks or months. The feces may have a "cow pie" consistency. Horses with the chronic form may steadily lose weight until they fall and cannot rise again. The acute form may end in recovery or may progress to the chronic phase. Salmonellas may be difficult to detect in the feces of animals with chronic salmonellosis but there may be up to 3×10^5 organisms per gram in the feces of acute or peracute cases.

Recovered animals usually have high O and H titers.

S. abortusequi apparently is spread mainly in the pasture. Infective discharges from aborting animals contaminate the grass, which then is eaten by susceptible animals. Abortion can readily be produced in mares by mixing pure cultures with their feed and by injecting cultures intravenously. Just before the act of abortion occurs, the affected mare usually shows fever and other signs of a general reaction. Some believe that the mare suffers a brief period of septicemia. If so, it disappears and the only lesions found after the abortion are in the fetal membranes, which are edematous and frequently show hemorrhages and areas of necrosis.

The specific organism may easily be cultivated by ordinary cultural methods from the placenta, fetus, or uterine exudate. Agglutinins are produced in the course of the infection and are useful for diagnosis. H agglutinins are indicative of recent infection. Bacterins have been successfully used to protect mares against abortion (9, 14). According to Good and Corbett (8), normal animals may agglutinate the specific organism in dilutions of 1:200 and occasionally as high as 1:300. Infected animals usually agglutinate in dilutions from 1:500 to 1:5,000.

Swine Salmonellosis

The most important *Salmonella* serotypes that cause disease in swine are *S. choleraesuis* and *S. typhimurium.* In Britain and Ireland, *S. dublin* and a variety of non-host-adapted serotypes are becoming more frequent causes of the disease in pigs (22). *S. derby, S. newport,* and *S. anatum* are common non-host-adapted serotypes in swine in the United States.

The reservoir of *S. choleraesuis* is probably the mesenteric lymphoid tissue of carrier swine which periodically shed the organism. Shedding occurs for about 3 months after recovery from the disease, but a few swine continue to harbor and shed the organism indefinitely (26). It survives well in manure, and persistence for up to 20 weeks in slurry has been reported (12). Thus contamination of buildings is important in the epidemiology of the disease caused by this and by other serotypes. Feed is not a usual source of *S. choleraesuis* but is an important source of *S. typhimurium* and other serotypes.

Paratyphoid is the disease in swine caused by *S. choleraesuis*. Most cases of the disease in the United States and Europe are caused by the monophasic (6,7:—1,5) hydrogen sulfide-positive (Kunzendorf) type. The other types, *S. typhisuis* and *S. choleraesuis* (diphasic), are rarely isolated. The disease occurs in pigs of all ages but is most common in fattening pigs after weaning. Stress of various kinds is an important predisposing factor. The organism was called the "hog cholera bacillus" by Salmon and Smith (19) because infection by hog cholera (swine fever) virus was invariably followed by a secondary invasion of *S. choleraesuis*.

The acute disease is characterized by purplish areas on the ears, rump, and abdomen, high fever, anorexia, and death in 1 to 3 days. At postmortem examination, petechiation and other signs of septicemia are present. Pneumonia may also be observed. A less acute form is characterized by foul-smelling diarrhea, which may result in eventual death or extreme loss of condition. In chronic cases, thickening of the intestine and mucosal necrosis are caused by secondary invasions of *Fusobacterium* and *Bacteroides* sp.

Salmonellosis caused by *S. dublin* is characterized by enteritis and meningoencephalitis (17). Disease caused by *S. typhimurium* and other serotypes is usually enteric and/or septicemic.

Antibody responses in infected swine are not consistent or predictable enough to be useful in diagnosis of carriers. Fecal cultural procedures are not reliable either, since the organism is difficult to isolate from feces and is frequently present in mesenteric lymph nodes but absent from the intestinal lumen (16).

A live avirulent strain of *S. choleraesuis* is available in Europe as a vaccine against paratyphoid (21) and has been shown to reduce mortality. Results on some premises have been disappointing, possibly because levels of natural exposure were too great and occurred before vaccinal immunity had adequately developed.

Ovine Salmonellosis

Abortion in sheep during the last 2 months of pregnancy caused by *S. abortusovis* occurs in England (11) and parts of Europe. It is not found in the United States. This organism also causes congenital infections, as a result of which lambs may be born weak and die or develop enteritis a few days after birth and die.

S. typhimurium and *S. dublin* cause disease where flock management practices are poor (7). The source of infection for sheep flocks may be infected cattle pastured on the same land. Salmonellosis in sheep is similar to that in cattle.

Canine and Feline Salmonellosis

Clinical salmonellosis is uncommon in dogs and cats, although a variety of serotypes may be carried (2) by normal animals.

Timoney *et al.* (24) have described a nosocomial outbreak of *S. typhimurium* gastroenteritis and septicemia in young cats in a veterinary hospital where the mortality was 61 percent.

Avian Salmonellosis

S. pullorum and *S. gallinarum* cause *bacillary white diarrhea* or *pullorum disease* and *fowl typhoid,* respectively, in chickens. A variety of other non-host-adapted serotypes, most of which are feed-borne, also cause infections and disease in poultry. In broiler flocks infections are very common but clinically inapparent and are of significance only from the standpoint of subsequent contamination of carcasses for human consumption.

Salmonella infections of chicks may be derived from fecal soiling of eggs, ovarian infection, other diseased chicks, feed, and contaminated surroundings. Thus the epidemiology can be quite complex.

S. pullorum. *S. pullorum* has been isolated from turkeys, chickens, a pheasant, canaries, a parrot, a calf, swine, a dog, a fox, a mink, a cat, a chinchilla, and man (6). It occurs most frequently in chickens, less often in turkeys, and rather infrequently in man, although one rather large outbreak of gastroenteritis involved over 400 men. It is highly fatal if cultures are fed to young chicks during the first few days of life, and particularly if the chicks are allowed to become chilled by a lowering of the temperature of the brooder house. Older chicks become progressively harder to infect in this way, but occasionally even adult birds may be killed. Old birds can be infected by subcutaneous or intravenous injection. In these cases the infection may remain localized, or septicemia may result. Large doses, given intraperitoneally, will kill guinea pigs.

In its natural host, pullorum disease proceeds in cycles. The infection is carried in the ovaries of some hens (Figure 7.3), but there are no symptoms to indicate this fact. Some of the eggs laid by such hens will contain the organism in their yolks. If these eggs are incubated, many will fail to hatch, but the ones that do will give rise to chicks that harbor the infection in their yolk sacs. Some of these chicks appear not to be seriously harmed by the presence of the organism and become in turn ovarian carriers of the disease as adults. Others, especially those that are shipped very young and those that are chilled or otherwise devitalized, may become ill from an acute diarrhea accompanied by septicemia. The diarrheal discharges are highly contagious for the other chicks, and soon a large part of the birds associating with a few sick ones are infected with the disease. In incubator-raised chicks the disease is especially malignant, for the infected down from a few diseased chicks will be blown around the entire machine by the fan circulating the air, and all or many of the chicks will contract the disease by inhaling the organism.

The affected chicks huddle near a source of heat, they do not eat, they appear sleepy, they may show diarrhea, and they usually die within a few hours. The lesions vary according to the method of infection. Chicks infected by inhaling the organism usually show caseous areas in the lungs. Similar caseous areas often are seen in the wall of the gizzard and in the heart muscle. The losses vary greatly depending upon how the chicks are handled. It

not infrequently occurs that a hatcheryman will have no trouble in chicks that he raises himself but there will be great losses in other chicks of the same lot that are shipped to distant points.

Eradication of the disease is based on serologic detection and elimination of carrier breeder hens and fumigation of eggs at incubation.

Agglutination tests are used in pullorum disease control. The birds are bled from the wing vein into small vials. The antigen is a suspension of *S. pullorum*. Three methods of performing the test are in use.

1. *The tube method.* This is the older and standard test. The serum is separated from the clot. The test may be set up in a number of tubes, using decreasing concentrations of serum, but usually, to save expense, only a single tube is used. Into the clean, dry tube 0.05 ml of undiluted serum (some merely add one drop without bothering to measure the quantity more accurately) is placed. The suspension of bacilli (antigen) is then pipetted into the tube and caused to mix with the serum. If 1 ml of antigen is used, a dilution of 1:20 is obtained; if 1.5 ml, 1:30; if 2 ml, 1:40. Birds that react in dilutions of 1:25 or higher are regarded as infected.

Some chicken sera yield a flocculent, fatty material that floats on the surface of the fluid. This interferes with the reading of the test. These cloudy reactions can be avoided by making the antigen alkaline (pH 8.0) by the addition of NaOH just before the tests are set up.

Figure 7.3. Pullorum disease in the chicken ovary. The diseased ovary is depicted on the left. On the right is a normal ovary for comparison. The ova of the diseased bird are small, misshapen, discolored, and sometimes hemorrhagic.

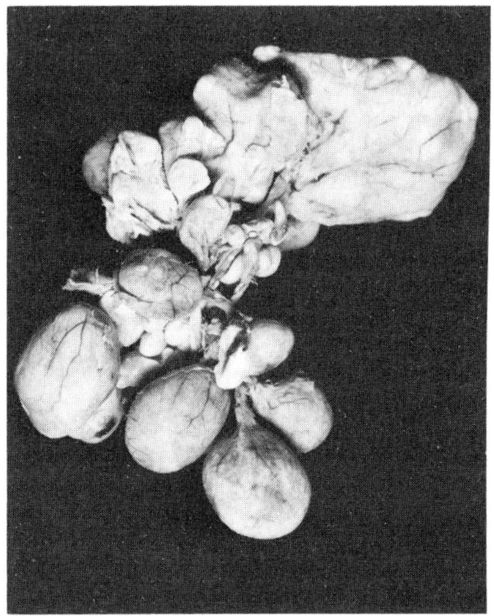

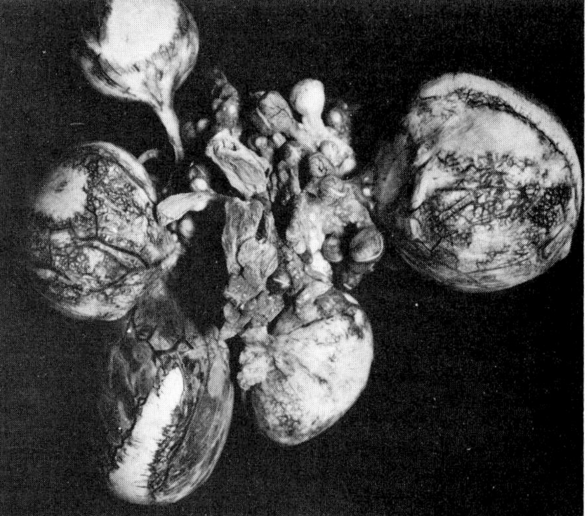

2. *The serum-plate method.* This is done in the same way as the plate method for brucellosis in cattle. When done by experienced operators, it is as accurate as the tube method.

3. *The whole-blood-plate method.* This method can be used while the birds are being held to await the outcome of the test. A drop of blood is collected on a clean glass slide and immediately mixed with a drop of the concentrated stained antigen that has been especially prepared for this test. The accuracy of the test may not be as great as that of the other methods, but it is the most widely used method.

Marked advances have been made in eradicating pullorum disease in many countries.

S. gallinarum. *S. gallinarum* causes fowl typhoid in turkeys and chickens. Its distribution is limited almost entirely to these fowls, and its occurrence is considerably less than that of *S. pullorum, S. typhimurium, S. oranienburg, S. bareilly,* and other feed-borne serotypes. Because it is traditionally an infection of barnyard flocks, its incidence has been greatly reduced by changes in poultry husbandry, and also by the eradication of *S. pullorum,* which, because of common antigens (Table 7.1), cross-reacts with *S. gallinarum* in the plate test.

Fowl typhoid affects adult birds. The symptoms are those of an acute septicemic disease, that is, wasting, weakness, drowsiness, and diarrhea. There is rapidly developing anemia and a leukocytosis. In many cases the birds are found dead under the roosts in the morning before any symptoms have been noticed. The lesions consist of thin anemic blood, multiple small necrotic areas in the liver and heart, and an enlarged spleen. The best means of making a diagnosis is the isolation of *S. gallinarum*.

Carcasses of birds that died of fowl typhoid have yielded viable bacteria from the liver up to 11 days and from the bone marrow up to 25 days after death. The organisms have also been obtained from maggots feeding on the carcasses (13).

Some workers have isolated *S. gallinarum* from diseased ovaries of hens, from eggs, and from outbreaks of typical bacillary white diarrhea in chicks. On the other hand, outbreaks of disease in adult birds which resemble fowl typhoid in every way have been attributed to *S. pullorum*.

S. typhimurium. *S. typhimurium* is a common salmonella infection of poultry in regions where pullorum disease has been controlled. It can cause severe losses in young birds. The disease is known as *paratyphoid* and is manifested by enteritis, diarrhea, and septicemia in severe cases. The organism can localize in the ovary and be transmitted in the egg.

In pigeon lofts, losses from *S. typhimurium* often are very great. The losses are in the squabs, which either die soon after hatching or develop swollen wing joints that render them unable to fly. The joint swelling is caused by the collection of a gelatinous exudate in the joint capsule. In this exudate the organism is readily found by making cultures. The adult stock shows no evidence of the disease ordinarily, but when it is destroyed for examination the ovaries of some of the females are found to be diseased. The organism can be found in many of the developing yolks and presumably passes in this way into the egg and then into the developing embryo. The pigeon fancier often calls this disease *megrims*. Cultures from pigeons usually lack the somatic antigens.

The serologic detection of carriers of *S. typhimurium* is more difficult than in the case of *S. pullorum* infection because many infected birds may be serologically negative.

Hinshaw and McNeil (10) reported on the use of the agglutination test in an attempt to eradicate *S. typhimurium* infection from turkey flocks. They found that the use of an H (flagellar) antigen and an O (somatic) antigen in separate tests at a 1:25 finding dilution enabled them to reduce markedly the *S. typhimurium* infection in a community, but they doubted that they could eliminate it entirely by testing alone. For more details see DeLay *et al.* (4). According to Sieburth (20), the indirect hemagglutination test which employs chicken erythrocytes that have been exposed to *S. typhimurium* antigens is useful in detecting infected birds.

Many other so-called exotic salmonella serotypes that are derived from feed are frequently isolated from broiler flocks and from eggs, although *Salmonella* contamination of the latter in New York State has greatly declined (1). Contamination of poultry meats is of great public health significance because many cases of human salmonellosis are derived from this source in the United States and elsewhere each year.

S. arizona **(Arizona Group).** *S. arizona* was previously named *Paracolon arizona,* and, later, *Arizona hinshawii.* It differs from other salmonellas mainly in being a slow lactose fermenter. More than 200 different serotypes have been described. The epidemiologically significant serotypes in turkeys (in which arizonosis is an important disease) are 7: 1,2,6, and 7: 1,7,8.

The disease in turkeys resembles that caused by other *Salmonella* sp. and is characterized by enteritis and/or septicemia (15, 25). The organism may localize in the ovary and egg transmission may result. Chronically infected birds may develop nervous symptoms and cateracts.

Diagnosis of *Salmonella* Infections

Isolation of the causative organism is by far the most certain means of diagnosis. However, repeated isolation attempts, involving large amounts of sample in enrichment broths, may be necessary. Shedding of the organism in feces may be intermittent and at a low level.

S. choleraesuis must be isolated directly on nonselective media since enrichment media and selective agents are toxic for it. There is an excellent review of culture methods for the detection of salmonellas in specimens from animals (3).

Serologic methods are most reliable when applied to entire herds or flocks, or when acute and convalescent sera are tested. Antibody responses are much more consistent in animals that have suffered invasive infections, such as bacteremia or septicemia.

Chemotherapy of *Salmonella* Infections

Strains of *S. typhimurium* that are resistant to many antibiotics have become very frequent in animals in the United States (23) and have severely compromised the efficacy of antimicrobial therapy. The decision to administer antibiotics to animals with salmonellosis has to be carefully taken because use of an antibiotic to which the salmonella is resistant may convert a local enteric infection into a septicemia (24) by destroying the protective colonic indigenous flora and thereby allowing unrestricted multiplication of the salmonellas.

A further disadvantage of antimicrobial therapy of enteric salmonellosis is that the number of animals that shed and the duration and amount of shedding may be increased if the *Salmonella* strain involved is resistant to the antibiotic used (5).

Chloramphenicol, gentamicin, and trimethoprim-sulfadiazine combination are effective for parenteral treatment of systemic salmonellosis but should be used only to treat the bacteremic or septicemic forms of the disease.

REFERENCES

1. Baker, Goff, and Timoney. Poultry Sci., 1979, *59,* 289.
2. Borland. Vet. Rec., 1975, *96,* 401.
3. Culture methods for the detection of animal salmonellosis and arizonosis. Iowa State Univ. Press, Ames, Iowa, 1976.

4. DeLay, Jackson, Stover, Jones, and Worcester. Jour. Am. Vet. Med. Assoc., 1955, *127,* 435.
5. Dixon. Brit. Med. Jour., 1965, *2,* 1343.
6. Edwards, Bruner, and Moran. Ky. Agr. Exp. Sta. Bull. 525, 1948.
7. Findlay. Vet. Rec., 1978, *103,* 114.
8. Good and Corbett. Jour. Inf. Dis., 1913, *13,* 53.
9. Good and Dimock. Jour. Am. Vet. Med. Assoc., 1927, *71,* 31.
10. Hinshaw and McNeil. Proc. U.S. Livestock Sanit. Assoc., 1943, *47,* 106.
11. Jack. Vet. Rec., 1968, *82,* 558.
12. Jones. Brit. Vet. Jour., 1976, *132,* 284.
13. Jordan. Brit. Vet. Jour., 1949, *110,* 387.
14. Koon and Kelser. Jour. Am. Vet. Med. Assoc., 1922, *62,* 193.
15. Kowalski and Stephens. Avian Dis., 1968, *12,* 317.
16. McCaughey, McClelland, and Roddy. Vet. Rec., 1973, *92,* 191.
17. McErlean. Vet. Rec., 1968, *82,* 257.
18. Morse, Duncan, Page, and Fessler. Cornell Vet., 1976, *66,* 198.
19. Salmon and Smith. Report on swine plague. U.S. Bur. Anim. Indus., 2nd Ann. Rpt., 1885.
20. Sieburth. Jour. Immunol., 1957, *78,* 380.
21. Smith. Jour. Hyg. (London), 1965, *63,* 117.
22. Thomas. Vet. Bull., 1977, *47,* 731.
23. Timoney. Jour. Inf. Dis., 1978, *137,* 67.
24. Timoney, Niebert, and Scott. Cornell Vet., 1978, *68,* 211.
25. West and Mohanty. Avian Dis., 1973, *17,* 314.
26. Zagaevskii. Veterinariya (Moscow), No. 9, 15.

THE GENUS *PROTEUS*

Organisms of the genus *Proteus* are readily differentiated from the salmonellas by their ability to decompose urea. Another characteristic of *Proteus* strains is their tendency to *swarm* on solid media. This may be defined as progressive surface spreading by bacteria from the parent colony. Among motile *Proteus* cultures this spreading growth over the surface produces a uniform layer hardly distinguishable from the medium and makes the isolation of other enteric bacteria from a mixed culture very difficult. They are highly motile by means of peritrichous flagella (Figure 7.4).

Organisms of the *Proteus* group are widely distributed in nature. Though often demonstrable in the feces of animals, especially in dogs and hogs, they rarely are found in large numbers except when the normal intestinal mechanism is deranged. They may be associated with diarrhea in young animals, with otitis externa (*P.*

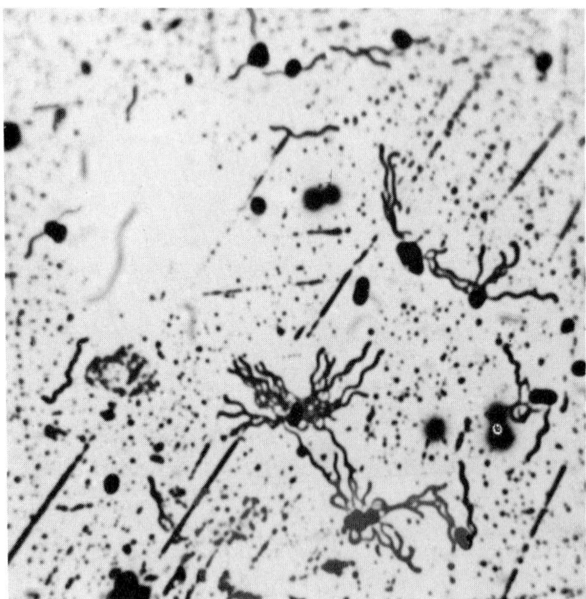

Figure 7.4. *Proteus mirabilis* showing peritrichous flagella. Leifson stain. × 1,400.

mirabilis) in the dog, and with urinary-trace infections in spayed bitches.

They are also important in spoilage of meat and carcasses because they grow and spread readily on moist surfaces at low temperatures.

Swarming of *Proteus* sp. can be prevented by use of 6 percent agar, or by the addition of 8 mg of sulfadiazine to the medium.

THE GENUS *YERSINIA*

This genus is named after the French bacteriologist Yersin, who first isolated *Y. pestis,* the cause of plague, in 1894. There are three species, *Y. enterocolitica, Y. pestis,* and *Y. pseudotuberculosis.*

Yersinia enterocolitica

This organism is ubiquitous and in recent years has been isolated with increasing frequency from alimentary tract disturbances in man and from cattle, swine, meats, shellfish, and ice cream (2). The serotypes found in swine and in man are similar (1), but the role of animals as a source of human infection is unknown. Most human cases appear to be associated with consumption of food contaminated by human carriers.

REFERENCES

1. Esseneld and Goudzwaard. Contrib. to Microbiol. and Immunol., 1973, *3,* 99.
2. Morris and Feeley. World Health Org. Bull., 1976, *54,* 79.

Yersinia pestis

SYNONYMS: *Pasteurella pestis,* plague bacillus

This organism is the cause of *plague* or *pest* of man. Time after time in past centuries plague spread over Europe from its endemic centers in Asia, destroying millions of people and spreading terror among the population. The disease became known as the *black death.* In warm climates the disease usually assumes the *bubonic* forms, so called from the swollen lymph nodes, known as *buboes,* which characterize it. In cold climates the disease is apt to take the pneumonic form, a much more fatal and contagious type.

Bubonic plague is not a disease of any of the domestic animals. It occurs naturally in rodents, especially in rats, in which it spreads rapidly at times. The disease in rats is quite similar to that in man and the mortality is about as great. The infection spreads from rat to rat, and from rat to man, through the agency of the rat flea (*Xenopsylla cheopis*). In recent times it has often been observed in plague centers that great human epidemics have been preceded by great rat epidemics.

In addition to rats, the disease also occurs naturally in marmots, ground squirrels, and other rodents. Unlike the rat, these creatures often live in areas sparsely inhabited by man. When plague spreads in such areas, it is known as the *sylvatic* form. In some of the wild animals that do not live in close association with man, plague has a much greater tendency to assume the more highly contagious pneumonic form than it does in the rat, and the disease contracted from them by man is also more likely to assume the pneumonic form.

Most cases of plague occur in the so-called plague centers of Asia (India, Burma, China, and Manchuria), but there are endemic foci in Africa, South and North America, and Hawaii. Western Europe has been practically free from the plague since the middle of the 18th century. It is believed that the first occurrence of this disease in the Western Hemisphere was a case in 1899 in Brazil. It appeared in San Francisco in 1900, probably brought in by oriental rats. A second epidemic was reported in San Francisco in 1907. In 1914 plague struck the Gulf states (Texas, Louisiana, and Florida), and in 1924 it broke out in Los Angeles.

About 1908 it was discovered that plague infection

existed in ground squirrels and other wild rodents in California. By 1960 it was known to be present in 17 of the western states as far east as North Dakota, Kansas, Oklahoma, and Texas. In this area, pockets of enzootic and epizootic plague have been found in 38 species of wild rodents. Of these, 11 rodent genera (including two of rabbits) are recognized to be of major importance in the ecology of sylvatic plague (4). During the years 1900–1951 there were 523 cases of plague in man and 340 deaths in the United States. These were found in 36 counties located in 12 states (8).

Morphology and Staining Reactions. The plague bacillus is a bipolar staining rod (0.5 by 1.5 μm) which resembles *Pasteurella multocida* (Figure 7.5). It may be readily stained with ordinary stains, and the bipolar appearance is easily demonstrated if diluted stains are used. The organism is Gram-negative, and capsules are not ordinarily developed. In media containing 3 percent salt solution great pleomorphism is exhibited, and this characteristic is used for diagnostic purposes.

Cultural Features. The growth on most media resembles that of the hemorrhagic septicemia organisms but is a little more luxuriant. Colonies on agar become a little larger, and they develop a little more rapidly. Gelatin is not liquefied; milk is slightly acidified but not coagulated. Indol is not formed. Acid but no gas is formed from glucose, levulose, maltose, galactose, and mannitol. Lactose, sucrose, dulcitol, raffinose, and inulin are not attacked.

There are three physiological types. Type I does not ferment glycerol but reduces nitrate, type II ferments glycerol and reduces nitrate, and type III ferments glycerol and does not reduce nitrate. Type I is responsible for sylvatic or wild-rodent plague in the western United States (1).

The organism grows best at temperatures somewhat below that of the body. It grows poorly when the temperature is below 20 C and above 38 C. It is nonhemolytic and forms a toxin that appears to be intermediate between endotoxin and exotoxin. It can be prepared in soluble form by phage lysis and differs from other endotoxins in that it is readily transformed into toxoid by formalin (1). The organism also produces a spreading factor and a coagulase (7).

According to Rockenmacher (9), catalase determinations can be used to distinguish between virulent and avirulent strains of *Y. pestis,* the former being able to decompose hydrogen peroxide more rapidly than the latter. Hudson *et al.* (5) claim that the FA technique is superior to animal inoculation in detecting *Y. pestis* in animal tissues.

Resistance. The plague organism does not exhibit any marked resistance to deleterious influence. Its life outside the animal body is precarious, and it seems to disappear speedily from soil, water, and buried cadavers. It can survive for months in the dried carcasses of small animals.

Pathogenicity for Experimental Animals. *Y. pestis* is pathogenic for rodents. The disease may be diagnosed by inoculating guinea pigs subcutaneously or, when specimens have undergone gross contamination and decomposition, by rubbing the material on the freshly shaved abdomen; the plague bacilli penetrate the minute abra-

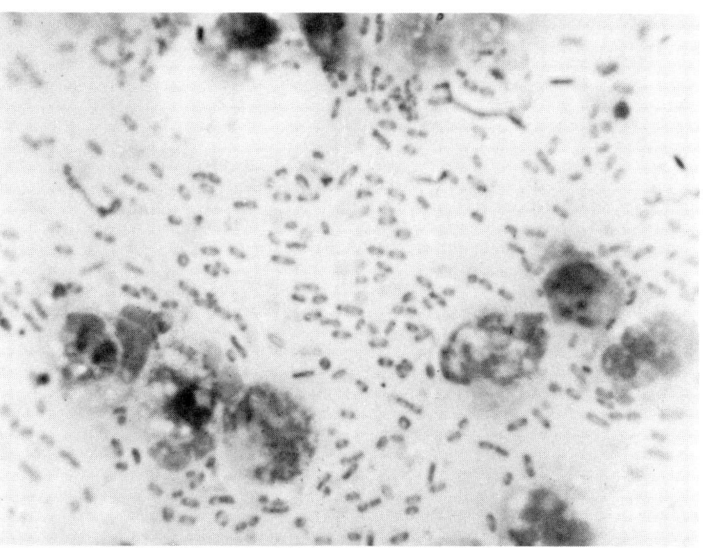

Figure 7.5. *Yersinia pestis* in a splenic smear. Note the bipolar staining rods. Gram stain. × 1,200.

sions while the contaminants do not. The animals die in 2 to 5 days; postmortem findings are characteristic and include subcutaneous and general congestion, congested spleen, granular liver, and pleural effusion. The bacilli may be found in spleen films and elsewhere, and cultured. For safety's sake it is important that the animal be freed of ectoparasites before inoculation.

According to Jawetz and Meyer (6), chick embryos of 12 to 14 days' incubation are highly susceptible to infection with virulent *Y. pestis* organisms, but newly hatched chicks are very resistant to plague infection, probably through the action of a cellular mechanism that is activated at hatching time. Hyperimmune plague antiserum of known protective value for mice is incapable of protecting chick embryos against an infective dose of *Y. pestis*. This is taken to indicate that a cellular defense mechanism must be present for antiserum to exert its protective action. In the absence of such a mechanism only the antitoxic, but not the anti-infectious, activity of antiserum becomes evident.

Immunity. Many vaccines have been used in preventing plague in man. The most widely used of these is Haffkine's vaccine, in which virulent cultures are grown for several weeks and then killed with heat and phenol. This vaccine contains the products of autolysis of the organism as well as intact bacilli. It has been used very successfully in India as a prophylactic procedure. During World War II the United States Army used formalin-killed, virulent plague bacilli with apparent success. The use of living avirulent strains has been investigated with encouraging results by Grasset (3) in South Africa.

Chemotherapy. Sulfadiazine and streptomycin appear to be effective in treating plague (2). It has also been shown that Aureomycin, Chloromycetin, and Terramycin are useful as therapeutic agents.

Control Measures. In dealing with plague, dependence is largely placed upon warfare on rats. Ratproofing of buildings, wharves, and ships has done much to keep the disease down and to prevent its spreading to parts of the world where it has not previously existed. Shipping from plague centers is subjected to cyanide fumigation before cargoes are discharged in plague-free areas in order to destroy the rats that may have found their way aboard.

REFERENCES

1. Burrows, William. Textbook of microbiology, 20th ed. W. B. Saunders, Philadelphia and London, 1973.
2. Frobisher, Martin, Ronald Hinsdill, Koby Crabtree, and Clyde Goodheart. Fundamentals of microbiology, 9th ed. W. B. Saunders, Philadelphia and London, 1974.
3. Grasset. Trans. Roy.Soc. Trop. Med. and Hyg., 1946, *40*, 275.
4. Hubbert, Goldenberg, Kartman, and Prince. Jour. Am. Vet. Med. Assoc., 1966, *149*, 1651.
5. Hudson, Quan, and Kartman. Jour. Hyg. (London), 1962, *60*, 443.
6. Jawetz and Meyer. Am. Jour. Path., 1944, *20*, 457.
7. Jawetz and Meyer. Jour. Immunol., 1944, *49*, 15.
8. Link. U.S. Public Health Service Monograph no. 26, 1954.
9. Rockenmacher. Proc. Soc. Exp. Biol. and Med., 1949, *71*, 99.

Yersinia pseudotuberculosis

SYNONYMS: *Bacterium pseudotuberculosis rodentium, Corynebacterium rodentium, Pasteurella pseudotuberculosis*

This organism is the cause of a plaguelike disease of guinea pigs, sometimes of rats, and occasionally of other rodents, which has been called *Pasteurella pseudotuberculosis*. The organism has little importance in animal pathology except in stocks of guinea pigs, although rare infections with it have been reported in cattle, sheep, goats, horses, pigs, foxes, mink, rabbits, chinchillas, birds, monkeys, and man. In 1940 it was found by Beaudette (1) in a blackbird, and in 1944 it was isolated by Rosenwald and Dickinson (12) from sick and dead turkeys. This organism resembles that of plague so closely, and the lesions in guinea pigs are so similar, that it is easy to confuse one with the other. In fact, an organism isolated from a rabbit in Alaska in 1965, and identified as *Y. pestis* was eventually established as a strain of *Y. pseudotuberculosis* (9).

Morphology and Staining Reactions. This organism varies from coccoid to bacillary forms 5 μm or more in length. They generally appear singly; occasionally they are in chains. Bipolar staining can sometimes be noted. This organism is somewhat larger than the hemorrhagic septicemia bacilli. It is Gram-negative, non-acid-fast, and not encapsulated.

Cultural Features. *Y. pseudotuberculosis* is motile at 18 to 26 C but not at body temperatures.

On plain agar good growth occurs without the addition of serum or other enrichment. Blood agar shows no evidence of hemolysis. The colonies are small, translucent, and granular. In old colonies the centers are raised and more opaque than the periphery, which frequently shows radial striations. The consistency is soft and butyrous.

Growth in broth is fairly good. There is moderate turbidity in 24 hours at 37 C, but later the growth sediments into a viscid mass. A surface ring usually appears. On potato there is a thin growth which is cream-colored at first, later becoming yellow, and then brown. Litmus milk slowly becomes alkaline. Indol is not formed. Acid but no gas is formed from glucose, maltose, mannitol, salicin, arabinose, xylose, rhamnose, and glycerol. Sucrose is sometimes fermented. Lactose, raffinose, dulcitol, and sorbitol are not attacked.

Based on O antigens, there are five somatic groups of organisms. The same H antigen is found in all strains with one exception. A common somatic antigen exists in Group II and the *Salmonella* Group B. Ransom (10) has indicated that the organism also shares two envelope and one somatic antigen with *Y. pestis*. According to Mair (5) the majority of strains prevalent in England and Europe belong in serologic type 1.

Pathogenicity. The disease is most often seen spontaneously in stocks of guinea pigs. The affected animals sicken, lose weight, develop diarrhea, and die in 3 to 4 weeks. In such animals the mesenteric lymph nodes are greatly swollen and caseous, and there may be nodular abscesses in the intestinal wall originating in follicles. Similar nodules usually stud the liver and spleen thickly. Outbreaks of pseudotuberculosis have been encountered in chinchilla colonies (4) and in mink, and the organism has been isolated from a bovine (6) and an ovine (17) fetus. In cattle it has also been associated with pneumonia as well as with abortion (3), and it has caused infection in cats, characterized by abdominal and urinary disturbances (7). It is a relatively common disease of captive birds and can cause outbreaks, although usually of sporadic occurrence (2). Oxytetracycline is effective in control of the disease.

According to Thal (15), there are toxic and atoxic strains of *Y. pseudotuberculosis,* the toxic ones producing an exotoxin that is thermolabile and transferable to a toxoid that stimulates the production of antitoxin. The existence of the toxin explains certain differences in the susceptibility of laboratory animals. Guinea pigs succumb easily to infection with virulent strains, but mice are more resistant. For white rats only toxic strains are pathogenic.

Mode of Transmission. Natural infection is supposed to occur through ingestion of the causative organism because primary localizations appear in the intestinal wall and the mesenteric lymph nodes.

Diagnosis. *Y. pseudotuberculosis* resembles *Y. pestis* in cultural characteristics and in the disease it produces in guinea pigs. However, it can be differentiated from the latter by its avidity for urea and ability to grow well on desoxycholate citrate agar, while *Y. pestis* fails to attack urea and grows poorly on desoxycholate citrate agar. Phage typing and inability to cross-immunize also identify the species.

Immunity. Thal (15) has found a live avirulent culture that is capable of producing a solid immunity in guinea pigs against virulent strains. Intranasal instillation has produced satisfactory results (16).

The Disease in Man. Although the disease is rare in man, *Y. pseudotuberculosis* can produce severe and fatal infections (8). The symptoms and anatomical changes simulate those caused by enteric fever, tularemia, and tuberculosis (11, 13). The organism is fairly resistant to penicillin and streptomycin, but is sensitive to sulfa drugs (14).

REFERENCES

1. Beaudette. Jour. Am. Vet. Med. Assoc., 1940, *97,* 151.
2. Harcourt-Brown. Vet. Rec., 1978, *102,* 315.
3. Langford. Can. Vet. Jour., 1969, *10,* 208.
4. Laughton, Till, and Noble. Vet. Rec., 1963, *75,* 835.
5. Mair. Jour. Path. and Bact., 1965, *90,* 275.
6. Mair and Harbourne. Vet. Rec., 1963, *75,* 559.
7. Mair, Harbourne, Greenwood, and White. Vet. Rec., 1967, *81,* 461.
8. Meyer. Personal communication, 1957.
9. Quan, Knapp, Goldenberg, Hudson, Lawton, Chen, and Kartman. Am. Jour. Trop. Med. and Hyg., 1965, *14,* 424.
10. Ransom. Proc. Soc. Exp. Biol. and Med., 1956, *93,* 551.
11. Reimann. Am. Jour. Hyg., 1932, *16,* 206.
12. Rosenwald and Dickinson. Am. Jour. Vet. Res., 1944, *5,* 246.
13. Schütze. A system of bacteriology in relation to medicine. Med. Res. Council (Brit.), 1929, *IV,* 474.
14. Snyder and Vogel. Northwest Med., 1943, *42,* 14.
15. Thal., E., Untersuchungen über *Pasteurella pseudotuberculosis* unter besonderer Berücksichtigung ihres immunologischen Verhaltens. Berlingska Boktryckeriet, Lund, 1954.
16. Thal, Hanko, and Knapp. Acta Vet. Scand., 1964, *5,* 179.
17. Watson and Hunter. Vet. Rec., 1960, *72,* 770.

8 The Genus *Hemophilus*

Organisms in this genus are Gram-negative, minute to medium-sized coccobacilli or bacilli which may show a tendency to filament formation and pleomorphism. They are strict parasites of mucous membranes, and, given the right conditions, pathogenic species can cause disease in a variety of organ systems.

Most *Hemophilus* species require the presence of two growth factors in blood: X (hemin) and V (diphosphopyridine nucleotide, or DPN). The X and V factors are released from erythrocytes during the heating required to produce chocolate agar. The V factor may also be supplied by staphylococci; thus, when strains of *Hemophilus* that need V factor are grown beside staphylococci on solid agars, they grow much more luxuriantly. Colonies that flourish next to the source of V factor exhibit the phenomenon known as *satellitism*. Colonies further away tend to be much smaller or may even fail to show on the medium.

The *Hemophilus* species of importance as animal pathogens are *H. equigenitalis, H. gallinarum, H. parahemolyticus* (*pleuropneumoniae*), *H. suis,* and *H. somnus* (*agni*). *H. equigenitalis* and *H. somnus* are not listed in the eighth edition of *Bergey's Manual,* but because they are important pathogens for which there is a substantial literature, they will be described in detail in this chapter.

Another species, *H. ovis,* was isolated once in 1925 by Mitchell (2) from an outbreak of bronchopneumonia in sheep in Canada, and possibly a second time, in 1956, from a ewe with mastitis (6). These organisms have since been lost.

H. hemoglobinophilus (canis) is found on canine genitalia and has been associated with neonatal mortality in puppies (1), though it does not often produce disease.

Hemophilus equigenitalis

This microaerophilic organism was first described in 1977 by Platt *et al.* (4), Ricketts *et al.* (5), and Timoney *et al.* (14) from outbreaks of a highly contagious venereal disease on stud farms in Britain and Ireland. Another report (3) published in the same year described a clinically similar disease that occurred in Ireland in 1976—an indication that the infection was present for some time before the causative agent was described. The disease was named *contagious equine metritis* (CEM). In addition to its occurrence in Britain and Ireland, CEM has been confirmed in Australia, Belgium, France, Germany, and the United States.

Morphology and Staining Reactions. The organism is a Gram-negative, short rod, frequently categorized as a coccobacillus, with filaments 5 to 6 μm occasionally observed. It may show bipolar staining.

Cultural Features. Growth on chocolate agar usually takes 2 to 5 days and incubation should be performed in 5 percent CO_2 at 37 C. Limited growth of some strains occurs aerobically. The organism is a facultative anaerobe and excellent growth occurs in an atmosphere of 90 percent H_2 and 10 percent CO_2. The colonies are raised pinpoints, shining, smooth, butyrous, and gray (Figure 8.1). After prolonged incubation they become

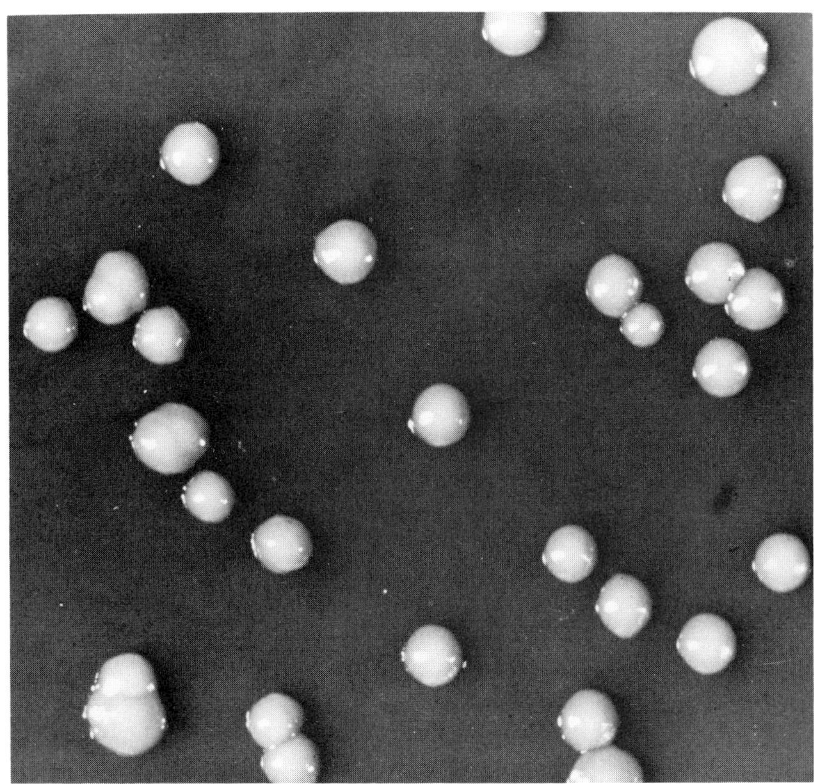

Figure 8.1. Colonies of *Hemophilus equigenitalis* on Eugon blood agar at 72 hours.

larger and more opaque. Good growth occurs in brain-heart infusion broth and in Robertson's cooked-meat medium.

H. equigenitalis is cytochrome oxidase-, catalase-, and phosphatase-positive but is otherwise unreactive biochemically. It is nonmotile with a DNA base composition of 36.1 percent GC (4). Strains exist that are sensitive or resistant to streptomycin.

The Natural Disease. Clinical symptoms associated with *H. equigenitalis* infection are seen only in the mare. The stallion is inapparently infected with the organism of CEM, which has a predilection for the folds and crevices in the mucous membrane surface of the penis and prepuce. No signs of any systemic disturbance have been observed in clinically affected mares.

The majority of mares involved in the outbreaks described in 1977 developed a profuse vulvar discharge with evidence of an endometritis, cervicitis, and/or vaginitis 2 to 12 days after being bred to an infected stallion. They returned to estrus after a shortened diestrous period. The discharge consists of a copious flow of thin grayish-white exudate, which pours out of the vulva, soils the hindquarters, and matts the tail hairs (Figure 8.2). Cases of inapparent *H. equigenitalis* infection have been reported in both barren and in-foal mares. Infection need not be incompatible with the maintenance of a nor-

Figure 8.2. Vulvar discharge from a mare affected with contagious equine metritis. (Courtesy Peter Timoney.)

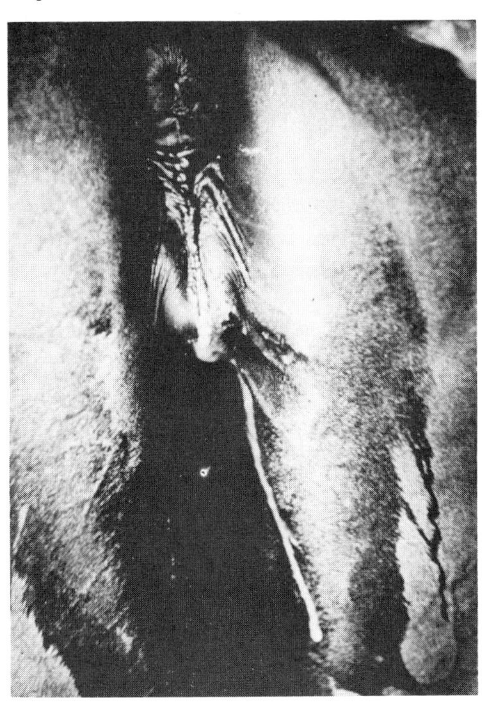

mal pregnancy and the birth of a healthy foal. The organism of CEM has been recovered from the placental membranes from known infected mares.

The disease is highly contagious and readily transmitted from mare to mare by an infected stallion, by contaminated instruments or materials, or by stud personnel.

Discharge from CEM-infected mares contains large numbers of neutrophils, some of which contain engested organisms. Untreated mares may continue to discharge for 10 to 11 days. The organism may be shed either constantly or intermittently for long periods after the discharge ceases and in many carrier mares is harbored in the clitoral sinuses (7). Shedding can be independent of the estrous cycle. *H. equigenitalis* can persist on the genitalia of infected stallions for extended periods of time.

Both local (13) and systemic antibodies are produced after infection and can be measured by the agglutination, antiglobulin, complement-fixation, and passive hemagglutination tests. These tests are unreliable for the detection of chronically infected mares, however, because many such animals do not have measurable antibody titers.

Mares that are reinfected during a subsequent breeding season exhibit a minimal clinical response, a lower carrier rate, and a lower antibody response than when infected for the first time (13). This suggests a local antibody effect which clears the infection before a systemic immune response can be stimulated.

Experimentally, *H. equigenitalis* has been transmitted to donkey mares (10) and to mice, rabbits, and guinea pigs (9). However, cattle, sheep, and pigs appear to be refractive to infection (12).

Diagnosis. Although the presence of large numbers of neutrophils in the characteristic profuse exudate, together with the presence of Gram-negative coccobacilli both intra- and extracellulary, is suggestive of CEM, isolation of *H. equigenitalis* is the only absolute means currently available of confirming CEM infection in either a mare or a stallion. Swabs from barren maiden or host-parturient mares should preferably be taken during estrus and should include a swab from the uterus or cervix and any discharge present and one from the clitoral fossa and sinus. The latter is the recommended sampling site in in-foal mares. The swabbing sites in the stallion comprise the urethral fossa, terminal urethra, and prepuce. All swabs should be transported to the laboratory in Amie's or Stuart's transport media and should be shipped frozen or refrigerated. Specimens should be plated out promptly on chocolate or Eugon agars in an atmosphere of 5 percent CO_2. Streptomycin (200 to 400 μg per ml) and fungizone (5 μg per ml) can be incorporated in the medium to suppress contaminants, but antibiotic-free medium should be inoculated at the same time because some strains of *H. equigenitalis* are streptomycin-sensitive. As the organism is very slow growing, plates should be examined daily for a week. Colonies usually are visible by the second or third day of incubation.

Of the serologic tests available, the complement-fixation test appears to be the most sensitive and specific in detection of carrier mares.

Chemotherapy and Control *H. equigenitalis* is sensitive to a wide range of antimicrobial agents including penicillin, ampicillin, neomycin, chloramphenicol, nitrofurazone, gentamicin, tetracycline, and chlorhexidine. Treated mares exhibit a rapid clinical response to therapy but may remain carriers of the organism. Local treatment of the external genitalia of CEM-infected stallions, on the other hand, has been very successful in clearing up the infection. The fertility of treated mares and stallions has not been found to be impaired following recovery from CEM.

Swerczek (8) has reported that surgical removal of the clitoral sinuses is effective in eliminating infection in certain carrier mares.

Artificial insemination using semen treated with antibiotics has also been shown to be a potentially useful method of control (11).

REFERENCES

1. Maclachlan and Hopkins. Vet. Rec., 1978, *103*, 409.
2. Mitchell. Jour. Am. Vet. Med. Assoc., 1925, *68*, 8.
3. O'Driscoll, Troy, and Geoghegan. Vet. Rec., 1977, *101*, 359.
4. Platt, Atherton, Simpson, Taylor, Rosenthal, Brown, and Wreghitt. Vet. Rec., 1977, *101*, 20.
5. Ricketts, Rossdale, Wingfield-Digby, Falk, Hopes, Hunt, and Peace. Vet. Rec., 1977, *101*, 65.
6. Roberts. Austral. Vet. Jour., 1956, *33*, 330.
7. Simpson and Eaton-Evans. Vet. Rec., 1978, *102*, 488.
8. Swerczek. Vet. Rec., 1979, *105*, 131.
9. Timoney, Geraghty, Dillon, and McArdle. Vet. Rec., 1978, *103*, 563.
10. Timoney, McArdle, O'Reilly, Ward, and Harrington. Vet. Rec., 1979, *104*, 84.
11. Timoney, O'Reilly, Harrington, McCormack, and McArdle. J. Reprod. Fert., Sup., 1979, *27*, 377.
12. Timoney, O'Reilly, McArdle, and Ward. Vet. Rec., 1978, *102*, 152.
13. Timoney, O'Reilly, McArdle, Ward, and Harrington. Vet. Rec., 1979, *104*, 264.
14. Timoney, Ward, and Kelly. Vet. Rec., 1977, *101*, 103.

Hemophilus gallinarum

SYNONYM: *Bacillus hemoglobinophilus coryzae gallinarum*

The name *H. gallinarum* was proposed in 1934 by Eliot and Lewis (15) for an organism that had been described first by De Blieck (12) in Holland under the name given above as a synonym. The latter is invalid because it is not a binomial. It is the cause of a serious and widespread disease of chickens known as *fowl coryza.* The organism is much like the influenza bacilli of man and swine in that it is frequently associated with virus infection.

Cultural Features. The organism is a facultative anaerobe that grows best on primary isolation when CO_2 is furnished. V factor, but not X factor, is required for growth. It is rather inactive biochemically. It does not produce indol or hydrogen sulfide. It does not change litmus or methylene blue milk or liquefy gelatin. It regularly ferments glucose and is irregular in fermenting mannose, galactose, levulose, maltose, sucrose, and dextrin (6). One percent sodium chloride is required in medium for growth.

In culturing *H. gallinarum,* Bornstein and Samberg (6) recommended the use of blood agar, incubated under increased CO_2 tension, or 7-day-old chicken embryos. The latter are inoculated in the yolk sac, and mortality results in 24 to 48 hours. The dead embryos are congested and present a heavy growth of the organism in both the yolk and the allantoic fluid. Here the organisms remain viable for 6 weeks under 5 C refrigeration as compared to 2 weeks in the case of blood agar. For isolation Bornstein and Samberg take material from facial swellings of cases of infectious coryza. The edematous area is swabbed with alcohol, the skin is pierced, and the fluid content is removed by pipette and streaked on blood agar.

Pathogenicity. The lesions produced in fowl by *H. gallinarum* are acute inflammation of the turbinates and sinus epithelium, disruption of the trachea without cellular infiltration, and acute air sacculitis characterized by swelling and heterophilic response (1). The exudate of natural cases of fowl coryza is highly infectious when introduced into the palatine cleft of susceptible birds. Filtrates of this material are not infectious except when coarse Berkefeld candles are used for the filtration and the filtrates are incubated for a time in the presence of fresh chicken blood. Pure cultures will reproduce the disease, and such cultures will retain their virulence for chickens after many generations in artificial media. Rabbits and guinea pigs are resistant to injections of pure cultures. Turkeys, pigeons, and many other species of birds are also refractory.

Raggi *et al.* (30) found that concurrent deposition of infectious bronchitis virus and *H. gallinarum* into the nostrils of 6-week-old White Leghorns produces a shorter incubation period, higher mortality, and severe macro- and microscopic lesions than can be instituted in birds inoculated singly with similar amounts of either one of these agents.

Concurrent infections by Newcastle disease or infectious laryngotracheitis viruses and by *Mycoplasma gallisepticum* also predispose to clinical infections by *H. gallinarum*.

Immunity. Hemagglutination-inhibiting (HI), agglutinating, and precipitating antibodies are formed in the sera of infected chickens, but the levels of these antibodies do not appear to affect the duration and severity of symptoms in experimentally infected chickens (19).

At least three immunotypes of *H. gallinarum* exist (33), and vaccinal immunity is immunotype-specific. However, birds which recover from infection by one immunotype are refractory to reinfection by a heterologous immunotype (32).

According to Page *et al.* (29), bacterins consisting of formalin-inactivated yolk-propagated cultures stimulate a high degree of immunity to the development of air-sac lesions and a limited but significant resistance to upper-respiratory-tract disease. There is evidence that recovered birds remain carriers of virulent bacilli, and it is in this manner that the disease appears to be propagated from year to year.

Hemophilus parahemolyticus (pleuropneumoniae)

This organism is the cause of *contagious pleuropneumonia* in swine, a disease of considerable economic importance in most swine-raising areas of the world. It causes disease by itself and does not require a concurrent virus infection, although a concurrent adenovirus infection has been observed in outbreaks in Saskatchewan (34).

Morphologic and Cultural Features. The organism forms stout rods or tangled filaments. It grows well on chocolate or blood agars and is V factor–dependent, and the majority of strains are beta-hemolytic on calf blood. Urease is produced, and xylose, ribose, glucose, fructose, mannose, sucrose, maltose, and mannitol are fermented. On the basis of the marked difference between the biochemical reactivity of strains of *H. parahemolyticus* of porcine and human origin, Kilian *et al.* (21) have proposed that porcine strains represent a different species which they have named *H. pleuropneumoniae*.

The Natural Disease. The organism may be carried in the tonsils and nasopharynx of normal swine. Disease is most common in winter. In chronically infected herds, piglets are usually affected during the later part of the suckling period, when colostral antibody has waned. The clinical symptoms are often vague and the lesions mild in such animals (23). Affected animals may not be detected until slaughter. In susceptible swine, the disease may have an acute form characterized by anorexia, emesis, fever, and hemorrhaging from the nose and mouth (34).

The lesions consist of an exudative and proliferative desquamative bronchopneumonia with fibrinous pleuritis. In more chronic cases there is a tendency for sequestration of the lesions. The lesions in the peracute form, and in the initial stages of less acute forms, include alveolar and interlobular edema with dilatation of lymph vessels, congestion, hemorrhage, and intravascular fibrinous thrombosis (18). These lesions appear to be a direct effect of the hemophilus endotoxin. A nodular form of chronic pneumonia due to *H. parahemoliticus* has also been described (8).

The antibody response in recovered carrier animals can be detected by either the complement-fixation or the agglutination test, the former being more sensitive and more reliable for the detection of infection (2).

Nielsen *et al.* (26) have used the complement-fixation test to control the disease in progeny testing stations. It was of value provided it was carried out within a week of the arrival of the pigs at the stations.

Strains of *H. parahemoliticus* from different regions are closely related antigenically. There are six serotypes based on the identification of heat-stable and heat-labile antigens (16).

Vaccination trials with bacterins have given good results (25, 38).

Hemophilus suis and *Hemophilus parasuis*

SYNONYM: *Hemophilus influenzae* var. *suis*

H. suis was first described by Lewis and Shope (22) in 1931. In subsequent studies Shope (35) clearly demonstrated that, whereas *H. suis* was relatively harmless to pigs when inoculated alone, it became highly pathogenic for susceptible swine when inoculated with influenza virus. The virus alone is also relatively harmless. Swine influenza is a disease produced only by the concerted action of the bacillus and the virus.

In 1969, Biberstein and White (4) described an organism isolated from swine that was identical to *H. suis* in all respects except that it was not X factor–dependent and produced porphyrin from D-aminolevulinic acid. This organism is ranked as a separate species in the eighth edition of *Bergey's Manual*. Because there appears to be a considerable overlap and an unclear distinction between the diseases produced by *H. suis* and *H. parasuis* and since many of the earlier isolations of *H. suis* in culture collections have proved to be V factor–dependent only, we have decided to discuss the two species together.

Morphology and Staining Reactions. *H. suis* and *H. parasuis* are Gram-negative coccobacilli with a tendency to filament formation in old cultures.

Cultural Features. Both *H. suis* and *H. parasuis* are V factor–dependent. *H. parasuis,* unlike *H. suis,* does not have a requirement for X factor. Both are urease-negative and produce small amounts of acid from maltose and sucrose. Serum is required for growth.

Epidemiology and Pathogenesis. Both *H. suis* and *H. parasuis* appear to be carried in the nasopharynx of many normal swine. Invasion by the virus of swine influenza, which usually begins to circulate actively in susceptible pig populations in the autumn, when temperatures may fall suddenly, predisposes swine to invasion by *H. suis*. Influenzalike symptoms result, with coughing, fever, inappetence, and, in severe cases, lobular pneumonia and death of the animal. The disease is highly contagious and spreads rapidly.

Both *H. suis* and *H. parasuis* have also been associated with a polyserositis syndrome in swine (*Glasser's disease*) in which there is fibrinous inflammation of the serous surfaces. Lesions are seen in the pericardium, pleura, peritoneum, joints, and, in severe cases, the meninges. There is no virus involvement in Glasser's disease, but stresses such as weaning and transportation are known to be predisposing factors.

Affected pigs may have swollen joints, lameness, symptoms of bronchitis and pleuritis, fever, and, occasionally, meningitis. The disease is fatal in a small proportion of affected animals.

Riley *et al.* (31) have described a fatal septicemia in swine that developed a few days after transportation and was shown to be caused by *H. parasuis*.

Immunity. There are three serotypes of *H. suis* based on the capsular polysaccharides. Nielsen and Danielsen (24) have protected swine against Glasser's disease with an autogenous bacterin prepared from a strain of *H. parasuis* isolated on the farm where the vaccine was used. Complement-fixing antibodies were formed in vaccinated pigs but not in unvaccinated littermates. Baehler *et al.* (3) have also reported success with a *H. parasuis* bacterin.

Diagnosis. *H. suis* and *H. parasuis* are usually isolated easily from lesions in acute cases by streaking material on chocolate agar and then inoculating a *Staphylococcus* sp. across the center of the plate as a source of V factor.

The three species of *Hemophilus* that may be isolated from respiratory and other lesions in swine may be differentiated as shown in Table 8.1.

Hemophilus somnus (agni)

H. somnus is the cause of infectious meningoencephalitis in cattle, a disease which was first reported in feedlot cattle in California in 1960 (20). Since then, the disease has been reported throughout the United States, Canada, and parts of Europe. Infections of the bovine genital tract and abortion caused by *H. somnus* have also been reported (9, 14, 37).

Morphologic Features. *H. somnus* is a very small, Gram-negative, nonmotile coccobacillus.

Cultural and Biochemical Features. The organism on primary isolation is CO_2-dependent and although not responsive to X and V factors, it has a strict requirement for unknown factors in blood and yeast. It also exhibits satellitism when grown near a suitable feeder bacterium. Colonies on blood or chocolate agar are minute and nonhemolytic. The organism is oxidase-positive.

The Natural Disease. *H. somnus* is known to colonize the respiratory tract of calves after natural exposure and subsequently to be transmitted horizontally to other animals (11). In feedlot cattle the disease is usually seen 1 to 2 weeks after shipping (28) during periods of wet weather. Lateral spread of infection among feedlot cattle is uncommon (28). The season of the year or antibiotic administration does not influence the occurrence of the disease (10). Infection is believed to occur via the respiratory route.

Affected animals exhibit weakness, fever, staggering, stiffness, knuckling of the fetlocks, dyspnea, somnolence—hence the name *H. somnus*—erratic behavior, paralysis, and sudden death. The mortality among affected animals may be very high (13).

The lesions consist of a fibrinous meningitis with arterial thrombosis and necrosis. Hemorrhages on serous surfaces and in muscles are widespread. The lymph nodes are enlarged, dark, and edematous, and the brain contains hemorrhagic areas (Figure 8.3) that may be a few centimeters in diameter. A suppurative polyarthritis may also be present.

Fibrin thrombi occur in the vessels of the brain and meninges, and there are multifocal areas of necrosis and infiltrations of polymorphonuclear cells (36).

Immunity. Exposed but unaffected animals become seropositive (20). Immunizing antigens occur in the protein, whole cell, and sonicate but not in the crude polysaccharide fractions of the organisms (27).

Bacterins have been shown to promote a protective immunity (17, 39) in calves.

Chemotherapy of Hemophilus Infections. Most *Hemophilus* sp. are sensitive to the tetracyclines, streptomycin, penicillin, ampicillin, erythromycin, and chloramphenicol. Sulfachloropyridazine, by itself or in combination with dihydrostreptomycin, and sulfadimidine have been shown to prevent spread of coryza in chickens but were not effective in eliminating infection from all birds (7). Bornstein and Samberg (6) found that streptomycin was very

Table 8.1. Characteristics of *Hemophilus* sp. from swine (5)

Characteristic	*H. parahemolyticus* (*pleuropneumoniae*)	*H. parasuis*	*H. suis*
V factor-dependent	+	+	+
X factor-dependent	−	−	+
Urease	+	−	−
Porphyrin (from D-aminolevulinic acid)	+	+	−
Serum required	−	+	+

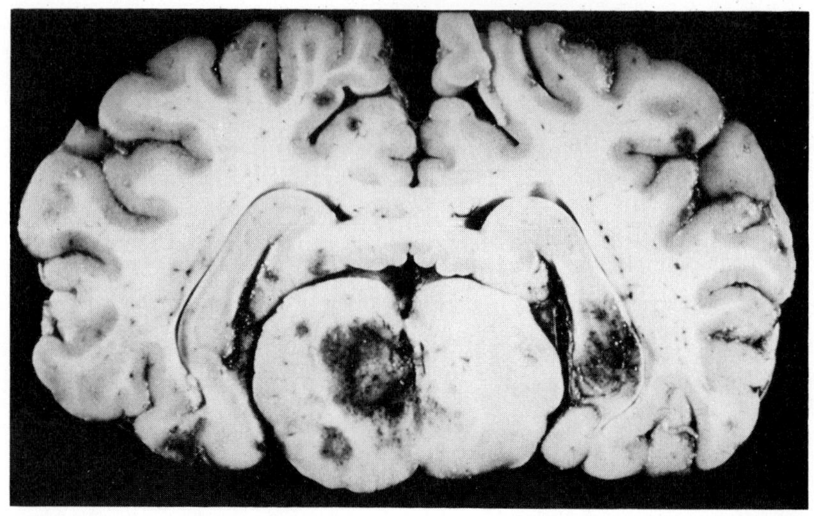

Figure 8.3. Hemorrhagic areas in the brain of a steer with infectious meningoencephalitis caused by *Hemophilus somnus*. (Courtesy Joseph Kowalski.)

effective in treating adult chickens but less so for young birds.

REFERENCES

1. Adler and Page. Avian Dis., 1962, *6,* 1.
2. Bachman. Schweiz. Arch. f. Tierheilk., 1972, *114,* 362.
3. Baehler, Burgisser, Meuron, and Nicolet. Schweiz. Arch. f. Tierheilk., 1974, *116,* 183.
4. Biberstein and White. Jour. Med. Microbiol., 1969, *2,* 75.
5. Biberstein, Gunnarsson, and Hornell. Am. Jour. Vet. Res., 1977, *38,* 7.
6. Bornstein and Samberg. Am. Jour. Vet. Res., 1954, *15,* 612.
7. Buys. Jour. S. Afr. Vet. Med. Assoc., 1972, *43,* 383.
8. Chan, Yamamoto, Konishi, and Ogata. Jap. Jour. Vet. Sci., 1978, *40,* 103.
9. Chladek. Am. Jour. Vet. Res., 1975, *36,* 1041.
10. Corstevet, Panciero, Rinker, Starks, and Howard. Jour. Am. Vet. Med. Assoc., 1973, *163,* 170.
11. Crandell, Smith, and Kissel. Am. Jour. Vet. Res., 1977, *38,* 1749.
12. De Blieck. Tijdsch. v. Diergeneesk., 1931, *58,* 310.
13. Dirksen, Kaiser, and Schels. Prakt. Tierärztl., 1978, *59,* 766.
14. Dreumel and Kierstead. Can. Vet. Jour., 1975, *16,* 367.
15. Eliot and Lewis. Jour. Am. Vet. Med. Assoc., 1934, *84,* 787.
16. Gunnarsson, Harnell, and Biberstein. Am. Jour. Vet. Res., 1978, *39,* 1286.
17. Hall and Williams Smith. Vet. Med./Small Animal Clin., 1977, *72,* 1368.
18. Hani, Konig, Nicolet, and Scholl. Schweiz. Arch., f. Tierheilk., 1973, *115,* 19.
19. Intani, Sugimon, and Katagiri. Avian Dis., 1977, *21,* 1.
20. Kennedy, Biberstein, Howarth, Frazier, and Dungworth. Am. Jour. Vet. Res., 1960, *21,* 403.
21. Kilian, Nicolet, and Biberstein. Int. Jour. Syst. Bact., 1978, *28,* 20.
22. Lewis and Shope. Jour. Exp. Med., 1931, *54,* 361.
23. Nielsen. Nord. Vet., 1975, *27,* 319.
24. Nielsen and Danielsen. Nord. Vet. Med., 1975, *27,* 20.
25. Nielsen. Nord. Vet. Med., 1976, *28,* 337.
26. Nielsen, Thomsen, and Vesterlund. Nord. Vet. Med., 1976, *28,* 349.
27. Noyer, Ward, Saunders, and MacWilliams. Can. Vet. Jour., 1977, *18,* 159.
28. Olander, Gallina, Beckwith, and Morrow. Proc. Ann. Meeting U.S. Animal Health Assoc., 1970, *74,* 589.
29. Page, Rosenwald, and Price. Avian Dis., 1963, *7,* 239.
30. Raggi, Young, and Sharma. Avian Dis., 1967, *11,* 308.
31. Riley, Russell, and Callinan. Jour. Am. Vet. Med. Assoc., 1977, *171,* 649.
32. Rimler, Davis, and Page. Am. Jour. Vet. Res., 1977, *38,* 1591.
33. Rimler, Davis, and Page. Am. Jour. Vet. Res., 1977, *38,* 1587.
34. Schiefer, Moffat, Greenfield, Agar, and Majka. Can. Jour. Comp. Med., 1974, *38,* 99.
35. Schope. Jour. Exp. Med., 1931, *54,* 349 and 373.
36. Smith and Biberstein. Cornell Vet., 1977, *67,* 300.
37. Waldham, Hall, Meinershagen, Cord, and Frank. Am. Jour. Vet. Res., 1974, *35,* 1401.
38. Weng, Hsu, and Liu. Jour. Chinese Soc. Vet. Sci., 1976, *28,* 337.
39. Williams, Smith, and Murdock. Am. Jour. Vet. Res., 1978, *39,* 1756.

9 The Genus *Pasteurella*

This genus is a heterogeneous group of usually bipolar bacteria that cause disease in a variety of animals. *Pasteurella multocida* is generally regarded as the type species although the name embraces a range of biotypes and serotypes. The eighth edition of *Bergey's Manual* lists *P. multocida, P. hemolytica, P. pneumotropica,* and *P. ureae* as official species. *P. anatipestifer,* a cause of septicemia in ducks and other fowls, is listed as species *incertae sedis*. In this chapter we will regard it as a species of *Pasteurella*.

Pasteurella multocida

In 1880, Pasteur (55) described the organism that causes cholera in fowls. Later it was learned that the fowl cholera bacillus could not be differentiated culturally from the organisms of rabbit septicemia, of swine plague, and of certain pneumonias of cattle. The apparent identity of these organisms and the similarity of the diseases produced by them in the various animal species led Hueppe (38) in 1886 to group them under one name, *Bacterium septicemiae hemorrhagicae*. Trevisan (66), the following year, proposed that the several disease-producing agents be recognized as separate species but that they be grouped in a single genus, *Pasteurella,* named in honor of Pasteur. Lignières (44) in 1901 applied the name *pasteurelloses* to the group of diseases caused by these organisms, a name that has come into rather common use.

Although it had been recognized that the cultural and biochemical features of the *Pasteurella* organisms isolated from birds, cattle, swine, sheep, rabbits, reindeer, American bison, and other wild animals were essentially identical, Flügge's (21) classification, established in 1886, was followed for years. According to his system, *P. aviseptica* caused fowl cholera, *P. suiseptica* caused swine plague, *P. lepiseptica* caused snuffles and pneumonia in rabbits, *P. boviseptica* caused pneumonia and sometimes septicemia of cattle, and *P. oviseptica* caused pneumonia in sheep.

Because these organisms cannot be differentiated from each other on any basis now known, including serological tests, Rosenbusch and Merchant (61) proposed, as Hueppe had many years before, that the hemorrhagic septicemia organisms of the various animals be recognized as a single species. Because Kitt (43) was the first to make the suggestion, they urged that the name of the species be *P. multocida,* derived by eliminating the middle name of the trinomial *Bacterium bipolare multocidum* which Kitt proposed. This has been adopted here.

Many years ago Moore (47) found members of the hemorrhagic septicemia group present on the mucous membranes of the respiratory tract of apparently normal cattle, sheep, swine, dogs, and cats. These observations were confirmed by Jorgensen (42) in cattle. One of the strains isolated by Jorgensen was tested on a cow after it was found to be of unusual virulence for rabbits. It proved to be highly virulent for the animal, destroying it with typical pasteurella pneumonia in 3 days following spraying of the culture into the nostrils. A majority of the strains isolated from mucous membranes of cattle were nonpathogenic, but this is not surprising because the majority of the strains derived from acute infections of cattle show little virulence for rabbits and other experimental animals.

Morphology and Staining Reactions. *P. multocida* is a very small ovoid rod about 0.3 μm wide by 0.4 to 0.5 μm long. When seen in carefully stained films from tissue, the ends of the rod are more deeply stained than the central portion, giving it a distinct bipolar appearance. This characteristic is not so marked in bacilli from cultures, and in any case it may be easily obscured by overstaining. Wright's or Giemsa's stain is recommended for demonstrating it, although careful staining with methylene blue usually is satisfactory. In the fresh material, unstained, the bipolar appearance usually can be seen. Pasteur referred to the fowl cholera bacillus as his "figure-of-eight bacillus."

The pasteurellas are Gram-negative and nonsporeforming. Many strains form a capsular substance when freshly isolated, but usually this property is quickly lost.

Cultural Features. Organisms of this group are easily cultivated on ordinary infusion agar, although growth is never luxuriant. Media made from meat extract is not suitable unless enriched with a little blood or serum.

In infusion broth, growth is manifested by slight clouding and a viscid sediment. Growth in broth is greatly increased by the addition of a few drops of sterile serum. Excellent growth is obtained on blood agar plates. The blood is not altered except that some strains may exhibit a slight greenish haze around the deep colonies. Gelatin is not liquefied. Milk supports growth but is only slightly changed; the litmus usually turns from a blue to a violet color. Indol is produced. Glucose, mannitol, and sucrose are fermented with acid, but no gas is produced. Lactose, maltose, and salicin are not attacked by most strains. Usually they are not soluble in ox bile; a few are easily dissolved. Nitrates are reduced to nitrites. Most strains produce indol, hydrogen sulfide, catalase, oxidase, and ornithine decarboxylase.

Biotypes. Frederiksen (22, 23) has proposed seven biotypes of *P. multocida,* based on fermentation of arabinose, xylose, maltose, trehalose, sorbitol, and mannitol. Strains from dogs constitute a biotype that is distinct from the other 6 and is characterized by failure to attack sorbitol and mannitol. Carter (15) has proposed another scheme of biotyping based on tests for hyaluronidase decapsulation, acriflavin flocculation, colonial iridescence, carbohydrate fermentation, mouse pathogenicity, and serum protection. Carter's proposed biotypes are: 1, mucoid; 2, hemorrhagic septicemic; 3, porcine; 4, canine; and 5, feline.

Other workers (24) have found that strains from dogs usually ferment maltose but not mannitol, whereas porcine strains give the opposite reactions.

Serologic Classification. On agar, colonies of *P. multocida* present dissociation patterns showing, for practical purposes, three principal colonial variants: (*a*) mucoid colonies that are large, flowing, of moderate virulence for mice, and not typable by the usual serologic methods; (*b*) smooth or fluorescent colonies that are medium-sized and discrete (they are quite virulent for mice and typable); and (*c*) rough or blue colonies that are small and discrete, low in virulence for mice, and autoagglutinable.

The mucoid colonies as well as the smooth types contain capsular material, but serologic typing depends on the presence of type-specific soluble antigen associated with the capsules of the smooth or fluorescent forms. By using these forms, Roberts (59), Carter (10), and others have established four serologic types, which Roberts labeled I, II, III, and IV and Carter B, A, C, and D, respectively. In so doing they used precipitation, capsular swelling, and hemagglutination tests. Carter recommends the hemagglutination test for identification of the serotypes. He employs human erythrocytes that have been exposed to extracts of smooth *Pasteurella* and tests them with known antisera. The use of hyaluronidase and extraction of the capsular antigens with normal saline has greatly simplified the identification of these antigens (14).

In addition to Carter types A, B, C, and D, another serotype, E, was found in cases of hemorrhagic septicemia in cattle in central Africa (12) in the early 1960s. Carter type C was also abandoned about this time because it proved unnecessary (13).

According to Carter (10, 11), types A and B predominate in cattle. Type A strains are most frequently associated with pneumonia. Type B strains are usually recovered from animals with epizootic hemorrhagic septicemia. Type A strains predominate as the cause of fowl cholera. Types A and D are most common in swine. Type D infections appear to be generally sporadic and have a wide host range, but most strains isolated from atrophic rhinitis of swine are either type D or mucoid.

P. multocida has also been shown to contain somatic and O antigens (51) of which at least 12 have been described. Numbers (arabic) are used to denote the different O antigens. The antigenic formula of each *P. mul-*

tocida serotype is written as a number (for the O antigen) and a letter (for the capsular antigen). Some of the more common serotypes causing disease in animals are shown in Table 9.1.

Resistance. Cultures of *Pasteurella* sp. die out quickly and transfers must be made at least twice each month. The organism is also readily killed by chemical and physical disinfectants.

Epidemiology and Pathogenesis. Strains of *P. multocida* are normally carried as commensals in the oropharynx of many animal species and cause disease only when certain predisposing factors allow them to multiply uncontrolledly and penetrate the physical and immunologic defenses of the respiratory tract. During this phase more virulent clones are apparently selected for and are propagated and later released to infect other host animals of the same species. These clones, however, are not usually virulent for other host species.

Important predisposing conditions in the several animal pasteurelloses include: fowl cholera—poor sanitation, poor ventilation, and overcrowding; pneumonia and shipping fever of cattle and sheep—exposure to cold, wet weather, transportation for long distances, crowding, exhaustion, and intercurrent infection with parainfluenza-3 virus; swine plague—other diseases such as swine influenza, malnutrition, and poor housing conditions.

In cattle there is a marked tendency toward a seasonal incidence of pasteurellosis that corresponds with the activity of certain respiratory virus and *Mycoplasma* infections. In the United States, this occurs in fall and early winter and is especially notable in large feedlot operations where many young susceptible cattle are regrouped together in early fall. In these populations respiratory viruses and mycoplasmas circulate rapidly and pave the way for secondary invasions by pasteurellas.

It is likely that primary infections by viruses and mycoplasmas predispose to secondary invasions by pasteurellas by impairing alveolar macrophage function, and by damaging the mucociliary mechanism in the trachea and bronchi. The local inflammatory effect they cause leads to increased fluidity of the mucus blanket with consequent sneezing and coughing, and, inevitably, formation of endogenous aerosols in the respiratory tree which can result in downward carriage of bacteria from the upper parts of the tract during inspiration.

Hemorrhagic septicemia of cattle, goats, and sheep usually takes the pectoral or pneumonic form. The affected animals suffer from very high temperature (106 to 108 F or higher), dysentery, edema, and, in advanced cases, cyanosis of the mucous membranes. They breathe with great difficulty in the later stages of the infection, and the death rate is high. The disease occurs in tropical areas of the world. Shipping fever occurs in cattle, sheep, and pigs after transportation in temperate zones and is characterized also by fever and bronchopneumonia.

The lesions in hemorrhagic septicemia include hemorrhages on serous surfaces, blood-stained fluid in the thorax and abdomen, enteritis, and edema in the subcutaneous tissues. Edema is characteristic of the less acute forms of the disease. Also, in subacute forms, lesions may be confined to the pectoral region and include fluid in the pleural and pericardial sacs. Areas of pneumonia are present in the lungs, together with greatly thickened septa.

Shipping fever in cattle caused by *P. multocida* is a bronchopneumonia with moderate amounts of fibrin on the lung surface. This is somewhat in contrast to the pneumonia produced by *P. hemolytica,* where amounts of fibrin are much greater and the lesions represent a true fibinous pleuropneumonia (63).

Swine plague usually consists of a fibrinous pneumonia accompanied in some cases by septicemia. Peracute cases have been described but they rarely occur.

The pneumonias that accompany low-grade cholera (swine fever) virus infections, or cholera infections in partially immunized animals, are frequently of this type. The lungs present a characteristic appearance, similar to those seen in this disease in rabbits and cattle. The anterior lobes are most often involved and frequently the

Table 9.1. Common serotypes of *P. multocida* in animals

Host	Disease	Serotypes encountered
Cattle	Hemorrhagic septicemia	6:B, 6:E
Chickens	Fowl cholera	5:A, 8:A
Turkeys	Fowl cholera	9:A
Pigs	Pneumonia	1:A, 3:A, 5:A, 1:D, 4:D, 10:D
Sheep	Pneumonia	1:D, 4:D

anterior portions of the diaphragmatic lobes as well. The lungs are firm and liverlike in consistency. The surface is covered with a serofibrinous exudate, and a turbid fluid containing flakes of fibrin is found in the thoracic cavity. The cut surface of the involved lung is firm and mottled in color, some lobules being dark red and others grayish. The lobules often are widely separated by the interlobular connective tissue which is distended by serofibrinous fluid.

Sautter *et al.* (62) reported a case of pasteurellosis in a sow in which the lungs were not involved. The outstanding gross lesions were vegetative endocarditis and evidence of bacteremia.

P. multocida type D may also be involved in the etiology of atrophic rhinitis in swine in synergism with *Bordetella bronchiseptica* (30) (see Chapter 10).

Fowl cholera, the pasteurellosis of birds, affects chickens principally, although ducks, geese, turkeys, swans, and other birds are susceptible. Wild birds frequently become infected and may, at times, be the source of infection for domestic flocks. In many cases the disease is peracute and manifested by an overwhelming bacteremia. Films of the blood or spleen pulp will then show large numbers of the minute, bipolar-staining organisms. Outbreaks generally begin in a few birds in apparently healthy flocks. The daily mortality in a flock usually rises sharply, the peak being reached as a rule within a few days (1). The fatalities vary from 10 to 75 percent.

The affected birds generally exhibit signs of depression, sleepiness, inappetence, and diarrhea. Death may occur within a few hours, or after 2 or 3 days. In some birds the course is much longer. Hendrickson and Hilbert (34) were able to cultivate the *Pasteurella* organism from the blood of chronically affected chickens, daily, for days and weeks. In one case this lasted as long as 49 days.

It has been suggested that the eye and skin abrasions are portals of entry for *P. multocida* in chickens (7).

The fowl cholera organism is frequently associated with chronic infections of the air sacs accompanied by accumulations of dry caseous material, with inflammatory processes in the wattles, especially of male birds, which frequently lead to necrosis, and with infections of the mucous membranes of the head, a condition commonly called *colds*. Also it is frequently found in the peritoneal cavity of young laying birds mixed with yolked material from ruptured ova. Whether the organism has anything to do with the rupture of the yolks, or is a secondary invader, is not known.

On the duck ranches of Long Island, cholera may take a heavy toll of the ducklings, which are raised in large numbers in very crowded, insanitary quarters. The necropsy findings usually consist of a few petechiae of the heart, a slightly swollen spleen, and perhaps a little reddening of the mucosa of the anterior part of the intestine.

Rabbit septicemia may be very acute, with hardly any premonitory signs. The causative organism can easily be found in films of the blood or spleen pulp after death. A more common form of the disease is less acute, the affected animals being clearly ill for some days during which they have fever, a nasal discharge of a seropurulent nature, inappetence, and finally difficult breathing. These animals suffer from a fibrinous pneumonia, the greater part of the lungs often being hepatized and the pleura covered with a fibrinous deposit. If such animals do not die within a few days, they become emaciated and usually are worthless afterward. *Snuffles* is the common name applied to a milder respiratory infection caused by this organism. This initially involves only the upper respiratory tract. Affected animals exhibit a mucopurulent exudate, which partially occludes the nares and frequently also the conjunctiva. The animals have difficulty in breathing. The noises made by a colony of affected animals are characteristic and are responsible for the common name of the disease. Some cases end in fibrinous pneumonia and death.

The lesions are minimal in peracute cases and generally are limited to a few petechiae on the heart and some of the serous membranes. In chronic cases the lesions are limited, as a rule, to the organs of the thorax.

In addition to the syndromes described above, *P. multocida* also causes a severe form of mastitis in ewes known as *bluebag* (68), which may occur sporadically or enzootically. Death may be a sequel to infection, and surviving ewes usually lose udder function.

Mastitis caused by this organism has also been reported in cattle (3, 67). The organism has caused purulent leptomeningitis in a dog. The condition was accompanied by signs of depression, anorexia, vomition, incoordination, and marked muscular twitching of the head and neck (60). *Pasteurella* sp. have been found in three horses, a pony, and a donkey in which death appeared to result from a *Pasteurella* septicemia (56).

Finally, it is not uncommon to find pure, or nearly pure, cultures of *Pasteurella multocida* in respiratory infections of calves. In some, the infection involves the upper part of the tract. The animals exhibit fever, inappetence, depression, and a mucopurulent nasal exudate. The mortality from this disease may not be very great. Frequently, however, in outbreaks of this disease in groups of calves, some develop pneumonia of the shipping fever type. They usually die.

Pasteurella hemolytica

Jones (40) in 1921 studied the organisms isolated from an outbreak of hemorrhagic septicemia in a large herd of cattle and found one that hemolyzed horse- and cow-blood cells. In other respects it was similar to *P. multocida,* but the possession of this distinguishing feature led to the name *P. hemolytica*. The organism does not produce indol. In addition to the sugars fermented by *P. multocida,* lactose and maltose are fermented by *P. hemolytica*.

Serologic Classification. Both somatic and capsular antigens are described (5, 6). The somatic antigen occurs in most strains of the species, while the capsular antigen is more strain-specific and more useful in classification. There are twelve known serotypes, designated 1–12.

Biotypes. Two biotypes, A and T, have been described (64). Biotype A ferments arabinose within 7 days and biotype T ferments trehalose within 2 days. The former is also more sensitive to penicillin.

Strains of *P. hemolytica* are usually designated by biotype and serotype, e.g., A 1.

Epidemiology and Pathogenesis. *P. hemolytica* is a common commensal of the nasopharynx of cattle, sheep, and goats. All twelve serotypes have been isolated from sheep, whereas in cattle serotypes 1 and 2 dominate in some regions (65, 71).

The same circumstances that predispose to disease-producing invasions by *P. multocida* are also important in disease production by *P. hemolytica*.

The number of calves carrying the organism increases greatly during outbreaks of shipping fever (36) and immediately after transportation (65). A single serotype may predominate for long periods in some herds (71), but two or more serotypes may occur in the same group of calves.

Variations in virulence occur among the serotypes, but the importance of these variations in outbreaks of respiratory disease is unknown. Infections by parainfluenza-3 (PI-3) or infectious bovine rhinotracheitis viruses have been shown in experiments to predispose calves to *P. hemolytica* pneumonia when the bacterial exposure was given at least 4 days after the viral agents (39, 45). In the case of PI-3 virus, the greatest effect of virus infection on clearance of *P. hemolytica* was observed when the bacterial challenge was given 7 days after the virus. The virus infection appears to impair the bacterial clearance abilities of the alveolar macrophages.

Affected calves exhibit severe dyspnea and fever. The course of the disease is more acute than that caused by *P. multocida*. The lesions are those of a fibrinous pleuropneumonia, which changes to a coagulative necrotic purulence in animals that survive to a later stage (16).

A similar disease is seen in feedlot cattle in the United States, where bacterial pneumonia is a major source of loss in feedlots.

P. hemolytica has also been reported as a cause of acute bovine mastitis (2, 3), and has caused lesions in the central nervous system of a calf (27).

In sheep, *P. hemolytica* is associated with two distinct syndromes, pneumonia and septicemia (25). The pneumonic syndrome is associated with biotype A and occurs as enzootics in flocks and sporadically in individual sheep. Organisms of biotype T cause an acute septicemic disease in sheep in the autumn, when their diet is improved by access to rape, turnips, or aftergrass. Interestingly, organisms of biotype T are the dominant form in the tonsils of adult healthy sheep, whereas they represent only a minor proportion of the total in the nasopharynx (26). There is evidence that in sheep (as in cattle), PI-3 virus and mycoplasmas are important in the pathogenesis of the pneumonia caused by *P. hemolytica* (17, 41).

The lesions in ovine pasteurellosis have been described by Harris (29). Hemorrhagic areas occur in the lungs, mainly on the periphery of the lobes. Petechiae may be found in the pericardium, and in some cases there is inflammation of sections of the small intestine. Affected animals cough, have a bilateral purulent nasal discharge, exhibit diarrhea, and are unthrifty. Harker (28) has also described lesions of inflammation, thickening, and edema in the wall and laminae of the abomasum of affected sheep.

Pasteurella pneumotropica

This organism was isolated by Olson and Meadows (54) from an infected cat-bite wound in a woman. It is a cause of pneumonia in mouse colonies and has been isolated from other in-contact laboratory rodents. It is also found in the pharyngeal area of cats.

It differs from *P. multocida* in its ability to ferment maltose and split urea and in being unable to ferment mannitol.

Pasteurella ureae

In 1966, Wang and Haiby (69) reported a case of human meningitis caused by *P. ureae*. They indicated that the organism was a variety of *P. hemolytica,* that it formed a distinct serologic group, that it was characterized by a strong urease reaction, and that recently isolated strains have all been of human origin.

Pasteurella anatipestifer

This organism is the cause of a septicemic disease of ducks known as *infectious serositis, new duck disease* (18), or *anatipestifer infection.* It has been described under the generic names of *Pfeifferella* (35) and *Moraxella* (8), but in the eighth edition of *Bergey's Manual,* it is placed in the genus *Pasteurella.* In morphology the organism is similar to *P. multocida.* In cultural features it differs in that it is able to liquefy gelatin as well as coagulated serum and egg. It does not ferment sugars. On primary isolation best growth is obtained if the infected material is seeded on medium that contains blood or serum and incubated under 10 percent CO_2.

Young ducks are most susceptible to infection and in field cases may show torticollis and extreme nervous signs. Tremors of the head and often loss of balance are seen. The mortality frequently is high. On postmortem examination infected ducks exhibit fibrinous pericarditis, perihepatitis with an enlarged liver, and splenitis. The air sac membranes usually are grossly thickened and opaque. Marshall *et al.* (46) have identified *P. anatipestifer* in smears of exudate from infected ducks by the FA technique. Although it has been stated that ducks and sometimes geese are the hosts of this organism, in 1970 Bruner *et al.* (9) found it in pheasants and Munday *et al.* (49) in a black swan. The infection has also been described in turkeys (33).

Pasteurellosis in Man

In 1952, Olsen and Needham (52) reviewed 21 cases of human pasteurellosis and added a series of 37 cases that they had examined at the Mayo Clinic. Reports compiled by 1970 (37) list 316 cases in man. Where no animal can be found, a reservoir of *P. multocida* infection in man with interhuman transmission is postulated. Suppurative diseases of the respiratory tract were most common, but wound infections, meningitis, abscesses, and septicemia were also observed. Many of the patients came from rural areas and most cases of wound infection resulted from animal bites. Such lesions frequently are slow in healing and present a dirty, watery discharge.

Immunity to *Pasteurella* Infections

The first bacterial vaccine ever used was prepared by Pasteur (55) in 1880 to prevent fowl cholera. This vaccine consisted of living cultures of two grades of virulence administered a few days apart. Although successful, it is no longer used.

A protective antigen occurs in the capsule of some *P. multocida* serotypes (57, 58). Mukkur (48) has shown that a glycoprotein of type A organisms is protective and elicits an agglutinating and bactericidal response in calves. Wei and Carter (70) have developed a live streptomycin-dependent vaccine for the prevention of hemorrhagic septicemia.

A variety of live vaccines against *P. multocida* have been developed for use in poultry (19, 32, 53). In turkeys, avirulent live vaccines administered in the drinking water may protect for up to 28 weeks after vaccination. Local antibodies are induced in tracheal secretions by the tenth day and persist for 6 weeks (20).

Bacterins may be cultures of the specific organism killed with heat or chemicals or a suspension of formalinized chicken embryo in which the bacterium has been propagated. They may also consist of the antigens absorbed by aluminum hydroxide from formalin-killed cultures. They are used on cattle and sheep 1 to 3 weeks before the animals are to be shipped in order to allow antibodies to form by the time they are needed.

In Africa the use of bacterins for control of hemorrhagic septicemia has given disappointing results (50), probably because the serotypes included in the vaccines were not the same as those causing disease.

Two kinds of immune serum are available for treating animals that are believed to be in the early stages of the disease. One is made from cattle, the other from horses. For use on cattle the homologous product is always preferable because fewer serum reactions will be obtained following its administration. Large doses of antiserum are useful in treating the disease in its early stages. If it is to be employed in a herd of cattle, it is advisable to take temperatures of all animals and to use large doses of the antiserum on those in which pyrexia is found. Smaller doses may be given to exposed animals that have normal temperatures. It is probably useless to give serum to animals in which pneumonia is fully developed.

Diagnosis of *Pasteurella* Infections

Pasteurellas are easily found in smears of pneumonic tissue but not in the blood or spleen of animals with *Pasteurella* pneumonias. In the septicemic pasteurelloses, the organism is present in the blood, spleen, and lungs.

Serologic methods of diagnosis are not routinely used. It has been suggested that increased antibody titers to *P. hemolytica* in older animals are evidence of a current or past pneumonic lesion.

Chemotherapy of *Pasteurella* Infections

Pasteurellas are sensitive to penicillin, tetracyclines, neomycin, chloramphenicol, streptomycin, sulfa compounds, and trimethoprim. Hawley (31) has treated calves with a tetracycline and antiserum combination and has observed dramatic recoveries.

R-factor mediated antibiotic resistance has been found in pasteurellas from cattle and poultry (4).

REFERENCES

1. Alberts and Graham. North Am. Vet., 1948, *29*, 24.
2. Andersen and Jensen. Dansk. Vet., 1977, *60*, 145.
3. Barnum. Can. Jour. Comp. Med. and Vet. Sci., 1954, *18*, 113.
4. Berman and Hirsh. Antimicrob. Agents and Chemother., 1978, *14*, 348.
5. Biberstein, Meyer, and Kennedy. Jour. Bact., 1958, *76*, 445.
6. Biberstein, Gills, and Knight. Cornell Vet., 1960, *50*, 283.
7. Bierer and Derieux. Poultry Sci., 1973, *52*, 2290.
8. Bruner and Fabricant. Cornell Vet., 1954, *44*, 461.
9. Bruner, Angstrom, and Price. Cornell Vet., 1970, *60*, 491.
10. Carter. Am. Jour. Vet. Res., 1955, *16*, 481.
11. Carter. Am. Jour. Vet. Res., 1957, *18*, 437.
12. Carter. Can. Vet. Jour., 1963, *4*, 61.
13. Carter. Vet. Rec., 1963, *75*, 1264.
14. Carter. Vet. Rec., 1972, *91*, 150.
15. Carter. Proc. 19th Ann. Meeting, Am. Assoc. Vet. Lab. Diagnosticians, 1977, p. 189.
16. Dao trong Dat and Schimmel. Arch. f. Exp. Vetmed., 1974, *28*, 303.
17. Davis, Dungworth, Humphrys, and Johnson. New Zeal. Vet. Jour., 1977, *25*, 263.
18. Dougherty. Cornell Vet., 1953, *43*, 421.
19. Dougherty, Saunders, and Parsons. Am. Jour. Path., 1955, *31*, 475.
20. Dua and Makeswaran. Avian Dis., 1978, *22*, 771.
21. Flügge. Die Mikroorganismen. F. C. W. Vogel, Leipzig, 1886.
22. Frederiksen. Jour. Gen. Microbiol., 1971, *69*, 8.
23. Frederiksen. Contrib. Microbiol. Immunol., 1973, *2*, 170.
24. Ghoniem, Amtsberg, and Bisping. Zentbl. Vet.-Med., 1973, *20B*, 310.
25. Gilmour. Vet. Rec., 1978, *102*, 100.
26. Gilmour, Thompson, and Fraser. Res. Vet. Sci., 1974, *17*, 413.
27. Goto and Itakura. Jap. Jour. Vet. Sci., 1975. *37*, 303.
28. Harker. Vet. Rec., 1974, *95*, 72.
29. Harris. Vet. Rec., 1974, *94*, 84.
30. Harris and Switzer. Am. Jour. Vet. Res., 1968, *29*, 777.
31. Hawley. Jour. Am. Vet. Med. Assoc., 1952, *121*, 371.
32. Heddleston, Rebers, and Wessman. Poultry Sci., 1975, *54*, 217.
33. Helfer and Helmholdt. Avian Dis., 1977, *21*, 712.
34. Hendrickson and Hilbert. Rpt. N.Y. State Vet. Coll. for 1930–31, p. 167.
35. Hendrickson and Hilbert. Cornell Vet., 1932. *22*, 239.
36. Hoerlein, Soxena, and Mansfield. Am. Jour. Vet. Res., 1961, *22*, 470.
37. Hubbert and Rosen. Am. Jour. Pub. Health., 1970, *60*, 1103.
38. Hueppe. Berl. klin. Schnschr., 1886, *23*, 753, 776, and 794.
39. Jericho and Langford. Can. Jour. Comp. Med., 1978, *42*, 269.
40. Jones. Jour. Exp. Med., 1921, *34*, 561.
41. Jones, Gilmour, and Rae. Jour. Comp. Path., 1978, *88*, 85.
42. Jorgensen. Cornell Vet., 1925. *15*, 205.
43. Kitt, Sitzungsher, and Geseelsch. J. Morph. und Phys. München, 1885, *1*, 240.
44. Lignières. Ann. Inst. Pasteur, 1901, *15*, 734.
45. Lopez, Thomson, and Savan. Can. Jour. Comp. Med., 1976, *40*, 385.
46. Marshall, Hansen, and Eveland, Cornell Vet., 1961, *51*, 24.
47. Moore. U.S. Dept. of Agr., Bur. Anim. & Indus. Bull. *3*, 1895.
48. Mukkur. Am. Jour. Vet. Res., 1978, *39*, 1269.
49. Munday, Corhould, Heddleston, and Harry. Austral. Vet. Jour., 1970, *46*, 322.
50. Mwangota, Muhammed, and Thomson. Cornell Vet., 1980, *70*, 27.
51. Namioka and Murata. Cornell Vet., 1961, *51*, 507.
52. Olsen and Needham. Am Jour. Med. Sci., 1952, *224*, 77.
53. Olson. Avian Dis., 1977, *21*, 178.
54. Olson and Meadows. Am. Jour. Clin. Path., 1969, *51*, 709.
55. Pasteur. Comp. Rend. Acad. Sci., 1880, *90*, 239, 952, and 1030.
56. Pavri and Apte. Vet. Rec., 1967, *80*, 437.

57. Penn and Nagy. Res. Vet. Sci., 1974, *16,* 251.
58. Penn and Nagy. Res. Vet. Sci., 1976, *20,* 90.
59. Roberts. Jour. Comp. Path. and Bact., 1947, *57,* 261.
60. Rogers and Elder. Austral. Vet. Jour., 1967, *43,* 81.
61. Rosenbusch and Merchant. Jour. Bact., 1939, *37,* 69.
62. Sautter, Pomeroy, and Fenstermacher. Jour. Am. Vet. Med. Assoc., 1957, *131,* 469.
63. Scheifer, Ward, and Moffat. Vet. Path., 1978, *15,* 313.
64. Smith. Nature, 1959, *183,* 1132.
65. Thomson, Benson, and Govan. Can. Jour. Comp. Med., 1969, *33,* 194.
66. Trevisan. Rendicants: Reale Instituto Lombardo di Scienze e Lettere, Milan, 1887, p. 94.
67. Tucker. Cornell Vet., 1953, *43,* 378.
68. Tunnicliff. Vet. Med., 1949, *44,* 498.
69. Wang and Haiby. Am. Jour. Clin. Path., 1966, *45,* 562.
70. Wei and Carter. Am. Jour. Vet. Res., 1978, *39,* 1534.
71. Wray and Thompson. Brit. Vet. Jour. 1973, *129,* 116.

10 The Genus *Bordetella*

There are three species in this genus: *Bordetella pertussis, B. parapertussis,* and *B. bronchiseptica.* Only *B. bronchiseptica* is important as a cause of disease in animals. All three species are related serologically (19) and produce a dermonecrotic toxin which is neutralized by *B. pertussis* antiserum. *B. bronchiseptica* causes disease in the respiratory tract of dogs, pigs, and laboratory rodents.

Bordetella bronchiseptica

This organism was first described by Ferry (11, 12) in 1910. It was isolated from the upper respiratory tract of a dog suffering from distemper and it was erroneously believed to be the causative agent.

Morphology and Staining Reactions. *B. bronchiseptica* is a small, Gram-negative bacillus that is motile by means of peritrichic flagella.

Cultural Features. The organism grows readily on ordinary laboratory media and on McConkey agar that contains 1 percent glucose. Characteristic blue-gray colonies are produced on this medium. Carbohydrates are not fermented; oxidase, catalase, and urease are produced; and most strains are hemolytic on blood agar. Tetrazolium is reduced to red, insoluble formazan, citrate is utilized, and most strains are sensitive to potassium tellurite (4). In litmus milk it produces a strongly alkaline reaction. Most strains exhibit D-mannose-insensitive hemagglutination of sheep erythrocytes (4).

There appears to be very little variation between strains from different host species (4).

Epidemiology and Pathogenesis. *B. bronchiseptica* is an obligate parasite of the upper respiratory tract of dogs, pigs, and rodents and has occasionally been found in other hosts as well. It is found mainly in young animals with, or recovering from, subclinical or clinical respiratory disease and is later cleared from the respiratory tract of the majority of these animals (3, 18). The extent to which carrier animals occur is not known. Bemis *et al.* (5) feel that the organism cannot be regarded as normal flora in the dog.

The Disease in Dogs. The role of *B. bronchiseptica* in canine respiratory disease has been debated for many years. Its importance as a secondary invader after distemper virus infection has long been known. In this situation the organism is important in the development of the bronchopneumonia which is often a fatal sequel to the virus infection.

The status of *B. bronchiseptica* as a primary pathogen has, however, been unclear until the use of specific pathogen-free dogs in recent studies (5) showed that it can cause a tracheobronchitis clinically similar to "kennel cough." Other workers (28, 30) reached the same conclusion from the results of experiments on normal puppies.

The naturally occurring disease has also been described in detail (3) in a closed breeding kennel where infection occurred shortly after weaning. Puppies shed the organism for 2 to 3 months but immune adult in-contact and exposed dogs did not harbor the infection. Affected pups had a moist, hacking cough which persisted for 1 to 2 weeks.

Infection has been shown to be transmitted by aerosol, and colonization and persistence of the bacterium in the trachea involve adhesion to tracheal cilia by means of fibrillar material (5).

Clinical recovery coincides with the appearance of local immunity, which reduces the numbers of the organism in the trachea, probably by prevention of adhesion. Total clearance of the organism does not occur until up to 3 months after infection. Recovered dogs maintain an immunity to reinfection for up to 14 months (5). Serum antibody does not appear to be important in local clearance of infection.

The inflammatory response is characterized by neutrophilic invasion of the ciliated respiratory mucosa, which remains intact. The neutrophils are highly efficient at ingesting and killing the organism (5).

The Disease in Pigs. *B. bronchiseptica* has been recovered from the lungs of young pigs (3 to 8 weeks of age) with respiratory disease (21). Many animals became chronically affected and stunted in growth. The involvement of primary virus infection in this disease has not been disproved, however.

The organism is a common inhabitant of the upper respiratory tract of swine, where it can be present in a carrier state or in association with upper-respiratory-tract disease characterized by sneezing, coughing, and a later deformity of the bony structures of the nose (known as *atrophic rhinitis*). This disease may result from infection by *B. bronchiseptica* alone (14, 25) or from a combined infection by *Pasteurella multocida* type D and *B. bronchiseptica* (13). Porcine cytomegalovirus has also been found in association with *B. bronchiseptica* in outbreaks of atrophic rhinitis but is not believed to be important in causing the lesions that result in atrophy of the turbinate bones (9, 23).

After infection with *B. bronchiseptica,* susceptible, nonimmune pigs exhibit rhinitis with degenerative changes in osteoblasts and osteocytes of the nasal turbinates, and their eventual atrophy. Advanced turbinate atrophy has been seen as soon as 3 weeks after experimental inoculation (29). However, turbinate atrophy induced in pigs a few weeks old may not persist until slaughter because turbinate regeneration apparently can occur in swine infected early in life (29).

Turbinate atrophy may also develop in pigs infected at 11 to 13 weeks (1), but the incidence of the disease is less than in pigs infected earlier.

Pigs with severe atrophic rhinitis exhibit shortening of the upper jaw and twisting of the snout to one side. However, lesions in the turbinates may be detected radiographically before gross clinical changes are evident (8).

Agglutinating antibodies appear in the serum of swine between 2 and 4 weeks after infection (7, 15) and persist for at least 4 months. Kong *et al.* (17) found that in pig populations where *B. bronchiseptica* infection was most frequent between 10 and 20 weeks of age, antibodies were not detectable until about 12 weeks of age. The frequency of positive titers (greater than 1:10) in herds increases steadily with advancing age (16).

Colostrum-deprived piglets develop turbinate atrophy more frequently than nondeprived animals, but colostral antibody may delay active antibody formation in passively immunized piglets (15). Sow vaccination has been shown to slightly reduce the incidence of the disease in herds with endemic infection (20).

Control of the disease in swine herds consists of elimination of infected carrier animals as detected by nasal swabbing (10), sow vaccination to protect piglets early in life, prophylactic tetracycline therapy during the first 12 days of life, and administration of immune serum to piglets (6). All of these measures are intended to reduce the numbers of *B. bronchiseptica* in the pig population so that piglets are exposed to minimal numbers of the organism.

The Disease in Laboratory Rodents. *B. bronchiseptica* is a common cause of bronchopneumonia, other respiratory infections, and septicemia in laboratory rodents (24).

Chemotherapy of Bordetellosis. Streptomycin and tetracycline have been shown to be effective in therapy of infected rats (22). Sulfamethazine at a level of 100 g per ton of feed cured swine of experimental nasal infections (26).

Aerosols of kanamycin, gentamicin, or polymixin B were effective in reducing populations of *B. bronchiseptica* in the airways of infected dogs and in producing clinical improvement (2).

R factor–mediated resistance to streptomycin, sulfadimethoxine, and an aminobenzyl penicillin has been found in strains from pigs in Japan (27).

REFERENCES

1. Backstrom and Bergstrom. Nord. Vetmed., 1977, *29,* 539.
2. Bemis and Appel. Jour. Am. Vet. Med. Assoc., 1977, *170,* 1082.
3. Bemis, Carmichael, and Appel. Cornell Vet., 1977, *67,* 282.

4. Bemis, Greisen, and Appel. Jour. Clin. Microbiol., 1977, *5,* 471.
5. Bemis, Greisen, and Appel. Jour. Inf. Dis., 1977, *135,* 753.
6. Bercovich and Oosterwoud. Tijdsch. V. Diergeneesk., 1977, *102,* 485.
7. Brassine, Dewoele, and Gouffaux. Res. Vet. Sci., 1976, *20,* 162.
8. Done. Vet. Rec., 1976, *98,* 23.
9. Edington, Smith, Plowright, and Watt. Vet. Rec., 1976, *98,* 42.
10. Farrington and Switzer. Jour. Am. Vet. Med. Assoc., 1977, *177,* 34.
11. Ferry. Am. Vet. Rev., 1910, *37,* 499.
12. Ferry. Jour. Inf. Dis., 1911, *8,* 399.
13. Harris and Switzer. Am. Jour. Vet. Res., 1968, *29,* 777.
14. Kemeny. Cornell Vet., 1972, *62,* 477.
15. Kemeny. Cornell Vet., 1973, *63,* 130.
16. Kemeny and Amtomer. Can. Jour. Comp. Med., 1973, *37,* 409.
17. Kong, Koshimizu, and Ogata. Jap. Jour. Vet. Sci., 1971, *33,* 17.
18. Koshimizu, Kodama, and Ogata. Jap. Jour. Vet. Sci., 1973, *35,* 223.
19. Leslie and Gardner. Jour. Hyg. (London), 1971, *31,* 423.
20. Pedersen and Barfod. Nord. Vetmed., 1977, *29,* 369.
21. Ray. Jour. Am. Vet. Med. Assoc., 1950, *116,* 51.
22. Rosen, Hunt, and Benorde. Jour. Am. Vet. Med. Assoc., 1950, *116,* 51.
23. Schoss. Deut. Tierärztl. Wchnschr., 1977, *84,* 413.
24. Smith. Jour. Med. Res., 1914, *24,* 291.
25. Switzer. Am. Jour. Vet. Res., 1956, *17,* 478.
26. Switzer. Vet. Med., 1963, *59,* 571.
27. Terrakado, Azechi, Ninomiya, and Shinuzu. Antimicrob. Agents and Chemother., 1973, *3,* 555.
28. Thompson, McCandlish, and Wright. Res. Vet. Sci., 1976, *20,* 16.
29. Tornoe and Nielsen. Nord. Vetmed., 1976, *28,* 233.
30. Wright, Thompson, Taylor, and Cornwell. Vet. Rec., 1973, *93,* 486.

11 The Genus *Moraxella*

Members of this genus have small, short, rod-shaped cells which occur in pairs and are therefore termed diplobacilli. *Bergey's Manual* (eighth edition) lists these species: *M. lacunata, M. liquefaciens,* and *M. bovis. M. bovis* is the only official species of veterinary importance, although a separate species affecting sheep (*M. ovis*) has been described (1).

Moraxella bovis

SYNONYM: *Hemophilus bovis*

This organism is the cause of *infectious keratitis* or *pinkeye* of cattle.

Morphology and Staining Reaction. *M. bovis* is a Gram-negative diplobacillus about 2 μm in length and 1 μm in width. It is nonmotile and does not form spores. Rough forms of the organism are fimbriated.

Cultural Features. The colonies after passage on cow-blood agar may be smooth, circular, translucent, and grayish in color and are beta-hemolytic. Convalescent and clinically normal carrier cattle frequently yield isolates that are rough, nonhemolytic, and corroding. Isolates on primary isolation media from acute clinical cases are also frequently of this type and are heavily fimbriated (17). Smooth strains are avirulent (17).

Serum or blood is necessary for good growth. Gelatin is liquefied but carbohydrates are not attacked. *M. bovis* is an aerobe and is oxidase-positive.

Epidemiology and Pathogenesis. Pinkeye occurs throughout the cattle-raising areas of the world and is most prevalent in the warmer months. Factors which enhance infection are solar radiation, dust, and intense fly activity. Transmission can occur by direct contact (7) and by mechanical transfer on the legs and mouth-parts of flies (*Musca domestica, M. autumnalis,* and *Stomoxys calcitrans*).

The infection is maintained between outbreaks in the conjunctiva and nares of carrier animals, where the organism may multiply and subsequently spread to uninfected cattle following exposure to sunlight or infection by other microbial agents such as infectious bovine tracheitis virus (12). The disease is highly contagious among cattle less than 2 years old but may also spread rapidly among older susceptible animals. During an outbreak most animals become infected, but clinical disease is more common in younger cattle (7).

Infectious keratitis is a common ailment of cattle in the range country of the western United States. It is seen most often in Hereford cattle in hot, dusty periods of the year. Beginning with photophobia and simple conjunctivitis, the inflammation later becomes purulent. Opacity of the cornea of the affected eyes usually develops, and frequently the inflammatory process invades the orbit and permanent blindness ensues. In the purulent discharge various pyogenic organisms may be found, particularly *Corynebacterium pyogenes.* These are secondary invaders. The infection may ascend the optic nerve and cause a fatal meningitis, but such instances are rare (10).

The pathogenesis of the keratitis is not completely understood. Henson and Grumbles (5, 6) have demonstrated a dermonecrotic toxin in the cell wall of *M. bovis* that after experimental corneal inoculation in calves produced lesions typical of those seen in the corneas of cattle with pinkeye.

Pugh *et al.* (13), however, have shown that there is a specific oculopathic substance in the cell sap of *M. bovis* that induces ocular pruritus and lacrimation in cattle.

Immunity. Immunoglobulins IgA, IgM, and IgG have all been detected in the lacrimal secretions of calves in a herd with enzootic pinkeye (11). The highest and most persistent titers to *M. bovis* were caused by antibodies of the IgG class, but these antibodies did not prevent clinical disease in the calves. Other studies have similarly failed to prove an association between antibodies and enhanced resistance (7).

However, Hughes and Pugh (8) have successfully stimulated protective immunity in calves by means of *M. bovis* bacterins. These vaccines did stimulate an increase in antibody titer. The incorporation of an adjuvant with the bacteria did not increase their immunogenicity (9). A pilus vaccine has also been shown to stimulate some protection in calves challenged with a homologous strain (15).

There is evidence (14) that vaccines must be polyvalent to succeed in the field because a variety of *M. bovis* strains apparently exist (16), and immunity is strain-specific.

Calves are not protected until about 4 weeks after vaccination, during which time they are liable to contract infection from carrier dams or other in-contact cattle.

Chemotherapy. Antibiotics are effective in treating pinkeye in cattle. Ellis and Barnes (3) recommended the use of tylosin tartrate solution at a concentration of 50 mg per ml, and Cooper (2) found 0.5 percent ethidium bromide eye ointment to be efficacious. Schrimsher (18) used a combination of methylprednisolone, penicillin, and dihydrostreptomycin in the treatment of pinkeye in cattle and in nonspecific keratitis in horses and claimed that in each case only one application was required.

Chloramphenicol has been found to be effective in eliminating *M. bovis* from eyes of affected cattle (4).

Antibiotic treatment of carrier animals to eliminate the organism has not been well studied, although it would be of great value in control of pinkeye in cattle populations.

REFERENCES

1. Calvi and Basso. Gaceta Veterinaria, 1977, *39,* 588.
2. Cooper. Vet. Rec., 1960, *72,* 589.
3. Ellis and Barnes. Vet. Med., 1961, *56,* 197.
4. Gallagher. Austral. Vet. Jour., 1954, *30,* 61.
5. Henson and Grumbles. Cornell Vet., 1960, *50,* 445.
6. Henson and Grumbles. Cornell Vet., 1961, *51,* 267.
7. Hughes and Pugh. Jour. Am. Vet. Med. Assoc., 1970, *157,* 443.
8. Hughes and Pugh. Am. Jour. Vet. Res., 1971, *32,* 879.
9. Hughes, Pugh, and Booth. Am. Jour. Vet. Res., 1977, *38,* 1905.
10. Jackson. Am. Jour. Vet. Res., 1953, *14,* 19.
11. Killinger, Wersiger, Helper, and Mansfield. Am. Jour. Vet. Res., 1978, *39,* 931.
12. Pugh, Hughes, and Packer. Am. Jour. Vet. Res., 1968, *29,* 2057.
13. Pugh, Hughes, and Schulz. Can. Jour. Comp. Med., 1973, *37,* 70.
14. Pugh, Hughes, Schulz, and Graham. Am. Jour. Vet. Res., 1976, *37,* 57.
15. Pugh, Hughes, and Booth. Am. Jour. Vet. Res., 1977, *38,* 1519.
16. Pugh, Hughes, and Booth. Am. Jour. Vet. Res., 1978, *39,* 55.
17. Sandhu, White, and Simpson. Am. Jour. Vet. Res., 1974, *35,* 437.
18. Schrimsher. Vet. Med., 1970, *65,* 169.

12 The Genus *Actinobacillus*

The genus *Actinobacillus* consists of pleomorphic Gram-negative nonmotile organisms which are catalase- and oxidase-variable and ferment sugars without gas production. Two species of importance as pathogens of domestic animals are described in the eighth edition of *Bergey's Manual*. These are *A. lignieresi* and *A. equuli*. Another species, *A. suis,* is listed as *incertae sedis,* while a fourth, *A. seminis* (1), a rare cause of ovine epididymitis, is regarded as being wrongly placed in the genus.

A new species, *A. salpingitis,* has been proposed for an "*Actinobacillus*like" organism causing salpingitis and peritonitis in chickens (13).

Actinobacillus lignieresi

This organism was first described by Lignières and Spitz (10, 11) in 1902. It had been isolated from Argentine cattle suffering from a disease which clinically resembled actinomycosis. Later actinobacillosis was recognized in Europe (6, 12), in the United States (24, 25), and in South Africa (18). It is quite common. It may be confused with actinomycosis.

Morphology and Staining Reactions. In the pus of the lesions of the disease the small rod-shaped organisms are encased in small cheeselike granules. These are quite similar to the "sulfur granules" of actinomycosis, but generally they are much smaller, measuring less than 1 mm in diameter (Figure 12.1). If these granules are picked out of the pus and crushed between slides, moderate magnification will show clublike bodies radiating out from the centers of the masses. Stains made from the crushed granules show small Gram-negative bacilli.

In cultures the organism exhibits considerable variation in morphology depending upon the medium used

Figure 12.1. *Actinobacillus lignieresi,* showing club-bearing rosettes in pus from a lymph node lesion. Unstained. × 720. (From Campbell, Whitlock, Timoney, and Underwood, *Jour. Am. Vet. Med. Assoc.*, 1975, *166,* 604.)

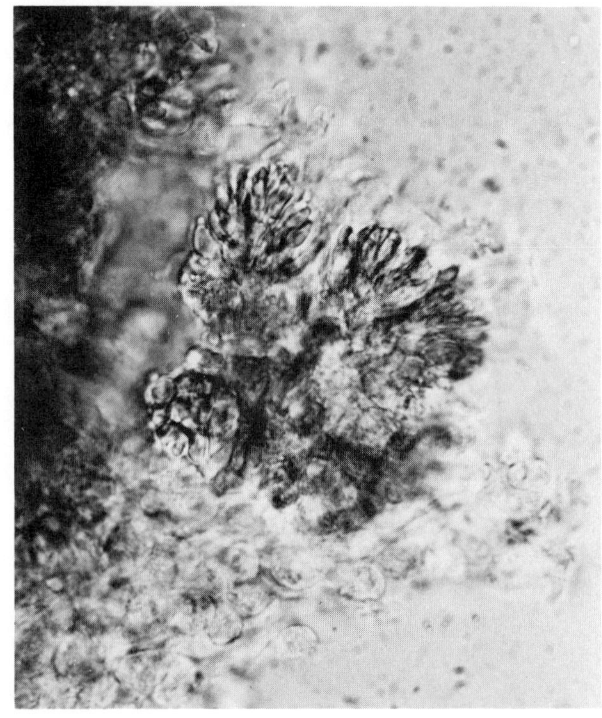

and whether surface or deep growth on solid media is examined. Diplococci and slender rods are seen in fluid cultures. Long curved forms are often seen in colonies growing in the depths of solid media. The bacilli are about 0.4 μm in width and 1 to 15 μm in length (Figure 12.2). They are nonmotile, stain with the usual dyes, and are Gram-negative.

Cultural Features. This organism is quite serophilic, and little growth occurs in most media unless some serum or blood is present. It is rather strongly aerobic, to the extent that growth practically always fails under anaerobic conditions. On the other hand, primary cultures in fluid media or in stabs in solid media are more apt to succeed than surface cultures. Primary cultures succeed best when they are incubated in an atmosphere consisting of 10 percent carbon dioxide.

In serum agar, delicate, naillike growths appear along the length of the stab. Surface colonies are bluish white and very delicate. They are smooth, glistening, convex, and vary from 0.5 to 1 mm in diameter. There is good growth in serum gelatin but the medium is not liquefied. Glucose serum broth usually shows a characteristic growth consisting of small grayish granules, which

Figure 12.2. *Actinobacillus lignieresi,* from a culture on serum agar incubated 24 hours at 37 C. × 1,400. (Courtesy L. R. Vawter.)

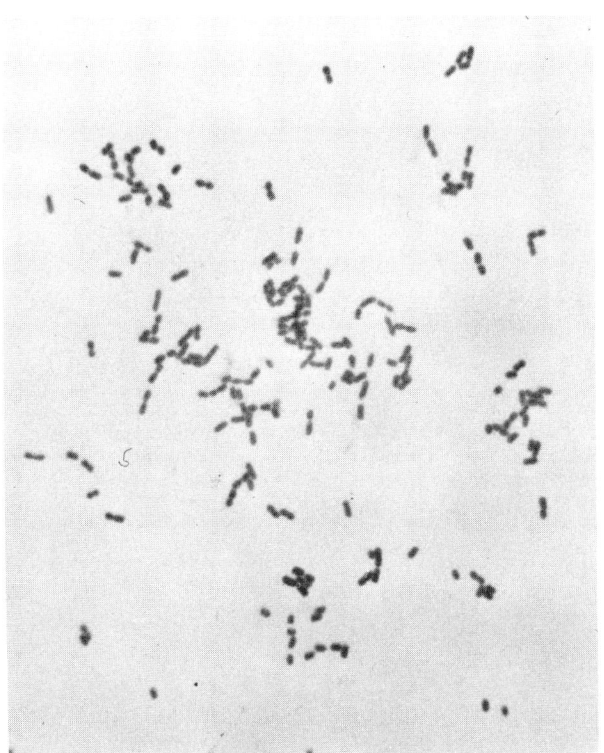

adhere to the sides of the tube but are easily broken loose by shaking. The remainder of the broth is clear. Litmus milk usually remains unchanged. Sometimes it develops slight acidity. Excellent growth occurs on coagulated blood serum. The medium is not softened or liquefied. When dissolved in serum broth, glucose, lactose, sucrose, maltose, raffinose, and mannitol are regularly fermented. Xylose is fermented irregularly. Arabinose, dulcitol, salicin, and inulin are not attacked. Indol is formed in small amounts. Cultures must be transferred at 4-day intervals; otherwise they lose viability.

Antigens. Six antigenic types can be distinguished by differences in heat-stable antigens (16). Cattle strains are usually type 1 and sheep strains are usually types 3 and 4. Heat-labile antigens also occur and are common to the various heat-stable antigenic types.

Epidemiology and Pathogenesis. *A. lignieresi* is a normal commensal of the buccal mucous membrane of cattle and sheep, and entry into the deeper tissues is a result of trauma or penetration by foreign material into the buccal epithelium.

The natural disease in cattle is manifested most commonly by slowly developing tumors, which may occur in any part of the body but are seen most frequently in the region of the lower jaws and neck (Figure 12.3). These are hard and often lobular. Sooner or later softened areas become evident, and these fluctuate upon pressure, indicating the presence of fluid, which is, in reality, a mucoid, nonodorous pus. This breaks through the skin, creating a deep ulcer which will not heal. In the meantime, the tumorous mass usually continues to enlarge and additional ulcers may form. A characteristic form of this disease is the so-called *wooden tongue* of cattle. In this disease the hard tumorous mass forms in the substance of the tongue, causing serious disability. Lesions in the internal organs, particularly of the lymphoid structures, the lungs, and the walls of the four compartments of the stomach, are not uncommon. Palotay (15) described three cases in cattle. One showed lesions in the subcutaneous tissue of the posterior limbs; in the submaxillary, internal iliac, and the prefemoral lymph glands; and in the ovaries. In another the tunics of the testicles were involved, and the third was evidenced by a large swelling in the middle posterior part of the thigh. Swarbrick (22) studied three atypical cases, one a circumscribed cutaneous lesion in the flank, one with urinary bladder involvement, and one a widespread infection in the head associated with multiple foreign bodies in the mouth.

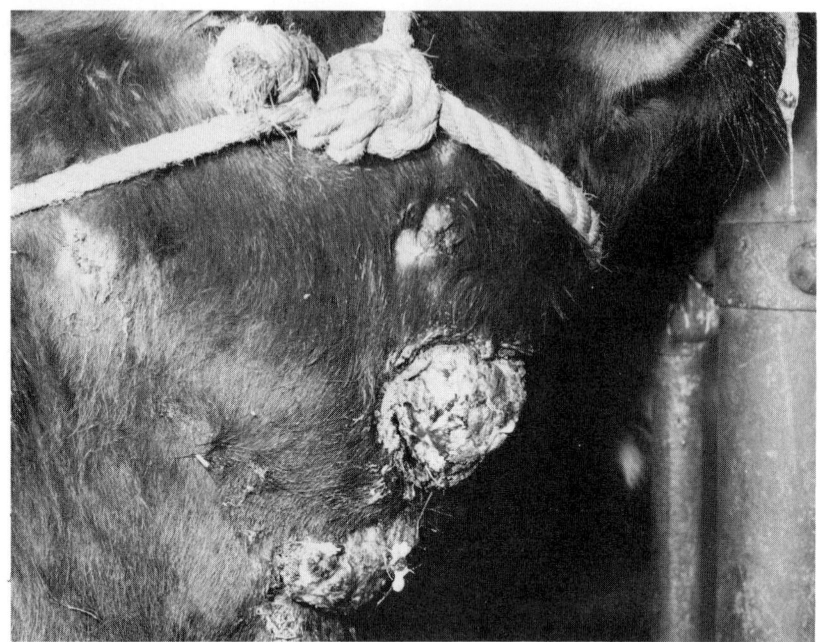

Figure 12.3. Actinobacillosis in a heifer. (From Campbell, Whitlock, Timoney, and Underwood, *Jour. Am. Vet. Med. Assoc.*, 1975, *166*, 604.)

Hebeler *et al.* (17) reported an outbreak in a dairy herd with about 7 percent morbidity and a high incidence of lesions of the skin and related lymph nodes rather than tongue or alimentary tract involvement. Campbell *et al.* (2) described an outbreak in a group of 52 heifers where the morbidity was 73 percent. An important predisposing factor in the outbreak was dry, stemmy haylage, which when eaten caused abrasions and penetrations of the buccal mucosa. Biopsies revealed some of this plant material imbedded in the lesions (Figure 12.4). Although the lesions of *A. lignieresi* tend to localize, generalized actinobacillosis has been observed in cattle (6).

This disease often is confused with actinomycosis. The true actinomycosis, which is caused by the "ray fungus," *Actinomyces bovis,* seldom occurs in the soft structures but is found mostly in the bone of the lower jaw.

Actinobacillosis occurs in sheep. According to Taylor

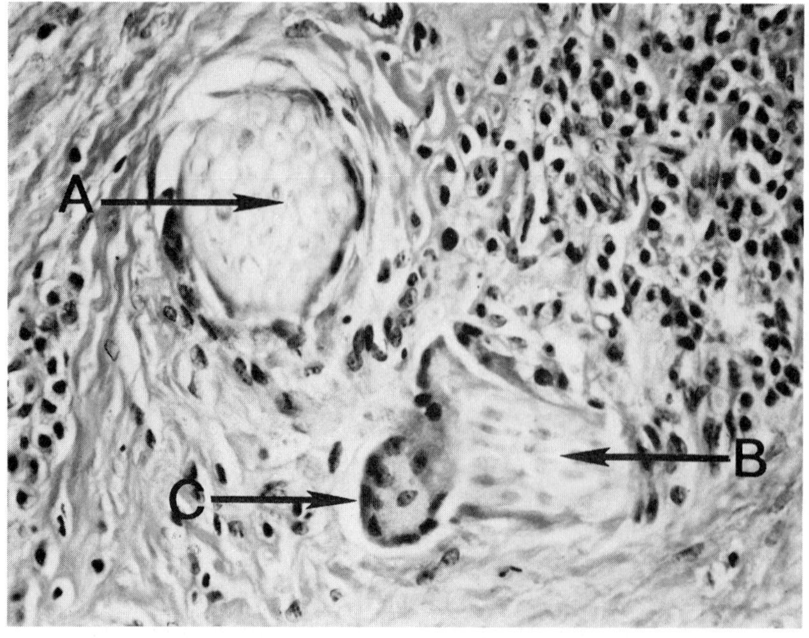

Figure 12.4. Plant material in a granuloma from which *Actinobacillus lignieresi* was isolated. The granuloma is transected by plant fibers (A and B). A giant cell is also present (C). (From Campbell, Whitlock, Timoney, and Underwood, *Jour. Am. Vet. Med. Assoc.*, 1975, *166*, 604.)

(23), it is fairly common in this animal in Scotland. Reports (8) indicate that lesions of the disease often are found in the head region with involvement of the cheeks, nose, lips, and lymph glands. Abscesses are seen in the soft palate, pharynx, and lungs. Skin lesions have also been reported. The organism has been described as the cause of mastitis in the ewe (9).

Sautter *et al.* (20) have noted a case of actinobacillosis in a dog, and Fletcher (15) reported a case in the tongue of a dog. Their isolates did not have all the characteristics of *A. lignieresi*. In 1969, Carb and Liu (3) found *A. lignieresi* to be the causative agent of a large, diffusely infiltrating granulomatous mass in the thigh of a 7.5-year-old Boston Terrier.

Immunity. Many normal cattle have specific agglutinins in their sera (15), which is presumably a result of the presence of the organism as a commensal in the buccal cavity. Affected cows may exhibit a significant rise in titer (4), but this reaction is not widely used in diagnosis.

The granulomatous nature of the lesion suggests that cell-mediated immunity is important in the host response, and possibly in resolution of the infection.

A report (17) on the use of formalinized bacterin during an outbreak of actinobacillosis in a herd of 543 cattle concluded that the vaccine reduced the number of cases that relapsed and prevented the occurrence of new cases.

Diagnosis. Gram-stained smears of sulfur granules will reveal club-bearing rosettes that contain central masses of Gram-negative rods and cocci.

Treatment. The infection, like actinomycosis, is iodine-sensitive, and local lesions may be successfully treated by injecting them with an aqueous solution of iodine (Lugol's solution). Clinical experience has shown that sodium iodide administered intravenously is highly successful in treating wooden tongue and other forms of actinobacillosis in which the lesions are inaccessible to local applications of iodine. *A. lignieresi* is very sensitive to the action of streptomycin, sulfonamides, particularly sulfapyridine, sulfamethazine, and sulfathiazole, and these substances may have value in treating the disease (21). It is also sensitive to tetracyclines and Chloromycetin (19).

REFERENCES

1. Baynes and Simmons. Austral. Vet. Jour., 1960, *36*, 454.
2. Campbell, Whitlock, Timoney, and Underwood. Jour. Am. Vet. Med. Assoc., 1975, *166*, 604.
3. Carb and Liu. Jour. Am. Vet. Med. Assoc., 1969, *154*, 1062.
4. Davies and Torrance. Jour. Comp. Path. and Therap., 1930, *43*, 216.
5. Fletcher. Vet. Rec., 1956, *68*, 645.
6. Franco. Vet. Med./Small Animal Clin., 1970, *65*, 562.
7. Hebeler, Linton, and Osborne. Vet. Rec., 1961, *73*, 517.
8. Johnson. Austral. Vet. Jour., 1954, *30*, 105.
9. Laws and Elder. Austral. Vet. Jour., 1969, *45*, 401.
10. Lignières and Spitz. Bull. Soc. Cent. Méd. Vet., 1902, *20*, 487.
11. Lignières and Spitz. Zentrbl. f. Bakt., I. Abt. Orig., 1903, *35*, 294.
12. Magnusson. Acta Path. et Microbiol. Scand., 1928, *5*, 170.
13. Mraz, Vladik, and Bobacek. Zentrbl. f. Bakt., 1976, *236A*, 294.
14. Nakazawa, Azuma, Yamashita, Iwas, and Uchimura. Jap. Jour. Vet. Sci., 1977, *39*, 549.
15. Palotay. Vet. Med., 1951, *46*, 52.
16. Phillips. Jour. Path. and Bact. 1967, *93*, 463.
17. Raducanescu, Mihailescu, and Anghelescu. Rev. Zootechnicsi Medicina Vet., 1972, *22*, 54.
18. Robinson. Jour. S. Afr. Vet. Med. Assoc., 1951, *22*, 85.
19. Sanders and Ristic. Jour. Am. Vet. Med. Assoc., 1956, *129*, 478.
20. Sautter, Rowsell, and Hohn. North Am. Vet., 1953, *34*, 341.
21. Smith. Vet. Rec., 1951, *63*, 674.
22. Swarbrick. Brit. Vet. Jour., 1967, *123*, 70.
23. Taylor. Jour. Comp. Path. and Therap., 1944, *54*, 228.
24. Thompson. Jour. Inf. Dis., 1933, *52*, 223.
25. Vawter. Cornell Vet., 1933, *23*, 126.

Actinobacillus (Shigella) equuli

SYNONYMS: *Shigella equirulis, Bacillus nephritidis equi, Bacterium viscosum equi, Bacterium pyosepticus equi, Shigella equi, Shigella viscosa*

A. equuli is a causative agent in purulent infections of the joints and in kidney abscesses in very young foals. It has also been found in adult horses. *A. equuli* was first described by Meyer (9), who found it in kidney abscesses in horses in South Africa and gave it the name *Bacillus nephritidis equi*. Magnusson (7), finding the organism in foals in Sweden and not realizing it was the same as the organism described by Meyer, named it *Bacterium viscosum equi*. McFadyean and Edwards (6) recognized that the two organisms were identical.

Because this organism has been renamed each time a new classification has appeared and because the names that have been applied to the disease produced are no longer valid we propose that the infection be named *equulosis*, a designation based on the specific part of the binomial and more likely to remain fixed.

Morphology and Staining Reactions. This is a small rod-shaped organism. Short chains and filaments are often seen. Capsules have been described, but generally it is believed to be noncapsulated. It is nonmotile, stains easily with the ordinary stains, and is Gram-negative.

Cultural Features. *A. equuli* grows readily in ordinary media, producing rather abundant growth. Colonies on agar plates are smooth, rather dry in appearance, and tough. Dissociation readily occurs, especially when the medium is acid and the incubation temperature high, the product being small, smooth, glistening colonies, some of which are dwarf types. On agar slants the growth is diffuse, grayish white, and very mucoid. A ropy sediment forms in broth, and old cultures become very cloudy and mucoid. A grayish pellicle sometimes appears. Gelatin stabs show a filiform growth. There is no liquefaction. Litmus milk is slowly acidified and sometimes coagulated. The uncoagulated cultures generally are very slimy. Indol is not formed and the Voges-Proskauer test is negative. No toxins are generated. Acid but no gas is formed from glucose, lactose, sucrose, galactose, maltose, raffinose, xylose, and mannitol. Freshly isolated cultures must be transferred at weekly intervals to maintain viability unless especially prepared medium is used (5). It is usually nonhemolytic, but hemolytic variants have been described (3).

Epidemiology and Pathogenesis. *A. equuli* commonly occurs in the tonsils and intestines of normal horses and causes disease only in animals debilitated by overtraining, parasitism, or exposure to bad weather. Platt (11) from a review of 61 cases of septicemia caused by *A. equuli* concluded that the organism was an opportunist which invaded foals that were congenitally defective in some way. Foals are infected either *in utero* or during or after birth. Dimock *et al.* (4) noted that the common verminous aneurysms of the mesenteric arteries often are infected with this organism, even when it cannot be demonstrated elsewhere. He believed that the larvae of *Strongylus vulgaris,* migrating from the intestinal lumen into the arteries, carry *A. equuli* with them and in this way set up infections in young susceptible animals. In prenatal infection it is possible that invasion of the fetal circulation by strongyle larvae from the dam may be a contributing factor.

In the past about 30 percent of the foals lost each season in the Bluegrass area of Kentucky died of *A. equuli* infection (4). These losses have been substantially reduced by use of antibiotics. About one-third of the foals that succumbed to equulosis died within the first 24 hours, and the majority succumbed prior to the 4th day following birth. In foals that died within the first 24 hours, the only visible lesion consisted of a severe enteritis. Rarely was there any evidence of nephritis. In foals which died at 2 or 3 days of age, the lesions observed at postmortem examination were more marked. These cases often exhibited a purulent nephritis, small abscesses being scattered throughout the cortex of the kidney. Many times the joints of the legs were affected. The joint lesions ranged from a slight increase in synovial fluid and congestion of the joint capsule to a purulent arthritis involving the joint cavity and tendon sheaths, with a great accumulation of fluid and extreme swelling. A few foals showed a severe purulent pleuropneumonia. The diagnosis was made by isolating the causative microorganism from the infected organs and joints of the diseased foal.

Adult horses are occasionally affected by an acute form of equulosis and are febrile, dysphagic, and salivate excessively.

Organisms closely related to if not identical with *A. equuli* have been isolated from endocarditis, septicemia, metritis, and arthritis in swine (2, 12, 13), from joints of rabbits (1), and from outbreaks of calf diarrhea (10). The exact relationship of these bacteria to *A. equuli* and the possibility that swine or other species of animals may act as carriers of the former needs further study.

Immunity. Specific treatment of foals with an antiserum prepared from *A. equuli* has been attempted but without encouraging results. After symptoms become evident, the prognosis is not good. Maguire (8) claimed that he obtained satisfactory protection by vaccinating pregnant mares.

Treatment. Streptomycin has been employed with very good results in preventing and treating equulosis in foals.

REFERENCES

1. Arseculeratne. Jour. Comp. Path. and Therap., 1962, *72,* 33.
2. Ashford and Shirlaw. Vet. Rec., 1962, *74,* 1417.
3. Carter, Marshall, and Jolly. New Zeal. Vet. Jour., 1971, *19,* 264.
4. Dimock, Edwards, and Bruner. Ky. Agr. Exp. Sta. Bull. 509, 1947.
5. McCollum and Doll. Cornell Vet., 1951, *41,* 11.
6. McFadyean and Edwards. Jour. Comp. Path. and Therap., 1919, *32,* 42.
7. Magnusson. Svensk. Veterinartijdskr., 1917, p. 81; Jour. Comp. Path. and Therap., 1919, *32,* 143.
8. Maguire. Vet. Rec., 1958, *70,* 989.

9. Meyer. Transvaal Dept. of Agr., Rpt. Govt. Bact., 1908–1909, p. 122.
10. Osbaldiston and Walker. Cornell Vet., 1972, *62,* 364.
11. Platt. Brit. Vet. Jour., 1973, *129,* 221.
12. Wetmore, Thiel, Herman, and Harr. Jour. Inf. Dis., 1963, *113,* 186.
13. Windsor. Vet. Rec., 1973, *92,* 178.

Actinobacillus suis

A. suis is not an official species in the eighth edition of *Bergey's Manual,* but because the name has widespread usage in the veterinary literature we will use it in the following description. The organism was first described in the early 1960s by van Dorssen and Jaartsveld (4) and by Zimmermann (5). Their isolations were made from a variety of lesions and from septicemic disease in pigs.

Morphology and Staining Reactions. The cells are rod-shaped, 0.5 to 3 μm in length, and occur singly, in filaments, and in masses. They are nonmotile and Gram-negative.

Cultural and Biochemical Features. The colonies are moderately sticky and may adhere to the agar surface. A viscous growth is produced in serum broth. Growth occurs on McConkey agar. Narrow, distinct zones of alpha hemolysis are produced on horse-blood agar and a wide zone of beta (complete) hemolysis is produced on sheep-blood agar. Hydrogen sulfide production is variable, indol and urease are not produced, and acid is evolved from glucose, lactose, arabinose, and salicin. Esculin is hydrolyzed.

Pathogenicity. Fatal acute septicemias in piglets aged 1 to 8 weeks have been shown to be caused by *A. suis* (1, 2, 5). Affected pigs develop rapid respirations and cyanosis of the extremities. At necropsy there may be a mucopurulent coating of the nasal mucosa, pleural edema, enlarged spleen, and a focal hepatic necrosis (1). A verrucous endocarditis and/or a pericarditis may also be present. Petechial hemorrhages may be found throughout the abdominal organs (2).

Pedersen (3) described a series of septicemic cases similar to the above in piglets but identified the causative organism as a nonhemolytic strain of *A. equuli*.

In older pigs, *A. suis* has been associated with arthritis, pneumonia, and subcutaneous abscesses (5). *A. suis* is pathogenic for mice (5), unlike *A. equuli* or *A. lignieresi*.

Chemotherapy. *A. suis* is sensitive to ampicillin, chloramphenicol, streptomycin, and tetracyclines (2), and these antibiotics should be useful in therapy and prevention.

REFERENCES

1. Lisen, Larsen, and Lium. Acta Vet. Scand., 1978, *19,* 313.
2. Moir, Randall, Thomas, Harbourne, McCrea, and Cowl. Jour. Comp. Path., 1974, *84,* 113.
3. Pedersen. Nord. Vetmed., 1977, *29,* 137.
4. Van Dorsen and Jaartsveld. Tijdschr. v. Diergeneesk., 1962, *87,* 450.
5. Zimmermann. Deut. tierärztl. Wchnschr., 1964, *71,* 457.

Actinobacillus salpingitis

Mraz *et al.* (4) have recently proposed that an *Actinobacillus*like organism they isolated from 25 outbreaks of disease in chickens and from the cloacae of healthy pullets be named *A. salpingitis*. Kohlert (3) had earlier reported the isolation of a similar organism from an outbreak of salpingitis and peritonitis in laying hens and named his isolate *Pasteurella salpingitis*.

The isolates of Mraz *et al.* (4) were hemolytic on sheep-blood agar, showed the basic properties of the *Pasteurella-Actinobacillus* group, and grew on McConkey agar containing crystal violet—the latter being a characteristic of *Actinobacillus*.

Other recent reports of *Actinobacillus*like organisms from salpingitis, airsacculitis, and bronchopneumonia in waterfowl include those of Bisgaard (1) and of Hacking and Siles (2).

REFERENCES

1. Bisgaard. Nord. Vetmed., 1975, *27,* 378.
2. Hacking and Siles. Jour. Wildlife Dis., 1977, *13,* 69.
3. Kohlert. Vet. Med., 1968, *23,* 132.
4. Mraz, Vladik, and Bobacek. Zentrbl. f. Bakt., 1976, *236A,* 294.

13 The Genus *Francisella*

Francisella tularensis

SYNONYMS: *Bacterium tularense, Brucella tularensis, Pasteurella tularensis*

This organism is the cause of tularemia, otherwise known as *deer-fly fever, rabbit fever,* and *Ohara's disease*. The disease affects various rodents, especially the wild cottontail rabbit, water rats, and beaver, and occasionally certain birds and sheep. It has been reported in the dog and in the coyote (19). Man becomes infected from some of these animals either through direct contact with them or their carcasses or through the agency of ticks, lice (27), or bloodsucking flies.

The disease was first recognized in ground squirrels in California by McCoy (21) in 1911. These animals become fatally infected with the lesions resembling those of bubonic plague, with which tularemia was at first confused. McCoy and Chapin (22) in 1912 isolated and described the causative organism. In 1914, Wherry and Lamb (32) found tularemia infection in man and reported it as the first recognized case.

Some years later Francis identified the organism as the cause of a serious disease of man in Utah. Francis (11) gave the name *tularemia* to the disease, the name being derived from Tulare County, California, from whence came the ground squirrels with which McCoy was working when the disease was discovered. For some years it was thought that the disease was confined to the United States, but it is now known to exist in the Scandinavian countries, in Soviet Russia, and in Japan. In these countries, as well as in the United States, the disease has become of considerable importance as a human infection.

Morphology and Staining Reactions. *F. tularensis* is a particularly small, nonmotile, poorly staining, bipolar rod. In older cultures bacillary forms up to 2 and even 3 μm in length may be seen. Coccoid forms usually are mixed with the bacillary types. Polar granules sometimes can be seen, but these do not regularly occur. The organism is Gram-negative; it stains with the usual stains. It has neither capsules nor spores.

Cultural Features. *F. tularensis* will not grow on ordinary agar or in plain broth. Media containing cystine or cysteine is necessary (12). This may be supplied by adding egg yolk or salts containing cystine or cysteine to ordinary types of culture media. Francis recommends a blood-cystine medium for the organism (12).

On suitable media *F. tularensis* develops readily, forming a smooth, viscous, grayish-white growth. It does not liquefy gelatin and grows poorly in milk. It forms acid but no gas from glucose, levulose, and glycerol.

Biochemical characterization is of little value in identification, which depends mainly on growth requirements, solubility in sodium ricinoleate and agglutination with specific antiserum or reaction with a fluorescent conjugate.

Epidemiology. The greatest reservoir of tularemia in the United States is the wild-rabbit population, especially in many midwestern states. It is from the handling of the carcasses of such rabbits that most of the human cases in this country originate. Of 266 authenticated cases of tularemia in California reported during the years 1927–1951, 81 percent were contracted from rabbits. Jack rabbits were involved more frequently than the cottontail. Cases are contracted from the bites of bloodsucking insects that have fed upon infected rabbits (15). Washburn and Tuohy (31) reported that tick-borne infection was almost twice as common in Arkansas as was rabbit-borne infection. Later it was shown by Calhoun (6) that the lone star tick (*Amblyomma americanum*) was the important carrier of *F. tularensis* in Arkansas and by Hopla (16) that the bacterium multiplied in this arthropod. The argasid ticks (4) as well as members of the genus *Dermacentor* (1) also can transmit tularemia. In general, strains of *F. tularensis* obtained from North American ticks, lagomorphs, and sheep are highly virulent and those from beaver, rodents, and water are less so (29).

The organism sometimes becomes prevalent in water holes and in small streams, being spread from the bodies of infected water animals such as water rats and beavers (9). Human cases have been reported from contact with such water (24).

There is serologic evidence that the western elk may be a significant reservoir in the United States (23). More than 50 percent of these animals are serologically positive.

The Disease in Animals. Parker and Dade (25) have reported severe losses in lambs pastured on land in Montana that is heavily infected with wood ticks, and have shown that this tick carries the infection. The ticks become infected by feeding upon wild rodents in which the disease is enzootic. Tularemia in range sheep is associated with stress of inclement weather, lambing, and ectoparasitism (3). Losses consist of unthriftiness and mortality. Normal sheep are resistant to challenge with virulent strains. The disease has been reported in epizootics in sheep in Idaho (13) and in Wyoming (28), in pen-raised beavers in Oregon (2), and in rabbits in South Carolina (20). It has occurred in cats and dogs. It has also appeared in calves and domestic chickens. It can infect practically all rodents and has been isolated from beavers, foxes, skunks, coyotes, bobcats, deer, snakes, quail, prairie chickens, pheasants, shrikes, ducks, gulls, hawks, owls, muskrats (water rats), monkeys (5) and mink (14).

The guinea pig is easily infected with this organism, and therefore is frequently used in diagnostic work. A generalized, fatal disease develops in which the most striking lesions are multiple necrotic areas in the liver and spleen. Great care must be taken when working with this disease, for many laboratory workers have contracted the infection (18). The organism is capable of entering the unbroken skin.

Immunity. One attack of tularemia gives a very solid and lasting immunity. Individuals who have suffered from the disease develop agglutinins that persist for long periods—sometimes for many years after all symptoms have disappeared. These agglutinins will react with *Brucella abortus*, and *Brucella* agglutinins will react with the organism of tularemia. The titer for the homologous organism is usually very much higher than it is for the heterologous; hence if both organisms are tested it is simple to judge which is specific.

Foshay *et al.* (10) prepared a vaccine from *F. tularensis* by oxidizing the bacterial growth in the presence of aqueous sodium nitrite and acetic acid. After 4 hours' treatment the bacteria were washed free of the acid and salts, phenolized, and standardized. This vaccine proved valuable in protecting against tularemia. Live avirulent vaccines have also been recommended for use (7, 30).

Chemotherapy. It is reported that the sulfonamides and penicillin have little effect on the course of tularemia infection. Streptomycin is very effective in treating this disease (8, 17, 26). Woodward *et al.* (33) indicate that Aureomycin also is useful in curing tularemia, and oxytetracycline has been used successfully by Frank and Meinershagen (13) in treating sheep.

REFERENCES

1. Allred, Stagg, and Lavender. Jour. Inf. Dis., 1956, *99*, 143.
2. Bell, Owen, Jellison, Moore, and Buker. Am. Jour. Vet. Res., 1962, *23*, 884.
3. Bell, Wikel, Hawkins, and Owen. Can. Jour. Comp. Med., 1978, *42*, 310.
4. Burgdorfer and Owen. Jour. Inf. Dis., 1956, *98*, 67.
5. Burroughs, Holdenried, Longanecker, and Meyer. Jour. Inf. Dis., 1945, *76*, 115.
6. Calhoun. Am. Jour. Trop. Med. and Hyg., 1954, *3*, 360.
7. Chamberlain. Appl. Microbiol., 1965, *13*, 232.
8. Chapman, Coriell, Kawol, Nelson, and Downs. Jour. Bact., 1946, *51*, 607.
9. Editorial. Pub. Health Rpts. (U.S.), 1940, *55*, 227.
10. Foshay, Hesselbrock, Wittenberg, and Rodenberg. Am. Jour. Pub. Health, 1942, *32*, 1131.
11. Francis. Jour. Am. Med. Assoc., 1922, *78*, 1015.
12. Francis. Pub. Health Rpts. (U.S.), 1923, *38*, 1396.
13. Frank and Meinershagen. Vet. Med., 1961, *56*, 374.
14. Henson, Gorham, and Shen. Cornell Vet., 1978, *68*, 78.
15. Hillman and Morgan. Jour. Am. Med. Assoc., 1937, *108*, 538.
16. Hopla. Am. Jour. Hyg., 1955, *61*, 371.

17. Howe, Coriell, Bookwalter, and Ellingson. Jour. Am. Med. Assoc., 1946, *132,* 195.
18. Lake and Francis. Pub. Health Rpts. (U.S.), 1922, *37,* 392.
19. Lundgren, Marchette, and Smart. Jour. Inf. Dis., 1957, *101,* 154.
20. McCahan, Moody, and Hayes. Am. Jour. Hyg., 1962, *75,* 335.
21. McCoy. U.S. Pub. Health Service Bull. 43, 1911.
22. McCoy and Chapin. Jour. Inf. Dis., 1912, *10,* 61.
23. Merrell and Wright. Jour. Wildlife Dis., 1978, *14,* 471.
24. Nikanorov. Abstract, Jour. Am. Med. Assoc., 1929, *93,* 696.
25. Parker and Dade. Jour. Am. Vet. Med. Assoc., 1929, *75,* 173.
26. Peterson and Parker. Pub. Health Rpts. (U.S.), 1946, *61,* 1231.
27. Price. Am. Jour. Hyg., 1956, *63,* 186.
28. Ryff, Michael, and Norton. Jour. Am. Vet. Med. Assoc., 1961, *138,* 309.
29. Thorpe, Sidwell, Johnson, Smart, and Parker. Am. Jour. Trop. Med. and Hyg., 1965, *14,* 622.
30. Tulis, Eigelsbach, and Hornick. Proc. Soc. Exp. Biol. and Med., 1969, *132,* 893.
31. Washburn and Tuohy. South. Med. Jour., 1949, *42,* 60.
32. Wherry and Lamb. Jour. Inf. Dis., 1914, *15,* 331.
33. Woodward, Ravy, Eppes, Holbrook, and Hightower. Jour. Am. Med. Assoc., 1949, *139,* 830.

14 The Genus *Brucella*

Within this genus are three closely related species that have been recognized for many years. They are *Brucella abortus*, *B. suis*, and *B. melitensis*. Two more species that possess characteristics much like those of *B. suis*—*B. canis* and *B. neotomae*—have now been established, and a sixth, *B. ovis*, whose relationship is less clear, has been included.

This important group causes *brucellosis* in domestic animals and man. After infection bacteremia is usually followed by localization of the bacteria in reticuloendothelial tissues, reproductive organs, and, less frequently, bones and joints. In cattle, sheep, and goats, lesions of the female reproductive tract may lead to the death of the fetus and its expulsion, thereby causing severe economic loss. The *Brucella* may also cause lesions in the male reproductive tract in cattle, sheep, goats, and dogs, as well as bursitis in the horse. Various wild animals have been identified as carriers of brucellae and in certain circumstances act as sources of infection for domesticated animals and man. Apart from the havoc that brucellosis can wreak on domesticated animals, it can be transmitted readily from animals to man and represents a real occupational hazard for veterinarians, slaughtermen, and farmers. In man, the chronic form of the disease can be particularly debilitating; it is characterized by intermittent chills and fever, or undulating fever, joint and muscle pain, and general malaise.

The first member of the genus *Brucella* was isolated in 1887 by David Bruce from the spleens of patients who died of Mediterranean fever. The organism was named *Brucella melitensis*. Ten years later a Danish veterinarian, Fredrick Bang, isolated a similar organism from an aborted bovine fetus and named it *Bacillus* (*Brucella*) *abortus*. The third major member, *Brucella suis*, was isolated in 1914 from an aborted porcine fetus. *Brucella ovis* and *B. canis* are relative newcomers, having been described within the past 25 years in Australia and America.

Differentiation of the Brucellae

Morphological and cultural features are not sufficiently characteristic to differentiate the six species of the genus *Brucella* and their various biotypes. Nor can the host from which the organism is isolated be entirely relied upon for identification, although each species does have a principal host, as presented in Table 14.1.

Having isolated a Gram-negative rod from a suspected case of brucellosis, one has to rely on the results of the series of laboratory tests outlined in Table 14.3 before final identification of the *Brucella* species and biotype can be made.

Gaseous Requirements. Strains of both *B. abortus* and *B. ovis* require an increased CO_2 tension to initiate growth on primary isolation. The other species do not have this requirement.

Biochemical Reactions. *B. abortus*, *B. suis* (3), and *B. neotomae* usually produce H_2S; the other species do not. *B. neotomae* and *B. ovis* do not produce oxidase; the others do. *B. ovis* is the only species that does not reduce nitrate.

Table 14.1. The species of *Brucella* and their principal hosts

Host	Principal pathogenic *Brucella* sp. isolated	Other pathogenic *Brucella* sp. isolated
Cattle	*B. abortus*	*B. melitensis* *B. suis*
Sheep	*B. melitensis* *B. ovis* (epididymitis)	*B. abortus*
Goat	*B. melitensis*	*B. abortus*
Horse	*B. abortus*	*B. suis*
Pig	*B. suis*	*B. melitensis* *B. abortus*
Dog	*B. canis*	*B. abortus* *B. melitensis* *B. suis*
Wood rat	*B. neotome*	
Human	*B. abortus* *B. melitensis* *B. suis*	*B. canis*

B. suis (9), *B. canis,* and *B. neotomae* are most active in urease production, while *B. ovis* is negative (5).

Dye Bacteriostasis. Huddleson (2), in 1928, devised a reasonably reliable system of differentiation by means of dyes. The dyes were added to a liver infusion agar. Basic fuchsin and thionin (certified dyes only) were used in final dilutions of 1:50,000. On these dye media, *B. melitensis* and *B. ovis* are not appreciably inhibited. *B. suis, B. canis,* and *B. neotomae* grow more readily on the thionin medium and *B. abortus* on the basic fuchsin. The scheme of separation is shown in Table 14.2.

These dyes are now normally used in graded concentrations of 10, 20, and 50 micrograms of dye per milliliter of medium (see Table 14.3). A plate of medium without dye is included as a control (7).

Bacteriophage Lysogeny. The Tbilisi (Tb) strain of bacteriophage is the reference strain used for typing brucella cultures. At the routine test dilution (RTD), which is the highest dilution of phage causing complete lysis of susceptible strains, this phage types only members of the species *B. abortus* and then only when they are of smooth or smooth-intermediate colony morphology (1). When the dose of phage is increased substantially, this phage will also type some biotypes of *B. suis* and *B. neotome* (see Table 14.3). The World Health Organization strains of *B. abortus* Strain 544 or *B. abortus* Strain 19 are used as propagating host organisms for this phage (4). Lysis by phage is particularly useful for the identification of *B. abortus* and is used in laboratories routinely faced with the identification of this species.

Table 14.2. Growth of *Brucella* sp. in dye media

Strain	Basic fuchsin	Thionin
B. abortus	+	−
B. suis	±	+
B. canis	±	+
B. neotomae	−	±
B. melitensis	+	+
B. ovis	+	+

+ = Good growth. ± = Slight growth. − = No growth.

Agglutination by Monospecific Serum. Smooth strains of *B. abortus, B. suis,* and *B. melitensis* possess two named antigens, A and M, present in different proportions. In *B. abortus,* A antigen predominates and in *B. melitensis,* M predominates. By cross-absorption, monospecific antisera are useful in the identification of species and biotypes of the genus as indicated in Table 14.3.

Substrate Oxidation. If a strain is not identified using the above tests, then it is sent to a reference laboratory where its ability to metabolize substrates by oxidation is determined. Using a Warburg respirometer to measure the isolate's ability to metabolize various amino acids and carbohydrates, one can ascertain the patterns of its oxidative metabolism and by comparison determine the identity of the species in question (see Table 14.3) (6, 8).

REFERENCES

1. Cottral, George E. (ed.) Manual of standardized methods for veterinary microbiology. Cornell Univ. Press, Ithaca, N.Y., 1978, p. 399.
2. Huddleson. Mich. Agr. Exp. Sta. Tech. Bull. 100, 1929.
3. Huddleson and Abell. Jour. Bact., 1927, *13,* 13.
4. Joint FAH/WHO Export Committee on Brucellosis. WHO Tech. Rpt. Ser. 289, World Health Org., Geneva, 1969, p. 9.
5. Jones, Zanardi, Leong, and Wilson. Jour. Bact., 1968, *95,* 625.
6. Meyer. Jour. Bact., 1961, *82,* 950.
7. Meyer. Adv. Vet. Sci., 1974, *18,* 231.
8. Meyer and Cameron. Jour. Bact., 1961, *82,* 387.
9. Pacheco and DeMello. Jour. Bact., 1950, *59,* 689.

Brucella abortus

SYNONYMS: *Bacillus abortus,* Bang's bacillus

Although *B. melitensis* is the type species of the genus, *B. abortus* is of major significance because of its widespread distribution and its ability to produce brucellosis in cattle. This disease is characterized by abortion in sexually mature cows and is thus an important cause of economic loss to the cattle industry around the world. The organism also infects the male reproductive organs and has been found to be associated with hygroma of the knee in cattle.

Cattle are the main reservoir for *B. abortus*, but it is also found in other species. In horses, *B. abortus* has been implicated in inflammations of the bursae located between the two attachments of the ligamentum nuchae. In fact, Roderick *et al.* (46) have shown that the injection of either *B. abortus* or *B. suis* in combination with *Actinomyces bovis* results in the conditions generally known as *fistula of the withers* and *poll evil*. *B. abortus* has been reported in sheep (32) and has been isolated from the uterine contents of aborting mares, from an aborted donkey (12), and from an aborted human fetus (8). However, it apparently does not play an important role in abortions in these species. It has appeared infrequently in chickens and dogs, in rare cases has caused canine abortion, and it has been isolated from the submaxillary lymph nodes of swine slaughtered in a packing plant (36). *B. abortus* has been described in bison, elk, and moose in Canada (10) and in a wide variety of free-living animals, including hares, foxes, reindeer, yaks, cows, rats, and mice, in various parts of the world.

In man, *B. abortus* causes a disease known as *brucellosis* or *undulant fever*, but it is not the only cause of this malady; some cases are caused by *B. suis*, *B. melitensis*, and *B. canis*.

Morphology, Staining Reactions, and Cultural Features. *B. abortus* is a short rod, or a coccobacillus, measuring 0.5 to 0.7 μm by 0.6 to 1.5 μm. The rods are frequently so short as to be easily mistaken for cocci. They are usually arranged singly, although in cultures short chains may form. Because it is a facultative intracellular bacterium, *B. abortus* is frequently found in clumps in smears made from exudates. *B. abortus* is Gram-negative and stains with ordinary stains although with some difficulty. It is not acid-fast but can resist decolorization with some mild acids; this properly provides the basis for some differential staining procedures.

It is nonmotile, does not form spores, and does not have a well-developed capsule, although poorly developed capsules have been demonstrated on freshly isolated strains using special stains.

Successful cultivation of *B. abortus* requires considerable care as it grows slowly and initially produces small colonies. It also needs increased tensions of CO_2 for primary isolation and is fastidious in its nutrient requirements. Various solid media with a beef, veal, or potato base are suitable for growing *B. abortus*. To this base 5 to 10 percent serum or blood must be added, and these must not contain anti-*Brucella* antibodies.

Tryptose agar, Albimi agar, and trypticase-soy agar have all been found to produce satisfactory growth when duly enriched with blood or serum. Growth is slow, the colonies being barely visible after 2 days and reaching maximum size only after 5 to 7 days. The isolates may be of the smooth type, characterized by round convex colonies with an entire edge, or they may dissociate to the rough type, characterized by large flat colonies with a dull granular appearance.

B. abortus is nonhemolytic. It is aerobic but it requires that 5 to 10 percent CO_2 be added to the air for initial isolation. Thus all isolations, whether in broth or on solid media, should be incubated in an incubator or in jars containing an atmosphere of 10 percent CO_2.

The organism grows rather scantily in fluid media, producing a faint clouding. Carbohydrates are not fermented and gelatin is not liquefied. The main biochemical characteristics of *B. abortus* are presented in Table 14.3, where they are compared with other members of the genus *Brucella*. Six species are recognized by the Subcommittee on Taxonomy of the Genus *Brucella*. Within the species *B. abortus* are nine biotypes segregated on the basis of conventional bacteriological methods (38). The recognition of such biotypes allows additional breakdown of the species, a useful device for epidemiological and other purposes.

Resistance. Apart from the risk of direct contact with infected animals, both man and animals can be infected indirectly. This raises practical questions concerning the resistance of *B. abortus*, located outside infected animals, to various environmental conditions. Table 14.4 summarizes studies on the survival times of *B. abortus* under different conditions. *B. abortus* is not very resistant to sunlight and drying. It survives better in winter than in summer, especially when protected from sunlight and drying by various means, for example under leaves or in a carcass.

The organism also survives in milk and dairy products (see Table 14.4), providing a source of infection for calves and humans. Fortunately, it is destroyed by pasteurization (5) and disinfectants.

Epidemiology and Pathogenesis. Despite a vigorous contemporary interest in brucellosis and worldwide research on some aspects of the disease, notably diagnosis and vaccination, there is still a dearth of information on the epidemiology of the condition. The disease can be

Table 14.3. Classification scheme for species and biotypes within the genus *Brucella*

				Growth on dyes							Agglutination by				
				Thionin			Fuchsin		Lysis by phage		Mono-specific sera				
Species	Biotype	CO_2 for growth	H_2S produced	10[a]	20	50	10	20	Routine test dilution (RTD)	$10^4 \times$ RTD	A	M	Anti-rough sera	L-Alanine	L-Asparagin
B. abortus	1	+,−	+	−	−	−	+	+	+	+	+	−	−	+	+
	2	+	+	−	−	−	−	−	+	+	+	−	−		
	3	+,−	+	+	+	−	+	+	+	+	+	−	−		
	4	+,−	+	−	−	−	+	+	+	+	−	+	−		
	5	−	−	+	+	−	+	+	+	+	−	+	−		
	6	−	−,+	+	+	−	+	+	+	+	+	−	−		
	7	−	−,+	+	+	−	+	+	+	+	+	+	−		
	8	+	−	+	+	−	+	+	+	+	−	+	−		
	9	−,+	+	+	+	−	+	+	+	+	−	+	−		
B. suis	1	−	+	+	+	+	−	−	−	+	+	−	−	+,−	−
	2	−	+,−	+	−	−	−	−	−	+	+	−	−	−	+,−
	3	−	−	+	+	+	+	+	−	+	+	−	−	+,−	−
	4	−	−	+	+	+	+	+	−	+	+	+	−	−	−
	5	−	+	+	−	−	+	−	−	−	−	−	+	+	+
B. melitensis	1	−	−	+	+	−	+	+	−	−	−	+	−	+	+
	2	−	−	+	+	−	+	+	−	−	+	−	−		
	3	−	−	+	+	−	+	+	−	−	+	+	−		
B. neotomae		−	+	+	−	−	−	−	−	+	+	−	−	+,−	+
B. ovis		+	−	+	+	−	+	+	−	−	−	−	+	+,−	+
B. canis		−	−	+	+	+	+	−	−	−	−	−	+	+	−

[a] Micrograms of dye per milliliter of medium.
[b] + = utilization rate above (QO_2N) rate of 50; − = no utilization; +,− = strain variability within species.
From Margaret E. Meyer, *Adv. Vet. Sci.*, 1974, *18*, 231.

considered worldwide in distribution although it has not been reported in every country. In the United States, cattle are the primary reservoir of infection, and this is probably true of other countries. *B. abortus* also infects sheep, goats, horses, and birds, but there is little direct evidence of substantial spread between species. Evidence of *Brucella* infection is found in several species of free-living animals, for example, bison, moose, and elk, in North America. Comingling of these species with cattle enhances the possibility of cross-infection, but there is no evidence that this represents a substantial source of infection for domesticated animals. In Africa, Thinn and Nauwerk (51) found large-scale involvement of game animals in the epizootiology of bovine brucellosis.

The primary source of interherd spread in cattle is an infected animal, whether recently exposed or a chronic carrier, which is introduced into or has contact with a susceptible herd. Such an animal sooner or later excretes *B. abortus* in its genital secretions after abortion or calving or in its milk or colostrum, providing a readily available source of infection for calves and adult cattle in the herd. In addition, calves of infected dams can become infected *in utero* (17, 42), bulls can transmit it by natural service, and it can be spread by artificial insemination of infected semen (4). Kerr and Rankin in 1959 (29) showed that the disease could be transmitted experimentally from udder to udder by a contaminated milking machine. These, however, are not major means of transmission of brucellosis in cattle under natural conditions.

The main portals of entry are the oral mucosa of calves drinking infected milk, the nasopharanyx and conjunctivae of cattle exposed to the organism, and occasionally the genital tract in both bulls and cows. Under experimental conditions the organism has been shown to penetrate the unbroken skin of guinea pigs (22) and cattle (11). After penetration of the host, *B. abortus* initially

Substrate oxidation[b]									
L-Glutamate	DL-Ornithine	DL-Citrulline	L-Arginine	L-Lysine	L-Arabinose	D-Galactose	D-Ribose	D-Glucose	i-Erythritol
−	−	−	+	+	+	+	+	+	+
		All *B. abortus* biotypes are identical							
−	+	+	+	+	+	+	+	+	+
+	+	+	+	+	+	+, −	+	+	+
+, −	+	+	+	+	−	−	+	+	+
+, −	+	+	+	+	−	−	+	+	+
+	+	+	+	+, −	−	+, −	+	+	+
+	−	−	−	−	−	−	−	+	−
+	−	−	−	+	+	+	+, −	+	+
+	−	−	−	−	−	−	−	−	−
−	+	+	+	+	+	+	+, −	+	+, −

localizes in the regional lymph node and then becomes generalized in the host's tissues. There it continues to develop in lymphoreticular tissue, producing a generalized infection which is not restricted to the udder, uterus, and associated nodes, although these organs do contain large numbers of bacteria and are prime sites for bacterial isolation.

B. abortus is a facultative intracellular bacterium and can survive and grow in host macrophages and epithelial cells. Smooth strains of the organism are more likely than rough strains to produce disease in both cows and bulls. It is thought that virulent strains have a protective outer protein coat, allowing them to survive intracellularly and to produce chronic generalized infection. This capacity permits the organism to evade the host's immune mechanisms and to survive for long periods. The organism therefore is able to await conditions conducive to proliferation, when it produces definitive clinical signs. Abortions in cows and epididymitis in bulls are the most obvious clinical signs of brucellosis. Preoccupation with abortion has led to an extensive search for the pathogenesis of the genital lesions and to some lack of appreciation for the generalized nature of the disease. Keppie *et al.* (27) demonstrated that the sugar alcohol erythritol was a powerful growth stimulant of *B. abortus* and that susceptible species such as cattle, sheep, goats, and pigs have much higher levels of erythritol in the placenta than brucellosis-resistant species such as man, rabbits, rats, and guinea pigs. The male genitalia of susceptible species also contain erythritol, accounting for the localization of infections in the male testes.

B. abortus preferentially utilizes *erythritol* over glucose, and the presence of erythritol in these tissues accounts, at least in part, for the massive proliferation of the organism in the genital tract of the male and the pregnant female (47, 53). *B. abortus* penetrates the

Table 14.4. Survival times of *B. abortus* under various environmental conditions

Medium	Temperature or season	Environmental conditions	Survival time (days)	Reference
Uterine exudate	February	Placed on ground	10	Cotton. Jour. Am. Vet. Med. Assoc., 1919, *55*, 504.
Placenta, fetal organs	Winter and spring	Covered with leaves in forest	135	Cotton. Jour. Am. Vet. Med. Assoc., 1919, *55*, 504.
Milk	15 C	Milk samples from infected cows	38	Huddelson, Hasley, and Torrey. Jour. Inf. Dis., 1927, *40*, 352.
Butter			142	Carpenter and Boak. Am. Jour. Pub. Health, 1928, *18*, 743.
Cheese	4.4 C		180	Gilman, Dahlberg, and Marquardt. Jour. Dairy Sci., 1946, *29*, 71.
Grass	10–70 F, February	0.6 in. rain	6	Ky. Agr. Exp. Sta. Bull. 43, 1931, p. 14.
	60–81 F, May	Sunny	<1	Ky. Agr. Exp. Sta. Bull. 43, 1931, p. 14.
	36–70 F, November		5	Ky. Agr. Exp. Sta. Bull. 43, 1931, p. 14.
Open plate cultures	October and November	Sunny	2–3	Ky. Agr. Exp. Sta. Bull. 43, 1931, p. 14.
Water	−40 C		800	Kuzdas and Morse. Cornell Vet., 1954, *44*, 216.
	37 C, 25 C, 8 C		57	
Infected guinea pig carcass	January (Wisconsin)	Placed on ground	44	Kuzdas and Morse. Cornell Vet., 1954, *44*, 216.
	June and August (Wisconsin)	Placed on ground	1	Kuzdas and Morse. Cornell Vet., 1954, *44*, 216.
	January (Wisconsin)	Buried	29	Kuzdas and Morse. Cornell Vet., 1954, *44*, 216.
Meat and salted meat	0–20 C		65	Prost. Ann. Univ. Marie Curie—Sklodowska, Lublin, Poland, 1957, *12*, 163.
Manure pit	158 F	In tubes at bottom of pit	<4 hours	King. Jour. Am. Vet. Med. Assoc., 1957, *131*, 349.
Manure pit		In tubes at top of pit	2	King. Jour. Am. Vet. Med. Assoc., 1957, *131*, 349.
In manure	12 C		250	Plommet. Anns. Recher. Vet., 1972, *3*, 621.

epithelial cells of the chorion and proliferates, producing a placentitis. An endometritis is produced with ulceration of the epithelial lining of the uterus. Lesions of the fetus include edema and congestion of the lungs along with hemorrhages of the epicardium and splenic capsule. Fetal death follows, and it is unclear whether this is attributable to the endotoxin of *B. abortus* or to interference with placental function. The presence of the organism induces an inflammation of the membranes; this interference with the circulation of the fetus may explain why abortion occurs. The fetus usually shows a dropsical condition, a fact which also points toward a circulatory disturbance. The organism may also be found, generally in pure culture, in the alimentary tract and in the lungs of aborted fetuses. The other tissues of the fetus usually are sterile. The location of the organism suggests that it is taken into the fetus by the swallowing of the amniotic fluid rather than through the bloodstream.

After calving or abortion, the organism does not usually persist long in the uterus. It may be recognized for a few days but later it seems to disappear. The presence of large amounts of erythritol in the pregnant uterus and its marked diminution after calving in the nongravid uterus may well explain this disappearance. Apart from the pregnant uterus and adjacent lymph nodes, the organism is frequently recognized in the udder. The organism survives in the reticuloendothelial system and the udder from one gestation period to the next. The infected udders cannot be detected clinically, but the organism may be isolated by inoculating the milk into guinea pigs. Experience has shown that nonpregnant animals which have high agglutinin titers toward antigens made from *B. abortus* usually have one or more infected quarters in their udders. Such animals usually are carriers for life, though a few are able to throw off the organism. Udder infection with members of the genus *Brucella* has considerable public health significance because organisms are discharged in the milk.

B. abortus may occasionally be isolated from the lymph nodes of the digestive tract and from the spleens of cattle. No lesions may be recognized in these organs, although *B. abortus* may be isolated occasionally from the bloodstream and from hygromas of the knee joints of cattle. In bulls, infection of the epididymis and testicle sometimes occurs. In these cases abscessation usually develops and the organs are destroyed. On the other hand, Rankin (43) has declared that bulls may become infected in calfhood and retain this condition into adult life, but are rarely responsible for the spread of disease to cows during natural service and that brucellosis is not an important cause of infertility in bulls.

When calves are fed upon infected milk, the organism can be found in the lymph glands of the digestive canal, but it generally disappears within a few weeks after the infected milk is withdrawn. Until sexual maturity is reached the genital organs seldom become involved.

B. abortus can infect horses but with much less frequency than cattle. In the horse, it frequently localizes in bursae, joints, or tendon sheaths and has been found in poll evil and fistulous withers, supra-atlantal bursitis, and supraspinous bursitis (46), as well as in lesions of the fetlock and sternum (52). It can also infect sheep (32), goats (16), and pigs (36) but much less frequently than other species of *Brucella*.

Immunity. Calves infected *in utero* or soon after birth ordinarily remain infected only for a short time unless they are raised on infected milk or kept in the presence of the infection. Within several weeks from the time they are removed from the presence of the infection, they usually free themselves of it and develop into uninfected cattle. There is evidence that calves infected with *B. abortus* at 7 months of age may become infected permanently (40), but serious disease does not usually appear until the animal reaches puberty, becomes pregnant, and the udder begins to function.

Adult animals that have never been in the presence of the organism are the most easily infected and the most likely to abort when infected. An animal that has aborted once or has been infected once as an adult, even though it may not have aborted, is not so readily infected a second time. A degree of immunity develops, therefore, as a result of the disease that has been overcome. This immunity frequently is not sufficient to prevent a second abortion, or even a third or a fourth. As a rule, most animals, after one or two abortions, will thereafter carry their calves to full term even though they may remain infected.

B. abortus is a facultative intracellular parasite similar in this respect to *Listeria monocytogenes* and *Mycobacterium tuberculosis*. Mackaness (33) demonstrated that resistance to *Listeria* was dependent, not upon antibodies, but upon the presence of specific lymphocytes which could activate macrophages and destroy the intracellular *Listeria*. It is now believed that immunity to *B. abortus* is dependent upon cell-mediated immunity; this is supported by the fact that passive transfer of immunoglobulin does not confer immunity and immune macrophages can produce a gradual fall in the number of organisms in the host. Fitzgeorge *et al.* (18) demonstrated that *B.*

abortus multiplied more slowly in the macrophages of vaccinated calves than in control animals, while Cunningham and O'Reilly (15) concluded that the presence of antibodies was a good indicator of infection. The presence of antibodies was, however, a poor indicator of the immune status of the host. Significant studies (26, 49, 50) have recently been published to substantiate the role of cell-mediated immunity in protecting the host against *B. abortus*. Specific T lymphocytes respond to *B. abortus* antigens and produce lymphokines, which in turn activate macrophages to the point where they can overcome the intracellular bacteria.

The search for an attenuated strain of *B. abortus* that would satisfactorily immunize cattle without having the undesirable effects of virulent strains has gone on for many years. The first success in this search came in 1930 when Buck (7) announced his *Strain 19*. A second was announced by McEwen and Priestley (37) in England when they described their *45/20 Strain*. A third is the *Mucoid ("M") Vaccine* of Huddleson (23).

Strain 19 Brucella abortus *vaccine*. This vaccine consists of a viable culture of a strain that was discovered to have practically no virulence for guinea pigs and cattle but to possess excellent immunizing properties. The strain has great stability; many deliberate attempts to change its virulence have failed, and it appears to have approximately the same properties now that it had in 1930.

Strain 19 is a smooth strain of *B. abortus*. It is not entirely lacking in virulence. Guinea pigs can be infected with it, but the lesions are minimal or absent and the organism eventually disappears from the tissues, leaving no recognizable lesions. Pregnant cattle can be made to abort by inoculating them with large doses of Strain 19. In these cases the vaccine organism can usually be demonstrated without difficulty in the fetal membranes and the fetus itself. Susceptible cattle, associating with those that have aborted as a result of inoculation with the vaccine strain, do not become infected. Much experience has shown that Strain 19 is never transmitted from one animal to another; that if any damage is done by the use of this vaccine, it is limited to the animal injected. Strain 19 is very rarely eliminated in the milk of vaccinated animals. It is capable of causing infections in man (2, 21, 48), though these usually are mild and result in recovery within a much shorter time than do infections with virulent strains. The vaccine, in view of its dangers for man, should be handled with caution.

The vaccination of calves 3 to 12 months old with Strain 19 is widely practiced in many parts of the world and has done much to reduce the ravages of brucellosis in cattle. Calfhood vaccination results in effective immunity for four or five pregnancies. According to Manthei (34), revaccination does not significantly enhance immunity. The vaccine therefore is administered as a single subcutaneous injection and with few exceptions is tolerated well by calves. It should not be used to vaccinate male calves because it may actually produce brucellosis and thereby affect the fertility of the animal (31). Antibodies can usually be demonstrated after about 10 days, and these increase to a maximum in about 2 to 3 months, after which the blood titers usually decrease. In 90 percent of the animals the titers 12 months later will have receded to a point below the diagnostic level. The immunity conferred by vaccination is not absolute. It is great enough, however, to protect the majority of young breeding animals through their period of greatest susceptibility to the disease.

The vaccination of adult cattle with Strain 19 is a matter over which there has been much controversy. It has been used widely enough to show that there is little danger in its use in adult animals, but it is not recommended for use in cattle in the later stages of pregnancy, although it seldom causes abortions. However, the immunity conferred by Strain 19 on other adult animals is beneficial. The principal and most practical objection to its use in adults is that it produces substantial levels of antibodies in their blood. These antibodies may persist for some time and make differentiation of vaccinated animals from naturally infected ones difficult using the current serological tests.

The McEwen 45/20 vaccine. McEwen and Priestley, working in the British Isles, discovered a rough strain of *B. abortus* that became progressively more pathogenic as it was passed in series in guinea pigs. The passage variant that served as a good immunizing agent, yet was not virulent enough to cause disease in cattle, was designated *45/20*. A rough type, it did not produce agglutinins in animals, and in this respect it had an advantage over Strain 19. It was tested extensively in the field in Great Britain with apparent success. In 1944 the Ministry of Agriculture and Fisheries discontinued further use of this vaccine, explaining that it did not immunize quite so well as Strain 19 and had a tendency to revert to the virulent form. Strain 19 is now used for official vaccinating in the British Isles, but a killed 45/20 adjuvant vaccine (K 45/20 A) has been developed and has gained acceptance as a suitable and efficacious alternative (1, 39).

Other vaccines have been examined as potential immunizing agents against *B. abortus*. The "M" vaccine of Huddleson (23), the *B. melitensis* strain H38 of Renoux (45), and recently a variety of soluble substances extracted from the cells of *B. abortus* (20, 35, 44) have all been used but have not yet found widespread acceptance.

Diagnosis. 1. *Clinical Means*. The presence of an infectious abortion may be suspected by clinical observation. There are causes of abortion other than *B. abortus;* therefore, it is not possible, without bacteriological or serological assistance, to be certain that this organism is the cause of the trouble.

2. *Isolation and Identification*. Isolation and recognition of *B. abortus* are often accomplished by direct culture on a basal medium such as tryptose agar or Albimi agar to which serum and selected antibiotics are added. The cultures are incubated at 37 C in an atmosphere of 10 percent CO_2 tension and are examined in 2 to 3 days. Final identification is made on the basis of the characteristics listed in Table 14.3. Serological typing of brucella strains and phage typing using the Tbilisi (Tb) strain of bacteriophage are useful aids to definitive identification of strains, but their use is restricted to specificially equipped reference laboratories.

Specimens should be examined from the following:

(*a*) The aborted fetus. Direct cultures will usually demonstrate *B. abortus* in the stomach content, the intestinal content, or the lung tissue.

(*b*) The placenta. Direct films from the outer surface of the chorion, especially from the margins of the characteristic thickenings, will usually suffice to make a positive diagnosis without the need for cultural methods. The organism occurs free or enclosed in epithelial cells. It is these intracellular organisms that can be recognized with certainty, even though many other bacteria may have invaded the placenta. New fetal membranes may be washed in water and rinsed in saline before attempts are made to culture the organism. After washing, obvious lesions are cut and the cut surface rubbed onto plates of selective media (30).

(*c*) The uterine exudate. After abortion or calving, when the placenta has been infected, *B. abortus* is present in the lochia and may be recognized by guinea pig inoculation. Within a few days, however, the organism seems to disappear and usually cannot be found in the uterus until the animal is again pregnant and reinfection of the organ occurs.

(*d*) Milk. When the udder is infected, *B. abortus* can be readily detected by the intraperitoneal injection of milk into guinea pigs or by direct cultural means.

(*e*) Abscesses. Direct cultures from abscesses of the

testicle and epididymis usually give pure cultures of *B. abortus,* and isolations have been made from hygromas in cattle and from infected bursae in horses. Isolation of *B. abortus* from infected tissue is not always easy, therefore, it is advisable to preserve aliquots for later reculturing, guinea pig inoculation, or serological examination.

3. *Inoculation of Guinea Pigs*. This is the most reliable method of detecting *B. abortus* in infected materials. Macerated tissue or fluid is inoculated into two guinea pigs which are killed 3 and 6 weeks later. Their sera is examined for the presence of antibodies and the following organs are cultured: spleen, liver, regional lymph nodes, and testicles.

4. *Fluorescent-Antibody Staining*. The direct examination of tissues with a fluorescent-antibody preparation can be an aid to diagnosis. This method is particularly useful for examining material that may be contaminated, such as placental membranes, cotyledons, or fetal or vaginal discharges.

5. *Serological Tests*. Both agglutination and complement-fixation tests have been used successfully for diagnosis. The former is as accurate as the latter and much simpler, making it the preferred method. The agglutination test may be conducted with serum, whole blood, vaginal mucus, whey, or milk.

(*a*) *Agglutination tests*. Two methods of conducting the test with blood serum are commonly used. The tube or "slow" method is regarded as the standard procedure, but the plate or "rapid" method, in competent hands, is probably as reliable.

The tube test. Serum is mixed, in small test tubes, with a suspension of a specially selected strain of *B. abortus*. Increasing dilutions of serum are placed in successive tubes beginning with a dilution of 1:50 and doubling the dilution in each successive tube (Figure 14.1). Complete agglutination in dilutions of 1:100 and higher may be considered positive, and lack of agglutination in 1:50, negative. Reactions in dilutions of 1:50 and no higher should be considered suspicious, with final judgment based upon the history of the animal and of the herd in which it has lived. The test should be repeated in 3 weeks; an increase in titer at that time would help clarify the status of a suspicious animal. The titer is dependent upon the concentration of antibody, the antigen concentration, and the test conditions. Clearly, these can be varied; for example, the antigen suspension may be diluted, thus altering the titer determined. Specifying the conditions of the test and the titers determined is

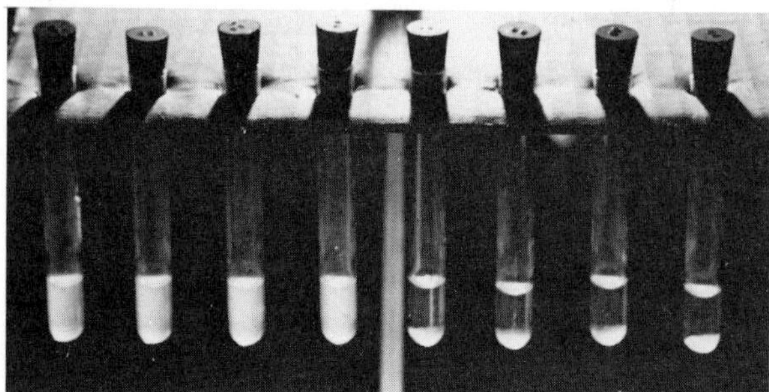

Figure 14.1. The tube agglutination test. Two tests are represented here. The four tubes on the left contain serum dilutions of 1:25, 1:50, 1:100, and 1:200. This serum is negative (devoid of agglutinins), indicated by the fact that the bacteria remain in suspension. The tubes on the right contain the same dilutions of a strongly positive serum, indicated by the fact that the bacteria have flocculated and settled to the bottom, leaving the fluid perfectly clear.

necessary. Whether the titer is described as positive or negative will vary, depending on the conditions of the test. In Britain, for example, a titer of at least 50 percent agglutination at 1:40 is considered positive.

The widespread practice of calfhood vaccination with Strain 19 has caused some modification of these interpretations. High titers persist in a few of these calves for years and such vaccinated animals are indistinguishable from animals currently infected with virulent field strains of *B. abortus*.

The plate or rapid test. The antigen for this test is a very heavy suspension of strains of *B. abortus* stained with gentian violet and brilliant green to make the test easier to read. The antigen is standardized, and should thus give results comparable to those of the tube method. Serum, whole blood, or whey may be used in this test. The test is done on a glass slide or plate and the reactions can be read in several minutes (Figures 14.2, 14.3). A fair degree of accuracy can be obtained by using whole blood instead of serum. The whole-blood method is often used for testing range cattle when it is desirable to hold the animals in chutes until the results are known. A drop of blood is collected on a glass slide from an incision in the end of the tail. A drop of antigen is mixed with the blood and the results are obtained in a few minutes.

The ring test. This agglutination test is done with milk. It was introduced in Germany in 1937 by Fleischhauer (19), who called it the *ABR* (Abortus, Bang-Ring) *test*. Used extensively in some of the Scandinavian

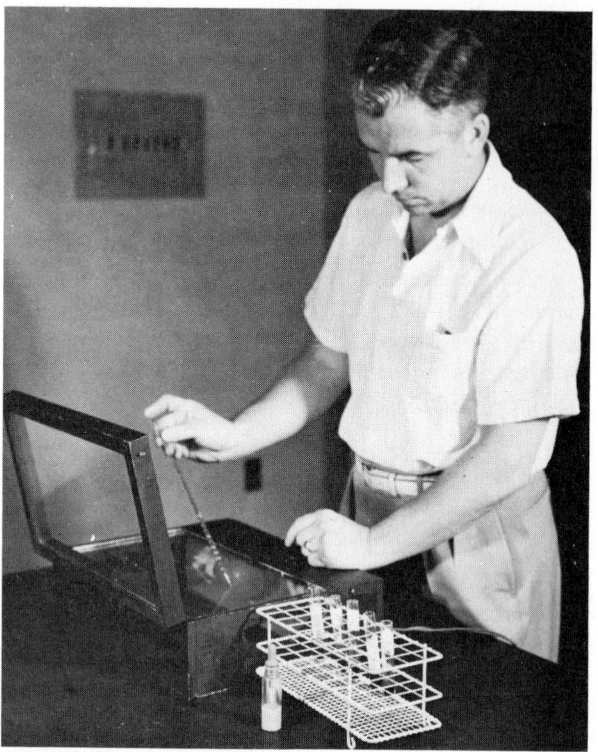

Figure 14.2. The rapid or plate agglutination test. This test may be carried out on an ordinary microslide or a piece of window glass. If many are conducted, it is convenient to use a special box, such as the one depicted here. It is made of wood, painted black inside and out. A portion of the top consists of a glass plate, marked into squares. The serum and antigen dilutions are made on this plate. A hinged cover can be closed over the tests to reduce the evaporation of fluid from the serum-antigen mixtures. An electric lamp on one side of the interior of the box provides oblique illumination, which facilitates reading of the tests; it also provides warmth, which hastens the reactions.

countries (6), it has also been widely adopted in the United States, especially for survey purposes.

The antigen most commonly used is a heavy suspension of *B. abortus* stained with hematoxylin. It is mixed with fresh milk in a tube in the proportion of one drop to each milliliter of milk. The mixture is then incubated in a water bath at 37 C for a period of 30 to 60 minutes.

The ring test depends upon the fact that clumps of agglutinated organisms are carried to the surface by the rising fat globules, whereas the unagglutinated ones are not so affected. A negative test is indicated by a column of milk of a bluish color—approximately the same color as before incubation—capped by a cream layer that is uncolored. A strongly positive test is indicated by a decolorized milk column capped by a bluish-violet cream

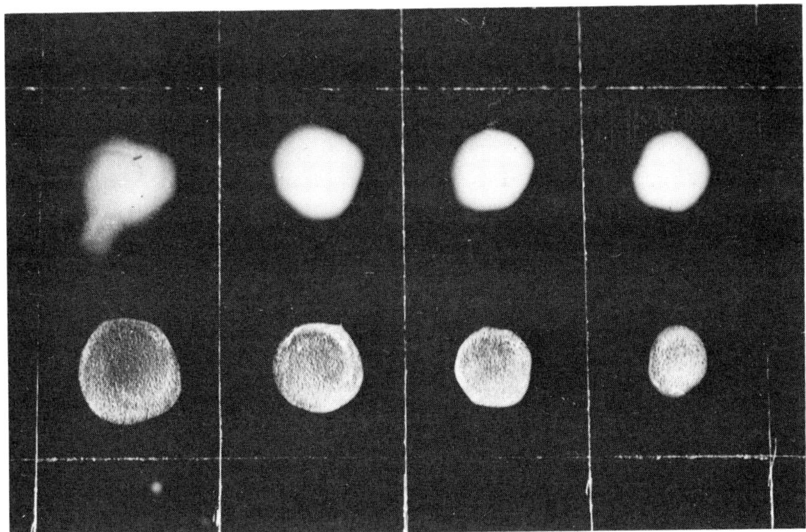

Figure 14.3. The rapid or plate agglutination test. Two tests are depicted, four dilutions of serum being tested in each case. These correspond to dilutions of 1:25, 1:50, 1:100, and 1:200, reading from left to right. The sample above is negative; the one below is positive in all dilutions.

layer. Intermediate reactions are indicated by slightly colored cream layers with incomplete decolorization of the milk.

This test often fails in samples from individual cows, especially when the percentage of fat is low and when the milk is thickened by mastitis or by decreased glandular activity. It cannot be done with colostrum or with skimmed or homogenized milk. Best adapted for composite or pooled milk samples, the test can be used on bulk sampled at milk-collecting stations in order to screen whole herds or areas quickly and economically. For this purpose it is more sensitive in detecting brucellosis than agglutination tests with whey, because dilution does not affect it as much. Not all cows are in milk production at any given time so ring tests should be made at 6-month intervals, or more often. Herds showing evidence of brucellosis are then blood-tested to identify the individual reactors so that they can be removed.

The Rose Bengal test. The Rose Bengal plate test is a rapid slide agglutination test in which the antigen consists of *B. abortus* stained with Rose Bengal. The test is rapid and cheap. It provides results comparable to the tube-agglutination and complement-fixation tests, and it gives negative reactions sooner in vaccinated calves, an advantage in distinguishing vaccinated from infected animals.

(*b*) *The card test.* In 1967, Nicoletti (41) recommended the use of the card test as a rapid, sensitive, and accurate means of screening for brucellosis, especially in range areas. The antigen is a stained, buffered whole-cell suspension of *B. abortus* strain 1119-3. The antibody source is plasma produced by the use of an anticoagulant and lectins, which produce rapid clumping of erythrocytes and allow rapid extraction of plasma. Only one antigen-plasma or serum dilution is made, and the results are read as positive or negative on this basis.

(*c*) *The complement-fixation test.* The technique of this test varies in different laboratories; in recent years it has been adapted to the microtiter system, requiring small quantities of reactants and allowing the test to be conducted on a large scale. Increasing in use, this test is particularly valuable in detecting chronically infected animals that no longer give a positive reaction in the agglutination test.

6. *Other tests.* A variety of tests have been used for the detection of brucellosis and none is perfect for all circumstances. None of the tests will detect animals recently infected and incubating the disease. Various devices, such as repeat testing, have been used to overcome these problems; however, the search continues for a better serological system which will not be subject to these inadequacies.

In 1967, Kerr *et al.* (28) used the antiglobulin test for the diagnosis of chronic cases of human brucellosis. They found that specific antibodies of the classes IgG and IgA will not cause agglutination of *B. abortus* cells, but will attach to them; subsequent agglutination can be developed using antiimmunoglobulin serum. Cunningham (13, 14) used a similar antiglobulin test to investigate serological responses to Strain 19 and 45/20 vaccines, and more recently Beh and Lascelles (3) found it a potentially useful test for differentiating vaccinated from infected cattle.

Various forms of radioimmunoassay tests (9, 54) and

different methods of performing lymphocyte blastogenesis tests (25, 26, 50) on *Brucella* antigens are presently being investigated. Both systems show promise but must be subjected to the rigors of extensive use in the field before their precise value is known.

Treatment. The organism's widespread distribution in the body and its ability to survive inside cells render present forms of chemotherapy ineffective.

Control. The economic losses from brucellosis have been substantial in the past and together with the hazards posed to human health have prompted many countries to impose national systems for the control and eradication of the disease. Many methods have been used for its control, but the following principles are usually incorporated, depending on local conditions of husbandry and the numbers of animals involved.

(*a*) Affected animals are detected and eliminated from the herd. Detection is usually done by serological methods, using the milk-ring test for rapid herd screening, followed by an agglutination test on each affected animal's serum. Slaughter of the affected animals may follow with indemnity paid by a regulatory agency.

(*b*) The resistance of the remaining animals or any replacements is increased by vaccination.

(*c*) General principles of hygiene are imposed to prevent spread or reintroduction of infection.

In herds that are only lightly infected, blood testing and removal of reactors may be begun immediately. If there is any danger of exposure, it is wise to conduct systematic calf vaccination as a protective measure. In heavily infected herds, in which many valuable animals would have to be removed, the so-called *test-and-slaughter* plan is not logical. In such herds it is best to advise systematic calfhood vaccination with Strain 19. If this is done for several years, clinical evidence of the disease generally disappears within 2 years, and at the end of a 5-year period natural attrition will have eliminated most of the chronically infected cows. Blood testing at this time usually will show few or no reactors, and these may then be eliminated. Calfhood vaccination is maintained in such a herd as long as there is a real danger of exposure to the disease from any source.

REFERENCES

1. Alton. Austral. Vet. Jour., 1978, *54,* 551.
2. Bardenwerper. Jour. Am. Med. Assoc., 1954, *155,* 970.
3. Beh and Lascelles. Res. Vet. Sci., 1973, *14,* 239.
4. Bendixen and Blom. Vet. Jour., 1947, *103,* 337.
5. Boak and Carpenter, Jour. Inf. Dis., 1931, *49,* 142.
6. Bruhn. Am. Jour. Vet. Res., 1948, *9,* 360.
7. Buck. Jour. Agr. Res., 1930, *41,* 667.
8. Carpenter and Boak. Jour. Am. Med. Assoc., 1931, *96,* 1212.
9. Chappel, Williamson, McNaught, Dalling, and Allan. Jour. Hyg. (London), 1976, *77,* 369.
10. Corner and Connell. Can. Jour. Comp. Med. and Vet. Sci., 1958, *22,* 9.
11. Cotton and Buck. Jour. Am. Vet. Med. Assoc., 1932, *80,* 342.
12. Crossman and Borson. Vet. Rec., 1968, *82,* 607.
13. Cunningham. Vet. Rec., 1967, *80,* 527.
14. Cunningham. Vet. Rec., 1971, *88,* 244.
15. Cunningham and O'Reilly. Vet. Rec., 1968, *82,* 678.
16. Doyle. Jour. Comp. Path., 1939, *52,* 89.
17. Fensterbank. Vet. Rec., 1978, *103,* 283.
18. Fitzgeorge, Solotorovsky, and Smith. Brit. Jour. Exp. Path., 1967, *48,* 522.
19. Fleischhauer. Berl. tierärztl. Wchnschr., 1937, *53,* 527.
20. Foster and Ribi. Jour. Bact., 1962, *84,* 258.
21. Gilman. Cornell Vet., 1944, *34,* 193.
22. Hardy, Jordan, Borts, and Hardy. Natl. Inst. Health Bull. 158, 1950.
23. Huddleson. Am. Jour. Vet. Res., 1947, *8,* 374.
24. Huddleson. Mich. Agr. Exp. Sta. Quart. Bull. 31, 1948.
25. Kaneene, Johnson, Anderson, and Muscoplat. Jour. Clin. Microbiol., 1978, *8,* 396.
26. Kaneene, Johnson, Anderson, Angus, Pietz, and Muscoplat. Am. Jour. Vet. Res., 1978, *39,* 585.
27. Keppie, Williams, Witt, and Smith. Brit. Jour. Exp. Path., 1965, *46,* 104.
28. Kerr, Payne, Robertson, and Coombs. Immunology, 1967, *13,* 223.
29. Kerr and Rankin. Vet. Rec., 1959, *71,* 224.
30. Kuzdas and Morse. Jour. Bact., 1953, *66,* 502.
31. Lambert, Deyoe, and Painter. Jour. Am. Vet. Med. Assoc., 1964, *145,* 909.
32. Luchsinger and Anderson. Jour. Am. Vet. Med. Assoc., 1967, *150,* 1017.
33. Mackaness. Jour. Exp. Med., 1962, *116,* 381.
34. Manthei. Jour. Dairy Sci., 1968, *51,* 1115.
35. Markenson, Sulitzeanu, and Olitzki. Brit. Jour. Exp. Path., 1962, *43,* 67.
36. McCullough, Eisele, and Pavelchek. Pub. Health Rpts. (U.S.), 1951, *66,* 205.
37. McEwen and Priestly. Vet. Rec., 1938, *50,* 1097.
38. Meyer. Adv. Vet. Sci., 1974, *18,* 231.
39. Morgan and McDiarmid. Vet. Rec., 1968, *83,* 184.
40. Nagy and Hignett. Res. Vet. Sci., 1967, *8,* 247.
41. Nicoletti. Jour. Am. Vet. Med. Assoc., 1967, *151,* 1778.
42. Plommet, Fensterbank, Renoux, Gestin, and Philippon. Anns. Recher. Vet., 1973, *4,* 419.
43. Rankin. Vet. Rec., 1965, *77,* 132.
44. Rasooly Boros and Gerichter. Israel Jour. Med. Sci., 1968, *4,* 246.
45. Renoux, Alton, and Amarasinghe. Archs. Inst. Pasteur Tunis, 1957, *34,* 3.
46. Roderick, Kimball, McLeod, and Frank. Am. Jour. Vet. Res., 1948, *9,* 5.

47. Smith, Williams, Pearce, Keppie, Harris-Smith, Fitz-George, and Witt. Nature, 1962, *193*, 47.
48. Spink and Thompson. Jour. Am. Med. Assoc., 1953, *153*, 1162.
49. Sukhodoeva and Nugmanova. Zh. Mikrobiol. 1979, *2*, 69. (Vet. Bull., 1979, *49*, no. 7, abs. 3797.)
50. Swiderska, Osuch, and Brzoska. Exp. Med. Microbiol., 1971, *23B*, 133.
51. Thinn and Nauwerk. Zentrbl. f. Vet.-Med., 1974, *21B*, 692.
52. Van der Hoeden. Tijdsch. v. Diergeneesk., 1930, *57*, 15.
53. Williams, Keppie, and Smith. Brit. Jour. Exp. Path., 1962, *43*, 530.
54. Wilson, Thornley, and Coombs. Jour. Med. Microbiol., 1977, *10*, 281.

Brucella suis

SYNONYM: Porcine type of *Brucella*

For some years this organism was thought to be identical with the one found in cattle, although several observers noted that the strain of porcine origin appeared to be more virulent for guinea pigs than the one commonly found in cattle. The lesions in guinea pigs caused by the bovine strain are proliferative in character, whereas those caused by infection with the porcine organism are both proliferative and degenerative; that is, the swine organism commonly produces abscess formation and the bovine does not. The bovine organism usually will not kill the guinea pig, or will do so only after a number of months, whereas the porcine variety will frequently cause death within 2 or 3 weeks. A common occurrence in guinea pigs inoculated with the porcine variety is the formation of abscesses behind the eyeball, causing the eye to protrude from the socket (22). *B. suis,* unlike *B. abortus,* does not require increased levels of CO_2 for its growth, and primary isolations can be made nonsupplemented in ordinary air. *B. suis* has recently been isolated from dogs in Germany. Two of the dogs had orchitis and epididymitis, and three bitches in the same kennel were infected (12).

B. suis has been isolated from wild hares in Denmark (2). They were believed to be the carriers involved in four enzootics of brucellosis in swine. It has also been isolated from three species of rats in Northern Queensland, Australia. The rats were trapped in areas frequented by wild pigs (8). Pregnant cattle exposed to *B. suis* by the intramammary route do not abort but develop severe mastitis, a high blood serum titer, and bacteremia, as indicated by recovery of the organisms from lymph nodes in widely scattered parts of the body (27).

Morphology, Staining Reactions, and Cultural Features. It is impossible to distinguish among the brucellae morphologically. The various characteristics used to differentiate *B. suis* from the other species of the genus are presented in Table 14.3. It will be noted that there are now five biotypes of *B. suis,* and metabolic profiles are used to help identify them. Differences among species of *Brucella* biotypes are often quantitative rather than qualitative, and inclusion of known reference strains in the tests is highly desirable.

Epidemiology and Pathogenesis. Brucellosis of swine occurs in most pig-raising countries. It occurs in the United States, but has not been reported in Canada or Great Britain. Its rate of occurrence in the United States has decreased substantially in recent years, but it still remains a health hazard for pigs and for butchers who process pig carcasses.

When porcine infections were first recognized, it was assumed that swine became infected through association with cattle or by drinking infected cows' milk. It is now known that *B. abortus,* the bovine type, is not highly pathogenic for swine, but that infections sometimes can be induced by feeding swine cows' milk contaminated with this organism (26).

B. suis is transmitted almost exclusively from pig to pig (9), spread by coitus or by the ingestion of feed contaminated by urine or genital excretions from infected sows and boars. Because of the current intensive methods of pig husbandry, spread is rapid in a susceptible herd. An outbreak of the disease is often followed by intermittent cases as susceptible newcomers contact chronically infected pigs.

Upon initial infection, *B. suis* is localized in the regional lymph nodes. There it proliferates and may cause bacteremia before producing generalized infection of the spleen, lymph nodes, joints, udder, and genitalia. As with *B. abortus, B. suis* is a facultative intracellular parasite and owes a great deal of its pathogenic properties to its ability to survive in the host's phagocytic cells. Erythritol has been shown to have a growth-stimulating effect upon *B. suis* and is found in the placenta of the sow and the seminal vesicles of the boar. Keppie *et al.* (19) suggest that the stimulatory action of erythritol on *B. suis* and its presence in these tissues explains the production of lesions in the male and female genital tracts. The clinical signs and lesions produced vary considerably, depending on the animal's age, previous exposure, and the organ or organs involved. The disease may affect suckling and weanling piglets, but it is more common in adults, where it produces abortion, metritis, spondylitis, lameness, and paralysis. Infections that localize in the bodies of the vertebrae (spondylitis), especially of the lumbar and sacral regions, are not uncommon (11). These sometimes are unsuspected and are found only after slaughter. More often signs of posterior paralysis caused by pressure from the necrotic tissue on the spinal cord are seen. According to Anderson and Davis (1), nodular spenitis in swine is associated with brucellosis and in the absence of other lesions justifies a presumptive diagnosis of this disease. Thomsen (24) claims that many cases show no symptoms and no gross lesions.

Brucellosis is an important disease of the reindeer (*Rangifer tarandus*) found in Russia, as well as in Alaska and Canada. *B. suis* biotype 4 has been isolated from infected animals; it causes bursitis, spondylitis, arthritis, and orchitis (7, 15). The same biotype of *B. suis* has been isolated from the larvae of the reindeer warble fly, and there is some speculation that this insect may act as a vector of the disease (25). Biotype 4 has also been isolated from wolves in Siberia and from sled dogs in Alaska fed on infected reindeer meat. This form of brucellosis is of particular interest and significance to the U.S.S.R. because of the large number of free-living reindeer and because of the importance of domesticated reindeer in that country's northern regions.

Immunity. Both field and experimental evidence indicate that swine immunity to brucellosis is very slight and that after a period of herd resistance, animals are again susceptible to the disease. Abortions do not usually occur after the first exposure, but most animals readily contract the disease when reexposed. Because *B. suis* is a facultative intracellular organism, cell-mediated immunity is likely to be important in protecting the host. Cameron *et al.* (6) suggested that the inbreeding of a particular group of Berkshire pigs established a strain of pig resistant to brucellosis, but this proposed genetic resistance has never been exploited. Nor is there a vaccine comparable to *B. abortus* Strain 19 available for protection against *B. suis*. Manthei (21) and Kernkamp and Roepke (20) have shown that Strain 19 does not immunize swine against *B. suis,* nor does it protect cattle against *B. suis* infection. In 1966, Edens and Foster (10) claimed that a vaccine containing endotoxin would produce suppression of infection with *B. suis,* but their claim has not been substantiated.

Diagnosis. Brucellosis in swine may be positively diagnosed by cultural methods and by the agglutination test (18). *B. suis* can readily be isolated from the blood, spleen, uterus, lymph nodes, and other organs of many cases, in addition to the uteruses and mammary glands of sows and the testes and semen of boars. The methods are the same as those used for *B. abortus* except that an increase of the CO_2 tension of the culture jar is unnecessary. The cultural characteristics of *B. suis* are given in Table 14.3.

The agglutination test is used as an aid to diagnosis, but it is not as reliable in swine as it is in cattle. Positive titers do not appear until 2 months after infection; many infected pigs have low titers, and nonspecific reactions occur, producing low titers. Hoerlein (13) claims that incubation of the tubes (standard *B. abortus* antigen is used) at 56 C for 16 hours will eliminate the nonspecific, but not the specific, reactions.

The agglutination test is valuable in determining whether or not infection exists in a herd. Hubbard and Hoerlein (14) consider a herd free of brucellosis if, on two consecutive tests of the entire herd, there are no pigs with titers greater than 1:100. They also suggest that animals in an infected herd with titers of 1:25 or higher be considered infected.

Treatment and Control. The facultative intracellular life style of the organism makes it a formidable subject for therapy. Trials with penicillin (4), streptomycin and sulfadiazine (16), and chlortetracycline (3) have all been fruitless.

In commercial swine herds the simplest way to eradicate the disease is to sell all stock for slaughter as they arrive at the proper age. When this is done, the premises are thoroughly cleaned and disinfected. After they have been kept free of all swine for at least 2 months (longer in winter), they may then be restocked from sources known to be brucellosis-free.

In breeding herds where blood lines must be preserved, Cameron (5) suggested a system endorsed by Hutchings and Washko (17) and Spink *et al.* (23). Pigs are raised from the infected unit. They are weaned at 8 weeks of age and tested individually by the agglutination test. If negative, they are removed from the infected herd, placed on clean ground, and raised in isolation from the main herd. All pigs are tested periodically. Any reactors are immediately removed. When of breeding age, they are bred to noninfected boars. The original herd is disposed of as soon as the replacement unit has grown to sufficient size. This plan is usually successful.

REFERENCES

1. Anderson and Davis. Jour. Am. Vet. Med. Assoc., 1957, *131*, 141.

2. Bendtsen, Christiansen, and Thomsen. Nord. Vetmed., 1956, *8*, 1.
3. Bunnell, Bay, and Hutchings. Amer. Jour. Vet. Res., 1953, *14*, 160.
4. Bunnell, Hutchings, and Donham. Am. Jour. Vet. Res., 1947, *8*, 367.
5. Cameron. Am. Jour. Vet. Res., 1946, *7*, 21.
6. Cameron, Gregory, and Hughes. Am. Jour. Vet. Res., 1943, *4*, 387.
7. Cherchenko and Bakaeva. Zh. Mikrobiol., 1962, *39*, 69.
8. Cook, Campbell, and Barrow. Austral. Vet. Jour., 1966, *42*, 5.
9. Cotton and Buck. Jour. Am. Vet. Med. Assoc., 1932, *80*, 344.
10. Edens and Foster. Am. Jour. Vet. Res., 1966, *27*, 1327.
11. Feldman and Olson. Arch. Path., 1933, *16*, 195.
12. Hellman and Sprenger. Berl. und Münch. tierärztl. Wchnschr., 1978, *91*, 385.
13. Hoerlein. Cornell Vet., 1953, *43*, 28.
14. Hubbard and Hoerlein. Jour. Am. Vet. Med. Assoc., 1952, *120*, 138.
15. Huntley, Phillip, and Maynard. Jour. Inf. Dis., 1963, *112*, 100.
16. Hutchings, Bunnell, and Bay. Am. Jour. Vet. Res., 1950, *11*, 388.
17. Hutchings and Washko. Jour. Am. Vet. Med. Assoc., 1947, *110*, 171.
18. Johnson and Huddleson. Jour. Am. Vet. Med. Assoc., 1931, *78*, 849.
19. Keppie, Williams, Witt, and Smith. Brit. Jour. Exp. Path., 1965, *46*, 104.
20. Kernkamp and Roepke. Jour. Am. Vet. Med. Assoc., 1948, *113*, 564.
21. Manthei. Am. Jour. Vet. Res., 1948, *9*, 40.
22. Moulton and Meyer. Cornell Vet., 1958, *48*, 165.
23. Spink, Hutchings, Mingle, Larson, Boyd, Jordan, and Evans. Jour. Am. Med. Assoc., 1949, *141*, 326.
24. Thomsen, Axel. Brucella infection in swine, Levin and Munksgaard, Copenhagen, 1934.
25. Vaskevich. Veterinariya (Moscow), 1972, *49*, 46.
26. Washko, Bay, Donham, and Hutchings. Am. Jour. Vet. Res., 1951, *12*, 320.
27. Washko and Hutchings. Am. Jour. Vet. Res., 1951, *12*, 165.

Brucella melitensis

SYNONYMS: *Micrococcus melitensis, Bacterium melitensis,* caprine type of *Brucella*

This organism was first isolated by Bruce (4) in 1887 from the spleen of a resident of the Island of Malta who had died from a disease known as *Malta fever* or *Mediterranean fever*. In 1905, Zammit (19) discovered that the source of the infection was milk from infected goats. The disease in goats, and to a less extent in sheep, is prevalent in southern Europe, in Mexico, and in certain areas of the southwestern part of the United States, where it appears to have been imported from Mexico. It has been prevalent in mohair goats owned largely by Indian tribes in northern Arizona and southern Utah. In 1946, Jordan and Borts (10) reported a number of human cases in Iowa in persons who had had no contact with goats or goat products. Borts *et al.* (3) succeeded in isolating *B. melitensis* from swine on a farm where a human infection had occurred. Since that time it has become evident that this type is well established in swine in the midwestern United States. Experimental infection has been induced in this animal by Beal *et al.* (2), and studies by Hoerlein (8) have led to the conclusion that the pathogenesis of *B. melitensis* for swine is similar to that of *B. suis*.

Carpenter and Boak (5) reported the finding of three strains of *B. melitensis* in cows' milk in central New York in 1934. In 1947, Damon and Fagan (6) isolated this type from a human case in Indiana. The patient was a farmer who owned a small herd of cows. Eight of the nine animals were positive to the agglutination test, and one animal had recently aborted. *B. melitensis* was found in the milk of one of these animals. It is interesting to note that Shaw (17) of the British Mediterranean Fever Commission isolated *B. melitensis* from the milk of two cows on the Island of Malta in 1905. In 1963 the organism was isolated from sheep in Argentina. It has been claimed that this was the first time *B. melitensis* was actually proved to cause natural ovine brucellosis in the Western Hemisphere (12).

In addition to goats, sheep, cattle, and swine, *B. melitensis* has been found in other populations of animals both free-living and domesticated. In 1952 it was found in wild hares shot in northern France (9). The infected animals were presumed to have contracted the disease from sheep and goats at pasture. *B. melitensis* has been isolated from camels (13), buffalo (14), and impala (15).

Morphology, Staining, Reactions, and Cultural Features. *B. melitensis* characteristically grows in the form of a small rod so short that it may be mistaken for a coccus.

The staining characteristics of *B. melitensis* are the same as those of the other brucellae. Morphologically these organisms are identical.

Differentiation of *B. melitensis* from the other species by any of the ordinary cultural features is not possible. Three biotypes of *B. melitensis* have been characterized. Special means of differentiating the brucellae are presented in Table 14.3.

Pathogenicity. *B. melitensis* is a facultative intracellular organism, and erythritol stimulates its growth (11). The disease produced in the goat appears to be quite like the corresponding infection in the cow. Abortions may occur. The udder becomes infected in a high percentage of cases, and the organism is shed in the milk. In many instances the effects upon the goat herd are so slight that the disease is not suspected until human infections are traced to it. Infections in sheep apparently are similar to those in goats. They are said to be common in southern Europe, but no cases have been reported in this species in North America.

Diagnosis. The diagnostic methods are the same as those used for brucellosis in other species. The agglutination test may be used, or the organism may be isolated by direct cultural means or through guinea pig inoculation. Alternatively, serological tests, including complement fixation, agar gel immunodiffusion, and the Rose Bengal plate test, are now available and give comparable results to the classic agglutination test (18). The complement-fixation test remained positive for a longer time than did the other tests after Waghela (18) infected goats with *B. melitensis*.

Immunity. It has been claimed that strains of *B. melitensis* have been used as a bacterin (killed adjuvant 53H38 vaccine) and as a vaccine (live avirulant Rev. 1 mutant vaccine) to induce a high degree of immunity in sheep (7) and goats (1). Strain 19 vaccine was less effective.

Chemotherapy. Treatment of experimental *B. melitensis* infection in mice with streptomycin combined with Aureomycin, Terramycin, or sulfadiazine eradicated the organism in the spleen of 99 out of 100 animals. Therapy with single drugs was definitely inferior (16).

REFERENCES

1. Alton. Jour. Comp. Path., 1966, *76,* 241.
2. Beal, Taylor, McCullough, Claflin, and Hutchings. Am. Jour. Vet. Res., 1959, *20,* 634.
3. Borts, McNutt, and Jordan. Jour. Am. Med. Assoc., 1946, *130,* 966.
4. Bruce. Practitioner, 1887, *39,* 161.
5. Carpenter and Boak. Jour. Bact., 1934, *27,* 73.
6. Damon and Fagan. Pub. Health Rpts. (U.S.), 1947, *62,* 1097.
7. Ghosh, Sen, and Singh. Jour. Comp. Path., 1968, *78,* 387.
8. Hoerlein. Am. Jour. Vet. Res., 1952, *13,* 67.
9. Jacotot, Vallée, and Barrière. Abstract in North Am. Vet., 1952, *23,* 169.
10. Jordan and Borts. Jour. Am. Med. Assoc., 1946, *130,* 72.
11. Keppie, Williams, Witt, and Smith. Brit. Jour. Exp. Path., 1965, *46,* 104.
12. Ossola, Szyfres, and Blood. Am. Jour. Vet. Res., 1963, *24,* 446.
13. Otgon. Zh. Mikrobiol., 1968, *8,* 120.
14. Sadykhov. Veterinariya (Moscow), 1968, *45,* 33.
15. Scheimann and Staak. Vet. Rec., 1971, *88,* 344.
16. Shaffer, Kucera, and Spink. Jour. Immunol., 1953, *70,* 31.
17. Shaw. Rpt. Comm. Appointed by the Admiralty, the War Office, and the Office of Civil Govt. of Malta for Investigations on Mediterranean Fever. London, 1907.
18. Waghela. Brit. Vet. Jour., 1978, *134,* 565.
19. Zammit. Rpt. Comm. Appointed by the Admiralty, the War Office, and the Office of Civil Govt. of Malta for Investigations on Mediterranean Fever. London, 1907.

Brucella neotomae

This organism was first isolated in 1957 by Stoenner and Lockman (5, 6) from the desert wood rat, *Neotoma lepida,* trapped alive in the Great Salt Desert of Utah. *B. neotomae* has been found subsequently in this species of rodent (7) and has not been recovered from any other naturally infected host (4). It is well tolerated by the wood rat, and upon experimental infection it persists for at least a year without producing significant lesions. The chief significance of *B. neotomae* is not its pathogenicity for animals but its role as a new and distinct species of the genus *Brucella.* The characteristics that differentiate it from other species are given in Table 14.3.

Brucellosis of Rodents. Rodents living on premises infected with *Brucella* sp. can become infected by exposure to the bacteria shed by infected domesticated animals. Such incidents have occurred in the past and have been self-limiting. The rodent population has not played a substantial role as a reservoir of infection for domestic animals. In recent years it has become obvious that various species of *Brucella* infect rodents in different parts of the world, including Kenya (2), the U.S.S.R. (3), and Australia (1).

REFERENCES

1. Cook, Campbell, and Barrow. Austral. Vet. Jour., 1966, *42,* 5.
2. Heisch, Cooke, Harvey, and DeSouza. East Afr. Med. Jour., 1963, *40,* 132.
3. Korol. Zh. Mikrobiol., 1964, *41,* 27.
4. Meyer. Adv. Vet. Sci., 1974, *18,* 231.
5. Stoenner and Lackman. Jour. Am. Vet. Med. Assoc., 1957, *130,* 411.

6. Stoenner and Lackman. Am. Jour. Vet. Res., 1957, *18*, 947.
7. Thorpe, Sidwell, Bushman, Smart, and Moyes. Jour. Am. Vet. Med. Assoc., 1965, *146*, 225.

Brucella ovis

The organism, a relative newcomer to the genus *Brucella,* was first isolated in 1953 by Buddle and Boyes (8) and described as *B. ovis* in 1956 (6). *B. ovis* causes epididymitis in rams, and since its early isolation in New Zealand and Australia it has been described in many of the world's sheep-raising countries: the United States, South America, South Africa, and the U.S.S.R. In addition to epididymitis in rams, the organism produces late abortions in females (28) and lowers flock fertility.

Morphology, Staining Reactions, and Cultural Features. *B. ovis* is a Gram-negative coccobacillus, although it is somewhat acid-fast under certain conditions of staining (29). It is nonmotile, nonencapsulated, and nonsporulating.

The organism requires enriched media and CO_2 for growth. Its main characteristics are presented in Table 14.3. It does not utilize erythritol or other carbohydrates. It is catalase-positive (18) and is both oxidase- and urease-negative (16). It grows equally well on basic fuchsin and thionin media.

Transmission and Pathogenicity. Under natural conditions only sheep are infected with *B. ovis.* Complete details concerning the method of spread are not known, but the disease can be produced in both rams and ewes during coitus, although ewes are quite refractory to this method of infection, and it may be transmitted from ram to ewe and thence to another ram via the ewe's vagina during the mating season. The organism can survive for some time on pasture, and ewes can be infected *per os,* but the means of spread within the ewe flock is still unclear.

Infection is followed by a transient systemic reaction with localization of the organism in the epididymis of the male. The systemic reaction is frequently inapparent and the tail of the epididymis is affected, often unilaterally. The ram may show no clinical signs at this time but secrete the organism in its semen for a prolonged period (12). In the epididymis a spermatocele forms and ruptures, and finally spermatic granulomas form with later testicular atrophy (3, 18). Such rams are of lowered fertility, and Shott and Young (27) speculated, but did not manage to prove, that the lesions may be due to an autoimmune response to the contents of the epididymal ducts released during bacterial infection.

The ewe appears to be somewhat less susceptible to infection by *B. ovis* (14), but lesions can be produced (22). They vary from a superficial purulent exudate on an intact chorioallatoic membrane to advanced fibrosis and necrosis of this membrane (21, 24).

Osburn and Kennedy (24) investigated the pathogenicity of the organism for lambs *in utero* and found that the lamb fetus may survive in the presence of infection. *B. ovis* can cause a placentitis which interferes with fetal nutrition, and Hughes (14) suggests that this may account for low birth weights in lambs. Frank abortion has not been the cardinal sign of this disease, but it has been reported under experimental conditions (5, 13), as well as under natural conditions in New Zealand (20, 28).

Immunity. In 1958, Buddle (7) advocated simultaneous vaccination with *B. abortus* Strain 19 and with a saline-in-oil adjuvant bacterin of formalinized *B. ovis* in order to protect rams against the development of clinical epididymitis. In 1963, Buddle and coworkers (9) indicated that two doses of the adjuvant *B. ovis* bacterin at an interval of 24 weeks was just as efficient as the Strain 19–*B. ovis* combination. Kater and Hartley (17) reported lameness in rams following vaccination by means of the simultaneous method. The ability of vaccines to provide immunity against naturally acquired infection has not been clearly established. There is evidence that agglutinin titers to *B. abortus* antigen persist for several years in vaccinated rams (26).

In California a *B. ovis* bacterin prepared as described by Biberstein *et al.* (2) has been used to vaccinate rams against the disease. The South Africans (30) have used live *B. melitensis* Rev. 1 vaccine to provide protection. Diaz *et al.* (10) demonstrated very substantial cross-reactivity between the antigens of *B. ovis* and *B. melitensis,* both rough and smooth types; this explains the use of the *B. melitensis* vaccine to control *B. ovis* infections.

Diagnosis. Diagnosis is accomplished by palpation of the testicles, culture of the semen, and demonstration of antibodies in the serum. Palpation is of limited value since many advanced cases show no palpable lesions of the testes. However, an enlarged epididymis with testicular atrophy is valuable in diagnosis. Culture of the semen is also an important adjunct to diagnosis and has been facilitated by the use of selective media modified for the growth of *B. ovis* (4, 15).

Drimmelen *et al.* (11) used a fluorescent antibody to detect the organism in a semen smear, and various serological tests have been used to detect antibodies in the serum of infected animals. Until fairly recently the complement-fixation test (1) has been the method, but Myers *et al.* (23) have developed an agar gel–diffusion test that is sensitive and simpler to perform, and Ris (25) has employed an indirect hemagglutination test. Jones *et al.* (15) have recently used a protein from *B. melitensis* in an allergic skin test for *B. ovis* infection; they recommend, however, that the test be used for diagnostic purposes on a herd basis.

In cases of abortion the organism can be cultured from the placental membranes and abomasal fluid of the fetus. The application of the fluorescent-antibody technique to films from these sources is also helpful.

Treatment and Control. *B. ovis* is reported to be sensitive to penicillin and streptomycin. Experimental infection has been successfully treated with Aureomycin and streptomycin. Streptomycin, alone and combined with sulfadimidine, is unsuccessful (19), and generally only valuable with rams in the early stages of infection. No extensive therapeutic trials have been reported, and attempts to treat chronic cases characterized by testicular degeneration are likely to prove fruitless.

The goal in controlling the disease is to prevent infection of young rams. This is achieved by isolating unaffected animals from infected ewes, and vaccination in instances where isolation is not possible.

REFERENCES

1. Biberstein and McGowan. Cornell Vet., 1958, *48,* 31.
2. Biberstein, McGowan, Robinson, and Harrold. Cornell Vet., 1962, *52,* 214.
3. Biberstein, McGowan, Alander, and Kennedy. Cornell Vet., 1964, *54,* 27.
4. Brown, Ranger, and Kelley. Cornell Vet., 1971, *61,* 265.
5. Buddle. New Zeal. Vet. Jour., 1955, *3,* 10.
6. Buddle. Jour. Hyg. (London), 1956, *54,* 351.
7. Buddle, New Zeal. Vet. Jour., 1958, *6,* 41.
8. Buddle and Boyes. Austral. Vet. Jour., 1953, *29,* 145.
9. Buddle, Calverley, and Boyes. New Zeal. Vet. Jour., 1963, *11,* 90.
10. Diaz, Jones, and Wilson. Jour. Bact., 1967, *93,* 1262.
11. Drimmelen, Botes, Claassen, Ross, and Viljoen. Jour. S. Afr. Vet. Med. Assoc., 1963, *34,* 265.
12. Hall. Austral. Vet. Jour., 1955, *31,* 7.
13. Hartley, Jebson, and McFarlane. New Zeal. Vet. Jour., 1954, *2,* 80.
14. Hughes. Austral. Vet. Jour., 1972, *48,* 12.
15. Jones, Dubray, and Morly. Anns. Recher. Vet., 1975, *6,* 11.
16. Jones, Zanardi, Leong, and Wilson. Jour. Bact., 1968, *95,* 625.
17. Kater and Hartley. New Zeal. Vet. Jour., 1963, *11,* 65.
18. Kennedy, Frazier, and McGowan. Cornell Vet., 1956, *46,* 303.
19. Kuppaswamy. New Zeal. Vet. Jour., 1954, *2,* 110.
20. McFarlane, Salisbury, Osborne, and Jebson. Austral. Vet. Jour., 1952, *28,* 221.
21. McGowan, Biberstein, Harrold, and Robinson. Proc. U.S. Livestock Assoc., 1961, *65,* 291.
22. Molello, Jensen, Fling, and Collier. Am. Jour. Vet. Res., 1963, *24,* 897.
23. Myers, Jones, and Varela-Diaz. App. Microbiol., 1972, *23,* 894.
24. Osburn and Kennedy. Pathol. Vet., 1966, *3,* 110.
25. Ris. New Zeal. Vet. Jour., 1964, *12,* 72.
26. Ris. New Zeal. Vet. Jour., 1967, *15,* 94.
27. Shott and Young. Cornell Vet., 1971, *61,* 281.
28. Simmons and Hall. Austral. Vet. Jour., 1953, *29,* 33.
29. Stamp, McEwen, Watt, and Nisbet. Vet. Rec., 1950, *62,* 251.
30. Van Heerden and Van Rensburg. Jour. S. Afr. Vet. Med. Assoc., 1962, *33,* 143.

Brucella canis

SYNONYM: Canine type of *Brucella*

During investigations in 1966 into outbreaks of abortions and whelping failures in dogs, a new Gram-negative coccobacillary organism was isolated in both the U.S.A (1, 13, 19) and Britain (15). In 1968 the organism was characterized and named *Brucella canis* by Carmichael and Bruner (4). Subsequently the Subcommittee on Taxonomy of the genus *Brucella* accepted *B. canis* as a provisional species of the genus (18) because of its biochemical characteristics and its DNA homology (11). This decision was not without its detractors (14), who would have it assigned as a biotype of *B. suis*.

Brucellosis in dogs caused by *B. canis* has been found in various breeds on several continents. It is widespread in dog-breeding establishments in the United States, but its precise incidence has not been determined. Morrisset and Spink (16) reported that in a given year 86 percent of the adult dogs in a kennel become infected and 38 percent of the females abort. *B. canis* is particularly well adapted to this species and is not readily transmitted to other animals, although it will infect man.

Morphology, Staining Reactions, and Cultural Features. The organism is a small rod-shaped bacillus similar to the other *Brucella* sp. in morphology and staining reactions. Unlike them, *B. canis* is inhibited by 10 percent CO_2. After several days of incubation, growth becomes quite mucoid (ropy in broth), a characteristic unusual for classic brucellae. Its cultural characteristics are shown in Table 14.3. *B. canis* does not utilize erythritol (12).

Pathogenesis. Infection can occur through all mucosae and by many routes of inoculation. Bacteremia follows, and though it may be intermittent, it is prolonged and may persist for 2 years after the initial infection (5). Infected dogs do not have elevated temperatures, and most show no clinical signs. Those that do have generalized lymphadenitis, splenitis, and embryonic deaths and abortions at approximately 50 days of gestation. Infected males have epididymitis, scrotal dermatitis, and testicular atrophy which is often unilateral. George (9) demonstrated sperm agglutination in the semen of infected dogs, phagocytosis of spermatozoa, and delayed skin hypersensitivity to testicular antigens, and suggested that autoallergy plays a role in the pathogenesis of *B. canis* infections and in male infertility.

Transmission occurs principally at the time of abortion, when many bacteria are shed in the persistent vaginal discharge. Transmission by this route may continue for 4 to 6 weeks after an abortion (3). Males harbor the organism in their genital tracts, from which it is shed intermittently, and it can be transmitted to the female by coitus.

Immunity. *B. canis* does not possess the smooth (O) antigens of *B. abortus* and *B. melitensis;* thus the usual bacterial suspensions available for diagnosis are of no value in the diagnosis of canine brucellosis. *B. canis* does share a close antigenic relationship with *B. ovis* (7), and suspensions of this organism have been used to diagnose canine brucellosis. Antibodies are produced against *B. canis* in infected animals. Their titers are high during periods of bacteremia but diminish rapidly when bacteremia ceases. No successful vaccines have been prepared against this agent. George, no doubt suspecting that stimulation of cell-mediated immunity was important in this disease, attempted to produce immunity with a live streptomycin-dependent mutant of *B. canis,* but he was unsuccessful (9). He did show that some resistance was produced to *B. canis* when animals were immunized with living *B. ovis,* and high levels of resistance were seen in dogs previously recovered from *B. canis* infection.

Diagnosis. Diagnosis is easy where there are clinical signs of abortion and infertility in females, and epididymitis in males. Diagnosis is also easy in kennel outbreaks where a number of animals are involved, but the individual animal that is infected, but appears normal, presents a diagnostic problem. Clinical signs; direct culture of blood, lymph nodes, or bone marrow; and serological tests are used in diagnosis. The latter include tube agglutination (2), complement fixation (6), agar-gel diffusion (17), and a rapid slide agglutination test (10). These tests are still not completely standardized between laboratories, and they are subject to occasional but important "false positives" and hard-to-interpret "low titers" and to the broad heterotypic reactivity shown by *B. canis* antigens. Flores-Castro and Carmichael (8), in a comparison of current methods for diagnosis in 1978, concluded that none of the serological procedures commonly used was, in itself, adequate to permit a definitive diagnosis in all cases and that isolation of *B. canis* from infected dogs is the only certain method of diagnosis.

Treatment and Control. There is currently no completely effective treatment for canine brucellosis. Although prolonged and intensive treatment with antibiotics has been attempted and some success is claimed for tetracycline hydrochloride, no documented evidence of the efficacy of any form of treatment has been published (3). Control in a breeding kennel is based on serological testing and if possible blood cultures of all animals. All animals that test positive are eliminated, leaving only *Brucella*-free animals to breed.

REFERENCES

1. Carmichael. Hounds and Hunting, 1967, *64,* 14.
2. Carmichael. Proc. U.S. Livestock Assoc., 1968, *71,* 517.
3. Carmichael. Theriogenology, 1976, *6,* 105.
4. Carmichael and Bruner. Cornell Vet., 1968, *58,* 579.
5. Carmichael and Kenney. Jour. Am. Vet. Med. Assoc., 1968, *152,* 605.
6. Deyoe, Billy L. Thesis, Iowa State Univ., Ames, Iowa, 1970.
7. Diaz. Jour. Bact., 1968, *95,* 618.
8. Flores-Castro and Carmichael. Cornell Vet., 1978, *68* supplement 7, 76.
9. George, Lisle W. Thesis, Cornell Univ., Ithaca, N.Y., 1974.
10. George and Carmichael. Am. Jour. Vet. Res., 1974, *35,* 905.
11. Hoyer and McCullough. Jour. Bact., 1968, *96,* 1783.
12. Jones, Zanardi, Leong, and Wilson. Jour. Bact., 1968, *95,* 625.
13. Kimberling, Ludisinger, and Anderson. Jour. Am. Vet. Med. Assoc., 1966, *148,* 900.
14. Meyer. Adv. Vet. Sci., 1974, *18,* 231.
15. Moore and Bennett. Vet. Rec., 1967, *80,* 604.
16. Morisset and Spink. Lancet, 1969, *8,* 1000.

17. Meyers, Jones, and Varela-Diaz. App. Microbiol., 1972, *23,* 894.
18. Subcommittee on Taxonomy of the Genus *Brucella.* Int. Jour. Syst. Bacteriol., 1971, *21,* 126.
19. Taul, Powell, and Baker. Vet. Med., 1967, *62,* 543.

Brucellosis (Undulant Fever) of Man

Historical Perspective. For more than a century a disease of man characterized by fever, chills, night sweats, and great weakness has been known in the Mediterranean countries. The causative agent of the disease was finally found in the blood of patients by David Bruce (2), a British military surgeon. The organism isolated was named *Micrococcus melitensis.* Because the work was done on the Island of Malta, the disease became known as *Malta fever.*

A commission headed by Bruce discovered in 1904 that the blood of many of the milking goats on the Island of Malta contained agglutinins for the Malta fever organism. It was soon learned that infection was widespread in these goats and that the organism was secreted in the milk (32). The goats showed little evidence of disease, but their milk was very dangerous for persons who had not become immunized to the organism by drinking it from early life. Army and Navy personnel sent to the island from other parts of the world suffered greatly from the disease, whereas the natives seldom were affected.

The organism of Malta fever has been known since 1886, that of contagious abortion of cattle since 1897, and that of swine abortion since 1914. The relationship of swine abortion to that of cattle was seen from the beginning, but not until 1918 was it known that *B. suis* and *B. abortus* had any relation to the agent of Malta fever. In the first place, Bruce described the Malta fever organism as a coccus, and its relationship to caprine abortion was not appreciated. In the second place, most of the active work on bovine abortion was done in parts of the world where the Malta fever organism was not known; consequently there were few workers who had worked with both organisms.

In 1918, Alice Evans (6) showed for the first time that the three organisms were quite similar in morphology and in cultural reactions. The work of Evans was confirmed by Meyer and Shaw (22), and the suggestion was made that the Malta fever and the abortion-producing organisms be grouped together under the name *Brucella,* in honor of Bruce, who discovered the first member. This suggestion met with general acceptance.

The discovery of the close relationship of the organisms of this new group immediately raised the question anew whether the abortion organisms might not at times be pathogenic for man. In 1924, Keefer (16) reported a case of Malta-fever-like disease in Maryland in a man who had apparently not been exposed to Malta fever. Evans determined the organism isolated from this man to be *B. abortus* rather than *B. melitensis.* In 1926, Carpenter and Merriam (4) reported two human cases of brucellosis in a rural area of New York; they supplied strong circumstantial evidence that the infections had been contracted by drinking infected raw cows' milk. Carpenter and others soon were able to demonstrate more cases of *B. abortus* infection of man contracted from cattle. Since that time several thousand cases of undulant fever in man, caused by infections derived from cattle and swine rather than from goats, have been found in the United States and elsewhere; and the disease became known as *brucellosis.* It apparently had gone undiagnosed in past years, or was wrongly diagnosed as typhoid fever, paratyphoid fever, la grippe, and the like.

***Brucella* Species Responsible for Human Infections.** It is clear now that the undulant fever complex may be induced in man by any of these three types of *Brucella.* In the United States most cases are caused by *B. abortus* and *B. suis.* This is because these types are more prevalent than *B. melitensis* in livestock. In the eastern part of the country human infections are mostly with *B. abortus,* whereas in the north central part of the country (the swine belt) *B. suis* infections probably outnumber those caused by *B. abortus. B. melitensis* infections are most common in Mexico and in certain small areas in the southwestern part of the United States. This type is also being found with considerable frequency in the midwestern states where the infection is apparently contracted from swine. In Alaska, clinical cases of brucellosis are appearing in the human population and there is evidence that the source of the disease is the caribou (the North American reindeer, *Rangifer tarandus*) infected by *B. suis* biotype 4.

In the decade since *B. canis* was first isolated, some 15 cases of human infections with this species have been recorded (1, 23, 29, 31). Half of these have involved laboratory personnel working with the organism, and most of the others have involved owners of infected pet dogs (3).

No cases of humans infected with *B. neotome* or *B.*

ovis have been reported. However, Gavrilov *et al.* (8) undertook a serological survey in the Kazakhstan area of Russia and found that 8 percent of the shepherds, 6 percent of the farm workers, and 1 percent of the veterinary students had antibodies against *B. ovis* in their sera. Robinson and Metcalfe (26) relate that Ris, a worker in the field of ovine brucellosis, reported a case of accidental inoculation with *B. ovis,* characterized by a mild illness and an antibody rise.

Sources of Human Infections. The principal sources of human infections, so far as they are known, are as follows:

1. *B. melitensis.* Most infections are contracted from the drinking of raw, infected goats' milk, or from eating certain cheeses made from such milk. Infections are also derived from direct contact with the infected secretions and excretions of goats and sheep. A few cases are known to have been contracted from swine and cattle. The organism produces a septicemia in pigs, and it has been recovered from hams from such pigs 21 days after they were placed in cover pickle. No isolations were made after the hams were smoked (14).

2. *B. abortus.* This type of infection is contracted by the drinking of raw, infected cows' milk. Reports from Italy have shown that eating certain cheeses made from unpasteurized cows' milk may result in infection. Apparently this rarely occurs and has not been reported in the United States. Infection may be contracted by direct contact with infected fetuses, membranes, and discharges of aborting cows. In the United States the disease is a rural one; city people usually drink pasteurized milk and have no direct contact with cattle. Most cases in city dwellers occur as a result of infections contracted during country vacations.

McCullough *et al.* (21) have recovered *B. abortus* from the submaxillary lymph nodes of slaughtered hogs. They have observed human brucellosis caused by *B. abortus* in packing-house workers, their exposure history implicated the hog as the source of infection.

3. *B. suis.* Infections of man with this type occur usually in two occupational groups, farmers who raise swine and workers in slaughterhouses who handle swine carcasses.

4. *B. canis.* Infections with this species have been reported in laboratory technicians and animal handlers in facilities where canine brucellosis is being studied. Other cases have been reported in owners of pet dogs infected with *B. canis.* The number of human cases diagnosed is likely to rise as the medical profession becomes more aware of the public health significance of this organism (3).

The Incidence of Human Brucellosis. Human brucellosis is almost never contracted from other humans. Infected animals are the reservoir of the disease; their elimination will effectively reduce the danger to man.

The number of human cases caused by *B. abortus* has been greatly reduced during the last two decades in the United States and in other countries with programs for control and eradication of the disease in cattle. Important in this respect is public awareness that human consumption of raw cows' milk is potentially dangerous, and insistence that all milk, even that of the highest quality, be pasteurized.

Human infections caused by *B. suis* have not decreased as much in areas of the United States where the organism has long been prevalent, probably because brucellosis in swine has not decreased as much as it has in cattle (11).

Although the susceptibility of the two sexes is about equal, at least two-thirds of the cases occurring in Iowa, according to Hardy *et al.* (9), were in men. These were partly *B. abortus* and partly *B. suis* infections. Iowa is largely a rural state and most of the cases were in farm families where the males usually handled the livestock. Direct contact is apparently more hazardous than the drinking of infected milk, because male infections are more common even in areas where the predominating type is *B. abortus.* Brucellosis, or undulant fever, may occur at all ages, but the greatest number of clinically recognized cases occur in the age group between 20 and 45 years (9). Infants, who consume a much larger volume of milk proportionally than adults, seldom become infected, although the disease has been recognized in children as young as 4 years of age.

Human infections from contact with infected animal tissues and secretions probably occur through the unbroken skin. Using guinea pigs as test animals, Hardy *et al.* (9) showed that brucellosis could be produced by dropping cultures onto abraded and even undamaged skin. Cotton and Buck (5) obtained similar results using cattle, so it seems reasonable to suppose that humans can be infected by this route. Kerr *et al.* (18) consider inhalation of infected dust from the environment contaminated by cattle with brucellosis a very potent method of infection, as are infections through the conjunctiva and accidental inoculation with *B. abortus* Strain 19 vaccine.

The high incidence of human cases in swine-slaughtering establishments in regions where swine infections are prevalent has pointed up the dangers in handling freshly slaughtered carcasses. As a rule, most cases in such plants occur in the personnel in the sticking and eviscerating rooms; those working in the cutting and packing departments usually escape. This indicates that the greatest hazard comes from contact with the blood and internal organs of the carcasses. It should be remembered that in swine the *Brucella* organisms frequently occur in the blood, and that the disease is more generalized than the corresponding one in cattle. It is true, also, that the *B. suis* type is more highly pathogenic for man than *B. abortus*. Both of these factors probably play a part in the difference between the hazards to man in handling swine and cattle carcasses. During an epidemic of brucellosis affecting 128 employees of a swine-slaughtering plant in Iowa, *B. suis* was isolated from the air of the establishment (10), suggestive evidence that air-borne transmission of the disease is also a very real possibility. Apparently, however, this is not the usual route of infection.

B. suis may retain its viability for as long as 3 weeks in fresh pork carcasses held at 40 F (13). In spite of this, no human cases have been traced to the handling of pork after it has been chilled. Perhaps this is because muscular tissue contains few organisms other than those in the blood vessels. Because carcasses are usually well bled, market pork contains few organisms.

Brucellosis, an Occupational Hazard for the Veterinarian. Veterinarians in country practice face brucellosis as an occupational hazard because their work often requires them to come in contact with infected secretions. Blood-test surveys made before 1940 indicated that a comparatively large percentage of veterinarians reacted positively (12). Many of these had no clinical history of the disease. At the time infection in students in veterinary colleges was not uncommon.

In a survey carried out in 1974 in New Zealand (26), Robinson and Metcalfe found antibody titers in 90 percent of the veterinarians sampled. The veterinarians who showed no evidence of *Brucella* antibodies were either recent graduates or involved in commerce, laboratory work, or teaching.

Kerr *et al.* (18) indicate that the practicing veterinarian is exposed to more viable *Brucella* organisms than other members of society, even in rural communities. They indicate that the veterinarian, in removing a retained placenta from a cow, a common procedure, comes in intimate contact with uterine discharges rich in organisms that can enter his body via the conjunctiva or the intact skin, or by inhalation. Wounds on the hands and arms are not uncommon during obstetrical procedures, and they make ideal sites of entry.

The other major source of infection for veterinarians is accidental inoculation with *B. abortus* Strain 19 while vaccinating cattle. In the course of vaccinating frisky young calves, the veterinarian may jab the needle into his thigh or scratch his thumb. Kerr *et al.* (18) reported that about one third of the veterinarians surveyed had inoculated themselves one or more times. Spink and Thompson (30) described the course of the disease in two veterinarians accidently inoculated with Strain 19. Spink (27) states that *B. abortus* Strain 19 probably does not cause chronic infections in humans but suggests caution in its use and prompt medical attention to accidental vaccination. It appears that this vaccine can cause severe effects in humans previously infected with *B. abortus*. The reactions are particularly severe when the vaccine is splashed into the eye of sensitized veterinarians.

Diagnosis of Human Infections. The acute disease is frequently overlooked or misdiagnosed. Patients frequently decide they have "influenza" or "chills" and recover. Even when a medical practitioner is consulted in the acute stage the disease may be misdiagnosed because of its sporadic nature and its vague signs. Diagnosis is based on the patient's history, clinical signs, isolation of the organism, and serological tests.

In the early, severe phase of the disease the individual is acutely ill, suffers from prostration and weakness, develops daily fever in the afternoon and evening, and suffers chills and night sweats during which the fever disappears only to have the cycle recur on following days. The intermittent fever is responsible for the name *undulant fever*. Such acute symptoms usually lessen after a few days, but, following an interval of varying length during which the patient feels better, another period of acute symptoms may appear. There may be several such remissions. The symptoms are the same, no matter which type of *Brucella* is the infecting agent. Infections with *B. melitensis* and *B. suis* are usually more severe than those with *B. abortus,* but this is not always the case. The mortality is low, but recovery from infections often is very slow. Many persons never fully recover from the effects of the disease.

The symptoms of chronic cases vary greatly, and this form of the disease is more difficult to diagnose. Usually the patient suffers from great debility, weakness, a low-grade remittent fever, and joint pains; there may be sweating, lassitude and malaise, gastritis, abdominal pain, skin rashes, headache, irratibility, depression, insomnia, arthritis, and backache. Kerr *et al.* (18) note that patients may be labeled "neurotic" because their complaints are hard to substantiate by laboratory tests.

An osteoarticular complication of brucellosis is the *melitococcic spondylitis* of man reported in Italy. *B. suis* has also been reported in septic arthritis of the hip. *Brucella* organisms have been implicated in cases of osteomyelitis (17) and in diseases of the nervous system (7). Perry (24) claims that calcific aortic stenosis is a residual lesion of brucellar endocarditis, chiefly caused by *B. abortus,* and Perry and Belter (25) have published a review on fatal brucellosis and heart disease.

Blood cultures, when positive, are diagnostic, but the isolation of the organism from the blood is usually difficult and often impossible, particularly when the offending organism is *B. abortus.* Greater success is achieved in the acute than in the chronic cases, but repeated attempts often have to be made, even in the acute forms.

Three serological tests have been used as an aid to diagnosis: the standard agglutination test, the antiglobulin test, and a complement-fixation test. The agglutination test has been used for years but it must be interpreted with great caution because it may produce aberrant results, such as occasional prozones, and "nonagglutinating" antibodies may be present, giving a negative test even in persons who have had the disease for a long time. Nevertheless it is useful, particularly in recently acquired acute cases of brucellosis (26). The antiglobulin test (Coomb's test) and a complement-fixation test (19) are supplementary, and while they too are subject to some variability in results, they are of value in the diagnosis of long-standing brucellosis.

Immunity. The brucellae are facultative intracellular bacteria, and although they stimulate the production of antibodies of the IgM and IgG classes, the cell-mediated immune response is probably essential for protection of the host. Killed bacterins are of questionable value and the use of live vaccines such as Strain 19 is fraught with considerable risk to humans.

In 1957, Zdrodowski *et al.* (33) reported on large-scale immunization of humans against melitensis brucellosis in the U.S.S.R. Their vaccines consisted of live cultures of either *B. abortus* Strain 19 or *B. abortus* Russian strain, and they claimed that the morbidity rate among various classes of people living in endemic areas was reduced by 3.3 to 11.2 times following vaccination. Strain 19 vaccine has been used in other countries where human cases have been prevalent and where the risk of contracting brucellosis is very high among laboratory technicians and researchers working with the organism (18).

Treatment. The intracellular nature of brucellae makes them relatively inaccessible to chemotherapeutic agents, and thus brucellosis, especially chronic brucellosis in humans, is often very refractory to treatment. In 1958 a joint FAO/WHO Expert Committee on Brucellosis recommended tetracyclines be given for 21 days. They also recommended that a combination of tetracycline and streptomycin be given for severe infections and for all *B. suis* infections (15). The Committee also suggested that chloramphenicol is of value but urged caution in its prolonged use. These recommendations have been corroborated by others (20, 28). Although these antibiotics often produce a good initial clinical response, a large percentage of patients suffer recurrence of the disease.

REFERENCES

1. Bleukenship and Sanford. Am. Jour. Med., 1975, *59,* 424.
2. Bruce. Practitioner, 1887, *39,* 161.
3. Carmichael. Theriogenology, 1976, *6,* 105.
4. Carpenter and Merriam. Jour. Am. Med. Assoc., 1926, *87,* 1269.
5. Cotton and Buck. Jour. Am. Vet. Med. Assoc., 1932, *80,* 342.
6. Evans. Jour. Inf. Dis., 1918, *22,* 580.
7. Fincham, Sahs, and Joynt. Jour. Am. Med. Assoc., 1963, *184,* 269.
8. Gavrilov, Bzhevskaya, Rementsova, Umanova, and Postricheva. Veterinariya (Moscow), 1972, *7,* 55.
9. Hardy, Jordan, Borts, and Hardy. Natl. Inst. Health Bull. 158, 1930.
10. Harris, Hendricks, Gorman, and Held. Pub. Health Rpts. (U.S.), 1962, *77,* 602.
11. Hendricks and Borts. Pub. Health Rpts. (U.S.), 1964, *79,* 868.
12. Huddleson, Irvin F. Brucellosis in man and animals. The Commonwealth Fund, New York, 1939.
13. Hutchings, Bunnell, Donham, and Bay. Proc. Am. Vet. Med. Assoc., 1950, p. 184.
14. Hutchings, McCullough, Donham, Eisele, and Bunnell. Pub. Health Rpts. (U.S.), 1951, *66,* 1402.
15. Joint FAO/WHO Expert Committee on Brucellosis. Third Report. WHO Tech. Rpt. Ser. 148, World Health Org., Geneva, 1958.
16. Keefer. Johns Hopkins Hosp. Bull., 1924, *35,* 6.
17. Kelly, Martin, Schirger, and Weed. Jour. Am. Med. Assoc., 1960, *174,* 347.
18. Kerr, Coghlan, Payne, and Robertson. Vet. Rec., 1966, *79,* 602.
19. Kerr, McCaughey, Coghlan, Payne, Quaife, Robertson, and Farrell. Jour. Med. Microbiol., 1968, *1,* 181.

20. Killough, Magil, and Smith. Jour. Am. Med. Assoc., 1951, *145,* 553.
21. McCullough, Eisele, and Pavelchek. Pub. Health Rpts. (U.S.), 1951, *66,* 205.
22. Meyer and Shaw. Jour. Inf. Dis., 1920, *27,* 173.
23. Munford, Weaver, Patton, Feeley, and Feldman. Jour. Am. Vet. Med. Assoc., 1975, *231,* 1267.
24. Perry. Jour. Am. Med. Assoc., 1958, *166,* 1123.
25. Perry and Belter. Am. Jour. Path., 1960, *36,* 673.
26. Robinson and Metcalfe. New Zeal. Vet. Jour., 1976, *24,* 201.
27. Spink, Wesley W. The nature of brucellosis. Univ. of Minnesota Press, Minneapolis, 1956, p. 113.
28. Spink, Hall, Shaffer, and Braude. Jour. Am. Med. Assoc., 1949, *139,* 352.
29. Spink and Morisset. Trans. Am. Clin. Climatol. Assoc., 1970, *81,* 43.
30. Spink and Thompson. Jour. Am. Med. Assoc., 1953, *153,* 1162.
31. Swenson, Carmichael, and Cundy. Ann. Int. Med., 1972, *76,* 435.
32. Zammit. Rpt. Comm. Appointed by the Admiralty, the War Office, and the Office of Civil Govt. of Malta for Investigation on Mediterranean Fever. London, 1907.
33. Zdrodowski, Vershilova, and Kotlarova. Jour. Inf. Dis., 1957, *101,* 1.

15 The Genus *Campylobacter*

This genus is composed of a group of short, curved, rigid rods, arranged singly or united into spiral forms. When they were first discovered, organisms in the genus *Campylobacter* were classified as vibrios on account of their curved shape and rapid motility. The name of the genus was in fact *Vibrio* for many years until it was found (26) that many of the member species were sufficiently different as to merit classification under the separate generic title *Campylobacter*. The term *vibriosis* is still applied to the diseases caused by pathogenic species of this genus.

General Characteristics of the Genus *Campylobacter*

Biochemically, species of *Campylobacter* are rather inactive, but all are oxidase-positive and some produce catalase. The latter characteristic is useful to separate the species into (*a*) a group of catalase-positive pathogenic members, and (*b*) a group of catalase-negative, mostly nonpathogenic members. The pathogenic *Campylobacter* have been further divided by their ability to grow at temperatures between 25 and 45 C.

Table 15.1 lists the *Campylobacter* sp. found in animals and man together with their more important characteristics. The thermophilic species do not grow at 25 but grow well at 42 to 45 C. In recent years they have been shown to be associated with acute enteritis in humans and dogs and may therefore have considerable zoonotic importance. However, much work has yet to be done to classify and categorize strains from enteritis cases in man and animals.

The morphologic and cultural features of the pathogenic *Campylobacter* sp. will be described together. The diseases caused in the various animal species will be covered separately.

Morphology and Staining Reactions. *C. fetus venerealis* and *C. fetus intestinalis* characteristically produce comma-shaped or S-shaped Gram-negative bodies (0.2 to 0.5 by 1.5 to 4.0 μm). The comma forms have a single polar flagellum while the S forms may have bipolar flagella. The catalase-positive species may show spiral formation when a number of S forms remain joined together. Cells in old cultures form coccoid or spherical bodies.

Cultural Features. Growth of *Campylobacter* sp. is microaerophilic to anaerobic. *C. fetus venerealis* and *C. fetus intestinalis* require an atmosphere of 10 to 20 percent CO_2. The oxygen concentration should be reduced to 5 percent or less. Optimum growth occurs at 37 C, on serum, blood agar, thiol agar, cystine-heart agar, and brain-heart infusion agar. Antibiotics such as novobiocin and bacitracin may be added to inhibit contaminants and allow growth of *C. fetus* (22).

Colonies usually are visible 2 days after inoculation. They are round, raised, and regular in shape and butyrous in consistency. They may be translucent at first but later become opaque. Colony diameter varies from 1 to 3 mm. Colonies of *C. sputorum bubulus* are characteristically greenish and surrounded by a zone of alpha hemolysis.

Carbohydrates are neither fermented nor oxidized, and neither gelatin nor urea is hydrolyzed. *C. fetus ven-*

Table 15.1. Some characteristics of the species of *Campylobacter* found in animals and man

Species	Serotype	Habitat	Disease	Catalase	Thermophilic (growth at 42 C)
C. fetus venerealis	A	Genital tract of cattle	Infertility and abortion in cattle	+	−
C. fetus intestinalis	A, B	Intestine of sheep and cattle	Abortion in sheep; occasional abortion in cattle	+	−
C. fetus intestinalis	C	Intestine of mammals and birds	Abortion in sheep; enteritis in dog and man	+	+
C. fetus jejuni	C				
C. sputorum mucosalis	Not known	Mouth and intestine of swine	Intestinal adenomatosis in swine	+	−
C. sputorum bubulus	Not known	Genital tracts of cattle and sheep	None produced	−	−

erealis is H_2S-negative (lead acetate paper), but the other species and subspecies are positive for this characteristic. It also is unique among the *Campylobacter* in being unable to grow in 1 percent glycine.

Antigens. *C. fetus venerealis* and *C. fetus intestinalis* have heat-stable somatic (O) antigens, flagellar (H) antigens, and heat-labile superficial protein antigens which mask the underlying O antigen. All strains of *venerealis* subspecies belong to serotype A, but *intestinalis* strains may belong to either A, B, or C.

Serotype C strains are thermophilic and have been isolated frequently from cases of enteritis in man and dogs.

C. fetus venerealis

The Disease in Cattle. *C. fetus venerealis* is an obligate parasite of the genitalia of the male and female. In the bull, infection involves the epithelium of the penis and the fornix of the prepuce. No lesions are produced. Transmission is by coitus or artificial insemination. The organism localizes in the anterior vagina and cervix but does not invade the uterus and oviducts until the progestational phase. A moderate endometritis and salpingitis then results and persists for several weeks to a few months (32). During this time the animal is infertile either because of failure of implantation or because of early abortion. Occasionally, though rarely, the pregnancy may continue to a later stage (5 to 7 months) before placental damage becomes sufficient to cause fetal death and abortion.

The inflammatory reaction in the cervical and endometrial mucosa involves a neutrophil invasion in the earlier stages. These cells are eventually replaced by foci of mononuclear cells.

Animals usually become fertile again within 5 months as a result of elimination of the infection from the uterus and oviducts. In some animals infection may persist in the cervicovaginal area for many months in spite of the presence of local antibodies. During this time the organism may exhibit a series of antigenic changes which allow it to survive and avoid the effects of local antibody production (4).

Immunity. The antibodies in the vaginal secretion are predominantly of the IgA class (3) and their effect is to immobilize the organism so that it cannot penetrate higher into the tract. These antibodies may persist for many months unlike antibodies of the IgM and IgG classes, which are present only for a short time. IgG antibodies, which have good opsonizing activity, are dominant in the uterine fluid, and their effect is to clear the organism from the uterus during the early convalescent phase.

Systemic vaccination with bacterins has been shown to be effective in preventing infertility in cattle (11) by stimulating antibodies of the IgG variety (3). When complete Freund's adjuvant is included with the bacterin, a heightened resistance is induced which will prevent not only infertility but the carrier state as well (33). Vaccination has been used to terminate natural infection in bulls (2).

C. fetus venerealis infection in cattle herds where natural breeding is carried on is self-limiting because of the normal immune response in infected animals. However, infection persists in some females and in the bull, and so clinical disease will continue to arise in susceptible virgin heifers and in newly introduced stock. Vaccination is important to protect these animals.

Laboratory Diagnosis. If the fetal membranes are available, a direct microscopic examination is made of the cotyledons. The finding of distinctly spiral-shaped organisms is regarded as positive evidence of the infection. Cultures are made, in serial dilution, on semisolid Bacto-thiol medium from stomach fluids, lungs, heart blood, amniotic fluid, and suspensions of ground cotyledons. The tubes are incubated under CO_2 tension at 37 C for 3 to 9 days and then examined for *C. fetus*. Careful culturing of cervicovaginal mucus, preputial samples, or semen by the millipore filter technic (21) will sometimes reveal the organism in infected animals. The use of the filter technique is less sensitive than direct culturing but has the advantage that it can be used with noninhibitory media. Inhibitory media that contain antibiotics such as novobiocin and bacitracin are very valuable for isolation from contaminated materials such as preputial scrapings (22).

In culturing these materials it is good practice to utilize both the filter technique and direct cultures onto inhibitory medium.

Serologic diagnosis of infection by the agglutination reaction on sera is unreliable because many infected animals do not develop detectable titers. Also, O antibodies to *C. fetus* are normally present in the sera of mature cattle (35).

The detection of agglutinating antibodies in cervical mucus is much more valuable in diagnosis but should be combined with mucus culture and be performed on a number of animals in a herd.

C. fetus intestinalis

The Disease in Cattle. *C. fetus intestinalis* is an occasional cause of abortion during the latter half of gestation in cattle. The disease is similar to that caused by *C. fetus venerealis*. The organism probably enters the animal by ingestion of infectious material.

The Disease in Sheep. Ovine infection by *C. fetus intestinalis* is contracted by ingestion of the organism (8). There is evidence that magpies (18), ravens (5), and other carriers (7) are concerned in spreading the disease, and it is possible that sheep are asymptomatic carriers (29). Venereal transmission does not occur. The organism localizes in the placentomes following a period of bacteremia (19), placentitis develops, and abortion occurs toward the end of the gestation period. Infection of ewes in the first half of the gestation period does not result in abortion. Only the heavily gravid animal is susceptible to bacterial invasion of its placenta and subsequent abortion.

Animals about to abort usually exhibit a vaginal discharge for several days beforehand.

In outbreaks of ovine vibriosis the percentage of ewes having abortions or immature lambs may be high. The pathological changes observed in naturally infected sheep are chiefly confined to the uterus, placenta, and fetus. The uterine wall as well as the fetal membranes are edematous. The fetus shows edema of the subcutaneous tissues, and the peritoneal, pleural, and pericardial cavities may contain blood-tinged fluid. The presence of necrotic spots in the liver has also been reported. As a rule, ewes do not abort in the year following an outbreak and appear not to carry the infection, but Smibert (29) was able to isolate *C. fetus intestinalis* from the fecal and intestinal contents of clinically normal sheep.

Vibrionic abortion has been reported in goats, (6) but the incidence of infection in these animals is unknown.

Ewes that abort usually recover completely and have a normal pregnancy in the next breeding season.

Immunity. Vaccination has been shown to be effective in the prevention of *C. fetus intestinalis* abortion in sheep flocks (30). Vaccinal immunity is serotype-specific; thus polyvalent vaccines that contain a number of the heat-labile antigens should be used. Thompson and Gilmour (31) have shown that good antibody responses to these different serotypes in a single vaccine can be obtained simultaneously. It has also been shown by this group of workers that vaccination at the beginning of an outbreak may have value in preventing later abortions in other members of the flock (10).

Williams *et al.* (34) have developed an *in vitro* bactericidal test that can be used to evaluate the immune response to bacterins.

Laboratory Diagnosis. *C. fetus intestinalis* can readily be seen in impression smears of fresh fetal cotyledons and stomach contents. The organism can also be cultured using the methods described above for *C. fetus venerealis*.

C. sputorum bubulus

C. sputorum bubulus is a very common commensal of the preputial epithelium of the bull (25). It can be distinguished from the pathogenic *C. fetus venerealis* by its failure to produce catalase.

C. sputorum mucosalis

This organism has been isolated from the oral cavity of swine (13) from a herd where a disease known as *porcine intestinal adenomatosis* had been diagnosed. More recently it has been shown to be important in the etiology of this disease in England (23) and of a similar disease in Australia (16).

Characteristics. *C. sputorum mucosalis* strains produce smooth entire colonies on blood agar, and appear as slender irregularly bent rods rather than spirals. They grow in 3.5 percent NaCl, are catalase-positive, produce a greenish pigment, and are resistant to nalidixic acid (40 μg per ml). However, much work remains to be done to develop methods for their isolation and differentiation from other similar organisms normally present in the pig's intestinal tract.

The Disease in Swine. Lawson *et al.* (14) have observed that the organism is associated with a group of porcine enteropathies where the primary lesion is adenomatosis, the lesion consisting of immature proliferating epithelial cells. The organism appears to be located within the apical cytoplasm of these cells (24).

In highly susceptible swine the disease may be characterized by a high mortality (15). However some degree of herd immunity usually exists which protects swine against the most severe form of the disease. In such herds, newly introduced nonimmune pigs are liable to be more severely affected.

Affected pigs do not thrive and their appetites are capricious. The lesions are found in the lower ileum and cecum and consist of proliferating epithelial cells throughout the entire depth of the mucosa. There is loss of villi and development of polypoid masses. In the absence of secondary infection most animals recover in about 6 weeks and the intestine is normal at slaughter.

C. fetus jejuni

The Disease in Man and Dogs. *C. fetus jejuni* is a thermophilic *Campylobacter* (table 15.1) that is being isolated with increasing frequency from cases of enteritis in humans (27). Infected dogs have been shown to be a source of infection for humans in some households (1). In these instances, affected persons had been in contact with diarrheic dogs. The disease in the dog has been described by Slee (28). Dullness, emesis, thirst, and bloody diarrhea were the signs observed, and the lesions at necropsy included a hemorrhagic enteritis, ascites, and congestion and mottling of the liver.

Recent observations indicate that both dogs and humans can be infected from contaminated pork and chicken carcasses.

The Disease in Cattle. *C. fetus jejuni* has been described by Jones *et al.* (12) as the causative agent of a disease in calves and older cattle which may occur in epidemic form during the autumn and winter months in stabled animals and is known as *winter dysentery* or *black scours*. The organisms are most abundant in the jejunum. The disease, which usually does not extend beyond the stage of simple, gastrointestinal catarrh, may in some instances be very severe. The exact role of *C. fetus jejuni* in winter dysentery is not definitely known. It is certain that other agents of as yet unknown identity can cause a similar disease.

Campylobacter Infection of Fowl

Avian vibrionic hepatitis has been described by Peckham (20) and Winterfield (36). It is an infectious disease of chickens characterized by degenerative changes in the liver and, less frequently, in the heart and other organs. Bile is a good source of the infective agent and it can be isolated in artificial media or by means of chicken embryos. The finding of *Campylobacter*like organisms by direct-phase microscopic examination serves as an aid in diagnosis.

Chemotherapy of *Campylobacter* Infections

Most strains of *Campylobacter* are sensitive to the tetracyclines, streptomycin, chloramphenicol, and macrolide antibiotics. Many strains are resistant to trimethoprim, novobiocin, polymixin B, and penicillin. Heifers and bulls have been successfully cleared of *C. fetus venerealis* infection by use of tetracyclines and streptomycin.

In dairy herds, antibiotic treatment of bull semen and use of artificial insemination is effective in preventing the disease (17). Feeding of tetracycline is effective in reducing abortion losses in sheep caused by *C. fetus intestinalis* infection but must be administered early in an outbreak to have any effect (9).

Furazolidone and erythromycin are effective therapeutic agents for avian vibrionic hepatitis.

REFERENCES

1. Blaser, Powers, Cravens, and Wang. Lancet, 1978, *2,* 979.
2. Bouters, De Keyser, Vandeplassche, Van Aert, Brone and Bonte. Brit. Vet. Jour., 1973, *129,* 52.
3. Corbeil, Schurig, Duncan, Corbeil, and Winter. Inf. and Immun., 1974, *10,* 422.
4. Corbeil, Schurig, Bier, and Winter. Inf. and Immun., 1975, *11,* 240.
5. Dennis. Austral. Vet. Jour., 1967, *43,* 45.
6. Dobbs and McIntyre. Vet. Bull., 1951, *21,* 720.
7. Firehammer, Lovelace, and Hawkins. Cornell Vet., 1962, *52,* 21.
8. Frank, Bailey, and Heithecker. Jour. Am. Vet. Med. Assoc., 1957, *131,* 472.
9. Frank, Baron, Meinershagen, and Scrinner. Am. Jour. Vet. Res., 1962, *23,* 985.
10. Gilmour, Thompson, and Fraser. Vet. Rec., 1975, *96,* 129.
11. Hoerlein and Kramer. Am. Jour. Vet. Res., 1964, *25,* 371.
12. Jones, Orcutt, and Little. Jour. Exp. Med., 1931, *53,* 853.
13. Lawson, Rowland, and Roberts. Vet. Rec., 1975, *97,* 308.
14. Lawson, Rowland, and Roberts. Res. Vet. Sci., 1977, *23,* 378.
15. Love, Love, and Edwards. Vet. Res., 1977, *100,* 65.
16. Love, Love, and Bailey. Vet. Rec., 1977, *101,* 407.
17. McEntee, Hughes, and Gilman. Cornell Vet., 1954, *44,* 395.
18. Meinershagen, Waldhalm, Frank, and Scrivner. Jour. Am. Vet. Med. Assoc., 1965, *147,* 843.
19. Miller, Jensen, and Gilroy. Am. Jour. Vet. Res., 1959, *20,* 677.
20. Peckham. Avian Dis., 1958, *2,* 348.
21. Plumer, Duvall, and Sheplar. Cornell Vet., 1962, *52,* 110.
22. Plastridge, Stula, and Williams. Am. Jour. Vet. Res., 1964, *25,* 710.
23. Roberts, Rowlands, and Lawson. Vet. Rec., 1977, *100,* 12.
24. Rowland and Hutchings. Vet. Rec., 1978, *103,* 338.
25. Samuelson and Winter. Jour. Inf. Dis., 1966, *166,* 581.
26. Sebald and Veron. Ann. Inst. Pasteur, 1963, *105,* 897.
27. Skirrow. Brit. Med. Jour., 1977, *2,* 9.
28. Slee. Vet. Rec., 1979, *104,* 14.
29. Smibert. Am. Jour. Vet. Res., 1965, *26,* 320.
30. Storz, Miner, Olson, Marriott, and Elaner. Am. Jour. Vet. Res., 1966, *27,* 115.
31. Thompson and Gilmour. Vet. Rec., 1978, *102,* 530.
32. Vandeplassche, Florent, Bonters, Huysman, Brone, and Dekeyser. Compt. Rend. Recherches, 1963, *29,* 1.
33. Wilkie and Winter. Can. Jour. Comp. Med., 1971, *35,* 301.
34. Williams, Renshaw, Meinershagen, Emerson, Chamberlain, Hall, and Waldholm. Am. Jour. Vet. Res., 1976, *37,* 409.
35. Winter. Jour. Immunol., 1975, *95,* 1002.
36. Winterfield. Jour. Am. Vet. Med. Assoc., 1959, *134,* 329.

16 The Genera *Fusobacterium* and *Bacteroides*

The Bacteroidaceae, a family of Gram-negative non-spore-bearing obligate anaerobes, inhabits the alimentary tract of man and animals and contains three genera—*Fusobacterium, Bacteroides,* and *Leptotrichia*. They are differentiated by gas chromatographic analysis of fatty acid formation from peptone or glucose. *Bacteroides* sp. produce major amounts of isovaleric and isobutyric acids. The major fermentation acids of *Fusobacterium* and *Leptotrichia* are butyric and lactic acids respectively.

Only *Fusobacterium* and *Bacteroides* contain species that commonly cause disease in the domesticated animals.

Fusobacterium necrophorum

SYNONYMS: *Bacillus diphtheriae vitulorum, Streptothrix cuniculi, Corynebacterium necrophorum, Cladothrix cuniculi, Bacterium necrophorum, Actinomyces necrophorus, Fusiformis necrophorus, Spheropherus necrophorus,* calf diphtheria bacillus, necrosis bacillus

This organism is found in necrotic lesions in warm-blooded animals. It produces the diseases commonly known under the collective name of *necrobacilloses.*

Morphology and Staining Reactions. In infected tissues this organism is ordinarily seen in the form of long filaments, but shorter elements and even coccoid forms occur. The rods are about 1 μm in width and may be in excess of 100 μm in length. In some cultures swollen rods are seen which may be nearly twice as thick as the usual forms. Freshly isolated strains growing in cooked-meat medium usually show a predominance of long filaments. The sides of these filaments are parallel and regular, and are either straight or form-sweeping curves. After prolonged artificial culture the predominating forms usually are short. Very young cultures stain uniformly as a rule, but the filaments in cultures older than 24 hours usually are vacuolated, that is, the stained portions are separated by sections that are almost or quite free of stain (Figure 16.1). The irregular distribution of cytoplasm along the filaments can easily be seen in un-

Figure 16.1. *Fusobacterium necrophorum* in a lung abscess in a calf. The long filaments with irregular distribution of chromatic material are characteristic. × 1,040.

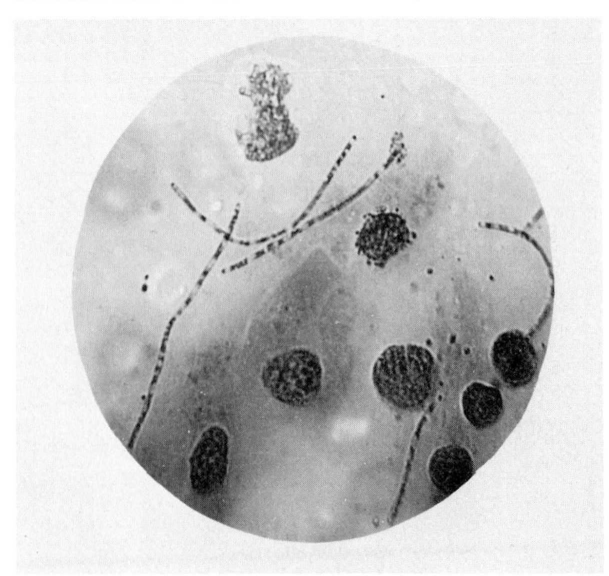

stained preparations. Some early authors have described branching, but most of those who have studied this organism agree that it does not branch. Flagella have not been demonstrated and motility is absent. Ordinary dyes stain young cultures readily. The organism is always Gram-negative.

Cultural Features. The necrosis bacillus is very sensitive to oxygen, and growth does not occur unless good anaerobic conditions are obtained. An atmosphere of 5 to 10 percent carbon dioxide enhances growth. Primary growths on solid media in anaerobic jars may fail because exposure to oxygen during the initial incubation phase and before anaerobiasis is fully established may fatally damage the cells. The optimal temperature is 37 C, and serum or blood, yeast extract, and a reducing agent such as cysteine are necessary for good growth. Cultures die rapidly after initial growth, even in cooked-meat or liver-brain medium. Thioglycollate medium, without enrichment, works well in maintaining stock cultures. Even in these media cultures die out in most cases within 1 or 2 weeks, although occasionally a strain will remain viable for several months. Tunnicliff (28) reports that a liver-brain medium to which calcium carbonate is added will retain viability for a year or more. Under favorable conditions acid and gas are formed from glucose, lactose, sucrose, maltose, and salicin. The amount of acid formed is not great and gas formation is limited. In cooked-meat medium covered with a vaspar seal (petrolatum and paraffin in equal parts), a large bubble of gas is regularly formed. Hemolysis of horse blood occurs. Serum gelatin is not liquefied and coagulated serum is not digested. In clear, solid media, colonies are fuzzy when the medium is fairly soft and dense when it is more solid. Colonies are rounded, gray, 1 to 3 mm in diameter. On sheep-blood agar, the selective isolation of *F. necrophorum* from tissues may be accomplished on the medium described by Fales and Teresa (7). This medium consists of an egg yolk agar base containing 0.02 percent crystal violet, 0.01 percent brilliant green and phenethyl alcohol, the latter to suppress Gram-negative facultative anaerobes. Under carbon dioxide incubation, colonies of *F. necrophorum* are blue, and are surrounded by opaque and clear zones. Antibiotics such as kanamycin, erythromycin, vancomycin, and bacitracin have also been used in selective media (1).

Cultures may be preserved by freezing at −70 C in calf serum or lyophilization in skim milk (7).

F. necrophorum can be differentiated from other species of *Fusobacterium* by indol production and formation of propionic acid from lactate. *Fusobacterium* may be differentiated from *Bacteroides* by failure of the former to synthesize 3-hydroxy fatty acids (12, 30).

Antigens. *Fusobacterium* does not cross-react serologically with *Bacteroides* (29) and fluorescent anti-sera against *F. necrophorum* do not react with other *Fusobacterium* species. Both heat-labile and heat-stable antigens are present in *F. necrophorum*, and there is considerable antigenic heterogeneity among strains. Feldman *et al.* (9) described four distinct antigenic groups among 14 strains of *F. necrophorum* from bovine liver abscesses.

Epidemiology and Pathogenesis. *F. necrophorum* is a commensal of the alimentary tract of many animal species and man. Infections in animals generally occur when they are kept in filthy surroundings, especially when there are accumulations of manure underfoot. It does not seem likely that the organism could multiply outside the body, but it undoubtedly remains viable in soil for short periods of time. Marsh and Tunnicliff (23) were able to demonstrate the organism in a wet pasture 10 months after sheep affected with foot-rot had run on it, but they could not demonstrate it after a second 10-month period. Under these conditions, which apparently were unusually favorable, the organism was able to survive through one winter in the rigorous climate of Montana.

The organism has little or no ability to invade normal epithelia but readily enters and multiplies in tissues damaged by trauma, virus infection, or maceration, or by other bacteria. In all species, the typical lesion is necrosis, abscess formation, and putrid odor. Bacteremia may occur in some instances, with dissemination to the liver and other organs. Strains of *F. necrophorum* contain a classical lipopolysaccharide endotoxin that is cell-wall associated and in which lipid A is a major toxic component (16). Other components of the organism also have toxic activity. Garcia *et al.* (15) have described a cytoplasmic proteinaceous toxin that has hemolytic activity and is protectively immunogenic, and Roberts (24) has described a leukocidin apparently distinct from this hemolysin. The leukocidin may be a significant virulence factor of *F. necrophorum* because the leukocytes of animals with relatively higher resistance to infection by the organism exhibit much less toxic effect following exposure to the leukocidin (25). Experimental infections of mice indicate that the organism multiplies in the liver, causing focal necrosis and accumulation of mononuclear cells including macrophages (17). The organism occurs within the macrophages, which are eventually killed by the leukocidin. Fales, Warner, and Teresa (6) have examined this toxic effect in isolated rabbit peritoneal macrophages and found that 90 percent of macrophages were killed within 6 hours. The cytotoxic effect of *F. necrophorum* for liver and other cells has not yet been fully defined but may be an effect of the endotoxin because the latter produces necrosis when inoculated intradermally into rabbits. In this connection, Berg (2) has observed that type A hemagglutinating strains of *F. necrophorum* belong to two groups, one of which is extremely virulent for mice and produces a potent leukocidin and a potent endotoxin. The second group, which is much less virulent for mice, has a potent leukocidin but very little endotoxin activity.

Cattle. Infection of the mouth and pharynx of calves (calf diphtheria) is an especially malignant form of necrobacillosis. The disease occurs usually in young calves that are bucket-fed under conditions of poor hygiene, but it has also been observed in cattle up to 2 years of age. The lesions may extend to the larynx, with subsequent aspiration of necrotic material into the lungs, resulting in fatal pneumonia.

Liver abscesses caused by *F. necrophorum* in cattle result in serious economic loss to the meat industry in many parts of the world. Lesions are often found in the liver as firm, dry, sharply circumscribed areas of a light yellow color, and sometimes as well-encapsulated abscesses. In the latter instance, other bacteria such as *Corynebacterium pyogenes* may also be present. Liver abscesses caused by *F. necrophorum* are especially common in feedlot cattle, and it has been proposed (26) that the organism enters the portal circulation from lesions on the rumenal epithelium and thence travels to the liver. The initial rumenal lesions may be caused by excessive acidity resulting from a high concentration diet (20).

Foot-rot, or foul in the foot, in cattle (Figure 16.2) has frequently been associated with *F. necrophorum,* but the role of the organism in the genesis of the lesions is uncertain. Berg and Loan (3) have isolated both *F. necrophorum* and *Bacteroides melanigenicus* in large numbers from biopsies of naturally occurring and experimentally produced lesions in cattle in the United States. In Britain, Thorley, Calder and Harrison (27) have reported *Bacteroides nodosus* in necrotic lesions of the interdigital skin in cattle.

Attempts to produce the disease experimentally with pure cultures of *F. necrophorum* have not been successful (10). However, typical foot-rot lesions were produced with a combination of fusiformlike organisms and staphylococci (18). It is probable that concurrent infection by *F. necrophorum* plus any of several other bacteria can produce foot-rot in cattle. Trauma and maceration are well-known predisposing factors. The milder form of the disease involves only the interdigital space where a fissure lined by foul-smelling necrotic tissues develops. In more severe lesions involving the laminar structures, bacteria found include *F. necrophorum, B. nodosus*, and *C. pyogenes.*

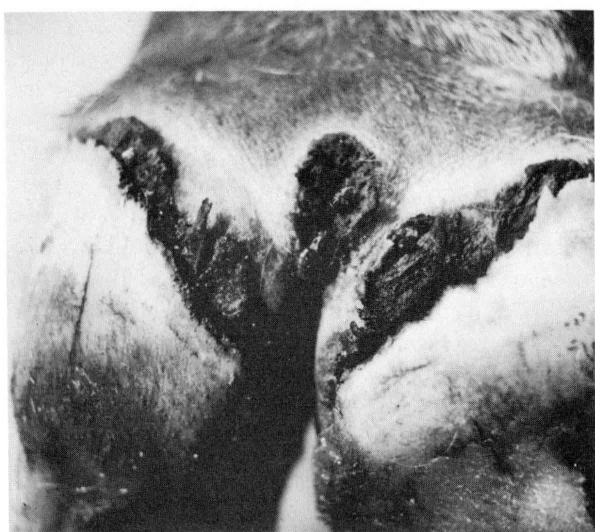

Figure 16.2. Bovine foot-rot.

Lesions associated with *F. necrophorum* have also been seen on the udder and teats of cattle. Uterine infections are not uncommon, and ulceration of the mucosa of the abomasum is often ascribed to this bacillus. The organism has been encountered in bovine mastitis and in rumenitis of calves reared on an early-weaning feeding system.

Sheep. F. necrophorum lesions in sheep are similar to those in cattle. The organism has been associated with the diseases known as ovine interdigital dermatitis, lip-and-leg ulceration, foot-rot, and infective bulbar necrosis (foot abscess) of ewes lambing in wet conditions. The most important bacterium in foot-rot of sheep, however, is *B. nodosus. F. necrophorum* is of importance in creating invasion sites for *B. nodosus, C. pyogenes* and *Spirocheta penortha,* which are also commonly found in lesions, as secondary invaders. Ovine interdigital dermatitis is a skin condition associated with an intense invasion by *F. necrophorum* of the posterior interdigital epidermis when subject to continuous wet conditions, and foot-rot associated with *B. nodosus* may be a sequel to this disease. Ovine foot abscesses are caused by *F. necrophorum* and *C. pyogenes* in synergy (24, 25). *F. necrophorum* facilitates the establishment and growth of *C. pyogenes* in the tissues through the leukocidal action of its exotoxin and prevention of phagocytosis, whereas *C. pyogenes* produces a macromolecular substance which stimulates the growth and invasiveness of *F. necrophorum*. *C. pyogenes* also contributes to the growth of *F. necrophorum* by removing O_2 and decreasing Eh.

Swine. In swine, *F. necrophorum* is associated with *ulcerative stomatitis* (sore mouth) and the condition known as *bullnose,* in which there is an infection of the subcutaneous tissues of the face, frequently originating in the wound made by the placing of a ring in the nose. It is also associated with necrosis of the epithelium and deeper layers of the intestines, a condition known as *necrotic enteritis*. Necrobacillosis has also been described in rabbits, where it involves the lips and mouth; in horses, where the lower posterior aspects of the legs may be involved (scratches); and in chickens, as a sequel to fowlpox virus infection (5).

Diagnosis. Gram-stained smears from the edges of lesions frequently reveal the organism. Cultures should be quickly made on suitable prereduced selective media, such as that of Fales and Teresa (7), and placed under anaerobiasis.

No serologic methods of diagnosis are available. Fluorescent antibody techniques have been tried on infected bovine livers, but proved difficult to interpret because fluorescence was also observed in healthy livers used to control the technique (13).

Immunity. Attempts to vaccinate animals with formalinized cell preparations and with culture filtrates of *F. necrophorum* have not been successful. Liver abscessation in cattle has been prevented by using a cytoplasmic fraction of sonically treated *F. necrophorum* (14). Precipitating antibodies were produced in almost all animals receiving the highest dose of vaccine, whereas only 35 percent of control cattle produced precipitins during the 6-month trial. Adult, healthy animals exhibit a high rate of seropositivity in the agglutination reaction, and young animals such as calves show little or no seropositivity (9). Thus, it appears that most animals, as they age and are exposed to the organism, develop antibodies. Furthermore, Feldman *et al.* (9) were unable to relate the presence and severity of abscessation to the magnitude of agglutinin titers, an indication that these antibodies are not important in protection against the disease.

Treatment. Reports on the use of the sulfonamides in the treatment of the necrobacilloses have indicated that certain members of this group of drugs are quite effective in treating these infections. Farquharson (8) reported marked success in treating calf diphtheria with sulfapyridine, and Hayes and Wright (19) found sulfamethazine to be exceptionally effective in treating an outbreak of this infection in 2,785 calves and feeder cattle. Foreman (11) reported that sulfapyridine is specific for all types of foot-rot in cattle, and Lebovit (21) showed that sulfathiazole injected intravenously produced very satisfactory results when used early in the course of the disease or in chronic cases. Leventhal and Easterbrooks (22) treated foot-rot in cattle with a combination of a multiple enzyme preparation (streptokinase, streptodornase, and human plasminogen) and tetracycline. They claimed marked success. Aureomycin has been recommended as effective in preventing the formation of liver abscesses in cattle. Spiramycin given at the rate of 10 mg per kg (20 percent solution intramuscularly) 4 times a year has been found to prevent foot-rot in cattle on premises where the disease was endemic (4). Larger amounts given in 2 doses 48 hours apart were also effective in treatment of acute foot-rot.

REFERENCES

1. Balows, Dehaan, Dowell, and Guze (eds.). Anaerobic bacteria: Role in disease. American Lecture Series in Microbiology No. 940. Proc. Int. Conf. on Anaerobic Diseases. Thomas, Springfield, Ill., 1975.
2. Berg. Unpublished data, cited in review by Langworth, Vet. Bull., 1969, *39*, 311.
3. Berg and Loan. Am. Jour. Vet. Res., 1975, *36*, 1115.
4. Chauvau and Royer. Bull. Mensuel Soc. Vet. Pratique de France, 1977, *61*, 255.
5. Emmel. Jour. Am. Vet. Med. Assoc., 1948, *113*, 169.
6. Fales, Warner, and Teresa. Am. Jour. Vet. Res., 1977, *38*, 491.
7. Fales and Teresa. Am. Jour. Vet. Res., 1972, *33*, 2317.
8. Farquharson. Jour. Am. Vet. Med. Assoc., 1942, *101*, 88.
9. Feldman, Hester, and Wherry. Jour. Inf. Dis., 1936, *59*, 159.
10. Flint and Jensen. Am. Jour. Vet. Res., 1951, *42*, 5.
11. Foreman. Jour. Am. Vet. Med. Assoc., 1946, *109*, 126.
12. Futsche and Boehmer. Zentrbl. f. Bakt., 1974, *226*, 248.
13. Garcia, Neil, and McKay. Appl. Microbiol., 1971, *21*, 809.
14. Garcia, Dorward, Alexander, Mogwood, and McKay. Can. Jour. Comp. Med., 1973, *38*, 222.
15. Garcia, Alexander, and McKay. Inf. and Immun., 1975, *11*, 609.
16. Garcia, Charlton, and McKay. Inf. and Immun., 1975, *11*, 371.

17. Garcia, Charlton, and McKay. Can. Jour. Microbiol., 1977, *23*, 1465.
18. Gupta, Fincher, and Bruner. Cornell Vet., 1964, *54*, 66.
19. Hayes and Wright. Jour. Am. Vet. Med. Assoc., 1949, *114*, 80.
20. Jensen and Mackey. Diseases of feedlot cattle. Lea and Febiger, Philadelphia, 1974.
21. Lebovit. Jour. Am. Vet. Med. Assoc., 1948, *112*, 453.
22. Leventhal and Easterbrooks. Jour. Am. Vet. Med. Assoc., 1956, *129*, 422.
23. Marsh and Tunnicliff. Mont. Agr. Exp. Sta. Bull. 285, 1934.
24. Roberts, Brit. Jour. Exp. Path., 1967, *48*, 665.
25. Roberts. Brit. Jour. Exp. Path., 1967, *48*, 674.
26. Smith. Am. Jour. Vet. Res., 1944, *5*, 234.
27. Thorley, Calder, and Harrison. Vet. Rec., 1977, *100*, 387.
28. Tunnicliff. Jour. Inf. Dis., 1938, *63*, 113.
29. Werner and Sebald. Ann. Inst. Pasteur (Paris), 1968, *115*, 350.
30. Werner. Zentrbl. f. Bakt., 1976, *228*, 73.

Bacteroides nodosus

SYNONYMS: *Actinomyces nodosus, Ristella nodosa, Fusiformis nodosus*

Bacteroides nodosus is an essential causal agent of foot-rot in sheep and was first described by Beveridge in 1941 in Australia (1).

Morphology and Staining Reactions. The organism is a large, rod-shaped bacterium characterized by the presence of terminal enlargements, usually at both ends. These enlargements are more pronounced in organisms seen in tissue smears than in those developing in culture. The rods usually are straight but may be slightly curved. They are 0.6 to 0.8 μm in diameter and 3 to 10 μm in length, although few are more than 6 μm long. In cultures the organisms tend to be shorter and in old cultures they may even be coccoid in form. They are nonmotile and do not form spores or capsules. They stain readily with all ordinary dyes. They are Gram-negative and non-acid-fast. Organisms stained with methylene blue often show one or several metachromatic granules, usually located at the ends of the rod.

Cultural Features. The organism is an obligate anaerobe. Growth is enhanced when 10 percent or more of carbon dioxide is introduced into the anaerobic culture jar. Growth occurs best at 37 C. At room temperature very slow growth occurs. Cultures grow best in neutral or alkaline media.

Practically no growth is obtained on any of the ordinary media unless horse serum is added to them in a proportion of 10 percent. Not all lots of horse serum prove satisfactory, and sheep serum not only failed to promote growth but actually inhibited it in the presence of horse serum. Rabbit and cow serum were not satisfactory.

Best growth was obtained on "V-F" agar, which is a peptic digest of beef muscle and liver. Veal infusion media were not very favorable even when horse serum had been added. Growth did not occur on inspissated horse serum or egg medium. Growth was never luxuriant in any fluid media, and ordinary types even with serum added often failed to promote growth. A simple medium recommended for the isolation of *B. nodosus* consists of pulverized, suspended sheep horn in an anaerobic medium with 10 percent CO_2 (14). A liquid medium used by Thomas (15) contained hydrolyzed sheep hoof as a basic ingredient.

On "V-F" agar plates containing horse serum and 0.1 cystein hydrochloride as a reducing agent, surface colonies are obtained. These are generally of a smooth surface, develop up to a diameter of 1 mm, and usually lie in small "etched" depressions in the agar surface. If blood is added to the medium instead of serum, no hemolysis is observed. Heavy inocula will often cause the curdling of milk after several days' incubation without change in reaction, and later the curd is digested. In cooked-meat media the fragments are partially digested. In old cultures tyrosine crystals are formed. None of the ordinary carbohydrates is fermented. Nitrates are not reduced but hydrogen sulfide is formed. A selective medium for isolation of *B. nodosus* has been described by Gradin and Schmitz (8). It contains 1 μg lincomycin per ml in Eugon agar with 0.2 percent yeast extract and 10 percent horse blood.

Natural Habitat. *B. nodosus* is an obligate parasite of the hoof of sheep, goats, and cattle. It survives for only a few days on pasture or in soil. The infection may be transmitted between cattle and sheep, but the disease is not transmitted to sheep from cattle under natural conditions (9). It is possible that the strains that occur in the hooves of cattle are less virulent for sheep.

Antigens. Both K (specific) and O (group) antigens have been described. The K antigen, a protein, is associated with the fimbriae and is the protective antigen (13). Egerton (7) examined the K antigens of the strains and found that each was serologically distinct, but all three strains possessed the same heat-stable or O antigens. The O antigen lipopolysaccharide is biologically, chemically, and ultrastructurally similar to that of the Enterobacteriaceae and consists of a polysaccharide joined to lipid A through an acid-labile 2-keto-3-deoxyoctonic acid link (12).

Epidemiology and Pathogenesis. Since the organism survives only in the hoof, carrier animals serve as sources for uninfected stock. The infection spreads rapidly when sheep are grazing lush, damp pasture in rainy weather. Thus, foot-rot is more common in late spring and early fall. Besides maceration of the feet due to wet conditions, minor wounds, abrasions from stony surfaces, and damage caused by migrating *Strongyloides* larvae are other predisposing causes of foot-rot in sheep.

Much of the recent definitive work on the pathogenesis of foot-rot in sheep has been done in Australia by Egerton, Parsonson, and Roberts (3, 4, 10). Invasion by *B. nodosus* of the interdigital epidermis is preceded by colonization of the stratum corneum by *F. necrophorum* apparently derived from feces. The latter organism damages the epidermis sufficiently to allow entry and multiplication of *B. nodosus*. *B. nodosus* has little inflammatory destructive action but produces a powerful protease which digests horn (2) and permits invasion of the epidermal matrix of the hoof. It is also

capable of slow persisting growth when nutrients are scarce and thus can sustain itself between the brief waves of growth of *F. necrophorum* and so persist in the lesion. Finally, it produces a heat-stable soluble factor that promotes the growth and invasiveness of *F. necrophorum*.

Although Beveridge (1) has indicated that *Spirochaeta penortha* is the accessory factor in producing foot-rot in sheep, Roberts and Egerton (10) have concluded that spirochetes and motile fusiforms are probably not essential to the pathogenesis of this disease but are derived from the environment. *Corynebacterium pyogenes* and other aerobic diphtheroids which usually have a superficial location in the lesion remove oxygen and reduce Eh, thus facilitating the growth of the anaerobes. The separation of horn in foot-rot is caused by lysis of the epidermal matrix as a result of the local inflammatory response to the infection and is not a result of direct bacterial attack (4).

The role of *B. nodosus* in the pathogenesis of foot-rot

Table 16.1. Involvement of Bacteroidaceae in diseases of the foot of cattle and sheep

Disease and host	Area affected	Bacteria and their role in pathogenesis	
1. Interdigital dermatitis (cattle, sheep)	Interdigital epidermis	*F. necrophorum*	Causes epidermal necrosis and secretes a leucocidal toxin which aids establishment of *C. pyogenes*.
		C. pyogenes	Elaborates a substance which stimulates growth of *F. necrophorum*. It also lowers Eh.
2. Scald (sheep)	Interdigital epidermis	*F. necrophorum*, *C. minutissime*	Causes epidermal necrosis and secretes a leukocidal toxin which may aid invasion by *C. minutissime*.
3. Foot-rot (sheep)	Laminar structure of hoof	*F. necrophorum*	Causes epidermal necrosis and makes way for entry of *B. nodosus*.
		B. nodosus	Secretes protease which digests epidermal matrix and facilitates entry of other bacteria. Secretes growth factor for *F. necrophorum*.
		C. pyogenes	As in No. 1.
		Spirochaeta penortha	Unknown, probably of minor significance.
4. Foot-rot, foul in the foot (cattle), heel abscess, infective bulbar necrosis (sheep)	Deeper tissues of the foot	*F. necrophorum*, *C. pyogenes*	As in No. 1.
5. Pododermatitis, stinky foot (cattle)	Interdigital epidermis (posterior region near bulbs of heel)	*F. necrophorum*, *F. nodosus*	As in No. 1.

in cattle is not as well defined as in sheep, but the organism has been recognized in bovine foot lesions in Australia (3), Holland (17), and Britain (16). Typical lesions in cattle displayed necrosis of the interdigital epidermis which became eroded. The posterior skin area between the claws showed a swollen grey seborrheic area with a pronounced foul odor. Cracking of the skin at its junction with the horn in the interdigital space was a common sequel. Also, the horn in the heel area sometimes became separated.

The involvement of Bacteroidaceae in diseases of the foot of cattle and sheep is summarized in Table 16.1.

Immunity. *B. nodosus* is excluded from the dermis by the bactericidal effects of serum and by phagocytes. After infection, IgG_1 antibodies are produced against the fimbrial antigen of the organism, and these antibodies, when present in high titer, are protective (13). Successful vaccines against ovine foot-rot must contain K antigen (5). Furthermore, Egerton, Morgan, and Burrell (6) found that there was a requirement for type-specific K antigen—a finding later confirmed by Egerton (7), who found three distinct and serologically different types of K antigen among ovine strains of *B. nodosus* in Australia. Immunity to foot-rot requires very high titer of antibody (5). This is so because in order to be effective against *B. nodosus* which is infecting the epidermal layers, antibodies in adequate concentration must diffuse out of the

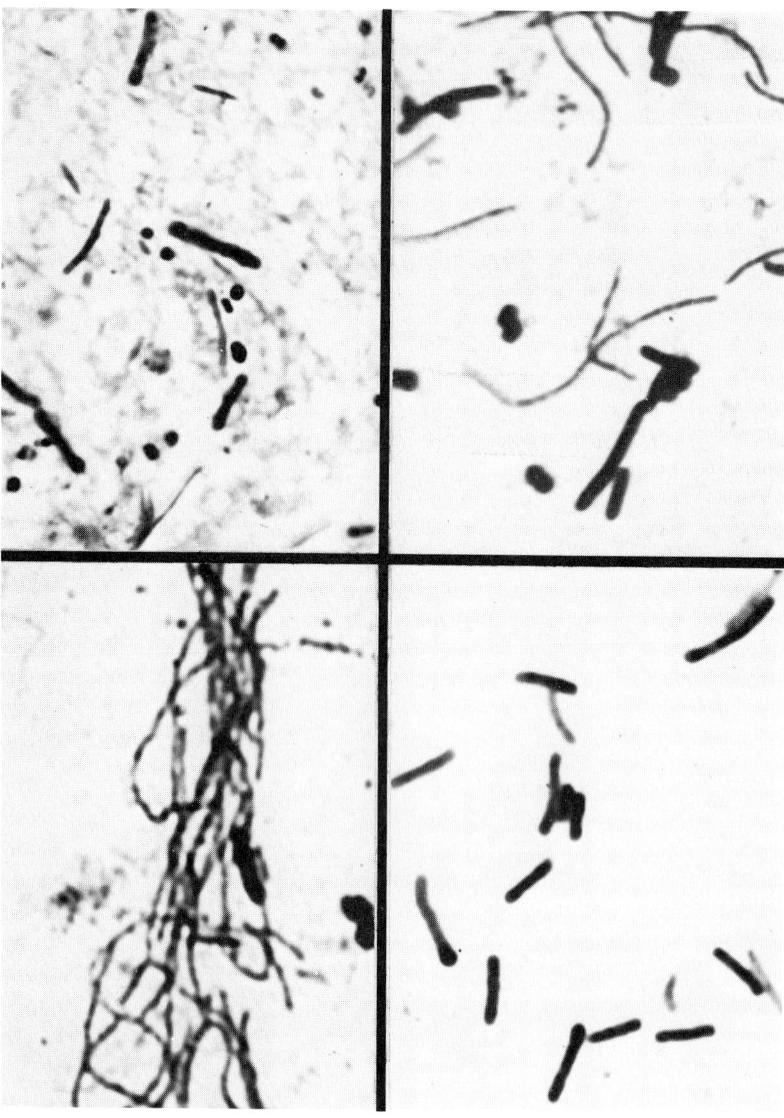

Figure 16.3. (*Upper left*) *Bacteroides nodosus* in a smear from a foot-rot lesion. Carbol fuchsin. × 1,500 (*Upper right*) Spirochetelike organism in a smear from a foot-rot lesion. Krajian silver stain. × 1,450. (*Lower left*) Mass of spirochetelike organisms in a smear from a foot-rot lesion. Krajian silver stain. × 1,450. (*Lower right*) *Bacteroides nodosus* from a 3-day-old colony on agar. Carbol fuchsin. × 1,450. (Courtesy H. Marsh and K. D. Claus, *Cornell Vet.*)

capillary bed beneath the stratum germinativum and through the nonliving layers of the epidermis toward the skin surface. Alum-precipitated anacultures are the form in which commercial vaccines are presented in Europe and Australia and must be administered twice at an interval of 4 to 6 weeks between doses. The agglutinin titers that result average about 1/15,000, and experimental trials (11) have indicated that the immunity thus stimulated will protect about 80 percent of the flock, assuming that other established methods of control, including routine foot care, are being carried out. The vaccine will not, of course, protect against foot lesions due to other microorganisms such as *Dermatophilus congolensis* or *Fusobacterium necrophorum* by itself. Booster doses of vaccine must be given to vaccinated sheep about 2 weeks before the expected occurrence of foot-rot each season.

Diagnosis. Smears prepared from the edges of lesions beneath the epidermal matrix and stained by Gram may reveal the characteristically shaped *B. nodosus* (Figure 16.3). It may be necessary to examine a number of smears to confirm the presence of the organism. Culture of *B. nodosus* from foot smears may be attempted on selective medium containing Eugon agar, 0.2 percent yeast extract, 10 percent horse blood and 1 μg lincomycin per ml (8).

Control and Treatment. Infected areas on the feet should be exposed by paring away the horn and allowing oxygen to penetrate the lesion. Topical chloramphenicol or tetracycline sprays may then be applied. Treated sheep and all others in the group are run through a foot bath containing 10 percent formalin, which disinfects the feet. The sheep are then released onto pasture that has not been grazed by cattle or sheep for 2 weeks previously. Vaccination is also advisable and should reduce the incidence to manageable proportions; it is beneficial even after foot-rot has appeared in the flock.

REFERENCES

1. Beveridge. Austral. Council Sci. and Indus. Res. Bull. 140, 1941.
2. Broad and Skerman. New Zeal. Jour. Ag. Res., 1976, *19,* 317.
3. Egerton and Parsonson. Austral. Vet. Jour., 1966, *42,* 425.
4. Egerton, Roberts, and Parsonson. Jour. Comp. Path., 1969, *79,* 207.
5. Egerton and Roberts. Jour. Comp. Path., 1971, *81,* 179.
6. Egerton, Morgan, and Burrell. Vet. Rec., 1972, *91,* 447.
7. Egerton. Jour. Comp. Path., 1973, *83,* 151.
8. Gradin and Schmitz. Jour. Clin. Microbiol., 1977, *6,* 298.
9. Laing and Egerton. Res. Vet. Sci., 1978, *24,* 300.
10. Roberts and Egerton. Jour. Comp. Path., 1969, *79,* 217.
11. Roberts, Foster, Kerry, and Calder. Vet. Rec., 1972, *91,* 428.
12. Stewart. Res. Vet. Sci., 1977, *23,* 319.
13. Stewart. Res. Vet. Sci., 1978, *24,* 14.
14. Thomas. Austral. Vet. Jour., 1958, *34,* 411.
15. Thomas. Austral. Vet. Jour., 1963, *39,* 434.
16. Thorley and McCalder. Vet. Rec., 1977, *100,* 387.
17. Toussaint, Ronen, and Cornelisse. Vet. Med. Rev., 1974, *2/3,* 223.

17 The Genera *Staphylococcus* and *Streptococcus*

THE GENUS *STAPHYLOCOCCUS*

The genus *Staphylococcus* belongs to the family Micrococcaceae which contains two other genera, *Micrococcus* and *Planococcus*. *Micrococcus* sp. are common in the environment, on skin, and on the mammary gland and frequently occur in specimens of milk and in swabs taken from epithelial surfaces. *Planococcus* occurs only in marine habitats.

Three species of *Staphylococcus* cause disease in animals: *S. aureus, S. epidermidis* (*albus*), and *S. hyicus*.

Staphylococcus aureus and *Staphylococcus epidermidis*

These two species were originally named because of the color of colonies, but this means of distinction is not valid because both species can give rise to either white or yellowish colonies.

Morphology and Staining Reactions. The pathogenic staphylococci appear as perfectly spherical organisms of uniform size (about 0.8 μm in diameter). In pus the organisms frequently are grouped in irregular masses that remind one of a bunch of grapes. This appearance caused Ogsten (36) to adopt the generic name for the group (*staphylo* [Gr.] = "bunch of grapes") (Figure 17.1). In fluid media the organisms usually appear singly, in small groups or in short chains. They are nonmotile, do not form spores, and usually do not possess capsular substance *in vitro*. The ordinary stains are readily taken, and young cultures always are Gram-positive. Older cultures lose part of their Gram-retaining ability. The acid-fast stain is not retained.

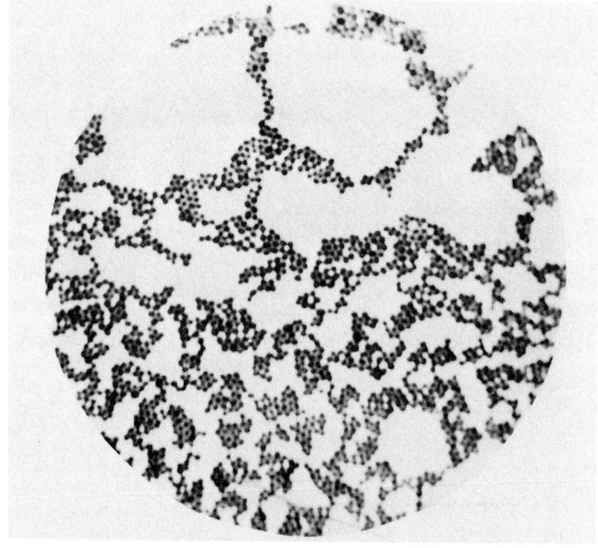

Figure 17.1. *Staphylococcus aureus,* a stained film from a 24-hour-old culture on slant agar, showing typical arrangement in grapelike masses. × 940.

Cultural and Biochemical Features. Colonies of pathogenic staphylococci are porcelain white or yellowish orange when growing on solid media. The orange-colored carotenoid pigment is best seen on media containing starch or fatty acids and that are rather dry, for example, coagulated blood serum. The orange-colored cultures are the most active biochemically, and their pathogenicity usually is greater. Their cultural features show quantitative rather than qualitative differences; hence they will be described together.

Broth is uniformly and rather heavily clouded. A moderate amount of rather viscid sediment forms in the bottom of the tube. The growth on agar is quite profuse, semitransparent, moist, and glistening. Gelatin is rapidly liquefied by freshly isolated strains of *S. aureus,* but the property is easily lost upon continued cultivation. *S. epidermidis* usually will not liquefy gelatin even when freshly isolated.

Some strains are strongly hemolytic; others have no action on blood. (Hemolysis will be discussed in greater detail under the heading "Toxins and Enzymes.") Litmus milk is reddened but frequently not coagulated. Acid but no gas is formed from glucose, lactose, sucrose, and mannitol by most cultures. In this group there is considerable variation in fermenting ability. Unlike many of the saprophytic micrococci, the pyogenic types are unable to utilize ammonium salts as a sole source of nitrogen. Nitrates usually are reduced. Certain strains of *S. aureus* produce bacteriocin (staphylococcin), an antibiotic that inhibits some Gram-negative but not Gram-positive bacteria (19). These strains are catalase-positive and can grow in the presence of a high salt concentration (7.5 to 10 percent sodium chloride).

The features by which *S. epidermidis* can be differentiated from *S. aureus* are shown in Table 17.1.

Resistance. Staphylococci are among the most resistant of non-spore-bearing organisms. Most strains are capable of resisting dehydration for long periods, they are relatively heat-resistant, and they tolerate the ordinary disinfectants better than the vegetative forms of most organisms. The use of staphylococci as indicators of swimming pool pollution has been suggested. They are more chlorine resistant than intestinal bacteria and their absence implies the lack of the enteric forms (17).

Table 17.1. Differentiation of *S. aureus* from *S. epidermidis* (*albus*)

Characteristic	*S. aureus*	*S. epidermidis* (*albus*)
Coagulase	+	−
Mannitol (anaerobically)	Acid	−
DNase	+	−
Biotin requirement	−	+
Cell-wall constituents		
Ribitol	+	−
Glycerol	−	+
Protein A	+	−
Alpha hemolysin	+	−

Cellular Antigens. Three important components of the cell wall of *S. aureus* are its peptidoglycan, ribitol, teichoic acids, and the precipitinogen protein A. *S. epidermidis* lacks Protein A and contains glycerol in place of ribitol; the teichoic acid complexes are covalently linked to the muramic acid mucopeptide of the cell wall. The immunological specificities of *S. aureus* and *S. epidermidis* reside in the teichoic acid moieties, which are termed polysaccharides A and B, respectively. Protein A is found only on strains of *S. aureus* and is a small basic protein (MW 13,000) which reacts with the Fc fragments of IgG molecules and is antiphagocytic and fixes complement. Over 30 type-specific agglutinogens have been found on *S. aureus,* but these are not used routinely because of nonspecific clumping effects exhibited by the organisms.

Other antigens associated with the outer cell are several capsular antigens which are antiphagocytic, and bound coagulase or clumping factor which acts on fibrinogen, causing the cells to aggregate in plasma.

Toxins and Enzymes. Staphylococci produce many extracellular toxins and enzymes, some of which may be important in the pathogenesis of disease. (These are listed in Table 17.2 for *S. aureus.*) The alpha hemolysin produces lysosomal disruption in leukocytes and is cytocidal for other cells; it is dermonecrotic when injected subcutaneously and is lethal for mice and rabbits when injected intravenously. It affects smooth muscle, leading to constriction, paralysis, and finally necrosis of smooth muscle cells in the walls of blood vessels. It plays an important role in the pathogenesis of gangrenous mastitis in the cow (9).

Alpha hemolysin also produces complete hemolysis of rabbit, sheep, and ox erythrocytes but has no effect on horse or human erythrocytes.

The beta hemolysin is a sphingomyelinase and produces incomplete hemolysis of sheep and ox erythrocytes at 37 C. After further storage at 4 C to 15 C, the incomplete hemolysis changes to complete, i.e., "hot-cold" lysis. There is evidence that beta toxin causes complete or partial masking of alpha toxin (29). When antibodies to beta toxin are present, the masking effect is neutralized and the alpha toxin is able to produce complete hemolysis. Beta hemolysin production is characteristic of staphylococci of animal origin. Its significance in pathogenesis is in dispute. Anderson (2) concludes that it is of little importance, but Naidu and Newbauld (35) have observed that inflammation and somatic cell re-

Table 17.2. Toxins and enzymes produced by *Staphylococcus aureus*

Toxin or Enzyme	Action
Toxins	
Alpha hemolysin	Hemolysis (sheep, rabbit); vasoconstriction and dermonecrosis
Beta hemolysin	Hot-cold hemolysis (sheep)
Gamma hemolysin	Weak hemolysis
Delta hemolysin	Dermonecrosis; destruction of leukocytes
Leukocidin	Leukocytic degranulation
Enterotoxin	Emesis and/or diarrhea
Enzymes	
Coagulase (free)	Clots purified fibrinogen in presence of CRF* from prothrombin
Hyaluronidase (spreading factor)	Hydrolyzes hyaluronic acid in intercellular ground substance
DNase	Hydrolyzes DNA
Fibrinolysin (staphylokinase)	Dissolves clots by activation of plasminogen
Lipase	Hydrolyzes bactericidal lipids of skin
Protease	Hydrolyzes proteins

*Coagulase reacting factor.

sponses were proportional to amounts of beta hemolysin infused into the bovine mammary gland.

The delta hemolysin is a phospholipase and is dermonecrotic. It is immunologically specific and will hemolyze human, rabbit, sheep, guinea pig, and horse erythrocytes. Because it migrates much more slowly through agar than alpha toxin, its effects take longer to be expressed.

An epsilon hemolysin is produced by *S. epidermidis* and lyses sheep and rabbit erythrocytes. It is immunologically distinct from the hemolysins of *S. aureus*. Enterotoxins, designated types A, B, C, and D (10), are elaborated by about 50 percent of coagulase-positive *S. aureus* of human origin that belong to phage groups III and IV. They cause acute gastroenteritis or so-called ptomaine poisoning in man.

Various starchy foods, spray-dried milk (3, 4), meat food products, and cold meats, especially ham, have been involved in staphylococcic food-poisoning outbreaks. Staphylococci will form enterotoxin when incubated in milk. That a high percentage of isolates from the bovine mammary gland produce enterotoxin was demonstrated by Bell and Veliz (5); hence it is possible that some food poisoning of man may be caused by the consumption of milk from cattle that are suffering from staphylococcic mastitis. Minett (33) and Crabtree and Litterer (12) suggest that this has occasionally happened. Enterotoxin-producing *S. aureus* are also common on poultry carcases (20). Except for very young kittens and suckling pigs that can be poisoned experimentally, domestic animals seem not to be susceptible to the enterotoxin. Rhesus monkeys are susceptible to the effects of enterotoxin B (25).

Of the many enzymes produced by staphylococci, coagulase has been the most studied. It causes plasma to coagulate, and its presence correlates well with virulence. However, virulent strains of coagulase-negative *S. aureus* frequently occur. The role of coagulase in pathogenesis is unclear, but it is known that coagulase is related to the organism's ability to grow well in serum and to withstand antibacterial factors. Its ability to coagulate plasma appears to be unimportant in pathogenesis in the bovine because the latter is deficient in the coagulase reacting factor (CRF), which is essential for coagulation to occur (15). Species with adequate levels of CRF may exhibit a small amount of intravascular clotting at the focus of infection (8).

Another enzyme, DNase, is usually present in coagulase-positive strains and can be used instead of coagulase as a criterion of potential virulence. Jasper (22) has shown this to be so for strains of staphylococci from cases of bovine mastitis.

Hyaluronidase, by degrading hyaluronic acid in the intercellular matrix, facilitates further spread of infection (14) and so conceivably contributes to the virulence of the producing organism.

Lipase production is important in skin invasion, and staphylococci that produce this enzyme are able to degrade bactericidal fatty acids on the skin surface.

Bacteriophage Typing of Staphylococci. A number of workers have investigated phage typing of *S. aureus* (7, 16, 41). The technique is used extensively for studying the epidemiology of staphylococcal infections in man. Nineteen phages are allocated into four groups (I, II, III, and IV) and two are unclassified. Most strains from humans are lysed by the phages of one group only, but strains from bovine and other animal sources cannot satisfactorily be typed according to the scheme devised for human strains. Evidently, strains from animals have a high degree of host specificity, and their phage lysis patterns are different.

Davidson (13) has devised a phage-typing scheme for bovine staphylococci, but neither this scheme nor the one devised for human strains is suitable for typing *S. aureus* from dogs (43).

Schemes for typing strains from poultry have also been reported (20, 39).

Pathogenesis. *S. epidermidis* is a normal commensal of the skin and mucous membranes of both man and animals. Colonization by *S. aureus* of the skin, nose, and oropharynx is also frequent in normal healthy animals. Penetration and lesion production by *S. aureus* and less frequently by *S. epidermidis* depend on a number of factors, such as skin trauma, the specific immune status of the animal, removal of other competing normal flora, the possession of lipase, and the existence of primary viral infections which cause skin lesions that are subsequently invaded by staphylococci.

The important factors involved in staphylococcal survival, multiplication, and lesion production after initial invasion are (*a*) resistance to phagocytosis as mediated by protein A and capsular material; (*b*) intracellular survival in phagocytic cells—strains of *S. aureus* may have enhanced intracellular survival abilities; (*c*) coagulase-mediated resistance to serum antibacterial factor; (*d*) hyaluronidase production, which aids spread of the infection; (*e*) the production of alpha toxin; (*f*) the production of other leukocidins; (*g*) the development of delayed hypersensitivity; and (*h*) adhesion to epithelial cells within the cavities of the bovine mammary gland (18).

Diseases Caused by *Staphylococcus aureus* and *Staphylococcus epidermidis*. *In horses.* Undoubtedly streptococci play a more important role in pyogenic infections of horses than the staphylococci. The latter are found frequently in miscellaneous infections, often in association with other organisms. *S. aureus* is usually found in pure culture in the peculiar disease known as *botryomycosis*. At one time this disease was thought to be caused by infection with an organism belonging to the higher fungi, but this idea has now been discarded. Botryomycosis usually begins, after castration of male animals, in the stump of the spermatic cord. The infected cord becomes greatly enlarged and sclerotic. Small pockets of pus are found here and there in the mass of new-formed tissue, and in the pus small granules resembling those of actinomycosis are found. When these granules are crushed, they yield masses of staphylococci embedded in a capsular material probably furnished by the host. Botryomycosis sometimes generalizes, in which case there is usually a fatal ending (32).

Bovine mastitis. *S. aureus* is frequently found in suppurative lesions in cattle and is especially significant as a cause of mastitis. In the more advanced dairying regions it is the most common pathogen of the bovine udder. Modern systems of housing and milking cows have favored this pathogen, which usually enters the udder via the teat canal. Transmission can occur between cows by means of the milking machine or the hands of the milker. In a minority of cases, the organism enters mammary tissue via wounds or lesions on the teat surface. After entry, the development, severity, and chronicity of the mastitis is related to such factors as the organism's adherence to the internal epithelial surfaces (18), the presence of antibody to alpha toxin, the number of neutrophils in the mammary secretion, the production of beta toxin and of coagulase, the frequency of milking out (40), and the ability of the organism to utilize nutrients within the udder and to multiply (2).

Phagocytosis and intracellular killing of staphylococci by leukocytes in the milk is inhibited by milk fat globules in the cells. Casein also inhibits intracellular killing (37, 38). The latter effect appears to be caused by a blocking of the bactericidal effects of the lactoperoxidase system and of histones (38). Although the efficiency of the intramammary phagocytic system may be reduced, it is still important in the mammary defense mechanism, because subclinical *S. epidermidis* infection is known to lessen the susceptibility of the udder to infection by either *Streptococcus agalactiae* or *Escherichia coli*. This diminished susceptibility is due to the increased leukocyte counts produced in response to the infection by *S. epidermidis*.

Another important factor in the pathogenesis of staphylococcal mastitis is the delayed hypersensitivity reaction (23). *S. aureus* does not always invade udder tissue, and the inflammation (mastitis) is apparently attributable to the immune response to the organism adhering to the internal duct and sinus epithelia.

S. aureus mastitis in cattle varies from subclinical to severely gangrenous. Most cases are of the subclinical chronic form, which, although quite inapparent, are of greatest economic significance because of losses in milk production.

Peracute gangrenous mastitis caused by *S. aureus* occurs in first-calf heifers in early lactation and results in loss of large masses of udder tissue. The alpha toxin is important in the development of the gangrene seen in this disease (9). This toxin damages the blood vessels, resulting in ischemic coagulative necrosis of adjacent tissue. The skin becomes purplish over the affected area and may eventually slough off. Affected animals have a high fever and may die of toxemia within a day or two. Chronic staphylococcal mastitis results in induration of the udder, occasional clots, and an increased cellularity of the milk.

Mastitis in other animals. Mastitis caused by *S. aureus* also occurs in sheep, goats, mares, sows, cats, and mink (42). The disease is usually acute but also occurs in a chronic form.

Tick pyemia of lambs. This disease occurs in Britain and Ireland and is associated with heavy infestations of 2 to 5-week-old lambs by the sheep tick *Ixodes ricinus* (44). During feeding, the tick inoculates *S. aureus,* which is already on the skin surface, into the deeper tissues, where it multiplies. Acute septicemia or bacteremia is often produced with toxemia, which rapidly kills the lamb. A less severe form of the disease results in abscesses in the kidneys, liver, joints, and the brain.

Canine pyoderma. S. aureus is the major bacterial pathogen of the canine skin, where such factors as trauma, dry skin, ectoparasitism, and matted, dirty hair may predispose to its invading the superficial and deeper layers of the skin. A number of different clinical entities are produced, including skin fold pyodermas that involve the face or genital-caudal area, impetigo, folliculitis, and furunculosis. Staphylococcal cellulitis of the deeper dermal layers is a frequent complication of demodectic mange. It is also found in the interdigital spaces of some breeds of dogs.

S. aureus is also a cause of external eye disease (34) and of urinary tract infections (11) in the dog. In the latter, the production of phosphatase and urease by *S. aureus* may play a role in calculus formation.

Of potential human health significance is the fact that there is considerable similarity (phage type, hemolysins) between a small percentage of coagulase-positive *S. aureus* from the nose and the tonsils of dogs and *S. aureus* strains from man (27).

Purulent synovitis in poultry. Serious losses in chickens (24) and turkeys (28) from a purulent synovitis have been caused by *S. aureus.* The infection causes lameness, swellings on the feet, and, occasionally, spondylitis. The strains which cause these infections are the same phage group as those found on the skin, and thus it is probable that the organism opportunistically enters birds whose resistance is compromised by such factors as concurrent viral infections or defects in husbandry.

Immunity. Repeated injections of heat-killed staphylococci will protect rabbits against otherwise fatal doses of *S. aureus.* Bacterins, especially autogenous bacterins, frequently appear to be of value in combating chronic infections in man. They are sometimes used on animals, although the results are not clear-cut. Immune serum has been used with similarly uncertain results. In one study (30) McDonald *et al.* found that repeated injections of bacterin produced long-term remissions in cats and dogs with dermatitis caused by *S. aureus.*

Special efforts have been made to devise systems of vaccinating dairy cattle to prevent staphylococcal mastitis. These have not been very successful. Toxoids that contain altered alpha toxin will stimulate production of antitoxin and are helpful in preventing acute gangrenous mastitis but have no apparent effect on the chronic form of the disease. There is some evidence that intramammary infusion of vaccine is more effective than parenteral administration (31). Staphylococcal toxoid is made by treating filtrates with 0.3 percent formalin for a few hours.

Diagnosis. *S. aureus* and *S. epidermidis* are readily recognized in smears from abscesses or from exudates, and cultures are easily made on sheep or cow blood agar. Coagulase and/or DNase activity should be checked for, as most pathogenic strains of *S. aureus* are positive for these enzymes.

Chemotherapy. Penicillin resistance caused by beta lactamase is now found in a substantial proportion of strains of *S. aureus* from animals (6, 21), so therapy must be based on the results of sensitivity testing. Lincomycin, erythromycin, and chloramphenicol are the best antibiotics for therapy of purulent staphylococcal lesions because there is good penetration into abscesses and minimal binding to purulent material. Nitrofurantoin, Fucidine and 2-chloro-4-phenyl-phenol are effective for topical application (1, 26).

REFERENCES

1. Andersen. Appl. Microbiol., 1963, *11,* 239.
2. Anderson. Brit. Vet. Jour., 1976, *132,* 122.
3. Anderson and Stone. Jour. Hyg. (London), 1955, *53,* 387.
4. Armijo, Henderson, Timothee, and Robinson. Am. Jour. Pub. Health, 1957, *47,* 1093.
5. Bell and Veliz. Vet. Med., 1952, *47,* 321.
6. Biberstein, Franti, Jang, and Ruby. Jour. Am. Vet. Med. Assoc., 1974, *164,* 1183.
7. Blair and Carr. Jour. Inf. Dis., 1953, *93,* 1.
8. Blobel and Berman. Jour. Inf. Dis., 1961, *108,* 63.
9. Brown and Sherer. Am. Jour. Vet. Res., 1958, *19,* 354.
10. Casman, Bennett, Dorsey, and Issa. Jour. Bact., 1967, *94,* 1875.
11. Clark. Vet. Rec., 1974, *95,* 204.
12. Crabtree and Litterer. Am. Jour. Pub. Health. 1934, *24,* 1116.
13. Davidson. Res. Vet. Sci., 1961, *2,* 396.

14. Duran and Reynals. Bact. Rev., 1942, *6,* 197.
15. Duthie and Lorenz. Jour. Gen. Microbiol., 1952, *6,* 95.
16. Edds and Saunders. Am. Jour. Vet. Res., 1966, *27,* 951.
17. Favero, Drake, and Randall. Pub. Health Rpts. (U.S.), 1974, *79,* 61.
18. Frost, Wanasinghe, and Woolcock. Inf. and Immun., 1977, *15,* 245.
19. Gagliano and Hinsdill. Jour. Bact., 1970, *104,* 117.
20. Gibbs, Patterson, and Thompson. Jour. Appl. Bact., 1978, *44,* 387.
21. Jasper. Calif. Vet., 1972, *26,* 12.
22. Jasper. Am. Jour. Vet. Res., 1973, *34,* 445.
23. Jones. Proc. Ann. Meeting U.S. Animal Health Assoc., 1974, *78,* 143.
24. Jungherr and Plastridge. Jour. Am. Vet. Med. Assoc., 1941, *98,* 27.
25. Kent. Am. Jour. Path., 1966, *48,* 387.
26. Kober. Berl. und Münch. tierärztl. Wchnschr., 1977, *90,* 401.
27. Live. Am. Jour. Vet. Res., 1972, *33,* 385.
28. Madsen. Turkey World, 1942, *17,* no. 2.
29. Marcia, Nagy, Vasru, and Klemm. Zentrbl. Vet.-Med., 1976, *23B,* 122.
30. McDonald, Greenfield, and McCausland. Can. Vet. Jour., 1972, *13,* 45.
31. McDowell and Watson. Austral. Vet. Jour., 1974, *50,* 533.
32. McFadyean. Jour. Comp. Path. and Therap., 1919, *32,* 73.
33. Minett. Jour. Hyg. (London), 1938, *38,* 623.
34. Murphy, Lavach, and Seserin. Jour. Am. Vet. Med. Assoc., 1978, *172,* 66.
35. Naidu and Newbauld. Zentrbl. Vet.-Med., 1975, *22B,* 308.
36. Ogsten. Arch. f. klin. Chirurg., 1880, *25,* 588.
37. Paápy and Guidny. Proc. Soc. Exp. Biol. and Med., 1977, *155,* 588.
38. Russell, Broker, and Reiter. Res. Vet. Sci., 1976, *20,* 30.
39. Shimizu. Am. Jour. Vet. Res., 1977, *38,* 1601.
40. Thomas, Neave, Dodd, and Higgs. Jour. Dairy Res., 1972, *39,* 113.
41. Torheim. Acta Path. et Microbiol. Scand., 1960, *49,* 397.
42. Trautwein and Helmboldt. Jour. Am. Vet. Med. Assoc., 1966, *149,* 924.
43. Wang. Jap. Jour. Vet. Sci., 1978, *40,* 401.
44. Watson. Vet. Rec., 1964, *76,* 743.

Staphylococcus hyicus

SYNONYMS: *Micrococcus hyicus, Staphylococcus epidermidis* (*albus*) biotype 2

This organism is the cause of *exudative epidermidis* of swine, a disease also known as *greasy pig disease* or *contagious impetigo*. Experimental transmission and characterization of the causative organism was achieved by Underhahl and his coworkers in 1963 (10).

Earlier, Sompolinsky (7) had concluded that the disease was caused by a coagulase-negative micrococcus which he named *Micrococcus hyicus*. Later, the organism was renamed *S. hyicus*. The eighth edition of *Bergey's Manual* does not list this organism as a separate species, and instead makes it a biotype 2 of *S. epidermidis* (*albus*). Because the name *S. hyicus* now has widespread usage in the veterinary literature we will use this name in the description of the agent and the disease it causes.

Morphology and Staining Reactions. The organism is a Gram-positive coccus (0.5 to 7.0 μm in diameter) which occurs as single cells, in pairs, and in short chains. There is no capsule (10).

Cultural and Biochemical Features. The colonies on blood agar are creamy white and circular. Rabbit erythrocytes are hemolyzed, but no hemolysis is seen on sheep blood agar. Coagulase is not usually produced, although Underdahl *et al.* (10) reported that some strains they examined were coagulase-positive. Phosphatase, gelatinase, hyaluronidase, and DNA are produced. Anaerobic growth occurs in thioglycollate broth.

Antigens. *S. hyicus* differs antigenically from *S. epidermidis* although some antigens are shared (3). Antiserum to *S. hyicus* that has been absorbed with *S. epidermidis* can be used to distinguish *S. hyicus* from nonpathogenic skin staphylococci.

Epidemiology and Pathogenesis. *S. hyicus* is highly contagious and easily spread from one group of pigs to another. Trading of animals has been shown to be an important factor in spread of the disease, which usually occurs about 2 weeks after an infected animal has been brought onto clean premises (8). Piglets between 1 and 7 weeks of age are usually affected, and both the morbidity and mortality are highly variable.

The organism enters via breaks in the skin barrier. Such lesions could be initiated by the sharp teeth of piglets competing for feeding space. The disease produced varies in severity from a form where the entire body becomes quickly covered with a moist, greasy exudate to a more chronic condition where the onset is slower and the skin is more wrinkled. The lesions appear a few days after experimental exposure and may first be present as vesicles on hairless skin surfaces, the coronary bands, and behind the ears. As the disease progresses over the body surface, the skin becomes thickened and layers of the epidermis may peel off. Milder forms of the disease may present as dandrufflike scaling or as reddish-brown spots on the ears and other body areas. Pigs begin to recover about 14 days after the lesions appear and are fully recovered in 30 to 40 days.

Histological examination of the skin of severely affected pigs reveals an accumulation of proteinaceous material, inflammatory cells, and bacteria over a parakeratotic layer (5). At necropsy, the ureters are enlarged and the kidneys cystic because of debris which accumulates and blocks urinary flow.

It has been suggested that the biotin requirement of affected swine is greatly increased by factors produced by *S. hyicus* and that biotin deficiency contributes to the lesions (9). Interestingly, Luke and Gordon (4) reported a good response to treatment with vitamin B supplements.

Diagnosis. Isolation of the causative organism can be made on the selective medium devised by Devriese (2). This medium contains potassium thiocyanate (30 g per liter) and polysorbate 80 (10 ml per liter). Final laboratory diagnosis must be based on the characteristics listed in Table 17.3.

Immunity. Piglets born to sows that have been actively or passively immunized are resistant to challenge (1). Sow vaccination should therefore be a useful means of controlling this disease. The specificity of the protective factors in immune serum has not yet been elucidated.

Chemotherapy. Penicillin, administered for 3 days to exposed pigs that had not yet shown lesions, has been effective in preventing exudative epidermitis (6). Once lesions have developed, antibiotic therapy is much less effective. The organism is sensitive to kanamycin, chloramphenicol, chlortetracycline, and nitrofurazone but is resistant to streptomycin, polymixin B, and sulfa compounds (11).

Table 17.3. The differentiation of *S. hyicus, S. aureus,* and other staphylococci and micrococci isolates from pigs (2)

Characteristic	*S. hyicus*	*S. aureus*	Other staphylococci and micrococci*
Coagulase (slide)	−	+	−
DNase	+	+	−
Hyaluronidase	+	+	−
Maltose	−	Acid	Acid (80%)
Mannitol	−	Acid	Acid (75%)
Polysorbate 80 reaction	+	+(86%)	−
Agglutination, with antiserum to *S. hyicus*	+	−	−

**Micrococcus* sp. are common commensals on the skin.

REFERENCES

1. Amtsberg. Berl. and Münch. tierärztl. Wchnschr., 1978, *91,* 201.
2. Devriese. Am. Jour. Vet. Res., 1977, *38,* 787.
3. Hunter, Todd, and Larkin. Brit. Vet. Jour., 1970, *126,* 225.
4. Luke and Gordon. Vet. Rec., 1950, *62,* 179.
5. Mebus, Underdahl, and Tweihaus. Path. Vet., 1968, *5,* 146.
6. Riet, Correa, Freitas, and Repiso. Veternaria (Montevideo, Uruguay), 1977, *4,* 25.
7. Sompolinsky. Schweiz. Arch. f. Tierheilk., 1953, *95,* 302.
8. Stuker. Schweiz. Arch. f. Tierheilk., 1976, *118,* 335.
9. Stuker and Glattli. Schweiz. Arch. f. Tierheilk., 1976, *118,* 305.
10. Underdahl, Grace, and Young. Jour. Am. Vet. Med. Assoc., 1963, *142,* 754.
11. Underdahl, Grace, and Tweihaus. Am. Jour. Vet. Res., 1965, *26,* 617.

THE GENUS *STREPTOCOCCUS*

The generic name *Streptococcus* was first used in 1884 by Rosenbach (17) to describe a spherical bacterium that grew in chains, which he had isolated from suppurative lesions in man. Since then, 21 separate species of *Streptococcus* have been described, as well as a number of distinct and partially defined strains for which species status has not been established.

Streptococci cause a variety of diseases of man and animals and are important saprophytes in milk and milk products. They are frequently present as parasites of the mucous membranes and intestines of animals and, given the appropriate conditions, may opportunistically produce disease.

The first systematic classification of the group was produced by Sherman in 1937 (19), who divided the streptococci into Pyogenic, Viridans, Lactic, and Enterococcus groups. The Pyogenic group included most of the pathogenic species; the Viridans group were chiefly characterized by the production of alpha hemolysis or greening on blood agar; the Lactic group was composed of strains associated with milk and having the ability to produce lactic acid in this substrate; and the Enterococcus group included strains which resembled *S. fecalis*—an intestinal inhabitant. Although Sherman's classification is no longer used in its entirety, the tolerance tests he used to establish his primary divisions are still useful in classification.

The present classification in *Bergey's Manual* (eighth edition) is based partly on tolerance tests and partly on biochemical behavior.

Serologic grouping is also of great importance in the identification of the streptococci. The majority of these organisms possess a dominant serologically active carbohydrate ("C substance") which is antigenically different from one species or group of species to another. In 1933, Lancefield (11), working with the precipitation test, used these antigenic differences to establish six groups (A to E and N), which were later found to correlate well with the groups in Sherman's (19) classification. As a result, many laboratories used the Lancefield grouping system as the principal identification method for the streptococci. Further serologic groups were added (F, G, H, K, L, M, O, P, Q, R, S, T, U, and V) as time passed, but no species designations were given the organisms of these newer groups.

It later became apparent that although streptococci such as *S. bovis* and *S. fecalis* could share the same group antigen (D), they were physiologically and taxonomically quite different. Recent work has shown that there can be considerable physiologic heterogeneity among organisms of a number of the other Lancefield groups as well (24). Thus the classification of the streptococci cannot be based solely on serologic grouping but must also include physiologic and biochemical criteria.

The carbohydrate or polysaccharide antigen that is the basis of the Lancefield grouping system is located in the cell wall in the case of groups A, B, C, E, F, G, H, and K. In groups D and N these antigens are teichoic acids that lie between the cell wall and the cell membrane.

The carbohydrate antigens of groups B and C streptococci—the groups that contain the majority of the animal pathogens—are rhamnose-glucosamine and rhamnose-N-acetylgalactosamine polysaccharides, respectively. The chemical nature of the carbohydrates in the other groups are listed by Deibel and Seeley (6).

Streptococcal species are important causes of mastitis in cattle, of strangles and a variety of other disease conditions in the horse, and of meningoencephalitis, arthritis, endocarditis, and cervical lymphadenitis in swine. Less frequently, they have been associated with septicemia in chickens and with respiratory and other infections in kittens and puppies. The more common streptococci that produce disease in animals are listed in Table 17.4.

Morphology and Staining Reactions. The chains of cocci may be short (diplococci) or they may be very long. Chain length depends upon species differences and upon the medium on which the culture is growing. Typical chain formation is best seen in fluid media; on solid media the chains become so entangled that their demonstration is difficult.

The individual cells of streptococci are seldom perfectly spherical, and frequently there is considerable variation in the size and shape of the elements in a single culture. Sometimes the cells are flattened from side to side; more often they are elongated. In fact, certain animal strains of streptococci may be so pleomorphic on primary isolation that they can readily be mistaken for short rods. Usually a few transfers on artificial media will bring forth the typical coccus form. Spores are never formed. With rare exceptions they are nonmotile. A number of species form definite capsules when developing in tissues or in culture media containing blood serum. Such strains show the mucoid or the matt types of colony formation rather than the smooth (glossy) or the rough forms usually produced. Most streptococci are Gram-positive. In old cultures many Gram-negative forms are commonly found. They are easily stained with all the usual dyes. They are never acid-fast.

Cultural Features. The streptococci are among the more fastidious bacteria with respect to nutritive requirements. They usually will not grow on meat extract media, and growth ordinarily is poor even on infusion media unless it is enriched by the addition of blood, ascitic fluid, or similar substances. However, horse meat infusion agar, without enrichment, has proved to be an excellent medium for the isolation of animal strains of streptococci (1).

All streptococci produce small, delicate, translucent colonies of a diameter of about 1 mm on solid media. Heavy inoculations give confluent growths that are nearly transparent. The surface of the growth is smooth and glistening, and the margins of individual colonies are perfectly circular. Deep colonies in agar usually are lenticular in shape. In softer media they may be globular. In size they may be hardly large enough to be easily visible with the naked eye. When growth is obtained on gelatin, it consists of a string of delicate beads along the line of the stab, with little or no growth on the surface, and in most cases without evidence of liquefaction.

In fluid media, growth usually is a little more abundant than in solids. In broth there may be a faint cloudiness or the medium may remain perfectly clear except for a fluffy sediment in the bottom of the tube. The appearance usually gives an accurate clue as to whether the coccus is growing in short or long chains; the short-chain type causes uniform clouding, whereas the long-chain type quickly sediments. All streptococci grow well in milk. With few exceptions the milk is soured through the formation of lactic acid from the milk sugar. Most strep-

Table 17.4. Characteristics of the streptococci that cause disease in animals

Species or group	Disease	Hemolysis	Lancefield group	Fermentation of				Hydrolysis of		CAMP test
				Trehalose	Sorbitol	Lactose	Inulin	Sodium hippurate	Esculin	
S. agalactiae	Mastitis in cow, ewe, and goat	Narrow beta or absent	B	+	−	+	−	+	−	+
S. dysgalactiae	Mastitis in cow, ewe, and goat	Alpha	C	+	±	+	−	−	−	−
S. equi	Strangles in horse	Beta	C	−	−	−	−	−		
S. equisimilis	Cervicitis and abscesses in horse; arthritis in swine	Beta	C	+	+	±	−	−		
S. zooepidemicus	Mastitis in cow; cervicitis and metritis in mare; wound infections in horse	Beta	C	−	+	+	−	−		
S. uberis	Mastitis in cow	Absent	Unknown	+	+	+	+	+	+	±
Group E (*S. infrequens*)	Cervical lymphadenitis in swine	Beta (slow)	E	+	±	−	±	−		
Group L (rarely found)	Mastitis in cow; endocarditis in swine	Beta	L	+	−	+	−	±	−	
S. suis type 1	Meningoencephalitis and arthritis in piglets	Beta (horse blood)	D(S)	+	−	+	+	−	+	−
S. suis type 2	Meningoencephalitis and arthritis in piglets	Alpha	D(R)	+	−	+	+	−	+	−

tococci grow readily under aerobic as well as anaerobic conditions. There are some strains, however, that grow only under anaerobic conditions. They are unique among bacteria, able to grow aerobically, and unable to synthesize heme compounds. They are therefore incapable of synthesizing cytochromes and of oxidative phosphorylation via a cytochrome-mediated electron transport chain. Because of this, the cytochrome inhibitor, sodium azide, is widely used in media for the selective isolation of streptococci from contaminated specimens.

They are catalase-negative. Sugars are fermented by all streptococci. The end product is largely dextrorotatory lactic acid. Gas is produced by only a few streptococci and by none of the types that are of importance in pathology.

Physiological Characteristics. The growth range of streptococci varies from below 10 C to above 45 C. The pathogenic types have a much narrower range than this.

The resistance of streptococci to heat is not great. The pathogenic types are usually killed by temperatures well below those used for pasteurization (ca. 63 C for 30 minutes). It is well known, however, that the milk-souring types are not wholly destroyed by pasteurization, and some of the intestinal types have rather unusual resistance. *S. thermophilus* grows at 50 C. Likewise, resistance to drying and to chemical disinfection is not very great. However, when cultures are rapidly and completely dried, they often remain viable for very long periods of time; hence it is possible that streptococci withstand drying better than is generally supposed.

Habitat. The streptococci are found on the mucous membranes of men and animals, in various suppurative processes in these hosts, and in milk and milk products. It is frequently said that these organisms exist principally as animal parasites. Stark and Sherman (21) have found *S. lactis* on growing vegetation and enterococci have been isolated from plants in a wild environment. This raises the question of whether these organisms may not occur more commonly on plants than has been hitherto supposed. In general, the increased growth on media enriched by blood or tissue extracts suggests that the streptococci are adapted for parasitic rather than saprophytic existence.

Hemolysis. The action of streptococci on horse erythrocytes is an important criterion in their identification. Many of the pathogenic strains produce hemolysins which completely lyse horse erythrocytes in fluid or agar media. This is beta hemolysis and is characterized by complete clearing of the zone surrounding colonies on blood agar. If the erythrocytes are at the bottom of a tube of fluid medium, a plume of free hemoglobin diffuses upward from the pad of cells.

Colonies of the alpha or viridans group at the end of 18 to 24 hours' incubation at 37 C show a slight or marked discoloration of a narrow zone of blood cells immediately surrounding the colony. The discoloration is easily seen with the naked eye. Under the microscope it can be seen that the erythrocytes in the discolored zone are intact. If incubated for a longer period—especially at room temperature or lower—a clear zone appears outside the greenish area. Under the microscope it may be seen that the blood cells have dissolved. The cells of the discolored zone remain intact, however, no matter how long the incubation is continued.

Hemolysis is best interpreted from deep colonies in pour-plates, rather than from surface colonies of streaked plates.

Streptococcus agalactiae

SYNONYM: *Streptococcus mastitidis*

This organism is a common cause of bovine mastitis in the United States and in most areas of the world. In Britain, the organism is now much less frequently found as a cause of bovine mastitis than in other countries, including the United States (25). The reasons for this disparity are not fully understood. In Denmark, an eradication program (15) has reduced the infection rate to less than 1 percent in cows.

S. agalactiae also causes mastitis in sheep and goats.

Morphology and Staining Reactions. In secretions from infected udders, *S. agalactiae* usually appears in the form of long chains (Figure 17.2). In some samples these are numerous and easily found in stained films; in other cases, even though the milk may be markedly altered in appearance, the organisms may be so scarce as to be found with great difficulty. The organism is Gram-positive and is readily stained by all the ordinary stains.

Cultural Features. On blood agar, the most actively hemolytic strains produce hemolytic zones not more than 1 mm broad. Many strains produce only a suggestion of hemolysis on blood agar plates, and others produce none whatsoever. Some strains produce a suggestion of greenish discoloration without hemolysis on blood agar plates.

Growth in serum broth is granular or flocculent, the growth appearing in the bottoms of the tubes, the rest of

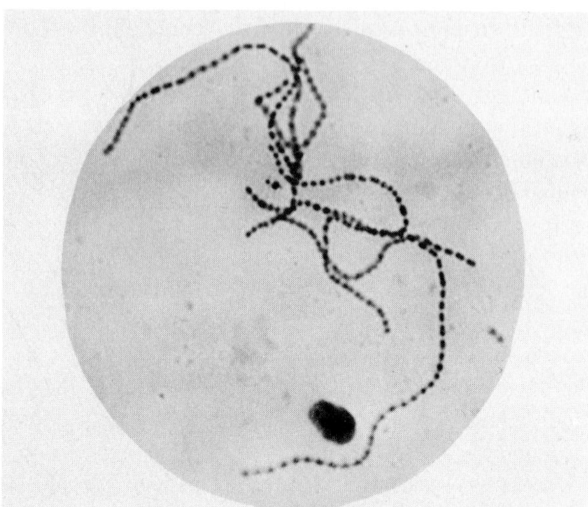

Figure 17.2. *Streptococcus agalactiae,* from a stained film made from a sample of mastitis milk which had been incubated overnight at 37 C. Similar chains are often found in the fresh udder secretion. Note that the chains consist of a series of paired organisms. This is characteristic but not diagnostic. × 1,050.

the broth remaining clear. Litmus milk, incubated at 37 C, is acidified and coagulated within 48 hours. There is slight reduction of the litmus at the bottoms of the tubes. At 10 C there is no observable growth in 5 days. Methylene blue milk is not reduced. In glucose broth the final hydrogen-ion concentration is from pH 4.4 to 4.7. Sodium hippurate is hydrolyzed. Glucose, lactose, sucrose, and maltose are regularly fermented; salicin is usually fermented, but not always. Inulin, mannitol, and raffinose are never attacked. Esculin is not broken down. Gelatin is not hydrolyzed. Many but not all strains of *S. agalactiae* produce a brick-reddish growth on solid media, especially when the medium contains starch.

About 90 percent of *S. agalactiae* strains tested by Gochnauer and Wilson (9) produced hyaluronidase.

The CAMP phenomenon. In 1944, Christie, Atkins, and Muench-Petersen (4) reported a lytic phenomenon produced by about 96 percent of the streptococci belonging to Lancefield's serological group B. This phenomenon is now referred to as the CAMP phenomenon. It was shown that culturing certain milk on cow blood agar plates yielded colonies of strongly hemolytic streptococci which, when subcultured, failed to show hemolysis. Reexamination of the original plates revealed the presence of many staphylococci of the alpha-beta type; that is, their colonies were in the center of a clear zone, which in turn was surrounded by a large darkened area where the staphylococcal beta toxin had altered, but not lysed, the cow red cells. Wherever there were colonies of the streptococci within these zones of darkening, they were surrounded by an area of complete hemolysis, but elsewhere on the plates they produced no distinct hemolysis.

Resistance. Resistance to heat, drying, and chemicals is not great. Most strains will withstand 50 C but not 60 C moist heat for 30 minutes. The organism is readily destroyed by pasteurization.

Antigens. The group antigen is located in the cell wall and is a rhamnose-glucosamine polysaccharide. At least five type-specific antigens (S) are described and are composed of glucose-galactose-N-acetyl-glucosamine polysaccharide. They are located on the outer envelope and are designated Ia, Ib, Ic, II, and III. Two antigenically related protein antigens are sometimes present also and are designated R and X. In New York State, type Ia *S. agalactiae* constitute about 70 percent of all isolates, and types II and III represent 17 and 10 percent, respectively. The type found varies in different areas (14).

Epidemiology and Pathogenesis. The habitat of *S. agalactiae* is largely confined to the mammary gland of the cow, sheep, and goat. Infection is spread between cows by means of the milker's hands or contaminated milking equipment. Sometimes the mouths of calves may serve as a mode of transfer to the immature mammary glands of their comrades when they suckle each other. The organism enters via the teat and colonization of the gland is favored by adhesion to the epithelia of the gland sinuses (8).

Multiplication of the organism on the surface of the teat and duct sinuses results in a slowly progressive inflammation and fibrosis of adjoining areas of the gland. The disease therefore begins insidiously and develops gradually. Older animals are more frequently affected. Excessive stripping may exacerbate the disease.

The milk, or udder secretion, becomes altered in varying degrees, sometimes showing little or no abnormality and sometimes showing flakes, stringy masses of fibrin, blood, and thick purulent material. In many cases the degree of alteration of the milk varies, being thick and purulent at one time and practically normal at another. The inflammation in the udder causes the formation of new interstitial tissue, and thus fibrosis changes the normal soft consistency of the gland to hardness, generally in the form of indurated masses that may not be seen but may be palpated.

Normal milk has a pH slightly on the acid side of neutrality, whereas blood serum is slightly alkaline. In inflamed udders the milk secretion is mixed with inflammatory exudate derived from the blood serum. The alkaline exudate causes the pH to shift to the alkaline side, and this fact is the basis of the color tests for mastitis. Unfortunately it happens that milk in the early and late stages of the lactation period is more alkaline than normal; hence the color tests are not safely used as the sole criterion of the existence of mastitis.

The number of leukocytes in milk coming from inflamed udders is much greater than the number found in normal milk, and usually exceeds 500,000 per ml. These cells can be counted directly during microscopic examination of stained films or electronically. Other methods of estimating numbers of cells include detection of DNA released from the cells by detergent lysis. This procedure is the basis of the California mastitis test (CMT) (18). Equal amounts of milk and an ionic surface-active agent consisting of a 3- to 5-percent concentration of alkyl arylsulfonate (pH 7.0) plus bromcresol purple indicator are mixed. Depending on the leukocyte count of the milk, the reaction varies from slight precipitation of amorphous material, which tends to disappear, to immediate development of a viscid gel. The bromcresol purple reveals abnormal alkalinity or acidity of the milk and provides a contrasting color.

The streptococci in most cases are difficult to demonstrate by direct methods, although frequently they can be found in the centrifuged sediment of the milk. To detect the organism it is best to culture the milk by streaking blood agar plates. Typical colonies are tested by the CAMP test, and subjected to biochemical studies.

In advanced cases, the secretion is much reduced in volume and is thin and watery. Thus herd infections by *S. agalactiae* can be a serious source of economic loss in dairy herds.

Immunity. Antibodies to the cellular antigens of *S. agalactiae* have been detected in the colostrum of first-calf heifers (3) in the absence of any signs of disease. Thus, cattle must have considerable exposure to the organism before they reach sexual maturity. Agglutinins for hematoxylin-stained *S. agalactiae* can be detected in milk from infected cows by a milk ring test (20).

Yokomizo and Norcross (27) have shown that antibodies to *S. agalactiae* type Ia belonging to immunoglobulin classes IgA, IgG, IgG_2, and IgM are present in colostrum. Most of the protective activity appears to be associated with IgM and IgA classes unlike the situation in human serum where protection is mediated by IgG class antibodies (23). Levels of IgA in the colostrum could be increased by previous intramammary vaccination. However, vaccination is not yet an effective means of controlling infection by *S. agalactiae* in dairy herds.

Chemotherapy in Control and Treatment. *S. agalactiae* is very sensitive to penicillin administered by intramammary infusion. Infected cows detected by the CMT and bacteriologic culture are segregated and treated with penicillin. This routine has been successfully used to reduce infection in herds in Britain, Denmark, and the United States (15, 25). Complete elimination of infection, however, has not been achieved, possibly because some herds become reinfected from human or porcine carriers. The epidemiologic significance of the latter as sources of infection for the bovine has not, however, been proved, although they have been shown to be carriers of group B streptococci.

Streptococcus dysgalactiae

S. dysgalactiae causes an acute, severe mastitis. The organism differs from *S. agalactiae* only in minor cultural particulars. It belongs to Lancefield's group C. The chains are usually short or medium in length. The colonies are usually nonhemolytic, and they often show a distinct greenish discoloration. Litmus milk is not always coagulated in 48 hours at 37 C. Methylene blue milk, however, is regularly reduced. The final pH in glucose broth varies between 5.3 and 5.0. It never goes below 5.0. Sodium hippurate is not hydrolyzed. This is perhaps the best single test for differentiating this species from *S. agalactiae*.

Epidemiology and Pathogenesis. Infection by this organism is much less frequent and more sporadic than that of *S. agalactiae*. The organism occurs on the skin of the udder and elsewhere and in the mouth. It multiplies in wounds and sores and may enter the udder via sores that involve the teat orifice. The mastitis produced is acute and painful and the secretion is purulent and yellowish in color. *S. dysgalactiae* produces hyaluronidase, which may contribute to its invasiveness either by itself or in synergism with *Corynebacterium pyogenes*. In summer mastitis these two organisms are frequently found together.

Damage to the affected quarter may result in complete loss of function. Hygienic control measures are not of any benefit in control, but treatment of teat wounds with antiseptic ointment may help to reduce numbers of the organism opportunistically multiplying in these sites, and so reduce the probability of teat invasion.

Streptococcus uberis

This organism also causes bovine mastitis and differs from *S. dysgalactiae* principally in the following details: It is nonhemolytic but may produce slight greening on blood agar; it is salicin-, esculin-, and hippurate-positive. It does not react in the Lancefield grouping system. A small number of strains are CAMP-positive.

Epidemiology and Pathogenesis. The organism has been found in the rumen, rectum, feces, and on the lips and skin of cattle (5). It multiplies in bedding. The disease is much more common in loose housed cattle than in animals on pasture. Infection of the udder is therefore related to the amount of environmental contamination.

The disease is usually acute but mild. More severe forms have been observed occasionally where infection was caused by encapsulated variants of the organism.

Control of this form of mastitis lies in improved environmental hygiene.

Streptococcus zooepidemicus

This organism is widespread in a variety of animal species. It is a normal commensal of the skin, upper respiratory mucosa (10), and tonsillar and associated pharyngeal lymphoid tissue of the horse (26). It produces either mucoid or matt colonies surrounded by a wide zone of hemolysis on blood agar. Sorbitol is fermented but not trehalose. Lactose fermentation is variable. *S. zooepidemicus* belongs to group C of the Lancefield typing system.

Antigens. Strains of *S. zooepidemicus* belong to at least 15 serotypes, the type-specific antigen being proteinaceous and trypsin-labile (12). Another proteinaceous trypsin-resistant antigen that is pepsin-labile has also been found but is of rare occurrence (2). It is found on *S. zooepidemicus* type 3.

Diseases caused by *Streptococcus zooepidemicus*. *In horses*. *S. zooepidemicus* is by far the most common cause of wound infections and is also a routine secondary invader following viral respiratory infections. It may invade the umbilical stump of the foal, causing omphalophlebitis, bacteremia, and polyarthritis. In the mare it may cause cervicitis and endometritis. This may be a sequel to vulvar deformity or to injury during parturition. Abortion may be caused when the organism is carried in the bloodstream to the placenta or enters the uterus from the distal genital tract (7).

In cows. Mastitis caused by this organism is usually acute and severe, and is often found in small, hand-milked herds where the milker takes care of other species on the farm. The organism enters via wounds on the teat or via a damaged meatus. Arthritis sometimes occurs in association with mastitis caused by *S. zooepidemicus*.

In sheep. Fibrinous pleuritis, pericarditis, and pneumonia have been reported in lambs (22).

In goats. Mastitis with eventual severe gland atrophy has occurred in goats (13). Hand stripping following machine milking was believed to have spread the infection.

In chickens. Fatal septicemia in chickens caused by *S. zooepidemicus* has been reported by Peckham (16).

REFERENCES

1. Bruner. North Am. Vet., 1949, *30*, 243.
2. Bryans and Moore. *In* Streptococci and streptococcal diseases, ed. Lewis W. Wannamaker and John M. Matsen. Academic Press, New York, 1972, pp. 327–37.
3. Campbell and Norcross. Am. Jour. Vet. Res., 1964, *25*, 993.
4. Christie, Atkins, and Muench-Petersen. Austral. Jour. Exp. Biol. and Med. Sci., 1944, *22*, 197.
5. Cullen and Little. Vet. Rec., 1969, *84*, 115.
6. Deibel and Seeley. *In* Bergey's manual of determinative bacteriology, 8th ed., ed. Robert E. Buchanan and Norman E. Gibbons. Williams & Wilkins, Baltimore, Md., 1974.
7. Dimock, Edwards, and Bruner. Cornell Vet., 1947, *37*, 89.
8. Frost, Wanasinghe, and Woolcock. Inf. and Immun., 1977, *15*, 245.
9. Gochnauer and Wilson. Jour. Bact., 1951, *62*, 405.
10. Kasai, Nobata, and Rya. Jap. Jour. Vet. Sci., 1944, *6*, 116.
11. Lancefield. Jour. Exp. Med., 1933, *57*, 571.
12. Moore and Bryans. *In* Equine infectious diseases, II. Proc. 2nd Int. Conf. on Equine Infectious Diseases, Paris, 1969, ed. J. T. Bryans and H. Gerber. S. Karger, Basel, Munich, and New York, 1970.
13. Nesbakken. Norsk. Vet. Tidsskr., 1975, *87*, 188.
14. Norcross and Oliver. Cornell Vet., 1976, *66*, 240.
15. Olsen. Proc. Int. Dairy Fed. Seminar on Mastitis Control, Reading University, 1975, pp. 410–21. International Dairy Federation, Brussels, Doc. 85, 1976.
16. Peckham. Avian Dis., 1966, *10*, 413.
17. Rosenbach. Mikroorganismen bei den Wundinfektionskrankheiten des Menschen. J. F. Bergmann, Wiesbaden, 1884.
18. Schalm and Noorlander. Jour. Am. Vet. Assoc., 1957, *130*, 199.

19. Sherman. Bact. Rev., 1937, *1*, 1.
20. Smith. Jour. Comp. Path. and Therap., 1954, *64*, 1.
21. Stark and Sherman. Jour. Bact., 1935, *30*, 639.
22. Stevenson. Can. Jour. Comp. Med., 1974, *38*, 243.
23. Stewardson-Krieger, Albrandt, Nevin, Kretschmer, and Gotoff. Jour. Inf. Dis., 1977, *136*, 649.
24. Wilson and Miles. *In* Topley and Wilson's Principles of bacteriology and immunity, vol. 1, 6th ed., Arnold, London, 1975.
25. Wilson and Salt. *In* Streptococci, ed. F. A. Skinner and L. B. Quesnel. Academic Press, New York, 1978, pp. 143–56.
26. Woolcock. Res. Vet. Sci., 1975, *18*, 113.
27. Yokomizo and Norcross. Am. Jour. Vet. Res., 1978, *39*, 511.

Streptococcus equisimilis

S. equisimilis is beta-hemolytic, although the zone of beta hemolysis is less than that produced by *S. zooepidemicus*. Colony morphology is similar to that produced by *S. zooepidemicus*. Acid is produced from trehalose but not from sorbitol. In contrast to strains from cattle, swine, and man, equine strains do not ferment lactose.

Antigens. The group antigen (C) is located in the cell wall, and there are four subtypes within the group. Type-specific protein antigens also exist.

Diseases Caused by *Streptococcus equisimilis*. *In swine*. *S. equisimilis* is the most frequent cause of suppurative arthritis in pigs from birth to 6 weeks of age (25). Infection is probably derived via the umbilicus from the genital tract of the sow because group C streptococci are common in its vaginal secretions. The disease is often confined to a single litter or to successive litters over a period of many months (38).

Clinical signs in piglets include inappetence, elevated temperature, roughened haircoat, lameness, and joint swelling. Necrosis of the joint surfaces may lead to permanent joint damage.

A microtiter complement-fixation procedure has been developed for the detection of antibodies. In immune swine sera these antibodies are predominantly IgG (37). Protection is not directly correlated with the antibodies, however, although their levels are a reliable measure of the immune status of groups of pigs (36). Experimental adjuvanated and extract vaccines for immunization of piglets from 3 weeks of age onward have been shown to stimulate a protective immunity (39).

In horses. *S. equisimilis* is rarely mentioned in association with disease in the horse. Bazeley and Battle (3) found that about 10 percent of streptococci from pathologic material were *S. equisimilis*. In a survey of equine tonsillar tissue and draining lymph nodes, Woolcock (42) found that about 4 percent of streptococci were *S. equisimilis*.

Streptococcus equi

S. equi is the cause of *strangles*, a severe purulent infection of the upper respiratory tract and draining lymph nodes of young horses. The organism has also been isolated from abscessed lymph nodes of burros (35).

Morphology and Staining Reactions. *S. equi* occurs in exudates and in fluid cultures in the form of long chains, and occasionally in short chains. Sometimes the chains are surrounded by definite capsular material. The organism is readily stained with the usual dyes and is Gram-positive when cultures are young. Old cultures retain the Gram stain poorly.

Cultural Features. This organism has a strong hemolytic toxin that causes it to show wide zones of beta-type hemolysis around colonies on blood plates and to hemolyze blood cells suspended in broth cultures. Acid is formed from glucose, sucrose, maltose, and galactose. *S. equi* does not ferment lactose and sorbitol, nor will it acidify milk. The colonies are either mucoid or matt on primary isolation. Spanier and Timoney (32) have shown that matt colonies are produced by strains lysogenized by bacteriophage. The matt condition is a result of phage-controlled hyaluronidase action on the hyaluronic acid capsule during the early growth phase.

Mucoid colonies are usually about 3 mm in diameter after 24 hours and adjacent colonies tend to run together. Matt colonies exhibit irregular surface folding and a "dried out" appearance.

Antigens. *S. equi* possesses the group C antigen as well as one species-specific, trypsin-labile protein antigen which, because of its similarity to the M proteins of group A streptococci, has been designated the M antigen. The M antigen is the protective antigen in *S. equi* (12, 40).

Epidemiology and Pathogenesis. *S. equi* is an obligate parasite of members of the Equidae. Transmission of the organism occurs by means of infective droplets or by direct or indirect contact. Outbreaks are usually seen in large groups of horses held together and often begin soon after the introduction of a carrier or infected animal which may be clinically normal. The site of carriage of the organism in carrier animals is not known.

The organism enters the nasopharynx, where initial

colonization and multiplication is probably favored by the M antigen, which is antiphagocytic and may also be responsible for adhesion of the organism to epithelial cells—a function known to be associated with M protein in group A streptococci (7). The presence of a hyaluronic capsule is also a vital virulence factor following invasion of the organism since it protects against phagocytosis. Nonencapsulated variants appear to have reduced virulence for the horse (42).

The disease is most common in horses less than 2 years old but can occur in older animals that have not had previous exposure to the organism or its antigens in the form of vaccination.

The incubation period is 3 to 6 days. The animal loses its appetite and is febrile. The normal mucosa appears dry at first, but later a serous and then a mucopurulent nasal discharge develops.

The mucosa is inflamed and there is abscessation of the lymph nodules of the pharyngeal region, which becomes very painful. The infection then spreads to the mandibular and parotid lymph nodes, which abscess and rupture to the surface in about 2 weeks from the onset of the first signs. Most animals recover completely after rupture of the lymph nodes. Sometimes the infection spreads to other areas of the body, resulting in generalized abscessation (*bastard strangles*). Involvement of vital structures or organs may result in death of the animal. Cardiac failure has been reported to be caused by myocarditis associated with *S. equi* infection (26). Laryngeal hemiplegia is a complication that may result from abscessation of the anterior cervical lymph node and involvement of the recurrent laryngeal nerve. Guttural pouch empyema has also been observed in experimentally infected horses (20).

Purpura hemorrhagica is another complicating aftermath of strangles and arises in a small percentage of animals that have recovered from the disease. Affected animals develop fever and edema of the dependent areas of the head and trunk and of the legs above the knee and hock. Punctate hemorrhages may also be found on the nasal mucosa. The primary lesion is necrosis of blood vessel walls. There is no evidence of thrombocytopenia. The pathogenesis of purpura hemorrhagica is not understood but is believed to involve an immune reaction because affected animals have very high antibody titers to the antigens of *S. equi* and the disease is often seen after a second natural exposure to the infection or after vaccination of animals that previously had the disease.

Immunity. Recovered animals are immune to further attacks. A bacterin prepared from log-phase growths of the organism was shown by Bazeley (2) in Australian field trials to stimulate a useful degree of protection. Later studies in the United States (4) confirmed that bacterins given in three intramuscular injections 1 to 2 weeks apart would protect the majority of horses. However, available vaccines often result in undesirable local and systemic reactions consisting of edema, induration, stiffness, and transient fever and neutrophilia. Purpura hemorrhagica follows vaccination in about 0.1 percent of inoculated animals (4).

The humoral immune response consists mainly of antibodies of the IgG class. Antibodies to the protective M antigen are measured by the chain-length assay and by the bactericidal index (40). Antibody titers after a course of three doses of vaccine decline in the 12 months post vaccination (41). Titers after natural infection decline much more rapidly.

Treatment. After strangles abscesses have drained, clinical signs disappear. Many experienced clinicians feel that antibiotics delay this process and may suppress or retard abscessation (6). Bastard strangles is believed to occur more frequently when horses with immature abscesses are treated with penicillin (4).

S. equi is very sensitive to penicillin, but use of this drug in strangles outbreaks is perhaps best reserved for prophylaxis of in-contact animals that have not yet developed symptoms.

Group E Streptococci (*Streptococcus infrequens*)

Cervical lymphadenitis, a contagious disease of swine, was first shown to be associated with group E streptococci in 1937 by Newsom (23). He named this disease *swine strangles* because of its similarity to equine strangles.

Group E streptococci isolated from this disease produce small, elevated, entire colonies. Slowly developing beta hemolysis on horse blood agar is visible in about 48 hours. Acid is produced from trehalose and, in the case of some strains, from sorbitol and inulin. There are five serotypes based on polysaccharide antigens, but type IV is most frequently isolated from cases of cervical lymphadenitis. Strains from swine may lack the type antigen, are capsulated, and produce streptodornase and a streptokinase specific for porcine plasminogen (10).

Epidemiology and Pathogenesis. The disease is common in the swine-raising areas of the midwestern United States but appears to be of infrequent occurrence elsewhere. Swine aged 9 to 14 weeks are more susceptible than other age groups. Carrier animals transmit the infection via nasal droplets. The organism is carried in the tonsil and possibly in other sites in carrier animals and is shed for long periods after clinical remission. It survives for extended periods in the soil (27).

The minimal infective dose of one group E strain for 12-week-old swine has been shown to be about 10^6 colony-forming units (1). The organism enters the mouth and/or nasal chambers and is followed by a rise in temperature and a leukocytosis 2 to 4 days after exposure. Lymph node enlargement is evident about 2 weeks later, and the abscessed nodes may eventually drain to the surface about 6 weeks after this. The mandibular lymph nodes are most frequently abscessed, followed by the retropharyngeals and parotids. The disease is frequently called *jowl abscessation* because of involvement of the mandibular lymph nodes. It is a cause of condemnation losses when meat is inspected and affected animals are often not detected until this time.

Immunity. Antibodies are formed in about 7 days (19) in response to infection and are detected by agglutination, precipitin, and passive hemagglutination tests (31). Immunity can be passively transferred by means of sera from convalescent cases (18).

Antibody to an antiphagocytic factor of the group E streptococci has been detected and shown to persist for at least 20 weeks (33).

Immunity to cervical lymphadenitis can be stimulated by an oral, avirulent, group E vaccine strain (11). Bacterins have been shown to be relatively ineffective in preventing abscessation, although they reduce the number and size of abscesses in affected pigs (15, 30).

Chemotherapy. Group E streptococci are usually sensitive to penicillin, tetracycline, chloramphenicol, and nitrofurazone. Feed additive use of tetracycline (50 parts per million) has been shown to prevent cervical lymphadenitis when applied continuously for 4 to 6 weeks after weaning (28).

Diagnosis. Procedures employing broth containing blood, azide, and crystal violet or penicillin and salt have been used for selective isolation of group E streptococci from tonsil swabs and biopsies (24). The fluorescent-antibody technique, however, is reported to be the most effective procedure for detection of these organisms from tonsil material (24, 29).

Streptococcus suis

S. suis belongs to Lancefield's serologic group D (8), although it has previously and erroneously been reported to belong to group S or to group R. Considerable difficulty may be encountered in grouping strains.

Strains of the organism (Types 1 and 2) have caused bacteremia, meningoencephalitis, and arthritis in swine in the United States (22), England (13, 34), the Netherlands (5), and Ireland (21). Disease occurs in 2- to 6-week-old piglets, although an outbreak in animals 10 to 14 weeks old has been reported (34).

The throat is the apparent route of entry (9), and the tonsil is the site of initial multiplication and colonization. The organism spreads in the bloodstream to the joints and brain. Affected swine are febrile and show nervous symptoms and lameness. Severe cases may die and animals that recover may develop chronic arthritis. Swine in the early stages respond well to penicillin. Convalescent serum has been shown to contain protective antibodies (8).

Group G Streptococci (*Streptococcus canis*)

Streptococci of this group are commonly found on canine mucous membranes. They produce wide zones of beta hemolysis on horse blood agar.

Metritis and vaginitis in the bitch have been associated with group G streptococci (16). Septicemia in puppies has also been caused by these organisms.

In the cat, group G streptococci have caused cervical lymphadenitis with abscessation, conjunctivitis, sinusitis, and leg abscesses (14).

Streptococcus bovis

This organism is always present in the mouths and intestinal tracts of cattle and, because of fecal contamination, is usually present in milk, where it may be mistaken for *S. agalactiae*. Feedlot bloat in cattle is believed to be caused by excess production of capsular polysaccharide from sucrose by *S. bovis*. This material increases the viscosity and the foaming properties of rumen contents. Antibody to the capsular material is secreted in the saliva and may be a factor in normal prevention of bloat (17). The ability of *S. bovis* to multiply rapidly and to ferment certain dietary starches to lactic acid gives it considerable importance in the etiology of lactic acidosis.

It does not hydrolyze sodium hippurate but does attack esculin, characteristics that differentiate it from the streptococci of bovine mastitis.

Streptococcus equinus

This organism is always abundantly present in the feces of horses. It was first isolated from air, undoubtedly because of the presence of dried horse manure, a situation which was formerly common in most cities. A striking characteristic of this organism is its inability to ferment lactose. It will be remembered that this also is true of *S. equi*. It does not grow well in milk and does not cause coagulation. It does not grow at temperatures lower than 20 C. *S. equinus* is not known to be pathogenic for animals.

Streptococcus lactis

This organism has no pathogenic properties, but because of its omnipresence in milk and milk products bacteriologists should be able to recognize it and differentiate it from other organisms that may be responsible for disease. *S. lactis* is the common milk-souring organism. In sour milk it usually occurs in short chains, whereas most pathogenic streptococci form long chains. This fact is of considerable differential value; however, it is not always a safe rule to follow. In culture media, particularly those that contain serum, this organism often forms long chains. A characteristic that has long been recognized is its rapid growth in milk. If litmus or other reducible dyes are present, the dye is reduced before coagulation occurs. The milk-souring *Streptococcus* grows at relatively low temperatures, and also at relatively high temperatures. Reduction and coagulation of litmus milk will occur at temperatures as low as 10 C. Esculin is almost always attacked.

The normal habitat of *S. lactis* has long been a mystery. Many workers have shown that it is not found in milk drawn aseptically from the udder; neither is it found in the mouths or intestines of cattle. It has, however, been found on vegetation. Once established in a dairy it flourishes. Its heat resistance may be a factor in its persistence in these environments.

REFERENCES

1. Armstrong, Boehm, and Ellis. Am. Jour. Vet. Res., 1970, *31*, 823.
2. Bazeley. Austral. Vet. Jour., 1940, *16*, 243.
3. Bazeley and Battle. Austral. Vet. Jour., 1940, *6*, 140.
4. Bryans and Moore. *In* Streptococci, ed. F. A. Skinner and C. B. Quesnel. Academic Press, New York, 1978.
5. De Moore. Antonie van Leeuwenhoek, 1963, *29*, 272.
6. Ebert. Vet. Med., 1969, *64*, 71.
7. Ellen and Gibbons. Inf. and Immun., 1972, *5*, 826.
8. Elliott. Jour. Hyg. (London), 1966, *64*, 205.
9. Elliott, Alexander, and Thomas. Jour. Hyg. (London), 1966, *64*, 213.
10. Ellis and Armstrong. Am. Jour. Vet. Res., 1971, *32*, 349.
11. Engelbrecht and Dolan. Vet. Med./Small Animal Clin. 1968, *63*, 872.
12. Erickson. Can. Jour. Comp. Med., 1975, *39*, 110.
13. Field, Buntain, and Dome. Vet. Rec., 1954, *66*, 453.
14. Goldman and Moore. Lab. Animal Sci., 1973, *23*, 565.
15. Gosser and Olsen. Am. Jour. Vet. Res., 1973, *34*, 129.
16. Hirsh and Wiger. Jour. Small Animal Pract., 1977, *18*, 25.
17. Horacek, Find, Tillinghost, Gettings, and Bartley. Can. Jour. Microbiol., 1977, *23*, 100.
18. Jenkins and Collier. Am. Jour. Vet. Res., 1978, *39*, 1181.
19. Jenkins and Collier. Am. Jour. Vet. Res., 1978, *39*, 325.
20. Knight, Voss, McChesney, and Bigbee. Vet. Med./Small Animal Clin., 1975, *70*, 1194.
21. McErlean. Irish Vet. Jour., 1956, *10*, 174.
22. McNutt and Packer. Vet. Stud., 1943, *6*, 68.
23. Newsom. Vet. Med., 1937, *37*, 137.
24. Riley, Morehouse, and Olsen. Am. Jour. Vet. Res., 1973, *34*, 1167.
25. Ross. *In* Streptococci and streptococcal diseases, ed. Lewis W. Wannamaker and John M. Matson. Academic Press, New York, 1972, pp. 339–46.
26. Rubarth. Svend. Milit. Sailsk. Kvortalsskr., 1943, *30*, 75.
27. Schmitz and Olsen. Proc. Ann. Meeting U.S. Animal Health Assoc., 1970, *74*, 257–67.
28. Schmitz and Olsen. Jour. Am. Vet. Med. Assoc., 1973, *162*, 55.
29. Schueler, Morehouse, and Olsen. Can. Jour. Comp. Med., 1973, *37*, 327.
30. Shuman and Wood. Cornell Vet., 1968, *58*, 21.
31. Shuman and Wood. Cornell Vet., 1970, *60*, 286.
32. Spanier and Timoney. Jour. Gen. Virol., 1977, *35*, 369.
33. Wessman, Wood, and Nord. Cornell Vet., 1977, *67*, 81.
34. Windsor and Elliott. Jour. Hyg. (London), 1975, *75*, 69.
35. Wisecup, Schroder, and Page. Jour. Am. Vet. Med. Assoc., 1967, *150*, 303.
36. Woods. Dissert. Abstr. Internatl., 1975, *36B*, 2102.
37. Woods and Ross. Inf. and Immun., 1975, *12*, 88.
38. Woods and Ross. Vet. Bull., 1975, *46*, 397.
39. Woods and Ross. Am. Jour. Vet. Res., 1977, *38*, 33.
40. Woolcock. Inf. and Immun., 1974, *10*, 116.
41. Woolcock. Austrl. Vet. Jour., 1975, *51*, 554.
42. Woolcock. Res. Vet. Sci., 1975, *19*, 115.

18 The Genus *Erysipelothrix*

Erysipelothrix rhusiopathiae

SYNONYMS: *Bacillus rhusiopathiae-suis, Bacterium erysipelatos-suum, Bacterium rhusiopathiae, Erysipelothrix insidiosa,* swine rotlauf bacillus

This organism, the only species in the genus, is the cause of *swine erysipelas,* long recognized as the most destructive disease of young pigs in many parts of continental Europe. For many years it was believed not to exist in the United States, although Moore (28) isolated a culture thought to be *E. rhusiopathiae* as early as 1892. In 1920, Ten Broeck (50) obtained the organism from the tonsils of 5 of 16 pigs affected with hog cholera in New Jersey. In 1921, Creech (7) succeeded in isolating it from the skin lesions of the *diamond skin disease,* a condition that had been recognized for years as similar to the mildest form of European swine erysipelas. This finding removed all doubt as to the presence of the disease in the United States. In 1922, Ward (63) called attention to the fact that a form of polyarthritis in swine in the United States is caused by this organism. In 1931 acute swine erysipelas with serious losses occurred in some isolated areas in South Dakota. Since that time it has been found in many areas of the United States. In some parts of the swine belt (South Dakota, Nebraska, Iowa) the disease has developed into one of the major problems of the industry, as it has been for many years in continental Europe.

In addition to swine, *E. rhusiopathiae* has been found in lambs suffering from polyarthritis, in calves suffering from a similar disease, in turkeys and ducks (40) suffering from acute septicemic infections, in wild and laboratory-bred mice (3), in the tonsils and on mucous membranes of apparently normal swine, in various decaying plant and animal tissues, on the skin of fresh and salt-water fish, and in skin lesions in man known as *erysipeloid.*

Morphology and Staining Reactions. Cells are Gram-positive but are easily decolorized and are short (0.5 to 2.5 μm), slender (0.3 μm) and show uneven staining. The rough form exhibits long filaments. There are no spores or flagella. The cell walls do not contain DL-diaminopimelic acid, which distinguishes them from those of *Listeria monocytogenes.*

Cultural Features. On solid media containing serum or blood, colonies are tiny, clear, and glistening. On blood agar there is first a greening and later a definite clearing around the colonies. In gelatin stabs, a "bottle-brush" growth is produced in 3 to 4 days. Gelatin is not liquefied. Hydrogen sulfide is produced, and most strains ferment glucose, lactose, and galactose with formation of acid.

Resistance. The organism is rather resistant to drying and to smoking, pickling, and salting. The remarkable life span of the erysipelas bacterium is shown by the fact that a 22-year-old erysipelas broth culture, not kept at low temperatures but exposed to the temperature variations of the seasons, was still able to kill mice and to produce in swine, percutaneously, a local skin reaction leading to immunization (65).

Once infected with the disease, farms usually experience recurrences of it from year to year, although Doyle (10) has stated that there is little evidence to support the view that *E. rhusiopathiae* remains viable for many months in the soil. Special soil conditions such as alkalinity may favor its survival. This has been observed in the Sid area of Yugoslavia where erysipelas is common in areas with alkaline but not in immediately contiguous areas with acid soils (16).

The bacterium survives for relatively long periods in putrefying flesh and in water. Cultures are destroyed by exposure to moist heat at 55 C for 10 minutes. The organism is quite resistant to phenol, a fact that can be used in isolating it from contaminated tissues.

Antigens. The various serotypes are classified in groups labeled A, B, C, D, E, F, G, and N. (There are both heat-stable and heat-labile antigens.) There is no clear relationship between serotype and host species, but group A organisms are more commonly isolated from septicemic erysipelas whereas group B occur more often in cases of arthritis in swine.

According to Gledhill (13), *Erysipelothrix* strains are qualitatively homogeneous as regards their antigens, the difference between serological groups arising from differences in the quantitative distribution of the antigens. Truszczynski (61) has demonstrated the presence of type-specific and species-specific antigens by means of the gel-diffusion precipitation test; the former occurred in acid extracts, broth cultures, and bacterial fractions, and the latter in broth cultures and bacterial fractions.

Pathogenesis of Septicemic Erysipelas in Swine. The source of the organisms that give rise to the first cases in outbreaks of erysipelas is uncertain. Many healthy swine carry the organism in their tonsils and reticuloendothelial tissues, and it is probable that stress, such as excessive heat and humidity, or other predisposing factors cause impairment of the antibacterial defense mechanism with subsequent multiplication of the organism in the animal's body. In this situation, infection is endogenous. The ubiquitous distribution of the organism in nature, however, suggests that the pig's habitat may also be an exogenous source of infection in some cases. In any event, once a pig becomes septicemic it sheds great numbers of organisms in the urine, feces, saliva, and vomitus, which leads to rapid spread among in-contact animals. Because the disease has been experimentally produced by the oral route of exposure and because the tonsil carrier state is so common among swine, it is likely that the majority of natural infections occur by the oral route. However, the disease can also be produced by skin scarification, suggesting that skin scratches may also contribute to spread of infection in groups of animals.

E. rhusiopathiae is a facultative intracellular parasite and exhibits a high rate of survival in pig neutrophils (52). It has been suggested that multiplication of the organism in, and subsequent killing of, phagocytes is the critical factor in determining the outcome of the infection (50). There is evidence that the reticuloendothelial (RE) system becomes blocked in acute erysipelas in swine (19). This blocking effect may in fact be simple depletion of viable phagocytes in the RE system.

The acute disease develops suddenly with high fever (106 F), prostration, conjunctivitis, and vomition in some cases. Areas of deep red to purple discolored patches may appear on the skin, particularly on the ears, abdomen, and insides of the legs. The spleen and lymph nodes are enlarged and reddened, and the mucosa of the stomach and small intestine is acutely inflamed, hemorrhagic, and sometimes ulcerated. The kidneys generally show cloudy swelling and often have ecchymotic hemorrhages. The mortality from this form of the disease is very high.

A less severe form of swine erysipelas is characterized by the formation of urticarial skin lesions that consist, in the beginning, of reddish or purplish rhomboidal blotches on the skin, several cm in diameter, principally on the abdomen. The shape of these blotches is like that of a diamond and has given the disease its common name, *diamond skin disease* (Figure 18.1). The urticarial areas later become necrotic; the affected skin dries into dense scabs, which finally peel off, leaving a bleeding area if removed too soon.

During the severe septicemic phase there is increased serum glutamic oxalacetic transaminase and a marked hypoglycemia of unknown origin (9). There is also increased erythrocyte destruction with a decrease in hemoglobin and packed cell volume.

A similar phenomenon occurs in experimental erysipelas in the mouse. Timoney and Shaw (unpublished data, 1975) have observed that plasma acid phosphatase and hemoglobin levels rise rapidly together about 36 hours after infection when bacterial numbers in the blood exceed 10^4 per ml.

In the late stages of the acute disease in the pig, nucleated erythrocytes appear. At death, the spleen is enlarged and pulpy—a condition consistent with hemolysis and stimulation of the hemopoietic system. Interestingly, *E. rhusiopathiae* has hemagglutinating activity for erythrocytes, and this has been shown to result in complement-dependent hemolysis following activation

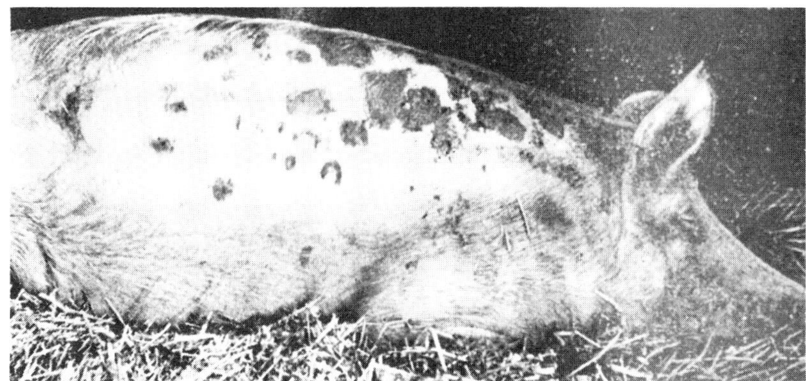

Figure 18.1. Diamond skin disease of the pig. Characteristic lesions of one type of swine erysipelas are visible. (Courtesy R. A. McIntosh.)

of the alternate complement pathway (8). The hemagglutinating activity is probably related to the high neuraminidase activity of virulent strains (31) which increases cell adhesiveness by removal of sialic acid residues which, in turn, removes negative charges on the erythrocyte surface. Neuraminidase appears to have other important but as yet unknown roles in the disease process. Neutralizing antibodies to the enzyme are present in high titer in commercial swine erysipelas antiserum (33) and are protective for mice (32). Also, there is a good correlation between virulence and neuraminidase production in strains of *E. rhusiopathiae* (22). It is possible also that neuraminidase activity is in some way involved in the generalized coagulopathy with the formation of hyaline thrombi in blood vessels, the thrombocytopenia, and the sticking of fibrin in joints, heart valves, and muscle that occur about 36 hours after swine are inoculated with the organism (65).

The high fever noted in erysipelas may be caused by the *Erysipelothrix* endotoxin—a glycoprotein of molecular weight of 31,700 (23). This substance also produces a shock effect in swine.

The chronic form of the disease nearly always takes the form of a vegetative endocarditis (Figure 18.2). The heart valves, particularly the mitral, are eroded and become so covered with fibrin deposits that their function-

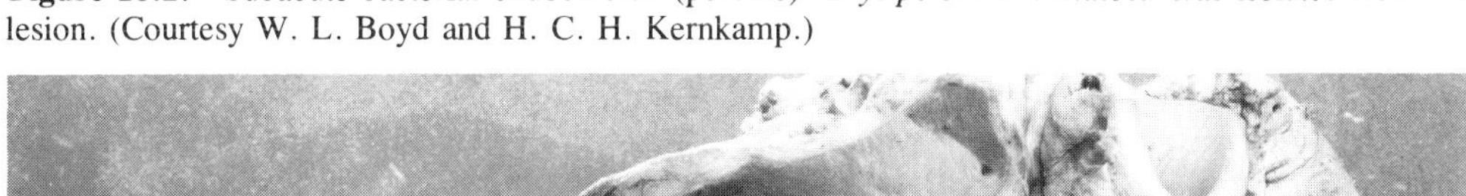

Figure 18.2. Subacute bacterial endocarditis (porcine). *Erysipelothrix insidiosa* was isolated from the lesion. (Courtesy W. L. Boyd and H. C. H. Kernkamp.)

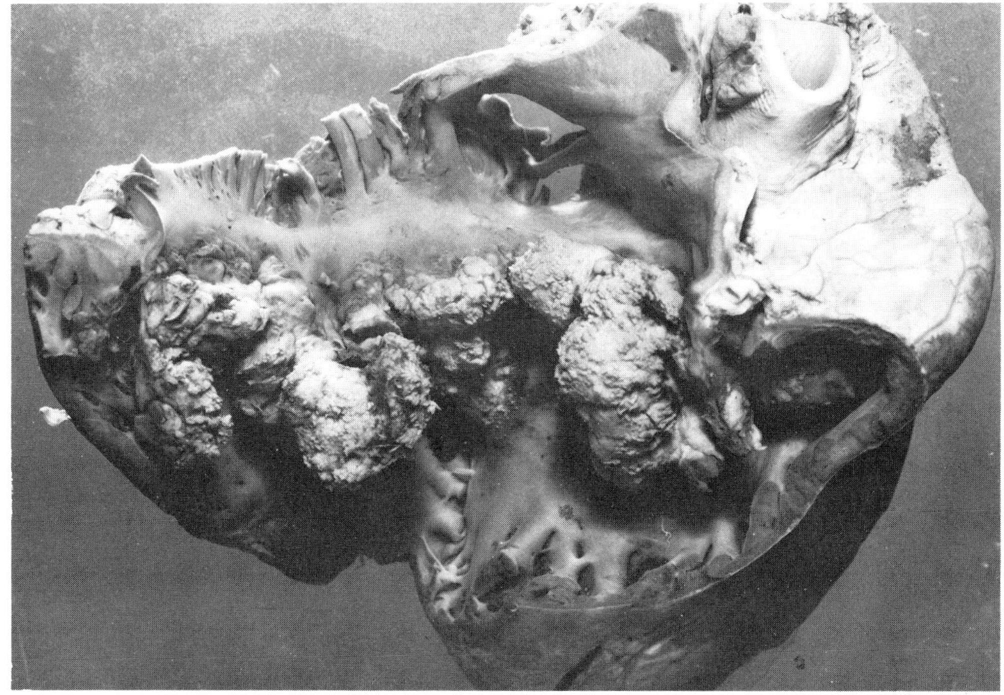

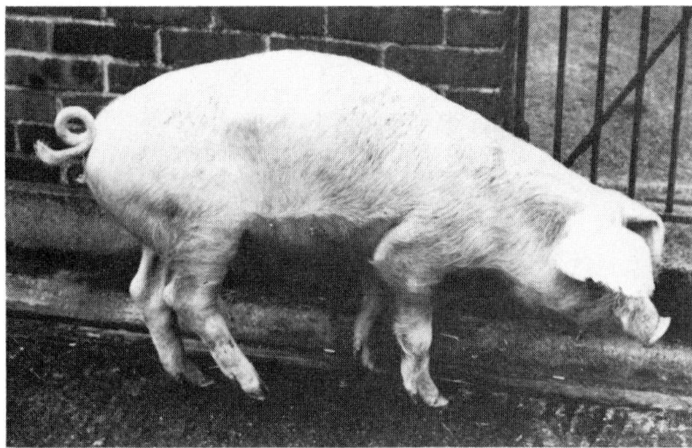

Figure 18.3. Erysipelothrix polyarthritis. Note the arched back, swollen right carpal region, and reluctance to bear weight on the right hind limb.

ing is seriously impaired. Affected animals invariably die from this condition sooner or later, and often suddenly.

Pathogenesis of *Erysipelothrix* Arthritis in Swine. The arthritic form of the disease generally occurs spontaneously in older animals, although arthritis may be a sequel to the more acute forms of the disease. The joints become enlarged and painful, the animals are reluctant to move (Figure 18.3), the gait is stilted, and they become stunted in growth. The synovial lining becomes hypertrophied, forming villous projections into the joint space (Figure 18.4). Erosions of the cartilage may result, and there is often a great increase in synovial fluid, which has a high content of neutrophils but is not grossly purulent. All diarthrodial joints may be affected, but arthritis is most noticeable in the limb joints.

In the early stages of the arthritis *E. rhusiopathiae* is readily cultured from affected joints. Later, the organism is harder to isolate, and a proportion of joints that have become chronically arthritic are seemingly culturally negative. This, together with the fact that the synovium in these cases is heavily infiltrated with mononuclear cells, including many plasma cells (Figure 18.5), has given rise to the concept that the pathogenesis of the chronic disease has an immunologic component (6). Other evidence supporting this concept included an apparent higher incidence of—and more severe—arthritis in vaccinated swine following challenge (11, 34), and the occurrence of autoantibody (rheumatoid factor) to complexed immunoglobulin in sera and synovial fluids of some chronically arthritic swine (48, 53). However, some workers (26, 49) feel that vaccination has no effect on the incidence of arthritis. These observations, together with the gross and microscopic morphologic similarities that exist between the disease in the pig and rheumatoid arthritis in man, led to the suggestion that erysipelothrix arthritis would be a useful model for the study of rheumatoid arthritis. However, erysipelas arthritis differs in some important ways from rheumatoid arthritis. Timoney and Berman (54) have shown that plasma cells in arthritic pig synovium contain antibody to *Erysipelothrix* and that some arthritic synovial fluids contain higher antibody titers to the organism than compan-

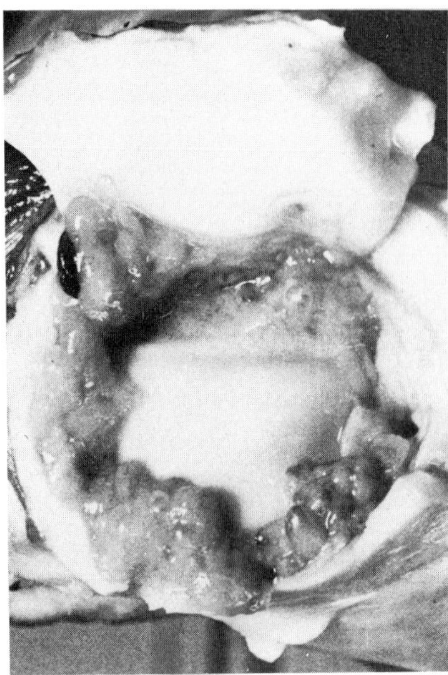

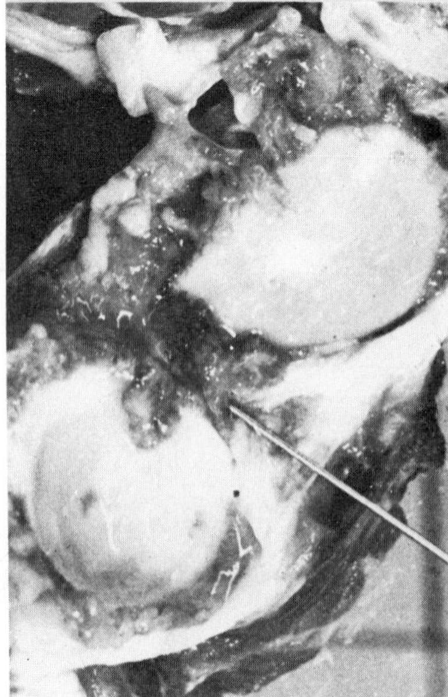

Figure 18.4. Erysipelothrix arthritis in a stifle (*left*) and a shoulder joint (*right*). Note the hyperemia and hypertrophy of the synovial membranes and the villous projection extending onto the joint cartilage.

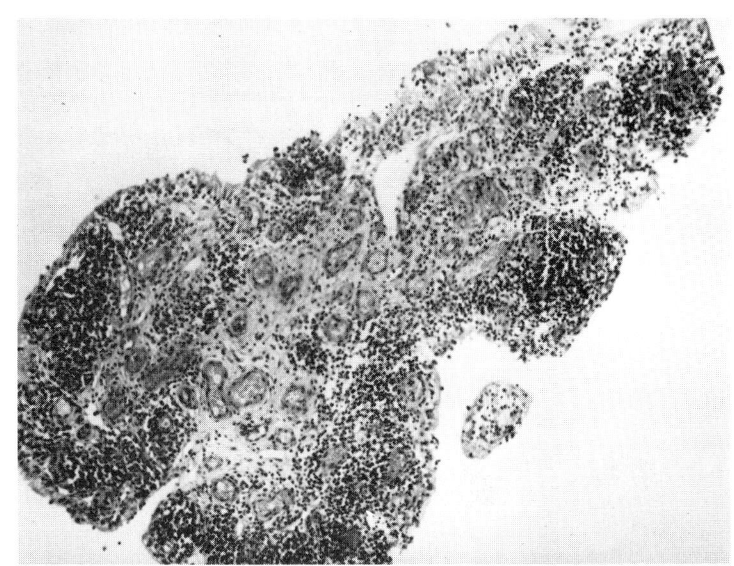

Figure 18.5. Erysipelothrix arthritis. A section of a hypertrophied villus showing cellular accumulations. These cells are mostly plasma and other mononuclear cells. × 110.

ion sera (53). Later, Timoney and Yarkoni (58) showed that levels of IgG were higher in arthritic fluids than in serum—further evidence of local antibody synthesis and proof of the immunocompetence of arthritic synovial tissue. Unlike rheumatoid arthritis in man, immune complexes seemed to play a minor role in the pathogenesis of the disease in swine since there was no evidence of complement depletion (56) or of selective release of lysozomal enzymes (lysozyme, acid phosphatase) into joint fluids (57). The latter might be expected to occur during phagocytosis of immune complexes. Instead, the cytoplasmic enzyme, lactic dehydrogenase, was present in amounts proportional to acid phosphatase levels—an indication of cell death and of a cytotoxic phenomenon. The cytotoxicity could be bacterial (47) and/or immunological. The latter possibility must be invoked for arthritic joints that no longer contain viable *E. rhusiopathiae*.

Schulz *et al.* (46) feel that fibrin deposition in the early stages is important in the pathogenesis of the chronic phase arthritis. They observed bacterial multiplication in the fibrin deposits (47). It is possible that the chronicity and eventual apparent autonomicity of the arthritis is caused by *Erysipelothrix* antigen that remains in organized fibrin deposits and continues to provoke a local immune response. *Erysipelothrix* antigens are known to persist in synovial tissue. White and Mirikitans (68) have shown persistence of a protein antigen, and Ajmal (1), using the fluorescent-antibody technique, has seen antigen in synoviocytes of arthritic joints.

Many joints heal spontaneously with the disappearance of infection, but animals with both infected and healed joints at the same time have been observed (54). This is a good indication of the need for the local presence of *E. rhusiopathiae* or its antigens to maintain the local immune/inflammatory response. The rheumatoid factor seen in some arthritic synovial fluids is probably a response to complexes of *Erysipelothrix* antigen and antibody. the rheumatoid factor oocurs in swine hyperimmunized with erysipelas vaccines (59) and has also been produced in rabbits and guinea pigs immunized with complexes of killed *E. rhusiopathiae* cells and homologous IgG antibodies isolated from pig serum. Thus, it seems that the rheumatoid factor is not of primary importance in the pathogenesis of chronic erysipelas arthritis.

Much of the joint destruction seen in infected joints is undoubtedly a result of enzymes released from neutrophils attracted by *E. rhusiopathiae* or its products. The chemotactic stimulus in arthritic joints that are culturally negative is as yet unknown.

Erysipelothrix **Infection in Other Animals.** *Sheep.* Poels (38) in 1913 described a polyarthritis in sheep caused by the swine erysipelas organism. The disease was first recognized in the United States by Ray (39) in 1930 and by Marsh (25), working independently. It has been described in Europe, Australia (69), and New Zealand.

The epidemiology of erysipelas in sheep is poorly understood. The condition is seen in lambs, beginning when they are 2 to 3 months of age. Docking and castration wounds may be the route of entry in lambs. In older sheep the organism may enter shearing wounds via contaminated sheep-dip solution. It is thought that the disease is also contracted through umbilical infection, but apparently this has not been proved. Affected animals develop a stiff gait, and eat well but do not thrive.

Advanced cases often get down and find difficulty in arising, but affected animals seldom die from the disease. Lesions are not present in the visceral organs; in fact they are found nowhere except in some of the joints of the legs. One joint or several may be affected. The involved joint usually is swollen and the joint capsule is thickened. Granulation tissue occurs on the inner surface of the capsule. The fluid is generally thin but pus cells are present in smears. The specific organism usually cannot be found in smears, but cultures are easily obtained. The organism is in every way typical.

Cattle. In 1953, Moulton *et al.* (30) reported an outbreak of arthritis in 6 out of 20 calves in a herd. The tibiotarsal, stifle, and carpal joints were involved. *E. rhusiopathiae* was isolated from one of the infected joints. A case of bovine encephalomeningitis has been attributed to this organism (66).

Birds. The swine erysipelas organism is pathogenic for turkeys, chickens, geese, ducks, mud hens, pigeons, parrots, quail, and many small wild birds and larger species often found in zoological parks. In this country the species most often and most seriously affected is the turkey. The first outbreak of this kind was recognized by Beaudette and Hudson (4) in 1936. In 1938, Van Roekel, Bullis, and Clarke (62) described three outbreaks occurring in Massachusetts, Vermont, and New York. Madsen (24), shortly before, described an outbreak in Utah. The disease is an important one economically both in this country and abroad.

Affected turkeys usually are adult, or nearing adult age. They exhibit a cyanotic skin that is most obvious as a "blue comb." The birds become droopy, develop diarrhea, and die. Frequently the male birds show the highest mortality. The lesions consist of massive hemorrhages and petechiae in the muscles of the breast and legs, also large hemorrhages on the various serous membranes, particularly those of the heart. Hemorrhages occur in the mucosa of the gizzard and of the small intestine, and the content of the intestine often is bloody. The liver and spleen are ordinarily congested and enlarged. The causative organism can easily be isolated from any of the tissues. In several reports on outbreaks in turkeys it was noted that the first cases appeared within a few weeks after the birds came in contact with sheep or a sheep range. Erysipelas has also caused heavy losses in fattening ducks raised on free ranges that included large areas of standing water (40).

Laboratory animals. White mice and pigeons are very susceptible to infection by inoculation and are commonly used in diagnostic work. After subcutaneous inoculation they usually die in from 18 hours to 4 days. Rabbits are not highly susceptible. Usually a local reaction occurs and the animal may die after 6 or 7 days. Guinea pigs are quite resistant. Inoculated mice usually show evidence of conjunctivitis, first serous and later purulent, which glues their eyelids together. They sit with arched backs and roughened hair and do not eat. The lesions consist of enlargement of the spleen, discrete grayish foci in the liver, and occasionally congestion of the lungs. The blood and spleen contain large numbers of organisms, many of which have been taken up by phagocytes. Pigeons that have been inoculated in the breast muscles show swelling and hemorrhagic inflammation around the point of inoculation. The spleen is swollen and the liver may show focal necrosis. The organism is abundant in the blood and tissues. Wayson (64) has given a good account of a natural outbreak of this disease in wild mice, and Balfour-Jones (3) has described an outbreak in a stock of laboratory mice.

Aquatic animals. E. rhusiopathiae (17) has been isolated from spleen and liver tissue of the caiman (*Caiman crocodilus*) and the American crocodile (*Crocodilus acutus*). It has produced an epizootic of septicemia in captive bottle-nose dolphins (12).

Man. Many cases of wound infection of the hands have been reported. In Europe most of the human cases have been attributed to the handling of infected swine and pork, but some have occurred in fishermen and fish dealers who have had no contact with swine. The disease has also been observed in veterinarians, laboratory technicians, slaughterhouse personnel, and veterinary students (21, 29, 71). The infection in man is known as *erysipeloid* to distinguish it from human erysipelas, which is caused by a hemolytic *Streptococcus.* The disease is rarely manifested by septicemia, which is likely to be fatal. The usual lesion is a localized, painful, purplish-red swelling on the finger or arm. The infection enters via small wounds or abrasions. The center of the lesion eventually becomes pale and the superficial skin in this area may die and slough. There is no suppuration. A complication of erysipeloid is arthritis in nearby joints in about 5 percent of cases. The lesions respond well to intramuscular penicillin.

Diagnosis. The differentiation of acute swine erysipelas from hog cholera (swine fever) in the field offers considerable difficulty, and even clinicians with great experience sometimes mistake one for the other. In cholera the affected animals are usually lethargic; in erysipelas they are usually bright and alert until shortly before death. Lameness is not common in cholera; it is frequent in erysipelas. Cholera-affected hogs usually will not eat for several days before death; erysipelas-affected animals frequently will continue to eat after hyperthermia and other symptoms are exhibited. Diarrhea is not as common in erysipelas as it is in cholera. The lesions often are not of great help in the differential diagnosis of these diseases. In erysipelas the spleen usually is slightly enlarged, tense, and bluish red in color, whereas in cholera it is usually unchanged, or it may present one or more wedge-shaped infarcts along its margin. In erysipelas the mucosa of the stomach is often highly inflamed, showing a dark bluish-red discoloration; this is not often found in cholera. The lymph nodes may or may not be congested, whereas they usually are hemorrhagic in cholera. Subserous hemorrhages of the epiglottis, trachea, kidneys, and urinary bladder may be found in both diseases but are ecchymotic in erysipelas and petechial in hog cholera.

Blood culture of sick pigs usually results in isolation of *E. rhusiopathiae* in 18 hours. There is a sensitive fluorescent-antibody test that makes confirmation of hog cholera infection possible in a few hours. Thus these diseases can readily and rapidly be distinguished by laboratory methods.

Serologic tests. Agglutination tests (42, 44) for erysipelas infection have been rather unsatisfactory because of the tendency of antigens to clump spontaneously and to give unclear end-points. A smooth culture that has been mouse- or pigeon-passaged should be used for preparation of antigen. A stained antigen for use in a rapid plate test has been described (15). A live antigen in a plate test has also been used and gives clearer end-points in titration work (55).

A growth-agglutination test (*Wachstumsprobe*) has been developed by Wellman (65) and is commonly used in Europe. This test has been improved by Nielsen (35), who incorporated the antibiotics of Wood's selective medium (70) in the system to inhibit contaminants in the test serum. However, the recent availability of inexpensive antibacterial filters for use with small fluid volumes should obviate the need for these antibiotics as serum samples could rapidly be filtered before being tested in the *Wachstumsprobe* test.

A modified complement-fixation test (18) and a passive hemagglutination test (41) have also been described for antibody to *E. rhusiopathiae*.

Chronically affected animals often have titers in excess of 1:640 in the agglutination test. Many infected animals, however, do not have detectable agglutinins yet are resistant to experimental infection. Presumably either very low agglutinin titers are protective or protective antibodies do not have agglutinin activity. The organism can persist in locations with high antibody titers, such as synovial fluids (53).

Immunity. Biological products available for immunization are antiserum, vaccine, bacterin, and culture-antiserum (simultaneous treatment).

Antiserum. Immune serum is of value both for prophylaxis and for treatment. For treatment, 10 to 30 ml of serum are injected as early in the course of the disease as possible. Losses may occur in spite of such procedure. For prophylaxis the serum is very successful, the principal disadvantage being that the immunity lasts only about 15 days. For animals weighing less than 100 pounds, 5 ml of the serum are sufficient. For large animals, an additional 1 ml is allowed for each 20 pounds in excess of 100 pounds of body weight.

Attenuated vaccines. The first attenuated vaccine against erysipelas was produced in 1883 by Pasteur and Thuillier (37). Attenuation of the culture for swine was accomplished by passing it through rabbits. In the course of time such cultures acquire great virulence for rabbits, but simultaneously they lose virulence for swine. Two stains are used, the most attenuated being injected first and the second about a week later. The procedure usually immunizes safely for periods of 8 months to 1 year, which ordinarily exceeds the average life span of swine. Breeding stock may require reimmunization after 1 year. This method is not wholly safe because vaccination erysipelas often occurs. For this reason it was not used in the United States for many years.

A number of other attenuated vaccines have been developed in recent years. One of these is the erysipelas vaccine avirulent (EVA) of Gray and Norden (14). It has been specially licensed by the U.S. Department of Agriculture and is available to veterinarians. EVA is a lyophilized single strain of *E. rhusiopathiae*. It is avirulent for mice, guinea pigs, pigeons, swine, turkeys, and man. The Swedish AV-R9 (43) vaccine is another attenuated strain that is commercially available in Europe. These attenuated vaccines when injected at the rate of 1 ml for pigs up to 100 pounds and 2 ml for pigs over this weight stimulated protection for up to 8 months. Breeding stock should therefore be immunized at least once each year. Attenuated vaccines can also be administered in the drinking water (36) and by aerosol (27). In swine immunized by these routes there is possibly a tonsillar blockade effect whereby the avirulent strain occupies the preferred colonization sites in the tonsils and prevents subsequent colonization by virulent strains, as well as stimulating an immune response. Response to attenuated vaccines is adversely affected by antibiotics parenterally and also by maternal antibody. Thus, pigs vaccinated too early in life may not develop an immune response to the vaccine.

The immunity stimulated by attenuated strains is cell-mediated. This has been shown by Timoney (51), who observed that macrophages from mice immunized with EVA vaccine exhibited enhanced microbicidal activity for *E. rhusiopathiae*. This finding is consistent with and explains earlier observations of Kuramasu *et al.* (20), who showed that the ability of mice to clear a challenge inoculum was present only so long as the vaccine strain persisted in their tissues. Presumably, the continued presence of the vaccine strain was necessary to maintain the cell-mediated immune response.

Killed vaccines (*adsorbed bacterins*). The first successful bacterins were produced independently in 1947 by Traub (60) and Dinter, who grew specially selected strains (B group) under conditions for optimum production of the soluble immunizing substance—a glycolipoprotein (67). These cultures were then formalinized and adsorbed and concentrated on aluminum hydroxide gel. For long-term protection, this bacterin is injected subcutaneously in 2 doses, 21 to 28 days apart. A single dose confers protection for up to 3 months and is usually sufficient for fattening swine vaccinated after weaning.

Poor response to erysipelas vaccination may be caused by low-level aflatoxin poisoning.

Arthritis and vaccination. There has been considerable debate as to whether vaccination increases the frequency and severity of arthritis. Experimentally, a higher frequency of arthritis has been observed in vaccinated swine that subsequently were challenged with virulent organisms (11). Undoubtedly, local infection by the organism is the primary cause of erysipelas arthritis. However, as discussed earlier, synovial tissue in this disease is immunocompetent; if the animal had previously been immunologically primed by exposure to *E. erysipelothrix* antigen in the form of vaccine, it is reasonable to expect that the response of immunocytes in the synovium to a second antigen exposure would be greater, with more severe tissue alteration and more severe clinical arthritis. Thus vaccination might appear to increase the frequency of arthritis.

Treatment. Penicillin is very effective in treating septicemic erysipelas (2, 5), and is also useful in diminishing the effects of local joint infections if given during the early, acute phase before joint destruction has occurred.

REFERENCES

1. Ajmal. Res. Vet. Sci., 1971, *12,* 403.
2. Aitken. North Am. Vet., 1949, *30,* 25.
3. Balfour-Jones. Brit. Jour. Exp. Path., 1935, *16,* 236.
4. Beaudette and Hudson. Jour. Am. Vet. Med. Assoc., 1936, *88,* 475.
5. Brown, Doll, Bruner, and Kinkaid. Jour. Am. Vet. Med. Assoc., 1949, *114,* 438.
6. Collins and Goldie. Jour. Path. and Bact., 1940, *50,* 323.
7. Creech. Jour. Am. Vet. Med. Assoc., 1921, *59,* 139.
8. Dinter, Diderholm, and Rockburn. Zentrbl. f. Bakt., 1976, *236A,* 583.
9. Dougherty, Shuman, Mullenox, Witzel, Buck, Wood, and Cook. Cornell Vet., 1965, *55,* 87.
10. Doyle. Vet. Rev. and Annot., 1960, *6,* 95.
11. Freeman. Am. Jour. Vet. Res., 1964, *25,* 589.
12. Geraci, Sauer, and Medway. Am. Jour. Vet. Res., 1966, *27,* 597.
13. Gledhill. Jour. Path. and Bact., 1945, *57,* 179.
14. Gray and Norden, Jr. Jour. Am. Vet. Med. Assoc., 1955, *127,* 506.
15. Grey. Vet. Med., 1947, *42,* 74.
16. Hajduk and Pukac. Vet. Glasnik, 1974, *28,* 369.
17. Jasmin and Baucom. Am. Jour. Vet. Clin. Path., 1967, *1,* 173.
18. Jeon, Cho and Oh. Korean Jour. Vet. Res., 1967, *7,* 1.
19. Jowtscheff. Monatsh. f. Vet.-Med., 1961, *16,* 216.
20. Kuramasu, Imamura, Sameshima, and Tajima. Zentrbl. f. Vet.-Med., 1963, *10B,* 362.
21. Klauder. Jour. Am. Med. Assoc., 1938, *111,* 1345.
22. Krasemann and Muller. Zentrbl. f. Bakt., 1975, *231A,* 206.
23. Leimbeck, Bohm, Ehard, and Schultz. Zentrbl. f. Bakt., 1975, *232A,* 266.
24. Madsen. Jour. Am. Vet. Med. Assoc., 1937, *91,* 206.
25. Marsh. Jour. Am. Vet. Med. Assoc., 1931, *78,* 57.
26. Mercy and Bond. Austral. Vet. Jour., 1977, *53,* 600.
27. Mohlmann, Stohr, Schultz, and Michael-Meese. Arch. f. Exp. Vetmed., 1972, *26,* 1.
28. Moore. Jour. Comp. Med. and Vet. Arch., 1892, *13,* 333.
29. Morrill. Jour. Inf. Dis., 1939, *65,* 322.
30. Moulton, Rhode, and Wheat. Jour. Am. Vet. Med. Assoc., 1953, *123,* 335.
31. Muller. Path. Microbiol., 1971, *37,* 241.
32. Muller. Med. Microbiol. and Immunol., 1974, *159,* 301.
33. Muller and Bohm. Berl. und Münch. tierärztl. Wchnschr., 1977, *90,* 314.
34. Neher, Swenson, Doyle, and Sikes. Am. Jour. Vet. Res., 1958, *19,* 5.
35. Nielsen. Acta Vet. Scand., 1969, *10,* 127.

36. Ose, Barnes, and Berkman. Jour. Am. Vet. Med. Assoc., 1963, *143*, 1084.
37. Pasteur and Thuillier. Comp. Rend. Acad. Sci., 1883, *97*, 1163.
38. Poels. Folia Microbiol., 1913, *2*, 1.
39. Ray. Jour. Am. Vet. Med. Assoc., 1956, *129*, 399.
40. Reetz and Schultz. Monatsh. f. Vet.-Med., 1978, *33*, 170.
41. Rhee and Lee. Res. Report, Off. Rural Development (Vet.) (Taiwan), 1971, *14*, 17.
42. Rice, Connell, Byrne, and Boulanger. Can. Jour. Comp. Med. and Vet. Sci., 1952, *16*, 209.
43. Sandstedt and Lehnert. Scand. Vet. Tidskr., 1944, *34*, 129.
44. Schoening, Creech, and Grey. North Am. Vet., 1932, *13*, 19.
45. Schulz, Drommer, Seidler, Ehard, Mickivitz, Hertrampf, and Bohm. Beitrage z. Path., 1975, *154*, 1.
46. Schulz, Ehard, Drommer, Seidler, Trautwein, Hertrampf, Giese, and Hazem. Zentrbl. f. Vet.-Med., 1976, *23B*, 617.
47. Schulz, Drommer, Ehard, Hertrampf, Leibold, Messow, Mumme, Trautwein, Uebarschar, Weis, and Winkelman. Deut. tierärztl. Wchnschr., 1977, *84*, 107.
48. Sikes. Ann. N.Y. Acad. Sci., 1958, *70*, 717.
49. Shuman, Wood, and Cheville. Cornell Vet., 1965, *55*, 387.
50. Ten Broeck. Jour. Exp. Med., 1920, *32*, 331.
51. Timoney. Res. Vet. Sci., 1969, *10*, 301.
52. Timoney. Res. Vet. Sci., 1970, *11*, 189.
53. Timoney and Berman. Am. Jour. Vet. Res., 1970, *31*, 1405.
54. Timoney and Berman. Am. Jour. Vet. Res., 1970, *31*, 1411.
55. Timoney. Jour. Comp. Path., 1971, *81*, 243.
56. Timoney. Am. Jour. Vet. Res., 1976, *37*, 5.
57. Timoney. Am. Jour. Vet. Res., 1976, *37*, 295.
58. Timoney and Yarkoni. Vet. Microbiol., 1976, *1*, 467.
59. Toshkov, Toshkov, Stoev, Soklova, and Karadjov. Acad. Bulg. Sci., 1968, *21*, 1101.
60. Traub. Monatsh. f. Vet.-Med., 1947, 10, 165.
61. Truszczynski. Am. Jour. Vet. Res., 1961, *22*, 846.
62. Van Roekel, Bullis, and Clarke. Jour. Am. Vet. Med. Assoc., 1938, *92*, 403.
63. Ward. Jour. Am. Vet. Med. Assoc., 1922, *61*, 155.
64. Wayson. Pub. Health Rpts. (U.S.), 1927, *42*, 1489.
65. Wellman. Jour. Am. Vet. Med. Assoc., 1955, *127*, 331.
66. Whaley, Robinson, Newherre, and Sippel. Vet. Med., 1958, *53*, 475.
67. White and Verwey. Inf. and Immun., 1970, 1, 387.
68. White and Mirikitans. Cornell Vet., 1976, *66*, 1976.
69. Whitten. Austral. Vet. Jour., 1952, *28*, 6.
70. Wood. Am. Jour. Vet. Res., 1965, *26*, 1303.
71. Wood. *in* Diseases transmitted from animals to men, 6th ed., ed. W. T. Hubbert, W. F. McCullock, and P. R. Schnurrenherger. Thomas, Springfield, Ill., 1975.

19 The Genus *Bacillus*

There are 48 species currently described in the genus *Bacillus,* but almost all are saprophytes and nonpathogenic for animals. The most important species is *B. anthracis,* the cause of anthrax in animals and man. *B. cereus* and *B. licheniformis* are occasionally isolated from cases of bovine mastitis and suppurative lesions in cattle and horses. They have almost no invasive ability by themselves and multiply only in tissues devitalized by injury or other infections.

Bacillus anthracis

B. anthracis causes the disease known as *anthrax* (German *milzbrand;* French *charbon*). Herbivorous animals are very susceptible to infection by *B. anthracis;* carnivorous birds are highly resistant. Cold-blooded animals are also resistant. The disease is often fatal in man, although he is not as susceptible as herbivorous animals.

Morphology and Staining Reactions. The anthrax bacillus is a large, Gram-positive rod about 1 μm in diameter and 3 to 6 μm long. In cultures it forms long chains which, unstained, appear as solid filaments because the square ends of the individual cells fit very closely together (Figure 19.1). In tissues long filaments are never seen, and the ends of the cells are rounded. Here the elements occur either individually or in short chains of 2 to 5 or 6 organisms and are regularly encapsulated, a single capsule enclosing as many organisms as remain in a chain (Figure 19.2). The capsules are well marked and can be stained rather readily. Spores are formed in abundance at 15 to 40 C when the organism is growing in the presence of air. Sporulation is inhibited by a high carbon dioxide tension such as occurs in dead carcasses; thus spores are rare in blood and internal organs.

Cultural Features. *B. anthracis* grows well on most laboratory media exposed to atmospheric oxygen. Growth occurs at temperatures from 12 to 44 C, with an optimum growth temperature of 37 C. Anaerobic conditions result in meager growths. Spores germinate when exposed to 65 C for 15 minutes and change into the vegetative bacillary form.

On agar plates the anthrax organism develops into characteristic "ground-glass" surface colonies. (Figure 19.3). The margins of these colonies are irregular and resemble, under low magnification, locks of wavy hair (Figure 19.4). It is for this reason that they are sometimes described as "Medusa-head" colonies, after the mythological maiden whose flowing locks were changed to serpents. Both the ground-glass and the Medusa-head appearance are caused by the fact that in such colonies the organism grows in the form of long filaments which lie in parallel wavy bundles like locks of a well-combed coiffure. Deep colonies are small, ragged, and stringy.

Other aerobic sporeforming bacilli whose surface colonies resemble *B. anthracis* form small, compact colonies in the depths of agar cultures and so may be distinguished from the latter by this characteristic.

On 50 percent serum agar in an atmosphere of 65 percent CO_2 *B. anthracis* produces smooth, mucoid colonies and the organism is capsulated. On blood agar,

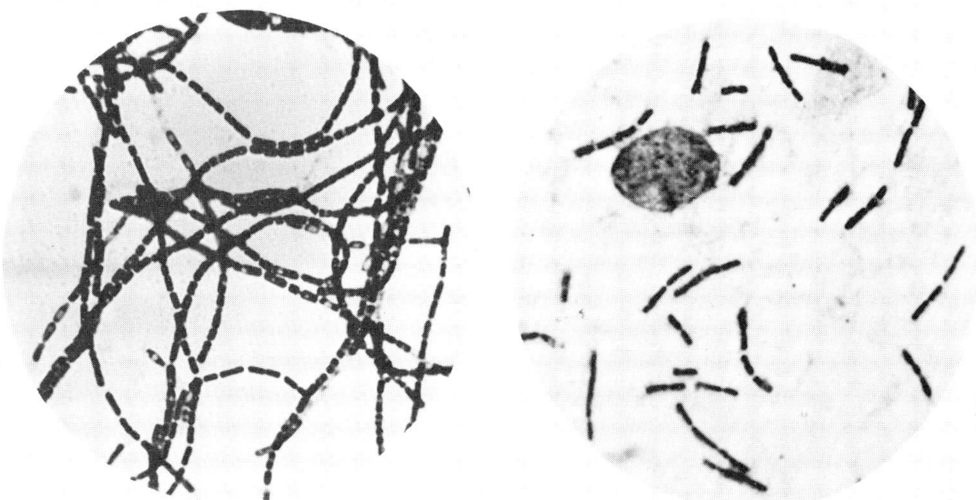

Figure 19.1 (*left*). *Bacillus anthracis,* a stained preparation from a 24-hour-old culture on solid media, showing arrangement of cells in long chains and the development of spores in many of the organisms. × 830.

Figure 19.2 (*right*). *Bacillus anthracis* in a bovine spleen. In tissues anthrax bacilli occur in short chains surrounded by a common capsule. The capsular material shows indistinctly in the illustration. It is responsible for the lack of sharpness of outline of the organisms. × 800.

only a narrow zone of hemolysis is produced, in contrast to other anthracoid *Bacillus* sp. which frequently produce a wide hemolytic zone.

Biochemically, *B. anthracis* is much less active than other similar but nonpathogenic *Bacillus* sp.; acid but no gas is produced in glucose, sucrose, maltose, and salicin (Table 19.1).

Resistance. The spores resist steaming or boiling at 100 C for 5 minutes, but are killed by autoclaving at 120 C for 20 minutes. They are also resistant to disinfectants such as 5 percent phenol or mercuric chloride. A 2 to 3 percent solution of formalin is effective if applied at a temperature of 40 C. A 0.25 percent solution is also effective when applied for 6 hours at 60 C.

Figure 19.3 (*left*). *Bacillus anthracis,* a surface colony on agar photographed by transmitted light showing the "ground-glass" appearance. × 6.4.

Figure 19.4 (*right*). *Bacillus anthracis,* an impression preparation from a colony on a gelatin plate. The habit of the bacilli of forming long filamentous chains that lie parallel accounts for the "Medusa-head" appearance of the colonies. × 170.

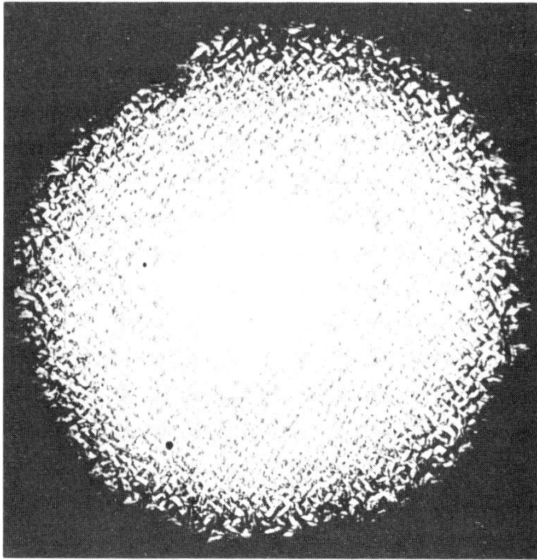

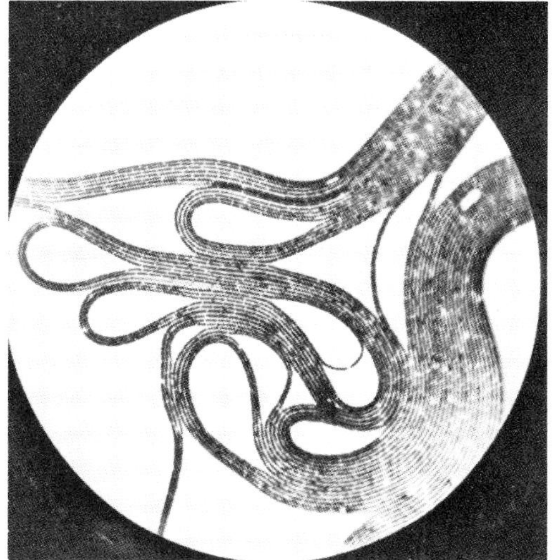

Table 19.1. Biochemical and other properties of *B. anthracis* and similar "anthracoid" *Bacillus* sp.

Property	*B. anthracis*	Other "anthrocoid" *Bacillus* sp.
Motility	Nonmotile	Usually motile
Hemolysis	Absent or slight	Wide zone
γ phage susceptibility	Susceptible	Not susceptible
Penicillin (0.5 units/ml) sensitivity	Sensitive (most strains)	Resistant
Litmus milk coagulation and peptonization	Slow	Rapid
Gelatin hydrolysis	Slow	Rapid
Methylene blue reduction	Slow	Rapid
Salicin (acid)	Slow	Rapid
Lecithinase production	Absent or slight	Marked
Pathogenicity for guinea pigs, mice	Pathogenic	Nonpathogenic

Disinfection of burlap feed bags contaminated with anthrax spores can be accomplished by exposing them to dielectric heat at 112.7 C for 30 minutes (4). The spores are not necessarily killed by the heat required to fix smears on microscope slides.

The vegetative phase of *B. anthracis* is killed in 30 minutes at 60 C and is quickly destroyed by enzymic action and the effects of putrefactive bacteria in decaying carcasses.

Spores have been shown to remain viable for over 50 years (25).

Epidemiology. The major naturally occurring anthrax areas of the world are found in the tropics and subtropics, e.g., India, Pakistan, Africa, and South America. The factors that determine this distribution are related to the circumstances and conditions that allow sporulation of *B. anthracis* in carcass discharges and subsequent vegetative multiplication in the soil. The principal areas of enzootic anthrax are in regions with alkaline soils with a high nitrogen level caused by decaying vegetation, alternating periods of rain and drought, and temperatures in excess of 15.5 C. Such areas have been described by Van Ness (26) as "incubator areas." Many of these areas are found along the Sedalia Cattle Trail in Oklahoma and were first seeded with *B. anthracis* from dying cattle in the 1800s. The basis of the "incubator area" concept of Van Ness is that temporary accumulation of water causes death of vegetation and increased humus when the temperature exceeds 15.5 C, thereby providing conditions for spore germination and vegetative multiplication. As the area dries out, resporulation occurs. Cattle then gain access to these sites, crop down to ground level, and so ingest the contaminated soils.

In the United States, endemic anthrax areas are found generally wherever there are soils rich in calcium and nitrogen, and with a periodic abundance of water. In 1955, Stein and Van Ness (21) reported the results of a 10-year survey of anthrax in the United States. From 1945 to 1954 losses among cattle, horses, mules, swine, and sheep were reported to be 17,604. These cases appeared in 3,447 outbreaks in 39 states. States reporting no cases were Arizona, Connecticut, Delaware, Idaho, Maine, New Hampshire, Rhode Island, Vermont, and West Virginia. States reporting 100 or more outbreaks were California (271), Illinois (205), Indiana (222), Iowa (133), Kansas (368), Louisiana (413), Missouri (267), New Jersey (114), Ohio (317), South Dakota (150), Tennessee (142), and Texas (288).

Sources of infection for animals other than the soils of "incubator areas" also exist and in some regions are far more important. In England, for instance, imported bone meals and vegetable proteins such as groundnut are an important source of infection for livestock. Wool and hair wastes, cleanings used in fertilizers, and tannery effluents may also be sources of infection. In the United States, animal feed is an unusual source of infection. One such epidemic occurred in 1952 in swine fed rations containing raw bone meal of foreign origin (8).

Affected animals shed large numbers of the organism, and other animals in the group are thereby exposed. Also, bloodsucking flies are known to transmit the infection. Carrion eaters have also been suspected of transporting the anthrax organism (7).

Pathogenesis. Natural infection of animals can occur via the skin or respiratory tract but usually occurs by ingestion of spores, which germinate, producing vegetative bacilli either in the mucosa of the throat or in the intestinal tract. A capsule (polyglutamic acid) is formed on the surface of vegetative cells and protects them from phagocytosis and lytic antibody. The organisms multiply in an edematous focus and then spread via the lymphatic channels to lymph nodes, where multiplication continues. The organism eventually invades the bloodstream and is filtered out in the spleen until the clearance capacity of the latter is exceeded. Uncontrolled multiplication continues in the blood until the animal dies. At death, 80 percent of the organisms are in the blood and 20 percent in the spleen. Death of the animal results from the effects of the extracellular toxic complex released by the organism (27). The toxic complex consists of three components (Factor I, edema factor; Factor II, protective antigen; and Factor III, lethal factor). The chemical nature and biologic significance of each of these is shown in Tables 19.2 and 19.3. These factors operate in combination and have little or no toxic action as single entities. Their total effect is to damage and kill phagocytes, increase capillary cell permeability (Figure 19.5), and damage the clotting mechanism. Capillary thrombosis occurs and there is leakage of fluid through the damaged capillary epithelium. Blood pressure falls and the animal lapses into shock. The toxic complex also blocks the opsonizing activity of the C′3 factor of complement and so phagocytosis is reduced. The net effect of the toxic complex on the animal is to produce edema, shock, and death. These effects can be neutralized by specific antiserum. A lethal quantity of toxin is elaborated some time before the organism attains the populations found when the animal dies (20). Thus antibiotic therapy must be initiated early in the course of the infection before a lethal concentration of toxin has been elaborated.

The manifestations of the disease depend upon the manner of infection. When it occurs through the internal organs (no visible evidence of a localization), its principal character is the sudden onset and rapidly fatal course. The peracute form that sometimes occurs in herbivora may terminate fatally in 1 or 2 hours, the acute form in less than 24 hours. The animals have a high fever and usually show bleeding from the body openings. The organism can be found in the excretions or in the blood in large numbers at the time of death, and its identification in stained films constitutes the simplest and most certain way of making an accurate diagnosis.

Localized anthrax is seen when infection has occurred through a wound in the skin. This form occurs naturally more often in man than in any of the domestic animals.

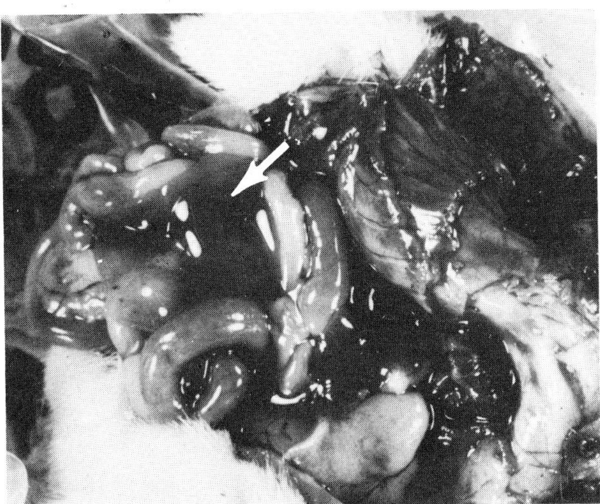

Figure 19.5. Anthrax in a mouse. Note the characteristic accumulation of gelatinous material (arrow) in the peritoneum. This is extravasated fluid which has clotted.

Cutaneous anthrax takes the form of a swelling of an edematous nature which is hot and painful at first but later becomes cold and painless. In man this type of anthrax lesion is called *malignant carbuncle,* because in its earlier stages it resembles a developing furuncle or carbuncle caused by *Staphylococcus aureus*. Recoveries in both animals and man are more frequent when the disease is localized than when it is septicemic. Localized infections often become generalized, however.

Anthrax in cattle, sheep, and horses usually appears in the spring and summer months, and most infections result from grazing on infected pastures. The cases usually are acute or peracute and most of them are fatal. Horses may exhibit signs of colic and edematous swellings of the throat, neck, and shoulders. In swine and dogs anthrax generally assumes a localized form with pharyngeal involvement and gastroenteritis. These animals are infected only by ingesting heavily contaminated feed, either the raw meat of other animals which have

Table 19.2. Components of toxic complex of *B. anthracis*

Component	Chemical nature
I (Edema factor)	Protein carbohydrate (chelator)
II (Protective antigen)	Protein, M.W. 100,000
III (Lethal factor)	Protein

Table 19.3. Toxic components of *B. anthracis* needed for lethality, edema, and immunogenicity

Components needed for		
Lethality	Edema	Immunogenicity
I + II	I + II	I + II
II + III	I + II + III	II + III
I + II + III		I + II + III

died of anthrax or, in the case of swine, infected bone or meat meal given as a feed supplement. In these cases the organism apparently enters the tissues from the upper part of the digestive tract, probably through the tonsils, and the disease is manifested by an inflammatory edema of the tissues of the head and neck. Often these regions become greatly distorted and swollen, and suffocation may occur through severe edema of the glottis. In these animals the infection occasionally localizes in the intestinal wall, the mesenteric lymph nodes, and the spleen.

A number of outbreaks of anthrax have occurred in mink, in which the mortality frequently is very heavy. The disease in this species is generally peracute and generalized. It occurs only when fresh meat from an infected carcass has been fed.

Generalized anthrax may easily be induced in susceptible animals by the inhalation of spores. In man, infections of this type occur among employees of plants in which hides, wool, and hair are processed, the spores being thrown into the air from the infected materials handled. The human form is a rapidly fatal malady known as *woolsorter's disease*.

Diagnosis. In some countries, anthrax is a notifiable disease; that is, state authorities must be informed of any reasonable suspicion of its presence. Diagnosis should be attempted by methods which result in the least amount of release of anthrax organisms to the environment. Exposure to atmospheric oxygen will cause formation of spores which will subsequently be extremely difficult to destroy. Thus samples of blood should be collected from a site such as an ear vein into a syringe and taken to the laboratory for preparation of smears for microscopic examination and for culture.

Direct microscopic examination of tissues and fluids is a simple and certain method when the animal has just died and putrefaction has not set in. The organism can be found in the bloodstream or in films from practically any organ when the disease has assumed the septicemic form. In the local forms the local edematous area must, of course, be examined. The organism is a relatively short, thick, Gram-positive rod, usually arranged in pairs or in chains of 3, 4, or 5 bacilli. Spores are not seen. With proper staining it may be observed that the chain of organisms is surrounded by a common capsule.

If putrefaction has begun, it is not always an easy matter to make an accurate diagnosis by the direct film method. Many of the anaerobic bacteria of decomposition resemble the anthrax bacillus quite closely. Usually these organisms are somewhat longer, and are arranged in chains longer than are formed by the anthrax bacillus in tissues. When many extraneous bacteria are present, it is better not to depend upon the direct microscopic method for making a diagnosis.

When the tissues and blood are fresh, there is no difficulty in cultivating the causative organism. If the tissues are decomposing, difficulties arise from two angles: first, the anthrax organism rapidly dies off and there may be few or no viable bacteria remaining and, second, other organisms that resemble the anthrax bacillus very closely may be present.

The characteristic "ground-glass" type of colony is searched for on plate cultures made from the organs or blood when the tissues are not absolutely fresh. Examinations of the peripheries of these colonies under moderate magnification should show no motile organisms when the plates are 18 to 24 hours old.

When animal feeds or other suspected substances are cultured, heating to 70 C for 10 minutes may be employed first in order to eliminate contaminating nonsporebearing organisms. Then the material may be plated in dilutions or injected into test animals. A method for isolating the organism from soil is also available (16). Burdon (5) has published methods for the positive identification of virulent strains without the use of motility or animal virulence tests, and Kinsely (15) has employed phenethyl alcohol and chloral hydrate in selective media to differentiate *B. anthracis* from *B. cereus*. The latter is similar to the anthrax organism, but is not pathogenic.

Specific strains of bacteriophage (gamma) are available which lyse *B. anthracis* and not other *Bacillus* sp. This test can therefore be used in identification of *B. anthracis* (3). A fluorescent-antibody test is also available for this purpose and can be applied directly to blood films (6) or to cultures grown on a sodium bicarbonate medium under CO_2 to allow capsules to develop.

Direct inoculation of guinea pigs with tissues, exudates, etc., is a reliable method of diagnosing the disease providing the material does not contain other organisms that destroy the experimental animal before the anthrax organism can be expected to make itself evident. Organisms of the malignant edema group frequently do this. If viable anthrax organisms are present and if the animal does not die from other causes earlier, it will usually die from anthrax 36 to 48 hours after subcutaneous injection. Occasionally death is as late as the 5th day after injection. The tissues of the guinea pig will be found swarming with the organism, and there will be a gelatinous infiltration under the skin at the point of inoculation.

The thermo-precipitation test (Ascoli test) is used very successfully in Europe for the detection of anthrax-infected hides. It may also be used with other tissues. The bit of hide or other tissue is extracted with water, either by boiling or with the aid of chloroform. In this way a clear fluid is obtained which should contain anthrax protein if the organism is present in the tissues. The fluid is layered in a very narrow tube with some of the precipitating serum (precipitin). The formation of a whitish ring at the line of juncture of the two fluids constitutes a positive reaction. The agar-gel precipitin technique has also proved useful for detection of anthrax antigen. In New York State, the Ascoli test is not approved as a diagnostic test for anthrax because of the possibility of cross-reactions with antigens from other *Bacillus* sp.

Comparative Efficiency of Anthrax Biologics. A study of the comparative value of the various products for producing immunity in previously unexposed animals was made by the U.S. Department of Agriculture (10). The findings indicated that spore vaccines, particularly when they are injected intradermally rather than subcutaneously, are the most effective agents for producing active immunity to anthrax. Well-marked immunity was also obtained with anthrax bacterin (washed culture) and anthrax spore vaccine in saponin. Aggressin was found to be inferior to the products named above, and bacterin made from whole culture (broth) had practically no value. Antianthrax serum immunized quickly and satisfactorily, but the duration of the immunity naturally was short. Because the South African avirulent anthrax vaccine is of more recent development, it was not included in this study, but results obtained from its use in South Africa and from trials in this country indicate it to be quite safe and very effective. Tests with the alum-precipitated protective antigens have indicated that they are effective in immunizing cattle, sheep, and man (12, 18, 19). For the best results two injections are recommended.

Chemotherapy in Anthrax. Antibiotics such as penicillin, lincomycin, dihydrostreptomycin and tetracycline are all effective in treating anthrax (1, 2, 13, 24). Results are most satisfactory in those species (swine, dogs, man) in which the disease runs a less acute course. The earlier treatment is begun, the better. In the herbivorous animals, the course often is too rapid; they are not recognized to be ill until near death, and treatment is ineffective. Recoveries have been effected in these species, however, as a result of antibiotic treatment even when bacteremia has developed. Exposed and incontact animals can be given long-acting depot preparations of penicillin to prevent development of the disease.

Immunity. The capsular polypeptide protects the organism from phagocytosis and naturally occurring lytic factors in serum, but antibodies to the capsule alone are not protective. The most effective vaccines require the presence of all three components of the toxic complex, although the somatic protein antigen (Factor II of the toxic complex) can be slightly immunogenic by itself. Antibodies to the toxic complex neutralize the effects of the toxin, including toxic damage to leukocytes (14). Thus the latter survive and phagocytose the invading bacteria. Bacteriolysis by natural and acquired lytic antibodies in conjunction with complement and lysozyme also occurs.

Vaccines. The first vaccine against anthrax was made in 1879 by Pasteur, who discovered that cultivation at 42 C reduced the organism's virulence. This vaccine was eventually superseded by spore vaccines which had better keeping qualities. Spore vaccines were prepared from avirulent noncapsulated variants. Later refinement involved the addition of saponin to delay dissemination of the spores into the tissues and allow an adjuvant effect (carbozoo vaccine).

The Sterne (22) vaccine is produced by growing virulent anthrax strains on 50 percent serum agar in an atmosphere of 10 to 30 percent CO_2. Rough, nonencapsulated dissociants which arise are then tested for loss of virulence by animal inoculation. Avirulent strains distinguished in this way are used for large-scale vaccine production. In 1946, Sterne (23) reported that more than 30 million doses of anthrax vaccine made as described above had been successfully used in South Africa. The same vaccine is employed for all domestic animals. In the United States, Personeus and colleagues (17) studied a vaccine made from a nonencapsulated variant of *B. anthracis* obtained from Onderstepoort, South Africa, and reported it to be excellent for protecting sheep and goats against anthrax.

One dose of vaccine will protect for one year and should be repeated annually.

Antianthrax serum. This may be produced from horses, cattle, or sheep. Horses and sheep produce the more potent sera. Horses are generally used because of the greater ease of immunization, i.e., they are less likely to die of anthrax during the immunization procedure and will yield much more serum.

Horses are first given the simultaneous treatment (serum and culture) for anthrax, followed by injections of small quantities of virulent cultures. Beginning with a 0.005-ml loopful, the dose is gradually increased at intervals of 3 or 4 weeks until finally whole-agar-slant cultures and even mass cultures of young virulent strains are used. All injections are given subcutaneously since there seems to be no advantage in intravenous injections.

In the past, antianthrax serum was used in treating herds where anthrax infection existed. All animals not showing fever or other signs of infection were given a 50-ml dose. Those showing a fever but no other symptoms were given from 100 to 300 ml. Animals severely infected with anthrax, if treated at all, were given larger doses. Frequently the administration of serum markedly alleviated symptoms in a few minutes. On the 2nd and 3rd day after treatment relapses sometimes occurred, in which case another dose of serum was administered. Animals that were severely infected and even showed bacilli in the blood sometimes recovered with serum treatment.

Within recent years some of the biological supply houses have announced the discontinuance of antianthrax serum because of its uncertain value.

Control Measures. In the infected areas of the United States vaccines are used in the control of anthrax (Figure 19.6). In certain regions the spore vaccine is injected intradermally, and in other sections subcutaneous inoculation of this vaccine combined with an adjuvant is preferred. Combinations of these methods sometimes are used, and, in endemic areas, original vaccination may be followed by a second, or even a third, dose of special, highly virulent vaccine. Favorable results have also been reported from areas where the South African variant vaccine and other recently developed immunizing materials have been used.

In the infected areas vaccination usually is carried out in the spring on horses, mules, cattle, sheep, and sometimes swine. A certain percentage of the animals will show severe or even fatal reactions to the vaccine. This is especially true among sheep. Such animals may be treated with penicillin, tetracycline, antiserum, or combinations of these substances.

Decontamination of imported protein supplements of animal origin is also important in control of anthrax in countries that must import livestock feeds.

The carcasses of animals that die of anthrax should be completely burned or buried very deeply in quick lime. Carcasses that are opened and the parts scattered provide an opportunity for sporulation of the anthrax bacillus,

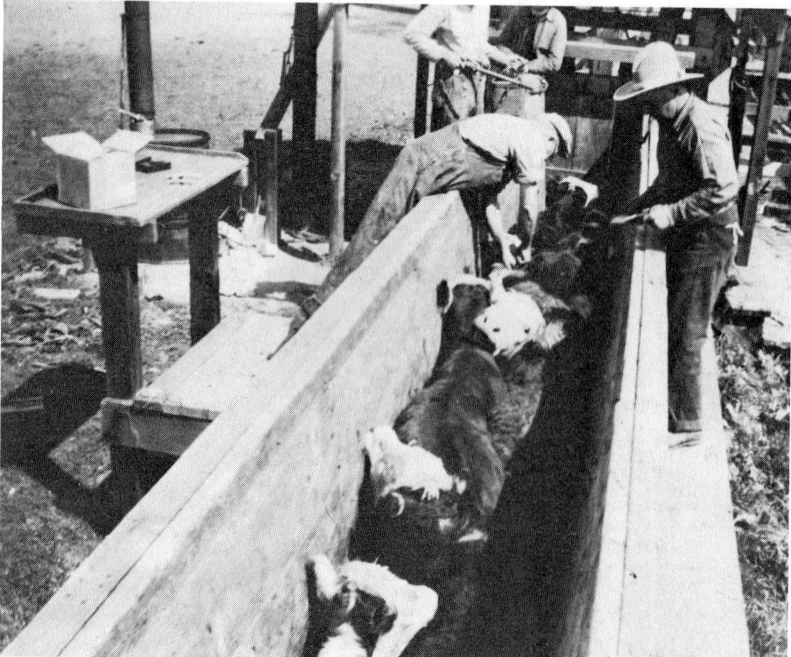

Figure 19.6. Vaccinating range cattle against anthrax. The use of such chutes for restraining semiwild range cattle is common practice. (Courtesy Jen-Sal Laboratories, Inc.)

and the spores remain viable in a contaminated area for years.

Treatment of Anthrax in Man. Anthrax in man may assume any of four forms: *(a)* the skin or cutaneous type (malignant carbuncle), *(b)* the pulmonary form (woolsorter's disease), *(c)* the intestinal form, or *(d)* the acute meningitis syndrome (11). The pulmonary and intestinal forms of the disease are usually quickly fatal. The fourth type was in the same category until penicillin was introduced.

Ordinarily serum has been used to treat human anthrax. It has been useful in curing the cutaneous form, but usually has not been administered quickly enough in the pulmonary or intestinal form to prevent fatalities. Furthermore, large doses of antianthrax serum given intravenously often cause serum sickness. A report by Ellingson, Kadull, Bookwalter, and Howe (9) indicates that penicillin has marked therapeutic value in curing anthrax infection. More recent reports substantiate their findings and also show that combinations of penicillin and sulfathiazole produce excellent results.

REFERENCES

1. Bailey. Jour. Am. Vet. Med. Assoc., 1953, *122,* 305.
2. Bailey. Jour. Am. Vet. Med. Assoc., 1954, *124,* 296.
3. Brown and Cherry. Jour. Inf. Dis., 1955, *96,* 34.
4. Bryan. Am. Jour. Vet. Res., 1953, *14,* 328.
5. Burdon. Jour. Bact., 1956, *25,* 71.
6. Cherry and Freeman. Zentrbl. f.Bakt., 1959, *175,* 582.
7. Cousineau and McClenaghen. Can. Vet. Jour., 1965, *6,* 22.
8. Editorial. North Am. Vet., 1952, *33,* 450.
9. Ellingson, Kadull, Bookwalter, and Howe. North Am. Vet., 1946, *131,* 1105.
10. Gouchenour, Schoening, Stein, and Mohler. U.S. Dept. Agr. Tech. Bull. 468, 1935.
11. Haight. Am. Jour. Med. Sci., 1952, *224,* 57.
12. Jackson, Wright, and Armstrong. Am. Jour. Vet. Res., 1957, *18,* 771.
13. Johnson and Percival. Jour. Am. Vet. Med. Assoc., 1955, *127,* 142.
14. Keppie, Harris-Smith, and Smith. Brit. Jour. Exp. Path., 1963, *44,* 446.
15. Kinsely. Jour. Bact., 1965, *90,* 1778.
16. McGoughey and St. George. Vet. Rec., 1955, *67,* 132.
17. Personeus, Cooper, and Percival. Am. Jour. Vet. Res., 1956, *27,* 153.
18. Puziss and Wright. Jour. Bact., 1963, *85,* 230.
19. Schlingman, Devlin, Wright, Maine, and Manning. Am. Jour. Vet. Res., 1956, *17,* 256.
20. Smith, Keppie, and Stanley. Brit. Jour. Exp. Path., 1955, *36,* 460.
21. Stein and Van Ness. Vet. Med., 1955, *50,* 579.
22. Sterne. Onderstepoort Jour. Vet. Sci. and An. Ind., 1937, *9,* 49.
23. Sterne. Onderstepoort Jour. Vet. Sci. and An. Ind., 1946, *21,* 41.
24. Sugg. Jour. Am. Vet. Med. Assoc., 1948, *113,* 467.
25. Umeno and Nobata. Jour. Jap. Soc. Vet. Sci., 1938, *17,* 87.
26. Van Ness. Jour. Am. Vet. Med. Assoc., 1956, *128,* 7.
27. Wright. *In* Microbiology 1975, ed. David Schlessinger. Am. Soc. Microbiol., Washington, D.C., 1975.

20 The Genus *Clostridium*

The anaerobic sporebearing organisms that are classed together under the generic name *Clostridium* are quite similar in morphology and staining qualities. All are rather large, rod-shaped, and Gram-positive when young. The rods usually are straight. Some species commonly appear in tissue fluids singly or in pairs, whereas others usually are found in long chains. The spores in most species are oval, are located somewhat centrally in the rod, and often are greater in diameter than the rod itself. Because of their great similarity in form, it is usually not possible to be certain of the identity of these organisms without studying their cultural and serological characteristics. In many instances the symptoms and lesions of the diseases produced by them are sufficiently characteristic to enable a reliable diagnosis to be made.

The application of the usual serologic tests to the intact clostridial cells has not been especially rewarding, because antigens common to the bacilli and their spores produce many cross-reactions. Ellner and Green (6), however, used soluble antigens from 10 species of pathogenic clostridia to divide these organisms into groups based upon the presence or absence of precipitin lines in agar-gel tests.

These organisms may be divided into two groups on the basis of their disease-producing mechanisms. The first consists of those species that have little or no power to invade and multiply in living tissues. Such organisms owe their pathogenicity to their power of forming powerful toxins, which are produced in localized areas or outside the body. The damage in these instances is almost wholly caused by the absorption of the toxin. The organisms of this group which will be described are *C. tetani* and *C. botulinum*. The second and larger group consists of species that have the power to invade and multiply in tissues. These organisms in most cases also produce toxins, but the toxins are much less potent than those of the first group and the damages to the tissues are not caused wholly by them. These organisms are sometimes referred to as the *gas gangrene* group because many of them are concerned in wound infections of the gas gangrene type in man. Wounds of animals sometimes become infected with pathogenic anaerobes, in which case the condition is similar to that of man. A number of these organisms, however, find their way into animal tissues through the digestive tract, and thus we have rapidly developing, highly fatal infections without the existence of wounds of the skin.

The number of species which has been found in these invasive infections of animals is large. The ones most frequently encountered are the only ones that will be considered here. These are:

Clostridium perfringens	The cause of lamb dysentery, "struck," and "pulpy kidney disease" of sheep, and occasionally of malignant edema infections of other species.
Clostridium hemolyticum	The cause of bacterial icterohemoglobinuria or "red water" of cattle.
Clostridium novyi	The cause of "black disease" of sheep and occasionally of

	malignant edema infections of other species.
Clostridium chauvoei	The cause of blackleg in cattle and sheep.
Clostridium septicum	The cause of braxy in sheep and of malignant edema infections in other species.
Clostridium colinum	The cause of ulcerating enteritis or "quail disease" of young game birds, turkeys, and chickens.

The nonpathogenic *Clostridium sporogenes* is also found in a considerable proportion of gas gangrene cases, but its contribution to the pathology of the disease is uncertain. Although *Clostridium bifermentans (sordelli)* produces a very potent toxin, it is encountered only sporadically in gangrenous infections of animals. Two outbreaks of *C. sordelli* infection in Rambouillet rams that occurred in Montana in 1962 were described by Smith *et al.* (28).

The sporebearing anaerobic bacteria cause animal diseases that are infectious without being contagious, that is to say, the diseases seldom if ever are transmitted from one animal to another. Most of these organisms have their habitat in the soil and intestine, and it is from soil, or from vegetation contaminated with intestinal contents, that the infections are derived. Epizootics seldom occur, although it is possible for them to happen when conditions become favorable for a large number of animals to become infected from the same source simultaneously.

THE TOXIN-FORMING, NONINVASIVE GROUP

Clostridium tetani

SYNONYM: *Bacillus tetani*

The causative agent of tetanus is the best known of all anaerobic sporebearing bacilli, principally because the symptoms of the disease are so well known and characteristic that it has not been confused with any other of the anaerobic infections. The organism was isolated in impure culture by Nicolaier (22) in 1884 from white mice that had been inoculated with garden soil. In 1889, Kitasato (14) obtained pure cultures by heating mixed cultures from infected wounds, thus destroying the ordinary bacteria of suppuration but leaving the heat-resistant tetanus spores. In the following year (1890) Von Behring and Kitasato (1) published their classical work announcing the discovery of bacterial toxins, of which the first was that of *C. tetani*.

Morphology and Staining Reactions. *C. tetani* is a straight, slender rod 0.4 to 0.6 μm in width and 2 to 5 μm in length. In both tissues and cultures it most often occurs singly, but sometimes chains of organisms forming long filaments are seen. In old cultures the rods and threads disappear, leaving the spherical spores. These spores are formed after 24 to 48 hours' incubation and appear in the ends of the rods, swelling them so they have the appearance of badminton rackets or drumsticks (Figure 20.1). In some media spores are formed in abundance; in others even after prolonged incubation they are few in number. Cultures are Gram-positive when young, but after a few days most of the cells become Gram-negative. Young cultures are actively motile by means of peritrichic flagella.

Cultural Features. The tetanus organism grows on all the ordinary media of the laboratory provided only that fairly good anaerobic conditions are maintained. It will grow in aerobic cultures in association with other aerobic organisms. Deep agar colonies are fluffy, cottony spheres. When blood is present, hemolysis occurs. Broth becomes slightly clouded but clears by sedimentation. Gelatin stabs first develop a spike of growth along the stab; next, cottony filaments extend from the stab at a right angle into the medium, giving a brushlike effect; then liquefaction and blackening of the medium occur,

Figure 20.1. *Clostridium tetani*, a stained preparation of a 48-hour-old culture in a meat-piece medium. The terminal spherical spores are characteristic. × 1,040.

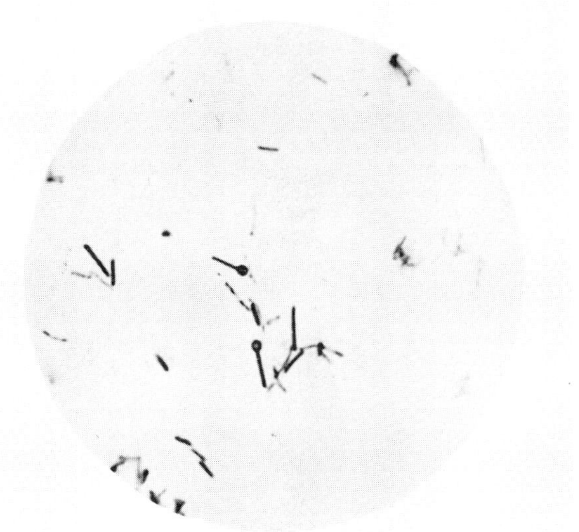

and gas bubbles are formed. Litmus milk is not usually changed. A soft clot may be formed. Coagulated blood serum is softened and in old cultures may be blackened but it is not liquefied. Cooked-meat medium and brain medium are not digested but become turbid and give off a very foul odor. Carbohydrates are not fermented, but glucose greatly favors growth in the simpler types of media. Growth occurs best at 37 C, but slow growth occurs at 20 C. Acetic, butyric, and proprionic acids are the principal fermentation products.

The organism may sometimes be isolated in pure culture from contaminated specimens by a light inoculation of a fresh blood agar plate. After incubation for 24 hours the plate should be checked for swarming, which will be evident as a thin veil of growth on the agar surface. Cells (Gram-positive rods) from the edge of the swarming area should be transferred to a tube of broth and to another blood plate containing 5 percent agar. After incubation, an isolated colony can be picked for further characterization.

Resistance. *C. tetani* spores are highly resistant and when protected from light and heat remain viable for years. Theobald Smith found a number of strains that resisted steaming at 100 C for 40 to 60 minutes. Five percent phenol is said to destroy tetanus spores in 10 to 12 hours; the addition of 0.5 percent hydrochloric acid may reduce the time to 2 hours. Boiling kills the spores of most strains in 15 minutes. Autoclaving at 120 C for 20 minutes is also sporicidal.

Natural Habitat. The organism of tetanus was found originally by Nicolaier (22) in garden soils, 12 out of 18 samples being positive. Fildes (9) in England, examined 70 soil samples, including both cultivated and uncultivated, and found 33 positive. Sanada and Nishida (26) have indicated that the higher the temperature applied to soil specimens the weaker the toxigenicity of *C. tetani* cultures isolated from them.

A number of workers have found the organism to be commonly present in horse manure. Some have found it in the feces of cows, sheep, dogs, chickens, rats, and guinea pigs, whereas others have failed to find it in some of these species, a fact which suggests that these animals may only be transitory hosts for the organism. Noble (23), for example, found it in 11 out of 61 samples of horses' feces, but failed to find it in 21 samples from cows. Human feces also are sometimes infected with tetanus bacilli. The experiences of various workers on this subject have differed widely, some being unable to find the organism in large series of cases, others finding it in a relatively large proportion. Ten Broeck and Bauer (30) demonstrated tetanus bacilli in the stools of 27 of 78 individuals living in Peking, China, and concluded that the organism must be living in the intestinal canal because certain individuals who had lived on an almost sterile diet for more than a month continued to yield several million tetanus spores per stool.

Antigens and Serologic Grouping. The serologic types of *C. tetani* have been categorized by Gunnison (10) and Mandia (17). A heat-stable glycopeptide antigen, designated IV,V, is shared by all strains, but a variety of different heat-labile flagellar or somatic antigens occurs. Smith (27) lists nine serotypes of *C. tetani*.

Epidemiology and Pathogenesis. Infections in all animals and man occur as a result of wound or umbilical contamination. Deep, penetrating wounds, the depths of which become necrotic, with reduced oxygen and lowered Eh, are the usual sites of multiplication of the organism, with subsequent toxin production. Washed spores injected into healthy tissue do not set up tetanus in the inoculated host.

C. tetani produces three toxins, *(a)* tetanospasmin, *(b)* hemolysin, and *(c)* a peripherally active nonspasmogenic toxin. The tetanospasmin is responsible for the characteristic clinical features of tetanus, and antibodies to the toxin are protective. The hemolysin causes local tissue necrosis and creates more favorable conditions for multiplication of *C. tetani*. It is hemolytic for erythrocytes and lethal in laboratory animals following intravenous administration.

Tetanospasmin is a protein with a molecular weight of 66,000 (monomeric form) or 132,000 (dimeric form) (31). It is destroyed by gastric juices, is heat-resistant, and is very poorly absorbed across mucous membranes. One mouse LD_{50} is equivalent to 2×10^{-8}mg. It is a protoplasmic toxin, its release requiring bacterial lysis. The receptor sites for the toxin in the body are quite well understood. The elegant studies of van Heyningen and Mellanby (31) have shown that it binds specifically to gangliosides in nerve tissue. Gangliosides are chloroform- and water-soluble mucolipids, containing sialic acid, stearic acid, sphingosine, galactose, acetylgalactosamine, and glucose. In nerve tissue the ganglioside is bound to the water-insoluble cerebrosides. Two molecules of ganglioside will bind to one molecule of toxin. The reaction is extremely difficult to reverse, and neutralizing antibody is ineffective once the toxin is bound.

The specific action of tetanospasmin appears to be to prevent the release of glycine—the transmitter substance for the inhibitory nerve network in the spinal cord (24).

This network prevents contraction of one muscle when its opposite-acting counterpart contracts. Thus, the effect of the toxin is to cause continuous stimulation and tetanic spasm of groups of muscles. Other effects include a paralytic action on the peripheral nerve system as well as an inactivating effect on the inhibitory system in the central nervous system. There is also an inhibitory effect on protein synthesis in the brain.

The action of the nonspasmogenic toxin is poorly defined. There is some evidence that it may play a role in the peripheral paralytic action of tetanus toxin.

There has been much debate about the manner by which tetanus toxin reaches the central nervous system, where its principal effects are produced. If a fatal dose of tetanus toxin is injected into the foot of a susceptible animal, the onset of the disease may be greatly delayed by severing the principal motor nerve trunks of that leg (18) or by infiltrating the nerve trunk with antitoxin (21). Fatal tetanus may be produced by injecting into one of the peripheral nerve trunks a dose of toxin which is not great enough to cause death when injected intravenously. These and many other similar experiments seem to indicate that the tetanus toxin is absorbed by the peripheral nerves and that most of it passes through the nerves centripetally until it reaches the motor cells of the anterior horn of the cord, at which time general symptoms of the disease make their appearance. Recent studies of Haberman and Wellhover (11) indicate that neuromuscular activity favors migration of the toxin, which can migrate along both motor axons and sensory nerves. There is preferential uptake of toxin via the ventral roots in the spinal cord. The toxin also accumulates selectively in the lumbar and cervical regions of the cord and in gray matter of the postpontine area of the brain stem. When the toxin travels up a regional motor nerve in a limb, tetanus develops first in the muscles of that limb, and then, as the toxin spreads upward, in the opposite limb, and subsequently in the muscles of the trunk. This is known as ascending tetanus.

Toxin can also circulate in the blood and lymph and produce tetanus first in the muscles supplied by the most susceptible motor nerve centers that serve the head and neck. The voluntary muscles of the forelimbs, upper trunk, and, later, the hind limbs are then involved. This form of tetanus is described as descending and is the form usually seen in man and horses. In descending tetanus the first symptoms involve the nictitating membrane which cannot be retracted and the facial and jaw muscles leading to *lockjaw* and *risus sardonicus* (Figure 20.2). The shorter the incubation period in tetanus, the worse the prognosis.

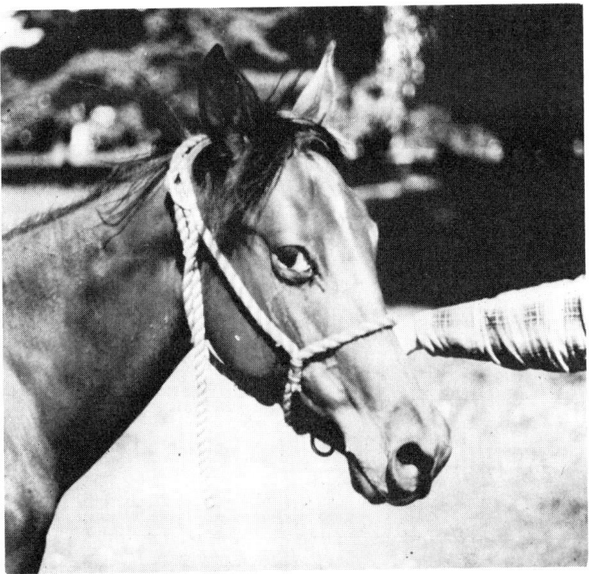

Figure 20.2. Tetanus in a horse. The membrana nictitans is visible and the nostrils are dilated because of tetanus of the facial muscles. (Courtesy William Rebhun.)

The symptoms of tetanus are similar in all animals. They consist of chronic or tetanic spasms of the muscles (Figure 20.3). Sometimes these begin in one part of the body, where the infected wound is located, but generally the disease extends to all parts.

Infections in horses occur most often as a result of nail wounds in the foot. In sheep the infection is seen most often after lambs are castrated or docked. In cattle it may be a puerperal infection following calving, or it may follow dehorning, castration, and nose ringing of bulls. Herd and Riches (12) and Wallis (32) have reported outbreaks of idiopathic tetanus in groups of heifers and have suggested that this condition was caused by an autointoxication resulting from massive multiplication of *C. tetani* in the forestomachs under certain unspecified conditions. In swine it is most frequently seen as a result of castration wound infection. The disease appears in dogs and cats, usually following wound infection (19). In all animals it may occur as a result of infection of otherwise trivial wounds, and even when no wounds can be found. Umbilical infections of newborn animals often occur.

Diagnosis. The symptoms of tetanus are so characteristic that laboratory examination of specimens is rarely performed. Microscopic examination of smears from infected wounds may reveal the characteristic "drumstick" appearance of the organism and its spore. *C. tetani*

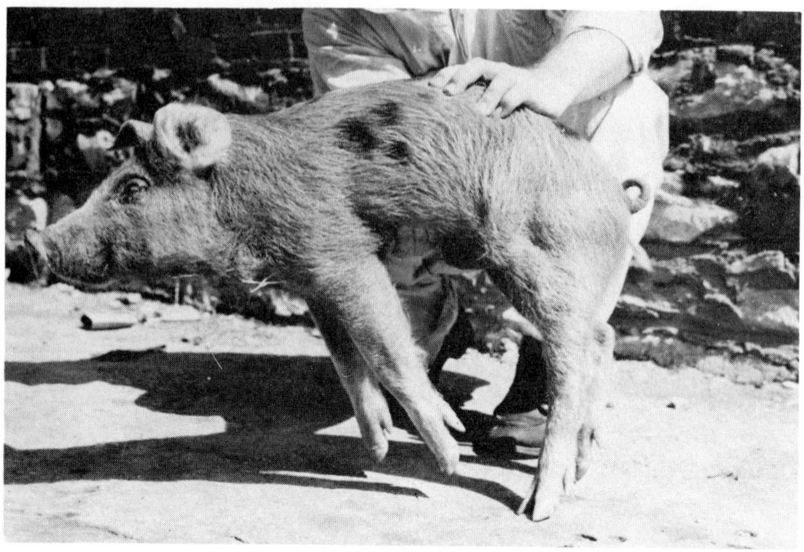

Figure 20.3. Tetanus in a pig. Tetanic spasms of the muscles manifested by rigidity of the parts is characteristic of tetanus in all animals. (Courtesy Jen-Sal Laboratories, Inc.)

may be isolated as described under "Cultural Features," above. Toxin present in the wound may be demonstrated by surgically excising the necrotic tissue and homogenizing it in some saline. The homogenate is centrifuged and 0.2 ml is injected into the hind-leg muscle of each of 4 mice. Two mice are also given antitoxin a few hours earlier. The mice are then observed for up to 3 days for development of tetanus in the unprotected group. If a large amount of toxin is present, the mice may be found dead after a few hours.

Immunity. Birds and other animals that are naturally resistant to tetanus have no antibodies in their tissues. The brain tissue of such animals, however, seems to have no affinity for the toxin, as was first demonstrated by Metchnikoff (20). The blood of most cattle contains neutralizing antibodies, and small amounts are found in the blood of sheep and goats. It has been suggested that perhaps this comes about from the activity of tetanus bacilli in the forestomachs of these ruminants. The blood of horses, dogs, pigs, and men does not normally contain antitoxin. The brain tissue of all susceptible animals possesses the power of uniting with tetanus toxin *in vitro*.

Tetanus antitoxin prepared from the sera of hyperimmunized horses may be used to protect passively animals that have received accidental or surgical wounds. Usually 1,500 units will protect an animal for 2 to 3 weeks.

When symptoms of tetanus have appeared, the efficacy of the antitoxin is much less than when it is used prophylactically. In animals already suffering from the disease, the antitoxin is administered as soon as possible and is given preferably in a single dose of from 100,000 to 200,000 units. In addition, adequate treatment includes large doses of penicillin and sedation. Animals frequently die in spite of such treatment. On the other hand, when the infected wound is thoroughly cleaned surgically and treated with antiseptics, and the animals are kept quiet in a darkened room, one-third or more of them will recover without treatment with antitoxin. The therapeutic effectiveness of tetanus antitoxin is markedly reduced by simultaneous administration of cortisone (4).

Vaccines against tetanus are made by incubating highly potent toxin with 0.4 percent formalin until the toxicity has been completely destroyed. The toxoid is then precipitated from solution with aluminum potassium sulfate (alum). The washed precipitate is then suspended in saline.

A single injection of this material will produce an appreciable degree of immunity, but experience has shown that it is best to give a second and a third dose at about 3-week intervals. Such animals will have sufficient antitoxin in their blood to protect them from natural infection for at least a year. Fessler (8) recommends that horses should be given two toxoid injections 6 to 8 weeks apart, followed by a booster dose 6 to 12 months later and then by annual booster injections. A similar regimen will be effective for other domestic animals. If dangerous wounds are contracted later, it is best to administer another dose at once. This will cause an immediate increase in antibodies. If the animal has not already had toxoid, the latter is useless in an emergency because the initial production of antitoxin is too slow. It has been established that a simultaneous injection of tetanus antitoxin and toxoid will not significantly reduce the efficacy of the former, but will markedly decrease the ability of the latter to produce active immunity.

Treatment. Many drugs have been used in the symptomatic treatment of tetanus. Karitzky (13) claimed that acidosis is the main cause of death in tetanus infection and that the treatment of acidosis markedly reduces the mortality rate in man. Couvy (5) reported success in treating tetanus of man by administering antiserum and urotropine. Sedatives, such as Mephenesin (2) and *d*-tubocurarine choloride (3), are recommended, and the tranquilizing drug chlorpromazine hydrochloride (16, 25) is also prescribed. In testing antibiotics on mice infected with tetanus, Taylor and Novak (29) concluded that Aureomycin, penicillin, and Terramycin reduced mortalities. Chloromycetin was of some value, antitoxin of little value, and polymyxin B ineffective. The tranquilizers diazepam (7-chloro-1,3-dihydro-1-methyl-5-phenyl-2H-1,4-benzodiazephin-2-one) and chlor diazepoxide (7-chloro-2-methyl-amino-5-phenyl-3H-1, 4-benzodiazepine 4-oxide) are highly recommended in treating tetanus (7, 15), and an evaluation of serologic and antimicrobial therapy in the the treatment of tetanus in the United States has been published by Young *et al.* (33).

REFERENCES

1. Von Behring and Kitasato. Deut. med. Wchnschr., 1890, *16,* 1113.
2. Boles and Smith. Jour. Am. Med. Assoc., 1951, *146,* 1296.
3. Booth and Pierson. Jour. Am. Vet. Med. Assoc., 1956, *128,* 257.
4. Chang and Weinstein. Proc. Soc. Exp. Biol. and Med., 1957, *94,* 431.
5. Couvy. Vet. Bull., 1948, *18,* 469.
6. Ellner and Green. Jour. Bact., 1963, *86,* 1098.
7. Femi-Pearse and Fleming. Jour. Trop. Med. and Hyg. (London), 1965, *68,* 305.
8. Fessler. Jour. Am. Vet. Med. Assoc., 1966, *148,* 399.
9. Fildes. Brit. Jour. Exp. Path., 1925, *6,* 62.
10. Gunnison. Brit. Jour. Exp. Path., 1937, *32,* 63.
11. Haberman and Wellover. *In* Radioactive tracers in microbial immunology. International Atomic Energy Agency, Vienna, 1972, pp. 67-76.
12. Herd and Riches. Austral. Vet. Jour., 1964, *40,* 356.
13. Karitzky. Arch. Klin. Chir., 1947, *260,* 1.
14. Kitasato. Zeitschr. f. Hyg., 1889, *7,* 225.
15. Lowenthal and Lavalette. Jour. Trop. Med. and Hyg. (London), 1966, *69,* 157.
16. Lundvall. Jour. Am. Vet. Med. Assoc., 1958, *132,* 254.
17. Mandia. Jour. Inf. Dis., 1955, *97,* 66.
18. Marie. Ann. Inst. Pasteur (Paris), 1897, *11,* 591.
19. Mason. Jour. S. Afr. Vet. Med. Assoc., 1964, *35,* 209.
20. Metchnikoff. Ann. Inst. Pasteur (Paris), 1898, *12,* 81.
21. Meyer and Ransom. Arch. Path. and Pharm., 1903, *49,* 369.
22. Nicolaier. Deut. med. Wchnschr., 1884, *10,* 842.
23. Noble. Jour. Inf. Dis., 1915, *16,* 132.
24. Osborne and Bradford. Nature, 1973, *244,* 157.
25. Owen, Leam, and Nestel. Vet. Rec., 1959, *71,* 61.

26. Sanada and Nishida. Jour. Bact., 1965, *89,* 626.
27. Smith, Louis. The pathogenic anaerobic bacteria, 2nd ed. Thomas, Springfield, Ill., 1975.
28. Smith, Safford, and Hawkins. Cornell Vet., 1962, *52,* 62.
29. Taylor and Novak. Antibiotics and Chemother., 1952, *2,* 517.
30. Ten Broeck and Bauer. Jour. Exp. Med., 1922, *36,* 261.
31. Van Heyningen and Mellanby. Microbial toxins, vol. 2A, ed. Kadis, Monte, and Ajl. Academic Press, New York, 1971.
32. Wallis. Vet. Rec., 1963, *74,* 188.
33. Young, LaForce, and Bennett. Jour. Inf. Dis., 1969, *120,* 153.

Clostridium botulinum

SYNONYM: *Bacillus botulinus*

As a disease of man botulism has been known for many years. The disease was given its name by Müller (19) in 1870. The causative agent was found in 1897 by Van Ermengem (9), who studied an outbreak occurring in Ellezelles, Belgium, in a group of persons who ate an imperfectly preserved smoked ham at a dinner. The organism was found in the ham and the tissues of one of the persons who died of the disease. The toxicogenic properties of the organism were recognized by Van Ermengem, also the fact that the toxin wrought its damage by attacking portions of the nervous system.

In Europe numerous outbreaks of the disease have occurred, the greater number being traced to hams, sausages, and other meat products. Beginning about 1919, a series of outbreaks have been recognized in the United States, but these have been traced, with but few exceptions, to canned vegetables. It has been shown by Meyer and Dubovsky (18) that the organism is commonly present in the soil in all parts of the world. Botulism is caused, therefore, by food materials that have been contaminated with soil, imperfectly sterilized, and then allowed to stand, with the air excluded, sufficiently long to allow the organism to generate its powerful toxin. The disease is an intoxication, almost never a bacterial infection, although there are a few reports of wound infection in man (6, 11). In one of these cases which terminated fatally the clinical course was strikingly similar to botulism, and *C. botulinum* Type A was isolated. In general, the organism does not appear to generate toxin in the alimentary tract but has been reported to do so in the crops of birds (7). More recently, botulism in infants resulting in sudden death has been shown to be caused by toxin production in the intestine (16).

Organisms causing botulism can be divided into proteolytic and nonproteolytic groups. The former is often designated *C. parabotulinum* and the latter *C. botulinum*. However, the serological specificity of the toxin is not always related to the proteolytic activity of the organism producing it. Strains that produce Type B toxin occur in both the ovolytic and nonovolytic groups. Because the type of toxin is of greater practical importance than proteolytic power, all toxicogenic strains are designated as *C. botulinum*.

Morphology and Staining Reactions. The types within the species cannot be distinguished on a morphological basis. All are relatively large rods which usually occur singly but may form short chains. They measure 0.5 to 0.8 μm in width and 3 to 6 μm in length. Motility occurs in young cultures, the cells being provided with peritrichic flagella. Spores form readily and abundantly. They are oval, are located centrally and excentrically, and cause slight bulging of the cells (Figure 20.4). The organism is Gram-positive, but in old cultures the cells usually decolorize.

Cultural Features. Colonies in deep agar are fluffy. Surface colonies are large and semitransparent with irregular edges. Better growths occur in media made from liver than in those made from muscle tissue. Gelatin is rapidly liquefied. Acid and gas are produced from glucose, levulose, and maltose. The fermentation of other sugars is variable from strain to strain and from type to type.

Figure 20.4. *Clostridium botulinum,* a culture in meat-piece medium incubated 48 hours at 37 C. × 1,040

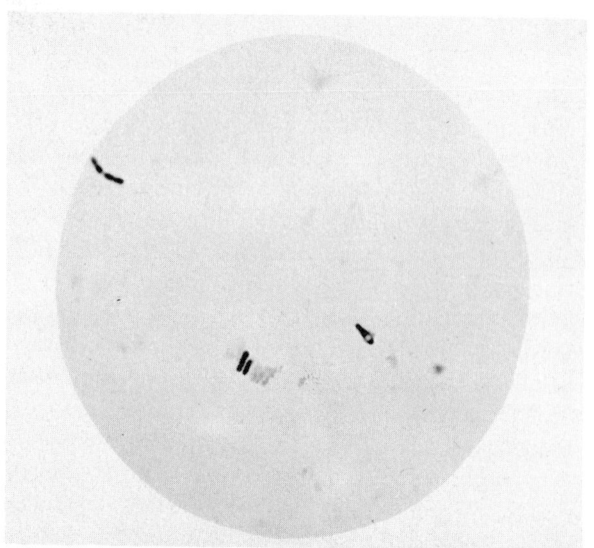

The nonproteolytic types (*C. botulinum*) acidify but do not coagulate milk. They do not liquefy coagulated blood serum or coagulated egg albumen, nor do they digest brain or meat medium. A narrow zone of hemolysis may be produced on horse-blood agar.

The proteolytic types (*C. parabotulinum*) slowly curdle milk and partially digest and darken the curd. When inoculated on coagulated blood serum or egg albumen, they digest and blacken these media and produce a putrefactive odor. They also digest and blacken brain or meat medium and emit putrefactive odors.

All organisms included in these species are strict anaerobes but are not otherwise fastidious in their growth requirements. They grow best at temperatures around 30 C but are capable of growing in a wide range of temperatures up to that of the body. The strains that are not proteolytic nevertheless give off a strong odor, which is suggestive of putrefaction but is not so powerful as that produced by the protein-liquefying types.

Resistance of the Organism. The spores are highly resistant and may withstand boiling for 30 minutes to several hours. Autoclaving at 120 C for 20 minutes is usually sufficient to kill most strains.

Serologic and Toxigenic Types. It appears that the species is rather heterogeneous serologically. According to Mandia (14) there are at least six serotypes of *C. botulinum* in his Group II of proteolytic clostridia, and antigens are shared by some strains with *C. sporogenes* (15). The antigenic configuration of strains bears no relationship to the toxin type produced, and because the latter is much more useful epidemiologically, strains of *C. botulinum* are classified according to the type of toxin produced. There are seven groups described on the basis of toxin type produced (Table 20.1).

Types A, B, E, and F are probably saprophytes of soil and aquatic sediments. Types C and D appear to be obligate parasites of the intestinal tracts of mammals and birds and occur in soil or aquatic sediments only as transients. In general, *C. botulinum* is most common in the northern hemisphere between the latitudes of 35 and 55 N.

Epidemiology and Pathogenesis. Botulism almost always arises from ingestion of food material contaminated with preformed toxin. The toxin may be elaborated in a decaying carcass which is ingested or indirectly causes contamination of another feedstuff. Fly larvae which develop on carcasses in which toxin has been produced may carry sufficient toxin to cause botulism in birds that feed on them. Another source is decaying vegetation at the edges of ponds and lakes which may provide an environment for toxin synthesis. Aquatic birds such as

Table 20.1. Distribution, hosts, and diseases associated with *C. botulinum* strains

Strain	Distribution*	Hosts affected	Disease
A	N. America (west)	Man Cattle, horses Chickens Mink	Botulism Forage poisoning Limberneck Botulism
B	N. America (midwest & east) Europe	Man Cattle, horses Chickens Mink	Botulism Forage poisoning Limberneck Botulism
C	N. America Australia Canada Europe	Ducks and other wild Avidae Man Mink	Limberneck, western duck disease Botulism
D	S. Africa	Cattle	Lamziekte
E	Russia N. America (Great Lakes)	Man	Botulism
F	Denmark N. America	Man	Botulism
G	N. America	Unknown	Unknown

*Places where disease due to this strain has been reported.

ducks that feed in these areas may develop botulism. Offals and fish meats are other well-known sources of botulinum toxin for mink and foxes, respectively.

Aphosphorosis may cause cattle and sheep to develop a depraved appetite for decaying carcasses, and this in turn may lead to the occurrence of botulism (20). Because of the lameness associated with the phosphorus deficiency, the disease in South Africa has been called *lamziekte* or the lame sickness. It occurs only in certain restricted areas on the range. A disease evidently the same as lamziekte occurs in certain parts of the Texas plains, where phosphorus deficiency exists and bone chewing is common. The symptoms are the same as those of the South African disease. *C. botulinum* Type D has been found in mud samples taken from lakes in the Zululand game parks of Africa (17). Carcasses buried in the litter of broiler houses have resulted in outbreaks of botulism Type C in broiler chickens (10). Levels of toxin in such carcasses can reach 10^6 mouse LD_{50} per g. In Holland, botulism in cattle has been caused by brewers' grains contaminated by *C. botulinum* Type B (6).

The spores of *C. botulinum* are distributed far more widely than the occurrence of botulism would suggest. This is so because a combination of circumstances is necessary for the occurrence of the disease. These are (*a*) contamination of a suitable substrate by the organism, (*b*) multiplication of the organism and production of its toxin, (*c*) survival of the toxin in the face of autolytic processes which might degrade it, and (*d*) ingestion of the toxin by susceptible animals.

The toxin is protoplasmic and is a protein of about 150,000 M.W. It usually exists as a complex consisting of toxin molecules and a hemagglutinin (500,000 M.W.) moiety. The toxins of nonproteolytic strains, including types C, D, E, and G, and a few strains of types B and F require digestion by proteolytic enzymes such as trypsin for full expression of toxic activity. The activated toxin may have a toxicity as high as 2.6 by 10^8 mouse LD_{50} per mg of N. Toxin production in *C. botulinum* Types C and D is phage-mediated.

Following ingestion, the toxin passes across the intestinal wall to the blood and the lymph. The hemagglutinin may serve to protect the toxin from the digestive processes prior to its passage into the bloodstream. Ruminal bacteria inactivate substantial quantities of ingested toxin (1), and so the oral lethal dose for cattle and sheep is much larger than when the toxin is administered by other routes. This observation is important in relation to handling of diagnostic specimens of rumen contents for assay for toxin: these should be frozen until assays are performed.

Once in the bloodstream the toxin is carried to the peripheral nervous system, where it binds at the neuromuscular junction. It causes paralysis of the cholinergic nerve fibers by blocking the release of acetyl choline. This action is presynaptic. The external effect in the animal is flaccid paralysis, which, when it progresses to involve the respiratory muscles, will result in the animal's death. Disturbances in vision also occur, there is difficulty in locomotion, the tongue often becomes paralyzed (Figure 20.5), swallowing becomes impossible because of pharyngeal paralysis, and respiratory paralysis finally terminates the disease. In poultry there is paralysis of the wings, legs, and neck and inability to retract the nictitating membrane (Figure 20.6). Posterior paralysis is a usual symptom in mink. Swine and carnivorous animals and birds are resistant to the effects of botulinum toxin. However, the disease has been reported in foxhounds (3).

Immunity. Homologous antitoxins protect animals very well against botulism. However, because of the sporadic and infrequent occurrence of the disease in birds in many areas, vaccination is not a universally routine practice. In high-risk regions such as South Africa and Australia and in certain populations such as mink or zoo animals exposed to circumstances of feed or environment that predispose to toxin in the feed, vaccination with formalinized, alum-precipitated toxoids is practiced. These have been used successfully in immunizing mink (2),

Figure 20.5. Paralysis of the tongue in a cow with botulism. Note the food material in the mouth which the animal was unable to swallow.

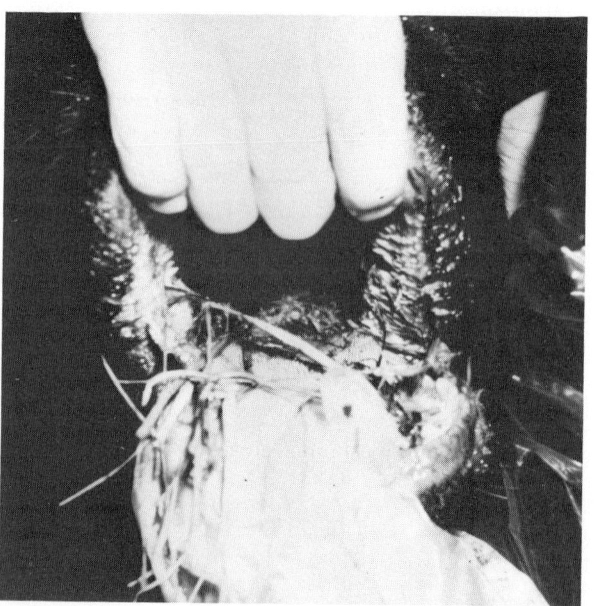

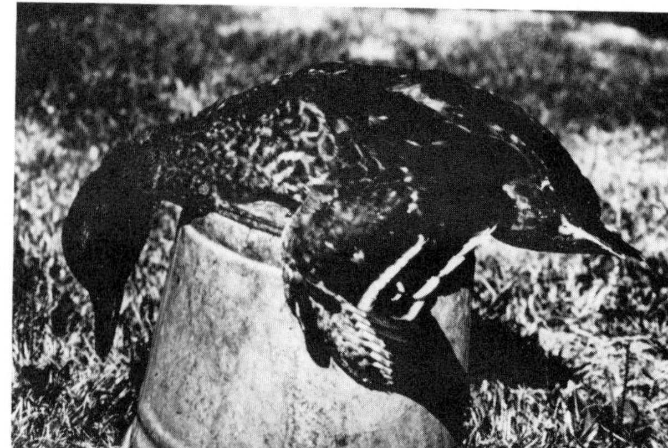

Figure 20.6. Limberneck in a duck. (Courtesy Dan Mills.)

horses (21), cattle, sheep, pheasants, and ducks (5). In some areas polyvalent toxoids are used for this purpose. In Australia nonimmune cattle and sheep are usually given a series of two injections and from then on a booster dose each year (4, 13). In South Africa (12) Types C and D toxoids have been shown to be most effective in a vaccination program when the primary and secondary inoculations are made with vaccines presented in water and oil emulsion and subsequent booster inoculations are performed with aqueous solutions.

Diagnosis. Diagnostic proof of botulism in animals centers on the demonstration of toxin in the serum, intestinal contents, and suspected foodstuff. Toxin in serum or filtered macerates of food or intestinal contents can be demonstrated by mouse inoculation. Mice passively protected with polyvalent antitoxin should also be inoculated. If botulinum toxin is present, only the unprotected mice should die. Levels of toxin in serum of affected animals are about 20 mouse LD_{50} per ml or lower. In the case of samples of intestinal contents or foodstuffs, the sample should be trypsinized before inoculation so that nontoxic precursor toxin can be activated.

Because the spores of *C. botulinum* are ubiquitous, their presence in specimens has very little diagnostic value.

Treatment. Attempts should be made to neutralize free toxin by the administration of polyvalent antitoxin. The response to antitoxin varies greatly depending on the toxin type, and is greatest for Type E. Efforts should also be made to empty the gastrointestinal tract of unabsorbed toxin by administration of purgatives.

Guanidine hydrochloride has been used in treatment of botulism because of an enhancing effect on the release of acetylcholine from nerve terminals (8). This drug and germine monoacetate (which acts in part postsynaptically to increase muscle tension by converting the single muscle action potential caused by a single nerve stimulus into a burst of repetitive potentials) have been shown to be helpful together in therapy of botulism.

REFERENCES

1. Allison, Malog, and Matson. Appl. and Envir. Microbiol., 1976, *32,* 605.
2. Appleton and White. Am. Jour. Vet. Res., 1959, *20,* 166.
3. Barsanti, Walser, Hatleway, Bower, and Cromwell. Jour. Am. Vet. Med. Assoc., 1978, *172,* 809.
4. Bennetts and Hall. Jour. Agr. (West Austral.), 1937, *14,* 381.
5. Boroff and Reilly. Jour. Bact., 1959, *77,* 142.
6. Breukink, Wagenaar, Wensing, Notermans, and Poulos. Tijdschr. Diergeneeskd. 1978, *103,* 303.
7. Dinter and Kull. Nord. Vet. Med., 1954, *6,* 866.
8. Duncan. *In* Microbiology—1975, ed. D. Schlessinger. Am. Soc. Microbiol., Washington, D.C., 1975, pp. 283–91.
9. Van Ermengem. Zeitschr. f. Hyg., 1897, *26,* 1.
10. Haagsma, Laak, and Ter. Tijdschr. Diergeneeskd., 1977, *102,* 429.
11. Hampson. Tijdschr. Diergeneeskd., 1951, *61,* 647.
12. Jansen, Knoetze, and Visser. Onderstepoort Jour. Vet. Res. 1976, *43,* 165.
13. Larsen, Nicholes, and Gebhardt. Am. Jour. Vet. Res., 1955, *26,* 573.
14. Mandia. Jour. Immunol., 1951, *67,* 49.
15. Mandia and Bruner. Jour. Immunol., 1951, *66,* 497.
16. Marx. Science, 1978, *201* (4358), 799.
17. Mason. Jour. S. Afr. Vet. Med. Assoc., 1968, *39,* 37.
18. Meyer and Dubovsky. Jour. Inf. Dis., 1922, *31,* 559.
19. Müller. Deut. Klin., 1870, *22,* 27.
20. Theiler *et al.* 11th and 12th Ann. Rpts., Dir. Vet. Ed. and Res., Union S. Afr., 1927, *2,* 821.
21. White and Appleton. Jour. Am. Vet. Med. Assoc., 1960, *137,* 652.

THE TISSUE-INVADING GROUP

Clostridium perfringens

SYNONYMS: *Clostridium welchii, Bacillus aerogenes capsulatus, Bacillus phlegmonis emphysematosae,* Welch bacillus, gas bacillus

The organism was first isolated and described by Welch and Nuttall (24) from a decomposing human cadaver in which the tissues were gaseous. It was named by them *Bacillus aerogenes capsulatus,* a term that does not conform to accepted rules of nomenclature and therefore is invalid. The name *Bacillus perfringens* was given the organism by Veillon and Zuber (23) in 1898. In 1900, Migula termed it *Bacillus welchii,* the name by which it is best known to American workers; however,

Veillon and Zuber's name seems clearly to have precedence, and it has been used in recent editions of *Bergey's Manual;* hence it will be used here. The term "Welch bacillus" will probably remain in use even if the formal name is divorced from Welch's name.

C. perfringens is widespread in the soil and is found in the alimentary tract of nearly all species of warm-blooded animals. It is frequently found as a postmortem invader from the alimentary tract in the tissues of bloating cadavers of man and animals. For this reason some caution is necessary in drawing conclusions based upon the presence of the organism in the tissues collected after death. It is found more often in the so-called gas gangrene infections of man than any other organism, although it generally is associated with other species of anaerobes in these processes. It is found also in malignant edemalike infections of animals, particularly sheep. Toxicogenic varieties of the organism are concerned in fatal toxemias in sheep, calves, young pigs, and man. These varieties are divided into five types, A to E, on the basis of the production of four major lethal toxins.

Morphology and Staining Reactions. *C. perfringens* occurs as thick, straight-sided rods, either singly or in pairs, seldom in chains. The individual cells are about 1.0 μm wide and 4 to 8 μm long. The spores are oval and small enough not to cause much swelling of the rods. Spores do not form in highly acid media: hence they are not apt to be found in media that contain fermentable carbohydrate. Strains vary in their ability to sporulate; in some cases it is difficult to find spores no matter what the nature of the culture medium. In old cultures pleomorphism may be found: clubbed types, ballooned cells, and filaments. Capsules are formed in tissues and in some types of culture media. There are no flagella; the organism is therefore nonmotile. Young cultures retain the Gram stain; older ones frequently decolorize.

Cultural Features. In deep agar, colonies are small and biconvex. If fermentable sugar is present, the medium will be fragmented and even blown out of the tube by the abundance of gas formed. If blood is present, it will be hemolyzed. Sharp hemolytic zones are formed around colonies on plates. In broth there is excellent growth, the fluid becoming greatly clouded. Gelatin is rapidly liquefied. In semisolid medium the avidity of *C. perfringens* for gelatin results in a type of growth that presents the illusion of motility. Coagulated egg medium and Loeffler's blood serum are not liquefied. There is good growth in cooked-meat medium, with considerable gas formation. The meat fragments are pinkish and not digested. A sour odor is emitted. A very characteristic reaction occurs in litmus milk—the "stormy" fermentation. The milk quickly coagulates and the curd is fragmented by active gas formation. Acid and gas are formed from glucose, levulose, galactose, mannose, maltose, lactose, sucrose, xylose, trehalose, raffinose, starch, glycogen, and inositol. Some strains attack glycerol and inulin. Fermentation products include acetic and butyric acids. The characteristics of *C. perfringens* and of the other tissue-invading clostridia are listed in Table 20.2.

Antigens and Toxins. Studies on serological relationships have indicated considerable heterogeneity within the species. Cross-reactions due to common capsular antigens have been found, and the use of the Quellung reaction and agar gel diffusion technique have demonstrated the sharing of common antigens among the five toxicogenic types. The production of four major toxins (alpha, beta, epsilon, and iota) is the basis of the classification of *C. perfringens*. These toxins are proteinaceous, enzymic in action, heat-labile, antigenic, and can be "toxoided" by the addition of chemicals which destroy their toxicity but not their antigenicity.

The major toxins associated with the five *C. perfringens* types and the diseases produced by them are listed in Tables 20.3 and 20.4. Other less important toxins produced include toxins with hyaluronidase, deoxyribonuclease, collagenase, and proteinase activities.

Epidemiology and Pathogenesis. *C. perfringens* is ubiquitous in nature and is part of the normal intestinal flora of healthy animals. Highly proteinaceous diets lead to great increases in populations of the organism in the gut. Type A strains are well adapted to survive in the soil, whereas Type B, C, D, and E strains appear to be more highly adapted to the intestine. Also, Type B and E strains have a much more distinct regional distribution than the other strains.

C. perfringens Type A. Type A *C. perfringens* causes a disease known as *yellow lamb disease,* which occurs in California and Oregon during spring when nursing lamb populations are at a maximum (14). Affected lambs are depressed, with pale mucous membranes, anemia, icterus, and hemoglobinuria and die within 6 to 12 hours of showing symptoms. Alpha toxin is produced in the small intestine, is absorbed into the circulation, and causes massive intravascular hemolysis and capillary damage.

The disease has also been reported in captive wild goats (19).

C. perfringens Type B. This type is usually found in the disease known as *lamb dysentery*. The disease is prevalent in the border country of England and Scotland,

Table 20.2. Characteristics of tissue-invading sporebearing anaerobes

Morphological and biochemical tests	*C. perfringens*	*C. hemolyticum*	*C. novyi*	*C. chauvoei*	*C. septicum*	*C. colinum*
Spores	Cent.	S.T.	S.T.	S.T.	S.T.	S.T.
Motility	−	+	+	+	+	+
Deep agar colonies	Lenticular	Lenticular	Lenticular	Pin point	Fluffy lenticular	Fluffy lenticular
Milk	Stormy ferm.	Coagulation	0	Coagulation	Coagulation	Coagulation
Gelatin	Gas liq., black	Gas liq.	Gas liq., black	Gas liq.	Gas liq.	Gas liq.
Glucose agar	Growth	Growth	Growth	No growth	Growth	Growth
Glucose	+	+	+	+	+	+
Lactose	+	−	−	+	+	−
Sucrose	+	−	−	+	−	+
Maltose	+	−	+	+	+	+
Galactose	+	−	+	+	+	−
Salicin	−	−	−	−	+	−
Pathogenic	+	+	+	+	+	+
Toxin formed	+	+	+	±	+	?
Liver surface smear	Single and short chains	?	Single and chains	Single	Single and filaments	Single and short chains

S.T. = Subterminal. Cent. = Central. 0 = No change.

Table 20.3 Characteristics of the major toxins of *C. perfringens*

Toxin	Properties	Mode of action	Effect in body
Alpha	Phospholipase (Lecithinase)	Hydrolyses lecithin complexes in mitochondria, cell membranes, blood phospholipids, and capillary endothelium	Hemolytic; leukocidal; increased capillary permeability due to endothelial damage; degeneration of muscle plasma membrane
Beta	Necrotizing, trypsin labile	Unknown	Necrosis of intestinal mucosa
Epsilon	Necrotizing and neurotoxic	Damages junctions between vascular endothelial cells of brain	Local liquefactive necrosis of brain tissue; necrosis of renal cortex; permeability of intestinal mucosa; increased perivascular edema produced in meninges and brain
Iota	Necrotizing, lethal; enzymic activation of prototoxin necessary	Unknown	Necrosis of intestinal mucosa

in Wales, and in South Africa and the Middle East. A similar disease was also described in Montana by Tunnicliff (22) in 1933. Lambs apparently become infected in the first days of life with Type B strains derived from their dams or from the environment. The organism multiplies to large populations in those lambs getting large quantities of milk. Beta toxin is produced and causes hemorrhagic zones and ulceration of the small intestine. Affected lambs die in a few hours after showing signs of abdominal pain, lack of interest in suckling, and continuous bleating.

Hemorrhagic enteritis of sheep, goats, calves, and foals caused by *C. perfringens* Type B has also been described (1, 6) and is reviewed by Roberts (17).

C. perfringens Type C. This type causes *enterotoxemia* in a variety of animal species. Hemorrhagic and necrotic enteritis in calves (8) and lambs (9) has occasionally been shown to be caused by the toxins of *C. perfringens* Type C. In lambs the disease resembles lamb dysentery. In calves, the disease is usually seen in animals that are healthy and vigorous and less than a week old. The hemorrhagic enteritis is caused by the beta toxin, which can sometimes be demonstrated in fresh intestinal contents. This toxin is very labile and easily denatured by enzymic action in the intestine, so failure to demonstrate it is not significant from the diagnostic standpoint.

Piglets aged 1 to 3 days may exhibit an acute hemor-

Table 20.4. The diseases in animals caused by, and the major toxins of, *C. perfringens* types A, B, C, D, and E

Type	Disease	Distribution	Toxins: Alpha	Beta	Epsilon	Iota
A	Yellow lamb disease	California	+*	–	–	–
B	Lamb dysentery	Europe, S. Africa	+	+*	+	–
	Hemorrhagic enteritis of sheep and goats	Middle East, Iran				
C	Necrotic enteritis (lambs, piglets, calves, chickens)	Worldwide	+	+*	–	–
	Struck (sheep)	England				
D	Enterotoxemia—"overeating disease," "pulpy kidney disease" (sheep)	Worldwide	+	–	+*	–
E	Enterotoxemia (lambs and calves)	United States, England, Australia	+	–	–	+*

*The most important toxin in the disease process.

rhagic enteritis with high mortality (5). Severe enteritis with patches of necrosis on the mucosa involving mainly the jejunum are seen at postmortem examination. Outbreaks of Type C enterotoxemia in chickens aged 6 to 12 weeks have also been described (16, 18). Affected birds exhibit weakness and dysentery. Beta toxin is apparently responsible for the intestinal lesions because it is found in the intestinal contents of affected birds. Predisposing causes of outbreaks include overcrowding and regrouping.

The disease of adult sheep called *struck* or *Romney Marsh disease* is also caused by *C. perfringens* Type C. The organism is present in the soil of the Romney Marsh areas of England, and presumably most sheep in the area become infected. The disease is seen in early spring. For reasons presently unknown, the organism multiplies in the abomasum and small intestine and produces beta toxin. The beta toxin causes necrosis of the mucosa of these regions. Dysentery or diarrhea are seldom present. In some cases, evidence of toxemia such as accumulation of fluid in the peritoneal and thoracic cavities is present without visible lesions in the intestinal tract. The beta toxin may be demonstrated in the fluids (21).

C. perfringens Type D. This type causes *enterotoxemia in sheep (pulpy kidney disease, overeating disease),* a disease that is common in most sheep-raising areas of the world. The organism is found in the soil and in the digestive tracts of most healthy sheep. Intensive sheep-raising systems, including feedlots, are particularly prone to outbreaks of enterotoxemia. During periods of high-level feeding of concentrates, the organism multiplies in the intestine and may produce lethal quantities of toxin.

The important toxin in this disease is the epsilon toxin, which requires trypsin activation. The toxin has a permease effect on the intestinal mucosa which enhances its own absorbtion. After absorbtion, foci of liquefactive necrosis, perivascular edema, and hemorrhages especially in the meninges are caused by the toxin (1). Receptor sites for the toxin occur on the vascular endothelium of the brain, where the toxin causes the intercellular junctions to break down and so allow escape of fluid (2). Hemorrhagic areas on the small intestine and petechiation of the endocardium may be present. Hyperemia and degenerative changes are found in the kidney cortex, which becomes soft and friable ("pulpy kidney") (Figure 20.7). Permeability changes affecting the vasculature of the serous surfaces of the peritoneum and pericardium are also reflected in effusions of straw-colored fluid into these cavities. Glucose is usually present in the urine in the bladder at death.

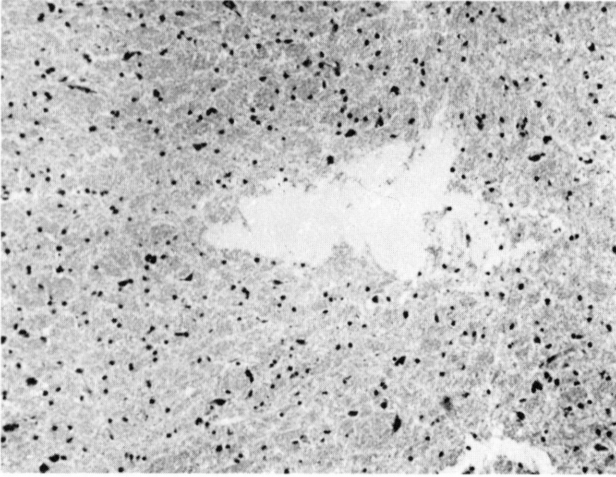

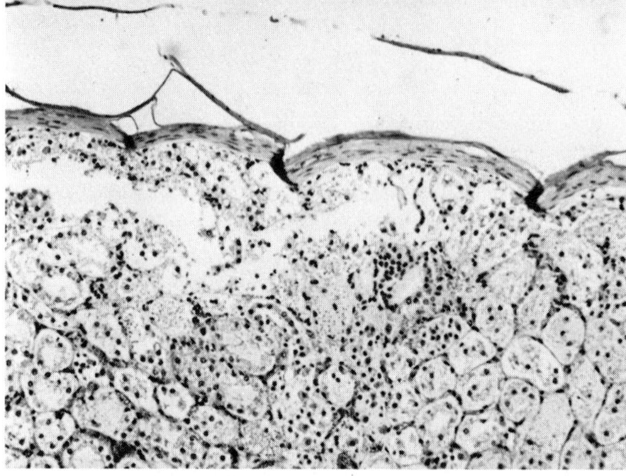

Figure 20.7. Lesions of enterotoxemia caused by *Clostridium perfringens* Type D in a lamb. The section of cerebrum (*upper*) shows an area of malacia; the section of kidney cortex (*lower*) shows necrosis of the tissues underlying the capsule. × 370.

Death of the animal may be sudden, or it may be preceded by dullness, retraction of the head, and convulsions with agonal struggling.

C. perfringens Type D enterotoxemia has also been reported in calves (7). The disease is similar to that in sheep, but some cases may exhibit a sudden onset of bellowing, manic charging about, and eventual convulsions and death.

C. perfringens Type E. This type is believed to have caused hemorrhagic, necrotic enteritis of calves in Australia (10). Both the organism and its toxin are also sometimes found in sheep or bovine intestines at postmortem examination where there are no signs of clostridial enterotoxemia (21).

Diagnosis of Clostridial Enterotoxemias. *C. perfringens* Type A is present in the muscles and organs of virtually all carcasses within a few hours of death unless they have been rapidly chilled. Thus, laboratory diagnosis of yellow lamb disease depends on demonstration of alpha toxin in intestinal contents and bloodstream of fresh carcasses. Large numbers of *C. perfringens* Type A will be found in the contents of the small intestine. Counts in this area normally are about 10^2 per ml.

In the case of lamb dysentery the mere presence of Type B organisms and/or beta toxin in intestinal contents or tissues of neonatal lambs is good evidence for a diagnosis of lamb dysentery.

Enterotoxemias in lambs and calves and struck in adult sheep are diagnosed in the laboratory by the demonstration of beta toxin in intestinal contents and serous exudates, and high counts of Type C organisms in the small intestine. The latter are differentiated from Type B strains by the production of epsilon toxin.

The mere presence of *C. perfringens* Type D or of its epsilon toxin in intestinal contents is insufficient evidence for a diagnosis of Type D enterotoxemia. This is so because of the widespread occurrence of Type D strains and because epsilon toxin may normally be present in the intestine but is not absorbed by the naturally resistant or the immune animal (21). Diagnosis of Type D enterotoxemia must be based upon (*a*) large numbers of *C. perfringens* Type D in the intestine; (*b*) epsilon toxin in the small intestine; (*c*) Type D organisms in the kidney and other parenchymatous organs at death; and (*d*) sugar in the urine. Sterne and Thomson (21) point out that the simultaneous presence of epsilon toxin in the intestine and sugar in the urine is pathognomic for Type D enterotoxemia.

Detection of Toxins. The toxins of *C. perfringens* are detected and identified by serum-neutralization tests in mice and guinea pigs. The procedures involved are described by Carter (3). Intestinal contents and other body fluids should be collected as soon after death as possible and 1 percent chloroform added as a preservative. Samples should be kept chilled during transport to the laboratory, where they are centrifuged and the supernatant (0.2 to 0.4 ml) injected intravenously into mice and intradermally into white skin areas of guinea pigs. Part of the sample should be treated with trypsin (1 percent trypsin powder, w/v) and left at room temperature for one hour to activate epsilon and iota and destroy beta toxins. The enzyme-treated solutions are then injected into a second group of mice and pigs. If toxin is present, the mice die in 4 to 12 hours. Guinea pigs are observed for 48 hours for the development of necrotic lesions at the site of inoculation. Simultaneously or after toxic activity has been detected, a third group of animals is inoculated with the toxic supernatants that have been reacted with antisera against Types A, B, C, D, and E. The neutralization tests are read over a 72-hour period and interpreted according to Table 20.5.

Table 20.5. Interpretation of serum neutralization tests for *C. perfringens* toxin

Antitoxin	Neutralizes	Toxins neutralized
Type A	Type A only	Alpha
Type B	Types A, B, C, and D	Alpha, beta, epsilon
Type C	Types A and C	Alpha, beta
Type D	Types A and D	Alpha, epsilon
Type E	Types A and E	Alpha, iota

Immunity. Type-specific alum-precipitated toxoids or formalinized toxoids are effective vaccines against the *C. perfringens* enterotoxemias. Types B and C vaccines or antisera will cross-protect because beta toxin is the important toxin in each. Thus either Type B or Type C antiserum can be used to passively protect against lamb dysentery.

Ewes should be vaccinated with either Type B or Type C vaccine in the fall and again a few weeks before lambing. Lambs will thereby be protected against lamb dysentery by colostral antibodies in the ewes' milk. Vaccination of ewes against Type D enterotoxemia will similarly result in passive protection of lambs (20). Lambs should be vaccinated at about 10 days and again 2 to 6 weeks later (13).

During an outbreak, toxoid and antiserum can be administered at the same time, followed by a booster inoculation of toxoid 4 weeks later (15).

Control and Treatment. Enterotoxemia can be prevented or outbreaks halted in older lambs by restriction of feed. The addition of sulfur to the ration has proved successful because it reduces food intake (7, 4). Chlortetracycline (22.5 mg per kg) in the feed will also prevent deaths (12). Specific antiserum is valuable in preventing further losses during outbreaks.

Because of the acute, rapid nature of the various enterotoxemias, treatment of affected animals is unlikely to be beneficial.

REFERENCES

1. Buxton, Linklater, and Dyson. Vet. Rec., 1978, *102*, 241.
2. Buxton and Morgan. Jour. Comp. Path., 1976, *86*, 435.

3. Carter. Diagnostic procedures in veterinary microbiology. Thomas, Springfield, Ill., 1973.
4. Christensen. Jour. Am. Vet. Med. Assoc., 1967, *111*, 144.
5. Field and Gibson. Vet. Rec., 1954, *67*, 31.
6. Frank. Am. Jour. Vet. Res., 1956, *17*, 492.
7. Griner, Aichelman, and Brown. Jour. Am. Vet. Med. Assoc., 1956, *129*, 375.
8. Griner and Bracken. Jour. Am. Vet. Med. Assoc., 1953, *122*, 99.
9. Griner and Johnson. Jour. Am. Vet. Med. Assoc., 1954, *125*, 125.
10. Hart and Hooper. Austral Vet. Jour., 1967, *43*, 360.
11. Hepple. Vet. Rec., 1952, *64*, 633.
12. Johnson. Jour. Am. Sci., 1956, *15*, 781.
13. Kennedy, Norris, Bechenhauer, and White. Am. Jour. Vet. Res., 1977, *38*, 1515.
14. McGowan, Moulton, and Rood. Jour. Am. Vet. Med. Assoc., 1958, *133*, 219.
15. Montgomerie. Vet. Rec., 1960, *72*, 995.
16. Parish. Jour. Comp. Path. and Therap., 1961, *71*, 405.
17. Roberts. *In* Diseases due to bacteria, ed. Stableforth and Galloway. Academic Press, New York, vol. 1, 1958, pp. 194–200.
18. Roberts and Collings. Avian Dis., 1973, *17*, 650.
19. Russell. Jour. Am. Vet. Med. Assoc., 1970, *157*, 643.
20. Smith and Matsuoka. Am. Jour. Vet. Res., 1959, *20*, 91.
21. Sterne and Thomson. Bull. Off. int. Epiz., 1963, *59*, 1487.
22. Tunnicliff. Jour. Inf. Dis., 1933, *52*, 407.
23. Veillon and Zuber. Arch. Med. Exp., 1898, *10*, 517.
24. Welch and Nuttall. Johns Hopkins Hosp. Bull., 1892, *3*, 81.

Clostridium hemolyticum

SYNONYMS: *Clostridium hemolyticus bovis, Bacillus hemolyticus*

This organism is closely related to *C. novyi* and is the cause of a disease of cattle, occasionally of sheep, commonly known as *red water disease*. It is also known as *hemorrhagic disease* and *infectious icterohemoglobinuria*. One case in a hog has been described by Records and Huber (6). Because of its similarity to *C. novyi* it has been claimed as *C. novyi* Type D (4).

Morphology and Staining Reactions. This organism is somewhat larger than most of the other tissue-invading anaerobic bacilli. It measures 1.0 to 1.3 μm in breadth and 3.0 to 5.6 μm in length. It has straight sides and rounded ends. It occurs singly, as a rule, but may form short chains in tissues and cultures. The spores are oval and are located subterminally. They cause bulging of the cells in which they lie. The cells are actively motile when young. Young cells are Gram-positive, but when they are more than 24 hours old they rapidly lose their ability to retain this stain.

Cultural Features. Deep agar colonies are lenticular at first, later becoming woolly. Little or no gas is formed unless fermentable sugar is added to the medium. When blood is present it is rapidly hemolyzed. Gelatin is liquefied in 2 to 4 days. Coagulated serum and egg media are not softened or liquefied. Cooked-meat media and brain media support good growth, but there is no digestion of the solids and no blackening unless iron salts are added. Even in the presence of an abundance of iron salts the blackening is but slight. Milk is not changed. Glucose and levulose are the only carbohydrates fermented. These are actively destroyed with the evolution of both acid and gas. Hydrogen sulfide is formed in large amounts in liver media and in media containing proteose-peptone. The methyl-red and Voges-Proskauer tests are negative, and nitrates are not reduced. Indol is formed in large amounts.

This organism is very exacting in its cultural requirements. Good anaerobic conditions are necessary, and the media must contain tryptophan for optimum growth and toxin formation. Acetic, propionic, and butyric acids are the principal fermentation products.

Antigens. Most strains share antigens with *C. novyi*, but no detailed serologic analysis has been made of *C. hemolyticum*. The principal toxin produced is a phospholipase.

Epidemiology and Pathogenesis. The organism was initially thought to be restricted to the Rocky Mountain region of the United States, but it was later found in the delta parishes of Louisiana, along the Gulf of Mexico, in Florida (2), Central Mexico, and as far away as Wales, New Zealand (3), Rumania, Turkey, and South America. A closely related organism has been isolated from a similar disease in Chile (8). The organism shows a predilection for alkaline water, and the disease is associated with pastures that contain swampy areas which continually maintain a pH of 8.0 or higher. In the United States the disease occurs principally during the summer and early fall months. It is believed that carrier animals may introduce the organism into uninfected areas (7, 9).

The site of toxin production is the liver. There is good circumstantial evidence that the tissue destruction caused by the migration of liver flukes provides a suitable microenvironment for germination of the spores of *C. hemolyticum*, with subsequent multiplication and toxin synthesis (Figure 20.8). This phase of the pathogenesis is similar to that of *C. novyi* Type B. The disease is unlikely to occur when fluke infestations are minimal. That

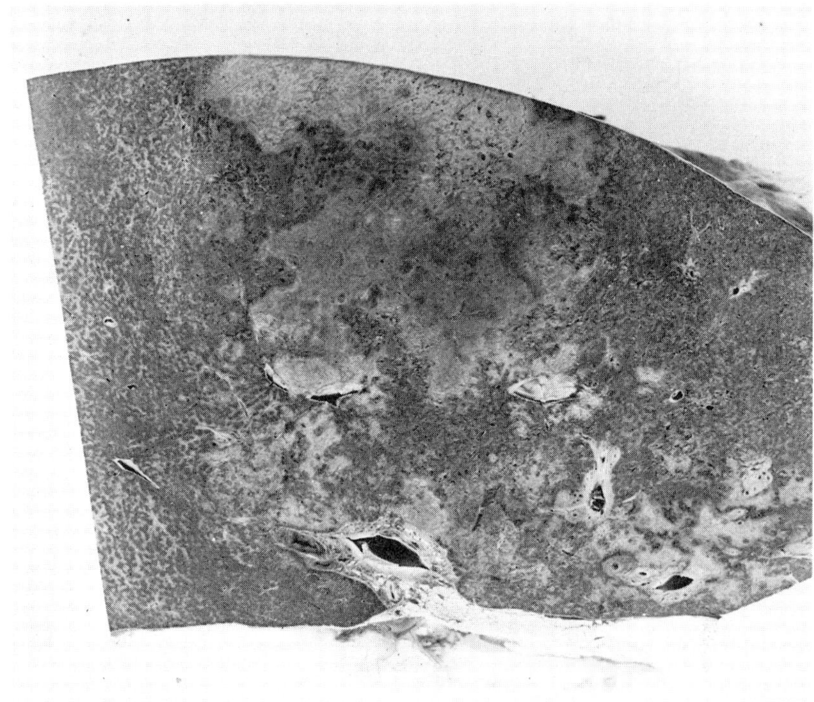

Figure 20.8. Massive infarct in a bovine liver caused by infection with *Clostridium hemolyticum*. This lesion is characteristic of the red water disease of cattle. (Courtesy Edward Records.)

damage to the liver is important in initiating bacterial multiplication, and toxin synthesis is illustrated by an outbreak of bacillary hemoglobinuria 2 to 3 days following liver biopsy of a group of cattle raised in an endemic area (5).

The phospholipase C released in the liver causes massive intravascular hemolysis and capillary damage. Hemoglobin is passed in the urine, and there is hemorrhage into the lumen of the intestine as a result of local capillary destruction.

The disease presents quite a uniform picture, which is readily recognized by those who have had experience with it. Appetite, rumination, lactation, and bowel movement suddenly cease, and the afflicted animal stands apart from the rest of the herd, presenting a picture of acute illness. The back is arched, the abdomen is tucked up, and it is difficult to make the animal move. Breathing is shallow, and there is grunting with each step. The temperature varies from 104 to 106 F in the early stages but becomes subnormal before death. The feces become deeply bile-stained or bloody. The urine is a dark-red or port-wine color, clear but foamy. The color is due to large amounts of hemoglobin. There are no intact erythrocytes in the urine. Sugar is absent, but albumin tests are strongly positive.

At the time when hemoglobinuria appears, as much as 40 to 50 percent of all of the erythrocytes of the body have been destroyed. The red cell count at this time may not be greater than 2,000,000 per mm^3 and the hemoglobin readings may be as low as 3.5 g per 100 ml of blood. The leukocyte count increases, sometimes to as high as 30,000 per mm^3. Death is caused by anoxemia because of the wholesale destruction of erythrocytes. The mortality is high, varying from 90 to 95 percent in untreated animals.

The most characteristic lesion is the large infarct that is always found in the liver. This is a mass of necrotic tissue, varying from 5 to 20 cm in diameter, often mottled, and usually lighter in color than the normal liver tissue. This lesion may be located in any part of the organ. It is formed as a result of an occluding thrombosis of one of the branches of the portal vein. The tissue has undergone coagulation necrosis. In the sinusoids of these areas great numbers of large rod-shaped bacteria containing subterminal or terminal spores may be seen (Figure 20.9).

Extensive hemorrhages are found on the serous membranes, in the subcutaneous connective tissue, and in the substance of the visceral organs. Acute degenerative changes occur in the organs, and the peritoneal and pleural cavities usually contain large quantities of hemoglobin-stained transudates. Besides the subserous hemorrhages that regularly occur in the intestinal wall, there is a severe hemorrhagic enteritis, the mucous

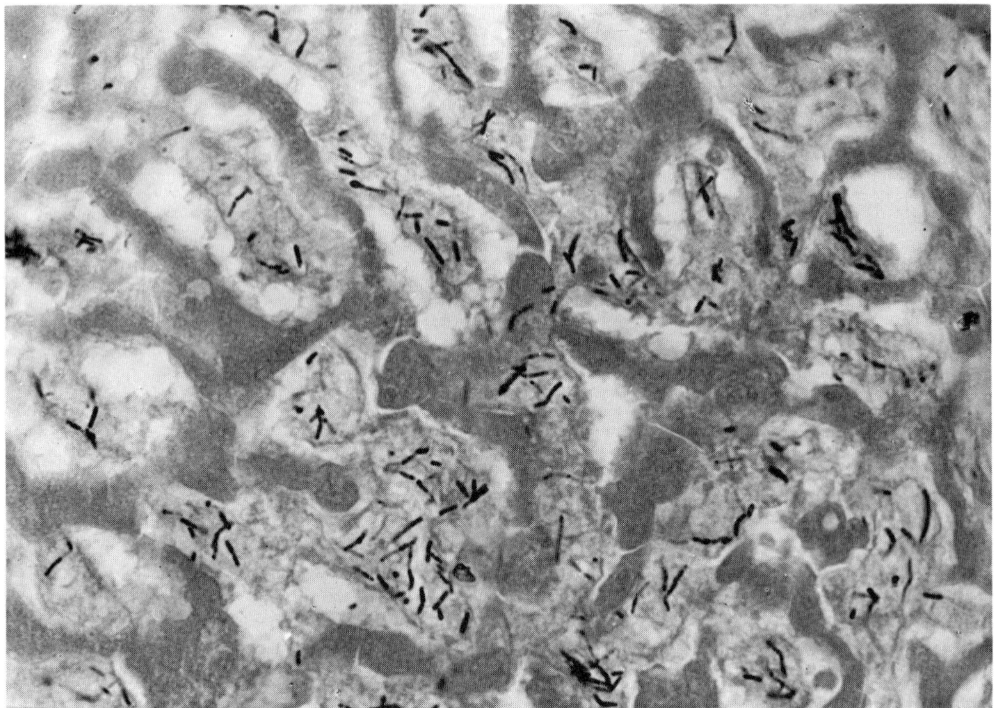

Figure 20.9. *Clostridium hemolyticum* in the characteristic liver infarct. A few of the organisms are beginning to form spores. × 750. (Courtesy Edward Records.)

membrance often being almost wholly undermined with extensive hemorrhage.

Rabbits, guinea pigs, and mice may be readily killed by toxin-containing cultures. Subcutaneous injection leads to the formation of a hemorrhagic, edematous area at the point of inoculation with little or no gas formation. Intravenous inoculation of rabbits usually leads to death in 2 to 4 hours with great blood destruction and hemoglobinuria.

Diagnosis. *C. hemolyticum* can be cultured from, and phospholipase C demonstrated in the liver lesion. Guinea pigs inoculated intramuscularly with homogenates of lesions die in 1 or 2 days.

Immunity. Alum-precipitated formalinized whole cultures of *C. hemolyticum* are used for immunization of cattle. Vaccination must be repeated every 6 to 12 months in endemic areas. Immunized animals produce agglutinating antibodies but very little antitoxin. Immunity to bacillary hemoglobinuria appears to be primarily antibacterial (1).

Treatment. Antiserum has been used for prophylaxis and therapy (10). For therapy, 500 to 1,000 ml must be used before the animal's body temperature recedes to subnormal. Whole-blood transfusions and fluid replacement should also be attempted.

Large doses of penicillin administered intravenously will inactivate *C. hemolyticum* in the liver and prevent further toxin synthesis.

REFERENCES

1. Claus and Macheak. Am. Jour. Vet. Res., 1965, *26,* 353.
2. McCain. Am. Jour. Vet. Res., 1967, *28,* 878.
3. Marshall. New Zeal. Vet. Jour., 1959, *7,* 115.
4. Oakley and Warrack. Jour. Path. and Bact., 1959, *78,* 543.
5. Olander, Hughes, and Biberstein. Path. Vet., 1966, *3,* 421.
6. Records and Huber. Jour. Am. Vet. Med Assoc., 1931, *78,* 863.
7. Safford and Smith. Proc. Am. Vet. Med. Assoc., 1954, pp. 159–161.
8. Smith, Louis. Introduction to pathogenic anaerobes. Univ. of Chicago Press, Chicago, 1954, p. 147.
9. Smith and Jasmin. Jour. Am. Vet. Med. Assoc., 1956, *129,* 68.
10. Vawter and Records. Jour. Am. Vet. Med. Assoc., 1929, *75,* 201.

Clostridium novyi

SYNONYMS: Novy's *Bacillus edematis maligni II, Clostridium edematiens*

This organism was first described by Novy (7), in 1894, who isolated it from a guinea pig that had been inoculated with unsterilized milk protein. It was lost sight of for many years until Weinberg and Séguin (14) rediscovered it in gas gangrene infections of man in 1915. They gave it the name *C. edematiens,* and this name is still used by most English and French workers. It is quite similar to *C. septicum* in its cultural features and in pathogenicity. There are three types—A, B, and C (11).

Morphology and Staining Reactions. This is one of the largest of anaerobic bacilli. It measures 0.8 to 1.0 μm in breadth and is from 3 to 10 μm long. The rods usually are quite straight and the ends rounded. The spores generally are present in abundance. They are located subterminally and are oval. Young cultures are motile by peritrichic flagella. Young cultures are Gram-positive; older cultures usually lose this property.

Cultural Features. This organism is more strictly anaerobic than most of the other clostridia. To obtain surface growth, the anaerobic apparatus must be in good working order. The organism requires cysteine in its reduced form. The reduced state can be maintained by the addition of 0.03 percent dithiothreitol to the medium (6). In deep agar cultures the colonies grow well, especially when glucose is present. The colonies vary in form, some being compact and of a yellowish tinge, others loose and woolly. The medium is disrupted by gas formation. On blood agar the colonies are surrounded by hemolytic zones. Gelatin is liquefied. Broth supports a poor growth, most of which sediments to the bottom. Litmus milk is reduced but not coagulated. Coagulated blood serum and egg albumen are not liquefied. There is good growth in cooked-meat medium. The meat fragments become reddish in color and a rancid smell is emitted. Acid and gas are formed from glucose, levulose, maltose, xylose, starch, and glycerol. Lactose, sucrose, mannitol, dulcitol, inulin, and salicin are not fermented. Principal fermentation products are acetic, propionic, and butyric acids.

Antigens. No detailed study of the serologic characteristics of *C. novyi* has been made. The organism shares somatic antigens with *C. hemolyticum*. The three immunologic types (A, B, and C) are based on the toxins produced (9, 11). These are listed in Table 20.6.

Epidemiology and Pathogenesis. *C. novyi* Type A occurs in the soil and in the intestinal tract of herbivorous animals. It may multiply in wounds contaminated by soil and cause gas gangrene. In yearling rams infections of the head and neck area result from the trauma of fighting and cause the condition known as *big head.*

After invasion, toxins are synthesized and released. In the case of Type A strains, the alpha toxin damages

Table 20.6. Toxins and diseases produced by and hosts of *C. novyi*

Type	Toxins produced	Disease	Hosts
A	Alpha, gamma, epsilon	Gas gangrene, Big head	Sheep and cattle, rams
B	Alpha, beta	Black disease	Sheep and cattle
C	—	Osteomyelitis*	Buffaloes

*Of questionable etiologic significance.

capillary endothelium at the site of invasion (4) and in the brain after absorption into the bloodstream. There is also damage to muscle, liver, and heart. Evidence for this is the elevation of intracellular enzymes such as lactic dehydrogenase and glutamic oxalacetic transaminase (10). Alpha toxins can be demonstrated in the lesions of affected animals (15).

Black disease or necrotic hepatitis of sheep, and, to a lesser extent, of cattle, occurs in Europe, Australia, New Zealand, and the United States. The disease is seen in areas where there is liver-fluke infestation. During periods of heavy pasture infestation by *Fasciola hepatica*, liver damage from the migration of immature flukes creates suitable foci for germination of spores of *C. novyi* Type B in the liver. The organism multiplies, producing large amounts of alpha and lesser amounts of beta toxin, which circulate in the bloodstream. The lethal effect of the alpha toxin results in the death of the animal. On postmortem, necrotic areas are found near the surface of the liver. Extensive subcutaneous blood-stained edema occurs under the skin—hence the name *black disease*. Other effects of the alpha toxin are seen in the serous cavities, where straw-colored fluid accumulates as a result of endothelial damage.

Byrne and Armstrong (3) reported two outbreaks of an alimentary-tract infection of Canadian cattle caused by *C. novyi*. They presented atypical symptoms of blackleg infection. In the first outbreak, 21 of 47 animals died. In the second, prompt diagnosis and the use of a bacterin containing *C. novyi* is given credit for limiting deaths to 2 in a herd of 50 cattle. Bourne and Kerry (2) have described cases of sudden death in sows from which *C. novyi* was isolated. The clinical signs and postmortem lesions resembled those seen in anthrax.

Diagnosis. The mere presence of *C. novyi* in liver tissue may not be sufficient evidence for a diagnosis of black disease because many healthy cattle and sheep in endemic areas harbor the organism in their livers (5).

The demonstration of alpha toxin in the lesion and in exudates is, however, excellent diagnostic proof (12). The fluorescent antibody test is a rapid and reliable means of demonstrating the organism in smears from lesions (1).

Immunity. Alum-precipitated formalinized whole broth cultures are effective when administered in two doses (13). Vaccination is usually carried out a short time before expected heavy fluke activity. During an outbreak of black disease hyperimmune serum can be administered for prophylaxis. Vaccination during this time will also reduce mortality following a lag period of 10 days.

Treatment. The practicality of treatment is questionable because of the rapid course of the disease. Depot preparations of penicillin administered parenterally might be useful in cattle, in which the disease has a slower progression than in sheep.

REFERENCES

1. Batty, Buntain, and Walker. Vet. Rec., 1964, *76,* 1115.
2. Bourne and Kerry. Vet. Rec., 1965, *77,* 1463.
3. Byrne and Armstrong. Can. Jour. Comp. Med., 1948, *12,* 155.
4. Elder and Miles. Jour. Path. and Bact., 1957, *74,* 133.
5. Jamieson. Jour. Path. and Bact., 1949, *61,* 389.
6. Moore. Jour. Gen. Microbiol., 1968, *53,* 415.
7. Novy. Zeitschr. f. Hyg., 1894, *17,* 209.
8. Oakley, Warrack, and Clarke. Jour. Gen. Microbiol., 1947, *1,* 91.
9. Oakley and Warrack. Jour. Path. and Bact., 1959, *78,* 543.
10. Pomberton, Matson, Laus, and Macheak. Clin. Chim. Acta, 1971, *34,* 431.
11. Scott, Turner, and Vawter. Proc. 12th Int. Vet. Cong., 1934, p. 168.
12. Sterne and Thomson. Bull. Off. Int. Epiz., 1963, *59,* 1487.
13. Turner. Austral. Council Sci. and Indus. Res. Bull. 46, 1930.
14. Weinberg and Séguin. Comp. rend. Soc. Biol. (Paris), 1915, *78,* 507.
15. Williams. Vet. Rec., 1962, *74,* 1536.

Clostridium chauvoei

SYNONYMS: *Bacillus chauvoei, Bacillus carbonis, Bacillus anthracis symptomatici, Clostridium feseri, Clostridium chauvei*

This organism is the cause of *blackleg* in ruminants. It occurs throughout the world and is a considerable source of economic loss, especially to cattle raisers. In cattle, the disease is also called *black-quarter, quarter ill,* or *symptomatic anthrax.* The disease has been reported in swine (14, 7) and in mink fed infected beef liver (10), but is of rare occurrence in species other than ruminants.

Morphology and Staining Reactions. This organism is seen in tissues and cultures as a straight, round-ended rod about 0.6 μm in width and from 3 to 8 μm long (Figure 20.10). It can be very pleomorphic, however. It usually appears singly or in chains of 3 to 5 organisms in the peritoneal exudate of inoculated guinea pigs, and this fact is useful in distinguishing it from *C. septicum* and other anaerobic bacilli which frequently occur in materials suspected of blackleg. The latter organisms usually occur in long chains. Spores are oval and appear excentrically, swelling the rods into lemon-shaped structures. Very young cultures are motile by means of peritrichic flagella. Pleomorphic cells stain somewhat unevenly. The Gram stain is positive when the cultures are young but erratic after they are a few days old.

Cultural Features. *C. chauvoei* is a little more exacting in its cultural requirements than are most of the organisms in this group. It is strictly anaerobic and will not grow on ordinary glucose agar except when tissues are carried over in the inoculum. The addition of blood or tissue makes ordinary broth and agar favorable for it. It will grow luxuriantly on all media made with a liver infusion base, without enrichment. It has a high requirement for cysteine.

Deep colonies on agar are delicate and compact, being irregularly spherical. When blood is present, there is evidence of slight hemolysis, but definite zones are not formed around surface colonies. In plain broth there is usually no growth unless blood or tissue has been carried over with the inoculum. In liver broth the fluid becomes

Figure 20.10. *Clostridium chauvoei,* a film from a brain-liver medium culture incubated 48 hours at 37 C. × 1,545.

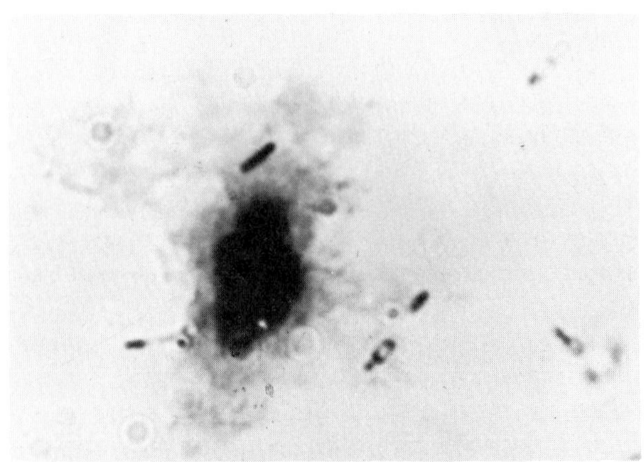

moderately clouded. Gelatin containing a little serum is slowly liquefied, and a few gas bubbles are formed. Growth on coagulated blood serum and coagulated egg is poor, and there is no liquefaction. Cooked-meat medium becomes pinkish, and the fluid is slightly clouded. Liver-brain medium gives excellent growth and is a good medium on which to maintain cultures. It is not digested. Acid and gas are formed from glucose, levulose, galactose, maltose, lactose, and sucrose. Inulin, salicin, mannitol, glycerol, and dextrin are not fermented. Cultures of this organism give off a characteristic odor by which experienced workers frequently can identify the species. The principal fermentation products are butanol and acetic and butyric acids.

Antigens. *C. chauvoei* strains have flagellar (designated by lower-case letters), somatic (arabic numerals), and spore (capital letters) antigens. Most strains share the same spore, somatic, and flagellar antigens (A:3:f). The spore antigen is shared with *C. septicum* (12).

Toxins are also produced and include alpha toxin with hemolytic and necrotizing activity, hyaluronidase, and deoxyribonuclease (8). Both soluble and insoluble protective antigens also occur. The soluble protective antigen is formed in conjunction with the alpha toxin from which it later dissociates (15). It is found in the supernatant of fluid cultures after 17 hours (6).

Epidemiology. The organism of blackleg exists in the soil. Whether it multiplies there, or whether it merely lives there in the spore form and multiplies in the intestinal canal of animals, is not known. In any case, it is known that when pastures or grazing grounds once become infected, the disease will reappear regularly in susceptible animals year after year.

Spring and fall are the seasons of greatest occurrence of blackleg in the United States. In Europe the disease is frequent in the summer months. The infection is most common on permanent pasture or wet bottom land, and certain pastures in a locality appear to be of especially high risk. Land cultivation diminishes this risk.

Cattle are susceptible at between 6 months and 2 years. Fat, thriving animals are much more likely to develop blackleg than stock that are unthrifty.

Pathogenesis. The mode of entry in cattle is uncertain because many cases of blackleg exhibit no external wounds that would explain entry of the organism from the exterior. It appears that entry is by the oral route during grazing. The organism multiplies in the intestine and then passes into the lymphatic and blood circulation. Muscle and liver tissue is thereby seeded by the organism, which remains dormant until the muscle mass is altered or damaged in some way that provides the right milieu for its growth. Kerry (9) has been able to demonstrate the organism in the livers and spleens of 20 percent of normal cattle, suggesting that the liver could serve as a source of the organism for muscle masses. It has also been suggested (13) that the organism may enter via the alveoli when the deciduous teeth are lost and that this is the reason for the occurrence of the disease in cattle 6 months to 2 years old. Lesions in the throat and neck are easily explained by this mode of entry. The muscles of the neck, throat, back, and abdomen may occasionally be affected.

In sheep, the disease often seems to be a wound infection, occurring after lambing, docking, and shearing (11). In Montana, infection has been reported in pregnant ewes soon after they were shorn. The organism was recovered from edematous fetuses in these ewes (4). When the organism begins to multiply, the necrotizing, leukocidic, and spreading effects of alpha toxin and hyaluronidase promote the development of the typical myonecrosis. The affected area is dark reddish brown to black in color. It has a crepitant, spongy texture because of entrapped gas and is dry on the cut surface. Leukocyte and platelet counts decrease and serum glutamic oxalacetic transaminase rapidly increase (2). Circulating toxin and tissue breakdown products lead to fatal toxemia with degenerative changes in the heart muscle and parenchymatous organs. In the later stages of the disease, there is a bacteremia also. The animal if seen before death will appear dull, lame, and usually standing away from the herd. The affected area is first swollen, painful, and crepitant. Later, sensation is lost and the skin becomes tighter. The animal dies in a day or two.

Diagnosis. The organism may be found in the heart blood, liver, and peritoneal fluid. However, cultural identification should always be performed because other clostridia pathogenic for guinea pigs (for example, *C. septicum*) can be secondary postmortem invaders of specimens of muscle.

A fluorescent antibody technique utilizing conjugates prepared from antisera against *C. chauvoei* and *C. septicum* and labeled with contrasting fluorescent dyes can be routinely used to distinguish between the two organisms (3).

Immunity. Currently used vaccines consist of formalinized whole cultures or anacultures to which alum may be added to increase antigenicity. Protection depends on the presence of the heat-labile soluble protective antigen (15). Some strains produce much more of this than others (5). Some immunity can be produced from injection of heated washed cells, indicating that somatic antigens are also important in protection.

By immunizing horses with washed cultures of the blackleg organism, a highly potent serum can be obtained that is useful, if used in large amounts, in protecting valuable calves when blackleg is present in a herd and in treating cases which have already developed.

Treatment. Penicillin is effective in treating blackleg if administered systemically and locally into the lesion while the latter is still in the early stages (1). Butler and Marsh (4) describe similar results for sheep. However, a large amount of muscle may eventually slough away, and the wound will require prolonged treatment. Also, the animal's body condition deteriorates considerably, and recovery may be slow. Thus, the decision to treat must be carefully made.

REFERENCES

1. Aitken. North Am. Vet., 1949, *30,* 441.
2. Barnes. Mechanisms of pathogenesis of clostridial myonecrosis. Ph.D. thesis, Univ. of Minnesota, 1963.
3. Battey and Walker. Jour. Path. and Bact., 1963, *85,* 517.
4. Butler and Marsh. Jour. Am. Vet. Med. Assoc., 1956, *128,* 401.
5. Chandler and Gulasekhuram. Austral. Jour. Exp. Biol. Med. Sci., 1970, *48,* 187.
6. Clans and Macheak. Am. Jour. Vet. Res., 1972, *33,* 1031.
7. Clay. Vet. Rec., 1960, *72,* 265.
8. Jayaraman, Lal, and Dhanda. Indian Vet. Jour., 1962, *39,* 481.
9. Kerry. Vet. Rec., 1964, *76,* 396.
10. Langford. Can. Vet. Jour., 1970, *11,* 170.
11. March. Jour. Am. Vet. Med. Assoc., 1919, *56,* 319; 1922, *62,* 217.
12. Moussa. Jour. Path. and Bact., 1959, *77,* 341.
13. Shaw. Agriculture, 1958, *65,* 138.
14. Sterne and Edwards. Vet. Rec., 1955, *67,* 314.
15. Veerpoort, Joubert, and Jansen. S. Afr. Jour. Agric. Sci., 1966, *9,* 153.

Clostridium septicum

SYNONYMS: *Vibrion septique, Bacillus septicus;* probably Ghon-Sachs bacillus; also erroneously, *Bacillus edematis-maligni, Bacillus edematis*

This organism was first identified by Pasteur and Joubert (5) in 1877 from carcasses of animals thought to have died from anthrax. *C. septicum* is generally called the *malignant edema bacillus* and the condition produced in animals is termed *malignant edema.*

Morphology and Staining Reactions. *C. septicum* is a rather large rod of the shape and size of the blackleg organism. It is 0.6 to 0.8 μm wide and 3 to 8 μm long. Usually it is straight and the ends are rounded. In cultures it often occurs singly or in short chains, but in animal exudates it appears in long chains. It has already been pointed out that the tendency of this organism to form long chains on the surface of the liver of inoculated guinea pigs is a feature by which it may be distinguished from *C. chauvoei,* which occurs singly or in very short chains. Young cultures show active motility because of peritrichic flagella. The spores are oval, occur excentrically, and swell the cells in which they are formed. It is Gram-positive, but, like most of the other organisms of this group, old cultures usually decolorize. It stains readily with all the usual stains.

Cultural Features. This organism grows readily in all ordinary media so long as good anaerobic conditions prevail. In its growth vigor it differs from the blackleg organism with which it is often confused, the latter being much more fastidious in its requirements than *C. septicum.*

Colonies in deep agar usually are cottony and filamentous. In blood agar plates the colonies are surrounded by hemolytic zones. Gelatin is liquefied and a few gas bubbles are formed in it. Plain infusion broth is lightly clouded. Litmus milk is coagulated, and some gas may be formed in the curd. The curd is not digested. Coagulated blood serum and coagulated egg albumen are not digested. There is good growth in meat medium and in brain-liver medium, but there is no digestion or darkening. Acid and gas are formed from glucose, levulose, galactose, maltose, lactose, and salicin. Sucrose and mannitol are not fermented.

Fermentation products are mainly acetic and butyric acids with small amounts of isobutyl, butyl and ethyl alcohols.

Antigens. Strains of *C. septicum* are serologically heterogeneous. By antigenic analysis of their somatic and flagellar agglutinogens they can be divided into six groups defined by two O and five H antigens (4). The possession of a common spore antigen renders the straight agglutination test useless as a means of distinguishing between *C. septicum* and *C. chauvoei,* but their toxins are specific. Protection against infection with *C. septicum* is afforded, for the most part, by immunization directed against the somatic antigens.

Epidemiology and Pathogenesis. *C. septicum* is common in soil and the intestinal tract of most animal species. After death it frequently invades the body tissues from the intestine. This is especially true for ruminants.

In the living animal, the organism may enter wounds, the umbilicus of lambs, or the abomasal lining of sheep. The latter disease is known as *braxy* or *bradsot* and causes heavy mortality among yearling sheep in hilly areas of Britain, Ireland, Norway, Iceland, and the Faroes. The circumstances which favor multiplication and invasion of the abomasal mucosa are not clear, although it is known that ingestion of frosted grass is frequently associated with the occurrence of braxy. It is possible that the icy feed material devitalizes the mucosa, allowing entry of the organism. Affected animals die very suddenly without previously showing symptoms, or after only a few hours of symptoms. The walls of the abomasum and the first part of the small intestine are edematous, hemorrhagic, and sometimes necrotic. The internal organs show only degenerative changes.

Wound infections in animals are known under the general name of *malignant edema*. Such infections are characterized by rapidly extending swellings, which are soft and pit on pressure. The diseased animals show fever and other signs of intoxication, and most of them die within a few hours or in 1 or 2 days. The affected tissues are infiltrated with large quantities of gelatinous exudate, most of which is in the subcutaneous and intermuscular connective tissue. The muscular tissue is dark red but, unlike blackleg, contains little or no gas. Infections in cattle sometimes resemble blackleg very closely. In recognition of this, the organism is referred to in German literature as the *parablackleg bacillus*. It is believed that in many cases cattle and sheep suffer from a mixed infection with blackleg and other anaerobic organisms, and that the organism of blackleg in such cases often is overlooked because it grows more delicately than the others and is crowded out of cultures (2).

C. septicum causes infections not only in cattle and sheep, which are also susceptible to blackleg, but also in horses and man, who are not susceptible to blackleg, and in swine, which are only slightly susceptible. Clostridial infections are generally considered to be of little significance in poultry, but *C. septicum* infection does occur in chickens (3, 6). In a broiler flock infected with this organism the birds showed varying degrees of depression, incoordination, inappetence, and ataxia. The mortality was about 1 percent.

C. septicum produces four toxins (alpha, beta, gamma, and delta), which are responsible for the tissue damage seen in braxy and malignant edema. The alpha toxin is a lecithinase and is necrotizing, lethal, and hemolytic. The beta toxin is a deoxyribonuclease and is leukocidal. The gamma and delta toxins have hyaluronidase and hemolysin activities, respectively. These toxins increase capillary permeability and cause myonecrosis and further spread of the infection along the fascial planes of muscle. The systemic effects of the toxins and tissue breakdown products result in a fatal toxemia in 2 to 3 days.

Guinea pigs are very susceptible to inoculation with *C. septicum*. The lesions in guinea pigs cannot be distinguished from those of blackleg. A blood-tinged gelatinous exudate is found beneath the skin at the point of inoculation, and the muscular tissue is dark red in color. Gas is not usually present in the tissues. The peritoneal cavity often is moist and may have a little more fluid in it than normal. The liver is lighter than normal, having a semicooked appearance, Stained films from the liver surface show long, jointed chains of cells.

Diagnosis. If *C. septicum* is the dominant organism in the lesion or in fresh pathological material, it is probably the etiologic agent. Once putrefaction has begun there is a good chance that *C. septicum* will be present in any case, as a result of postmortem invasion from the intestine; thus the diagnosis is less certain. Specimens should also be carefully checked for *C. chauvoei*. If present, the latter should preferentially be considered the etiologic agent (8).

The most rapid and efficient method of detecting *C. septicum* or *C. chauvoei* is the fluorescent antibody technique employing antisera conjugated with contrasting-colored fluorescent dyes (1).

Immunity. Animals may be immunized by injecting them with formalinized whole culture of *C. septicum*. This usually produces lifelong immunity (7). Immunity to *C. septicum* is primarily antibacterial rather than antitoxic. High-titer *C. septicum* antitoxin has been produced in horses but has little practical value in treating infections.

Treatment. Prompt systemic and local administration of penicillin may be effective. The tetracyclines have been used to treat chickens (6).

REFERENCES

1. Batty and Walker. Bull. Off. int. Epiz., 1963, *59*, 1499.
2. Breed. Jour. Am. Vet. Med. Assoc., 1937, *90*, 521.
3. Helfer, Dickinson, and Smith. Avian Dis., 1969, *13*, 231.
4. Moussa. Jour. Path. and Bact., 1959, *77*, 341.

5. Pasteur and Joubert. Bull. Acad. Med., II Ser., 1877, *6,* 781.
6. Saunders and Bickford. Avian Dis., 1965, *9,* 317.
7. Smith, Louis. Introduction to pathogenic anaerobes. Univ. of Chicago Press, Chicago, 1954, p. 147.
8. Sterne and Thomson. Bull. Off. int. Epiz., 1963, *59,* 1487.

Clostridium colinum

This organism was first recognized with certainty by Peckham (5) in 1959 as the cause of *ulcerative enteritis* or *quail disease*. This disease had been known for many years and was originally named because of the frequency with which it was seen in bobwhite quail. The disease also occurs in a wide variety of wild and domestic avian species.

Morphology and Staining Reaction. *C. colinum* occurs in tissues and culture as a Gram-positive rod about 1 μm in width and 3 to 4 μm in length. It has oval, subterminal spores, but sporulation is infrequent. Peritrichic flagella are present, but motility is difficult to establish conclusively because of gas production by the organism.

Cultural Features. The organism is difficult to culture on the usual media but grows readily on tryptose-phosphate-glucose-yeast agar or broth with 8 percent sterile citrated horse plasma added. The colonies on agar are 1 to 3 mm in diameter, semiconvex with a filamentous margin, semitranslucent, grayish, and glossy. Some strains are beta-hemolytic. Fructose, glucose, maltose, sucrose, raffinose, and trehalose are fermented. Acetic and formic acids are the principal fermentation products. Indol, hydrogen sulfide, urease, catalase, and lecithinase are not produced.

Epidemiology and Pathogenesis. The ecology of *C. colinum* has not yet been worked out. The disease has been described in game birds such as bobwhite quail, partridge, grouse, and young domestic chickens and turkeys. Natural infection occurs probably via the oral route. Experimentally, it has been shown that at least 10^6 organisms *per os* are required to produce the disease in quail (2). Chickens are much more resistant, and the disease in this host has been observed only after outbreaks of coccidiosis or infectious bursal disease (8). Overcrowding and poor sanitation have been noted to be predisposing causes in grouse (4). Intestinal contents are infective (7), and it must be presumed that the organism is shed in the feces. Quail that develop a chronic form of the disease have been shown to remain carriers of infection (1).

After oral infection the organism enters the intestine and then passes into the portal circulation and lodges in the liver, where diffuse liver necrosis is produced. The necrosis is centrilobular or diffuse pinpoint to coagulative, and many bacteria are present (3). The intestine becomes ulcerated along the lower third of its length. The ulcers vary from about 0.1 mm to 2 or 3 mm in diameter. In some birds, extensive spleen necrosis occurs. A toxin has not been implicated in the pathogenesis of *C. colinum* lesions (3). Birds may die in a day or two or linger for a week. Affected birds are inactive, sluggish, and anorexic. In the later stages they cannot move and die within a few hours. Chronically affected quail become emaciated and pass watery feces.

Diagnosis. The disease must be diagnosed by the isolation and identification of *C. colinum* from the lesions. No other diagnostic procedures are as yet available. The incorporation of polymyxin B (25 mcg per ml) in the isolation medium facilitates isolation from intestinal contents.

Treatment. The organism is sensitive to tetracyclines, penicillin, bacitracin, and furacin. Streptomycin is apparently effective in control of the naturally occurring disease (6), although the organism is resistant to this antibiotic *in vitro*.

REFERENCES

1. Bass. Proc. Soc. Exp. Biol. and Med., 1939, *42,* 377.
2. Berkhoff and Campbell. Avian Dis., 1974, *18,* 205.
3. Berkhoff, Campbell, Naylor, and Smith. Avian Dis., 1974, *18,* 195.
4. Le Dune. Vet. Med., 1935, *30,* 394.
5. Peckham. Avian Dis., 1959, *3,* 471.
6. Peckham. *In* Diseases of poultry, 9th ed., ed. Hofstad *et al.* Iowa State Univ. Press, Ames, Iowa, 1972.
7. Shillinger and Morley. Jour. Am. Vet. Med. Assoc., 1934, *84,* 776.
8. Wilter. Proc. 26th Northeastern Conf. of Lab. Workers in Pullorum Disease Control, June, 1952.

21 The Genus *Listeria*

There are four species described in the genus *Listeria* of which only one, *Listeria monocytogenes,* is pathogenic for warm-blooded animals.

Listeria monocytogenes

SYNONYM: *Listerella monocytogenes*

Morphology and Staining Reactions. This organism occurs in the form of small rods, 1 to 2 μm in length (Figure 21.1), which frequently show slight clubbing and therefore appear like diphtheroids. Coccoid elements are commonly found. Young cultures are motile by peritrichic flagella when grown at 20 to 25 C and exhibit a tumbling motility. Spores are not produced. It is Gram-positive and non-acid-fast. Gram-negative cells can usually be found in young cultures, and old cultures often are nearly wholly Gram-negative.

Figure 21.1. *Listeria monocytogenes,* a culture from a serum-agar slant incubated for 18 hours at 37 C. × 1,000.

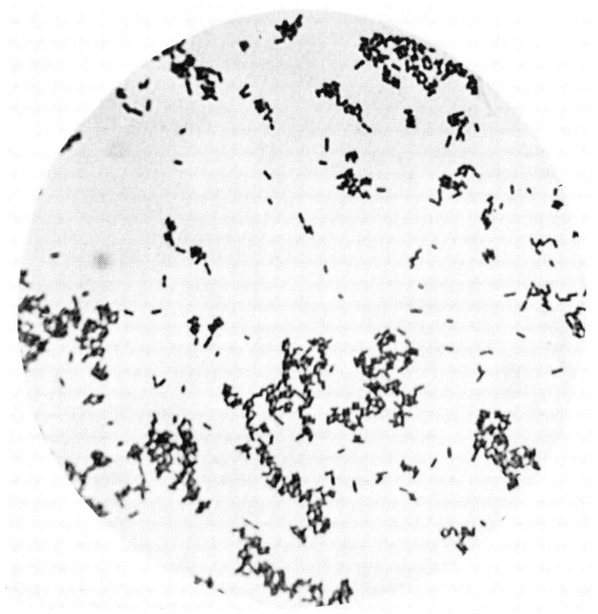

Culture Features. Growth occurs on most of the ordinary laboratory media, although it is never abundant. In general, the gross features of cultures resmble those of streptococci. The colonies may be seen after 24 hours' incubation at 37 C as minute points (deep colonies) and as small, flat, bluish-white, transparent surface colonies. The deep colonies are surrounded by narrow zones of hemolysis of the beta type (Figure 21.2) and this characteristic makes them conspicuous. The surface colonies seldom if ever exceed 1 mm in diameter and on clear solid media appear blue-green when illuminated by oblique light. Stab cultures in gelatin appear as an "inverted fir tree" growth or as a line of discrete colonies along the stab.

Acid without gas is formed from glucose, rhamnose, and salicin within 48 hours. Acid but no gas is sometimes produced in 3 to 10 days in arabinose, galactose, lactose, maltose, rhamnose, sucrose, dextrin, sorbitol, and glycerol. Hydrogen sulfide and indol are not formed. Unlike *Erysipelothrix rhusiopathiae, L. monocytogenes* produces catalase, and this test is a simple method of differentiating these organisms.

Resistance. *L. monocytogenes* is ubiquitous in nature and in animal and human feces. It survives for years in soil (4), milk, silage, and feces (9). A major factor in

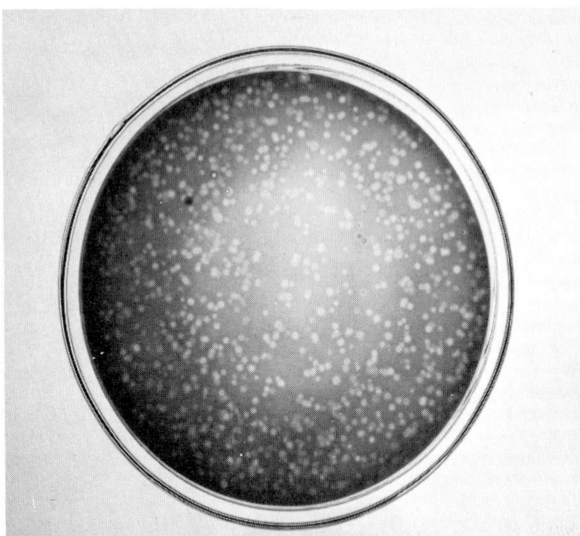

Figure 21.2. *Listeria monocytogenes,* a blood agar plate incubated at 37 C for 24 hours. The colonies are not discernible in the photograph. They are very minute, each being surrounded by a sharply defined but narrow zone of beta-type hemolysis.

survival is pH: above a pH of 5.0 the organism multiplies; below this figure, survival of the organism is poor (19). This effect appears to be associated with the lactic microflora in low-pH silage (12). It is more heat-tolerant than most other nonsporulating bacteria and has been shown to survive pasteurization by the low-temperature holding process (2). Pasteurization is unlikely to be effective if the number of organisms exceeds 1,000 per ml of milk.

Antigens. There are somatic ("O") and flagellar ("H") antigens expressed by *L. monocytogenes.* Fifteen O antigens (I to XV inclusive) and 4 H antigens (A to D inclusive) are described (32, 36). Serotypes are assigned according to the antigenic formula and are given arabic numbers and lowercase letters. There are seven serotypes and 11 subtypes. Cattle and sheep are commonly infected with serotypes 1 or 4b.

Epidemiology and Pathogenesis. Because the organism is widely distributed in soil, vegetation, and feces, most animals experience exposure to the organism during their lifetimes. Ruminants exhibit especially high rates of isolation of *L. monocytogenes* from their feces—a reflection of their exposure to large quantities of contaminated herbage. The organism is also commonly found in tissues, such as swine tonsils (15), and lymph nodes of apparently healthy animals (16). Also, many healthy animals are seropositive (16). *L. monocytogenes* is common in poor-quality silage where the pH is greater than 5.0, and ruminants fed on such material are much more likely to develop listeriosis (20). The same serotype has been found in silage and in tissues of affected animals fed this silage. The association of listeriosis with silage in Iceland was so striking that the disease in that country has been named *Votheysveiki* ("silage disease").

Intercurrent disease, climatic and other stresses, and pregnancy are important predisposing factors in the occurrence of listeriosis. Thus the disease is more common in sheep and cattle in winter and early spring. Viral damage to mucosal surfaces may also be a factor in allowing the organism to breach epithelial barriers. The organism is a facultative intracellular parasite, and stresses which diminish the host's immune competence may allow the parasite to escape from phagocytic cells and to multiply out of control and so cause disease.

The initial mode of entry of *L. monocytogenes* into the animal is usually ingestion, although infection has been demonstrated through the nasal mucosa and along branches of the trigeminal nerve (7). Direct infection of the conjunctiva in cattle has also occurred as a result of silage particles falling into the faces of browsing cattle (29). Entry of the organism through the intestinal epithelial barrier into the tissues is not well understood. Experimental intestinal infections (33) have indicated that the organism can enter and multiply in ileal cells and then pass directly from cell to cell. Infected cells eventually degenerate. This degeneration is potentiated by neutrophils which are attracted toward infected cells. Infection eventually involves the Peyer's patches and the liver. A bacteremic or septicemic phase may then develop, depending on the immune status of the animal.

In the pregnant animal, the organism may localize in the placentomes and then enter the amniotic fluid. The fetus aspirates the organism, which multiplies and kills it. Abortion then occurs. Abortions in cattle usually occur in the second half of pregnancy and in sheep and goats are seen at a late stage of gestation.

Primary listeric septicemia is much more common in young than in adult ruminants, whereas in monogastric animals, septicemia is the most common form of listeriosis irrespective of age (14). Death may occur suddenly or after an illness of a few days' duration characterized by depression, dyspnea, slobbering, nasal discharge, and lacrimation. At necropsy focal necrosis of the liver, spleen, and abdominal lymph nodes are seen. Enteritis and occasionally mycocardial necrosis occur. The pathogenesis of the focal hepatic necrosis has been studied by Siddique *et al.* (39), who observed that *L. monocytogenes* enters hepatic cells by endocytosis, where it is initially found in a membrane-bound vesicle. The hepatic cell dies, leading to multiple necrotic foci in the parenchyma. This toxic effect is poorly understood. Phospholipase and lipase activities have been associated with some strains of *L. monocytogenes* (21) and can cause cell membrane damage. Also, Watson and Lavizzo (41) have described hemolytic and lipolytic antigens that are toxic for mouse macrophages and may be similar to the enzymes described above.

Meningoencephalitis is perhaps the most easily recognized form of listeriosis seen in domestic animals. The name *circling disease* was given by Gill (11) in 1931 to this disease in sheep in New Zealand. The disease has since been observed in cattle and sheep in many parts of the world. Affected animals may move in circles in one direction, may exhibit unilateral facial paralysis, and have difficulty in swallowing. Fever, blindness, and headpressing are also commonly observed. The disease may progress until the animal is completely paralyzed and dies within 2 or 3 days. During these later stages, many animals make constant chewing motions.

In the encephalomyelitic form the cerebrospinal fluid may be cloudy because of an increased globulin and leukocyte content. There may be some congestion of the meninges. Usually the visceral organs show little or no evidence of disease. Sections of the brain of such animals show polymorphonuclear and mononuclear foci in the white matter of the cerebrum and cerebellum and perivascular cuffing with mononuclear cells (Figure 21.3). Areas of malacia occur in the pons and medulla oblongata (6), with loss of parenchyma and accumulations of macrophages. Bacteria are not found in the latter, but rather are seen in neutrophils in the area. The cause of the malacia is unclear, but possibly is caused by phospholipase released by the organism. Charlton and Garcia (7) have provided an excellent description of the histologic features of spontaneously occurring encephalitic listeriosis in sheep. Diffuse and focal intrafasicular and perineural accumulations of lymphocytes and plasma cells unilaterally involve the trigeminal nerve. Accumulations of *Listeria monocytogenes* in proximal parts of damaged cranial nerves and sometimes in intact nerve fibers was suggestive of centripetal migration of the organism along the trigeminal nerve to the brain (Figure 21.4). Charlton and Garcia postulated that further dissemination within the brain probably occurs by means of intra-asconal movement. Other workers have also suggested that the organism may enter the brain following entry through the mucosa of the nasopharynx and

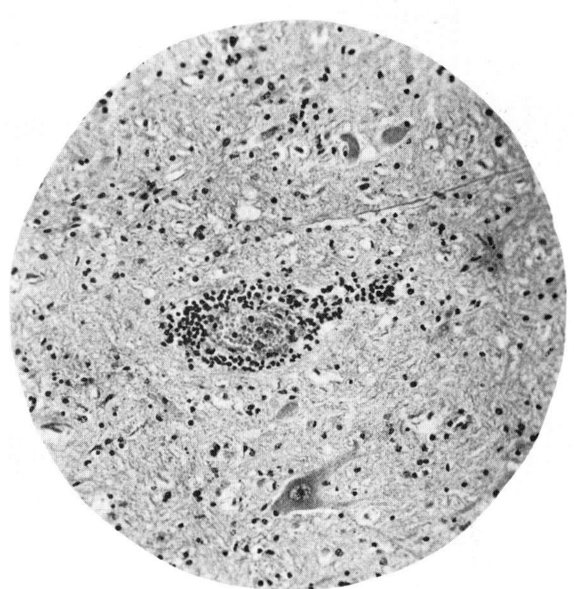

Figure 21.3. Listeriosis in the brain of a cow. The cells infiltrating the brain substance are both mononuclears and polymorphonuclears. There is marked perivascular cuffing. × 65. (Courtesy S. H. McNutt.)

upward migration along either the first cranial or the trigeminal nerve (1). However, listeric encephalomyelitis also has been frequently observed as a sequel to and in conjunction with septicemia; thus hematogenous spread of the organism to brain tissue must occur also.

Listeriosis in chickens sometimes exhibits distinctive features (13). Necrotic myocarditis may be observed, accompanied by fluid in the peritoneal and pericardial cavities, muscle edema, and focal necrosis of the liver. The septicemic disease is the form most often seen. Intercurrent diseases of bacterial, viral, and parasitic origin are important predisposing factors in the occurrence of listeriosis in poultry (32).

In horses, listeriosis usually presents the septicemic form. Emerson and Jarvis (10) described listeriosis in ponies where the symptoms were fever, mild colic, restlessness, depression, anorexia, jaundice, and reddish urine. McCain and Robinson (25) described two cases of the septicemic disease. The organism was isolated from blood, liver, and skeletal musculature. Many apparently healthy horses are serologically positive (23).

Listeriosis has been described in many other domestic and feral species, including rodents raised for food, laboratory use, or pelts. The disease is usually septicemic,

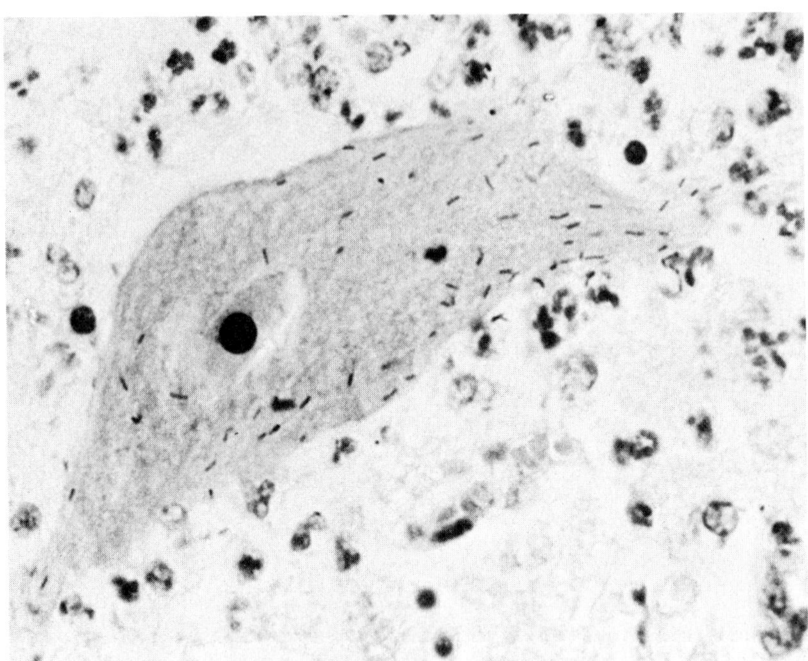

Figure 21.4. *Listeria monocytogenes* in a large neuron from an infected sheep. Giemsa stain. × 1,050. (From K. M. Charlton and M. M. Garcia, *Vet. Path.*, 1977, *14*, 297.)

but rabbits and chinchillas also have a characteristic hemorrhagic and necrotic metritis which may or may not be associated with abortion (14). Central nervous system involvement is occasionally observed. Conjunctival instillation of *L. monocytogenes* results in a purulent conjunctivitis in the rabbit and guinea pig—the Anton reaction. The organism rapidly enters conjunctival epithelial cells and thereafter is indirectly chemotactic to neutrophils.

In man, listeriosis is a cause of abortion, perinatal infection, septicemia, and meningoencephalitis. Persons with immunosuppressive underlying disorders are especially at risk (5) and usually exhibit a bacteremic form of the disease which in some cases may be complicated by meningitis. In contrast to ruminants, where the primary nervous lesion is encephalitis, nervous lesions in man primarily involve the meninges. The source of infection for man is unclear, but statistics on human cases indicate that animal contact is not an important factor (28). Some human infections may result from consumption of milk, because the organism may be shed from the bovine udder (16, 38). A high rate of seropositivity in the agglutination test has been recorded (17).

Immunity. Immunity to *L. monocytogenes* is cell-mediated by means of rapidly dividing, short-lived T lymphocytes (24, 30). Antibody, often at high titers, is produced by clinically affected animals but does not play an important role in resolution of the disease (16).

Antibodies may be detected by growth-inhibition (35), precipitin (8, 36), complement-fixation (36), passive-immunohemolysis (4), and hemagglutination tests (34). Because of cross-reactions with other organisms, a high rate of seropositivity in normal animals, and a lack of antibody responsiveness in many clinically infected animals, antibody titers are seldom measured. There are no vaccines in use in the United States. In Russia, an avirulent strain (AUF) is used in sheep and is reported to give 100 percent protection for 10 months (37).

Diagnosis. The encephalitic form of the disease is diagnosed by characteristic perivascular cuffing with mononuclear cells and focal necrosis in the pons, medulla, and anterior spinal cord. Brain tissue may be cultured directly on blood agar, but should also be macerated in nutrient broth, stored at 4 C, and subcultured onto colistin–nalidixic acid agar (CNA agar) at weekly intervals if the direct culture is negative. The organism is difficult to demonstrate in cerebrospinal fluid of ruminants with encephalitis, possibly because it is confined to lesions in the brain parenchyma.

Inhibitory solid and fluid media containing nalidixic acid, trypaflavine, and serum have been developed and are excellent for isolation from contaminated specimens (genital exudates, fetuses, feces, etc.). In the diagnostic laboratory of the New York State College of Veterinary Medicine, CNA agar is routinely and successfully used for diagnosis of listeriosis in the bovine and sheep.

The fluorescent-antibody technique (40) is rapid, but false-positives may occur because of cross-reacting antibodies in the conjugate. The occurrence of monocytosis is not useful in the diagnosis of listeriosis in ruminants because it is seen only in monogastric animals (14).

Treatment. Ampicillin and benzyl penicillin G exert a bacteriostatic rather than a bactericidal action on *L. monocytogenes*, but both are often therapeutically effective (22, 26). Treatment failures also occur. Intrathecal ampicillin has been used for treatment of listeria meningitis in man (22). Olafson (31) has treated circling disease of ruminants with sulfonamides with some success. Jensen and Mackey (18) have found penicillin and sulfanilamide and Bennett *et al.* (3) have found tetracyclines to be effective in the early stages of listeriosis in animals.

It appears that penicillin and gentamicin in combination have a bactericidal effect on *Listeria* and may be more effective therapeutically than either antibiotic used singly (27).

REFERENCES

1. Asahi, Hodosa, and Akiyama. Am. Jour. Vet. Res., 1957, *18,* 147.
2. Bearns and Girard. Can. Jour. Microbiol., 1958, *4,* 55.
3. Bennett, Russell, and Derivaux. Antibiotics and Chemother., 1952, *2,* 102.
4. Bind, Maupos, Chiron, and Raynaud. *In* Problems of listeriosis, ed. Malcolm Woodbine. Leicester Univ. Press, 1976, pp. 242–50.
5. Bottone and Sierra. Mount Sinai Jour. of Med., 1977, *44,* 42.
6. Charlton. Vet. Path., 1977, *14,* 429.
7. Charlton and Garcia. Vet. Path., 1977, *14,* 297.
8. Drew. Proc. Soc. Exp. Biol. and Med., 1946, *61,* 30.
9. Dykstra. *In* Problems of listeriosis, ed. Malcolm Woodbine. Leicester Univ. Press, 1976, pp. 71–73.
10. Emerson and Jarvis. Jour. Am. Vet. Med. Assoc., 1968, *152,* 1645.
11. Gill. Vet. Jour., 1931, *87,* 60; 1933, *89,* 258.
12. Gouet, Girardeau, and Riou. Am. Feed. Sci. and Technol., 1977, *2,* 297.
13. Gray. Avian Dis., 1958, *2,* 296.
14. Gray and Killinger. Bact. Rev., 1966, *30,* 309.
15. Hohne, Loose, and Seeliger. *In* Problems of listeriosis, ed. Malcolm Woodbine. Leicester Univ. Press, 1976, pp. 125–30.
16. Hyslop. *In* Problems of listeriosis, ed. Malcolm Woodbine. Leicester Univ. Press, 1976, pp. 91–103.
17. Jasinska, Lewandowsk, Sobiech, Adamczewski, and Radzimski. Weterinaria Westeryn gosp. Wroclaw, 1969, *24,* 53.
18. Jensen and Mackey. Jour. Am. Vet. Med. Assoc., 1949, *114,* 420.
19. Kahn, Seaman, and Woodbine. Zentrbl. f. Bakt., 1973, *224,* 355–361.
20. Kruger. Arch. f. Exp. Vetmed., 1963, *17,* 181.
21. Leighton, Threlfall, and Oakley. *In* Problems of listeriosis, ed. Malcolm Woodbine. Leicester Univ. Press, 1976, pp. 239–241.
22. Macnair, White, and Grahm. Lancet, 1968, *1,* 16.
23. Mayer, Seeliger, Sickel, and Kinzler. Berl. and Münch. tierärztl. Wchnschr., 1975, *88,* 345.
24. Mackaness. Jour. Exp. Med., 1966, *120,* 105.
25. McCain and Robinson. Proc. 18th Ann. Meeting Am. Assoc. of Vet Lab. Diagnosticians, Portland, Ore., 1975, p. 257.
26. Medoff, Kunz, and Weinberg. Jour. Inf. Dis., 1971, *123,* 247.
27. Mohan, Gordon, Beaman, Belding, Luecke, Edminton, and Gerhardt. Jour. Inf. Dis., 1977, *135,* 51.
28. Moore and Zehmer. Jour. Inf. Dis., 1973, *127,* 610.
29. Morgan. Vet. Rec., 1977, *100,* 113.
30. North. Jour. Exp. Med., 1973, *138,* 342.
31. Olafson. Cornell Vet., 1940, *30,* 141.
32. Patterson. Jour. Path. and Bact., 1940, *51,* 427.
33. Racz, Tenner, and Kaiserling. *In* Problems of listeriosis, ed. Malcolm Woodbine. Leicester Univ. Press, 1976, pp. 71–73.
34. Sachse and Potel. Zeitsch. Immunitaetisforsch Exp. Therap., 1957, *114,* 472.
35. Schafer. Inaugural diss. Tierärztl. Hochschule, Hannover, 1976.
36. Seeliger. *In* Listeriosis, 2nd ed. Hafner, New York, 1961.
37. Selivanov, Sedov, and Kotylena. Uchenye Zopiski Kazanskogo, Veterinarnogo Instituta, 1972, *112,* 123.
38. Sipka, Stajner, and Zakula. Wiener tierärztl. Monatsch., 1973, *60,* 50.
39. Siddique, McKenzie, Sapp, and Rich. Am. Jour. Vet. Res., 1958, *39,* 887.
40. Smith, Marshall, and Eveland. Proc. Soc. Exp. Biol. and Med., 1960, *103,* 842.
41. Watson and Lavizzo. Inf. and Immun., 1973, *7,* 753.
42. Welshimer. Jour. Bact., 1960, *80,* 316.

22 The Genus *Corynebacterium*

The genus *Corynebacterium* contains a large number of species and includes important animal parasites and pathogens, plant pathogens, and nonpathogenic bacteria. *Corynebacterium diphtheriae,* the cause of human diphtheria, is the type species of the genus, and other members have been traditionally described as diptheroid (diphtherialike) bacilli.

The corynebacteria are Gram-positive, at least when the cells are young, and they show a rather high degree of pleomorphism (different morphologies). They are straight to slightly curved rods with irregularly stained segments, and they sometimes have granules. They frequently show club-shaped swellings at one or both ends, giving rise to the name *Corynebacterium* (club bacterium). Snapping division produces angular and palisade (fence of stakes) arrays of cells, an arrangement that is not common in any other type of bacteria except the acid-fast organisms. The corynebacteria are not acid-fast and they do not form spores. The pathogenic species are nonmotile, aerobic, and facultatively anaerobic.

The traditional method of classifying these bacteria on the basis of their morphology has been recently questioned, because many other types of bacteria also become pleomorphic under conditions that make for unbalanced cell-wall synthesis (2). Microbiologists now suggest that the cell-wall composition is a more valid basis for classification. On the basis of the cell-wall sugars, lipids, and antigens, a close association can be demonstrated between the corynebacteria, the mycobacteria, and the nocardias. Using these criteria, the following species might validly be included in the genus *Corynebacterium: C. diphtheriae, C. bovis, C. equi, C. pseudotuberculosis* (*ovis*), and *C. renale.* On the other hand, *C. pyogenes* and *C. hemolyticum,* although they are pleomorphic, have different biochemical characteristics and different structural components, and they share a cell-wall antigen with streptococci of Lancefield's group G. For these reasons, reclassification of these two pathogenic species has been suggested (2).

Corynebacterium pyogenes

This species is aptly named *pyogenes* (pus producer) because it is frequently associated with the production of pus, particularly in ruminants. It is found in abscesses in cattle, sheep, goats, and swine, and occasionally in other animals, but it rarely affects man.

Morphology and Staining Reactions. *C. pyogenes* most often occurs as small slender rods, which frequently are slightly curved and often clubbed at one end (Figure 22.1). The individual elements are usually short, and some strains form chains that are hard to distinguish from streptococci. Wide variation in morphology exists between different strains, and between individual cells of a single strain. The organism is nonmotile and never forms a capsule. It is Gram-positive.

Cultural Features. Ordinarily there is no growth on plain agar or in plain broth unless a considerable amount of blood, tissue, or tissue debris is carried over in the inoculum. It grows readily in milk and on coagulated

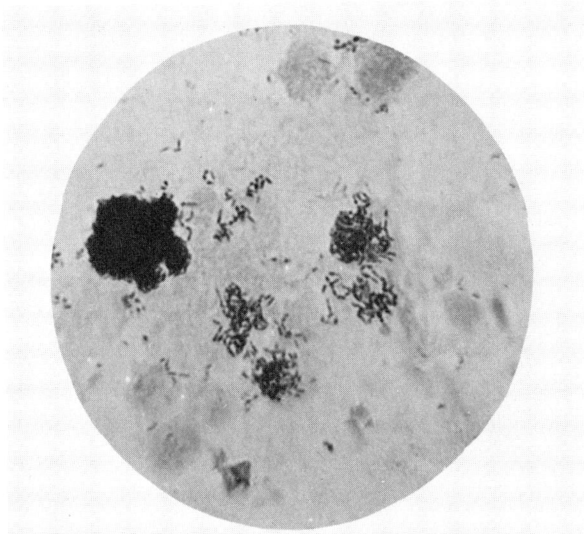

Figure 22.1. *Corynebacterium pyogenes*, a film from vegetations on the heart valve of a calf. × 1,030.

serum slants, where a trough of liquefaction develops along the lines of growth.

A few drops of blood or blood serum make all of the usual laboratory media favorable for the growth of this organism. In fluid media the growth is granular and sinks to the bottom of the tube.

Figure 22.2. *Corynebacterium pyogenes*, a blood agar plate incubated for 36 hours at 37 C. The colonies may be discerned as minute points surrounded by narrow zones of clear hemolysis. Blood plates incubated overnight may have numerous colonies on them, but they are likely to be overlooked unless they are inspected with great care because the hemolytic zones at that time have not appeared. At about 24 hours' incubation the hemolytic zones begin to appear, but they are not well developed until about 36 hours.

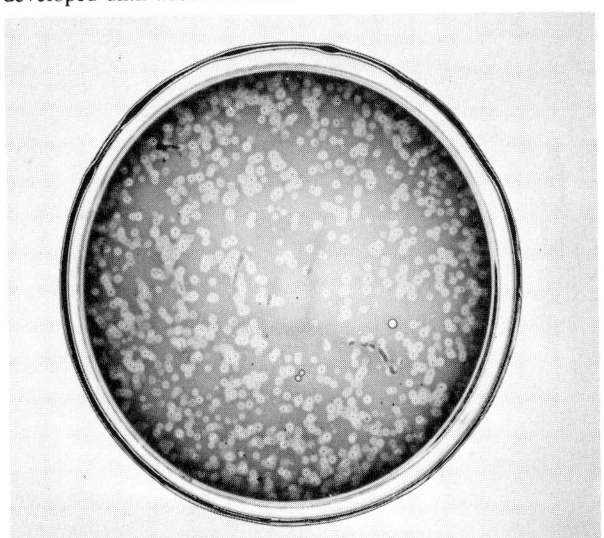

On blood agar plates the organism *C. pyogenes* is hemolytic and colonies are very small and translucent. After an 18-hour incubation at 37 C they may easily be overlooked, for at that time there is no evidence of hemolysis. After approximately 24 hours, hemolysis begins to be evident, making the colonies conspicuous. The zones of hemolysis are exceedingly clear but always narrow, seldom exceeding 2 mm in diameter (Figure 22.2).

Growth occurs best at body temperature. The minimum temperature of growth is about 24 C. The organism is aerobic and facultatively anaerobic. Indol, hydrogen sulfide, and nitrites are not produced. Gelatin is liquefied. An excellent description is given by Brown and Orcutt (3), and the organism's characteristic properties are shown in Table 22.1. An unusual strain, associated with bovine mastitis has been described by Afnan (1).

Resistance. *C. pyogenes* is a very delicate organism. It is easily destroyed by heat, drying, and ordinary disinfectants.

Pathogenicity for Experimental Animals. Guinea pigs, rats, and mice are quite resistant to infection. Subcutaneous injections of cultures produce abscesses, which usually develop slowly and become well encapsulated.

Rabbits are most susceptible. After intravenous injection no immediate effects are seen, but in 2 or 3 weeks the animals begin to lose weight and may become lame or paralyzed. Abscesses may develop in the kidneys, lymph nodes, or the muscular tissue, but more often they are found in the bones or joints. Paralysis usually is caused by the formation of an abscess in the vertebral column, which exerts pressure on the spinal cord.

According to Gwatkin (6), the superficial injection of a pure culture into the tongue of a calf resulted in the formation of a hard lump in the tissue beneath the inoculated area. This was accompanied by erosion of the mucous membrane and extrusion of pus. Rubbing the organisms on the tongue produced no lesions.

Corynebacterial Infections. *In Cattle*. Throughout the world, *C. pyogenes* is associated with pyogenic infections of cattle where it is commonly found in abscesses and purulent infections of various organs and tissues. These infections are usually sporadic. *C. pyogenes* may be the primary agent involved or it may occur in association with other bacteria and invade devitalized tissues. *C. pyogenes* is found in association with one distinct disease entity, summer mastitis in cattle. The organism is particularly common in pneumonias in calves and adult

Table 22.1. Differential characteristics of *Corynebacterium* sp. important in infectious diseases of domesticated animals

Characteristic	*C. pyogenes*	*C. renale*	*C. pseudotuberculosis (ovis)*	*C. equi*	*C. bovis*	*C. suis*†
Hemolysis	+	−	+	−	−	−
Catalase production	−	+	+	+	+	−
Liquefaction of inspissated serum	+	−	−	−	−	−
Casein hydrolysis	−	+	−	−	−	−
Pigment production	−	−	−	+ (pink)	−	−
Metachromatic granules	−	+	+	−	−	−
Acid from glucose	+	+	+	−	−	+
Acid from lactose	+	V	V	−	−	−
Acid from maltose	+	V	+	−	−	+
Acid from starch	+	V	+	−	−	+
Nitrate reduction	−	+	±*	+	−	−
Urease production	−	+	+	+	−	+

+ = positive reaction; V = variable reaction; − = negative reaction.
*Most isolates from horses and cattle are positive.
†*C. suis* is anaerobic.

cattle, where it is presumed to be a secondary invader and produces a suppurative pneumonia.

C. pyogenes can be found in a great variety of suppurative conditions in cattle. Abscesses caused by this organism usually develop slowly and often have heavy fibrous capsules. The pus may be thick, greenish white, and nonodorous, or it may be thin and fetid, especially when other organisms are present. Cardiac valvular vegetations are frequently associated with this organism, and it often causes destructive arthritis in calves. The organism has been found in the normal uterus, but it can produce endometritis and pyometritis in cattle, frequently accompanied by staphylococci and associated with calving, retained placenta, and proliferation of the bacteria during the luteal phase of the estrus cycle. *C. pyogenes* has been implicated as a cause of abortions in cattle (7) and seminal vesiculitis and lowered fertility in bulls. In addition to these sporadic supperative infections, *C. pyogenes* has been associated with a number of cases of generalized lymphadenitis in cattle in Scotland. These animals had generalized abscessation of the lungs, joints, and subcutaneous tissues of the legs and lumbar region. *C. pyogenes* was isolated in pure cultures from these lesions (5).

Mastitis. In Europe, mastitis in dairy cows and heifers which is caused by *C. pyogenes* has a marked seasonal incidence and is known as *summer mastitis*. Flies are thought to be important vectors of the organism—hence the high incidence at the height of the fly season—but they are not the sole vectors. In North America the seasonal incidence is not so marked and it is thought to be transmitted in another fashion or precipitated by unknown factors that cause the commensal organism to proliferate and produce mastitis.

The disease may be sporadic or involve a number of animals in the herd. Affected quarters usually suffer extensive permanent damage. *C. pyogenes* sometimes causes damage to the immature udders of young calves that are kept together and have developed the habit of suckling each other. In these animals secondary infections of the joints may result in suppurative arthritis, which usually leads to death.

In swine. The character and location of the lesions in swine are much like those in cattle. Generally in association with other pyogenic organisms, *C. pyogenes* is commonly found in suppurative pneumonias and, in fact, in nearly all suppurative conditions. Multiple joint involvement not infrequently occurs as a part of these infections. This often appears after farrowing, which probably means that uterine infections are the primary localizations. Stiffness of gait, lameness, progressive cachexia, pneumonia, and paralysis of the hindquarters are often seen.

In sheep and goats. Chronic purulent pneumonia and joint infections of sheep resulting in acute lameness are frequently caused by *C. pyogenes*. Its presence is associated with much connective tissue formation and with pleurisy, accompanied by an ill-smelling pleural exudate.

Cameron and Britton (4) have described a type of *C. pyogenes* infection in sheep fed upon large amounts of grain, especially barley, in which bilateral deep-seated chronic abscesses developed in the larynx. They were believed to be caused by abrasions resulting from gulping the grain. Affected lambs breathe with great difficulty, and the mortality rate is high.

In other animals. Zaki and Farrag (11) have reported *C. pyogenes* to be a rare cause of metritis in the horse and of pyometritis in the dog. It is commonly associated with pneumonia in the camel and has been isolated from traumatic reticulitis in the buffalo and from septicemias and suppurative lesions in birds held in captivity.

Mode of Transmission. *C. pyogenes* has a worldwide distribution in cattle and is known to live on the mucous membranes of healthy animals. Commonly found on the tonsils and in the retropharyngeal lymph nodes, it can also be isolated from the nasal cavities and the udders of apparently normal heifers (8). This organism is an opportunist that gains entry through the umbilicus in calves, through wounds and abrasions of the skin, and following traumatic reticulitis in adult cattle. Frequently a secondary invader in tissues devitalized by bacterial or viral infections, *C. pyogenes* has been reported to have a synergistic relationship with *Fusobacterium necrophorum* in mixed infections involving both organisms (10).

The mode of transmission of the organism is not always apparent. When it occurs in sporadic abscesses, it may follow existing tissue damage at a wound. However, the role of flies as vectors in mastitis is still debated, as is the possibility of invasion via the teat canal or by the hematogenous route.

Diagnosis. The presence of *C. pyogenes* in inflammatory exudates is best demonstrated by staining smears of the exudate and examining them for the presence of pleomorphic, Gram-positive rods, and by making cultures on blood agar plates. The culture should be incubated for not less than 36 hours at 37 C unless other organisms threaten to overrun the plate. The minute, distinctive colonies are surrounded by sharp, clear, narrow zones of hemolysis. These colonies should be picked up and transferred to blood agar slants. The subcultures can be identified by their action on litmus milk and especially by their ability to liquefy solidified blood serum slants. Failure to produce catalase and reduce nitrates are other identifying characteristics.

Immunity. Little is known about immunity to this organism. Although a large number of vaccines, toxoids, and antisera have been used to prevent and treat diseases caused by *C. pyogenes,* particularly summer mastitis, their efficacy is equivocal.

Chemotherapy. Although *C. pyogenes* is sensitive to penicillin and some of the other antibiotics *in vitro,* it usually will not respond *in vivo.* This probably is due to the tissue reaction, which walls off the organism and makes it inaccessible to antibiotics. The unsuitable environment within an abscess, replete with cell debris and rich in enzymes released from phagocytic cells, may also render antibiotics ineffective.

The Disease in Man. On rare occasions, *C. pyogenes* causes infection in man. It has produced sporadic infections in persons associated with animals—notably a fatal infection in a French shepherd and an osteomyelitis in a German horse dealer. Infection of human feet devitalized by frostbite, and vulvovaginitis in 32 Japanese women have also been attributed to *C. pyogenes* (9).

REFERENCES

1. Afnan. Vet. Rec., 1970, *86,* 229.
2. Barksdale. Bact. Rev., 1970, *34,* 378.
3. Brown and Orcutt. Jour. Exp. Med., 1920, *32,* 219.
4. Cameron and Britton. Cornell Vet., 1943, *22,* 265.
5. Cowie. Vet. Rec., 1962, *74,* 258.
6. Gwatkin. Can. Jour. Comp. Med. and Vet. Sci., 1952, *16,* 422.
7. Hinton. Vet. Bull., 1972, *42,* 753.
8. Mattermann and Horsch. Arch. f. Exp. Vetmed., 1977, *31,* 405.
9. Purdom, Seaman, and Woodbine. Vet. Bull., 1958, *4,* 55.
10. Roberts. Brit. Jour. Exp. Path., 1967, *48,* 674.
11. Zaki and Farrag. Vet. Med., 1955, *50,* 219.

Corynebacterium renale

SYNONYMS: *Bacillus renalis bovis, Bacillus pyelonephritidis bovis*

This organism is found principally in cattle, but it also has been seen in horses and sheep, and one case has been described in a dog (14). Female animals are affected much more commonly than males (2). The organism has been found only in the urinary tract, where it produces a diphtheritic inflammation of the urinary bladder, or the ureters, of the kidney pelvis, and frequently of the kidney tissue itself (4). The lesions are characteristic and are similar in the several species affected. The disease is known under several different names: *bacillary pyelonephritis of cattle, specific pyelonephritis of cattle, infectious pyelonephritis of cattle.*

Morphology and Staining Reactions. *C. renale* is a rather large diphtheroid bacillus. Individual organisms do not vary greatly in morphology, all being rather short stumpy rods that are usually a little thicker at one end than at the other (Figure 22.3). In exudates and in cultures, the organisms are found in clumps varying from a few cells to many hundreds. They are nonmotile, nonspore-

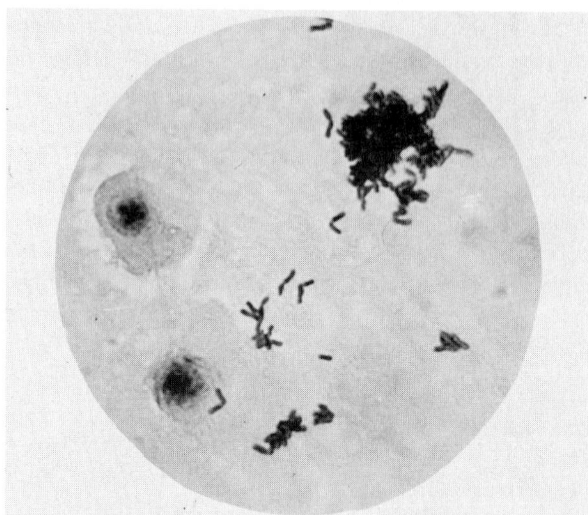

Figure 22.3. *Corynebacterium renale,* a film from urine of a naturally infected cow.

bearing, and nonencapsulated. Strongly Gram-positive, they stain readily with the usual stains. Bars and granules are sometimes seen when *C. renale* is stained with methylene blue.

Cultural Features. Growth occurs in all of the ordinary laboratory media but is greatly favored by a little blood or serum. For isolation purposes blood plates are most convenient. After 24 hours' incubation at 37 C, *C. renale* colonies are observed as minute opaque bodies. After 48 hours the colonies become larger than those of streptococci, but smaller than those of staphylococci. The older colonies are opaque and ivory-colored, and the margins are uneven. Their surfaces look dull, and they do not lyse the blood cells.

In broth and other liquid media there may be slight clouding, but most of the growth appears in the form of a granular sediment. A characteristic reaction is seen in litmus milk. It begins with the reduction of the litmus in the bottom of the tube, followed by the formation of a soft curd, which is slowly digested. The medium is alkaline at all times. Finally the medium separates into a dark red fluid and a heavy sediment. The main differential characteristics of *C. renale* are presented in Table 22.1.

Lovell (11) called attention to a characteristic reaction of *C. renale* when grown on agar to which 10 percent sterilized skim milk had been added. The colonies develop with a cream-to-yellow pigmentation, and after 48 hours each colony is surrounded by a wide halo or zone of translucency. Later these zones become indistinct. Apparently they are caused by digestion of the suspended casein molecules. The reaction is not diagnostic, but because it is given by most strains of *C. renale* and seldom by other diphtheroids, it does have diagnostic value.

Coagulated blood serum and gelatin support good growth of this organism, and neither medium is softened or liquefied. Good growth occurs in sterile bovine urine, and the reaction becomes strongly alkaline because of the production of ammonia from urea. This organism is a powerful urea splitter; therefore, the urine of infected animals is always strongly alkaline. Certainly, part of the bladder irritation found in association with pyelonephritis is caused by the ammoniacal fermentation of the urine in the bladder.

Early attempts were made (6) to classify the diphtheroids associated with pyelonephritis in cattle into distinctly different species on the basis of the organisms, their habitats and cultural characteristics. *C. renale* emerged as the predominant organism associated with pyelonephritis. Recently, Yanagawa *et al.* (16) extracted antigenic fractions from cells of *C. renale* and divided 78 strains into three types. All isolates from cattle fell into type III.

Resistance. No records of resistance tests have been found. Laboratory strains die out quite easily, however, so it is safe to say that *C. renale*'s resistance to physical and chemical factors is slight.

Pathogenicity for Experimental Animals. *C. renale* is only slightly virulent for laboratory animals. Enderlen (3) produced pyelonephritis in two rabbits by injecting large doses of bacterial suspensions intravenously after ligating the ureters. He, and many others using other methods, failed to induce infections in this species and in guinea pigs. Lovell and Cotchin (12) were successful in infecting some of a series of white mice by intravenous injection. More recent experimental studies in mice (15) failed by this route, indicating that mice are more easily and consistently infected via the urinary tract (see Figure 22.4).

Attempts to produce the disease in cattle have usually failed when the organisms were given by routes other than the urinogenital tract. When cultures are injected into the urinary bladder by way of the urethra, success is not always attained, although the disease has been unquestionably established in this way by several groups of workers, such as Jones and Little (10) and Feenstra *et al.* (5). Controversy exists as to whether the disease is hematogenous in origin or strictly localized in the urinary tract, which is invaded through the urethra. Present evidence, derived mainly from studies in experimental ani-

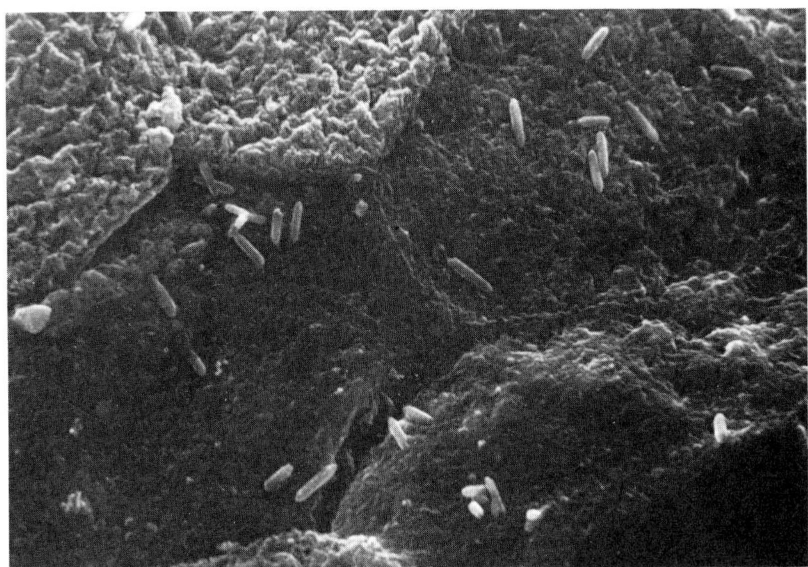

Figure 22.4. *Corynebacterium renale* attached to the mucous membrane of the urinary bladder of a mouse during an experimental infection. × 1,060. (From E. Honda and R. Yanagawa, *Am. Jour. Vet. Res.*, 1978, *39*, 155.)

mals, favors the theory that the infection ascends the urogenital tract. That the disease is much more common in cows than in bulls supports this concept, in that the shorter and wider urethra of the cow favors the entrance of the infecting organism from the outside.

The Natural Disease. In natural infections the urinary bladder is always involved, including one or both ureters in most cases, and usually one or both kidneys (1). The walls of affected bladders are thickened and the mucosa is superficially ulcerated and covered with a slimy secretion mixed with shreds of tissue and fibrin. Petechiae and larger hemorrhages are usually present in the bladder wall, and small clots of blood often are found in the bladder content. The affected ureters become enormously distended, and the mucosa usually contains necrotic areas, or is necrotic in its entirety. The kidneys often are greatly enlarged, and in extreme cases most of the kidney substance may undergo necrosis. More often the kidney pelvis is enlarged, the papillae are necrotic, and abscesses form throughout the kidney structure. The content of the affected pelvis consists of a grayish, slimy, nonodorous exudate, mixed with fibrin, small blood clots, necrotic tissue, and calcareous material.

Great numbers of the characteristic diphtheroid bacilli may be found both free and bound in the fragments of necrotic tissue in this exudate. These generally occur in clumps, arranged in palisade and radiating fashion. Quite often streptococci are found in this exudate also.

The urine, voided in small amounts at frequent intervals because of the bladder irritation, contains much albumin, leukocytes, fibrin, epithelial debris, and usually small bright-red blood clots.

Mode of Transmission and Pathogenesis. Jones and Little (10) and others have reported finding *C. renale* in many apparently normal cattle. These findings are more numerous in herds where clinical cases have been recognized, but the organism has often been found in herds in which the disease has never been recognized. This strongly suggests that this organism is quite widely distributed and that sporadic cases are caused by predisposing factors other than the actual presence of *C. renale*. The following have been suggested as contributors to the production of disease: the presence of pili on the *C. renale,* enhancing the organism's chances of colonizing the bladder (9), differences in virulence between serotypes (7), and the association of pyelonephritis with pregnant and parturient animals, suggesting that the anatomical and physiological changes may predispose the animal to the condition.

The available evidence indicates that the bacterium is spread from animal to animal by contamination of the urinogenital orifices with urine from diseased or carrier animals. In herds in which the adult cows are stanchioned, neighboring cows are often infected, probably by switching tails contaminated with infected urine.

Diagnosis. The symptoms of pyelonephritis are quite characteristic in most cases. For laboratory confirmation, a sample of urine should be collected in a sterile bottle. If, as is generally the case, it contains blood clots or bits of necrotic tissue, films may be made from these on slides and stained with the Gram technique. The characteristic clumps of short, stubby, Gram-positive organisms is presumptive evidence. If clumps are not present, the sample may be centrifuged and the sediment examined microscopically. For final confirmation, the sediment should be streaked on an agar plate, with or without enrichment. After 24 to 36 hours' incubation at 37 C a search for characteristic colonies should be made. Final confirmation depends on the organism's conformity with the biochemical characteristics listed in Table 22.1. Diagnosticians must be on their guard against confusing morphologically similar organisms with *C. renale*. Diphtheroid organisms are often present on skin and mucous membranes.

Immunity. A number of serological tests, including agglutination, indirect hemagglutination, agar-gel diffusion, and others (8) have been used for the detection of antibodies against *C. renale* in experimental studies. None is used for routine diagnostic purposes. Little is known about immunity to *C. renale*, although recent studies of cattle suggest that an antibody response is present in cows with pyelonephritis and urethritis but none in cases of cystitis alone (7). Without treatment, recoveries almost never occur after the disease is well established. There are no biological products of value in this disease.

Chemotherapy. Until the appearance of antibiotic therapy there were no forms of treatment that materially affected the course of the infection. *C. renale* is sensitive *in vivo* and *in vitro* to penicillin, and there are many reports of apparent cures with large doses. However, because of the nature of the later lesions and the difficulties of early diagnosis, unless the animal is unusually valuable, slaughtering for beef is often advisable. In some cases, treated animals have relapsed after a few weeks or months; in other cases the cure appears to have been complete (13).

Control Measures. As soon as cases are recognized, the animals should be segregated from other susceptible stock, treated with penicillin, or slaughtered. Treated animals should be carefully watched for a year or more for a return of the symptoms.

The Disease in Man. As far as is known, this organism is not pathogenic for man.

REFERENCES

1. Boyd. Cornell Vet., 1918, *8*, 120.
2. Boyd and Bishop. Jour. Am. Vet. Med. Assoc., 1937, *90*, 154.
3. Enderlen. Deut. Zeitschr. f. Tiermed., 1891, *17*, 325.
4. Ernst. Zentrbl. f. Bakt., I Abt. Orig., 1905, *39*, 549; 1906, *40*, 79.
5. Feenstra, Clark, and Thorp. Mich. State Coll. Vet., 1945, *5*, 147.
6. Feenstra, Thorp, and Clark. Jour. Bact., 1945, *50*, 497.
7. Hiramune, Inui, and Murase. Am. Jour. Vet. Res., 1971, *32*, 237.
8. Hiramune, Inui, and Murase. Res. Vet. Res., 1978, *13*, 82.
9. Honda and Yanagawa. Am. Jour. Vet. Res., 1978, *39*, 155.
10. Jones and Little. Jour. Exp. Med., 1925, *42*, 593; 1926, *43*, 11; 1930, *51*, 909.
11. Lovell. Jour. Comp. Path. and Therap., 1946, *56*, 196.
12. Lovell and Cotchin. Jour. Comp. Path. and Therap., 1946, *56*, 205.
13. Morse. Cornell Vet., 1948, *38*, 273.
14. Olafson. Cornell Vet., 1930, *20*, 69.
15. Shimono and Yanagawa. Inf. and Immun., 1977, *16*, 263.
16. Yanagawa, Basri, and Otsuki. Jap. Jour. Vet. Res., 1967, *15*, 111.

Corynebacterium pseudotuberculosis

SYNONYMS: The Preisz-Nocard bacillus, *Corynebacterium ovis*

This organism causes *caseous lymphadenitis*, a disease prevalent in sheep and goats in many parts of the world. It also causes disease in horses, camels, deer, and mules, and rarely in cattle and men. The lesions produced in all species usually involve suppuration and necrosis of the lymph nodes.

Morphology and Staining Reactions. The organism is a pleomorphic rod, frequently so short that it may be mistaken for a coccus. In the caseous pus from lymph nodes it sometimes occurs as rod forms that quite closely resemble the organism of human diphtheria. It forms no spores and is nonmotile. It retains the Gram stain but is not acid-fast.

Cultural Features. *C. pseudotuberculosis* will grow on all the ordinary media, although not luxuriantly. The colonies on agar grow slowly and take several days to reach maximum size when incubated at the optimum temperature (37 C). When fully developed they have papilliform centers surrounded by concentric rings that parallel the irregular margin. The color is grayish or yellowish and the surfaces are dull and dry. When touched with the needle, they fragment easily. Entire smaller colonies may be pushed around the surface of the medium as if they were flakes of wax. The differential characteristics of *C. pseudotuberculosis* are given in Table 22.1.

The organism produces an exotoxin which is lethal when injected into guinea pigs and rabbits (6). Jolly (14) reported that the exotoxin of *C. pseudotuberculosis* increased the permeability of the vascular bed. More recent studies (7) have indicated that this toxin is a phospholipase D which attacks the sphingomyelin of the erythrocytes and the endothelial cells of blood vessels.

Pathogenicity for Experimental Animals. By inoculation *C. pseudotuberculosis* is pathogenic for horses, cattle, sheep, goats, rabbits, guinea pigs, and mice. Fowls are refractory.

Guinea pigs are highly susceptible to *C. pseudotuberculosis* infection. The disease is characterized by abscesses in the liver, spleen, and kidneys, and it progresses rapidly to death (5). Intraperitoneal inoculation of guinea pigs with large doses produces rapid intoxication and death from peritonitis. Smaller doses or less virulent strains have a tendency to localize in the scrotal sac, producing orchitis and, later, abscesses. Inoculation of the organism into mice results in the production of caseous abscesses in the internal organs, notably the liver, kidney, and spleen.

The Natural Disease. *In sheep and goats.* Caseous lymphadenitis, prevalent in sheep and goats in many parts of the world, is primarily a wound infection and starts with local inflammation at the site of entry of the organism, often going unnoticed, and proceeds to the regional lymph node, which slowly enlarges and becomes filled with pus. The pus is greenish and nonodorous. Initially, it may be thin, but eventually it is thick and caseous and may become arranged in concentric layers resembling an onion. The superficial nodes are often affected. In sheep, superficial nodes close to shearing wounds may be enlarged and abscessed, and in goats the superficial nodes of the head and neck are most often affected. In both species, deep abscesses may be found in the lungs and the mediastinal or mesenteric lymph nodes. Animals that appear quite normal are often found at slaughter to be rather badly affected. Eventually they become emaciated and weak and die.

In horses. C. pseudotuberculosis has been known for some time as the cause of *ulcerative lymphangitis,* a condition similar to cutaneous glanders (farcy) in the horse. Nodules appear on the legs and break down to form ulcers, which exude a thick greenish pus usually mixed with blood. They are located most often around the fetlock. These lesions fill with cicatricial tissue and heal after a time, but others appear nearby. Some cases heal spontaneously within a few weeks, but most progress slowly for months or even years.

Recently, Hughes and Biberstein (13) and Knight (16) have described a second disease entity caused in horses by this organism. It is characterized by large, painful abscesses in the pectoral, lower abdominal, and inguinal regions. These occur typically in the adult horse, develop slowly, run a course of several months, and recur after opening and draining.

In cattle. Judging from the paucity of reports, it is probable that the disease does not often occur in cattle. Kitt (15) found it in a case of bronchopneumonia in a cow and Hall and Stone (11) in a calf. Reportedly, a considerable number of cases of the so-called skin-lesion tuberculosis in Utah contain the organism (9).

Mode of Transmission and Pathogenesis. In the sheep and the goat, caseous lymphadenitis commonly spreads directly from an open abscess and enters the new host through a skin abrasion. Because the organism can survive in the environment, spread may also occur indirectly, and animals may become infected from heavily contaminated sheep resting areas, hay racks, and the like. Shearing wounds in sheep and butting abrasions in goats facilitate entry. In some instances the organism may penetrate the abraded buccal mucosae or be inhaled and produce pulmonary abscesses.

The distribution of the lesions of ulcerative lymphangitis on the fetlock of the horse supports the contention that skin abrasions are important in this disease. However, the seasonal incidence of pectoral and other abscesses in horses suggests that the organism is borne by arthropods in this condition (16).

Once *C. pseudotuberculosis* has gained entry into the host, it adopts the status of a facultative intracellular parasite. The following factors are thought to contribute to its ability to survive in the host and produce abscesses (at least in the sheep and goat): an exotoxin (14) which increases vascular permeability, a heat-stable pyogenic factor (5) which attracts leukocytes, and the presence of a large amount of surface lipid (8) toxic for phagocytes. The lipid is also thought to allow the organism to survive unharmed in phagolysosomes of the host's phagocytic cells and produce an abscess in the regional node or be carried to another site.

Diagnosis. The appearance of the lesions in sheep and goats is quite characteristic, and the organism can usually be isolated without difficulty from the abscesses in large numbers. The dry scaly colonies, which cause hemolysis on blood agar plates, are easily recognized. Animals devoid of abscesses of the superficial lymph nodes but having abscesses deep in their body cavities still present a great diagnostic dilemma.

Immunity. Antibodies are produced in response to infection with *C. pseudotuberculosis.* Various serological tests have been used to detect the antibodies, to confirm the diagnosis, and to detect the inapparent carrier. These tests include: bacterial agglutination (2), toxin neutralization in mice (1) and rabbits (10), and an antihemolysin-inhibition test (21). (Certain strains of *Staphylococcus aureus* can lyse erythrocytes. This hemolysis can be inhibited by the exotoxin of *C. pseudotuberculosis,* and this hemolysin inhibition, in turn, can be blocked by antibodies to the exotoxin, providing a specific means of identifying these antibodies. This system is known as antihemolysin inhibition.)

None of these tests enjoys widespread acceptance. Knight (17) has recently described a serological method for the detection of *C. pseudotuberculosis* infections in horses that relies on the ability of *C. pseudotuberculosis* toxin to lyse erythrocytes pretreated with filtrates from *C. equi*. This lysis can be inhibited by antibodies to *C. pseudotuberculosis* and hence used as a method of detecting horses previously exposed to the organism.

Although many biological agents, including killed and autogenous bacterins, have been used in attempts to produce artificial immunity to this organism, none has yet proved efficacious. The facultative intracellular nature of this organism suggests (3) that cell-mediated immunity and agents that stimulate its production, such as attenuated live vaccines, are likely to be necessary for protection against *C. pseudotuberculosis*.

Chemotherapy. Although antibiotics can be effective against *C. pseudotuberculosis in vitro,* the diseases it causes are refractory to antibiotic therapy. This is because *C. pseudotuberculosis* is a facultative intracellular parasite and relatively inaccessible to antibiotics. The nature of the lesion—a caseous abscess with a good capsule—is not very conducive to antibiotic penetration and persistence. Antibiotics have been found to be ineffective *in vivo* except in very slight infections (19). In treating chronic abscesses in horses, Ichthyol ointment is recommended to hasten maturation (13). When mature, the abscess is incised, drained, and flushed with an antiseptic. This procedure usually brings prompt recovery.

Control Measures. Methods presently used for control consist of isolation of infected animals, especially those with open abscesses, prevention of wounds, and application of general principles of hygiene and disinfection to prevent spread to other animals.

The Disease in Man. In 1966, Lopez *et al.* (18) reported the first case of *C. pseudotuberculosis* in man. The clinical picture consisted of fatigue, muscular aches, tenderness and enlargement of the liver, and localized lymphadenopathy. Conclusive bacteriologic identification of the microorganism was established in specimens obtained by lymph-node aspiration and surgical excision of the involved lymph node. Examination of the node revealed a pathologic process manifested by focal areas of chronic inflammation. There were nests of epithelioid cells, surrounded by fibroblastic reaction, and a chronic sclerosing lymphadenitis. More recently, sporadic human cases have been reported in Australia (4, 12, 20).

REFERENCES

1. Abdel Hamid. Res. Vet. Sci., 1975, *18,* 223.
2. Awad. Am. Jour. Vet. Res., 1960, *81,* 251.
3. Ayers. Jour. Am. Vet. Med. Assoc., 1977, *171,* 1252.
4. Battey, Tonge, Horsfoll, and McDonald. Med. Jour. Austral., 1968, *2,* 540.
5. Bull and Dickinson. Austral. Vet. Jour., 1935, *11,* 126.
6. Carne. Jour. Path. and Bact., 1940, *51,* 199.
7. Carne and Onon. Nature, 1978, *271,* 246.
8. Carne, Wickham, and Kater. Nature, 1956, *178,* 701.
9. Daines and Austin. Jour. Am. Vet. Med. Assoc., 1932, *80,* 414.
10. Doty, Dunne, Hokanson, and Reid. Am. Jour. Vet. Res., 1964, *25,* 1679.
11. Hall and Stone. Jour. Inf. Dis., 1916, *18,* 195.
12. Hamilton, Perceval, Aarons, and Goodyear. Med. Jour. Austral., 1968, *2,* 356.
13. Hughes and Biberstein. Jour. Am. Vet. Med. Assoc., 1959, *135,* 559.
14. Jolly. Jour. Comp. Path., 1965, *75,* 417.
15. Kitt. Monatsh. f. prakt. Tierheilk., 1890, *1,* 145.
16. Knight. Jour. Am. Vet. Med. Assoc., 1969, *155,* 446.
17. Knight. Cornell Vet., 1978, *68,* 220.
18. Lopez, Wong, and Quesada. Am. Jour. Clin. Path., 1966, *46,* 562.
19. Maddy. Jour. Am. Vet. Med. Assoc., 1953, *122,* 257.
20. Rountree and Carne. Jour. Path. and Bact., 1967, *94,* 19.
21. Zaki. Res. Vet. Sci., 1968, *9,* 489.

Corynebacterium equi

This organism was first described and named by Magnusson (17) in southern Sweden in 1923 as the causative agent of a purulent pneumonia in goals. It was subsequently found in foals in Australia (6), the United States (11), and India (20). Over the same time span the organism was isolated from the lymph nodes of pigs (1, 9, 14, 19), where its role in disease is still controversial. It has been isolated from two cases of pyometra in cattle (10), from a water buffalo (21) that had aborted, and from a sheep in Australia (22) with chronic pneumonia.

Morphology and Staining Reactions. *C. equi* is a rather large organism that shows considerable pleomorphism, ranging from coccoid forms to bacillary forms. On solid media the form usually is coccoid; in fluids it usually is bacillary. Sometimes short chains are found in fluid media. Metachromatic granules can usually be demonstrated, especially in cultures grown in milk. Growth on solid media is abundant; the colonies are moist and mucoid in appearance. This appearance suggests that *C. equi* is a good capsule former, a hypothesis that a number of authors support. Karlson *et al.* (15), however, were unable to convince themselves that capsules were present.

This organism is Gram-positive and it stains readily with other dyes. A number of authors claim that acid-fast forms are demonstrable in old cultures, but several other workers have been unable to confirm this. Spores are not formed.

Cultural Features. Good growth occurs on all the ordinary media. After 2 days' incubation, colonies on the surface of agar plates measure nearly 1 cm in diameter and are raised, moist, translucent, and regular in outline. At first they are white, but a rose-pink color soon appears. Old cultures are distinctly pinkish, especially those developing on potato. There is a rather poor growth in milk, without coagulation or other evidence of change in the chemical composition. *C. equi* ferments no carbohydrates, does not form indol, and is not hemolytic (see Table 22.1).

Resistance. *C. equi* is moderately resistant to heat and to some chemical reagents. It requires exposure to 60 C for 1 hour before it is killed. Cotchin (9) found that it would successfully resist the action of 2.5 percent oxalic acid for 1 hour; he made use of this property for isolating it from tissues contaminated with other bacteria. A new selective medium has been devised by Woolcock *et al.* that facilitates the isolation of *C. equi* (26).

Bruner and Edwards (4), using complement fixation, demonstrated that *C. equi* possesses a species-specific antigen. Using bacterial agglutination tests (5), the species can be divided into four serologic groups. Cultures from the genital tract of mares, from aborted equine fetuses, from foals with pneumonia, and from the submaxillar lymph node of pigs belonged to the same serologic group.

Natural Infections. *In foals.* The organism causes pneumonia in foals at 2 to 5 months and older. Outbreaks characteristically occur where a number of mares are congregated and foal. Pneumonia is the most common sign shown by affected foals; they may be anorectic, have a nasal discharge, and, less frequently, show signs of arthritis and diarrhea (7). The mortality rate is high (64 percent), and necropsy frequently reveals a bilateral suppurative bronchopneumonia with necrosis and infiltration of macrophages. Lymphadenitis is common, and there may be abscessation of the lymph nodes. In contrast to strangles, the lymph nodes of the head are seldom involved in this process.

Although pneumonia in the foal is the most common disease entity with which *C. equi* is associated, the organism has also been found in internal abscesses with pleurisy in foals (3) and in uterine infections in mares (5). The organism has been isolated from two cases of enteritis in foals, where it was found in association with focal necrosis and thickening of the intestinal tract (8).

In swine. The infection in swine occurs in the lymph nodes and particularly in those of the cervical region. Holth and Amundsen (14), who first found the organism in swine in Norway, believed that it caused a tuberclelike disease. This view was also taken by other Scandinavian workers, notably Plum (19), who confirmed the Norwegian findings. Karlson *et al.* (15) in the United States, do not accept this view because they were able to demonstrate the organism in approximately as many apparently normal as diseased lymph nodes. They believe the acid-fast organisms that the European workers describe as acid-fast forms of *C. equi* are, in reality, tubercle bacilli with which the organism develops concurrently. They believe, on the basis of their findings, that the organism is relatively if not wholly nonpathogenic, and that when gross lesions are evident it is because tubercle bacilli are present as well as *C. equi*. Cotchin (9), who carried out a similar survey in pigs in England, isolated *C. equi* and tubercle bacilli from some suspected tuberculous sublimaxillary lymph nodes and *C. equi* from one normal lymph node. He also concluded that *C. equi* was not associated etiologically with the tuberculouslike lesions observed.

Transmission and Pathogenesis. Little definitive information currently exists concerning the habitat, mode of transmission, and pathogenesis of diseases caused by *C. equi*. In a survey of 127 horses in Australia the organism was found in the feces of 90 (26), suggesting that it is a common commensal of the horse. It is also believed that the organism exists in the soil (16) and is transmitted to animals mostly by inhalation and perhaps by ingestion (23).

The organism does not appear to produce a potent exotoxin. Researchers have speculated that *C. equi* may also be a facultative intracellular parasite capable of survival inside the host's macrophages, accounting for its distribution in lymphatic tissue and macrophages (8, 16).

Diagnosis. The organism is a Gram-positive pleomorphic rod; however, caution is advised in direct microscopic examination of pus, as *C. equi* may appear spheroidal and be confused with staphylococci.

In neither horses nor swine can the presence of this

organism be more than suspected before a bacteriological examination with isolation of the organism is made. Sippel *et al.* (24) have recovered three species of the genus *Corynebacterium* from the lungs of foals: *C. equi, C. pseudotuberculosis,* and *C. pyogenes*. They claim that the clinical appearance of these infections is quite similar, making the three diseases difficult to distinguish.

Immunity. *C. equi* has type-specific antigens which fall into major groups; there is some cross-reactivity within groups, but the type-specific antigens do not cross-react with the antigens of other corynebacteria or related organisms. These type-specific antigens are thought to be fairly superficial and are probably capsular in origin. Species-specific antigens can also be demonstrated, although they are thought to be less superficial in distribution and do not cross-react with the antigens of other corynebacteria.

Magnusson (17) encountered difficulty in producing high antibody titers to *C. equi* in experimental animals. Convalescent horses lack measurable agglutinating antibodies, and, to date, no practical methods of immunizing against this organism have been developed.

Chemotherapy. There is little information on this subject. Britton (3) reported failure in treating an infected foal with sulfanilamide and sulfaquinoxaline. Doll and Dimock (12), in a study of penicillin dosage and blood levels for horses, reported that the penicillin resistance of *C. equi* is so great that dosage for maintaining effective blood levels is impractical.

Control Measures. There are no known methods of preventing infections with *C. equi* except by using general sanitary measures, which may minimize but will not eliminate infections. Mares should be removed from infected premises before foaling.

The Disease in Man. In recent years several cases of infection with *C. equi* have been reported in humans undergoing immunosuppressive therapy (2, 13, 18, 25) for malignant neoplasms. Pulmonary abscesses developed in all patients, some of whom were bacteremic. Almost all the patients had contact with animals.

REFERENCES

1. Bendixen and Jepsen. Medlemsblad f. d. Danske Dyralegeforning, 1938, *21,* 401.
2. Berg, Chmel, Mayo, and Armstrong. Am. Jour. Clin. Path., 1977, *68,* 73.
3. Britton. Cornell Vet., 1945, *35,* 370.
4. Bruner, Dimock, and Edwards. Jour. Inf. Dis., 1939, *65,* 92.
5. Bruner and Edwards. Jour. Inf. Dis., 1939, *65,* 92.
6. Bull. Jour. Comp. Path. and Therap., 1924, *37,* 294.
7. Burrows. Jour. Am. Vet. Med. Assoc., 1968, *152,* 1119.
8. Cimprich and Rooney. Vet. Path., 1977, *14,* 95.
9. Cotchin. Jour. Comp. Path. and Therap., 1943,*53,* 298.
10. Craig and Davies. Vet. Jour., 1940, *96,* 417.
11. Dimock and Edwards. Ky. Agr. Exp. Sta. Bull. 333, 1932.
12. Doll and Dimock. Jour. Am. Vet. Med. Assoc., 1946, *108,* 209.
13. Golub, Falk, and Spink. Ann. Inter. Med., 1967, *66,* 1174.
14. Holth and Amundsen. Norsk Vet. Tidsskr., 1936, *48,* 2.
15. Karlson, Moses, and Feldman. Jour. Inf. Dis., 1940, *67,* 243.
16. Knight. Jour. Am. Vet. Med. Assoc., 1969, *155,* 446.
17. Magnusson. Arch. f. Tierheilk., 1923, *50,* 22.
18. March and von Graevenitz. Cancer, 1973, *32,* 147.
19. Plum. Cornell Vet., 1940, *30,* 14.
20. Rajagopalan. Indian Jour. Vet. Sci., 1937, *7,* 38.
21. Rajagopalan and Gopalakrishnan. Indian Jour. Vet. Sci., 1938, *8,* 225.
22. Roberts. Austral. Vet. Jour., 1957, *33,* 21.
23. Roberts and Polley. Equine Vet. Jour., 1977, *9,* 159.
24. Sippel, Keahey, and Bullard. Jour. Am. Vet. Med. Assoc., 1968, *153,* 1610.
25. Williams, Glamigan, and Campbell. Ann. Thorac. Surg., 1971, *12,* 471.
26. Woolcock, Farmer, and Mutimer. Jour. Clin. Microbiol., 1979, *9,* 640.

Other Corynebacteria of Veterinary Interest

Corynebacterium bovis. This organism, whose differential characteristics appear in Table 22.1, occurs in bovine milk taken from healthy udders, and it has also been found in the reproductive tracts of cows and bulls. It appears to be a saprophyte but on occasion has been associated with cases of bovine mastitis (1, 2).

Corynebacterium suis. *C. suis* is a urea-splitting, anaerobic corynebacterium (see Table 22.1) that has been associated with pyelonephritis and cystitis in sows in England. Affected sows show characteristic signs of vaginal discharge and urine turbidity a month after service.

Corynebacterium Associated with Ovine Posthitis. Southcott, in Australia, isolated a diphtheroid from the preputial lesions of a wether with ovine posthitis, characterized it as a *Corynebacterium,* and successfully reproduced the lesions of ovine posthitis ("sheath rot," "pizzlerot," "balanitis") with this organism. He could readily detect the organism in well-developed cases of preputial ulceration in sheep and cattle and considered its ability to hydrolyze urea important in its pathogenicity (3, 4).

REFERENCES

1. Cobb and Walley. Vet. Rec., 1962, *74,* 101.
2. Duckitt, Seaman, and Woodbine. Vet. Bull., 1963, *33,* 67.
3. Southcott. Austral. Vet. Jour., 1965, *41,* 193.
4. Southcott. Austral. Vet. Jour., 1965, *41,* 225.

23 The Genus *Actinomyces*

Most species produce a true mycelium that fragments into elements of irregular size and may exhibit angular branching. They are non-acid-fast and nonmotile and usually grow as facultative anaerobes. They are usually carboxyphilic. The cell wall contains neither diaminopimelic acid nor arabinose.

The three species of *Actinomyces* that commonly cause disease in domesticated animals are *A. bovis, A. viscosus,* and *A. suis.*

Actinomyces bovis

SYNONYMS: *Streptothrix actinomyces, Discomyces bovis, Nocardia bovis, Streptothrix israeli,* and others

This organism is the cause of the common disease of cattle known as *actinomycosis* or *lumpy jaw.* Human infections occasionally occur, the manifestations being similar to those in cattle.

It should be pointed out that conditions that resemble actinomycosis clinically, and are often called *actinomycosis,* are caused by other organisms, particularly *Actinobacillus lignieresi* and *Staphylococcus aureus.* The true actinomycosis of cattle usually is an affection of the bony structures, particularly the mandible or lower jaw (15). Pulmonary actinomycosis in swine has been reported by Vawter (16) and *A. bovis* has been isolated from a bovine lung (1).

In the study of equine poll evil and fistulous withers which appear to be inflammations of the supraatloid and supraspinous bursa, respectively, Roderick, Kimball, McLeod, and Frank (11) regularly have isolated *A. bovis* and *Brucella abortus. Brucella suis* has also been obtained from these lesions and injections of either *B. abortus* or *B. suis* combined with *A. bovis* into the supraspinous bursa of experimental horses produces a bursitis apparently identical with field cases.

Morphology and Staining Reactions. In the "sulfur granules" in the tissues, *A. bovis* is seen as a tangled mass of filaments around the periphery of which is a considerable mass of acidophilic capsular material. The filaments stain Gram-positively, and also retain the usual basophilic stains. When stains are made of crushed granules, a great diversity of forms, resembling a mixed infection, is seen. They are coccoid, rods of varying size, filaments, branching forms, club-shaped forms, and spiral elements (Figure 23.1). Actually all of these are forms of the one organism. In cultures it usually appears in the form of diphtheroid bacilli when young (Figure 23.2); older cultures may show filaments of all kinds. When grown in an atmosphere of carbon dioxide, branching filaments and clubs are frequent (Figure 23.3).

Cultural Features. *A. bovis* frequently is regarded as an obligate anaerobe. This conception is false. Growth cannot be obtained on the surface of solid media incubated in the air, but it may be obtained when the media are enclosed in a tight vessel into which 10 to 15 percent carbon dioxide is introduced. When shake cultures are made in media, growth does not occur on the surface. The optimum zone, in this case, is about 1 mm below the surface, but scattered colonies usually are found throughout the depths of the medium. Cultures some-

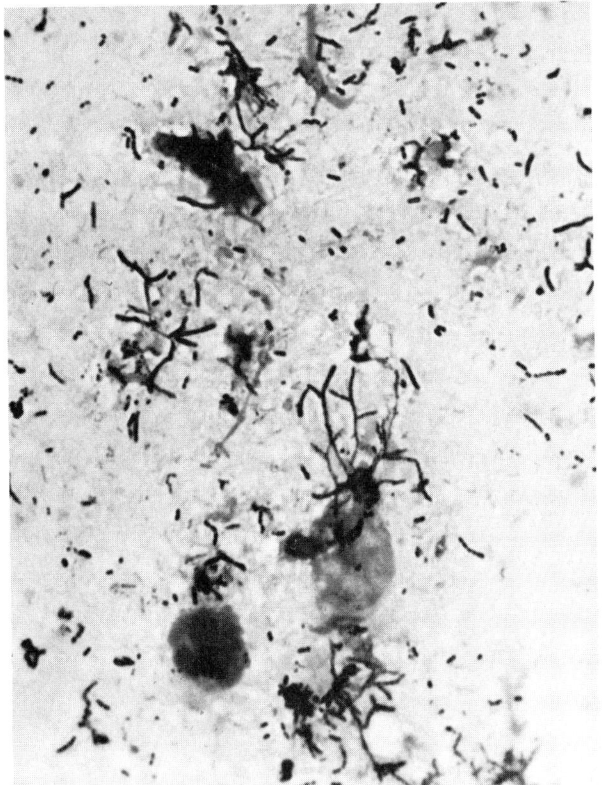

Figure 23.1. *Actinomyces bovis,* showing branched filaments and coccoid bodies in actinomycotic pus. × 1230. (Courtesy L. R. Vawter.)

times will develop on the surface if the tubes are hermetically sealed, a procedure which results in an increase in the carbon dioxide content of the imprisoned air.

A. bovis is a serophilic organism, i.e., little or no growth can be obtained in ordinary media unless animal fluids are present. It does not grow at temperatures very much below those of the animal body. It is catalase-negative.

In stab cultures in serum agar a nodular growth occurs along the lower parts of the stab. There is no growth on the surface or in the upper centimeter of the stab. In shake cultures small, biconvex colonies appear throughout the medium except in the upper layer. Growth on serum agar slants will occur only if the tubes are incubated in a carbon-dioxide-containing atmosphere, or anaerobically.

The growth in serum broth is not abundant. If incubated in the air the medium should be in tall columns, and it should be heated shortly before the serum is added and inoculation is made. The growth is in the form of granules, which collect along the sides of the tube and in the bottom. The fluid is clear except for the granules.

Loeffler's blood serum slants are good for isolation providing they are incubated in a carbon dioxide jar. Growth is evident after 2 or 3 days in the form of fine

Figure 23.2 (*left*). *Actinomyces bovis,* showing diphtheroid forms in a culture on Loeffler's blood serum incubated for 7 days at 37 C under increased CO_2 tension. × 980. (Courtesy L. R. Vawter.)

Figure 23.3 (*right*). *Actinomyces bovis* from a serum-broth culture incubated 6 days at 37 C. Clubs, filaments, and diphtheroid forms are present. × 980. (Courtesy L. R. Vawter.)

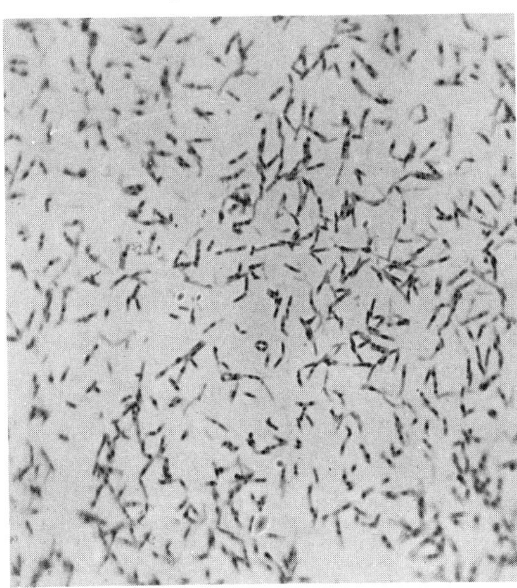

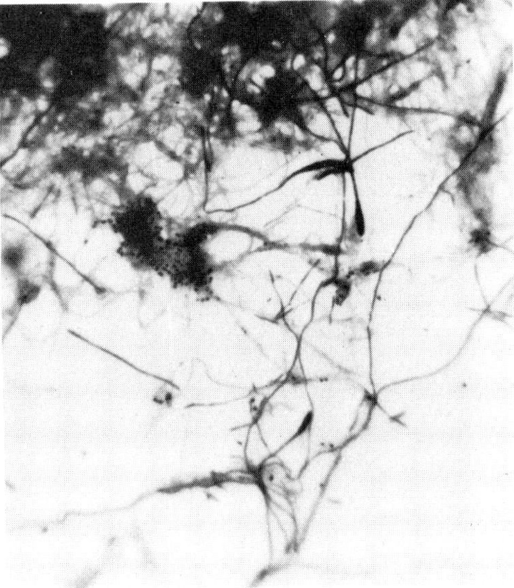

colonies which may easily be scraped off the medium. After 5 or 6 days' incubation at 37 C the colonies will have reached maximum size, which is about 0.5 mm in diameter. The condensation water at the bottom of the slant usually contains excellent growth in the form of a slimy deposit.

On blood agar plates the colonies are small and nonhemolytic.

Little growth occurs in milk unless serum is added to it. In serum milk there is little change in the appearance of the medium. Sometimes the litmus is bleached in the bottom of the tube.

No growth occurs in gelatin unless serum is added. Serum gelatin is not liquefied.

In serum-containing broth under a vaseline seal, glucose, levulose, maltose, galactose, sucrose, and salicin are slowly fermented without gas formation. Fermentation end products include acetic, formic, lactic, and succinic but not propionic acids.

The cell wall peptidoglycan contains alanine, glutamic acid, lysine, and aspartic acid. Arabinose does not occur.

Serologic Grouping. *A. bovis* belongs to group B of the classification of *Actinomyces* of Slack and Gerencser (13). There are two serotypes, 1 and 2.

Epidemiology and Pathogenesis. The organism is apparently a normal and obligate parasite of the oropharynx and digestive tract. It opportunistically invades the deeper tissues of the jaw via wounds or dental alveoli, or in association with entry of foreign materials such as pieces of wood or wire. In the mandible a rarefying osteomylelitis is produced (Figure 23.4). There is characteristically a formation of soft granulation tissue both here and along the lower esophagus and reticulum in those rare cases of visceral involvement. This tissue develops necrotic areas filled with pus, which may discharge to the surface via fistulous tracts. Later, the connective tissue hardens into dense tumorlike masses. A thick, mucoid, tenacious, greenish-yellow, nonodorous pus is characteristic of the disease. The pus contains cheeselike granules varying in size up to 3 or 4 mm in diameter. These are the colonies of the organism and are commonly called *sulfur granules* (Figures 23.5 and 23.6).

If these granules are examined in the fresh condition, simply by pressing a clean cover glass on them, the ray-fungus appearance can be easily discerned This is the most rapid way to make a definite diagnosis. The borders of the crushed granules show radiating, swollen, clublike filaments (Figure 23.7). The clublike forms are not seen in stained preparations of the pus, as a general rule, but can be observed in histologic sections.

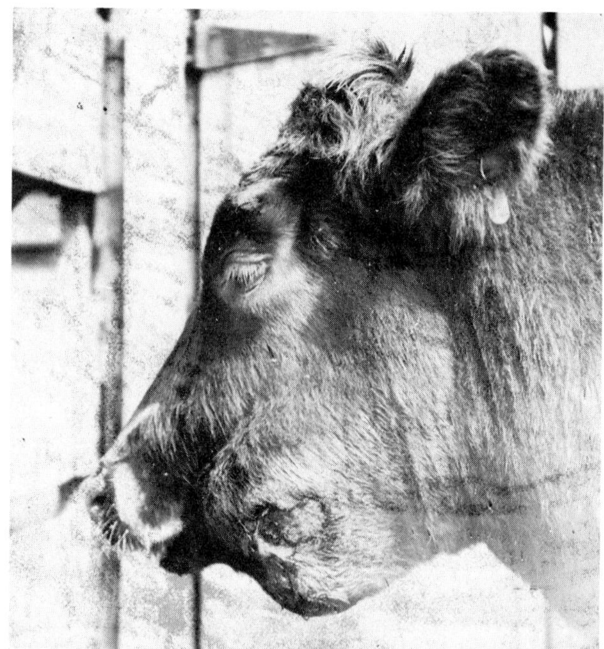

Figure 23.4. Bovine actinomycosis. This is a case of true actinomycosis, involving the bone of the jaw and caused by *Actinomyces bovis*.

Sulfur granules are found in the pus of actinobacillosis, and also in those actinomycosislike lesions that are caused by staphylococci. Fresh impression preparations show radiating, clublike forms, not unlike those of true actinomycosis. The sulfur granules in the nonactinomycotic lesions usually are much smaller than those of true actinomycosis, and frequently are so small that they are difficult to find on gross examination. The granules may be differentiated by making stained preparations: true actinomycosis shows Gram-positive elements, short rods, filaments, and branching forms; actinobacillosis shows small Gram-negative rods; and staphylococci show their typical morphology. When making such examinations it is well to select the granules from the pus, wash them, and crush them on clean slides. If the slide is made at random from the pus, no organisms at all may be found. The granules can usually be obtained rather easily by placing some of the pus in a tube of broth or salt solution, shaking the tube to dissolve the mucin that holds the pus together, pouring the solution into a flat dish, and searching for the granules, which do not break up.

A. bovis infection occurs more commonly in cattle than in other animals, and in the bovine species lesions

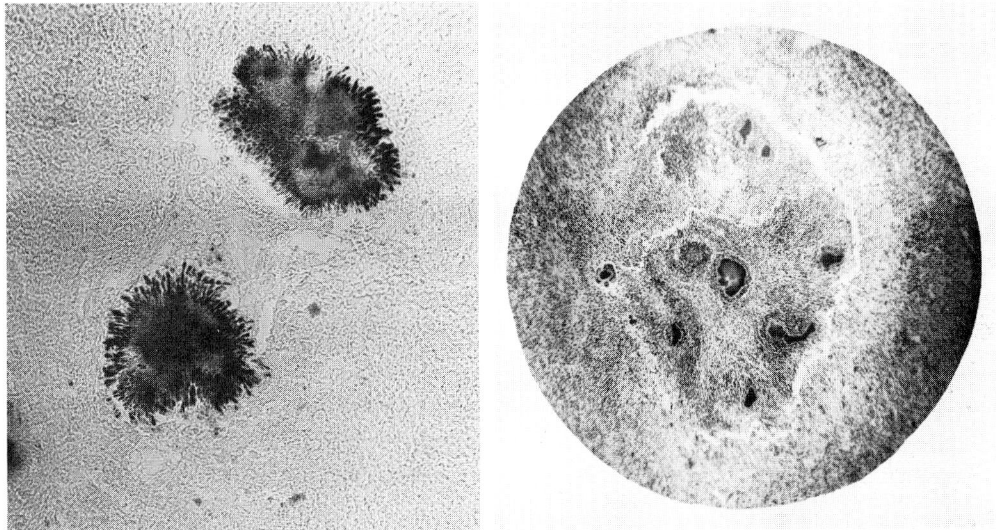

Figure 23.5. (*left*). *Actinomyces bovis,* showing sulfur granules in pus of a bone lesion. Picrofuchsin stain. × 330. (Courtesy L. R. Vawter.)

Figure 23.6. (*right*). Actinomycotic lesion, showing sulfur granules embedded in pus in center of the lesion. The greater part of the actinomycotic nodule consists of granulation tissue. × 82.

Figure 23.7. *Actinomyces bovis,* showing clubs and sulfur granules in pus of a bone lesion. Unstained. × 490. (Courtesy L. R. Vawter.)

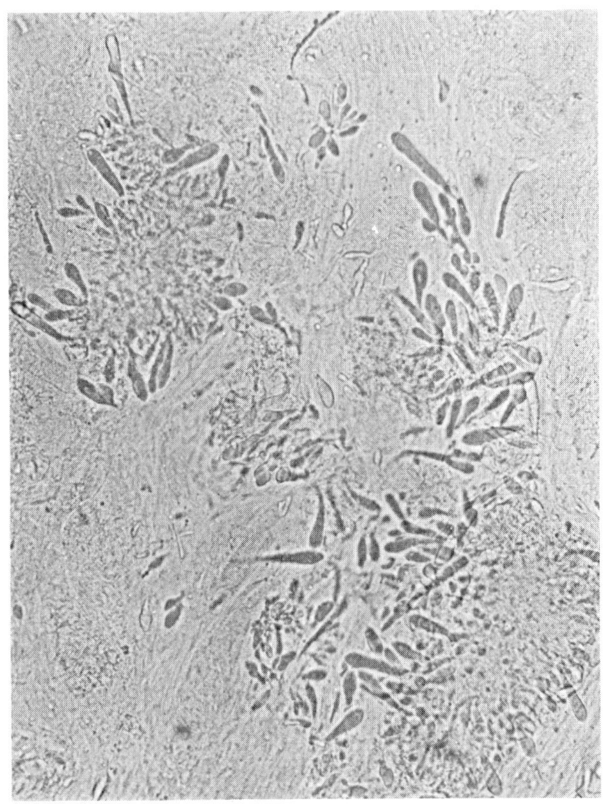

are seen most frequently in the bones of the face and jaw. That it does occur at times in other tissues is known. Kimball *et al.* (5) have found it in the bovine testis, where it causes orchitis.

In 1953, Ryff (12) described a case of encephalitis in a deer due to *A. bovis*. In 1952, Burns and Simmons (2) reported a case of actinomycotic infection in a horse. The intermandibular space of this animal was affected. Cases of actinomycosis in the dog have also been recorded. In one case *A. bovis* was isolated from lung tissue (9). In a second case the right cheek bones of the animal were involved (8), and in a third the infection was localized in the osseous tissue of the mandible (10).

Immunity. The mononuclear response and the granulomatous nature of the lesion suggests that cell-mediated immunity is important in the host response to infection. This has not been studied, nor has any attempt been made to develop a vaccine.

Treatment. This infection is iodine-sensitive. Local lesions are treated with Lugol's solution, and sodium iodide is administered intravenously for internal lesions. A report by Chanton, Hollis, and Hargrove (3) on the treatment of human cases of actinomycosis indicates that penicillin and sulfadiazine therapy is effective. Lane and colleagues (7) used Terramycin in treating orocervical actinomycosis, with apparent success. Other reports indicate that Aureomycin and penicillin have therapeutic value in treating experimentally infected mice (4) and that the results obtained by treating actinomycosis of the bone in cattle with streptomycin are extremely encouraging (6). Suter (14) studied *in vitro* development of resistance of *A. bovis* to antibiotics and concluded that none resulted on exposure to erythromycin, carbomycin, and penicillin, while treatment with oxytetracycline, tetracycline, chloramphenicol, and dihydrostreptomycin produced a slow and moderate buildup of resistance.

REFERENCES

1. Biever, Robertstad, Van Steenbergh, Scheetz, and Kennedy. Am. Jour. Vet. Res., 1969, *30,* 1063.
2. Burns and Simmons. Austral. Vet. Jour. 1952, *28,* 34.
3. Chanton, Hollis, and Hargrove. South. Med. Jour., 1948, *41,* 1022.
4. Geister and Meyer. Jour. Lab. and Clin. Med., 1951, *38,* 101.
5. Kimball, Twiehaus, and Frank. Am. Jour. Vet. Res., 1954, *15,* 551.
6. Kingman and Palen. Jour. Am. Vet. Med. Assoc., 1951, *118,* 28.
7. Lane, Kutscher, and Chaves. Jour. Am. Med. Assoc., 1953, *151,*986.
8. McGaughey, Bateman, and Mackenzie. Brit. Vet. Jour., 1951, *107,* 428.
9. Menges, Larsh, and Habermann. Jour. Am. Vet. Med. Assoc., 1953, *122,* 73.
10. Migliano and Stopiglia. Jour. Am. Vet. Med. Assoc., 1951, *118,* 52.
11. Roderick, Kimball, McLeod, and Frank. Am. Jour. Vet. Res., 1948, *9,* 5.
12. Ryff. Jour. Am. Vet. Med. Assoc., 1953, *122,* 78.
13. Slack and Gerencser. Jour. Bact., 1970, *103,* 265.
14. Suter. Antibiotics and Chemother., 1957, *7,* 285.
15. Vawter. Cornell Vet., 1933, *23,* 126.
16. Vawter. Jour. Am. Vet. Med. Assoc., 1946, *109,* 198.

Actinomyces viscosus

A. viscosus causes periodontal disease and subgingival plaques in hamsters fed a high-carbohydrate diet (4, 7). Recently it has been recognized as a cause of abscessation in dogs (2, 3) and cats (1). Infections by this organism have probably been frequently diagnosed as nocardiosis because of the lack of club formation in the sulfur granules found in the lesions.

Morphology and Staining Reactions. *A. viscosus* produces a diphtheroidal form that resembles *Corynebacterium* sp., and a filamentous form similar to that of *A. bovis*. The cells are Gram-positive. Both the diphtheroid and filamentous forms are found together in sulfur granules. They are non-acid-fast and nonmotile.

Cultural and Biochemical Features. Microcolonies on brain-heart-infusion agar incubated in CO_2 for 24 hours have a dense center with a filamentous fringe. After 3 to 4 days' incubation the colonies are circular, convex, smooth, glistening, and cream to white in color. In liquid media, a viscous sediment develops which gives a viscous rope when swirled. The organism is catalase-positive, unlike other members of the genus. Nitrate is reduced, H_2S is produced in triple sugar iron agar, and esculin is hydrolyzed. Glucose is fermented, resulting in production of acetic, lactic, and succinic acids. Gelatinase and urease are not formed.

Epidemiology and Pathogenesis. The habitat of *A. viscosus* is probably the oropharynx and digestive tract where the organism is an obligate parasite. It opportunistically invades wounds in dogs, possibly as a result of the tendency of these animals to lick wounded areas, or as a result of simple extension from the oropharyngeal area. Most infections are seen in large hunting dogs, and there is a consistent history of trauma of the infected sites. They frequently result in abscesses or pedunculated cysts around the head and neck. Love (5) has described a case of ascites in the dog, where *A. viscosus* was isolated from the ascitic fluid. A case of *A. viscosus* infection in the cat has also been described (1), where a suppurative granulomatous lesion was produced in the tail and anal area.

Granules found in the lesions consist of soft irregular masses of filaments and diphtheroidal forms in an acidophilic matrix (6). There are no clubs.

Diagnosis. Large amounts of purulent exudate must be cultured because the causative organism may be infrequent. Since the lesions often involve skin areas, secondary contamination with other bacteria can complicate interpretation of the culture. Detailed biochemical testing of isolates will be necessary to identify an isolate as *A. viscosus* (2).

Treatment. The organism is sensitive to penicillin, chloramphenicol, erythromycin, and oxytetracycline. Antibiotics may have to be given for several weeks to effect a cure. Very extensive, fistulated lesions do not respond well to therapy.

REFERENCES

1. Bestetts, Buhlman, Nicolet, and Frankhauser. Acta Neuropath., 1977, *39,* 231.
2. Davenport, Carter, and Patterson. Jour. Clin. Microbiol., 1975, *1,* 75.
3. Georg, Brown, Baker, and Cassell. Am. Jour. Vet. Res., 1972, *33,* 1457.
4. Jordon and Keyes. Archs. Oral Biol., 1964, *9,* 401.

5. Love. Austral. Vet. Jour., 1977, *53,* 107.
6. Sneath. Jour. Gen. Microbiol., 1957, *17,* 184.
7. Socransky, Hubersak, and Propas. Archs. Oral Biol., 1970, *15,* 993.

Actinomyces suis

Actinomycosis of the mammary gland of cows is a relatively common disease that has long been thought to be caused by *A. bovis*. However, detailed investigations of isolations of *Actinomyces* sp. from swine have indicated that they differ consistently in some important respects from classical *A. bovis* strains. Swine isolates produce granular colonies with filamentous offshoots, do not produce H_2S, and may utilize adonitol, inulin, raffinose, and xylose; they also differ antigenically from *A. bovis* and *A. israeli* (3, 4, 5). These authors propose therefore that the species *A. suis* be established for the organism commonly isolated from actinomycosis of the swine mammary gland. The eighth edition of *Bergey's Manual* gives this organism the status of *species incertae sedis*.

Morphology and Staining Reactions. Short, Gram-positive forms are present on initial isolation, giving rise to branched filaments on subculture. The cells in smooth colonies are of medium length and uniform thickness with variable staining characteristics. Cells from rough colonies exhibit long, curved, swollen V- and Y-shaped forms with frequent branching.

Cultural and Biochemical Features. Granular microcolonies with filamentous offshoots are produced. As the colonies enlarge, smooth-rough and rough colonial forms may occur. On serum agar colonies are white and on blood agar are brown to reddish brown.

A. suis is catalase-, indol-, gelatinase-, and H_2S-negative; does not reduce nitrate; and ferments adonitol inulin, raffinose, and xylose. In agar gel precipitin tests, the organism was antigenically different from *A. bovis, A. israeli, A. naeslundi,* and *A. propionicus* (3).

Epidemiology and Pathogenesis. Little is known about the habitat of *A. suis,* but it is likely that it is a parasite of the oropharynx of swine and opportunistically invades wounds on the mammary gland. The sharp teeth of piglets frequently cause superficial wounds of the mammary skin during suckling, and it is probable that infection occurs in this way. After entry the organism produces a typical actinomycotic granuloma, resulting in enlargement, induration, and eventual escape of pus that contains typical sulfur granules.

Treatment. *A. suis* is very sensitive to penicillin, erythromycin, and chloramphenicol and less sensitive to chlortetracycline and streptomycin. It is resistant to polymixin B (2). Treatment is more likely to be successful when the lesions are less than fist size. If large lesions are present, surgical excision with antibiotic therapy is necessary, but relapses are frequent (1).

REFERENCES

1. Bethke and Buschmann. Deut. tierärztl. Wchnschr., 1972, *79,* 238.
2. Franke. Deut. Tierarztl. Wchnschr., 1971, *78,* 524.
3. Franke. Zentrbl. f. Bakt., 1973, *223,* 111.
4. Grasser. Zentrbl. f. Bakt., 1962, *184,* 478.
5. Grasser. Zentrbl. f. Bakt., 1963, *188,* 251.

24 The Genus *Nocardia*

In this genus several species are pathogenic for cattle, dogs, cats, marsupials, and man, causing tuberculosis-like diseases or ulcerative lesions. Most are soil saprophytes. In early stages of growth on culture media these microorganisms form a mycelium that is not septate, but eventually the filaments form transverse walls and break up into coccoid cells. Most forms produce aerial hyphae. Members of the genus are nonmotile, aerobic, Gram-positive, and do not form endospores. Their colonies may be rough or smooth, of a soft to a doughlike consistency, or compact and leathery. Many species of the nocardiae form pigments of a blue, violet, red, yellow, orange, or green color, although most of the cultures are colorless. Some are acid-fast, and the small coccoid forms cannot be distinguished with certainty from acid-fast bacilli. This fact should be remembered by those who are dealing with materials that may have been contaminated with soil. Some of these forms have proved pathogenic for experimental animals when cultures were injected, and it is possible that occasional spontaneous animal infections may be caused by such organisms. Two of the acid-fast members of the genus which have been involved in diseases of animals are *N. farcinica,* and *N. asteroides.*

Nocardia farcinica

SYNONYMS: *Actinomyces farcinicus, Streptothrix farcinica, Streptothrix nocardii, Actinomyces nocardii,* and others.

This organism is the causative agent of a disease of cattle in tropical countries first described in France under the name *farcin-de-boeuf* (bovine farcy) (6). The disease is said to be enzootic on the island of Guadeloupe in the French West Indies. It is not known to exist in North America. The taxonomic status of the causative organism is confused. Ridell (7) studied 34 strains of *N. farcinica* using agar gel precipitin tests, ability to grow in 7 percent NaCl at 45 C, and production of arylsulfatase. He decided that about two-thirds of these strains belonged to the genus *Mycobacterium* and the remainder to *Nocardia*. Berd (2) found that five African strains of *N. farcinica* were distinct from either of two groups of the *N. asteroides* strain. Immunological evidence that *N. farcinica* and *N. asteroides* strains are different has also been obtained (4).

Thus further work needs to be done in Africa to resolve the question of the precise identity of the pathogen involved in bovine farcy. It is possible that a similar disease has been produced by two different organisms, one belonging to the genus *Mycobacterium,* the other to *Nocardia*.

Morphology and Staining Reactions. Stained films show filaments varying in length and averaging perhaps 0.3 μm in width. Branching is frequently seen. The filaments easily break into fragments, many of which resemble bacilli. These elements are Gram-positive, and most of them retain the acid-fast stain (3).

Cultural Features. Growth on solid media resembles that of many of the saprophytic actinomycetes which are so common in garden soil. Growth occurs readily on plain agar slants. Small ragged colonies quickly coalesce to form a tough, yellowish white, dry pellicle, which becomes wrinkled and powdery. The powdery appearance indicates that aerial hyphae are formed. In broth the growth occurs principally as whitish granules, although small islands of growth may appear on the surface. Gelatin is not liquefied and milk is not changed. An abundant, dull pellicle forms on the surface of potato slants. No pigment is formed. Growth is best at 37 C but also occurs at 45 C. *N. farcinica* contains nocardomycolic acids and is positive for acetamidase and for ethanolamine assimilation. Acid is not produced from rhamnose, as it is by most strains of *N. asteroides*.

Epidemiology and Pathogenesis. Little is known of the epidemiology and pathogenesis of bovine farcy. The occurrence of lesions on the limbs, particularly the prescapular area, suggests that the organism enters via soil or environmental contamination of superficial wounds. Tick bites may also be a route of entry (1). Entry is followed by a local subcutaneous cellulitis which spreads along local lymphatic channels to regional lymph nodes. The lesions may break through the skin, forming sinuses communicating with cold abscesses. The disease is chronic, and eventually lung involvement may occur, after which the animal becomes emaciated and dies. Cultures are easily obtained from the freshly opened nodules.

Diagnosis. Smears from pus are stained by the Gram and Ziehl-Nielsen methods. The organism appears as masses of fine branching filaments which tend to stain uniformly when the smear is taken from a young lesion. In many cases ovoid enlargements are seen along the course of the filaments, giving them a beaded appearance. In older lesions the organism appears to break into small coccal forms (5).

Confirmation of diagnosis can be made by guinea pig inoculation. The animal usually dies within 10 to 20 days. Necropsy shows general emaciation and numerous tuberclelike nodules scattered over the surface of the peritoneum.

Immunity. There are no vaccines. Some infected animals react in the tuberculin test.

Treatment. The parenteral administration of sodium iodide is recommended.

REFERENCES

1. Al Janabi, Branagan, and Danskin. Trop. An. Health and Produc., 1975, *7*, 205.
2. Berd. Am. Rev. Resp. Dis., 1973, *108*, 909.
3. Henrici and Gardner. Jour. Inf. Dis., 1921, *28*, 232.

4. Magnusson and Mariat. Jour. Gen. Microbiol., 1968, *51*, 151.
5. Nasis. Vet. Rec., 1961, *73*, 370.
6. Nocard. Ann. Inst. Pasteur, 1883, *2*, 293.
7. Ridell. Int. Jour. Systematic Bact., 1975, *25*, 124.

Nocardia asteroides

SYNONYMS: *Cladothrix asteroides, Streptothrix eppingeri, Actinomyces asteroides*

N. asteroides is an opportunistic pathogen which is being isolated with increasing frequency from cases of bovine mastitis and from granulomatous lesions of the subcutis and thoracic organs of dogs and cats. In man the infection is often a complication of neoplasia or immunosuppression.

Morphology and Staining Reactions. *N. asteroides* forms long, filamentous, branching cells which tend to break into coccoid or bacillary forms after 4 days' incubation. It is Gram-positive and some stains are acid-fast.

Cultural and Biochemical Features. The organism is aerobic and produces raised, heaped, folded granular colonies with irregular borders. Yellow-orange pigment formation is common. Acid is produced from D-fructose and D-glucose, dextrin, and mannose. Nitrate is reduced and urease but not gelatinase is produced. Its optimum growth temperature is 28 to 30 C. Casein is not hydrolyzed.

Epidemiology and Pathogenesis. *N. asteroides* is a soil saprophyte and is therefore widely distributed in the environment. Entry of the organism occurs via wounds, ingestion, and inhalation. The cutaneous form of the disease is characterized by pyogranuloma formation and tracts which drain pus to the surface. Infection of the respiratory tract in dogs and cats results in pleural effusion and pyothorax. The exudate usually has the appearance of tomato soup. Sulfur granules may be uncommon. Systemic nocardiosis in dogs is sometimes accompanied by pyrexia, emaciation, coughing, and nervous signs—symptoms indistinguishable from those of distemper.

Such cases may in fact be mixed infections involving both distemper virus and *N. asteroides*—the latter being an opportunistic invader that has taken advantage of the immunosuppressive effects of the virus infection (4). The organism has also been isolated from lesions in the central nervous system of the dog at necropsy (21) and from cases of vertebral osteomyelitis (16) in this species.

There are many other reports of the disease in dogs (5, 6, 7, 14, 17).

Feline nocardiosis is less common than the disease in the dog and has been reviewed by Frost (10). Akun (1) has described cases involving the submandibular lymph gland, the pleura, and the lungs.

The disease has also been diagnosed in equine mandibles where it was associated with bilateral anomalies of the inferior dentition (25). The infection has also been described in swine (12).

Numerous reports of bovine mastitis caused by *N. asteroides* exist (2, 8, 9, 11, 18, 20). The organism is a common contaminant of the skin of the udder and has been found in bulk tank milk (9). Entry apparently occurs via contaminated infusion equipment during therapy of other forms of mastitis. The organism then multiplies in the already devitalized tissue, producing a purulent granulomatous inflammation. Systemic signs may or may not be present. Diffuse fibrosis or discrete hard nodules may be felt in the affected areas. An enzootic of nocardia mastitis in a dairy herd in California has been described by Pier, *et al.* (18). In this outbreak the disease was acute, with high fever. Most cases developed soon after calving. Nocardia-infected cows should be culled because of permanent loss of mammary function and the risk of their becoming permanent shedders of the microorganism (11).

Immunity. Immunity to *N. asteroides* has not been extensively studied but probably involves principally the cell-mediated response. Pier *et al.* (19) have prepared a nocardial antigen from *N. asteroides* and claim that it can be used in allergic, precipitin, and complement-fixation tests to detect present or previous nocardiosis in cattle.

Diagnosis. The organism appears as Gram-positive, branched, slender filaments (0.5 to 1.0 μm). The organism is partially acid-fast, and this characteristic is best demonstrated when alcohol is omitted from the staining procedure. Specimens must also be cultured and the causative organism isolated and identified.

Treatment. *In vitro* drug sensitivity tests are not accurate guides to the therapy of nocardiosis. For instance, sulfonamides are inactive against most strains *in vitro* yet are very successful in therapy. Great variability in minimum inhibitory concentration of a wide variety of antimicrobials has been observed (3). Marked synergy of erythromycin and ampicillin has been observed *in vitro* (3). These workers also reported minocycline was the most effective drug *in vitro*. Reports by Runyon (22) and Strauss *et al.* (24) indicate that sulfadiazine is effective in animal protection tests, but Aureomycin, Chloromycetin, and streptomycin give only partial protection. Sapegin and Cormack (23) treated two cases of canine nocardiosis with Hibitane (bis-*p*-chlorophenyldeguanidohexane) and reported good clinical recovery. Other reports have indicated that benzalkonium chloride (15) and the combination of cycloserine and sulfonamides (13) are effective.

REFERENCES

1. Akun. Deut. tierärztl. Wchnschr., 1952, *59,* 202.
2. Awad. Vet. Rec., 1960, *72,* 341.
3. Bach, Sabath, and Finland. Antimicrobiol. Ag. Chemother., 1973, *3,* 1.
4. Blake. Jour. Am. Vet. Med. Assoc., 1954, *125,* 467.
5. Bohl, Jones, Farrell, Chamberlain, Cole, and Ferguson. Jour. Am. Vet. Med. Assoc., 1953, *122,* 81.
6. Brodey, Cole, and Sauer. Jour. Am. Vet. Med. Assoc., 1955, *127,* 433.
7. Christensen and Clifford. Am. Jour. Vet. Res., 1953, *14,* 298.
8. Ditchfield, Butas, and Julian. Can. Jour. Comp. Med. and Vet. Sci., 1959, *23,* 93.
9. Eales, Leaver, Swan, and Wellington. Austral. Vet. Jour., 1964, *40,* 321.
10. Frost. Austral. Vet. Jour., 1959, *35,* 22.
11. Fuchs and Boretius. Arch. f. Exp. Vetmed., 1972, *26,* 683.
12. Gottschalk, Correa, Correa, and Compos. Arquinos do Instituto Biologico., (S. Paulo), 1971, *38,* 167.
13. Hoeprich, Brandt, and Parker. Am. Jour. Med. Sci., 1968, *255,* 208.
14. Johnston. Jour. Path. and Bact., 1956, *71,* 7.
15. Merkal and Thurston. Am. Jour. Vet. Res., 1968, *29,* 759.
16. Mitten. Jour. Small Anim. Prac., 1974, *15,* 563.
17. Moss. Jour. Am. Vet. Med. Assoc., 1956, *128,* 143.
18. Pier, Gray, and Fossatti. Am. Jour. Vet. Res., 1958, *19,* 319.
19. Pier, Thurston, and Larsen. Am. Jour. Vet. Res., 1968, *29,* 397.
20. Pier, Willers, and Mejia. Am. Jour. Vet. Res., 1961, *22,* 698.
21. Rhoades, Reynolds, Rahn, and Small. Jour. Am. Vet. Med. Assoc., 1963, *142,* 278.
22. Runyon. Jour. Lab. and Clin. Med., 1951, *37,* 713.
23. Sapegin and Cormack. North Am. Vet., 1956, *37,* 385.
24. Strauss, Kligman, and Pillsbury. Am. Rev. Tuberc., 1951, *63,* 441.
25. Tritschler and Romack. Vet. Med., 1965, *60,* 605.

25 The Genus *Mycobacterium*

The family Mycobacteriaceae contains one genus, the genus *Mycobacterium*. The members of this genus are aerobic, slightly curved or straight rods, which sometimes branch. Filaments may be produced under some conditions, but these fragment into rods or cocci when disturbed. They are acid-alcohol-fast at some stage of growth and have an unusually high lipid content. They are hard to stain by Gram's method but are usually considered to be Gram-positive.

The genus contains strains which grow rapidly (7 days) and strains which grow slowly (2 to 6 weeks), as well as strains which cannot be grown *in vitro*. Because bacterial species have been traditionally differentiated on the basis of their morphological and physiological characteristics, it is clear that a genus containing strains with such diverse growth rates and requirements has been very difficult to classify. In the past, taxonomists have given an individual organism different names because of difficulties in developing clear-cut systems for classifying, naming, and identifying these organisms (8). These problems have still not been resolved. The eighth edition (1974) of *Bergey's Manual* (68) lists 40 species in the genus *Mycobacterium* while other authorities (8) listed only 22 species in 1974. While several unresolved problems in taxonomy still exist, it is agreed that the genus *Mycobacterium* contains a number of species of acid-fast bacteria which are saprophytic, as well as other species, notably *Mycobacterium tuberculosis, M. bovis, M. avium,* and *M. paratuberculosis,* that are pathogenic for animals, causing tuberculosis and Johne's disease.

It is now evident that there are a large number of acid-fast bacteria that do not cause classical tuberculosis or Johne's disease. Many are saprophytic, but some can cause disease in domesticated animals and man, and the designation "saprophytic," "atypical" or "anonymous" is no longer satisfactory. Runyon (66) in 1959 proposed a system of four groups for classifying the mycobacteria, including *M. tuberculosis*. The groups are based upon growth rate and pigment production, and the system is still used in some laboratories.

Group I contains the photochromogenic strains that grow slowly and produce a yellow pigment only when exposed to light. This group contains *M. tuberculosis* and such organisms as *M. ulcerans* and *M. marinium* (*balnei*), producers of skin ulcers, as well as *M. kansasi,* an acid-fast bacillus capable of causing pulmonary disease in man.

Group II contains the scotochromogenic strains that grow slowly and form an orange-yellow pigment both in the light and dark. These are the organisms that frequently occur in adenitis in children but are rarely found as independent causes of pulmonary disease and are usually considered to be saprophytes.

Group III are the nonchromogenic strains that grow slowly, do not produce pigment, have smooth colonies, and are resistant to isoniazid. These bacteria are highly pleomorphic and produce *Nocardia*like filaments. They occasionally cause pulmonary disease in humans. Another organism that has been associated with progressive pulmonary disease in man is *M. xenopei* (14). Actually it does not quite fit in any group, but Runyon placed it in Group III even though it is pigmented.

Group IV is reserved for the rapid growers. Most of

these belong to the *M. fortuitum* subgroup, organisms that will not grow at 45 C, and to the *M. phlei* and *M. smegmatis* subgroups. *M. fortuitum* is pathogenic for man and the lower animals. It has been implicated in a serious epizootic of bovine mastitis in a large Oregon dairy herd (56).

Although much has been done to classify and name the strains of mycobacteria, a number of unresolved taxonomic dilemmas still confront the bacteriologist who isolates one of them from a lesion in a domesticated animal. Despite Runyon's four groups and the 40 named species in *Bergey's Manual,* problems and contradictions still exist in identifying and naming these ''atypical'' species.

The Tubercle Bacilli and Tuberculosis

Tuberculosis was described more than 2,000 years ago, and bone lesions found in Egyptian mummies proved that it existed among people long before that. Quite naturally there was much confusion between tuberculosis and other diseases of man in ancient and medieval times, and this confusion lasted until after the middle of the 19th century. Many early writers claimed the disease to be infectious, but others regarded it as a form of malignant tumor and noninfectious until after the causative agent had been found and experimentation had removed all doubt as to its nature. Although he was not the first to claim infectiousness, Villemin (84) demonstrated, in 1865, that tuberculous tissue from man and cattle produced the disease in rabbits by inoculation.

The tubercle bacillus probably was first seen in tissues by Baumgarten (4) in 1882. In the same year Koch (37) succeeded in demonstrating the organisms in diseased tissues by staining them with alkaline methylene blue and counterstaining with Bismarck brown (vesuvin). With this method the tubercle bacilli remained blue while all other organisms and tissues lost the blue and took on the brown color of the counterstain. Koch also found that the organism could be cultivated in pure culture on a medium consisting of coagulated bovine serum. With such cultures he readily reproduced the disease in experimental animals and thus removed all doubt as to its etiological relationship. His final report on his work was published in 1884 (38).

The Types of Tubercle Bacilli. Villemin (84) showed that tuberculosis could be produced in rabbits by inoculating them either with sputum from human cases or with tissue from nodules that occur on the chest wall of tuberculous cattle. He believed, therefore, that the diseases of man and cattle were identical and caused by a single virulent agent. This belief was also held at first by Koch because, after demonstrating tubercle bacilli in human tissues, he found what appeared to be the same organism in tissues of tuberculous cattle. Rivolta (65), however, in 1889 showed that the organism that affects birds was not identical with those affecting mammals, and Smith (73) in 1898 pointed out certain differences in cultural characteristics and pathogenicity between the types ordinarily found in man and those usually found in cattle.

A number of types of tubercle bacilli are now known to be responsible for tuberculosis in animals. The human type, *M. tuberculosis,* causes tuberculosis in humans but can also cause disease in pigs, monkeys, and occasionally in cattle, dogs, and parrots. The bovine type, *M. bovis,* is closely related to the human type and is considered by some (7) to be a subspecies of *M. tuberculosis.* It causes tuberculosis in cattle, pigs, horses, man, and occasionally in cats and sheep. The avian type, *M. avium,* differs from the mammalian types in many respects and produces disease primarily in birds and occasionally in pigs, cattle, sheep, and man. The murine type, *M. murium* or the vole bacillus, differs from the others in many respects and is virtually nonpathogenic for man and domesticated animals. The cold-blooded types include *M. piscium, M. marinium,* and *M. platypoecillis.* They occur in fish and other cold-blooded animals.

Morphology and Staining Features. *M. tuberculosis* in both tissues and cultures is a slender, rod-shaped organism. It shows considerable pleomorphism. Were it not for its acid-fastness it might be classed in the diphtheroid group. Granules are often evident in stained preparations. In general, the *human* type (Figures 25.1 and 25.2) is more apt to be beaded and the cells are usually longer than the *bovine* type (Figure 25.3). The latter usually is rather short, relatively plump, and solid staining. The *avian* type (Figures 25.4 and 25.5) is more variable than either of the mammalian types, sometimes appearing in the form of long beaded rods and at other times as very short, solid-staining forms. The difference in morphology is not a sufficient basis upon which to differentiate one type from another.

All forms are strongly acid- and alcohol-fast, and they are Gram-positive. The acid-fast characteristic aids in finding tubercle bacilli in tissues and exudates since it is possible to stain them differently from other bacteria, tissue cells, and tissue debris.

Cultural Features. Koch first cultivated tubercle bacilli on bovine blood serum that had been coagulated with heat. He was not able to induce the organism to

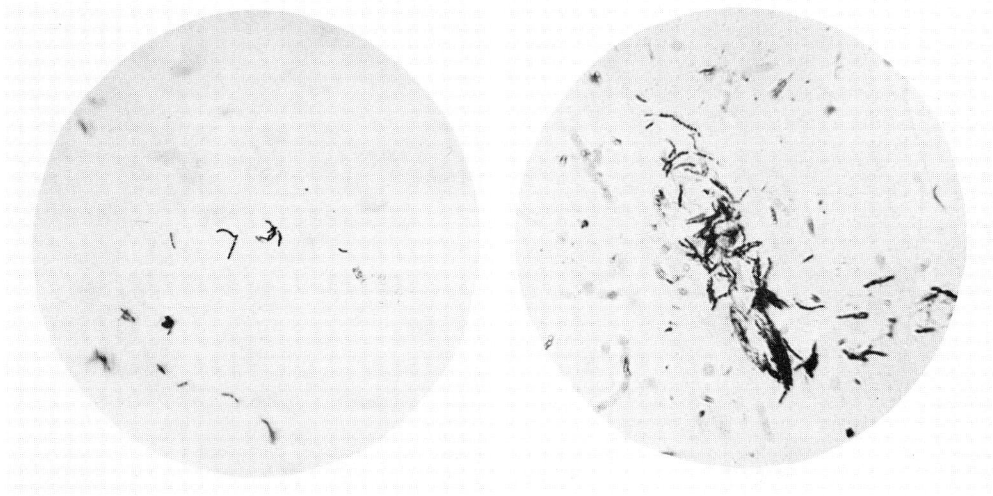

Figure 25.1 (*left*). *Mycobacterium tuberculosis* in the sputum of a consumptive patient. × 770.
Figure 25.2 (*right*). *Mycobacterium tuberculosis* from a culture on glycerol-egg medium incubated 6 weeks at 37 C. × 770.

grow on any of the common laboratory media. In 1902, Dorset (13) introduced the use of coagulated egg medium. Many modifications of the original formula have been made, and these continue to be our best media for isolating tubercle bacilli from infected tissues. Excellent media may be made by adding yolk material to basic media solidified with agar. Many of the egg media contain dyes which act as inhibiting agents for other bacteria frequently associated with tubercle bacilli in the materials cultured. Glycerol in egg medium favors the growth of the human but not of the bovine type of bacilli.

Figure 25.3. *Mycobacterium bovis,* from a culture on Dorset's egg medium incubated 6 weeks at 37 C. These long beaded forms are seen only in cultures. In tissues this type ordinarily is solid-staining and shorter than the other types. × 1,030.

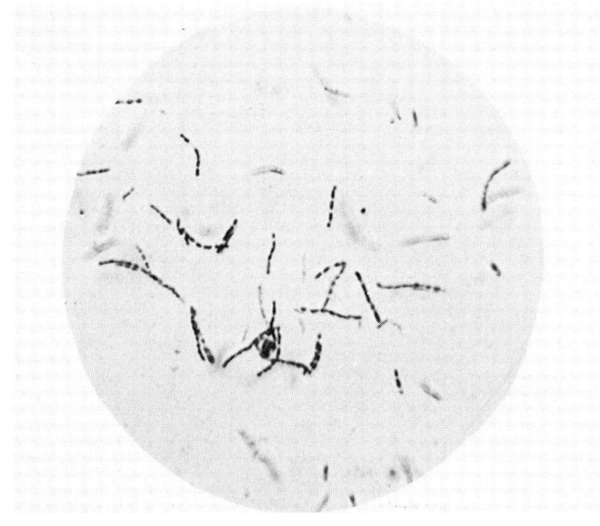

These complex organic media will support the growth of small inocula of mycobacteria. Lowenstein-Jensen is one such medium which contains eggs, glycerol, and malachite green. Stonebrink's medium (77) contains no glycerol; this favors the growth of the human but not of the bovine type of bacilli, and so it is usually used for the isolation of *M. bovis*.

On solid media tubercle bacilli multiply slowly. The avian type multiplies much faster than either of the mammalian, and the human develops much more readily and faster than the bovine. English workers have used the terms *eugonic* and *dysgonic* in referring to the ease with which mammalian bacilli can be cultivated, the first term being equivalent in general to the human and the latter to the bovine type.

All tubercle bacilli are aerobic in nature. Growth does not occur under anaerobic conditions, and it is inhibited even when the culture tubes are sealed so that the amount of available air is limited. Growth occurs only at temperatures close to that of the body.

On solid media it is not possible to differentiate between the human and bovine types of cultures by the appearance of the growth. Primary cultures usually require from 3 to 4 weeks' incubation at 37 C before colonies can be detected with the naked eye. The colonies appear first as minute dull flakes, which gradually thicken into dry, irregular masses that stand high above the surface of the medium. The color is slightly yellow, but if exposed to light it gradually changes through shades of deep yellow to a brick red. When cultures have become accustomed to growing on media, confluent growth develops over the entire surface. This has the appearance of

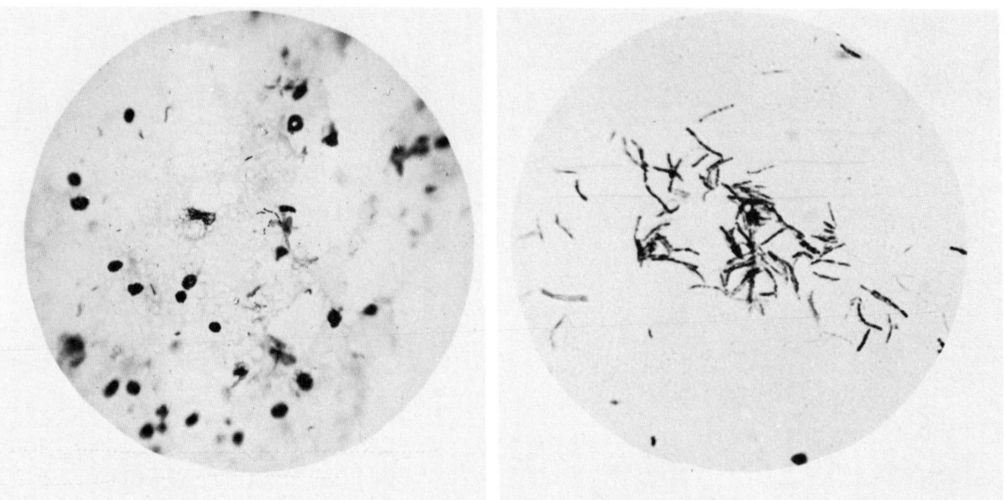

Figure 25.4 (*left*). *Mycobacterium avium,* a film from a liver lesion of a naturally infected chicken. × 360.
Figure 25.5 (*right*). *Mycobacterium avium,* from a culture on Dorset's egg medium which had been incubated 6 weeks at 37 C. × 770.

rough, waxy blankets, which after several weeks' incubation become thick and wrinkled. Where this blanket reaches the margin of the medium's surface, it often crowds up the side of the glass container for an appreciable distance. Old, isolated colonies on solid media become so firm and so loosely attached to the medium that they may be made to skate around with the inoculating loop, or, if the tubes are shaken vigorously, the dry growth often breaks loose and rattles.

M. avium presents a different appearance. The primary colonies are smooth and shiny. They develop much more rapidly than the mammalian types and are not so fastidious in their nutritive requirements. Colonies usually may be detected in less than a week and are well developed at 2 weeks. The colonies are soft in consistency. They cannot be pushed around the surface nor shaken loose as can the other types. When heavily inoculated, the surface blanket is moist, soft, and not greatly wrinkled. The color is a light cream but, like the mammalian types, it becomes yellowish, pinkish, and even dull reddish if incubated in the presence of light.

Theobald Smith (74) early pointed out a growth character by which the mammalian types generally may be differentiated from each other. This depends upon the fact that the human type utilizes glycerol very actively, whereas glycerol utilization by the bovine type is limited.

More rapid tests *in vitro* have been used by Harrington and Karlson (30). They found that the human type produced niacin and nicotinamidase and reduced nitrate to nitrite, whereas the bovine type did not. The growth of the human type was inhibited by nicotinamide, but not by the thiophene-2-carboxylic acid hydrazide, whereas the opposite was true for the bovine type.

On fluid media, except those in which special wetting agents are included, growth is restricted to the surface. The mammalian types present a very dry, rough surface; the avian is much softer, moister, and less wrinkled. Beneath the pellicle, mammalian cultures usually show a perfectly clear medium with little or no sediment (Figure 25.6); the avian cultures generally show considerable mucoid sediment, and stalactites of a slimy nature often extend downward from the pellicle when the cultures become old. When exposed to light, all types of tubercle bacilli gradually change from a creamy color, through shades of tan, to a reddish tan.

In 1945, Dubos (15) described a method by which diffuse growths of all types may be obtained in liquid media. The method hastens multiplication and is adequate for primary isolations from infected tissues. Certain complex lipids have the property of stimulating tubercle bacilli, and at the same time they serve as wetting agents which coat the bacterial cells, causing them to break apart and become dispersed in the fluid instead of adhering to each other in waxy masses that float on the surface. The agent that Dubos found adapted best to this use is a synthetic, nonionic compound consisting of esters of long-chain fatty acids and of polyhydric alcohols called *Tween*. There are several Tweens; the one best adapted for this use is *Tween 80*. Dubos and Middlebrook (16) showed that Tween 80 has toxic as well as stimulating properties, especially for mammalian types. This toxic action can be neutralized by adding a serum albumin fraction, which also serves as a growth stimu-

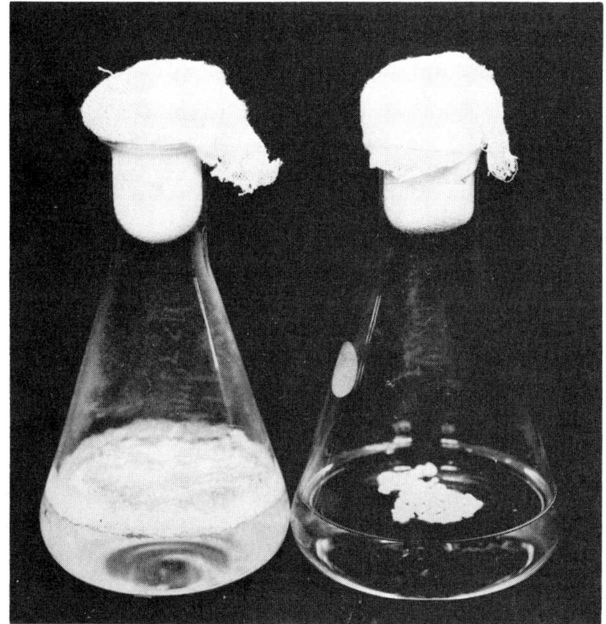

Figure 25.6. *Mycobacterium bovis,* a growth on glycerol broth. The culture in the right-hand flask is about 2 weeks old; that in the left is about 2 months old. Growth appears as a dull-grayish-white pellicle, which finally covers the surface of the fluid medium, becomes thick, opaque, and folded into creases, and pushes up on the sides of the flask at the margins. The fluid remains perfectly clear.

lant. Several fluid media for cultivating tubercle bacilli have been developed incorporating Tween 80.

The discovery that traces of free fatty acids inhibit the growth of mammalian tubercle bacilli suggested an explanation for the observation that many media will support growth of these organisms when the inoculum is large but will not do so when it is small. Obviously, a good medium for isolating these organisms from tissues where they are present, usually in relatively small numbers, is one that contains all the necessary nutrients and at the same time is relatively free of inhibiting substances. Cummings, Drummond, and Lewis (12) have shown that heating increases the ether-soluble material in several kinds of egg media. About twice as much is present when these media are coagulated in the autoclave at 100 C as when they are inspissated at 85 C. The latter, therefore, makes a much better medium than the former. Oleic acid–albumin media (16,64) will support the growth of mycobacteria even when small inocula are used. Relatively simple synthetic media will also support mycobacterial growth, and if fatty acids restrict the growth of small inocula, that effect can be overcome by the addition of serum or albumin (64).

Moore (52) and Fite and Olson (22) have shown that all three types of tubercle bacilli can be cultivated on the chorioallantoic membrane of the developing chick embryo. Characteristic lesions are produced, and these are associated with rapid multiplication of the bacilli. There are some differences in the appearance of the lesions depending upon the type of the infection, but these are not sufficiently distinctive to enable differentiation to be made.

Differentiation of the Types of Tubercle Bacilli. Identification of the types of tubercle bacilli cannot be based upon the host from which they are isolated. Microscopic examination may reveal the organism's type, but this is not entirely reliable as the sizes and shapes of the types vary considerably. Cultural features generally will serve to differentiate the avian from the mammalian, but distinguishing between *M. tuberculosis* and *M. avium* on cultural grounds is quite uncertain. The most satisfactory method is based upon pathogenesis for experimental animals, although this too can produce equivocal results. Strains that have grown in unusual hosts are especially variable in their pathogenicity for experimental animals.

Relative Virulence for Laboratory Animals. *M. avium* is usually highly pathogenic for chickens and rabbits. It is nonpathogenic for guinea pigs as a rule. Local lesions are frequently produced in this species of animal, but only rarely does the disease become generalized. *M. tuberculosis* and *M. bovis* are almost wholly nonpathogenic for chickens, but most strains will produce in guinea pigs progressive infections that lead to death from generalized tuberculosis. These features serve to distinguish the avian-type bacillus from the mammalian types (see Table 25.1).

The differentiation of *M. tuberculosis* from *M. bovis* is more difficult. On the whole, the bovine type is perhaps a little more virulent for guinea pigs than the human type, as measured by the rapidity of the development of the lesions and the time of death of the animals, but this difference is too slight to make it useful in differentiating the types. In the rabbit, however, there is generally an appreciable difference in the virulence of the two types, as was first pointed out by Smith (73).

Table 25.1. Relative virulence for laboratory animals of the types of tubercle bacilli

Type	Guinea pig	Rabbit	Chicken
M. tuberculosis	+	±	0
M. bovis	+	+	0
M. avium	±	+	+

When this animal is given a small dose of bovine-type tubercle bacilli of normal virulence, a progressive disease is set up which leads to its death in 3 weeks to 3 months. A dose of the same size of human-type bacilli of normal virulence usually produces only local lesions, from which the animal recovers. At the end of 3 months rabbits that have been inoculated with human material usually not only are living but have gained weight and appear to be thriving (54).

Cell Structure and Resistance. The mycobacteria have a rather thick cell wall which has a very high lipid content (60 percent) in contrast to the cell walls of the Gram-positive (<5 percent) and Gram-negative (20 percent) bacteria. This lipid coat probably accounts for their acid-fast staining characteristics and for their ability to withstand killing by acids or alkalies. It may also account for their relatively slow growth by impeding the uptake of nutrients and for the parasite's successful survival against the host's defenses.

Tubercle bacilli do not form spores and they exhibit only moderate resistance to heat. They are destroyed by pasteurization. Resistance to desiccation is fairly great. Direct sunlight is rapidly fatal to them. To most disinfectants the resistance is somewhat greater than that exhibited by nonsporing organisms. This is especially true of resistance to acids and alkalies. This property is often used in isolating tubercle bacilli from sputum or exudates contaminated by other bacteria. In moist soils, manure heaps, and old strawstacks, tubercle bacilli may remain alive for very long periods. Schalk, *et al.* (69) were able to show that avian-type tubercle bacilli would remain viable in heavily infected plots of ground for periods as long as 4 years, and in buried fowl carcasses for more than 2 years.

Virulence of *M. tuberculosis*. *M. tuberculosis* does not possess exotoxins, capsules, or noteworthy extracellular enzymes to account for its virulence. It has proved difficult to identify factors that clearly differentiate virulent and avirulent strains without doing pathogenicity tests on experimental animals. One of the organism's major characteristics is the large amount of surface lipid material referred to above. One of these surface lipids, 6,6'-dimycolyltrehalose, has been isolated and called "cord factor" because its presence causes the organism to grow in cords in liquid culture. This cord factor is abundant in virulent strains and its removal renders them avirulent. It is currently felt that the cord factor may contribute to the organism's virulence but is not the sole factor involved.

M. tuberculosis is readily taken up by host macrophages, but unlike most bacteria it can survive and grow intracellularly in these phagocytic cells. The organism has the ability to prevent the fusion of the cell's lysosomes with the phagosome and thus it avoids intracellular digestion and killing (24). Goren *et al.* (25) have recently shown that sulfatides from *M. tuberculosis* accumulate in the lysosomes, which then do not fuse with the cell's phagosomes. This "antifusion" effect prevents the access of lysosomal enzymes to the bacteria in the phagosome. This effect may well prove to be a major virulence factor for *M. tuberculosis,* since its success as a parasite depends on its ability to survive in host cells.

The Pathogenesis of Tuberculosis. The outcome of any microbial infection is dependent upon the balance struck between the virulence of the organism and the efficacy of the host's defense mechanisms. This is particularly well demonstrated in tuberculosis, where the virulence of the organism, the dose and site of infection, and the host's natural and acquired immunity all contribute substantially to the outcome, which can vary from complete resolution in a short time to progressive chronic pneumonia and death of the host.

The name *tuberculosis* is derived from the Latin word *tuberculum,* which means a small lump or nodule. It is an apt name because the disease is characterized by the formation of small masses of inflammatory tissue, or tubercles, in the organs where the bacilli encounter phagocytic cells which engulf and carry them into the lymphatic vessels of the region. The initial, or primary, lesions may develop where invasion of tissue first occurred, or in the lymph nodes which drain that area. The bacilli are always arrested for a time by these nodes, and tubercles are formed in them. In the more resistant species and individuals, the lesions may be confined for long periods, even for the life of the individual, in these nodes. The disease is then said to be localized or arrested. In the more susceptible, the disease progresses by the escape of bacilli through the lymphatics to the next series of nodes, where secondary foci develop. If the disease continues to progress, the organisms eventually reach the bloodstream, by which they are scattered to all parts of the body. Such individuals are said to be suffering from generalized tuberculosis.

Tubercles have a characteristic microscopic structure by which they may be tentatively identified. Initially they consist of aggregations of macrophages which have migrated to the site of bacterial infection. As these are frustrated in their attempts to destroy the tubercle bacilli, more macrophages migrate to the site. These may be attracted by products of the specific immune response, such as lymphokines, and they mop up the cell debris. Lymphocytes and leukocytes also migrate to the site and contribute to the cellular infiltrate.

Stimulated by the tubercle bacilli in their centers, these tubercles continue to enlarge. Shortly they may be seen with the naked eye as translucent, pearly structures like small grains of tapioca. As growth of the tubercles continues, necrosis begins in their centers, and the pearl appearance gives way to yellowish-white opaqueness (Figure 25.7). Generally about this time another type of cell appears in the lesion—giant cells of the Langhans type. These are formed from macrophages either by fusion or by continued growth and multiplication of nuclei without division of cytoplasm. They become quite large and conspicuous. Their cytoplasm is clear and their nuclei, numbering from 2 or 3 or 10 or more, are arranged in the form of a crescent, or half-circle, around the periphery of one side of the cell. Tubercle bacilli frequently can be seen lying within the cytoplasm of these cells. As the tuberculous mass grows and the necrotic center becomes larger and larger, macrophages and giant cells can generally be found just outside the advancing necrotic front.

Old tuberculous masses may be very large. They may involve entire lung lobes and large areas of the liver and spleen, and they may cause lymph nodes to become 20 times as large as normal. The central parts of such lesions usually consist of very dry, cheesy material in which calcium deposits often appear, so that they make a gritty sound when they are incised. Such lesions often become surrounded by dense connective tissue.

Figure 25.7. A very early tubercle in the lung of a rabbit caused by *Mycobacterium avium*. The structure is typical of all primary tubercles regardless of the type of bacillus concerned. The central area of necrosis is surrounded by a layer of macrophages which make up the greater part of the field. The periphery of the lesion consists of fibroblasts and lymphocytes. Giant cells appear a little later near the margin of the necrotic area. × 110.

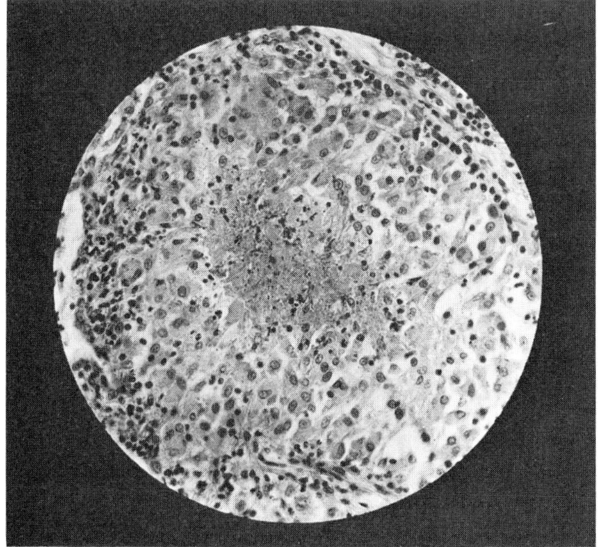

When tuberculous necrosis occurs in the lungs, the process often causes perforation of the bronchi and bronchioles, in which case the caseous material escapes into the air passages and is coughed up. The sputum thus becomes purulent and it contains tubercle bacilli, often in large numbers. Individuals that discharge bacilli in air droplets during coughing are called *open cases,* and the sputum is highly infectious. Man often expectorates, thus grossly contaminating his environment. Animals swallow such sputum, but the organisms escape in the feces and thus infect their surroundings. Frequently in man but rarely in animals, the discharge of tuberculous pus from lung abscesses leaves large cavities with exposed blood vessels. These may rupture, allowing blood to escape into the air passages. Hemoptysis, or bleeding into the air passages, may be so severe in man as to lead to death; this condition is unusual in animals because cavitation rarely occurs, even when the lesions become very large.

Tuberculosis in Animals, including Man. *Cattle.* In adult cattle, the lesions of tuberculosis are usually found in the lungs and the lymph nodes of the head and thorax. Most infections seem to be contracted by inhalation, but undoubtedly some occur through ingestion of the organism. In recently infected animals, the bronchial, mediastinal, submaxillary, and retropharyngeal nodes more often exhibit visible lesions than the lungs, but this may well be because small pulmonary lesions are not readily found. The lung lesions usually take the form of caseocalcareous masses located in the anterior lobes. Some are so small that they can easily be overlooked; others involve entire lobes (Figure 25.8). Active lesions may show hyperemia around the periphery of the caseous masses. Old, inactive lesions may become very calcareous and heavily encapsulated. Tubercle bacilli are often difficult to demonstrate by microscopic means, especially in the older lesions, but cultural methods and guinea pig inoculation usually succeed.

Tuberculous pleuritis or peritonitis is relatively common where tuberculosis of cattle is prevalent. In this form of the disease large masses of smooth grapelike bodies cover the serous surfaces. Often the lung tissue

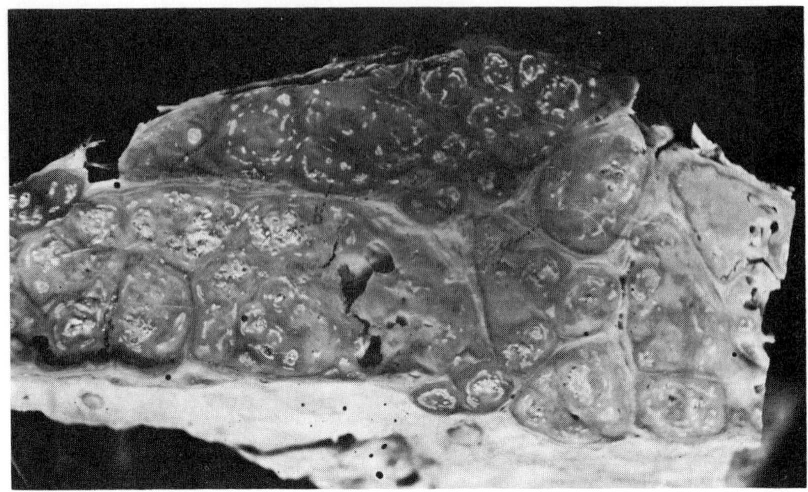

Figure 25.8. Advanced tuberculosis in the lung of a cow. The entire diaphragmatic lobe is involved in the tuberculous process. There is extensive necrosis and fibrosis. The necrotic tissue contains large amounts of calcareous material.

itself is not so seriously involved as its serous surface. In a majority of cases of lung tuberculosis in cattle, however, the disease causes massive adhesions of the lungs to the chest wall, the fibrous tissue being so strong that the lungs cannot be removed from the cavity unless they are cut out. Less often involved in adult cattle are the liver, the spleen, and the mesenteric lymph nodes. Udder infection is found in less than 1 percent of all cases, even those that are fairly advanced. In these cases the lesions, like those found elsewhere, may be nodular, or they may involve large areas of tissue. When large areas are involved, bacilli are shed into the lactiferous ducts, and the milk from such animals may contain large numbers of organisms. This milk is very dangerous for man, especially children, and for other animals when it is consumed in a raw state. Calves fed on milk containing tubercle bacilli usually show primary lesions in the abdominal cavity rather than the thorax. In these cases the mesenteric lymph nodes may become greatly enlarged and hardened, and the liver and portal lymph nodes usually are involved. Lung lesions, if present, are secondary. Calves may also be infected by inhalation, in which case the distribution of lesions is like that in most adults. A good description of the lesions of tuberculosis in cattle is given by Stamp (76).

Avian-type tubercle bacilli may be found in lesions in cattle in areas where tuberculosis in poultry is prevalent. These organisms are picked up from the soil, which is polluted by infected chickens. The lesions are usually found in the lymph nodes that drain the alimentary canal. They may have no effect on the health of the animals but are important in that such animals will regularly react to avian tuberculin and johnin and thus may be mistaken for cases of paratuberculosis or Johne's disease. Such animals also occasionally react to mammalian tuberculin. *M. avium* has occasionally been isolated from lung lesions in cattle (55), from milk (42, 78), and rarely from a cow with generalized avian tuberculosis (80).

In Denmark, Plum (57), Bang (2), and others have found cases of infectious abortion in cattle apparently caused by avian-type tubercle bacilli. In these instances tuberculous lesions are found in the uterine wall and in the placenta. The diagnosis of such cases can readily be made by examining the placenta, or the uterine discharge following abortion. The lesions may remain in the uterine wall from one gestation period to the next, and such animals may continue to abort. The organisms are not usually found in any other body organs or tissues, except occasionally in the mesenteric lymph nodes, a fact which suggests that the disease may be contracted through the digestive tract. Although avian tuberculosis is common in some parts of the United States where there are also many dairy herds, this form of the disease has been reported only once (20).

Swine. Swine are subject to infection with all three types of tubercle bacilli, and the incidence of each type depends upon the locality in which the animals live and the character of their feed. The human-type infection, for example, almost always occurs in swine that are fed on garbage (swill). Where tuberculosis is prevalent in cattle, most of the infections in swine come from that source. In the corn belt of the United States, which might also be called the swine belt, the vast majority of cases are of the avian type, the reason being that tuberculosis in chickens is prevalent in this area, whereas bovine tuberculosis is almost nonexistent (17). Generally speaking, *M. bovis* is capable of causing a more serious form of the disease than either of the other two types. Infections with the bovine organism generally are progressive and will lead to the eventual death of the animal. The life span of most swine is short, not over 8 or 9 months. Such animals do not live long enough to become active spreaders of the disease; hence, the disease is contracted more from the environment than from other swine.

Lesions of tuberculosis, regardless of type, are found more often in the abdominal cavity of hogs than is the case in cattle. Infections are contracted most commonly by ingestion; thus the primary lesions are found in the lymph nodes of the head and of the abdominal cavity *(tuberculous adenitis)*. In human-type infections the lesions are seldom found in any other locations and they are usually of minimal size. In *M. avium* infections, the majority show only adenitis, but a few cases may exhibit lesions in the liver, spleen, and lungs. The bovine type more often involves the visceral organs. Extensive lung lesions resembling those of cattle are not uncommon. Lesions are frequently found in the liver, and *M. bovis* may produce a large, prominent, fluid-filled lesion in the spleen.

Horses. Horses are relatively susceptible to infection with bovine-type tubercle bacilli, but cases are infrequently encountered except when the animals live in very intimate association with tuberculous cattle.

The lesions of equine tuberculosis are most frequent in the lymph nodes of the pharyngeal region and in those of the mesentery, but lung, liver, and spleen lesions are not rare (Figure 25.9). In some cases the lesions appear very much like those in cattle, there being both caseation necrosis and calcification in the older lesions. In many instances, however, they do not have the usual appearance but consist of yellowish-white masses of rather soft tissue which have the appearance of a tumor. Necrosis is not obvious to the naked eye, nor is there any calcification.

Many strains of tubercle bacilli isolated from horses are of reduced virulence for experimental animals, and some are nearly avirulent. Reports on avian-type tuberculosis in the horse are rare, but Lesslie and Davies (43) described a case in which this type produced lesions in the lymph glands, lungs, and skin.

Sheep and goats. This disease is rather rare in sheep and goats (45). In sheep most of the infections that have been typed abroad were found to be of the bovine type, but in the United States most have proved to be avian in origin (31). These cases have been found in areas of the country where avian tuberculosis is common, but bovine tuberculosis is rare. Lesions of the lungs and thoracic lymph nodes were found in all cases; a majority showed liver tubercles, and the spleen was involved in about one-half of the cases.

The data on tuberculosis in goats is very meager, suggesting that the goat is relatively resistant to infection. Soliman *et al.* (75) described an outbreak in goats in 1953 in England. Out of 41 animals examined in a flock, 32 showed macroscopic lesions. The lesions were mainly intestinal and the disease was of a progressive nature only in young kids. The type of the organism

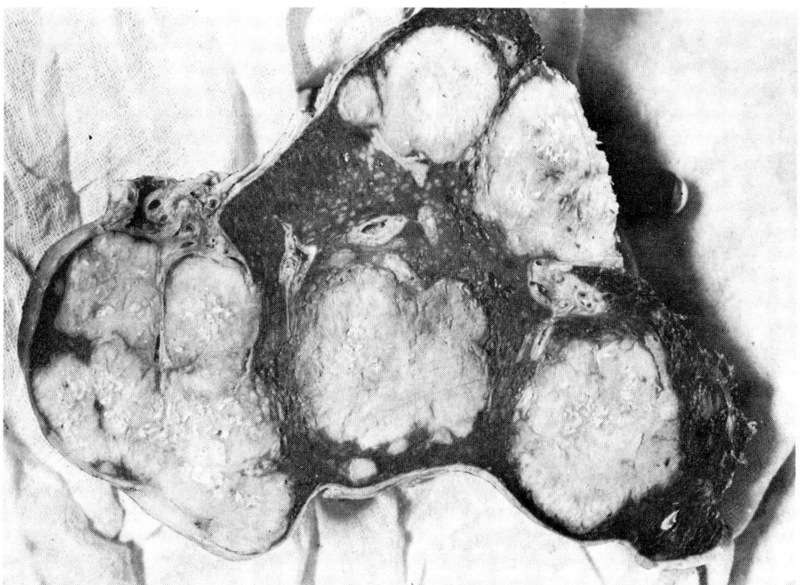

Figure 25.9. Tuberculosis of the spleen in a horse. Lesions in horses often resemble tumors, being white or gray in color, uniform in consistency, and lacking obvious gross evidence of necrosis.

causing the infection was not determined. A brief review of tuberculosis in goats was given, and although it appears that the bovine type has been concerned in most known cases of tuberculosis in this animal, the avian type has also been implicated.

Dogs and cats. Cases of tuberculosis in dogs (53) and cats are not usual in the United States but appear to be more common elsewhere. Dogs are susceptible to both human- and bovine-type infections, but the majority of cases have been shown to be caused by the human type. Many cases have been reported in which small lap dogs have obviously been infected by their tuberculous masters. Cats, on the other hand, appear to be very resistant to human-type infections and seldom are infected by tuberculous owners. They are quite susceptible to bovine-type infections, however, and usually contract the disease by drinking milk from tuberculous cows. Hix *et al.* (33) have reported a case of avian-type infection in the cat, and Wilkinson (87) described a granuloma associated with the human type.

Verge and Senthille (83) reviewed all reported cases of dog and cat tuberculosis from all parts of the world in which the infecting organism had been typed. Their findings are reported in Table 25.2.

In dogs, the disease usually involves the thoracic organs primarily. Lesions elsewhere are infrequent. In cats, the primary lesions are usually in the abdominal organs but the lungs often become involved secondarily.

Chickens. Chickens are not susceptible to mammalian tubercle bacilli; all cases are caused by avian-type organisms. Infections are contracted by ingestion of bacilli from infected soil and water. The organism is sometimes found in eggs laid by tuberculous hens, and this may occasionally account for the way the disease enters previously uninfected flocks. It has already been pointed out that *M. avium* persists for long periods on infected premises.

Table 25.2. Types of tubercle bacilli affecting dogs and cats (naturally occurring cases)

Animal species	Human No.	Human %	Bovine No.	Bovine %	Avian No.	Avian %
Dogs	389	65.7	189	32.0	2*	0.3
Cats	6	4.6	125	95.4	0	0.0

*One of these cases was credited to an author who denies having reported such a case; therefore it must be regarded as an error.

Unlike mammals, birds seldom suffer from tuberculosis of the lungs. The lesions occur in the intestinal tract, in the liver and spleen, and frequently in the bones and joints.

Intestinal ulcers may be found in any part of the intestine. They are readily found as tumorlike masses on the outside of the gut measuring up to 4 or 5 cm in diameter. When incised they are found to be filled with caseous material, which is discharged through a relatively small ulcerated passage into the lumen of the intestine. Great masses of bacilli are ordinarily demonstrated with ease in this material, and it is these bacilli, discharged with the feces, which contaminate the soil.

Liver lesions are always found in infected birds (Figure 25.10). These appear as caseous areas, varying in size, distributed throughout all parts of the organ.

The spleen is generally enlarged, showing moderate to marked hypertrophy. Instead of the normal, smooth surface, tuberculous spleens usually become nodular. When incised, a few large caseous masses may be seen or large numbers of very minute foci.

Infected joints are swollen and contain caseous material. Tubercle bacilli may be found in abundance in this material and, in fact, in all tuberculous lesions in birds.

Figure 25.10. Tuberculosis of the liver in a chicken. Gross lesions in cut section (*upper*). Lesions as seen from the surface (*lower*).

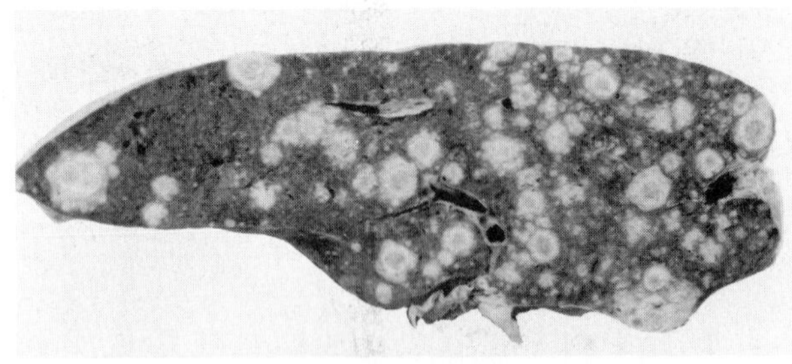

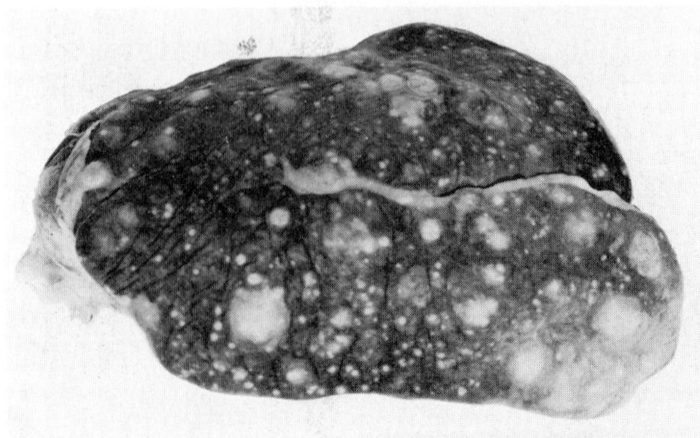

Tuberculosis in birds develops rather slowly. Well-developed lesions seldom are found in birds less than 1 year of age, and such birds seldom become spreaders during the first few months of the course of the infection. The disease is manifested by loss of body weight, listlessness, and weakness. The owners frequently refer to the disease as "going light." Lameness, caused by bone and joint lesions, is frequent.

Birds other than chickens. Tuberculosis occurs in turkeys, pigeons, pheasants, ducks, and geese, as well as in many wild birds. The disease in these species is essentially like that in chickens. Ducks and geese are not infected as often as chickens, pheasants, and turkeys. In 1966, Bickford *et al.* (6) investigated the epizootiology of tuberculosis in starlings on a farm in Indiana where there was a high incidence of avian tubercle bacilli in the swine. Of 125 starlings examined, 7 had gross tubercles in the liver, and 1 also had lesions in the spleen and intestines.

Wild animals. Tuberculosis in wild animals is not common except when they are in captivity. The disease has been found on several occasions in wild birds (5, 49) living a natural life. It has been described in free-living African (Cape) buffalo (28), and there have been a considerable number of reports of the disease in wild deer. Cases in deer are caused in almost all instances by *M. bovis,* and infection results from association with cattle on pasture or by browsing on land used for pasturing cattle. It is not unlikely that some of the "breaks" in tuberculosis-free herds are caused by the introduction of the disease by infected wild deer.

Tuberculosis among wild field mice (voles) occurs in England. The vole bacillus is different from the types previously described. It is discussed on page 265.

Zoo animals. Tuberculosis has always been one of the major problems of zoological parks. Even in countries where the disease has been eradicated for decades in cattle, infections with *M. tuberculosis* and *M. bovis* occur in zoo ruminants and pose a threat to human and animal health. This is particularly true when details about tuberculosis in zoos are withheld for the sake of public relations (70).

The most severe losses have been among birds, but extreme care is necessary to control the disease among members of the monkey family. The human type causes losses among apes and the bovine type among reindeer and other ruminants. The latter has been found in an outbreak in mink on a fur-raising farm (61), but avian-type tuberculosis also occurs in this animal (29, 88). Both bovine- and avian-type tuberculosis have been reported in captive kangaroos (81). The human-type bacillus has caused tuberculosis in a captive rhinoceros (58) and the disease has been described in the elephant (72). Tubercle bacilli of the cold-blooded type cause serious losses among reptiles and amphibia.

Tuberculosis continues to be a major threat to the world's zoos. For an excellent and detailed account of this specialized subject the reader is referred to the proceedings of a recent symposium edited by R. J. Montali (51).

Human tuberculosis. The most common form of tuberculosis of man is *pulmonary consumption.* This disease primarily affects the lungs and pleura and the associated lymph nodes. In many individuals the disease becomes arrested early and no symptoms are induced. Such individuals will, however, react to tuberculin, and x-rays may show one or several small encapsulated and calcareous lesions. In other cases, the disease spreads from the original focus and causes large exudative and destructive lesions. The victim suffers from a low-grade, intermittent fever, weakness, shortness of breath, a hacking cough, loss of weight, and finally emaciation. Large amounts of purulent sputum are raised, and this often is very rich in tubercle bacilli. This type of tuberculosis is caused in most cases by *M. tuberculosis.* The disease is transmitted from man to man, animal infections playing little part, except when *M. bovis* is involved. Griffith (26) in England and workers in the Scandinavian countries, where bovine tuberculosis formerly was prevalent, showed that from 1 to 6 percent of human pulmonary infections were caused by the bovine type. This situation does not exist in the United States, where bovine tubercle infection is now comparatively rare.

Extrapulmonary tuberculosis of man is often caused by *M. bovis.* These infections occur more often in children than in adults and are caused by the drinking of infected cows' milk. They involve the lymph nodes of the pharyngeal region and the abdominal organs instead of the organs of the thorax. Bovine tubercle bacilli are often found in infections of the bones and joints, of the skin, and in tuberculous meningitis. These forms of tuberculosis are caused more often by bacilli of the human type than by those of the bovine type except, possibly, the infections of the neck glands, in which the bovine type may be more frequent than the human type. Because bovine tuberculosis has been reduced in incidence in many parts of the world, and because a large part of all milk consumed is pasteurized, surgeons have noted that those forms of tuberculosis in which the bovine-type bacillus frequently occurs are becoming rare.

It has been generally believed that human beings are not susceptible to infection with the avian-type tubercle bacillus. This matter was critically reviewed in 1947 by Feldman (17), who concluded from the evidence that authentic cases had occurred. Feldman *et* al. (18) in 1949 added another case in which the evidence seemed to be quite clear. In this instance a child showed extensive lung lesions. Some of the previously described cases were also of a serious nature. It must be accepted that, although the avian tubercle bacillus ordinarily has little virulence for man, infections do occur. A study made in 1957–1964 by Kubin *et al.* (41) in Czechoslovakia on 9 cases revealed the seriousness of the disease's clinical course.

Infectivity of the Three Main Types of Tubercle Bacilli for the Domesticated Animals and Man. The natural host of *M. tuberculosis* is man, of *M. bovis* is cattle, and of *M. avium* is birds, yet all appear in foreign hosts, often producing serious diseases. Some species of animals are susceptible to infection with only one type, but others may be infected with two or all three. This creates a rather confusing situation. In general, *M. tuberculosis* is capable of invading a number of species of animals but of producing progressive disease only in the dog and rarely in the cat. *M. avium* is more cosmopolitan because it is capable of causing serious infections not only in birds but in swine and sheep, and rarely in man. *M. bovis* is the most cosmopolitan because it can produce serious disease in all domesticated animals, except birds, and in man.

I. Pathogenicity of *M. bovis*.
   a. For cattle. Causes a progressive and destructive disease.
   b. For horses. Causes a progressive disease.
   c. For swine. Highly infective. The disease is progressive and fairly frequent where swine associate with tuberculous cattle.
   d. For sheep and goats. Progressive infections occur but are relatively rare.
   e. For dogs. Causes progressive infections, but this type is not as common in dogs as in man.
   f. For cats. Causes a progressive disease. Most common type in cats.
   g. For birds. Not infective. Naturally occurring cases unknown.
   h. For man. Causes a progressive disease, especially in children. Most cases involve the lymph nodes and abdominal organs rather than lungs, but pulmonary cases are not rare.

II. Pathogenicity of *M. tuberculosis*.
   a. For cattle. Causes only minimal lesions in the lymph nodes. Of no importance except that animals will react to tuberculin. Careless caretakers suffering from pulmonary tuberculosis may cause many animals to become sensitized to tuberculin.
   b. For horses. No cases reported but it is probable that horses would react like cattle.
   c. For swine. Lesions confined to lymph nodes of the alimentary tracts. Minimal in nature and not important.
   d. For sheep and goats. No cases reported.
   e. For dogs. Progressive tuberculosis produced. Mostly infection contracted from tuberculous owners.
   f. For cats. Apparently highly resistant, but a few cases on record.
   g. For birds. All birds, except members of the Psittacidae (parrot family), are resistant. Cases reported in parrots of tuberculous owners.

III. Pathogenicity of *M. avium*.
   a. For birds. All birds thought to be susceptible. Disease occurs mostly in domesticated and wild birds kept in captivity.
   b. For cattle. Persistent uterine infections that result in abortions. Minimal lymph node lesions, of little importance except that animals react to tests made with avian tuberculin and johnin when paratuberculosis or Johne's disease are suspected.
   c. For horses. Cases have been reported. Of little importance.
   d. For swine. Lesions usually but not always confined to lymph nodes. This is by far the most common type of tubercle infection of swine in the United States.
   e. For sheep. May produce progressive disease. Lesions occur in lungs as well as lymph nodes. Most cases of tuberculosis in sheep in the United States in recent years have been caused by this type. Not a common disease, however, because sheep do not usually associate with tuberculous chickens.
   f. For goats. Rare cases reported. May produce progressive disease.
   g. For dogs and cats. Unusual, but rare cases occur.
   h. For man. Infectivity is low but a few cases of pro-

gressive tuberculosis have been shown to be due to this type.

Routes of Infection in Tuberculosis. The localization of the lesions in tuberculosis depends in considerable degree upon the manner in which the infection enters the body. There are several routes of entry.

1. *Inhalation.* The fact that tubercle lesions in adult human beings and cattle occur more frequently in the chest cavity than elsewhere suggests that infection commonly occurs through inhalation. Experiments by McFadyean (46) and others have shown that infections can be easily produced in guinea pigs by spraying them with tubercle bacilli. This fact and the knowledge that in pulmonary tuberculosis both man and cow cough into the air droplets containing tubercle bacilli that can readily be inhaled by others near them, is convincing evidence. Lung infection can also be produced experimentally by causing susceptible animals to inhale tubercle bacilli suspended in dust. Ravenel and Reichel (62) many years ago showed that tubercle bacilli suspended in butter could be found in the lacteals shortly after feeding; hence it appears to be possible for these organisms to reach the lungs, in some cases at least, without leaving lesions in the digestive tract.

2. *Ingestion.* Ingestion of tubercle bacilli in considerable numbers in infected milk readily produces tuberculosis in young animals. In these cases lesions usually occur in the lymph nodes of the alimentary canal, tuberculous ulcers frequently are found in the intestine, and lesions occur in the liver and spleen more frequently than in the organs of the chest. Before pasteurization of skim milk and whey became the general practice, many calves and pigs were infected with tuberculosis by these products. Human beings and animals affected primarily with pulmonary tuberculosis often develop intestinal lesions from swallowing quantities of infective sputum. Infection in birds is nearly always the result of ingestion of organisms picked up with the feed from the ground.

3. *Wound infection.* Tuberculosis of the skin occasionally occurs in man but is very rare in animals. In man the disease has been called *pathologists's* or *prosector's wart* because it often begins in skin wounds apparently contaminated with tubercle bacilli while handling infected tissues. The lesion may be caused by human or bovine tubercle bacilli, which usually are of attenuated virulence from residence in the skin (27).

An ulcerous skin lesion that sometimes occurs on the lower extremities of man is also caused by an acid-fast microorganism known as *M. ulcerans*. This organism prefers to grow at temperatures lower than 37 C and is antigenically distinct from other pathogenic species of *Mycobacterium*. Experimentally it produces ulcerative skin lesions in rats, mice, and calves (19, 82). It has caused udder infection in dairy cattle.

Tuberclelike skin lesions of cattle are quite common. It is a form of lymphangitis, associated with acid-fast bacteria (see page 278). Although many have referred to these lesions as *skin tuberculosis,* most workers have failed to isolate tubercle bacilli from them or to infect experimental animals. Their tuberculous nature has not been proved, and epidemiological evidence suggests that the causative agent is not the tubercle bacillus.

4. *Congenital tuberculosis.* A few instances have been described in which newborn calves were infected with generalized tuberculosis. In these instances a tuberculous lesion developed in the placenta, and this eroded into the fetal blood vessels, thus showering the fetal tissues with organisms. Such animals die shortly after birth.

Diagnosis. The diagnosis of tuberculosis in animals after death is seldom difficult because the lesions present a characteristic appearance. In cases of doubt the causative organism can be demonstrated in stained films or cultures or by the inoculation of experimental animals. Diagnosis during life is more difficult. The disease may be suspected, but means other than clinical examination are usually required to make a positive diagnosis. Bacteriologic examinations during life are possible, but difficult, in animals. In tuberculous cattle careful examination or culture of milk after it has been centrifuged may be useful in diagnosing udder infection (47). Aids in detecting and identifying tubercle bacilli now being used are the fluorescent-antibody (FA) technique (23); the use of para-aminobenzoic acid medium (34); guinea pig inoculation, a procedure believed to be superior to culture; microscopic examination of cultures (67) and typing with specific bacteriophages (3, 63).

Culture of specimens. All species of mycobacteria are pathogenic for humans; therefore, great care should be taken in handling suspect material, from taking the sample on the farm or slaughterhouse to final identification in the laboratory. A good description of the precautions necessary and the culture procedures used is included in the *Manual of Standardized Methods for Veterinary Microbiology* (11). Good lesions should be taken for culture, usually including the regional lymph node. They are digested with papain and extracted with pentane before being cultured on Stonebrink's or Lowenstein-Jensen medium, and examined for 8 weeks.

Serological tests for tuberculosis. Researchers have attempted to apply the complement-fixation and other serological tests to the problem of diagnosis in cattle but have failed because the reactions are nonspecific. Tuberculous animals usually will react, but a considerable number of apparently noninfected animals also react. It is probable that cattle are often sensitized by acid-fast organisms other than tubercle bacilli, and that this negates the value of the test. A test based on the hemolysis of sheep erythrocytes, coated with an extract of the human-type tubercle bacillus, which occurs if appropriate antibodies and guinea pig complement are present, is sometimes used along with the tuberculin tests (21). This hemolytic test is supposed to give fewer false positive reactions in tuberculosis-free herds, but like the other serological tests it is nonspecific.

In recent years, with the elucidation of the important role that T lymphocytes and their associated lymphokines play in immunity to facultative intracellular bacteria, such as the mycobacteria, a number of new tests have been used in an attempt to improve the diagnosis of tuberculosis. Pritchard *et al.* (59) used lymphocyte blastogenesis to identify pigs with *M. avium* infections, and Little and Naylor (44) used the leukocyte migration-inhibition test in cattle. Thoen *et al.* (79) used an enzyme-labeled antibody test to identify chickens as early as 2 weeks after experimental infection with *M. avium*. These tests are very sensitive and potentially useful. Time alone will tell if they are specific and practical enough to stand up to the rigors of field use.

The tuberculin tests. For the diagnosis of tubercle infection in animals, tuberculin tests are the most reliable. These tests are used extensively on cattle, swine, and chickens, and occasionally on other species. When testing for the mammalian types of tuberculosis, tuberculin made from either human- or bovine-type tubercle bacilli can be used. When testing for the avian type of tuberculosis, tuberculin made from bacilli of that type must be used. Animals may be tested with both types simultaneously when the intradermal method is used.

Tuberculin is a protein, or mixture of proteins, produced by tubercle bacilli during growth. It is contained in any aqueous extract of the organisms and is present in any medium upon which tubercle bacilli have grown. Old tuberculin (OT) is a glycerol broth filtrate that has been concentrated tenfold by evaporation. Purified protein derivative of tuberculin (tuberculin PPD) is a soluble protein fraction prepared from a synthetic medium in which the mycobacterium has been grown.

It was first discovered by Koch that tuberculin was highly toxic for tuberculous but nearly innocuous for normal animals. When tuberculin is injected into animals harboring one or more tubercles, a *general reaction* manifested by fever and constitutional symptoms occurs if the dose is sufficiently large. If the animal is destroyed at the height of the reaction, it will be found that an inflammatory reaction has occurred around the tubercles present in the organs. This is termed the *focal reaction.* When sufficient tuberculin is used, tuberculous animals sometimes react so violently as to die. If the tuberculin is injected into a tissue from which it is not quickly disseminated, such as the dense layers of the skin, *a local reaction* at the point of injection becomes manifest. This local reaction is important in many of the tuberculin tests now used in animals and man.

Animals that become infected with tubercle bacilli or that develop tuberculosis have a marked cell-mediated immune response to the organism when re-exposed to it or to tuberculin. This response occurs at the site where the tuberculin (antigen) and the host's T lymphocytes interact. Lymphokines are released from the T lymphocytes, and these in turn attract a large number of cells to the site, producing a delayed hypersensitivity or, in this case, the tuberculin reaction. This marked reactivity and the associated cellular infiltration and firm swelling are exploited in the tuberculin test.

Application of Tuberculin Tests in Animals. The tuberculins used on animals are relatively concentrated. Those used on man are greatly diluted because it is considered unwise to incite constitutional reactions for fear of stimulating the progress of the disease itself. Because reacting animals are ordinarily destroyed when they are found to be reactors to the tests, there is no reason to fear severe reactions. Concentrated tuberculin will give reactions in some cases when weaker solutions fail.

There are three basic methods of applying tuberculin as a diagnostic agent: the *intradermal* or intracutaneous method; the method of applying the tuberculin to the mucous membranes of the eye, the *ophthalmic method;* and the method of subcutaneous administration, sometimes called the *thermal test.* A thermal intravenous test has been used rarely and without marked success to supplement the intradermal tuberculin test.

1. *The intradermal test.* This test is now extensively used on cattle, swine, chickens, and man. A small quantity, usually not more than 0.1 ml, of tuberculin is injected into the deeper layers of the skin (dermis) with a

fine hypodermic needle introduced nearly parallel to the skin surface. In routine work in cattle in the United States the site of injection is usually the thin, hairless skin on the undersurface of the tail near its base (Figure 25.11). In swine the skin of one of the ears is usually injected, and in chickens the margin of one of the wattles. Positive reactions are indicated by firm, warm swellings at the point of injection. The reactions in cattle are judged on the 3rd day, sometimes a little later. The same period is used for tests in swine, but reactions in chickens are best judged in about 48 hours.

In Britain it has long been customary to inject tuberculin into the thick skin of one side of the neck, the area having been clipped previously. The reaction is judged by the increase in skin thickness as determined by calipers. This method has not become popular in this country because it requires more time to conduct.

A modification of the intradermal tuberculin test for cattle is the *Stormont test*. This was developed by Kerr *et al.* (36) in Northern Ireland. It involves two injections of tuberculin into the same skin site, 7 days apart. The tests are read within 24 hours after the second injection. The authors claim that initial sensitization of the skin by the primary injection gives a sharper reaction to the second. The results of comparative tests—the single intradermal method measured against the double method—were analyzed statistically by Priestley (60). It was claimed that, in measuring the results against the finding of lesions in the slaughtered animals, the Stormont test had an error of only 1.8 percent, whereas the single injection method showed 18.9 percent error on a group of over 300 animals. Although this procedure was employed in Britain for a time, it has now been discontinued.

Tuberculin testing of dogs and cats has not been widely practiced in the United States. Granting that the intradermal method is helpful, the BCG vaccine (see page 263) provides an additional diagnostic aid (32). This vaccine is injected subcutaneously, and the dog or cat that produces an early reaction at the site of inoculation should be regarded as a tuberculous suspect.

2. *The ophthalmic test*. This test is sometimes used on cattle. A concentrated tuberculin (Koch's OT) is instilled into the conjunctival sac with a fine brush or with a medicine dropper. A positive reaction is indicated by an inflammation of the conjunctiva during the course of which pus is formed and appears at the inner canthus. One instillation of tuberculin serves to render the eye more sensitive to another; hence it is common practice to sensitize the eye by one treatment and to repeat the treatment 2 or 3 days later. The reaction is observed and judged after the second instillation. The inflammation and appearance of the exudate are prompt. The test is usually read 4 to 6 hours after the application of the second dose of tuberculin.

3. *The thermal test*. This was once the standard method of testing cattle for tuberculosis but has been largely replaced by tests that require less time. The tuberculin (10 percent Koch's OT, 2 ml or more) is injected subcutaneously after several temperatures have been taken at 2-hour intervals to make certain that the animal is not suffering a fever from some other cause. After 8 hours, temperatures are again taken at 2-hour intervals through the 16th or 18th hour after the injection. A typical reaction consists of a rise in temperature of at least 2 degrees F, which appears between the 8th and 18th hours and subsides within 24 hours.

The Reliability of Tuberculin Tests on Animals. Tuberculin is regarded as a highly accurate diagnostic agent when it is properly used and the results are properly

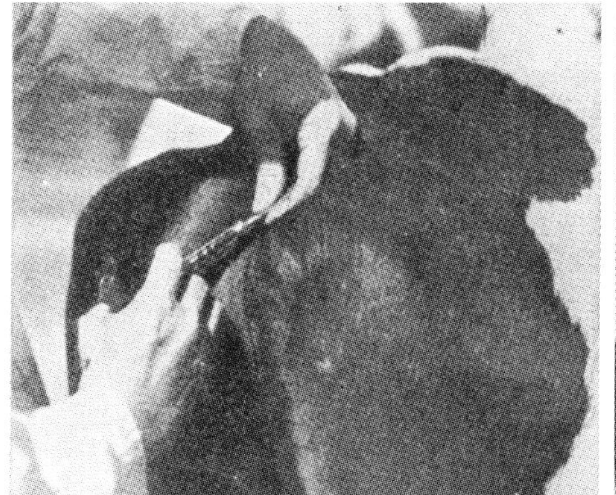

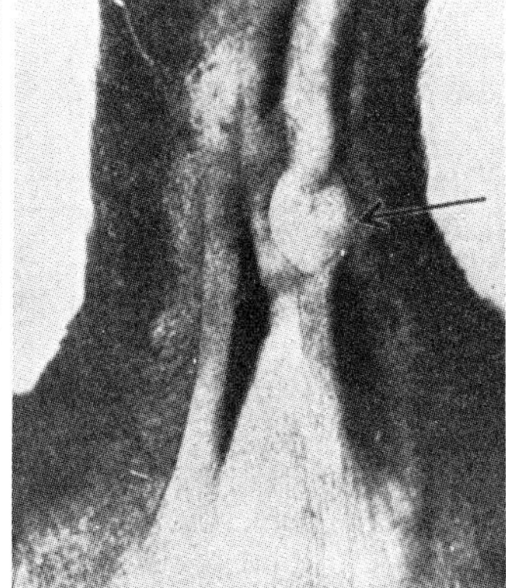

Figure 25.11. The intradermal tuberculin test in cattle. (*Left*) Making the intradermal injection into the right tail fold. (*Right*) Typical swelling at the point of injection 72 hours later. (Courtesy E. T. Faulder.)

interpreted. It is not infallible, however, particularly in cattle. No matter how carefully it is used, some errors occur. When lesions of tuberculosis are extensive, the tissues often are so saturated with tuberculoprotein as to make them insensitive to tuberculin; in advanced cases of the disease, therefore, the tuberculin test often is falsely negative.

On the other hand, a certain number of animals that give positive reactions to tuberculin fail to show lesions at autopsy. Such cattle are called NVL (No Visible Lesion) or NGL (No Gross Lesion) cases. The cause of these reactions has never been determined, but several plausible hypotheses have been offered:

1. That many such animals are in the early stages of the disease, at which time reactions to tuberculin will occur though there are no visible lesions.

2. That many animals have small lesions that may be located in parts of the carcass not ordinarily examined in routine meat inspection.

3. That animals which have been in contact with avian tubercle bacilli will ordinarily exhibit slight or no visible lesions but some will react to tuberculin. Also, cattle may be sensitized to tuberculin by contact with human tubercle bacilli. It is possible to produce tuberculin sensitivity in guinea pigs by oral administration of killed *M. tuberculosis* (86), and this leads to speculation that similar reactivity may appear in other animals.

4. That some, perhaps many, animals come in contact with acid-fast organisms other than tubercle bacilli that are able to sensitize them to tuberculin. For instance, experiments in calves have shown that *Nocardia farcinica* may sensitize these animals to avian or mammalian tuberculin or both (1). Certainly the potential role of scotochromes in producing skin sensitivity in man deserves further investigation.

Immunity in Tuberculosis. That a form of immunity does occur in the course of tubercle infection was first shown in the so-called *phenomenon of Koch*. Koch (40) observed that guinea pigs already infected with a low-grade tubercle infection reacted differently to a second inoculation of a culture of high virulence than animals which had not suffered the primary infection. The animals that were already infected proved to be refractory to the second dose. Whereas the previously normal animal developed an acute, progressively fatal disease, the previously infected developed only a swelling at the point of inoculation. This became a local abscess, which opened to the surface and sloughed away the necrotic tissue and the virulent bacilli without involvement of the neighboring lymph nodes. Much later Calmette and Guerin (9), using a dose of virulent tubercle bacilli intravenously which produced acute, fatal, miliary tuberculosis in normal cattle, found that tuberculin-reacting cattle (infected) could not be so killed. These animals showed an immediate reaction from which they rapidly recovered, and then they continued unaffected on their course of life. These experiments show that a new, more acute infection cannot be superimposed upon one already established; that a chronic disease is a protection from a more acute form.

It has become clear over the past decade that this phenomenon is a cell-mediated rather than a humoral immunity. The initial infection with *M. tuberculosis* stimulated the production of substantial numbers of T lymphocytes specifically sensitized to the antigens of *M. tuberculosis*. On later exposure, or re-exposure, to the bacilli these specific T lymphocytes proliferate and produce lymphokines which, among other useful properties, have the ability to activate macrophages. While the macrophages of normal animals readily ingest mycobacteria, they also allow mycobacteria to grow intracellularly. However, macrophages from tuberculous animals can be activated by lymphokines to destroy the bacilli more effectively. While this chain of events is initiated by the specific interaction between T lymphocytes and the antigens of the tubercle bacilli, the increased bactericidal capacity of the macrophages is nonspecific; that is, the activated macrophages have an increased number of lysosomes and are capable of destroying other facultative intracellular bacteria such as *Brucella* and *Listeria*. The activation of macrophages is short-lived, lasting only a few weeks unless sustained by further T cell stimulation and lymphokine release. This in turn is dependent upon the availability of antigen from virulent tubercle bacilli or from a modified live vaccine strain of the organism.

In the course of infection with tubercle bacilli, the host becomes sensitized to the antigens of the organism and develops a delayed form of hypersensitivity to these antigens. This is most easily demonstrated by a positive skin test to tuberculin. The localized hypersensitivity reaction produced is dependent upon the same cellular events as those responsible for the cell-mediated immunity described above. However, in this instance they are restricted to the local site of tuberculin deposition and the result is used for the detection of animals infected with *M. tuberculosis*.

Antibodies are formed during the course of infections with tubercle bacilli. They can be detected by a variety of serological tests including precipitation, complement fixation, and hemagglutination. They are usually found in low titer in tuberculous animals, and bear no relation to the state of resistance of the individual. These antibodies are not bactericidal *in vivo,* even in the presence of complement; while they do opsonize the tubercle bacilli and facilitate phagocytosis, this process merely enables the bacilli to enter cells, where they may grow.

Artificial Immunization. Because of its great importance, no doubt more attempts have been made to find immunization methods for tuberculosis than for any other disease of man or animals. Unfortunately these methods have not met with a large measure of success. The earlier attempts at immunization have been reviewed by Mohler and Schroeder (50). The matter will not be discussed in detail here, but a few of the products tried will be described briefly.

1. Tuberculin. This name has been given to a variety of aqueous extracts of tubercle bacilli. Tuberculin was first made by Koch (39) in the hope that it would have immunizing value, but these hopes have not been realized. In the course of the work of testing it on patients, its diagnostic value was discovered and it is for this purpose that it is used today.

2. Killed tubercle bacilli. When large numbers of tubercle bacilli, killed by heat or chemicals, are deposited in tissues, tuberculous tissue is produced around the deposit and abscessation is likely to occur. When used as vaccines, therefore, the dosage must be kept small. There is evidence that such vaccines enhance the resisting power of experimental animals somewhat, but the products have never been of service in practical work.

3. Living cultures. Numerous experiments with attenuated tubercle bacilli and with acid-fast organisms other than tubercle bacilli as vaccines for enhancing the resistance of animals to tuberculosis have been tried but with little success until recently. Perhaps the best known of these vaccines that have now been discarded was the *bovovaccine* of Von Behring, a vaccine which was widely heralded for protecting cattle. The nature of the vaccine was not disclosed for a long time but finally it became known that it consisted of a virulent strain of human tubercle bacilli. The vaccine will indeed confer a rather strong resistance on cattle, and with little damage to them, but the method was discarded with the discovery that some of the vaccinated cattle were eliminating human tubercle bacilli in their milk.

BCG vaccine. BCG stands for *bacillus of Calmette and Guerin* (9). These French workers cultured a bovine-type tubercle bacillus continuously on a bile-saturated medium for 13 years, during which the culture was renewed 70 times. Under these conditions it gradually changed in physical characteristics and diminished in virulence until, at the end of the period, it had completely lost its tuberculogenic properties. For many years this culture has been used as a vaccine on many kinds of animals, monkeys, and man. It has proved to be quite harmless, and it confers an appreciable, but not absolute, resistance to tuberculosis in the injected animal.

To be effective it must be given before virulent tubercle infection has occurred. This means that it must be given very early in life, in most instances. It can be given to very young calves in areas in which bovine tuberculosis is prevalent to reduce their susceptibility to tuberculous infection. It is used rather widely on human infants born into tuberculous environments. Such infants usually successfully resist infection that destroys many not so protected (35). It is also used on adults negative to the tuberculin test who are likely to be heavily exposed to *M. tuberculosis* in their work or travel. It is thought that the immunity conferred by the vaccine is transient, lasting only as long as the vaccine organisms persist in the tissues—usually not longer than a few months. Virulent infection contracted during this period is successfully resisted, and the lesions are walled off and arrested. These lesions constitute a protecting mechanism thereafter.

BCG as an immunopotentiating agent. In addition to its use as a vaccine for tuberculosis, BCG has been used in recent years to nonspecifically stimulate the host's resistance against various targets, notably tumors. It has been found that BCG will, under certain circumstances, render the host more resistant to solid tumors and even leukemias. The basis for this phenomenon is not entirely clear; it may merely cause T lymphocytes to activate macrophages; it may act as an adjuvant or it may produce some measure of cross-reactivity with the tumor. In any event, it is now being used on an experimental basis for the nonspecific enhancement of the host's resistance, particularly in instances where cell-mediated immunity is thought to be important.

Treatment of Tuberculosis. The search for an agent that could safely be used to treat tuberculosis in man and animals was a long, diligent, and fruitless one until the 1940s, when streptomycin was found to be effective for treatment of the disease in lower animals. Since that time substantial advances have been made in the treatment of human tuberculosis. The subject is vast, involving largely the treatment of humans, and is beyond the scope of this book. The drugs used for the initial treatment of humans include isoniazid, rifampin, streptomycin, and ethambutol. Although isoniazid and rifampin are very effective, they are often used in combinations of two or even three drugs. This reduces the possibility that drug-resistant strains of the tubercle bacilli will emerge during the course of treatment, which might continue for years before satisfactory remission occurs.

Because of the risk that tuberculosis will spread to man, an animal in which it is detected is usually destroyed rather than treated. In countries where bovine tuberculosis is still a serious problem, however, treatment with isoniazid may be used. This too is fraught with some danger; Corrêa and Corrêa (10) noted the emergence of isoniazid-resistant strains of *M. bovis,* one of which had been isolated from a cow treated with isoniazid for 6 months. To prevent the development of tuberculosis in calves exposed to heavily infected cattle, Seelemann *et al.* (71) recommend the feeding of "Ferroteben" (a complex iron salt of *o*-oxybenzal-isonicotinic acid-hydrazid) at the rate of 10 mg per kg of body weight. Merkal and Thurston (48) found benzalkonium chloride to be bactericidal for saprophytic mycobacteria.

Control Measures. *In cattle.* BCG vaccination is used abroad to a limited extent to reduce the ravages of tuberculosis, but principal dependence everywhere is placed on the tuberculin test and the elimination of reactors for controlling this disease. In many countries the tuberculin test is being used systematically and country-wide not only to control but also to eradicate the disease.

The Federal-State Cooperative Plan for the Eradication of Bovine Tuberculosis, also called the Accredited Herd Plan, was launched in the United States in 1917 and is similar to eradication plans used elsewhere. The plan called for every bovine animal in the country to be subjected to tuberculin tests; those that reacted were to be removed and slaughtered. All slaughtered animals were subjected to veterinary meat inspection examinations to determine the extent of the development of the disease in each case and to ascertain whether or not any portions of the carcasses might be salvaged for human food. Before condemned animals were slaughtered, their market value was determined and the owners were reimbursed for their losses from the public treasuries.

The Accredited Herd Plan has been very successful. In 1922 an estimated 4.0 percent of all cattle in the country were infected with tuberculosis; by 1940 the estimated number had been reduced to about 0.46 percent. The incidence of this disease had been reduced in less than 20 years by more than 85 percent. In January 1965 New Hampshire became the first state to attain an Accredited Tuberculosis-Free status. Maine achieved this goal in October 1967. Bovine tuberculosis has ceased to be an important public health or economic problem in this country, but the disease has not been eradicated, and it is clear that efforts will have to continue for a considerable time before this objective is reached. Systematic testing of all cattle must continue so that all centers of infection may be detected and stamped out. We now have a highly susceptible bovine population in which the disease could spread quickly.

Instructions for the *TB Manual* of the USDA, dated 11 December 1968, state: "When the presence of *M. bovis* has been confirmed by culture on any premises, liquidation of the herd remains the procedure of choice. Otherwise, the herd shall remain in quarantine until it has passed two negative tuberculin tests at intervals of at least 60 days and an additional two negative tuberculin tests at intervals of 6 months, the total quarantine period to be not less than 16 months after the last reactor has been disclosed. The entire herd must be included in three of the four required tests."

In poultry. The stamping out of tuberculosis in poultry is in many ways more difficult than in cattle because of widespread soil contamination. The disease is no longer a serious problem to commercial poultry raisers, largely because of their general practice of selling off all old birds annually and using as laying birds only those that were hatched the previous spring. Because tuberculosis develops slowly, very few birds less than 1 year old will develop "open" cases. Where this practice is used consistently, the disease tends to disappear from infected premises. The disease is serious principally in the barnyard flocks. Such birds often range over the entire farm and are allowed to live for several years. Under such conditions advanced cases of the disease occur, and the premises are constantly reinfected.

The tuberculin test is useful in detecting infected flocks as well as infected birds. The removal of such birds will not eliminate the disease from the flock, because it is impossible to disinfect the soil. If only a few affected birds are found, it is advisable to remove them and to retest the flock repeatedly at intervals of 1 or 2 months. If the percentage of reactors is high, slaughter of all birds is advisable before starting a new flock in new or thoroughly disinfected buildings located on soil that has not previously been occupied by birds. The owners

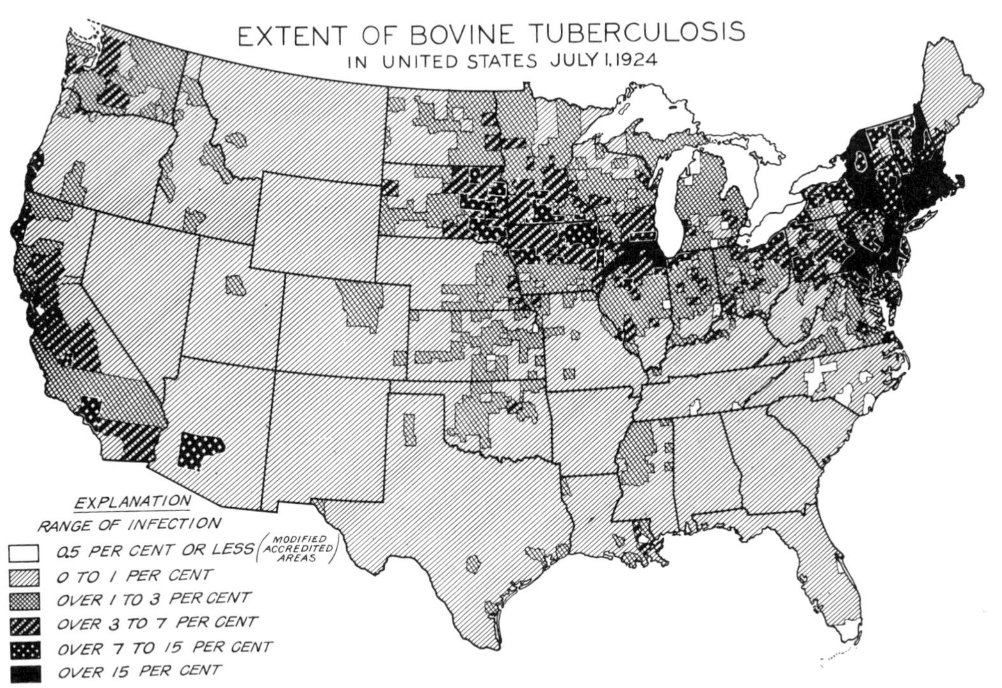

Figure 25.12. This map showing the extent of bovine tuberculosis in the United States in 1924 conveys a good idea of the distribution of the disease before much progress had been made in the work of eradication.

should be advised to eliminate the old flock annually and replace it with young birds.

In man. The elimination of tuberculosis from cattle has removed the hazard of bovine-type infection of man in the United States. Tuberculosis of the human type has been greatly reduced by education, early diagnosis, and hospitalization. The family continues to be the most important epidemiologic unit in the development of tuberculosis, and the adult members of the family are the most significant segment, both as sources of infection and as victims. The incidence of tuberculosis among employees and nurses at sanitoria remains high, and cases among medical students are more numerous than among young adults in general. Control of the disease must center on reducing infection in these professionals. BCG vaccination has some value, but isolation, sanitation, and other factors must also be utilized.

In other animals. Because the three principal reservoirs of tubercle infection are man, cattle, and poultry, the disease will disappear in other species as soon as these reservoirs are drained.

Mycobacterium microti (The Vole Bacillus)

This organism was isolated by Wells (85) from wild voles (*Microtus agrestis*) caught in various parts of England. The disease closely resembles tuberculosis. The caseous lesions contain masses of acid-fast organisms that differ from previously known tubercle types. The disease itself is of little importance, but the causative agent serves to immunize animals against tuberculosis, and there is considerable interest in it for use as a practicable vaccine for both man and animals.

Morphology and Staining Features. The vole bacillus is much longer and more slender than human tubercle bacilli. Some organisms show granules and vacuolization along their entire length. Many cells assume S-shaped forms. Others are sickle- or spiral-shaped. Branched forms have not been seen. It is strongly Gram-positive and acid-fast. Like tubercle bacilli, it does not stain well with ordinary stains.

Cultural Features. Cultures grow very slowly. On the best media, colonies are usually not seen until after a month's incubation at 37 C. They will not grow at room temperature. Nonglycerolated egg medium is good for isolation. The colonies appear as pearly white conical or granular masses. The organism grows very well on potato after becoming adapted to growth on artificial media, but it will not grow on glycerol-egg or glycerol-agar media. It will grow as small filmy flakes on the surface of tryptinized broth but not on plain broth. A fine deposit forms in the depths of the fluid.

Pathogenicity for Experimental Animals. Relatively large doses (0.1 to 1.0 mg) injected intravenously in rabbits cause death from acute miliary tuberculosis. Small intravenous doses, or doses given subcutaneously, generally produce only trivial local lesions in which the bacilli gradually perish. Relatively large doses injected intraperitoneally in guinea pigs cause a generalized disease resembling acute tuberculosis. If the dose is not too large, the lesions in the organs tend to retrogress and the bacilli die out. When 1 to 5 mg of vole bacilli are injected intraperitoneally in white rats, lung lesions similar to those produced by other tubercle bacilli are produced. The rats usually do not die, and the organism has been found in the spleen of such animals for as long as 493 days. Noncaseous lesions resembling tubercles are found in the liver, spleen, and lymph nodes of golden hamsters inoculated subcutaneously. Fowls show no ill effects from inoculation with large doses of vole organisms, but the organism can be found as long as 4 months later in the spleen.

REFERENCES

1. Awad. Jour. Comp. Path. and Therap., 1958, *68,* 324.
2. Bang. Maanedskr. f. Dyrlaeger, 1920, *31,* 415.
3. Bates and Fitzhugh. Am. Rev. Resp. Dis., 1967, *96,* 7.
4. Baumgarten. Zentrbl. med. Wissenschr., 1882, *20,* 257 and 337.
5. Beaudette and Hudson. Jour. Am. Vet. Med. Assoc., 1936, *89,* 215.
6. Bickford, Ellis, and Moses. Jour. Am. Vet. Med. Assoc., 1966, *149,* 312.
7. Bradley. Am. Rev. Resp. Dis., 1972, *106,* 122.
8. Bradley and Bond. Advs. Appl. Microbiol., 1974, 18, 131.
9. Calmette and Guerin. Ann. Inst. Pasteur, 1924, *38,* 371; 1926, *40,* 89.
10. Corrêa and Corrêa. Arquivos do Inst. Biológ., São Paulo, 1973, *40,* 205.
11. Cottral, George E. (ed). Manual of standardized methods for veterinary microbiology. Cornell University Press, Ithaca, N.Y., 1978, p. 537.
12. Cummings, Drummond, and Lewis. Pub. Health Rpts. (U.S.), 1948, *63,* 1305.
13. Dorset. Am. Med., 1902, *3,* 555.
14. Doyle, Evander, and Gruft. Am. Rev. Resp. Dis., 1968, *97,* 919.
15. Dubos. Proc. Soc. Exp. Biol. and Med., 1945, *58,* 361.
16. Dubos and Middlebrook. Am. Rev. Tuberc., 1947, *56,* 334.
17. Feldman. Ann. N.Y. Acad. Sci., 1947, *48,* 469.
18. Feldman, Hutchinson, Schwarting, and Karlson. Am. Jour. Path., 1949, *25,* 1183.
19. Feldman and Karlson. Am. Rev. Tuberc., 1957, *75,* 266.
20. Fincher, Evans, and Saunders. Cornell Vet., 1954, *44,* 240.
21. Fisher and Gregory. Austral. Vet. Jour., 1951, *27,* 25.
22. Fite and Olson. Pub. Health Rpts. (U.S.), 1944, *59,* 1423.
23. Gilkerson and Kanner. Jour. Bact., 1963, *86,* 890.
24. Goren. Ann. Rev. Microbiol., 1977, *31,* 507.
25. Goren, D'Arcy Hart, Young, and Armstrong. Proc. Natl. Acad. Sci., 1976, *73,* 2510.
26. Griffith. Jour. Comp. Path. and Therap., 1928, *41,* 122.
27. Griffith. Jour. Hyg. (London), 1957, *55,* 1.
28. Guilbridge, Rollinson, McAnulty, Alley, and Wells. Jour. Comp. Path. and Therap., 1963, *73,* 337.
29. Hall and Winkel. Jour. Am. Vet. Med. Assoc., 1957, *131,* 49.
30. Harrington and Karlson. Am. Jour. Vet. Res., 1966, *27,* 1193.
31. Harshfield, Roderick, and Hawn. Jour. Am. Vet. Med. Assoc., 1937, *91,* 323.
32. Hawthorne and Lauder. Am. Rev. Resp. Dis., 1962, *85,* 858.
33. Hix, Jones, and Karlson. Jour. Am. Vet. Med. Assoc., 1961, *138,* 641.
34. Hok, Seng, Yen, and San. Am. Rev. Resp. Dis., 1966, *94,* 620.
35. Holm. Pub. Health Rpts. (U.S.), 1946, *61,* 1298.
36. Kerr, Lamont, and McGirr. Vet. Rec., 1946, *58,* 443 and 451.
37. Koch. Berl. klin. Wchnschr., 1882, *19,* 221.
38. Koch. Mittheilung. Gesundheitsamte, 1884, *2,* 1.
39. Koch. Centrbl. f. Bakt., 1890, *8,* 563.
40. Koch. Deut. med. Wchnschr., 1891, *17,* 101.
41. Kubin, Krumi, Horak, Lukavsky, and Vanek. Am. Rev. Resp. Dis., 1966, *94,* 20.
42. Lesslie and Birn. Vet. Rec., 1967, *80,* 559.
43. Lesslie and Davies. Vet. Rec., 1958, *70,* 82.
44. Little and Naylor. Brit. Vet. Jour., 1977, 133, 374.
45. Luke. Vet. Rec., 1958, *70,* 529.
46. McFadyean. Jour. Comp. Path. and Therap., 1910, *23,* 239.
47. Maitland. Jour. Hyg. (London), 1950, *48,* 397.
48. Merkal and Thurston. Am. Jour. Vet. Res., 1968, *29,* 757.
49. Mitchell and Duthie. Am. Rev. Tuberc., 1929, *19,* 134.
50. Mohler and Schroeder. Proc. Am. Vet. Med. Assoc., 1909, p. 252.
51. Montali, Richard J. (ed.). Mycobacterial infections of zoo animals. Proc. symposium Nat. Zoological Park. Smithsonian Inst. Press, Washington, D.C., 1978.
52. Moore. Am. Jour. Path., 1942, *18,* 827.
53. Olsson. Cornell Vet., 1957, *47,* 193.
54. Park and Krumwiede. Jour. Med. Res., 1911, *20,* 313; 1912, *22,* 109.
55. Pearson and McGowan. Brit. Vet. Jour., 1958, *114,* 477.
56. Peterson. Jour. Am. Vet. Med. Assoc., 1965, *147,* 1600.
57. Plum. Acta Path. et Microbiol. Scand., 1938, Sup. 37, 438.
58. Powers and Price. Jour. Am. Vet. Med. Assoc., 1967, *151,* 890.
59. Prichard, Thoen, Himes, Muscoplat, and Johnson. Am. Jour. Epidemiol., 1977, *106,* 222.

60. Priestley. Vet. Rec. 1946, *58*, 455.
61. Pulling. Jour. Am. Vet. Med. Assoc., 1952, *121*, 389.
62. Ravenel and Reichel. Jour. Med. Res., 1908, *13*, 1.
63. Redmond and Cater. Am. Rev. Resp. Dis., 1960, *82*, 781.
64. Reed and Morgante. Am. Jour. Med. Sci., 1956, *231*, 320.
65. Rivolta. Gior. di Anat. e Fisol., 1889, *1*, 122.
66. Runyon. Med. Clin. N. Am., 1959, *43*, 273.
67. Runyon. Am. Jour. Clin. Path., 1970, *54*, 578.
68. Runyon, Wayne, and Kabuca. Mycobacteriaceae. *In* Bergey's manual of determinative bacteriology, 8th ed., ed. Robert E. Buchanan and Norman E. Gibbons, Williams and Wilkins, Baltimore, 1974, p. 681.
69. Schalk, Roderick, Foust, and Harshfield. N. Dak. Agr. Exp. Sta. Tech. Bull. 279, 1935.
70. Schliesser. *In* Proc. Symposium Natl. Zoological Park. Smithsonian Inst. Press, Washington, D.C., 1978, p. 29.
71. Seelemann, Buschkiel, and Rackow. Zentrbl. Vet.-Med., 1957, *4*, 80.
72. Seneviratna, Wettimuny, and Seneviratna. Vet. Med., 1966, *61*, 129.
73. Smith. Jour. Exp. Med., 1898, *3*, 451.
74. Smith. Jour. Med. Res., 1905, *7*, 253; 1905, *8*, 405.
75. Soliman, Rollinson, Barron, and Spratling. Vet. Rec., 1953, *65*, 421.
76. Stamp. Vet. Rec., 1944, *56*, 443.
77. Stonebrink. Proc. Tuber. Res. Comm., 1957, *44*, 67.
78. Stuart and Marshall. Vet. Rec., 1952, *64*, 309.
79. Thoen, Eacret, and Hines. Avian Dis., 1978, *22*, 162.
80. Thordal-Christensen. Nord. Vetmed., 1952, *4*, 577.
81. Tilden and Williamson. Jour. Am. Vet. Med. Assoc., 1957, *131*, 526.
82. Tolhurst, Buckle, and Wellington. Jour. Hyg. (London), 1959, *57*, 47.
83. Verge and Senthille. Rec. Med. Vet., 1942, *118*, 49.
84. Villemin. Comp. rend. Acad. Sci., 1865, *61*, 1012.
85. Wells. Brit. Jour. Exp. Path., 1938, *19*, 324.
86. Whitehead and Corson. Cornell Vet., 1962, *52*, 36.
87. Wilkinson. Vet. Rec., 1964, *76*, 777.
88. Wilton and Vance. Can. Jour. Comp. Med. and Vet. Sci., 1959, *23*, 256.

Mycobacterium paratuberculosis

SYNONYMS: *Mycobacterium johnei*, *Mycobacterium enteritidis*, Johne's bacillus, bacillus of Johne's disease

This organism causes disease in cattle, sheep, goats, llamas, and some wild ruminants. It has been reported in the European red deer (87) and has been described in horses and a donkey (44). In English-speaking countries the disease is usually known as *Johne's disease*. It is also known as *paratuberculosis, chronic bacterial enteritis, chronic hypertrophic enteritis,* and a number of colloquial names. The causative organism was first recognized in Germany by Johne and Frothingham (30) in 1895, who saw it in the tissues of diseased cattle. These workers mistook the organisms for avian tubercle bacilli and thought they were dealing with an isolated, atypical case. Later it was recognized that many cases of this disease occurred. They were regarded as atypical tuberculoses until 1905, when Bang (1) in Denmark showed that it could readily be transmitted to other cattle and that the disease was not a form of tuberculosis but a separate entity. *Mycobacterium paratuberculosis* was first isolated and grown in artificial media by Twort (84) in 1911. Many others have isolated the organism from cattle since that time by using a special technique developed by Twort.

Howarth (27), Dunkin (9), McEwen (52), and others who have worked with sheep and goats have failed in their attempts to isolate *M. paratuberculosis* from these species using the technique that generally succeeds with cattle material. In 1945, Taylor (79) claimed to have cultivated the organism in 4 out of 15 attempts. All four animals from which cultures were derived came from a single farm. McEwen (52), Hagan (19), and Levi (49) found no difficulty in infecting sheep with material from cattle, and all were able to recover the organisms in culture. Taylor's original successes may have been with a strain of this type. Later Taylor (82) isolated a strain from sheep in Iceland and two from sheep in Scotland. One of the Scottish strains was considered to be the classical bovine type and the other was a highly pigmented strain. The Icelandic strain was similar to the classic variety. Taylor stated that growth of the Icelandic and pigmented strains, hitherto said to be resistant to artificial cultivation, was obtained on media that contained 60 percent egg yolk and that both were probably varieties of the classical type. He also showed that these two strains were capable of producing clinical Johne's disease in cattle and that they retained their cultural characteristics after one passage through cattle (83). It seems reasonable to conclude that the same species of organism is found in cattle, sheep, and goats, but that unrecognized host factors render cultivation from sheep and goats more difficult than from cattle. In 1965, Stuart (78) recovered a pigmented variant of *M. paratuberculosis* from an experimentally infected cow. It differed from the pigmented sheep strains only in some cultural characteristics.

Morphology and Staining Reactions. *M. paratuberculosis* appears in both tissues and cultures as a short, thick rod measuring about 0.5 by 1.0 μm. It is considerably smaller than any of the tubercle bacilli. In tissues and feces it commonly appears in clumps, some containing a great many organisms. This arrangement is an aid in its identification. It is strongly acid- and alcohol-fast and Gram-positive. It has neither spores nor capsules. In tissues it develops intracellularly in the macrophages and giant cells which appear at the site of localization.

Cultural Features. The causative agent of Johne's disease was first obtained in artificial culture by Twort (84) in 1911. This worker succeeded in obtaining growth, after earlier workers had failed, by incorporating in his media a suspension of heat-killed acid-fast organisms of other species. Although unable to isolate the "essential substance," Twort correctly inferred that it was contained in extracts of acid-fast organisms and was essential for the growth of *M. paratuberculosis*.

In 1953, Francis *et al.* (12) isolated from *M. phlei* a substance which they named *mycobactin*. They claimed that this material occurred in relatively high concentration (1 percent of dry weight) in this organism and that it possessed most if not all of the "essential substance." They succeeded in isolating their factor as a crystalline aluminum complex and also in an amorphous metal-free form. Recently Merkal and Curran (56) have suggested that the mycobactin dependence of newly isolated strains of *M. paratuberculosis* reflects the organism's inability to extract sufficient ferric ion from the medium. Other mycobacteria such as *M. phlei* produce mycobactin that does sequester sufficient iron, hence promoting the growth of the Johne bacillus.

Primary cultures of the Johne organism grow very slowly on all media, much more slowly than tubercle bacilli. On Dorset's egg medium, fortified with about 5 percent by weight of the moist cells of one of the rapidly growing saprophytic acid-fast organisms, the organism can be grown without great difficulty from infected lymph nodes, where it often exists in the absence of other bacteria. The cultures must be incubated at 37 C for about 6 weeks before evidence of growth appears. During the period of incubation the tubes must be partially closed so that evaporation will not cause dehydration of the media. Growth appears in the form of very small, dry, irregular colonies, not unlike primary cultures of mammalian tubercle bacilli. When these are subcultured on fresh media of the same type, a confluent growth is obtained. This usually is visible after 2 or 3 weeks' incubation but reaches its maximum only after 5 or 6 weeks.

Other media recommended for the primary culture of the Johne bacillus are Taylor's modification of Finlayson's egg medium (81) and Smith's modified Dubos' solid and liquid media (75). For primary cultivation of *M. paratuberculosis,* Merkal *et al.* (58) advocate the use of benzalkonium chloride as a decontaminant followed by inoculation onto modified Herrold's medium (an egg-yolk agar plus mycobactin). Organisms accustomed to growth in the laboratory are dry and flaky and of a cream color. Even after many years of artificial culture, the organism will give little or no growth on most of the media that serve for tubercle bacilli if the essential supplement is not added. Meager growths may occur, but they will fail after two or three transplants on the same unfortified medium.

It is usually difficult to grow this organism on fluid media. On ordinary glycerol broth to which mycobactin has been added in the form of the killed cells of *M. phlei,* growth is always poor. After several months' incubation, small floating islands of growth may develop, and there may be considerable sediment in the bottom of the flasks, but complete pellicles are rarely formed. Synthetic media, especially those of Long (50) and Dorset *et al.* (6), and Smith's modified Dubos' liquid medium are much more successful. It is generally necessary to add mycobactin to these media in the beginning, but after a few generations many strains can be induced to grow without it. Strains adapted to such media often grow profusely and heavily. These growths resemble those of mammalian tubercle bacilli, being dry, rough, folded pellicles with clear underlying medium.

Resistance. The organism of Johne's disease has about the same degree of resistance to deleterious influences as tubercle bacilli. It is resistant to acids and alkalies and to antiformin. These substances are used to treat contaminated tissues and fecal material in order to eliminate other bacteria when cultures are made. Lovell *et al.* (51) found that cultures remained viable in sterilized water for more than 9 months. Cultures were recovered from intestinal scrapings suspended in unsterilized river water for 163 days. Bacilli stored first at −14 C for 5 months, then at 4 C for 5 months, and finally at 38 C for 8 months were still viable (41). The organism remains alive for 15 weeks when kept in feces at −70 C but there is a substantial loss of viability (70).

Naturally infected feces showed viable bacilli when exposed to atmospheric conditions but kept moist for as long at 245 days. *M. paratuberculosis* has also survived for several weeks in cattle and pig slurry (89). The organism is highly resistant to penicillin (75) and chloramphenicol (88); these antibiotics are sometimes added to culture media to prevent growth of other contaminating bacteria.

Pathogenicity for Experimental Animals. Because of the difficulty of growing *M. paratuberculosis* in culture and the long incubation period of the naturally occurring disease, early investigators made many attempts to develop a model of Johne's disease in small experimental animals. Francis (11), in England, reported apparent success in infecting very young mice (13 to 14 days old) and young hamsters by feeding them with massive doses of cultures of *M. paratuberculosis*. Chandler (5) also infected mice, and Gilmour *et al.* (16) studied the pathogenesis of Johne's disease in orally dosed hamsters. It appears that the use of such animals in diagnostic work is limited, especially in cases where relatively small numbers of organisms are encountered, but these experimental animals have recently been used for studying the pathogenesis of Johne's disease. In 1971, Madge (54) demonstrated that mice infected with *M. paratuberculosis* had lesions in the intestinal tract and suffered from maladsorption of glucose and other substances. Larsen and Miller (42) used hamsters to study the effects of dexamethasone on animals experimentally infected with *M. paratuberculosis*.

Experimental infections have been established in calves (18), sheep (34), and pigs (32) by oral administration of large doses of Johne's bacilli. Calves have also been infected by inoculation of the bacillus by the subcutaneous and intravenous routes (43). The disease has also been induced in colts by intravenous inoculation (44).

The Natural Disease. Johne's disease is prevalent in France, Belgium, Holland, Denmark, Russia, and the British Isles. The disease occurs throughout the United States and Canada, but it does not appear to be a serious problem in many areas. The disease is probably more prevalent than was formerly believed owing to the development of increasingly efficient means for its detection and perhaps to an actual increase in the disease. Taylor (80) cultured the ileocecal lymph nodes of 243 adult cattle slaughtered routinely in an abattoir in England for Johne's bacilli. He succeeded in isolating cultures from 37 animals, an incidence of 15 percent. He concludes that this high percentage indicates that the infection is much more prevalent in England than clinical cases would suggest. Rankin (65) recovered *M. paratuberculosis* from lymph nodes of 6 and 7.5 percent of two groups of apparently normal English cattle. The corresponding figure for cattle from Ireland slaughtered in England was 0.8 percent. He also identified a culture of this species taken from a mesenteric lymph gland of a horse that had shown no clinical signs of illness (66).

In all the countries mentioned, the infection is best known in cattle, but it also occurs in sheep. We have even less information about its distribution in sheep than we have in cattle. It has been identified in both sheep and goats in the United States.

Calves and adult cattle can be infected by mouth if they ingest a sufficient number of organisms. *M. paratuberculosis* has a predilection for the intestinal tract, where it produces lesions and signs of enteritis (14, 18, 62). Lesions in the intestinal mucosa are produced a few months after infection; the organism is excreted in the feces and may also be transported to other parts of the body in macrophages.

Cattle seldom develop symptoms of Johne's disease after 5 years of age, and most cases appear in 2- and 3-year-old females. The disease most often becomes apparent in the early part of the first or second lactation period. The greatest losses occur among high-producing animals. The strain of lactation breaks down the resistance of the animal to an infection that previously had been latent. The organism lodges in the intestinal canal and the lymph nodes of the mesentery. The lower end of the small intestine, the cecum, and the beginning of the colon are the parts most often involved, but advanced cases may show lesions in all parts of the alimentary canal from the stomach to the anus. The lesions in the intestinal wall take the form of a thickening that may be very obvious or very slight. This thickening is caused by the proliferation of great masses of epithelioid cells in the lower layers of the mucosa and the submucosa (see Figure 25.13). Unlike tubercle infections, there are no tubercles and no necrosis. The epithelium always remains intact, but it is often thrown into deep folds that cannot be flattened by stretching of the gut wall. The mesenteric lymph nodes never show great enlargement or necrosis, but they are often slightly enlarged. Sometimes the lymphatics on the serous surface of the affected bowel become filled with epithelioid cells which convert the usually inconspicuous channels into glassy, tortuous cords along the mesenteric attachment. Great numbers of small acid-fast organisms usually can be easily demonstrated in films made from scrapings from the cut surface of the thickened portion of the intestinal wall, or from that of the lymph nodes which drain the affected areas. The organisms are usually found in clumps, and many of them are located intracellularly. In sections, most of the organisms are present in the epithelioid cells (see Figure 25.14). Large giant cells, of the type seen in tubercles, are usually conspicuous in sections (see Figure 25.15).

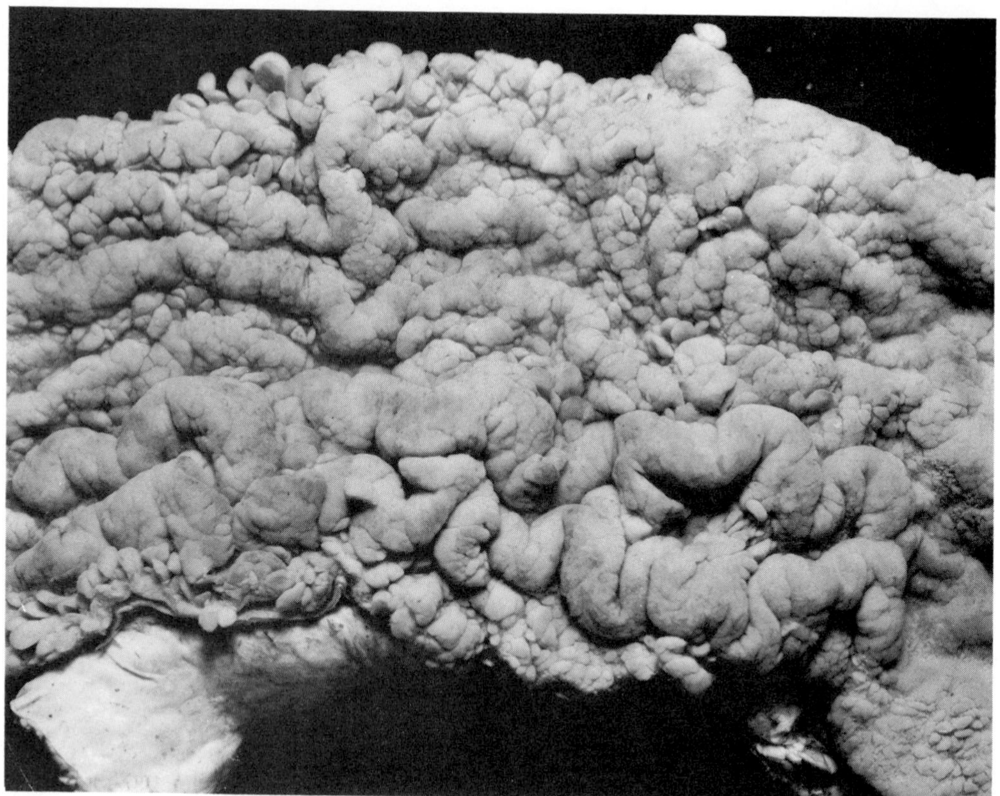

Figure 25.13. Johne's disease, showing the mucous membrane of a portion of the ileum. The wall is greatly thickened by large deposits of epithelioid cells in the subepithelial tissue of the mucosa. The irregular folds and plaques are characteristic. There is a complete absence of ulcers and necrosis.

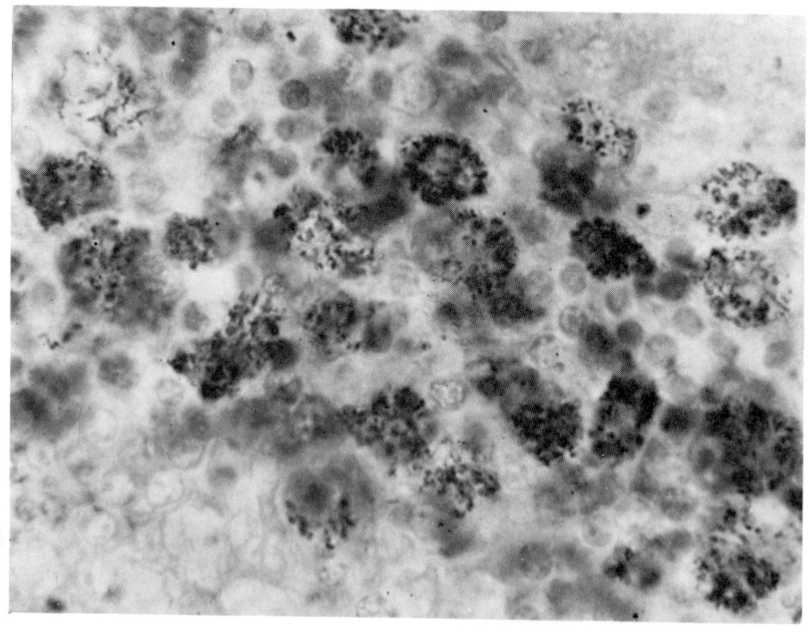

Figure 25.14. Johne's disease, showing epithelioid cells in the mucous membrane of a rapidly progressive case of the disease. The cells are packed with masses of *Mycobacterium paratuberculosis.* This preparation had been stained with the Ziehl-Neelsen technique for acid-fast bacteria. In preparations stained with hematoxylin and eosin these cells appear quite normal. × 890.

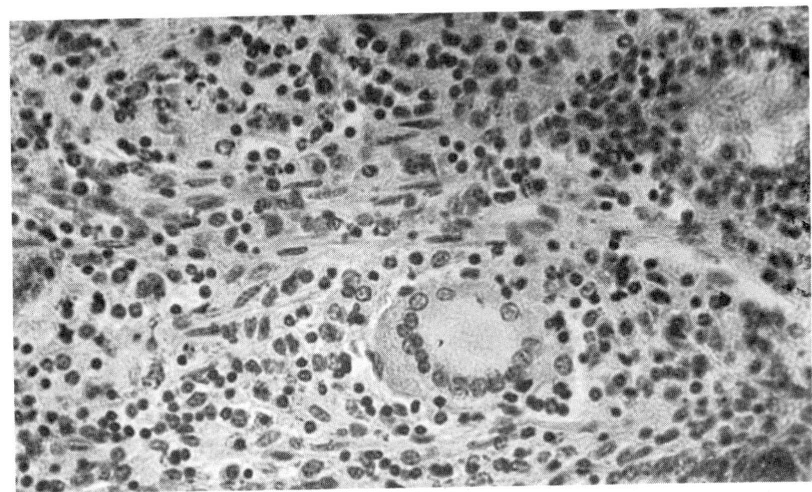

Figure 25.15. Johne's disease, a section through the subepithelial tissue of the mucosa of the small intestine of an acute case, showing the epithelioid cells that infiltrate this tissue and cause thickening of the mucosa. A typical giant cell is shown. × 540.

Lesions in other organs are rare. Organisms sometimes can be demonstrated in the liver but lesions are absent. Although reports of uterine infection in cattle are few, Pearson (63) records two cases in cattle in England in which infection occurred in the uterine mucosa, and in one of these a congenital infection of the fetus was found, the organism being isolated from the ileocecal lymph nodes and bowel of the fetus, and in 1967, Kopecky *et al.* (37) found 18 cases of uterine infection among 148 culls of a 1,000-cow dairy herd in which paratuberculosis was a problem. Fourteen of these 18 positive specimens came from cows that presented no clinical evidence of Johne's disease. It is possible that transuterine infection is not as uncommon as originally believed. Doyle (8) examined the udder tissue of 34 cows clinically affected with Johne's disease and obtained positive cultures from the udders of two. He concluded that the excretion of Johne's bacilli in the milk is rare and probably occurs only in the fulminating type of infection. In old cases of Johne's disease, calcareous plaques often can be found in the large blood vessels near the heart (13, 19). Organisms cannot be demonstrated in these lesions, which are believed to be caused by metabolic disturbances occasioned by the disease.

Larsen and Kopecky (39) examined the genital organs of six bulls having clinical signs of paratuberculosis and found Johne's bacilli in these organs from all six animals.

The symptoms of Johne's disease are quite variable. It is clear that many animals harbor the disease, and probably spread infection, without showing any definite evidence of malfunction. It is clear, also, that many infected animals recover from the disease. Allergic tests indicate that infected herds usually include many infected animals that never show evidence of the disease. The usual history of an infected herd is that losses are never heavy at any one time, but new cases continue to appear from time to time and the losses over a period of years may be considerable. Evidence indicates that factors other than the organism itself are responsible for the clinical cases. Smythe (76) in England has pointed out that, although the infection may exist in herds that are raised on alkaline soils, high in lime, the disease does not usually seriously affect them. When such animals are moved to acid soils, they often develop clinical symptoms shortly thereafter. Jansen (29) has pointed out the same thing in Holland, it has been observed in France, and there is similar evidence in the United States. The disease persists in regions of Wisconsin with acid soils but not in regions with alkaline calcareous soils (36). It seems likely that some soil deficiencies may have an important effect upon the development of the disease. Corresponding to this is the old observation that the disease, in young heifers in which it has been latent, often appears suddenly during the early part of the lactation period—a time when the animal's mineral balance is suffering strain.

The initial symptoms are vague. One of the earliest is edema of the intermandibular space. General unthriftiness quickly becomes evident. The hair coat becomes dry, and the skin loses its normal pliability. Diarrhea begins and frequently is very profuse. The body temperature at this time is normal. The gluteal muscles begin to shrink, and the tail and hind legs become soiled with the liquid feces. If the scouring continues, dehydration occurs and general emaciation develops. The animal stands listlessly, the postorbital fat disappears, and the eyes sink into their sockets (see Figure 25.16). Death may occur within a week from the time the diarrhea begins. On the

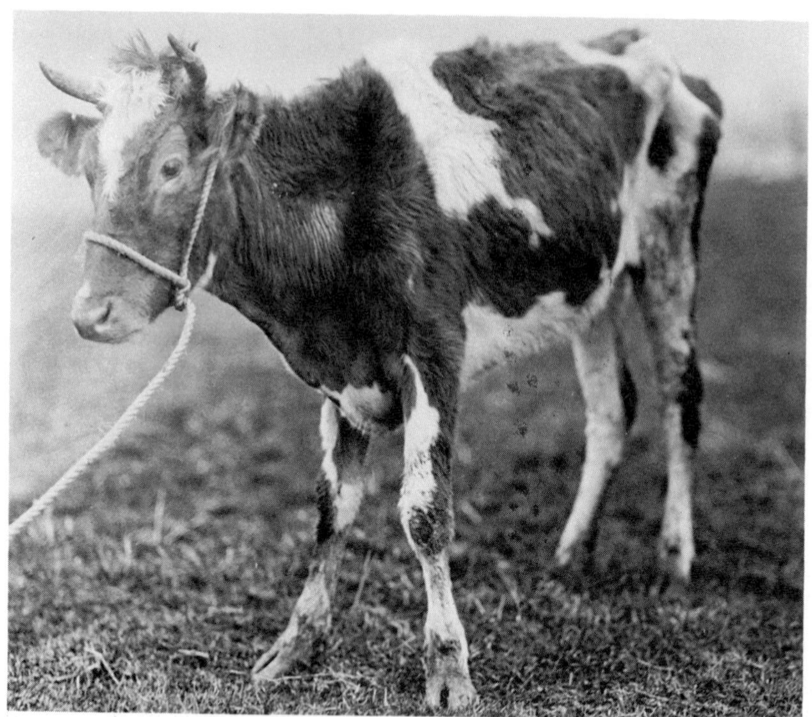

Figure 25.16. An advanced case of Johne's disease. The animal is emaciated, has a rough dry coat, a harsh skin, is constantly scouring, and is so weak that it must brace its legs to keep from falling. This animal had been artificially infected slightly more than 1 year previously by being fed material that contained the organism.

other hand, many animals after scouring for a few days will cease to do so, their appetite will return, and their condition may improve greatly. Such improvement may last only a short time and be followed by a second attack of scouring, or it may be permanent. Some cases will apparently recover completely only to break down during the early part of the next lactation period (21).

The foregoing description has dealt with the disease in cattle. In sheep and goats the symptoms and lesions are similar. The disease apparently may be more acute in these animals than in cattle. The lesions frequently are not conspicuous. Instead of great bowel-wall thickening, often there may be no observable thickening, but petechial hemorrhages may be seen. In the goat, granulomas have been observed in the mesentery (48). In some cases, however, the thickening is marked and similar to that seen in cattle. A study by Stamp and Watt (77) of the pathology of Johne's disease in sheep as it occurs in Scotland also indicates that the lesions vary from insignificant to characteristic masses of epithelioid and giant cells which may undergo encapsulation, necrosis, caseation, and calcification. They suggest that the pigmented variety of *M. paratuberculosis* is more virulent for sheep than is the classical strain. Nakamatsu *et al.* (61) conducted a histopathological study on 45 naturally infected goats and determined that the lesions were located mainly in the intestines and regional lymph nodes. They concluded that certain remote lesions occurring in the kidneys, walls of capillaries, and connective tissues were of an allergic nature rather than the result of direct contact with *M. paratuberculosis*.

Mode of Transmission. Experimentally it is easy to produce infections in young calves by drenching them with infected materials. Very large doses will usually produce clinical symptoms in from 6 to 18 months if the animal is infected before it is 1 year old. Older animals can be readily infected by mouth with large doses of material, but they do not usually develop clinical symptoms and they often throw off the infection completely. Factors other than the virulence of cultures determine whether or not the clinically obvious disease will be produced.

Although it would appear that the natural route of infection is via the mouth, it is evident that transuterine infection must be considered, and there is also the possibility that the infected bull may be the agent that transmits the disease to the cow (37, 39, 63). Exposure of calves to an environment naturally contaminated with *M. paratuberculosis* usually leads to the development of infected animals, whereas exposure of adult cattle to the same conditions seldom does (68, 69). Young calves can also be infected by inoculation by the subcutaneous and intravenous routes (43).

Diagnosis. Several methods are available for detecting the presence of this disease in animals, although none is completely accurate or entirely satisfactory for detecting infected animals that do not show clinical signs of the disease. The principal methods are as follows:

1. *Clinical methods.* Mature animals which persistently exhibit diarrhea and become emaciated should be looked upon with suspicion. If such animals die or are slaughtered, a portion of the lower end of the small intestine should be sent to a laboratory to be examined for the presence of the organism and lesions typical of Johne's disease.

2. *Examination of feces.* Positive diagnoses may be made in many cases by staining fecal samples. Small shreds of mucus should be sought and spread on new, chemically cleaned slides, which are stained with the Ziehl-Neelson technique. The specific organism is quite small and has a tendency to occur in clumps. It must be distinguished from larger acid-fast organisms, which are common in cattle feces.

Harding (25) stained tissue sections with auramine-rhodamine dye and used fluorescent microscopy to detect the organisms. This system has been extended and is presently used by some laboratories to examine feces for the presence of *M. paratuberculosis.*

The organism is fastidious and grows slowly. However, recent improvements in culture methods (58, 59) have made the cultural examination of feces a useful, if slow and painstaking, system of detecting the organism. The technique consists of cutting down contaminating organisms with benzalkonium chloride and then culturing the sample on special media containing mycobactin—for example, Herrold's medium. The cultures are incubated and examined for three months. Although this system of diagnosis is slow, it is now widely used and has the advantage of not giving false positive results.

3. *Scrapings from the rectal mucous membrane.* In a limited number of advanced cases, the disease spreads to the lower bowel and even the rectum. In such cases the thickened rectal mucosa may be recognized by palpation. If no thickening is recognized, a bit of the mucosa may be obtained for microscopic examination. The fragment should be well rinsed with clean water, placed on a slide, and crushed. Films made from the crushed fragment then are stained for acid-fast organisms. It should be kept in mind that acid-fast bacteria occur in the feces of all cows and that these must be differentiated from the bacillus of Johne's disease. The Johne bacillus is smaller than most of the saprophytic forms, and it occurs in characteristic clumps. An experienced observer usually can be sure of the identification of the organisms seen.

4. *The allergic tests.* In 1909, before the bacillus of Johne's disease had been cultivated artificially, Oluf Bang (2) called attention to the fact that many infected animals would react to avian tuberculin administered subcutaneously. This test was used by many workers with fairly satisfactory results. One of Twort's first efforts after obtaining pure cultures of the organism causing Johne's disease was to make a product analogous to tuberculin for use in diagnosis. Since that time johnin and avian tuberculin have been used in a variety of test systems to detect animals with Johne's disease, based on the assumption that such animals will produce some manifestations of delayed hypersensitivity when challenged with johnin or avian tuberculin. While these tests are of some value in determining the existence of the disease in a herd, none of them is specific enough to confirm Johne's disease.

(a) The allergic skin test. In this test johnin is injected intradermally into the suspect animal. Johnin (35) is a substance similar to tuberculin which is extracted and purified from the medium on which *M. paratuberculosis* has been grown. The test is read at 48 hours, by which time a sensitized animal shows a substantial infiltration of cells into the site of johnin deposition, producing a thickening of the skin. While some authorities (26) advocate the use of the intradermal johnin test as a useful means of identifying infected animals before the onset of clinical disease, others (47) consider it to be of doubtful diagnostic value.

(b) The systemic test using intravenous johnin. The reaction following the intravenous injection of johnin and avian tuberculin is the same. Normal animals, if not overdosed, show little or no reaction. Diseased animals usually begin to show signs of discomfort within an hour or so. There is depression, the animal ceases to eat, the head is held low, the hair coat stands on end, and the animal may shiver. Some animals begin to scour profusely, and this may last for several days. The fever curve begins from the 3rd to the 5th hour after injection of the test material and reaches its height from the 5th to the 8th hour, depending upon the size of the dose and the potency of the test fluid. After the peak has been reached, the temperature usually falls quickly to normal by the 10th or 12th hour (22). A temperature rise of 1.5 degrees F is significant, and Larsen (38) considers the test valuable for the differentiation of Johne's disease from other kinds of diarrhea in cattle.

The intravenous injection of johnin produces a substantial change in the distribution of lymphocytes and neutrophils in sensitized animals, increasing neutrophils and decreasing lymphocytes. In sensitized animals the ratio of neutrophils to lymphocytes 6 hours after injection is more than twice that before injection (55).

The potency of the early johnins was low. When it was learned how to cultivate *M. paratuberculosis* in synthetic media without the addition of extracts of other acid-fast organisms, and when profuse growths were produced, much better allergic products were obtained. With such products attention was turned to the application of the intradermal test. McIntosh and Konst (53) in Canada, and a number of English workers have produced potent johnin and have devised methods of obtaining standardized products. Undoubtedly these are more potent and more specific than the earlier products used, and, according to Sikes (74), the intradermal johnin test when properly applied is a highly efficient biological test for sensitivity to *M. paratuberculosis* infection in cattle. He cautions against repeated tests in the same site, claiming that such procedure results in negative tests in infected animals. A new site for each test is best; otherwise let 20 weeks elapse between tests.

Unfortunately, all johnins fail to elicit reactions in some cases of the disease. Also, they cause reactions in cattle that appear to be noninfected, but on this score the fault, in many cases at least, is that there are no methods to confirm the presence of the disease at autopsy. In some cases the lesions are so slight or so inconspicuous that they are very difficult to find. In herds in which occasional clinical cases are occurring, it is not uncommon to find a considerable number of reacting animals. Many of these animals, if not destroyed as a result of the test, live their normal life spans without exhibiting symptoms and frequently fail to react on tests administered later. This is part of the evidence that adult animals often harbor the infection without showing it, and that they often free themselves of it spontaneously.

Allergic tests are of value in determining the existence of the disease in herds. Positive results indicate that some of the animals may be infected and suggest that some of the more specific tests should be carried out on the herd.

5. *Serological tests*. Hagan and Zeissig (23) found that the complement-fixation test could be used for the diagnosis of Johne's disease in cattle. The antigens were made from tubercle bacilli and therefore were nonspecific. They would be of little value in animals sensitized by any other acid-fast organisms, including tubercle bacilli. In their experimentally infected cattle, the complement-fixation test became positive as early as the allergic tests, and long before clinical symptoms appeared, and it remained positive in animals so debilitated from the disease that they would no longer react to allergic tests. It was in such cases that the test was believed to have its principal value. It was obvious, however, that many animals that probably were not infected with Johne's disease reacted, presumably because of sensitization with heterologous antigens. Sirgurdsson *et al.* (73), working with sheep in Iceland, also found the test of value. Their antigen was made by extracting the affected intestinal mucosa of animals suffering from the disease, and it may be regarded as specific. They examined a flock of 55 sheep of which 31 were proved at autopsy to have been infected. Of these, 30 had reacted strongly to the test. Four others that had been strongly positive serologically did not show lesions. Of 118 sheep from a noninfected area which were tested, only 4 reacted, and these rather weakly. Only about 50 percent of 39 infected animals in their experimental flock reacted to intradermal tests with a johnin PPD (Purified Protein Derivative). As a result they were inclined to regard the serological test as much more reliable in sheep than the allergic one.

The complement-fixation test may not become positive until the infection is well developed; the titer may drop when clinical signs of disease become apparent, and there is still considerable doubt about the ability of the test to detect infected animals and carriers (33). Despite these reservations, the complement-fixation test is still the most widely used serological test for the diagnosis of Johne's disease.

Larsen *et al.* (45) sensitized sheep erythrocytes with johnin (PPD) and used these cells in hemagglutination tests. They found that the test was not specific; that animals sensitized with Johne's bacilli as well as with other species within the genus *Mycobacterium* reacted. The fluorescent-antibody test (15, 17), the agar-gel diffusion test (55), and counterimmunoelectrophoresis (60) have also been used in efforts to diagnose Johne's disease, but it appears that cultural examination of fecal specimens is of more value than serologic procedures in detecting paratuberculous cattle before they develop clinical signs of the disease.

With the recent elucidation of the role of lymphocytes and cell-mediated immunity in diseases caused by facultative intracellular bacteria such as *M. paratuberculosis*, the application of these cellular events to the diagnosis of infection has been vigorously investigated. In the area of Johne's disease, Bendixen (3) developed a leukocyte-migration test, and various investigators (4, 31) have studied lymphocyte blastogenesis, but the results are still too preliminary for these tests to be generally used and evaluated.

Immunity. Animals that develop clinical evidence of Johne's disease seldom recover fully. Often they improve temporarily and seem to be fully recovered only to suffer a recurrence after days, weeks, or months. One animal observed by Hagan and Zeissig (24) remained well for 5 years after having suffered severely from the disease during its first and second lactation periods. Minimal lesions were found at autopsy. It has already been pointed out that many more animals react to allergic tests than ever show symptoms and that in these asymptomatic animals the disease develops only to a limited extent and then is often thrown off.

A definite age immunity exists in this disease (20). Artificial infection by drenching with massive doses of infective material succeeds readily in calves but usually fails to produce clinical disease in older animals. Calves that are introduced into infected surroundings after they are 6 months of age seldom develop into clinical cases, though they may become allergic reactors, indicating that they harbor infection. Rankin (67) has estimated that the intravenous dose of *M. paratuberculosis* necessary to produce disease in a 1-month-old calf is about 5 mg of cultivated organisms weighed wet.

The actual mechanisms of resistance to Johne's disease are unknown. The B cells respond to the organism with the production of specific antibodies, but their role in protection is unclear. Merkal *et al.* (57) postulated that the humoral response was responsible for an immediate form of hypersensitivity—the release of histamine—and thus for the production of diarrhea. They also postulated a role for T lymphocytes in the pathogenesis of Johne's disease, suggesting that their products were responsible for the production of fever, emaciation, and anemia.

Cell-mediated immunity is likely to be as important in protecting the host against *M. paratuberculosis* as against other mycobacteria and facultative intracellular bacteria. However, there is little information available on the role of cell-mediated immunity in the intestinal tract, and its significance in Johne's disease has still to be elucidated.

Vallée and Rinjard (85) in 1926 began a series of experiments in France to determine whether Johne's bacillus might be used as a vaccine to protect cattle. It was found that subcutaneous injection of this organism mixed with mineral oil and pumice produced dense tumors at the point of inoculation and that these remained for many months. Large doses injected without oil usually ulcerate and discharge fairly promptly. In a report published in 1934 (86), these authors state that over 12,000 animals had been vaccinated, that the vaccine had had no untoward effects, and that it was believed to have given an appreciable protection against the disease. Doyle (7) tested the method in England and found it to be highly efficient against natural infection under field conditions. Sigurdsson (71) vaccinated lambs with heat-killed *M. paratuberculosis* suspended in mineral oil and concluded that the bacterin provoked a satisfactory resistance to subsequent infection. By 1960 about 450,000 sheep had been vaccinated by this method, obtaining excellent protection (72).

More recently Huitema (28) used a vaccine consisting of killed bacteria mixed with a liquid paraffin adjuvant, and Larsen *et al.* (40) prepared a vaccine of fractionated and homogenized bacteria administered in Freund's adjuvant. However, all vaccines still have serious drawbacks: their efficacy is hard to evaluate in the field and in lab animals; many produce unsightly nodules at the vaccination site; and vaccinated animals develop hypersensitivity to johnin and the tuberculins (38).

In countries where vaccination is practiced, 1 dose is given at 1 week of age. This seems to inhibit the intracellular multiplication of the organism, lower the level of the organisms shed, and prevent most cases of clinical disease in infected herds (33).

Chemotherapy. Numerous chemotherapeutic agents have been tried in the treatment of Johne's disease. So far none has influenced the course of the disease to any marked degree (33), although streptomycin, viomycin, and isoniazid are effective *in vitro* against the organism (10, 46, 64).

The Disease in Man. There are no reports of human infections.

Control Measures. The control of Johne's disease is an unsolved problem, mainly because of the difficulty in detecting carrier animals and because of the long period of covert infection. It spreads insidiously through movement of cattle and sheep, in which the disease is latent. Before animals are imported into uninfected regions, johnin testing is advised, since most animals in the latent stages of the disease will react. In recent years culturing all the animals on a routine basis—e.g., every 6 months, with the elimination of shedders and their calves—has become increasingly used as a means of control in individual herds.

It is clear that most clinical cases, which are undoubtedly the most serious spreaders of infection, are infected in early calfhood; therefore, protection of the young calves is indicated. These should be removed from their dams as soon as possible and raised separately, in different barns and on different pastures. The infection can be eliminated from a farm where there has been an outbreak in sheep by disposing of all the sheep and leaving the area free from sheep or cattle for 1 year before restocking. The success reported by Sigurdsson (72) in the vaccination of lambs warrants the use of bacterin, especially in areas where the disease is prevalent.

Testing with avian tuberculin or johnin, with elimination of reactors, is obviously a wasteful procedure because many reactors will never develop the disease. If they are few in number, this method may be tried, and sometimes it succeeds. In other herds, new reactors will continue to be encountered on each of many successive tests. Furthermore, clinical cases frequently develop in such herds between tests, an indication that the tests miss some cases.

REFERENCES

1. Bang. Berl. tierärztl. Wchnschr., 1906, p. 759.
2. Bang. Zentrbl. f. Bakt., I Abt. Orig., 1909, *51,* 450.
3. Bendixen. Am. Jour. Vet. Res., 1977, *38,* 2027.
4. Buergelt, Hall, Merkal, Whitlock, and Duncan. Am. Jour. Vet. Res., 1977, *38,* 1709.
5. Chandler. Jour. Comp. Path. and Therap., 1962, *72,* 198.
6. Dorset, Henley, and Moskey. Jour. Am. Vet. Med. Assoc., 1926, *70,* 373.
7. Doyle. Vet. Rec., 1945, *57,* 385.
8. Doyle. Brit. Vet. Jour., 1954, *110,* 215.
9. Dunkin. Jour. Comp. Path. and Therap., 1935, *48,* 236.
10. Ford. Brit. Vet. Jour., 1952, *108,* 411.
11. Francis. Brit. Vet. Jour., 1943, *53,* 140.
12. Francis, Macturk, Madinaveitia, and Snow. Biochem. Jour., 1953, *55,* 596.
13. Gifford, Eveleth, and Gifford. Vet. Med., 1942, *37,* 416.
14. Gilmour. Vet. Rec., 1965, *77,* 1322.
15. Gilmour. Res. Vet. Sci., 1971, *12,* 295.
16. Gilmour, Campbell, and Brotherston. Jour. Comp. Path. and Therap., 1963, *73,* 98.
17. Gilmour and Gardiner. Jour. Comp. Path., 1969, *79,* 71.
18. Gilmour, Nisbet, and Brotherston. Jour. Comp. Path., 1965, *75,* 281.
19. Hagan. Symposium series, Am. Assoc. Adv. Sci., 1937, *1,* 69.
20. Hagan. Cornell Vet., 1938, *28,* 34.
21. Hagan and Zeissig. Rpt. N.Y. State Vet. Coll. for 1927–28, p. 150.
22. Hagan and Zeissig. Jour. Am. Vet. Med. Assoc., 1929, *74,* 985.
23. Hagan and Zeissig. Jour. Am. Vet. Med. Assoc., 1933, *82,* 391.
24. Hagan and Zeissig. Jour. Am. Vet. Med. Assoc., 1935, *87,* 199.
25. Harding. Jour. Comp. Path. and Therap., 1957, *67,* 180.
26. Hole and McClay. Vet. Rec., 1959, *71,* 1145.
27. Howarth. Jour. Am. Vet. Med. Assoc., 1932, *81,* 383.
28. Huitema. Off. internat. Epizoot., 1967, *68,* 743.
29. Jansen. Jour. Am. Vet. Med. Assoc., 1948, *112,* 52.
30. Johne and Frothingham. Deut. Zeitschr. f. Tiermed., 1895, *21,* 438.
31. Johnson, Muscoplat, Larsen and Thoen. Am. Jour. Vet. Res., 1977, *38,* 2023.
32. Jørgensen. Acta Vet. Scand., 1969, *10,* 275.
33. Julian. Can. Vet. Jour., 1975, *16,* 33.
34. Kluge, Merkal, Monlux, Larsen, Kopecky, Ramsey, and Lehmann. Am. Jour. Vet. Res., 1968, *29,* 953.
35. Konst and McIntosh. Can. Jour. Comp. Med., 1958, *22,* 157.
36. Kopecky. Jour. Am. Vet. Med. Assoc., 1977, *170,* 320.
37. Kopecky, Larsen, and Merkal. Am. Jour. Vet. Res., 1967, *28,* 1043.
38. Larsen. Jour. Am. Vet. Med. Assoc., 1973, *163,* 902.
39. Larsen and Kopecky. Am. Jour. Vet Res., 1970, *31,* 255.
40. Larsen, Merkal, Kopecky, and Booth. Am. Jour. Vet. Res., 1969, *30,* 2167.
41. Larsen, Merkal, and Vardaman. Am. Jour. Vet. Res., 1956, *17,* 549.
42. Larsen and Miller. Am. Jour. Vet. Res., 1978, *39,* 1866.
43. Larsen, Miller, and Merkal. Am. Jour. Vet. Res., 1977, *38,* 1669.
44. Larsen, Moon, and Merkal. Am. Jour. Vet. Res., 1972, *33,* 2185.
45. Larsen, Porter, and Vardaman. Am. Jour. Vet. Res., 1953, *14,* 362.
46. Larsen and Vardaman. Am. Jour. Vet. Res., 1952, *13,* 466.
47. Larsen, Vardaman, and Merkal. Am. Jour. Vet. Res., 1963, *24,* 91.
48. Lenghaus, Badman, and Gillick. Austral. Vet. Jour., 1977, *53,* 460.
49. Levi. Jour. Comp. Path. and Therap., 1948, *58,* 38.
50. Long and Seibert. Trans. Nat. Tuberc. Assoc., 1926, p. 270.
51. Lovell, Levi, and Francis. Jour. Comp. Path. and Therap., 1944, *54,* 120.
52. McEwen. Jour. Comp. Path. and Therap., 1939, *52,* 69.
53. McIntosh and Konst. Can. Jour. Pub. Health, 1943, *34,* 557.
54. Madge. Compar. Biochem. and Physiol., 1971, *40a,* 649.
55. Merkal. Compar. Biochem. and Physiol., 1973, *163,* 1100.
56. Merkal and Curran. Appl. Microbiol., 1974, *28,* 276.
57. Merkal, Kopecky, Larsen, and Ness. Am. Jour. Vet. Res., 1970, *31,* 475.
58. Merkal, Kopecky, Larsen, and Thurston. Am. Jour. Vet. Res., 1964, *25,* 1290.
59. Merkal and Larsen. Am. Jour. Vet. Res., 1962, *23,* 1307.
60. Muhammed, Tadayon, and Cheema. Vet. Rec., 1978, *102,* 401.

61. Nakamatsu, Fujimoto, and Satoh. Jap. Jour. Vet. Res., 1968, *16*, 103.
62. Payne and Rankin. Res. Vet. Sci., 1961, *2*, 175.
63. Pearson. Vet. Rec., 1955, *67*, 615.
64. Rankin. Vet. Rec., 1953, *65*, 649.
65. Rankin. Vet. Rec., 1954, *66*, 550.
66. Rankin. Jour. Path. and Bact., 1956, *72*, 689.
67. Rankin. Jour. Path. and Bact., 1959, *77*, 638.
68. Rankin. Jour. Path. and Bact., 1961, *71*, 10.
69. Rankin. Jour. Path. and Bact., 1962, *72*, 113.
70. Richards and Thoen. Jour. Clin. Microbiol., 1977, *6*, 392.
71. Sigurdsson. Jour. Immunol., 1952, *68*, 559.
72. Sigurdsson. Am. Jour. Vet. Res., 1960, *80*, 54.
73. Sigurdsson, Vigfusson, and Theodors. Jour. Comp. Path. and Therap., 1945, *55*, 268.
74. Sikes. Am. Jour. Vet. Res., 1953, *14*, 12.
75. Smith. Jour. Path. and Bact., 1953, *66*, 375.
76. Smythe. Vet. Rec., 1935, *15*, 85.
77. Stamp and Watt. Jour. Comp. Path. and Therap., 1954, *64*, 26.
78. Stuart. Brit. Vet. Jour., 1965, *121*, 332.
79. Taylor. Jour. Comp. Path. and Therap., 1945, *55*, 41.
80. Taylor. Vet. Rec., 1949, *61*, 539.
81. Taylor. Jour. Path. and Bact., 1950, *62*, 647.
82. Taylor. Jour. Path. and Bact., 1951, *63*, 323.
83. Taylor. Jour. Comp. Path. and Therap., 1953, *63*, 368.
84. Twort. Proc. Roy. Soc. Med., 1911, Series B, *83*, 158.
85. Vallée and Rinjard. Rev. gén. méd., vét., 1926, *35*, 1.
86. Vallée, Rinjard, and Vallée. Rev. gén. méd., vét., 1934, *43*, 50.
87. Vance. Can. Vet Jour., 1961, *2*, 305.
88. Wullepit. Vlaamsch Diergeneesk. Tijdschr., 1977, *46*, 185.
89. Zorawasi, Karpinski and Schwarek. Medycyna Weterynaryjna, 1978, *34*, 528.

Mycobacterium lepraemurium (The Acid-Fast Organism of Rat Leprosy)

In a rat-destruction campaign waged in Odessa in 1901 Stephansky (12) found about 5 percent of the animals to be suffering from a disease which resembles human leprosy, particularly in the fact that the lesions contain large numbers of acid-fast organisms and are not bound together in clumps and masses as in human leprosy(7). The disease has been seen in other parts of the world (9), but usually only a fraction of 1 percent of the population is involved. In some cases there is enlargement of the lymph nodes, particularly those of the axillary and inguinal regions. The glands become enlarged and hardened but do not suppurate. Myriads of acid-fast bacilli, usually located intracellularly in large cells which probably are epithelioid in nature, can be found in such glands (Figure 25.17). In other cases the disease affects the skin and subcutaneous tissue and sometimes the underlying

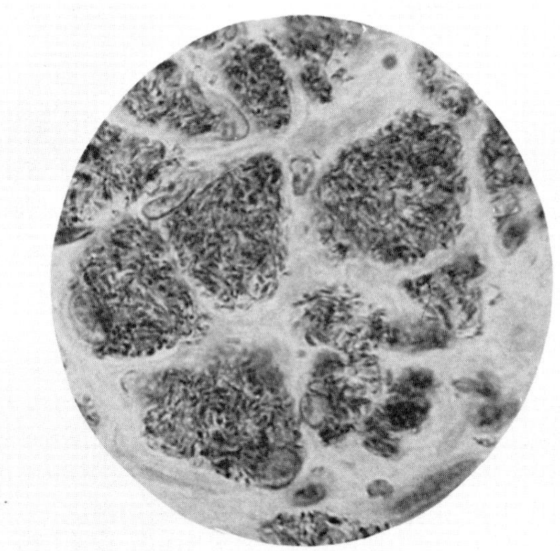

Figure 25.17. The acid-fast organism of rat leprosy. Large epithelioid-type cells are located in the granulomatous lesion of the subcutaneous tissue and packed with the acid-fast lepra bacilli. × 1,030.

muscle. The hair is lost from such areas, and sometimes ulcers are formed from which a thick discharge, rich in bacilli, exudes. In the granulation tissue which forms beneath the skin, bacilli are plentiful. Lesions in the internal organs are rare, except that nephritis usually exists, in which cases bacilli cannot be demonstrated in the kidneys.

Although lesions were induced in rats, mice, and hamsters by injecting infected tissues, isolated cultures failed to reproduce the disease and apparently the bacillus of rat leprosy was not cultured on artificial media for many years. In 1962, Rees and Tee (10) succeeded in cultivating *M. lepraemurium* in rat fibroblasts and studied the mycobacterial antigens of the bacilli. In 1966, Kato and Gozsy (4) achieved limited multiplication of the rat leprosy bacillus by employing an alkaline (pH 8.4) galactomannan-containing medium alone or in parabiosis with a feeder strain *(Torula minuta)*. Hyperosmolarity (NaC1, 2 percent) enhanced multiplication in both cases.

The rat leprosy organism probably has no relation to that of human leprosy, inasmuch as rats are resistant to inoculation with leprous tissue from man. In recent years granulomatous lesions have been described on the skin of cats; it appears that this condition, cat leprosy, is also caused by *M. lepraemurium*.

Cat Leprosy. In 1962 Brown, May, and Williams (1) described a nontuberculous granuloma in cats in New Zealand. The condition, which resembled rat leprosy and is now called *feline* or *cat leprosy,* has been described in Australia (5), Britain (14), Holland (8), Canada (11), and the United States (3). The granulomas are usually found in the skin, most frequently the skin of the head and limbs. The skin may ulcerate, and occasionally the subcutis and peripheral lymph nodes are also affected (13). The characteristic distribution of lesions has led to the suggestion that the disease is transmitted by the bites of infected rats or cats. Examination of a smear made from these lesions or from the regional lymph node will usually reveal large numbers of acid-fast bacilli, many located inside macrophages.

The organism of cat leprosy can be differentiated from *M. tuberculosis* by its inability to grow on the media used to culture the tubercle bacilli (11). The agent has not yet been grown on artificial media, but it can be grown on tissue cultures of rat cells and will reproduce the lesions of rat leprosy when inoculated into rats, mice, and guinea pigs (5, 8). The organism of cat leprosy has been shown in skin tests to have a very similar antigenic composition (6) and similar growth characteristics (2) to *M. lepraemurium*. The present evidence, therefore, indicates that it is very similar, if not identical, to *M. lepraemurium* (6).

REFERENCES

1. Brown, May, and Williams. New Zeal. Vet. Jour., 1962, *10,* 7.
2. D'Arcy Hart and Rees. Int. Jour. Leprosy, 1968, *36,* 83.
3. Frye, Carney, and Loughman. Vet. Med. Sm. Anim. Clin., 1974, *69,* 1271.
4. Kato and Gozsy. Jour. Bact., 1966, *91,* 1859.
5. Lawrence and Wickham. Austral. Vet. Jour., 1963, *39,* 391.
6. Leiker and Poelma. Int. Jour. Leprosy, 1974, *42,* 312.
7. Lowe. Int. Jour. Leprosy, 1937, *5,* 311.
8. Poelma and Leiker. Int. Jour. Leprosy, 1974, *42,* 307.
9. Rabinowitsch. Zentrbl. f. Bakt., I Abt. Orig., 1903, *33,* 577.
10. Rees and Tee. Brit. Jour. Exp. Path., 1962, *43,* 480.
11. Schiefer, Gee, and Ward. Jour. Am. Vet. Med. Assoc., 1974, *165,* 1085.
12. Stephansky. Zentrbl. f. Bakt., I Abt. Orig., 1903, *33,* 481.
13. Thompson, Little, and Cordes. New Zeal. Vet. Jour., 1979, *27,* 233.
14. Wilkinson. Vet. Rec., 1964, *76,* 777.

Acid-Fast Bacilli Associated with Ulcerative Lymphangitis in Cattle, "Skin Tuberculosis"

In the course of the work of eradicating bovine tuberculosis in the United States, much attention has been given to a condition that occurs in many parts of the country to which the name *skin tuberculosis* was early attached. Traum (12) appears to have been the first to call attention to the fact that these lesions sometimes caused cattle to react to the tuberculin test. Animals in some areas are more often affected with these lesions than those in others, and the distribution of cases does not correspond to the distribution of orthodox tuberculosis. The condition is not caused by tubercle bacilli.

The lesions usually occur in the skin of the lower parts of the legs. Their frequent occurence at these sites has led to the suggestion that the acid-fast organisms invade the host via wounds, abrasions, or scratches inflicted by thorny plants. The lesions first appear as nodules that seem to be attached to the skin but are actually located in the subcutaneous tissue. In the course of time these nodules usually soften and ulcerate through the skin. In the meantime, other nodules often appear along the course of the lymphatics. It is not uncommon to see animals having from 4 to 5 to as many as 25 nodules, many of which have broken through the skin (Figure 25.18). After discharging their contents, the lesions usually heal. In some cases, instead of discharging, the lesions coalesce forming large dense masses consisting largely of connective tissue in which areas of suppuration occur. The pus may be fluid, pasty, or dry, inspissated, and calcareous. The neighboring lymph nodes usually do not become involved, unlike the situation which invariably occurs in the presence of true tubercle infection.

The histological structure of these nodules resembles that of tuberculous tissue. Acid-fast bacilli that cannot be distinguished morphologically from bovine tubercle bacilli can be found in most cases, although usually they are not numerous. Many workers (1–3, 5, 6, 10, 12) have studied these lesions, but none has succeeded either in obtaining cultures of the acid-fast organism or in causing infections in laboratory animals. Although many have tried to trasmit this condition, the only successful effort appears to be that of Hedström (4). He used finely dispersed tissue material taken from skin lesions in their early stage of development. Animals were injected,

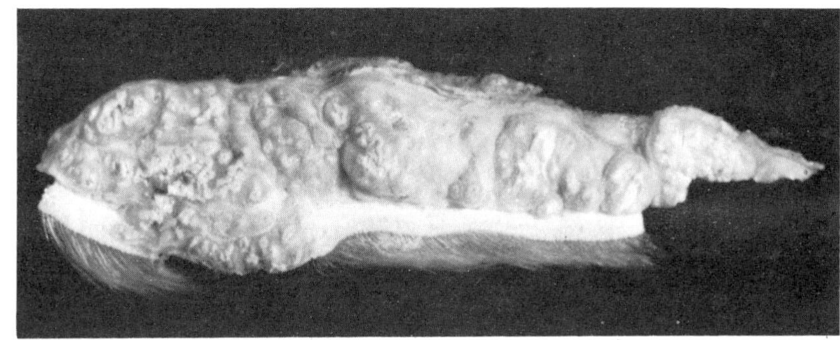

Figure 25.18. Acid-fast lymphangitis, cross section of gross lesions in the subcutaneous tissue of a cow. Note ulceration through skin. Reduced one-half.

either intracutaneously or subcutaneously into several places on the lateral surface of the neck and on the lateral sides of the forelimb. Six weeks after the inoculations the skin where the intracutaneous injections were made showed small, solid swellings, which gradually increased, later became node-forming, and finally reached the size of a hazelnut about 6 months after the inoculation. Where the tissue material was injected subcutaneously no reaction was observed.

Several workers have occasionally isolated cultures of acid-fast bacilli, but the strains isolated have the characteristics of saprophytes, that is, they have been incapable of producing more than an abscess at the point of inoculation (12).

Animals affected with these lesions do not always react to tuberculin, and when reactions occur, they are somewhat atypical in many instances. Such animals may react at one time and fail to react at another. When the lesions are removed surgically, gradual loss of sensitivity occurs. The disease is not a serious one, *per se,* although the blemishes produced are distasteful to owners of fine cattle. The most serious feature about them is the fact that they confuse the diagnosis so far as tuberculosis is concerned. Reactions to tuberculin cannot be safely ascribed to the presence of such lesions unless the history of the animal makes the occurrence of genuine tuberculosis in the same animal highly improbable, for the lesions are found in tuberculous as well as in nontuberculous cattle. Identical lesions have been described in English cattle by Robertson and Hole (10) in 1937, in Danish cattle by Götzsche and Plum (1) in 1938, in Swedish cattle by Krantz (5) in 1938, and in Swiss cattle by Thomann (11) in 1949. As early as 1913 Perard and Ramon (7) described a similar if not identical condition in France.

In 1960 Ressang and Titus (9) reported a case of buffalo leprosy in a Holstein-Friesian cow. The leprosy nodules were located mainly in the lower part of the left hind- and right front-leg. It seems that a disease known as buffalo leprosy is not uncommon in water buffaloes in Indonesia, but cattle ordinarily are not affected. From descriptions of the disease and from the results obtained in transmission experiments by Ressang and Sutarjo (8) it is not entirely clear whether buffalo leprosy is a distinct entity or part of the acid-fast ulcerative lymphangitis complex.

REFERENCES

1. Götzsche and Plum. Maanedskr. f. Dyrlaeger, 1938, *50,* 33.
2. Hagan. Cornell Vet., 1929, *19,* 173.
3. Hastings, Beach, and Weber. Jour. Am. Vet. Med. Assoc., 1924, *66,* 36.
4. Hedström. Collected papers from the State Vet. Med. Inst. Stockholm, 1949, p. 180.
5. Krantz. Skandi. Vet. Tidskr., 1938, *28,* 20.
6. Mitchell. Jour. Am. Vet. Med. Assoc., 1928, *73,* 493.
7. Perard and Ramon. Comp. rend. Soc. Biol. (Paris), 1913, *65,* 133.
8. Ressang and Sutarjo. Commun. Vet., 1961, *5,* 89.
9. Ressang and Titus. Commun. Vet., 1960, *4,* 47.
10. Robertson and Hole. Jour. Comp. Path. and Therap., 1937, *50,* 39.
11. Thomann. Schweiz. Arch. Tierheilk., 1949, *91,* 237.
12. Traum. Jour. Am. Vet. Med. Assoc., 1916, *49,* 254; 1919, *55,* 639.

The Saprophytic Acid-Fast Bacilli

Acid-fast organisms belonging to the mycobacteria are widespread in nature. Nearly all soils harbor them (1), and they are common on vegetation and in the alimentary tracts of herbivorous animals. They have also been found on the mucous membranes and skins of animals. They have been isolated from cases of bovine mastitis (5, 6, 8). Affected animals may or may not react to tuberculin tests. They show granulomatous lesions in the udders and it appears that the condition may result because of a lack of aseptic technique in giving udder infusions of oily therapeutic preparations.

For the most part the organisms seem to be harmless, although abscesses and tubercles may be produced by injecting them into animals. They frequently show a very close resemblance to tubercle bacilli but may be distinguished from them by lack of pathogenicity for animals, rapid manner of growth on culture media, and the fact that they will grow well at room temperature. Most of these organisms will develop luxuriantly on plain glycerol agar, on plain agar, or on solutions of simple mineral salts. They grow on fluid media in the form of pellicles, in most instances, and produce filtrates that resemble tuberculin. Usually these filtrates will not give reactions in animals affected with tuberculosis but will in animals that have been inoculated with the homologous organisms.

The studies of Thomson (7), Gordon (2), and Gordon and Hagan (3) have made it clear that many of the acid-fast organisms that have been isolated from a variety of sources by different persons in the past and have been endowed with different names, depending usually upon the source from which they were obtained, are in reality alike. Thus of a collection of 331 strains, most of which had been isolated by the authors from soil and water but which included about 50 named strains of other authors, the greater part fell into three principal groups. Gordon and Smith (4) restudied 124 strains in 1953 and concluded that 62 percent belonged in two species which they designated *M. smegmatis* and *M. phlei*.

M. fortuitum is sometimes grouped with these organisms because it is also a rapid grower; however, *M. fortuitum* fails to grow at 45 C, whereas *M. phlei* and *M. smegmatis* will do so. It also possesses a higher order of virulence for mice. Other cultures are regarded at present merely as "saprophytic acid-fast bacilli."

REFERENCES

1. Frey and Hagan. Jour. Inf. Dis., 1931, *49*, 497.
2. Gordon. Jour. Bact., 1937, *34*, 617.
3. Gordon and Hagan. Jour. Bact., 1938, *36*, 39.
4. Gordon and Smith. Jour. Bact., 1953, *66*, 41.
5. Richardson. Vet. Rec., 1970, *86*, 497.
6. Stuart and Harvey. Vet. Rec., 1951, *63*, 881.
7. Thomson. Am. Rev. Tuberc., 1932, *26*, 162.
8. Tucker. Cornell Vet., 1953, *43*, 576.

26 The Genus *Dermatophilus*

In 1958, Austwick (5) reviewed the histories of *streptothricosis, mycotic dermatitis,* and *strawberry foot-rot* and concluded that the causal organisms were congeneric. He proposed that *Dermatophilus,* the earliest generic name, be used for them and recognized three species: *D. congolensis* from streptothricosis in cattle, *D. dermatonomus* from mycotic dermatitis in sheep, and *D. pedis* from strawberry foot-rot in sheep. He also suggested that these organisms be assigned to the family Dermatophilaceae and placed in the order Actinomycetales. In 1964, Gordon (8) studied members of the genus *Dermatophilus* and decided that all isolates can be accommodated in the species *D. congolensis,* with *D. dermatonomus* and *D. pedis* falling into synonymy. This conclusion was supported by serologic studies by Roberts (25) in 1965. Accordingly, we will consider *D. congolensis* to be the cause of the diseases commonly known as *cutaneous streptothricosis, mycotic dermatitis, lumpy wool, strawberry foot-rot,* and *cutaneous actinomycosis.*

Dermatophilus congolensis

SYNONYMS: *Actinomyces congolensis, Streptothrix bovis, Tetragenus congolensis, Dermatophilus dermatonomus, Nocardia dermatonomus, Polysepta dermatonomus, Dermatophilus pedis, Polysepta pedis, Rhizobium pedis*

This organism is the cause of cutaneous streptothricosis in cattle, horses, sheep, goats, deer, elands, and rabbits. It was first described by Van Saceghem (31), in 1915 in the Belgian Congo. The disease is most common in Africa, but similar cases have been described in Europe, Australia, New Zealand, India, and North and South America (4). It is widespread in the United States and Canada.

Morphology and Staining Reactions. *D. congolensis* produces characteristic narrow, tapering filaments with lateral branching at right angles. Septa are formed in transverse horizontal and vertical planes and give rise to parallel rows of coccoid cells that form motile flagellate zoospores (Figure 26.1). Both mycelia and spores are Gram-positive.

Cultural Features. The organism grows well at 37 C. Colonies on solid media are grayish white, becoming yellowish with age, and sometimes viscous and adherent to the medium. They may be smooth, moist, mucoid, and not adherent. *D. congolensis* coagulates milk, usually liquefies gelatin slowly, and may produce a pellicle on liquid media. It ferments glucose and mannitol with acid production. It is variable in its ability to attack dextrin, galactose, levulose, and sucrose. It does not attack arabinose, dulcitol, lactose, or sorbitol.

Antigens. All strains of *D. congolensis* that have been studied appear to have similar somatic antigens, hemolysins, and precipitinogens. Flagellar antigens exhibit considerable variability, but there is some sharing of flagellar antigen between isolates (25).

The soluble antigens responsible for the delayed hypersensitivity reaction seem to be similar in a variety of isolates (25).

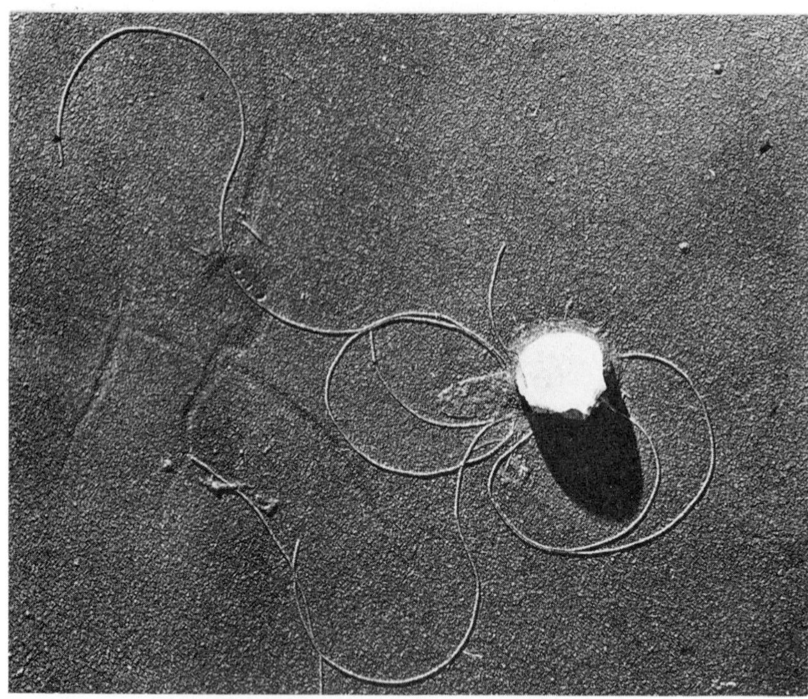

Figure 26.1. Electron micrograph of *Dermatophilus congolensis* showing flagella. × 26,800. (Courtesy I. Grinyer.)

Epidemiology. *D. congolensis* is an obligate parasite of the skin of cattle, sheep, deer, and other species. The organism does not survive in the soil (23). The infective form of the organism is the motile zoospore which is released when infected skin becomes wet. The life span of the motile zoospore is only a few hours, but dried spores can survive for long periods. Infection is spread by contact, by the splashing effects of heavy rain, and by insect activity. Infection is maintained on carrier animals where small lesions persist (6) for long periods. The hair follicles are possible sites where infection persists in carrier cattle (6). There is a definite correlation of the incidence of cutaneous streptothricosis with wet weather—the disease in tropical Africa is closely associated with the rainy season. Cases in deer and horses in New York State are more numerous after wet summers.

Besides rainfall, other predisposing environmental factors are the activities of ticks and blood-sucking flies and thorny bushes or any overhanging branches where cattle congregate. In some areas of Africa, pecker birds are involved in the spread of infection.

Lumpy-wool disease in sheep is more frequent during periods of mild wet weather, and strawberry foot-rot is similarly a disease seen during wet summers.

Pathogenesis. Entry of zoospores which reach the skin of a new host into the deeper layers of the epidermis is dependent on loss of the sebaceous film on the surface of the stratum corneum (24). The mechanical obstacle that this film presents to entry of the infective stage is greatly reduced by the macerating effects of rain. A similar effect is produced on the stratum corneum. Trauma caused by insect and tick bites and by shearing (sheep) also is important in entry of the organism.

The zoospores are chemotactically responsive to CO_2 diffusing out through the skin. They germinate and a hyphal branch penetrates the epidermis. The hyphae branch laterally and invade the hair or wool follicles. The dermis is not invaded. Neutrophils collect beneath the infected epidermis, and a serous exudate accumulates and leaks to the surface. A new layer of epidermis is formed as the older layer above deteriorates, a process that continues and eventually results in formation of a thick scab. Infection of newly forming epidermis occurs from organisms already in the follicular sheath.

The restriction of *D. congolensis* to the epidermis is due to a factor produced by the neutrophils that have gathered in the dermis (25). It is also probable that the basement membrane of the epidermis is a natural barrier to dermal invasion.

Streptothricosis as it usually is seen in cattle, horses, deer, and at times in sheep is characterized by small, confluent, raised, and circumscribed crusts composed of epidermal cells and coagulated serous exudate with embedded hairs appearing on the skin of the back of infected animals. The lesions may be local or become progressive and sometimes fatal. The disease is essentially an exudative dermatitis followed by extensive scab formation (Figure 26.2).

The extent to which the disease occurs in cattle varies considerably in different parts of Africa. In East Africa the disease is of relatively little economic importance, but in Nigeria losses due to death or culling are substantial (17). In some herds, 4 percent of cattle have to be culled because of the disease. There are also substantial losses because of damage to hides and poor growth rates.

The first signs of mycotic dermatitis in sheep are the appearance of small areas of hyperemia, which persist for 10 to 14 days and are followed by the formation of crusts. Masses of amber-colored crust material may mat the wool fibers, but usually the crust separates from the skin surface and remains as a zone of hardened exudate or is cast off. Removal of the scab from an active lesion leaves a concave, raw, and moist area. Progressive lesions may result in death and may cause serious losses in lambs.

The organism also causes strawberry foot-rot in sheep. It was described by Harriss (9) in 1948 in Scotland, where it has been called *proliferative dermatitis in sheep* and was believed for a time to be caused by a virus (1). Employing the organism derived from sheep, Abdussalan and Blakemore (1) were able to infect rabbits and guinea pigs by skin scarification. Papules appeared on the 2nd day after several rabbit passages; originally the incubation period was 5 days. Scabs were soon formed. These dropped off in about 2 weeks, leaving smooth, hairless skin. Material from the fourth rabbit passage produced the disease in sheep and goats.

The natural disease in sheep begins with the appearance of dry scabs located on the legs at any point between the coronet and the knee or hock. Papules preceding the scalp formation were not observed. It was thought that mechanical injury to the skin from prickly plants probably preceded the formation of lesions. The local lesions show a tendency to spread until sometimes almost the entire skin area of the lower portions of the legs is involved. More often the lesions, after reaching 2 to 4 cm in diameter, heal without further spread. The affected areas become denuded of hair or wool. When the areas are large, the exudate mats the hair and forms a hard, dry casing over the region. This usually can be easily stripped off, leaving a mass of granulation tissue that has the appearance of a strawberry, hence the origin of the common name of the disease. The lesions may remain for long periods, but usually they heal within 5 to 6 weeks. The secondary infection rarely invades deeper structures, and usually the animal does not become lame. When lameness occurs, it is because the interdigital space has been invaded. There is little evidence of systemic reaction, although affected animals often do not gain weight as they should. The lesions usually heal without scar formation. They have not been seen on the face, lips, or wooled portions of the body in the natural disease. By inoculation it is possible to produce lesions on the lips, but these do not progress far and they heal rapidly.

Figure 26.2. Horse showing dermatophilosis (streptothricosis.)

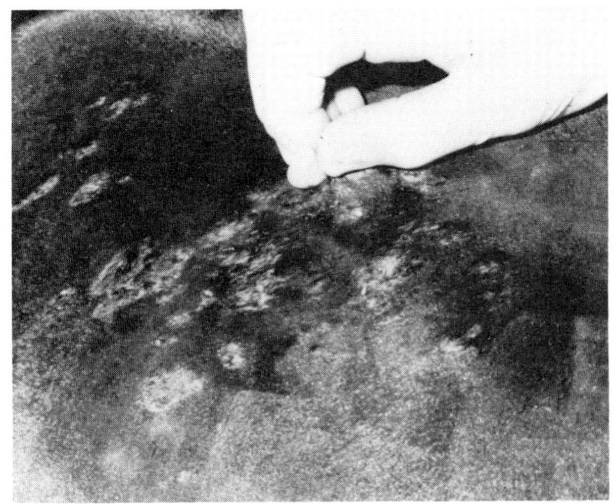

After being placed on infected pastures, the animals usually manifest the disease in 2 to 4 weeks. The longest period between exposure and appearance of symptoms has been 98 days for lambs and 117 days for adult sheep. By inoculation into the scarified skin, typical lesions are produced much earlier.

The mortality is very low but the morbidity is high. Most of the sheep on infected pastures contract the disease.

Dermatophilosis in horses is usually sporadic in occurrence. However, Pascoe (18) has described an unusual outbreak in Australia, where 68 of 278 horses involved had lesions on the coronets and pasterns. The disease was termed *aphis* or *greasy heel* and resembled the disease in England known as *mud fever*. *D. congolensis* was isolated from the lesions. Most horses recovered within 7 days.

Immunity. The immune response to *D. congolensis* involves both the formation of antibodies and the development of cell-mediated immunity, as evidenced by the delayed hypersensitivity reaction. In sheep, the antibody to somatic antigen is bactericidal following phagocytosis of zoospores by neutrophils. Flagella and natural agglutinating antibodies appear to have no significance in protection (27). Circulating acquired antibodies do not appear to influence or diminish lesions in experimentally infected rabbits treated with methotrexate (15). Thus, the antibody response does not appear to play a significant role in protection against *D. congolensis* (19).

The appearance of delayed hypersensitivity coincides with an accelerated infiltration of the lesion by neutrophils accompanied by decreased hyphal penetration of follicle sheaths and earlier healing (26). The mechanism underlying this phenomenon is not understood. In sheep, delayed hypersensitivity appears in 4 or 5 days, at just about the time that acute primary infections show signs of being overcome (28).

In sheep, vaccination increases the resistance of freshly scarified skin but does not appear to have any effect on natural infection. Vaccines have also been used in an attempt to protect cattle. In a field trial in the southern region of Chad, young cattle appeared to be protected following intradermal vaccination with young live culture (22).

Diagnosis. Smears prepared from moistened scab material and stained by methylene blue or Gram stains will usually reveal the typical branched filaments dividing both transversely and longitudinally. A fluorescent antibody technique has also been developed (20) and is particularly useful when the scabs have deteriorated as a result of secondary bacterial contamination. Polymixin B in the isolation medium has been found to reduce growth of contaminants (3).

Treatment and Control. *D. congolensis* is sensitive *in vitro* to tetracyclines, chloramphenicol, penicillin, and streptomycin (21). It is resistant to kanamycin, polymixin B sulfate, bacitracin, and sulfonamides (2). For cattle, intramuscular penicillin (5,000 units per kg) for five days or 75,000 units per kg in a single injection is sometimes effective (16). Penicillin and streptomycin have a synergic action against *D. congolensis* in sheep and have been shown to be effective in treatment of lumpy-wool cases (29). Other researchers (30, 13) have similarly shown that penicillin and streptomycin can produce marked improvement in cattle and sheep. However, Oduye (16) warns that in West Africa, at least, antibiotic therapy is effective only in a limited number of cases.

According to Kammerlocher and Mammo (11) fulvicin administered orally and 1 percent gentian violet in alcohol and 5 percent salicylic acid in alcohol applied topically all proved to be effective during a 30-day treatment period. For successful topical therapy, removal of scabs and exudate from all lesions prior to treatment is essential. Aluminum potassium sulfate (alum) has been used in a dip for sheep with beneficial results (10); copper naphthenate (37.5 percent concentration) has been recommended as a topical medication for horses (12). Intravenous sodium iodide and/or oral administration of potassium iodide have been found to be beneficial in cattle in Nigeria (16).

Chemical defleecing of sheep with cyclophosphamide (25 mg per kg) given in a drench has been found to be a valuable adjunct in therapy (14). Other means of control include dipping to reduce skin trauma from tick and insect activity.

Finally, it has been suggested (7) that selective breeding of cattle using bulls known to transmit a low susceptibility to dermatophilosis would be a valuable long-term control measure. Interestingly, natural genetic selection must already have occurred in parts of Africa since a number of local cattle breeds (Ndoma, Muturu, Baole) are resistant to dermatophilosis.

REFERENCES

1. Abdussalan and Blakemore. Jour. Comp. Path. and Therap., 1948, *58,* 333.
2. Abu-Samra, Imbali, and Mahgoub. Brit. Vet. Jour., 1976, *132,* 627.
3. Abu-Samra and Walton. Sabouraudia, 1977, *15,* 23.
4. Ainsworth and Austwick. Fungal diseases of animals. Commonwealth Agricultural Bureaux, Bucks., England, 1959. pp. 73–79.
5. Austwick. Vet. Rev. and Annot., 1958, *4,* 33.
6. Bida and Dennis. Res. Vet. Sci., 1977, *22,* 18.
7. Dumos, Lhoste, Chabeuf, and Blancou. Rev. Elev. Med. Vet. Pays Trop., 1971, *24,* 349.
8. Gordon. Jour. Bact., 1964, *88,* 509.
9. Harriss. Jour. Comp. Path. and Therap., 1948, *58,* 314.
10. Hart and Tyszkiewicz. Vet. Rec., 1968, *82,* 272.
11. Kammerlocher and Mammo. Vet. Med., 1965, *60,* 65.
12. Kaplan and Johnston. Jour. Am. Vet. Med. Assoc., 1966, *149,* 1162.
13. LeRoux. Jour. S. Afr. Vet. Med. Assoc., 1968, *39,* 87.
14. McIntosh, Smith, and Cunningham. Austral. Vet. Jour., 1971, *47,* 542.
15. Merkal, Richard, Thurston, and Ness. Am. Jour. Vet. Res., 1972, *33,* 401.
16. Oduye. World Animal Review, 1975, No. 16, 13.
17. Oduye and Lloyd. Brit. Vet. Jour., 1971, *127,* 505.
18. Pascoe. Austral. Vet. Jour., 1972, *48,* 32.
19. Perreau and Chambron. Rev. Elev. Med. Vet. Pays. Trop., 1966, *19,* 263.
20. Pier, Richard, and Farrell. Am. Jour. Vet. Res., 1964, *25,* 1014.

21. Plowright. Jour. Comp. Path. and Therap., 1958, *68*, 133.
22. Provost, Touade, Guillaume, Peleton, and Danisou. Bull. Epiz. Dis. of Africa, 1976, *22*, 223.
23. Roberts. Austral. Jour. Agric. Res., 1963, *14*, 386.
24. Roberts. Austral. Jour. Agric. Res., 1963, *14*, 492.
25. Roberts. Nature, 1965, *206*, 1068.
26. Roberts. Brit. Jour. Exp. Path., 1966, *47*, 9.
27. Roberts. Brit. Jour. Exp. Path. 1966, *47*, 372.
28. Roberts and Graham. Austral. Vet. Jour., 1966, *42*, 74.
29. Roberts. Jour. Comp. Path., 1967, *77*, 129.
30. Shotts, Jr., Tyler, and Christy. Jour. Am. Vet. Med. Assoc., 1969, *154*, 1450.
31. Van Saceghem. Soc. de Path. Exot. Bull., 1915, *8*, 354.

PART III

THE MYCOPLASMAS

27 The Genus *Mycoplasma*

The mycoplasmas are the simplest and tiniest self-replicating prokaryotes and are separated from the Eubacteria into a separate class, the Mollicutes. They have no cell wall and contain only the minimum in metabolic and physical structure for growth and multiplication.

The term *pleuropneumonialike organisms* (PPLO) was applied to mycoplasmas for many years because the first isolations were made by Nocard in 1898 from cases of contagious bovine pleuropneumonia (45). The term PPLO is no longer used, having been replaced by the title *Mycoplasma*.

In 1923, Bridré and Donatien (9) cultivated an organism closely related to the causative agent of pleuropneumonia from the joints of goats that suffered from a disease known as *contagious agalactia*. In 1934, Shoetensack (60) found an organism belonging to this group in dogs suffering from distemper. Dogs frequently carry *Mycoplasma* spp. in their respiratory and genital tracts, the organisms usually being more prevalent if some pathological condition is present. *Mycoplasma* spp. have also been found in cats. In 1952, Markham and Wong (39) proved that *Mycoplasma* spp. were of etiologic significance in chronic respiratory disease in chickens and infectious sinusitis of turkeys. Saprophytic and parasitic strains have been isolated from the bovine genital tract, from the lungs of calves with respiratory disease, from the udders of cows with mastitis, from the arthritic joints of calves and adult cattle, and from the eyes of cattle with conjunctivitis (27). *Mycoplasma* spp. have also been recovered from cases of atrophic rhinitis in swine, although they are of doubtful etiologic significance in this disease. *M. hyopneumoniae, M. hyorhinis*, and *M. hyosynoviae* are causes of enzootic pneumonia and of arthritis in swine. In mice, *M. neurolyticum* produces "rolling disease"—a disease of the nervous system. Thus a variety of important diseases are caused in animals. Table 27.1 is a list of these diseases.

GENERAL CHARACTERISTICS OF THE GENUS *MYCOPLASMA*

Morphology and Staining Reactions. The mycoplasmas are extremely pleomorphic and may appear as cocci, filaments, spirals, ring forms, globules, and granules. This plasticity in shape is a result of the lack of a cell wall. The basic cell shape is the coccus, and filament formation is a consequence of a fast growth rate in which genome replication precedes and outstrips cytoplasmic division (51). The filamentous form tends to be transitory and changes eventually into chains of cocci.

The ability of the living *Mycoplasma* cell to change shape is probably caused by the presence of contractile material such as actinlike proteins (26, 42). The gliding motility exhibited by some mycoplasmas, including *M. gallisepticum*, may have its basis in this contractile material (51). *M. gallisepticum* also has a polar bleb which is adhesive and serves as a fulcrum during movement.

The mycoplasmas are Gram-negative, but this stain is not satisfactory in routine work with these organisms. They are stained by Giemsa, Castaneda, Dienes, or

Table 27.1. The pathogenic *Mycoplasma* spp. and the diseases they cause in domestic animals

Species of Mycoplasma	Host	Disease
M. mycoides	Cattle	Contagious bovine pleuropneumonia
M. bovigenitalium	Cattle	Mastitis, vulvovaginitis
M. agalactiae var. *bovis*	Cattle	Mastitis
M. canadense	Cattle	Mastitis
M. bovirhinis	Cattle	Bronchopneumonia
M. agalactiae	Goat, sheep	Contagious agalactia, arthritis, conjunctivitis
M. capri	Goat	Contagious caprine pleuropneumonia
M. hyopneumoniae (*suipneumoniae*)	Pig	Enzootic pneumonia
M. hyorhinis	Pig	Arthritis, polyserositis
M. hyosynoviae	Pig	Arthritis
M. felis	Cat	Conjunctivitis
M. gallisepticum	Chicken, turkey, other birds	Chronic respiratory disease
M. synoviae	Chicken, turkey	Synovitis, air-sacculitis, myocarditis

methylene blue methods. The minute organisms (0.2–0.5 μm) stain pink or purple.

Cultural Features. Mycoplasmas require cholesterol in the medium if growth is to occur. The related genus, *Acholeplasma,* does not have this requirement. Cholesterol functions as a regulator of membrane fluidity during changes in growth, temperature, or in the fatty acid composition of membrane lipids (51). Serum or ascitic fluid (10 or 20 percent by volume) is added to fluid or agar media to supply cholesterol and other nutrients. Other ingredients of *Mycoplasma* media include yeast extract (10 percent), deoxyribonucleic acid, and penicillin and thallous acetate to control bacterial contaminants. The final pH is adjusted to between 7.0 and 8.0.

Fabricant and Barber (24) recommend the following media because of their wide range of applicability. In each case the broth form of the medium is listed first, the agar-plate form second. In evaluating them it is advisable to use each medium both by direct plating and by plating after 3 days of incubation at 37 C in the corresponding broth medium. All plates are examined after 6 days of incubation at 37 C in a candle jar with added moisture. The media are (*a*) BS and BA (23), Difco heart infusion broth or agar supplemented with 10 percent swine serum and bacterial inhibitors; (*b*) II and IIP (22), which are the same as BS and BA except that they are supplemented with 10 percent yeast extract (Chanock type); (*c*) C and CP (11), Difco PPLO broth or agar supplemented with 20 percent horse serum and 10 percent yeast extract (Chanock type); (*d*) RYE and RYEP (55), homemade rabbit infusion supplemented with 10 percent rabbit serum and 10 percent yeast extract (Chanock type); and (*e*) VFS and VFSP medium (13, 65), a peptic digest of beef and beef liver made with pig stomach as the source of pepsin; this medium is never autoclaved but sterilized by filtration.

Olson *et al.* (46) and Frey *et al.* (25) have developed specific media for the pathogenic avian mycoplasmas. These media were later modified by Adler *et al.* (1), who substituted nicotinamide for nicotine adenine dinucleotide.

Other substances that have been added to *Mycoplasma* media for the isolation and culture of specific strains include vaginal mucus (*M. bovigenitalium, M. agalactiae*), avian allantoic fluid (*M. capri*), and swine gastric mucin (*Acholeplasma granularum*).

During incubation, plates or tubes should be sealed to prevent drying. After 2 to 7 days' incubation at 37 C the characteristic colonies may be seen. These are from 10 to 600 μm in diameter and transparent, with a yellowish center (Figure 27.1). They may be seen with a hand lens under reflected light or, better, under the 16-mm objective of the microscope with oblique illumination. Some mycoplasmas will hemolyze erythrocytes in the medium.

In liquid medium growth appears as a faint clouding. Growth of most mycoplasmas in all types of media is aerobic. A few strains grow better in microaerophilic conditions (64).

Most pathogenic mycoplasmas from animals ferment glucose, maltose, and fructose. Nonfermenting strains produce ammonia from arginine.

Mycoplasmas may also be propagated in embryonated eggs or in cell-culture systems. Many strains grow more profusely in these systems than in cell-free media. Chick

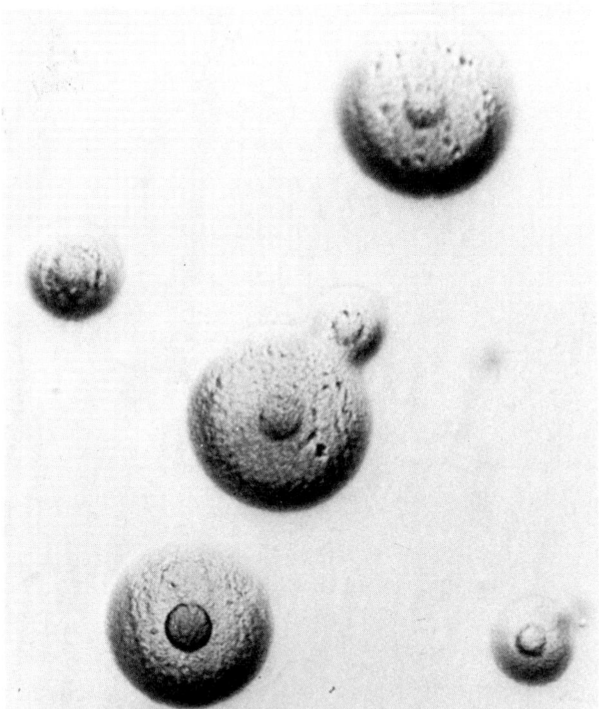

Figure 27.1. Colonies of *Mycoplasma gallisepticum*. × 200. (Courtesy M. S. Hofstad, *Cornell Vet.*)

embryo inoculation is particularly valuable for the growth of fastidious strains.

Identification. Identification of *Mycoplasma* isolates frequently is complicated because a large proportion of the cultures derived from mucous membranes will contain more than one species of *Mycoplasma*. It is impossible to characterize accurately, identify, or classify such cultures until they are purified. At the present time no completely dependable means exist for culture purification. The presently accepted procedure of cloning (colony picking) three times from terminal dilutions is no guarantee of culture purity. However, Yoder (70) has described a technique for obtaining pure cultures that is superior to those previously available.

The fluorescent-antibody (FA) technique has been used both for detecting the presence of mycoplasmas and also for identification (12). Complement-fixation (CF) and agar-gel diffusion tests have shown serologic relationships among human mycoplasmas (62), and Lemcke (38) used CF tests to distinguish 17 serotypes from 82 cultures derived from man, mammalian cell cultures, laboratory rats and mice, cattle, goats, poultry, embryonated eggs, and sewage. The serotypes of human and lower animal origin were largely host-specific. A useful tool in serotyping isolates is the metabolic-inhibition test (2, 50)

Other characteristics used in identification include special growth requirements, colonial and cell morphology, and biochemical reactions (63).

Resistance. Mycoplasmas are very susceptible to heat and drying, and are killed in a few minutes by a temperature of 60 C. They remain viable for long periods in frozen tissue.

MYCOPLASMA INFECTIONS OF CATTLE

Mycoplasma mycoides subsp. *mycoides*

SYNONYMS: *Asterococcus mycoides*, *Bovimyces pleuropneumoniae*, organism of contagious bovine pleuropneumonia.

This organism is the cause of a destructive disease of cattle which has been known to occur in Asia, Africa, and Australia for more than 200 years. From time to time in the past it has spread over the greater part of Europe. In the early part of the 19th century it became widespread in Europe, and from there it was disseminated to South Africa, Australia, and the United States in exported cattle. According to Moore (40) contagious bovine pleuropneumonia (CBPP) was imported into the United States in 1843, 1847, and 1859. It was restricted to some of the eastern states until 1883, when it appeared in Ohio. By 1886 it had reached a few herds in Illinois, Kentucky, and Missouri. Its spread led to the establishment in 1884 of the Bureau of Animal Industry of the U.S. Department of Agriculture. In 1887, Congress made funds available to the Bureau to deal with the disease. During the next 5 years it was hunted down, all affected animals were destroyed, and in September 1892 the Secretary of Agriculture proclaimed the country to be free of the disease. It has not occurred in the United States since March 1892, and in Britain since 1898. The disease is still present in Spain and Portugal, Africa, Australia, India, and possibly other regions of the Far East.

Epidemiology and Pathogenesis. *M. mycoides* is an obligate parasite of cattle and is usually transmitted by droplet inhalation. Close and prolonged contact is required for successful transmission. The organism has also been shown to survive in hay kept in the shade for at least 216 hours (67), and animals fed contaminated hay seroconverted. Although none died, some of these animals had lesions of CBPP at slaughter (69). Urinary shedding occurs and may contribute to the spread of infection. Transplacental infection has been observed also.

Animals that develop subclinical disease and those that recover are both very important in the epidemiology of CBPP because they constitute a clinically inapparent reservoir of infection which can thus spread insidiously. The natural disease spreads slowly and is difficult to eradicate. Walker (66), who worked on CBPP in Nairobi, found that 58 percent of the cattle in a large infected herd had not contracted the infection after a period of 7 months.

The disease may be quite acute, proving fatal within a week, or it may be chronic. It may become arrested by walling off infected lung foci, in which case the animal may appear to have recovered but the sequestration is likely to break down at any time, perhaps weeks or months later, with an extension of the disease, the reappearance of symptoms, and the discharge of virulent material. The movement of such animals into new herds and the reopening of the lesions thereby spreads the disease.

The pleural cavity of acutely infected animals contains a great deal of fluid—as much as 15 or 20 liters. The surface of the lung is injected and covered with a thin deposit of fibrin. The subpleural tissue is thickened and filled with fluid (Figure 27.2), and the same kind of fluid distends the interlobular septa. When the affected lobes are incised, these fluids run out, coagulating after a few moments' exposure to the air.

The pneumonia begins as nodules or foci, which spread until entire lobes are involved. These areas are hepatized and are bright red, brownish red, or grayish in color depending upon the stage of the process. The surface of the cut section presents a marbled effect, the varicolored lobules being separated from each other by wide bands of infiltrated interlobular tissue (Figure 27.3). Necrosis occurs in chronic cases, large portions of lung tissue often being necrotic and sequestered by connective tissue.

Bacteremia often occurs during the acute phase of CBPP and may result in placental localization with abortion or joint involvement with synovitis. There is a neutropenia and a lymphocytosis (56). The mortality varies from 10 to 90 percent. About 50 percent of exposed cattle develop clinical symptoms, and a smaller percentage become infected without clinical illness. Animals that recover are unthrifty and may continue to carry and shed the organism. They are immune to reinfection (68).

Diagnosis. *M. mycoides* may be isolated from tissues collected at necropsy on agar containing serum, ox heart and liver digest, penicillin, and thallous acetate. An FA procedure is also available to detect the organism in tissues. Field detection of infected animals depends heavily on serologic methods. These include the CF test, which is particularly sensitive for the diagnosis of infections in the acute, earlier stages. An agar-gel diffusion precipitation test is also useful in detecting acute infection. It has special application in the slaughterhouse, where it can be

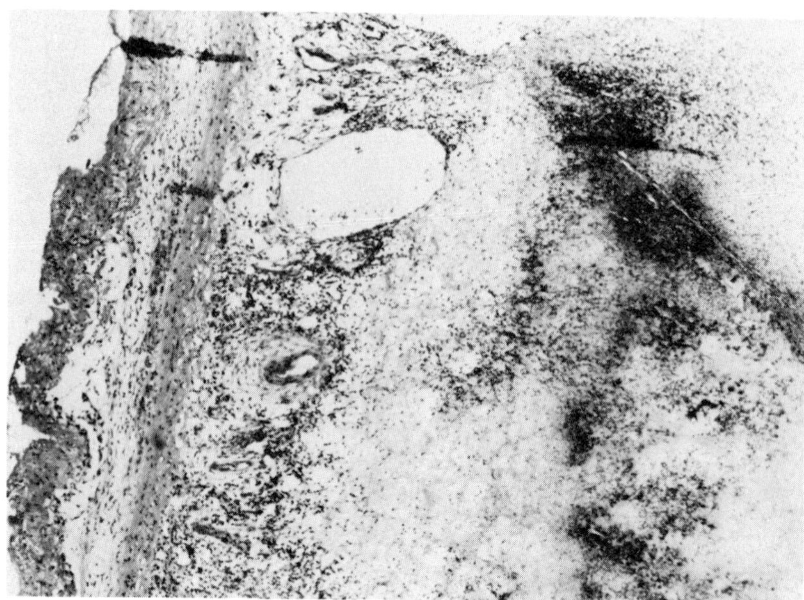

Figure 27.2. Photomicrograph of the greatly thickened pleura from a steer with contagious bovine pleuropneumonia. The thickening is due to severe edema and leukocyte infiltration. From the pleural lining inwards, there are fibrin and leukocytes, edematous connective-tissue infiltrated by leukocytes, dilated lymphatics, and then an area of necrotic edematous connective tissue and necrotic inflammatory cells. × 105. (Courtesy Charles A. Mebus, Plum Island Animal Disease Center, USDA.)

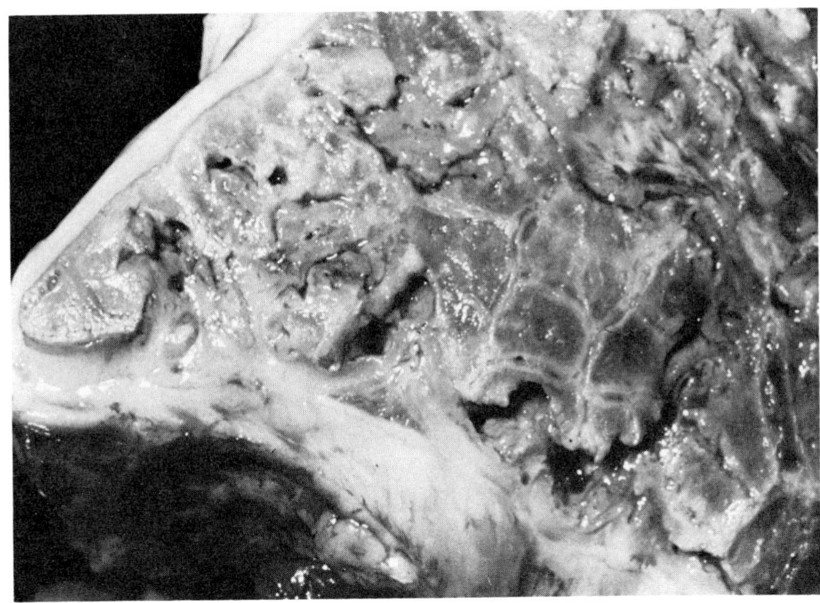

Figure 27.3. Cut surface of a lung from a steer affected with contagious bovine pleuropneumonia. The pleura is greatly thickened by connective tissue and the lung parenchyma is necrosed. The necrotic lobules are separated by zones of infiltrated interlobular tissue. (Courtesy D. A. Gregg, Plum Island Animal Disease Center, USDA.)

used to reveal antigen in suspect lesions. An allergic skin test is available and is most reliable in detecting chronic infection. The dominant immune response at this stage of the infection is cell-mediated (54). Also, circulating antigen combines with antibody in the serum at this time and so makes its detection more difficult. Gourlay (27) has reported that later in the acute stage the CF and agar-gel tests detected 100 percent of his CBPP cases, the slide-agglutination test 72, and the allergic test 68. In the late chronic stages none of the tests was entirely satisfactory, the allergic test detecting 74, the CF 72, the slide-agglutination 35, and the agar-gel 21 percent.

Newing and Field (43) developed a whole blood rapid-slide test for diagnosing CBPP which has since been modified to incorporate a stained antigen to be used on serum instead of blood. This test fails to detect about 25 percent of acute cases and more than half of cases in the chronic phase.

Immunity. Animals that have recovered from the disease cannot be infected again for a long period of time. Methods of artificial immunization have been used for many years in badly infected areas. The earlier method consisted in the subcutaneous injection, usually in the tail, of pleural fluid. This method gives protection from the lung disease, but reactions are often severe and some animals even die from the inoculation.

In 1952 and 1953, Sheriff and Piercy (57, 58) isolated and adapted their Tanganyika (TI) strain of CBPP to embryonated hens' eggs. After 9 transfers in eggs a lyophilized vaccine was made. It is a living product that retains its viability for years when stored at low temperatures. The vaccine has been tested rather widely and appears to be highly effective in immunizing cattle against CBPP (30, 47, 49). Priestley (48) recommends that 0.5 percent agar be incorporated when reconstituting the vaccine. This acts as an adjuvant and induces rapid and solid immunity.

The disease has been eradicated from many countries by detecting and slaughtering all infected herds, but this is practical only in areas where most herds are not already infected. Vaccination is practiced in Africa and Australia, where the disease is enzootic.

Chemotherapy. Sulfonamide drugs and antibiotics have little or no effect on this organism. In fact these drugs are frequently used to suppress the growth of extraneous bacteria when attempts are made to isolate *M. mycoides*.

Mycoplasma bovigenitalium

This *Mycoplasma* was first isolated in England in 1947 (20) from the genital tracts of heifers and from the seminal fluid of bulls. Since then *M. bovigenitalium* has been observed in bovine genital tracts throughout the world (28).

It is not usually found in virgin heifers (21). In cows it causes a granular vulvovaginitis (2), which can also be experimentally produced by inoculating the scarified vaginal mucosa with cultures. Edward and Fitzgerald (21) reported its isolation from cows with infertility problems but its exact role in infertility is as yet undefined.

In the udder, *M. bovigenitalium* may produce a mastitis characterized by firm, swollen but relatively painless quarters, reduced milk flow, and a thick yellow secretion. The leukocyte count is increased and the organism can be demonstrated in stained smears of the secretion (15, 61). Complement-fixing antibodies are produced locally and in the serum some weeks after infection. Counter (14) has described a severe outbreak of mastitis involving heifers and dry and nonlactating cows. *M. bovigenitalium* and *Acholeplasma laidlawii* were isolated from 15 of 53 animals. Many of the affected cows lost udder function permanently. Mastitis caused by *M. bovigenitalium* appears to be rare.

Bulls frequently shed the organism in their semen (21). The source of these organisms could be the seminal vesicle (3), since the organism has been frequently isolated from this site in bulls with chronic seminal vesiculitis (6). Furthermore, the organism is capable of producing seminal vesiculitis when experimentally inoculated into the seminal vesicles (7). The natural route of invasion and the extent to which infection in the bull contribute to infertility are unknown.

Mycoplasma agalactiae var. *bovis*

SYNONYMS: *Mycoplasma bovis, Mycoplasma bovimastitidis*

M. agalactiae var. *bovis* causes an acute, rapidly spreading mastitis in dairy herds and has been observed in the United States (10, 31), Europe (17, 53), Australia (13), and Japan (59).

Epidemiology and Pathogenesis. The origin of outbreaks is unknown, but poor husbandry appears to be important in their spread because milking cows are often infected in all 4 quarters whereas dry cows are infected in only 1 or 2. Experimentally, infection can be transmitted through the teat canal (31). The organism is shed in the milk and also in the urine and feces of experimentally infected cows (34).

Systemic signs are usually absent, although some infected cows may develop a transient fever. A leukopenia may appear, however, and the mastitis is characterized by a sharp drop in milk production and extremely swollen udders that are not painful. The supramammary lymph nodes may be enlarged and firm. The secretion varies in appearance. It may be slightly yellow and, on standing, deposit a fine sediment on the bottom of the container. In some cases the milk is definitely watery, with flakes and a few clots, and in others contains large yellow-white caseous chunks or pus. Cell counts in milk can be as high as 100 million per ml (10), and the neutrophil is the dominant cell. The California milk test (CMT) is usually 3+ a few days after infection. Casein nitrogen is greatly increased (52), which is not the case in most other forms of mastitis.

M. agalactiae var. *bovis* can be seen in Giemsa- or methylene blue–stained smears of milk and appears as ring or pleomorphic coccobacillary forms, tiny branched or beaded filaments, or amorphous clumps (36).

Affected quarters may contain nodules, abscesses, and purulent material in pockets and in plugs in the collecting ductules. The organism is present as discrete microcolonies in the affected gland (37). Bennett and Jasper (5) suggest that the interaction of the immune defense in the gland with these organisms is responsible for the tissue damage. Lymphocytes and other mononuclear cells infiltrate a week after infection and the secretory parenchyma is replaced by granulation tissue, which in turn becomes fibrosed (37). Milk production, therefore, is permanently lost.

The organism may be shed for about 2 months from affected quarters.

M. agalactiae var. *bovis* has also caused severe arthritis and tendovaginitis in calves and cows (35) and in feedlot cattle (32). In some outbreaks there is an association with respiratory disease in calves (41). It has also been isolated from the genital tract of normal cows (35).

Immunity. The following serologic methods are used to measure antibody response to *M. agalactiae* var. *bovis:* complement fixation, growth and film inhibition, indirect hemagglutination, agar-gel diffusion, and single radial hemolysis. These tests are reviewed by Boughton (8).

Chemotherapy. *M. agalactiae* var. *bovis* is sensitive to tetracycline, tylosin, novobiocin, kanamycin, and nitrofurazone. However, field experience has indicated that treatment of affected quarters is usually ineffective.

Mycoplasma canadense

This rarely found *Mycoplasma* has been isolated from cases of bovine mastitis in California (19) and England (29). In the English outbreak, Gourlay *et al.* (29) reported that the organism caused a nonacute mastitis in a closed herd of 250 cows. The infection continued to spread despite apparent successful treatment with oxytetracycline, and some treated cases relapsed.

Mycoplasma bovirhinis

M. bovirhinis is a common parasite of the bovine respiratory tract. It has been reported from the United

States, Europe, and Australia (28), and although most isolations have been made from animals with respiratory disease (16, 44), the organism is also frequently found on the respiratory mucosae of normal animals. *M. bovirhinis* is not a primary pathogen (18) and its as yet ill-defined role in respiratory disease is believed to be secondary to other agents. Calves can be successfully immunized against colonization by the organism (33). The antigen must first be inoculated intramuscularly and then intratracheally to induce a local immunity.

REFERENCES

1. Adler, Damassa, and Field. Avian Dis., 1974, *18,* 568.
2. Afshar, Stuart, and Huck. Vet. Rec., 1966, *78,* 512.
3. Afshar. Vet. Bull., 1975, *45,* 211.
4. Barber and Fabricant. Jour. Bact., 1962, *83,* 1268.
5. Bennett and Jasper. Am. Jour. Vet. Res., 1978, *39,* 417.
6. Blom and Erno. Acta Vet. Scand., 1967, *8,* 186.
7. Blom, Erno, and Birch-Anderson. Acta. Path. et Microbiol. Scand., 1973, *81B*, 176.
8. Boughton. Vet. Bull., 1979, *49,* 377.
9. Bridré and Donatien. Comp. rend. Acad. Sci., 1923, *177,* 841.
10. Carmichael, Guthrie, Fincher, Field, Johnson, and Lindquist. Proc. Ann. Meeting U.S. Livestock Sanit. Assoc., 1963, *67,* 220.
11. Chanock, Hayflick, and Barile. Proc. Natl. Acad. Sci., 1962, *48,* 41.
12. Clark, Bailey, Fowler, and Brown. Jour. Bact., 1963, *85,* 111.
13. Cottew. Austral. Vet. Jour., 1970, *46,* 378.
14. Counter. Vet. Rec., 1978, *103,* 130.
15. Davidson and Stuart. Vet. Rec., 1960, *72,* 766.
16. Davies. Jour. Comp. Path., 1967, *77,* 353.
17. Davies and Boughton. Vet. Rec., 1976, *99,* 322.
18. Dawson, Stuart, Darbishire, Parker, and McCrae. Vet. Rec., 1966, *78,* 543.
19. Dellinger, Jasper, and Ilic. Cornell Vet., 1977, *67,* 351.
20. Edward, Hancock, and Hignett. Vet. Red., 1947, *59,* 329.
21. Edward and Fitzgerald. Vet. Rec., 1952, *64,* 395.
22. Fabricant and Freundt. Ann. N.Y. Acad. Sci., 1967, *143,* 50.
23. Fabricant. *In* The *Mycoplasmatales* and the L-phase of bacteria, ed. L. Hayflick. Appleton-Century-Crofts, New York, 1969, pp. 621–41.
24. Fabricant and Barber. Proc. Ann. Meeting U.S. Animal Health Assoc., 1969, *73,* 573–81.
25. Frey, Hanson, and Anderson. Am. Jour. Vet. Res., 1968, *29,* 2163.
26. Ghosh, Maniloff, and Gerling. Cell, 1978, *13,* 57.
27. Gourlay. Jour. Comp. Path., 1965, *75,* 97.
28. Gourlay. Jour. Am. Vet. Med. Assoc., 1973, *163,* 905.
29. Gourlay, Wyld, Burke, and Edmonds. Vet. Rec., 1978, *103,* 74.
30. Gray and Turner. Jour. Comp. Path. and Therap., 1954, *64,* 116.
31. Hale, Helmboldt, Plastridge, and Stula. Cornell Vet., 1962, *52,* 582.
32. Hjerpe and Knight. Jour. Am. Vet. Med. Assoc., 1972, *160,* 1414.
33. Howard, Gourlay, and Taylor. Vet. Microbiol., 1977, *2,* 29.
34. Jain, Jasper, and Dellinger. Cornell Vet., 1969, *59,* 10.
35. Jasper. Jour. Am. Vet. Med. Assoc., 1967, *151,* 1650.
36. Jasper, Jain, and Brazil. Jour. Am. Vet. Med. Assoc., 1966, *148,* 1017.
37. Kehoe, Norcross, Carmichael, and Strandberg. Jour. Inf. Dis., 1967, *117,* 171.
38. Lemcke. Jour. Hyg. (London), 1964, *62,* 199.
39. Markham and Wong. Poultry Sci., 1952, *31,* 902.
40. Moore. Pathology and differential diagnosis of the infectious diseases of animals, 4th, ed. Macmillan, New York, 1916, p. 412.
41. Moulton, Boidin, and Rhode. Jour. Am. Vet. Med. Assoc., 1956, *129,* 364.
42. Neimark. Proc. Natl. Acad. Sci., 1977, *74,* 4041.
43. Newing and Field. Brit. Vet. Jour., 1963, *109,* 397.
44. Nicolet and De Meuron. Zentrbl. Vet.-Med., 1970, *17B,* 1031.
45. Nocard, Roux, Borrel, Salimberi, and Dujerdin-Beaumetz. Ann. Inst. Pasteur, 1898, *12,* 240.
46. Olson, Kerr, and Campbell. Avian Dis., 1963, *7,* 310.
47. Priestley. Jour. Comp. Path. and Therap., 1955, *65,* 168.
48. Priestley. Vet. Rec., 1955, *67,* 729.
49. Priestley and White. Vet. Rec., 1952, *64,* 259.
50. Purcell and Chanock. Med. Clin. North Am., 1967, *51,* 791.
51. Razin. Microbiol. Rev., 1978, *42,* 414.
52. Resmini and Ruffo. Latte, 1969, *43,* 720.
53. Rinaldi, Carbio, Guallini, and Redaelli. Atti. Soc. ital. Sci. vet., 1969, *22,* 796.
54. Roberts,Windsor, Masiga, and Kariavu. Inf. and Immun., 1073, *8,* 349.
55. Sabry. M.S. thesis, Cornell Univ., 1968.
56. Sharma, Vyas, Vyas, Chowhan and Jatkar. Indian Jour. An. Sci., 1978, *48,* 108.
57. Sheriff and Piercy. Vet. Rec., 1952, *64,* 615.
58. Sheriff and Piercy. Proc. 15th Internat. Vet. Cong., Stockholm, 1953, *1,* 333.
59. Shimizu and Nogatomo. Jap. Jour. Vet. Sci., 1977, *39,* 581.
60. Shoetensack. Kitasato Arch. Exp. Med., 1934, *11,* 277.
61. Stuart, Davidson, Slavin, Edgson, and Howell, Vet. Rec., 1960, *75,* 59.
62. Taylor-Robinson, Somerson, Turner, and Chanock. Jour. Bact., 1963, *85,* 1261.
63. Timms. Vet. Bull., 1978, *48,* 187.
64. Turner. Jour. Path. and Bact., 1935, *41,* 1.
65. Turner, Campbell, and Dick. Austral. Vet. Jour., 1935, *11,* 63.
66. Walker. A system of bacteriology. Med. Res. Council (Brit.) 1930, *7,* 322.
67. Windsor and Masiga. Bull. Animal Health Produc. in Africa, 1977, *25,* 357.
68. Windsor and Masiga. Res. Vet. Sci., 1977, *23,* 224.

69. Windsor and Masiga. Res. Vet. Sci., 1977, *23,* 230.
70. Yoder. Am. Jour. Vet. Res., 1975, *36,* 560.

MYCOPLASMA INFECTIONS OF GOATS AND SHEEP

Mycoplasma mycoides var. *capri*

SYNONYMS: *Capromyces pleuropneumoniae, Asterococcus mycoides* var. *capri*

This organism causes contagious pleuropneumonia in goats, a disease similar to CBPP in cattle. It occurs in the Mediterranean region, Africa, Asia, Mexico, China, and the USSR. It was described in the Sudan as early as 1902 (25). In the Near East and in the savannah zones of Africa it is a common disease in goats. An organism similar to *M. mycoides* var. *capri* was isolated from a goat in Connecticut in 1969 (22).

The epidemiology, pathogenesis, and pathology of the disease in the goat are similar to those of CBPP. The infection is transmitted by the respiratory route via inhalation of droplets. The organism may easily be demonstrated in the tissues and fluids of acute cases but is difficult to find in chronic lesions. Diagnosis by serologic means (the CF test) is not satisfactory because many chronically infected animals do not have detectable antibodies. However, recent work (26) indicates that serology may be more reliable in acute infections with strain F38 in Kenya.

Mycoplasma agalactiae

SYNONYMS: *Borrelomyces agalactiae, Anulomyces agalaxiae, Capromyces agalactiae,* organism of contagious agalactia of sheep and goats

The disease caused by this organism is known to occur in parts of southern Europe, northern Africa, Asia, and the USSR. It differs serologically, culturally, and biochemically from *M. mycoides* var. *capri* or var. *mycoides* (11).

The causative organism was first isolated and studied by Bridré, Donatien, and Hilbert (6) in 1923. It is spread by ingestion and by entry into the teat meatus. It can be found in the blood in the early stages of the disease.

The name suggests that the disease is localized in the udder and is misleading in this respect. Actually it is a generalized disease that affects males and females alike. The principal lesions are located in the joints, the eyes, and in the mammary glands of females. The disease may be acute but usually is chronic. The involved joints may become ankylosed but usually do not. The mastitis is manifested by the usual symptoms, and milk secretion diminishes and even ceases. Pregnant females often abort. Chronically affected animals become weak and emaciated. The mortality rate is low. Subclinical cases may continue to shed the organism for several months.

Most attempts to immunize goats have proved rather disappointing, but Foggie *et al.* (12) claim that they were able to protect this animal against challenge inoculation by vaccinating with a live culture, attenuated by 40 passes on selective agar. Hyperimmune serum gives only transient protection. Mycoplasmas have also been implicated in the etiology of edema disease in goats in the Near East.

MYCOPLASMA INFECTIONS OF SWINE

Mycoplasma hyopneumoniae

SYNONYM: *Mycoplasma suipneumoniae*

This organism causes enzootic pneumonia of pigs (EPP) (18), a disease that has also been called *virus pneumonia of swine, infectious pneumonia of pigs,* and *ferkelgrippe*. EPP occurs wherever swine are raised and causes heavy economic loss because affected animals gain weight more slowly and exhibit inefficient food conversion. Switzer (39) has estimated that between 35 and 60 percent of swine slaughtered in the midwestern United States have lesions of EPP.

Epidemiology and Pathogenesis. *M. hyopneumoniae* is host-specific and survives only briefly in the external environment (5). At one time it was believed that herds that were free of infection based on clinical and pathologic criteria would remain free of the disease if they remained closed to all except swine derived from EPP-free herds or animals raised in isolation following caesarian section (47). Experience in England, however, has, indicated that EPP-free herds do experience breakdowns (16) where the origin of infection is unexplained.

The organism is spread in aerosols generated by infected pigs and can be transmitted in this way from sows to their pigs. It is also introduced into herds by the purchase of infected stock. Pigs usually show signs of infection by *M. hyopneumoniae* at 3 to 10 weeks of age. After an incubation period of 8 to 14 days, infected pigs may suffer from a transient diarrhea and then develop a dry cough that may last for a few weeks or persist indefinitely. Affected pigs eat well but are unthrifty and gain weight at a reduced rate. The worst affected may suffer severe stunting. Many infected animals may be clinically normal but have pronounced lung lesions at slaughter.

The lesions of EPP are hepatized, purplish, or grayish pneumonic areas in the apical and cardiac lobes of the lung. Secondary bacterial invasions of pneumonic areas may occur. Histologically, the lung lesions are characterized by mononuclear cell accumulation and peribronchiolar lymphoreticular hyperplasia.

Infected animals may continue to shed the organism. Development of a cell-mediated response is greatly delayed in infected pigs and does not appear until 15 to 20 weeks after inoculation (1). This immunosuppression may explain the chronicity of the disease. Complement-fixing, precipitating, and growth-inhibitory antibodies are produced some weeks after infection, but tests based on the presence of these antibodies are not reliable for the detection of infected individuals. Complement-fixing antibodies are probably not involved in resistance to infection (39). Recovered swine are resistant to reinfection (17), indicating that protective immunity does develop in EPP.

Diagnosis. The indirect hemagglutination (17) and CF tests are useful in the detection of infected herds (37). Switzer (39) has observed that the CF test is positive in twice as many swine as have lesions of EPP at slaughter.

The organism may be demonstrated easily in Giemsa-stained touch preparations of lung lesions (19), where it appears as ring and bipolar forms.

A highly efficient medium for the isolation of the organism from lung tissue has been developed by Goodwin (15). It contains 30 percent serum that includes one-third by volume rabbit antiserum to *M. hyorhinis*. The latter is a common contaminant or secondary invader of lesions, which, if allowed to grow, multiplies to the exclusion of *M. hyopneumoniae*. In liquid culture the organism appears as cocci on fine branching filaments or as globular structures (microcolonies). It is apparently nonmotile (19). The colonies on solid media are about 400 μm in diameter after incubation for 7 to 10 days. They are convex and do not have a nipple.

Besides the laboratory methods described above, herd diagnosis of EPP also relies heavily on the gross and microscopic pathologic appearance of the lesions at slaughter and the clinical and epidemiologic features of the disease in the herd.

Chemotherapy. *M. hyopneumoniae* is sensitive to tetracycline, lincomycin, tylosin, and tiamulin (38). However, antibodies have little effect once the disease process has begun. Switzer (39) has noted that tetracycline will inhibit lesion development if administered at the time the pigs are infected but does not affect lesions if given later.

Mycoplasma hyorhinis

M. hyorhinis is a common inhabitant of the nasal cavities of normal pigs but also sporadically causes acute polyserositis in pigs less than 6 weeks old. It has been frequently isolated from the turbinates of pigs with atrophic rhinitis, where it is apparently a secondary invader in the wake of infection by *Bordetella bronchiseptica*. It is also commonly found in the nasal cavities and in lung lesions of EPP in association with *M. hyopneumoniae*, the isolation of which it complicates (15). Gois *et al.* (14) found that 70 percent of nasal swabs from pigs from herds affected with EPP were positive for *M. hyorhinis*. The isolation rate declined with increasing age.

Infections by *M. hyorhinis* develop during the first few weeks of life. Initial invasion of the respiratory tract is usually subclinical. If these pigs are stressed, bloodstream invasion may occur, with subsequent localization of the organism on serous surfaces including the synovial membranes.

The polyserositis caused by *M. hyorhinis* is comprised of a serofibrinous synovitis and arthritis, pericarditis, pleuritis, and peritonitis. Roberts *et al.* (31) have described the pathology of the arthritis. The synovial membrane shows mild hyperemia and hypertrophy of the synovial villi associated with a yellowish coloration of the synovial membrane. Histopathologically, these changes are characterized by hypertrophy of the synovial villi, hyperplasia of synovial cells, and lymphocytic infiltration concentrated in nodular foci. The synovial fluid is increased in volume and contains flecks of fibrin. Affected pigs are stiff and reluctant to stand or move. Recovery is slow but often is complete without permanent damage to the joint. Complement-fixing antibodies develop within 2 weeks of infection and persist for at least 6 months (33).

Chemotherapy. *M. hyorhinis* is sensitive to tylosin and lincomycin. Treatment is effective in the early stages of infection.

Mycoplasma hyosynoviae

This *Mycoplasma* causes a polyarthritis in young swine over 10 weeks of age. Methods for its isolation and identification have been described by Ross and Karman (34) and by Gois and Taylor-Robinson (13). It requires sterols, does not ferment glucose or hydrolyze urea, and utilizes arginine.

Epidemiology and Pathogenesis. The principal reservoir of *M. hyosynoviae* is the adult carrier animal. The organism persists in the tonsil and is shed in the nasal and pharyngeal secretions (35). Stress is an important predisposing cause of outbreaks and there is a breed susceptibility: Hampshire swine develop a more severe disease following infection than do other breeds (36).

As a result of stress (regrouping, change of feed, housing, transportation) the infection in the tonsil becomes bacteremic and enters the joints, where it causes synovitis, synovial effusion, and villous hypertrophy. There is minimal damage to cartilage. Affected swine become stiff, lame, and have difficulty in rising. The organism is rapidly cleared from affected joints, and complete recovery occurs after a few weeks in most cases.

Diagnosis. The organism can be demonstrated only during the acute phase of the arthritis (32). Complement-fixing antibodies develop about 10 days after infection. These antibodies are present also in pharyngeal carriers (35).

Chemotherapy. *M. hyosynoviae* is sensitive to tylosin and the tetracyclines. These drugs may be effective in preventing or treating outbreaks.

MYCOPLASMA INFECTIONS OF POULTRY

Mycoplasma gallisepticum

In 1943, Delaplane and Stuart (10) described chronic respiratory disease (CRD) of chickens and isolated an agent that could be propagated in embryonated chicken eggs. Six years later Hitchner (21) also used this technique to propagate an agent that was present in infectious sinusitis of turkeys (IST). It was soon discovered that these agents are constantly found both in sinusitis of turkeys and CRD of chickens. In 1952, Markham and Wong (27) referred to them as PPLO and ascribed to them an etiologic role in both diseases.

The organism involved was later named *Mycoplasma gallisepticum*. CRD is found wherever poultry are raised intensively and has been described in pheasants, pigeons, and partridges as well as in chickens and turkeys. In turkeys the disease is commonly called *infectious sinusitis of turkeys* (IST).

Epidemiology and Pathogenesis. *M. gallisepticum* is commonly spread by infectious aerosol, by contact, and by egg transmission (7) following infection of the egg during formation in the ovary. It has also been spread in contaminated virus vaccines. Concurrent infections by bacteria such as *Hemophilus gallinarum* and *Escherichia coli* or viruses such as infectious bronchitis virus predispose to development of CRD and to increases in its severity. The organism is ovoid in shape with a polar bleb which serves as an adhesion organ to respiratory epithelium (9). Adhesion to cells involves neuraminic acid moieties.

CRD in chickens is typically a disease with a long incubation period (1 to 3 weeks) and a long course. It is accompanied by tracheal râles, nasal discharge, and coughing. Feed consumption is reduced, egg production may be lowered, and the birds lose weight. In chicks the disease often takes the form of a simple coryza. Gross lesions are associated with the presence of mucoid to mucopurulent exudate in the trachea, bronchi, air sacs, and nasal passages. Instances of synovitis involving the synovial membranes of the joints, tendovaginal sheaths, and bursae have been noted. Microscopically, the mucous membranes are thickened, hyperplastic, and infiltrated with mononuclear cells.

In turkeys IST is characterized by swelling of the infraorbital sinuses. These are filled with a thick mucoid exudate. In some cases conjunctivitis and inflammation of the air sacs are observed. The disease runs a chronic course and affected birds lose weight. The death rate usually is not high, but failure to gain weight may cause considerable economic loss. The lesions are progressive and much more extensive than those of CRD, with severe involvement of the nasal passages, sinuses, lungs, and air sacs. Synovial and joint lesions have also been seen.

Diagnosis. The history, lesions observed, and cultural and serologic procedure are used in combination for diagnosis. The rapid serum plate (RSA) and tube agglutination tests, the hemagglutination-inhibition (HI) test, the complement-fixation test, electrophoresis of cell proteins, and immunofluorescence have been used for serologic diagnosis and identification of isolates. The RSA and HI tests in particular have been widely and successfully used for detection of infection in eradication programs.

The organism may be cultured in media such as the "C" medium of Olson *et al.* (29) or in later modifications of this medium (3).

Treatment and Control. *M. gallisepticum* is susceptible to many antibiotics *in vitro*. Of these, tiamulin and tylosin have been reported to be most effective in preventing and eradicating CRD and IST (4). Antibiotic treatment of hatching eggs has proved an efficacious and practical method of producing *Mycoplasma*-free chicks. Through the studies of Chalquest and Fabricant (8) and Levine and Fabricant (24) an egg-dipping procedure has been developed that consists essentially of immersing prewarmed eggs in chilled antibiotic solutions. Under field conditions tylosin has been the most effective antibiotic used in this process. Treatment of chickens and turkeys, although often clinically effective, is of limited value because *Mycoplasma* are not completely eliminated from the birds.

Yoder (45) recommends preincubation heat treatment of hatching chicken eggs to inactivate mycoplasmas. He suggests maintaining an internal egg temperature of 46 C for 12 to 14 hours to inactivate both *M. gallisepticum* and *M. synoviae*.

Medication of breeder flocks reduces or eliminates egg infection but gives best results when applied early in the course of the disease.

Mycoplasma synoviae

M. synoviae is a cause of infectious synovitis and airsacculitis in chickens and turkeys. The broiler breeds are more susceptible to synovitis than the laying breeds. The disease causes losses through condemnations at meat inspection and poor weight gains. Infection by *M. synoviae* has become increasingly more important as the eradication of *M. gallisepticum* has progressed (42).

The morphologic and cultural features of *M. synoviae* are similar to those of *M. gallisepticum* and have been described by Olson (28). It ferments glucose and maltose and has a specific requirement for coenzyme I (DPN) and for nicotine adenine dinucleotide (NAD). There appears to be a single serotype (30) that contains 3 subtypes (44).

Epidemiology and Pathogenesis. *M. synoviae* is an obligate parasite of the chicken and turkey and is distributed widely wherever poultry are intensively raised (42). The most frequent source of infection is infected eggs, natural infection in this case being transmitted vertically. The organism is therefore a potential contaminant of vaccines propagated in eggs, and lateral spread can occur by this means. The organism is also shed from the respiratory tract of infected birds and can spread by contact or infectious aerosol to other birds kept nearby (20). Airsacculitis is most extensive at low ambient temperature regardless of humidity conditions. At moderate ambient temperature the incidence is greater when humidity is low than when it is high (46).

Invasion by the respiratory route usually results in air sac inflammation whereas intravenous inoculation of the organism commonly results in synovitis. Interestingly, lymphocytes have been shown to be necessary for the development of macroscopic lesions of synovitis (23).

Mixed infections of *M. synoviae* and viruses such as infectious bronchitis virus result in more severe respiratory lesions. Thus vaccination with infectious bronchitis or Newcastle Disease virus when *M. synoviae* infection is spreading greatly increases the frequency and severity of air sac inflammation.

Clinical manifestations of infectious synovitis include swollen joints and tendon sheaths which contain a creamy white viscid purulent exudate. The hocks, the feet, and the bursa on the breast are most commonly affected. Signs of airsacculitis include slight rales. The linings of the air sacs are thickened with a whitish yellow exudate. There may also be endocarditis, valvular lesions, and anemia. The latter is probably due to the hemolytic effect of hydrogen peroxide, produced by *M. synoviae* that have adhered to the erythrocytes. Timms (42) has written an excellent review of the pathogenesis and pathology of infection by *M. synoviae*.

Immunity. B lymphocytes are correlated with the development of resistance to lesions whereas T lymphocytes are necessary for the development of macroscopic synovitis (23). A cell-mediated response develops during the second week of infection (43), and its effect in lesion development may be cytotoxic. Rheumatoid factor is produced during the course of the disease and is a response to complexing of the host's immunoglobulin to *Mycoplasma* antigen.

Diagnosis. Infection is usually detected by the RSA and the HI tests (42). The organism can be isolated on media containing NAD and differentiated from *M. gallisepticum* by serologic methods using specific antisera (42).

Chemotherapy and Control. The organism is sensitive *in vitro* to tylosin, tetracyclines, lincomycin, tiamulin, and nitrofuran (furaltadone). Administration of antibiotics in feed or water is effective in reducing egg infection in breeder flocks and in controlling synovitis and air sac inflammation in broilers when started early in the course of the disease (2).

Serologic detection and elimination of infected birds from breeding flocks and heating infected eggs to 46 C before incubation (45) or dipping infected eggs in antibiotic are also important in preventing vertical transmission of infection.

MYCOPLASMA INFECTIONS OF CATS

Mycoplasma felis

This organism has been shown to cause conjunctivitis in kittens, with possible involvement of the lower respiratory tract under favorable conditions (40, 41).

REFERENCES

1. Adegboye. Res. Vet. Sci., 1978, *25,* 323.
2. Adler. Proc. 19th West. Poult. Dis. Conf. Calif., 1970, pp. 3–4.
3. Adler, Damassa, and Field. Avian Dis., 1974, *18,* 568.
4. Baugha, Alpaugh, Linkenheimer, and Maplesden. Avian Dis., 1978, *22,* 620.
5. Betts, Whittlestone, and Beveridge. Vet. Rec., 1955, *67,* 685.
6. Bridré, Donatien, and Hilbert. Comp. rend. Acad. Sci., 1923, *177,* 841.
7. Carnaghan. Jour. Comp. Path. and Therap., 1961, *71,* 279.
8. Chalquest and Fabricant. Avian Dis., 1959, *3,* 257.
9. Clyde. *In* Microbiology, ed. David Schlessinger. Am. Soc. of Microbiology, Washington, D.C., 1975, pp. 143–46.
10. Delaplane and Stuart. Am. Jour. Vet. Res., 1943, *4,* 325.
11. Edwards. Vet. Rec., 1953, *65,* 873.
12. Foggie, Etheridge, Endog, and Arisoy. Jour. Comp. Path., 1970, *80,* 345.
13. Gois and Taylor-Robinson. Jour. Med. Microbiol., 1972, *5,* 47.
14. Gois, Carny, and Veznikova. Documenta Vet., 1975, *8,* 205.
15. Goodwin. Vet. Rec., 1976, *98,* 260.
16. Goodwin. Vet. Rec., 1977, *101,* 419.
17. Goodwin, Hodgson, Whittlestone, and Woodhams. Jour. Hyg. (London), 1969, *67,* 193.
18. Goodwin, Pomeroy, and Whittlestone. Vet. Rec., 1965, *77,* 1247.
19. Goodwin, Pomeroy, and Whittlestone. Jour. Hyg. (London), 1967, *65,* 85.
20. Hemsley. Brit. Vet. Jour., 1965, *121,* 76.
21. Hitchner. Poultry Sci., 1949, *28,* 106.
22. Jones and Barber. Jour. Inf. Dis., 1969, *119,* 126.
23. Kune, Kawkuho, Morita, Hayatsu, and Yoshioka. Am. Jour. Vet. Res., 1977, *38,* 1595.
24. Levine and Fabricant. Avian Dis., 1962, *6,* 72.
25. Lindley. Jour. Am. Vet. Med. Assoc., 1967, *151,* 1810.
26. MacOwan and Minette. Vet. Rec., 1977, *101,* 380.
27. Markham and Wong. Poultry Sci., 1952, *31,* 90.
28. Olson. "*Mycoplasma synoviae* infection." *In* Diseases of poultry, ed. M. S. Hofstad, B. W. Calnek, C. F. Helmholdt, W. M. Reid, and H. W. Yoder. Iowa State Univ. Press, Ames, 1973, pp. 320–31.
29. Olson, Kerr, and Campbell. Avian Dis., 1963, *7,* 310.
30. Olson, Kerr, and Campbell. Avian Dis., 1964, *8,* 209.
31. Roberts, Switzer, and Ramsey. Am. Jour. Vet. Res., 1963, *24,* 19.
32. Ross. Ann. N.Y. Acad. Sci., 1973, *225,* 359.
33. Ross, Dale, and Duncan. Am. Jour. Vet. Res., 1973, *34,* 367.
34. Ross and Karman. Jour. Bact., 1970, *103,* 707.
35. Ross and Spear. Am. Jour. Vet. Res., 1973, *34,* 373.
36. Ross, Switzer, and Duncan. Am. Jour. Vet. Res., 1971, *32,* 1743.
37. Schuller, Swoboda, and Baumgartner. Wiener tierärztl. Monatsch., 1977, *64,* 236.
38. Stipkovitz, Laher, Schutze. Deutsche tierärztl. Wchnschr., 1978, *85,* 464.
39. Switzer. Jour. Inf. Dis., 1973, *127,* S 59.
40. Tan. Jap. Jour. Exp. Med., 1974, *44,* 235.
41. Tan and Miles. Res. Vet. Sci., 1974, *16,* 27.
42. Timms. Vet. Bull., 1978, *48,* 187.
43. Timms and Cullen. Brit. Vet. Jour., 1974, *130,* 75.
44. Weinack and Snoeyenbos. Avian Dis., 1976, *20,* 253.
45. Yoder. Avian Dis., 1970, *14,* 75.
46. Yoder, Drury, and Hopkins. Avian Dis., 1977, *21,* 195.
47. Young and Underdahl. Jour. Soc. Farm Mgrs. and Rural Appraisers, 1956, *20,* 63.

PART IV

THE RICKETTSIAE

28 The Rickettsiaceae

In the eighth edition of *Bergey's Manual* a group of small rod-shaped, coccoid, and often pleomorphic microorganisms that occur intracellularly as elementary bodies, but may occasionally be extracellular, are placed in the order Rickettsiales. The rickettsiae are true bacteria possessing a typical structure and most of the enzymes. They are usually nonfilterable and Gram-negative, and can be cultivated outside the host only in living tissues, embryonated chicken eggs, or rarely in media containing body fluids. They are associated with reticuloendothelial, vascular cells, or erythrocytes in vertebrates and also in invertebrates which may act as vectors. They cause diseases in man and animals. Rickettsiae seldom kill invertebrate hosts.

THE FAMILY RICKETTSIACEAE

The rickettsiae comprise a group of small, bacterial organisms that are commonly found in the tissues of arthropods. In 1909 Ricketts saw and described the one that causes Rocky Mountain spotted fever of man. He demonstrated that the disease was transmitted to man by ticks, principally *Dermacentor andersoni,* and showed that the infection occurs commonly in the tick, the human infections being merely incidental. During Ricketts's studies of typhus in 1910 he contracted the disease and died. Another scientist, Von Prowazek, who was one of the early workers in this field, also died of typhus, and in 1916 Da Rocha-Lima named the causative agent of louse-borne typhus fever *Rickettsia prowazeki.* It is the type species of the group.

Morphology and Staining Reactions. Rickettsiae are small bacteria with a typical cell wall. In some instances there is a great deal of pleomorphism; in others they are quite uniform in size and shape. Most of them occur in groups in the cytoplasm of the parasitized cells; sometimes they occur intranuclearly. Nearly all measure less than 0.5 μm in diameter. They stain poorly with ordinary dyes, but can be well and characteristically stained by May-Gruenwald-Giemsa, Gimenez, and Macchiavello stains. *Rickettsia tsutsugamushi* cannot be stained by Macchiavello stain and requires a modification of the standard Gimenez staining procedure for success. With Machiavello and Gimenez stains the rickettsiae stain bright red against a blue (Macchiavello) or greenish (Gimenez) background. By the modified Gimenez staining procedure *R. tsutsugamushi* organisms appear reddish-black against a green background. With Gram's stain they are negative.

Cultural Features. Most species of rickettsiae have been cultivated successfully in tissue culture. A few, including *Rickettsia melophagi,* a nonpathogenic form found in the sheep ked, are said to have been cultivated in special lifeless laboratory media, but none of the pathogenic forms except *Rickettsia quintana* has been cultivated in the absence of living cells. They can readily be propagated in chicken embryos and in tissue cultures. Although they may be grown on the chorioallantois of the developing chick embryo, a more successful method of growing rickettsiae has been devised by Cox (2). It consists of cultivation in the yolk sac of a developing hen's egg. It was demonstrated by Rabinowitz, Aschner, and Grossowicz (9), however, that growth of *R. prowazeki* could be obtained by inoculating the yolk sac of dead embryos. In this case 3-day-old embryos were killed by chilling. Upon reincubation at 37 C, living cells could be demonstrated for as long as 16 days, and apparently the rickettsiae grew in these cells.

Rickettsiae contain enzymes concerned with metabolism. They can oxidize intermediate metabolites and can convert glutamic acid into aspartic acid. When stored at 0 C rickettsiae lose their biological activity due to the progressive loss of nicotinamide adenine dinucleotide (NAD). These properties including toxicity, hemolytic activity, infectivity, and respiratory activity can be restored by subsequent incubation with NAD. Purified rickettsiae may also lose their biological activity if they are starved by incubation for several hours at 36 C. This can be prevented by the addition of glutamate, pyruvate, or adenosine triphosphate (ATP). During the starvation process the ATP level falls to zero while the level rises again on addition of glutamate.

Rickettsiae may be preserved in infected tissues stored at −20 C or lower and also in the lyophilized state for several months.

Pathogenicity. The rickettsiae appear to be well-established parasites of arthropods (6). Some are transmitted transovarially in ticks, but do not seem to be pathogenic for them. Certain types are pathogenic for the body louse. They also appear to be reasonably well adapted to animals, especially rodents, which may constitute a reservoir of infection in nature. Many varieties of rickettsiae on intraperitoneal inoculation into male guinea pigs will produce a febrile attack within 7 to 12 days, which may be accompanied by orchitis. The disease in the guinea pig often is not fatal. Other laboratory animals such as dogs, cats, rabbits, rats, and mice are more resistant and may show no febrile or other reaction to injection, although the organism may become established and persist for months. According to Price (8), guinea pigs that are infected intraperitoneally with a strain of rickettsiae of low virulence are protected against a simultaneous injection of a highly virulent strain, providing the less virulent strain is given in about 10 to 30 times the concentration of the more virulent one. This is known as the rickettsial-interference phenomenon. Infection with Q fever, scrub typhus, and epidemic typhus protects guinea pigs against a virulent strain of spotted fever under the same conditions.

The rickettsiae cause a number of diseases in man and in animals. These infections will be discussed below under the headings "Human Rickettsial Diseases" and "Animal Rickettsial Diseases."

Diagnosis. The diagnosis of rickettsial diseases is based on recovery of the causative agent from acute phase blood specimens in a suitable host or on a fourfold or greater increase in agglutinin or complement-fixing antibody titer between acute and convalescent phase serums.

Guinea pig and chicken embryo inoculations usually are employed in isolating rickettsiae. At present the complement-fixation test seems to be the most accurate means of differentiating the various types (1). Several agglutination and toxin-neutralization systems have been developed for research purposes. Each species has group-distinctive antigens which do not cross-react with antiserums to other groups; however, the rickettsiae of the spotted-fever and typhus-fever groups share common antigens which cross-react in the complement-fixation test only with other members of their respective groups.

The most reliable serological results are obtained with ether-extracted antigens prepared from yolk sacs of embryonated chicken eggs containing maximum growth of rickettsiae (10). Except for *Rickettsia akari,* members of the spotted-fever group achieve maximum growth in 5-day-old embryos inoculated with a dose calculated to destroy most embryos by the 4th day after inoculation into the yolk sac. Inoculated eggs are incubated at 33.5 C for 48 hours after death of embryos before yolk sacs are harvested. Maximum yields of *R. prowazeki* and *Rickettsia typhi* are achieved in 5-day-old embryos maintained at 36.5 C that were inoculated into the yolk sac with a dose calculated to cause death in 60 to 70 percent of the embryos between the 8th and 9th days after inoculation. Maximum growth of *Coxiella burneti* is obtained when given an inoculum producing 50 percent embryo mortality one day earlier. Yolk sacs are harvested from surviving embryonated eggs and from embryos not dead for more than 6 hours. Infected yolk sacs are stored at −20 C to −70 C for subsequent antigen preparation.

Ether extraction of infected yolk sacs is used for the preparation of rickettsial antigens. Yolk sacs are emulsified in a Waring blender with sufficient 0.66 M phosphate-buffered saline, pH 5.8, to make a 20 percent suspension. The material is held overnight at 4 C after the addition of formalin adequate to make 0.2 percent concentration. This suspension is mixed with 1.5 volumes of ether in a separatory funnel, shaken several times during the day, and permitted to separate overnight at 4 C. The aqueous phase containing the antigen is removed and residual ether removed by vacuum. Antigen activity is then assayed by cross-box titration against three specific antiserums with adequate controls to evaluate anticomplementary activity. This activity can be removed sometimes by one or more additional ether extractions.

According to Van der Scheer, Bohnel, and Cox (11), soluble antigens can be prepared from infected yolk sacs by ether extraction, followed by treatment with benzene, and precipitation with sodium sulfate. Complement fixation with this antigen does not always distinguish between European and murine typhus.

In 1915 Weil and Felix found that the serum of patients with typhus fever agglutinated certain strains of *Proteus* bacteria. Apparently these *Proteus* strains possess somatic (O) antigens in common with the rickettsiae. This reaction (Weil-Felix) is not specific, but it has proved useful in serological diagnosis and identification of rickettsial infections.

The identification of *Rickettsia rickettsi* in a film from the gut tissues of the wood tick, *Dermacentor andersoni*, can be established by means of the fluorescent antibody technique (FAT). The indirect fluorescent antibody method has been used to demonstrate *R. tsutsugamushi* in smears of the serum from patients with scrub typhus. Some cross-reactions are observed in FAT because some rickettsial organisms share common antigens.

The cultivation of live rickettsia in the laboratory, particularly during centrifugation, and also in infected animals is hazardous. Consequently, laboratory and animal personnel should be vaccinated and adequate facilities available for isolating and studying these pathogens.

Immunity. Recovery from an attack of rickettsial disease usually confers a solid and lasting immunity. Vaccines against these diseases are now being prepared by injecting the yolk sac of developing chick embryos. The rickettsiae are concentrated by a process of grinding, washing, and centrifugation and then purified by the removal of yolk lipids and tissue debris (3). The infected yolk sac material usually is formalinized before the concentration procedure is started. Craigie claims that the ethyl ether used in the process is bactericidal for rickettsiae (3).

Antibodies after vaccination initially are IgM, later IgG.

Treatment. Streptomycin, Aureomycin, Chloromycetin, Terramycin, and para-aminobenzoic acid (PABA) have been reported to be highly effective in treating rickettsial diseases (4, 5, 7).

REFERENCES

1. Bengston and Topping. Am. Jour. Pub. Health, 1942, *32*, 48.
2. Cox. Science, 1941, *94*, 399.
3. Craigie. Can. Jour. Res., 1945, *23* (Sect. E), 104.
4. Fellers. U.S. Armed Forces Med. Jour., 1952, *3*, 665.
5. Haig, Alexander, and Weiss. Jour. So. Afr. Vet. Med. Assoc., 1954, *25*, 45.
6. Huff. Quart. Rev. Biol., 1938, *13*, 196.
7. Ley and Smadel. Antibiotics and Chemother., 1954, *4*, 792.
8. Price. Proc. Soc. Exp. Biol. and Med., 1953, *82*, 180.
9. Rabinowitz, Aschner, and Grossowicz. Proc. Soc. Exp. Biol. and Med., 1948, *67*, 469.
10. Stoenner, Lackman, and Bell. Jour. Inf. Dis., 1962, *110*, 121.
11. Van der Scheer, Bohnel, and Cox. Jour. Immunol., 1947, *56*, 365.

HUMAN RICKETTSIAL DISEASES

The human rickettsial diseases, with some exceptions, are clinically similar, characterized by fever, skin rashes, or dark blotches resulting from lesions of the blood vessels and nervous symptoms. They may be divided into five groups (see Table 28.1) on the basis of clinical data, insect vectors, locality, serology, and other factors. Both man and domestic and wild animals are susceptible to diseases of all five groups, and various biting insect vectors may transmit each type.

Typhus Fever

Typhus is found in central Europe, in South and Central America, and in Asia, Russia, Africa, and the United States. Mortality may be as low as 5 percent or as high as 70 percent. The blood of patients is infectious, but the organisms have not been seen in the blood.

The European type, the classic form of typhus, is transmitted by the human body louse (*Pediculus vestimenti*). The reservoir of infection is not definitely known. It is not transmitted transovarially in lice, and infected lice usually die within 2 weeks. The disease may be maintained in endemic form by mild infections, or possibly man may act as an asymptomatic carrier. It has spread to the Atlantic seaboard of the United States, where it appears in a mild form sometimes called *Brill's*

Table 28.1. Human rickettsial diseases

Disease group	Geographic distribution	Causative organism	Major vectors	Primary natural hosts	Suggested experimental hosts
I. Spotted fever group					
Spotted fever	North and South America	*Rickettsia rickettsi*	*Dermacentor andersoni* *D. variabilis* *Rhipicephalus sanguineus* *Amblyomma americanum* *A. cajennense*	Many species of feral mammals, chiefly rodents; dogs; birds	Male guinea pigs, *Microtus* sp., and fertile hens' eggs
Siberian tick typhus	Siberia	*R. siberica*	*Dermacentor nuttalli* *D. silvarum* *D. marginatus* *D. pictur* *Hemaphysalis concinna* *H. punctata*	Many species of feral mammals, chiefly rodents	Male guinea pigs and fertile hens' eggs
Rickettsial pox	Russia North America	*R. akari*	*Allodermanyssus sanguineus*	*Mus* species and *Rattus* species	Mice and fertile hens' eggs
North Queensland tick typhus	Australia	*R. australis*	*Ixodes holocyclus*	Small marsupials and rats	Mice and fertile hens' eggs
Fievre boutonneuse	Mediterranean area of Africa and Europe	*R. conori*	*Rhipicephalus sanguineus*	Dogs and small feral mammals	Male guinea pigs and fertile hens' eggs
South African tick-bite fever	South Africa		*R. appendiculatus*		
Indian tick typhus	India		*Hemaphysalis leachi*		
Kenya tick typhus	Africa		*Amblyomma hebraeum*		

II. Typhus fever group					
Epidemic typhus (European type)	Worldwide (colder climates)	*R. prowazeki*	*Pediculus humanus* *Amblyomma variegatum* *Hyalomma* spp.	Man (cattle, sheep and goats?)	Male guinea pigs, cotton rats, and fertile hens' eggs
Murine typhus	Worldwide (warmer climates)	*R. typhi*	*Xenopsylla cheopis*	*Rattus norvegicus*	Male guinea pigs and fertile hens' eggs
New typhus member	North America	*R. canada*	*Hemaphysalis leporispalustris*	Man and rabbits	Rabbits and fertile hens' eggs
III. Scrub typhus	Eastern and southern Asia Islands of southwest Pacific	*R. tsutsugamushi*	*Leptotrombidium akamushi* *L. deliensis*	Many species of small feral mammals, chiefly rodents	Mice, cotton rats, and fertile hens' eggs
IV. Q fever	Worldwide	*Coxiella burneti*	Chiefly airborne, also found in many species of ticks	Cattle, sheep, goats, and many species of feral mammals	Guinea pigs, hamsters, and fertile hens' eggs
V. Trench fever	Europe North Africa Mexico North America	*R. (Rochalimaea) quintana*	*Pediculus humanus*	Man, voles	Laboratory-reared body lice, voles

Modified slightly from a table supplied by Herbert G. Stoenner, Rocky Mountain Laboratory, Hamilton, Mont.

disease (35). Brill's disease also occurs in Europe, and Murray *et al.* (24), after studying 26 cases in Yugoslavia, which is a louse-borne typhus zone, concluded that they had obtained further support for Zinsser's hypothesis that man is the interepidemic reservoir of epidemic typhus fever.

Murine typhus, which prevails in the southern United States and in Mexico, is a disease associated with rats (22). It is transmitted to man by the rat flea (*Xenopsylla cheopis*) and the rat louse (*Polyplax spinulosa*). In an epidemic it may be transmitted from man to man by the human louse.

The European type is called *Rickettsia prowazeki,* while the murine type is called *R. typhi*. A third type, *R. canada,* produces a febrile illness in man that resembles Rocky Mountain spotted fever in man (6). The three may be differentiated by the complement-fixation test.

Rocky Mountain Spotted Fever

Clinically the disease resembles typhus. However, there appear to be at least three forms of the disease: (*a*) the eastern form, occurring in the eastern United States, less frequently fatal, and transmitted by the dog tick (*Dermacentor variabilis*); (*b*) a more highly fatal form occurring in the Rocky Mountain area and transmitted by the sheep tick (*Dermacentor andersoni*); and (*c*) a Brazilian form (São Paulo typhus) transmitted by a tick (*Amblyomma cajennense*). The ticks probably maintain the disease among dogs, rabbits, field mice, sheep, etc., by their bites, and in the western form at least transmit the infectious agent to their progeny (27). The rickettsiae of spotted fever usually are called *Rickettsia rickettsi*.

In 1976 Sexton *et al.* (32) surveyed Mississippi dogs for Rocky Mountain spotted fever antibodies and for tick parasites infected with rickettsiae of the spotted fever group. Of 116 serum samples, 53 (46 percent) had CF antibody titers greater than 1:8, as compared with only 1 (5 percent) of 21 samples from a group of dogs from metropolitan Chicago. *R. rickettsi* was demonstrated in only 1 of 129 *Dermacentor variabilis* removed from Mississippi dogs, whereas 167 (19 percent) of 884 *Rhipicephalus sanguineus* from these dogs harbored spotted fever rickettsiae. The clinical and clinicopathologic changes and the pathogenesis of experimental studies with *R. rickettsi* in dogs were described by Keenan *et al.* (17, 18). The syndrome varied in severity from a mild febrile exanthema to death within 6 days after inoculation. The severity was dose-related and the sign of illness comparable to infection in man.

Rickettsia conori infection occurred in a young dog from Tunisia. The dog had fever and inappetence and also vomited. It responded favorably to daily intramuscular injection of 400 mg of oxytetracycline for one week (8).

Other rickettsial diseases that may be included in the spotted fever group are Marseilles fever, Kenya fever, South African tick-bite fever, rickettsialpox, Bullis fever, North Queensland tick typhus, Indian tick-bite fever, and Russian tick-bite fever.

Scrub Typhus

SYNONYMS: Mite typhus, tsutsugamushi disease

This disease, resembling typhus clinically, is found principally in Japan, Malaya, and the islands of the South Pacific. The common transmitting agent (*Trombicula akamushi*) is much like the American "chigger." Rodents serve as a reservoir for the disease (1). The causative agent is *Rickettsia tsutsugamushi*.

Trench Fever

SYNONYMS: Wolhynian Fever, shin bone fever, five-day fever

This disease occurred in World War I in the armies in France, Mesopotamia, and Salonika (2). According to Jacobi (15), it appeared in World War II in the German Army in Russia. Usually it produces a high fever of the relapsing type, and the most constant symptom is pain in the legs. Natural transmission is through the human body louse, *Pediculus humanus*. The cause is *Rochalimaea quintana*.

Q Fever

SYNONYM: Nine-mile fever

This is a febrile disease of man resembling influenza. It is an acute and specific rickettsial infection of variable severity and duration. Its clinical course is characterized by sudden onset, severe headache, malaise, and patchy infiltration of the lungs. It is distinguished from most other rickettsial diseases of man by the failure of patients to develop a cutaneous rash.

Q fever was first described as a human disease in 1937 in Queensland, Australia, and its etiologic agent was named *Rickettsia burneti* by Australian workers (10, 11, 7). In 1938 Davis and Cox (9) recovered a *Rickettsia* from infected ticks at Nine-Mile Creek, Montana, which upon subsequent study proved to be *R. burneti*. In *Ber-*

gey's Manual this organism now bears the name *Coxiella burneti*. The disease appears to be quite common all over the world, usually masquerading as "flu" or atypical pneumonia. A fever in man may also be associated with hepatitis, pericarditis, meningitis, arthritis, orchitis, epididymitis, phlebitis, esophagitis, and arteritis.

C. burneti is a bipolar rod, 0.24 by 1 μm (see Figure 28.1). It occurs intracellularly in the cytoplasm of infected cells and possibly extracellularly in infected ticks. Some observations suggest existence of a smaller filterable stage, but its true nature has not been identified. Strains newly isolated from animals and ticks are characteristically in phase I, which reacts only with antibodies in late convalescent-phase serums. With repeated passage in embryonated chicken eggs the organism converts to phase II, which reacts with antibodies of early convalescent-phase serums.

The phase I *C. burneti* antigen isolated by phenol extraction is a complex lipopolysaccharide (LPS) molecule containing substances similar to LPS from other Gram-negative bacteria (31). Phase I *C. burneti* are more resistant to phagocytosis than are phase II organisms (16, 19).

Figure 28.1. Smear of yolk-sac culture of embryonated hen's egg with *Coxiella burneti*. Macchiavello stain. × 1,290. (Courtesy Herbert G. Stoenner, Rocky Mountain Laboratory, Hamilton, Mont.)

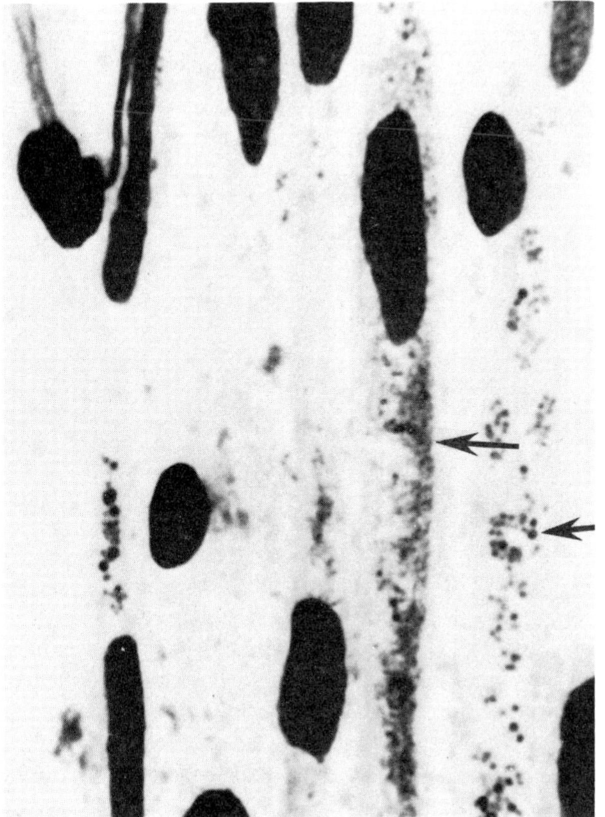

The prevalence of infection with *C. burneti* among domestic animals is determined by examining serums by the complement-fixation, capillary-tube agglutination, or radioisotope precipitation (RIP) tests. These techniques measure different antibodies, so complete agreement cannot be expected. Complement-fixing antibodies are associated with 19S macroglobulins while RIP antibodies seem to occur in the 7S gamma globulins. Furthermore, the rate of antibody response to *C. burneti* and the persistence of antibodies vary in different animal species. The RIP test is the most sensitive and will detect antibodies for longer periods after the infection has occurred than do other tests. Infection rates among herds of dairy cattle are most easily determined by testing individual or pooled milk samples by the capillary-tube test.

Q fever is essentially an occupational disease, being limited almost entirely to livestock attendants, farm residents, and laboratory personnel. According to Derrick (12), it is a natural infection of certain wild animals, especially bandicoots in Australia, and is transmitted in nature by ticks. These ticks spread the infection to cattle, which sometimes develop a mild illness. Cattle ticks become infected by feeding on infected cattle. It is then possible that feces deposited on the skins of the animals by the infected ticks may be a source of infection for man. Infection also occurs in such domestic animals as sheep, goats, dogs, cats, and donkeys, as well as in domestic fowl and pigeons. The organisms have been demonstrated in the wool, in birth fluids, in the feces, and in the placental tissues of naturally infected sheep. Apparently *C. burneti* produces only mild or inapparent illness in domestic animals in most instances, but they act as reservoirs of the organism. Herd-to-herd transmission among cattle has been demonstrated (28), and dairy farmers and meat packers from areas where there is evidence of Q fever infection in the cattle show serum antibodies against *C. burneti* (20). Infection in a dairy herd may be followed by excretion of rickettsiae in the milk for as long as 32 months (14).

Epidemiological evidence points to the spread of infection by the inhalation of dust contaminated with infected secreta or excreta of diseased animals or ticks. The fact that outbreaks of Q fever in men who have no contact with livestock sometimes follow dust storms adds weight to this theory (33). The organism has also been found in cow's milk, where it may survive ordinary pasteurization. It is claimed that a temperature of 145 F for 30 minutes will kill *C. burneti,* whereas 143 F for the same period of time is not sufficient (13). The disease rarely spreads from man to man, although this mode of transmission has been reported. The role of ticks in the spread of Q fever is uncertain, but six strains of ticks common in various parts of the world have been shown to harbor *C. burneti.* Certainly it is not dependent on arthropod transmission in the infectious cycle. Leibisch (21) in Germany observed that the two peaks in the prevalence of Q fever in man (April and September) correspond to periods of activity of adult *Dermacentor marginatus.* Russian investigators (26) have suggested Q fever is transmitted by *Ixodes persulcatus* and *Ixodes trianguliceps* to cattle and sheep in Udmurtskaya USSR. The virulence of the organism can be enhanced by residence in the tick *Alveonasus canestrinii* (25). Although antibodies to *C. burneti* have been detected in birds, their role in the transmission is unclear. On occasion brucellosis and Q fever have occurred in the same cows.

Vaccination appears to have some value in the control of the disease among occupationally exposed individuals and among infected livestock (34). Extended studies by the California group (4, 5) using a phase I formalin-inactivated Q fever vaccine proved the effectiveness of this biologic in the immunization of dairy cattle. Further, their field trials indicated vaccination greatly reduced the shedding of the organism in the milk of dairy cows. Sadecky *et al.* (29, 30) also showed that the administration of a formalin-inactivated phase I *C. burneti* vaccine in naturally infected ewes and cows eliminated the shedding of the organism in the milk. Formalin-inactivated epidemic typhus and Q fever vaccines administered as a mixture have produced an immunity to both organisms in guinea pigs and in man (23).

Results of oral chemotherapy studies in cows and guinea pigs suggest that in some cases chlortetracycline may suppress rather than eradicate the Q fever agent (3).

REFERENCES

1. Ahlm and Lipschutz. Jour. Am. Med. Assoc., 1944, *124,* 1095.
2. Arkwright, Bacot, and Duncan. Jour. Hyg. (London), 1919–20, *18,* 76.
3. Behymer, Ruppanner, Riemann, Biberstein, and Franti. Folia Veterinaria Latina, 1977, *7,* 64.
4. Biberstein, Crenshaw, Behymer, Franti, Bushnell, and Riemann. Cornell Vet., 1974, *64,* 387.
5. Biberstein, Riemann, Franti, Behymer, Ruppaner, Bushnell, and Crenshaw. Am. Jour. Vet. Res., 1977, *38,* 189.
6. Bozeman, Elisberg, Humphries, Runcik, and Palmer. Jour. Inf. Dis., 1970, *121,* 367.
7. Burnet and Freeman. Med. Jour. Austral., 1937, *1,* 296.
8. Clerc and Lecomte. Recueil de Med. Vet., 1974, *150,* 189.
9. Davis and Cox. Pub. Health Rpts. (U.S.), 1938, *53,* 2259.
10. Derrick. Med. Jour. Austral., 1937, *2,* 281.
11. Derrick. Med. Jour. Austral., 1939, *1,* 14.
12. Derrick. Jour. Hyg. (London), 1944, *43,* 357.
13. Enright, Sadler, and Thomas. Am. Jour. Pub. Health, 1957, *47,* 695.
14. Grist. Vet. Rec., 1959, *71,* 839.
15. Jacobi. Munch. med. Wchnschr., 1942, *89,* 615.
16. Kazar, Skultetyova, and Brezina. Acta Virol., 1975, *19,* 426.
17. Keenan, Buhles, Huxsoll, Williams, and Hildebrandt. Am. Jour. Vet. Res., 1977, *38,* 851.
18. Keenan, Buhles, Huxsoll, Williams, Hildebrandt, Campbell, and Stephenson. Jour. Inf. Dis., 1977, *135,* 911.
19. Kishimoto and Walker. Inf. and Immun., 1976, *14,* 416.
20. Kitze. Am. Jour. Hyg., 1957, *65,* 239.
21. Liebisch. Deut. Tierärztl Wchnschr., 1976, *83,* 274.
22. Maxcy. Pub. Health Rpts. (U.S.), 1926, *41,* 213.
23. Morris, Wisseman, Aulidio, Jackson, and Smadel. Proc. Soc. Exp. Biol. and Med., 1967, *125,* 1216.
24. Murray, Psorn, Djakovic, Sielski, Broz, Ljupsa, Gaon, Pavlevic, and Snyder. Am. Jour. Pub. Health, 1951, *41,* 1359.
25. Pautov and Morozov. Zhurnal Mikrobiologii, Epidemiologii i Immunobiologii, 1974, *8,* 29.
26. Pchelkina and Korenberg. Zhurnal Mikrobiologii, Epidemiologii i Immunobiologii, 1974, *5,* 123.
27. Philip. Pub. Health Rpts. (U.S.), 1933, *48,* 266.
28. Reed and Wentworth. Jour. Am. Vet. Med. Assoc., 1957, *130,* 458.
29. Sadecky and Brezina. Acta Virol., 1977, *21,* 89.
30. Sadecky, Brezina, Kazar, Schramek, and Urvolgyi. Acta Virol., 1975, *19,* 486.
31. Schramek and Brezina. Acta Virol., 1976, *20,* 152.
32. Sexton, Burgdorfer, Thomas, and Norment. Am. Jour. Epidem., 1976, *103,* 192.
33. Spicer, Crowther, Vella, Bengtsson, Miles, and Pitzolis Trans. Roy. Soc. Trop. Med. and Hyg., 1977, *71,* 16.
34. Wentworth. Bact. Rev., 1955, *19,* 129.
35. Zinsser. Am. Jour. Hyg., 1934, *20,* 513.

ANIMAL RICKETTSIAL DISEASES

Members of the rickettsiae afflicting domestic animals comprise a heterogenous group (Table 28.2) whose members share only a few common characteristics. The morphological and staining characteristics of the eight infectious agents are comparable. Vectors are involved in the transmission of the disease, and intermediate

Table 28.2. Animal rickettsial diseases

Disease	Geographic distribution	Causative organism	Major vectors	Natural hosts: cell or tissues affected	Suggested experimental hosts
Heartwater	East and south Africa	*Cowdria ruminantium*	*Amblyomma hebraeum, A. variegatum,* and other *Amblyomma* spp.	Sheep, cattle, goats, and some wild ungulates: vascular endothelium	Bluetongue-immune sheep and mice
Tick-borne fever (pasture fever)	Great Britain, Norway, Finland, The Netherlands, India	*Ehrlichia phagocytophila*	*Ixodes ricinus*	Cattle, sheep, bison, wild ungulates: primarily granulocytes	Cattle, sheep, guinea pig, mouse, and goats
Benign bovine rickettsiosis ("nopi," "nofel")	North and central south Africa, Middle East, Ceylon	*Ehrlichia bovis*	*Hyalomma excavatum* and other *Hyalomma* spp.	Cattle: lymphocytes and monocytes	Cattle, sheep, and monkey
Benign ovine rickettsiosis	North and central Africa	*Ehrlichia ovina*	*Rhipicephalus bursa*	Sheep: lymphocytes and monocytes	Sheep
Canine ehrlichiosis	Worldwide	*Ehrlichia canis*	*Rhipicephalus sanguineus*	Domestic and wild Canidae: lymphocytes and monocytes	Babesia-free dogs
Equine ehrlichiosis	California (USA)	*Ehrlichia equi*	—	Horse and burros: primarily granulocytes	Horse, donkey, sheep, goat, dog, monkey, and cat
Bovine petechial fever, ondiri disease	Kenya	*Cytoecetes ondiri*	—	Cattle, sheep: primarily granulocytes	Cattle and sheep
Contagious ophthalmia	Africa, Australia, New Zealand, Europe, North and South America	*Colesiota conjunctivae*	Flies	Sheep, cattle, goats, swine, and chickens: conjunctival epithelium	Sheep, cattle, goats, swine, and chickens
Salmon poisoning syndrome	Northwestern United States	*Neorickettsia helminthoeca,* Elokomin fluke fever agent	*Nanophytes salmincola*	Dogs and wild Canidae: reticuloendothelial system, lymph nodes	Dogs and black bear

Modified from a table supplied by Herbert G. Stoenner, Rocky Mountain Laboratory, Hamilton, Mont.

hosts definitely exist for six of the animal rickettsial diseases. Except for *Colesiota conjunctivae* the disease in the natural hosts principally involves pathological changes in the blood vascular system. *C. conjunctivae* is limited to the conjunctival sac. Within the limits of our present knowledge each organism is immunologically distinct. Certain of these diseases have been studied extensively in their natural hosts, but their limited host ranges have proved to be a handicap. None of the organisms has been cultivated in the embryonated hen's egg, and only *Cowdria ruminantium, Ehrlichia equi,* and *Ehrlichia phagocytophilia* cause disease or infection in laboratory animals. Difficulties in the preparation of antigens have forestalled the developments of serological tests for diagnosis and research.

There is no evidence that any of the animal rickettsial organisms listed in this section produces disease in man. *E. equi* does produce infection in nonhuman primates (rhesus, macaques, and baboons) (9).

Heartwater Disease

This disease is caused by *Cowdria* (*Rickettsia*) *ruminantium*. The organism was first described in 1925 by Cowdry (3), who was working at the time in South Africa. It is the cause of a disease of cattle, sheep, goats, and some wild ungulates commonly called *heartwater* because one of the characteristics of the disease is hydropericardium. This disease occurs in eastern and southern Africa. It has long been known in South Africa and is associated with the bont tick, *Amblyomma hebraeum,* and other *Amblyomma* species which are the transmitting agents (1).

Character of the Disease. Affected ruminants develop a high fever and show gastrointestinal and nervous signs. A high mortality is often reported in cattle, sheep, and goats, except in indigenous ruminants. The organism infects a variety of feral ungulates without necessarily causing overt disease. Capillaries may be occluded by swollen epithelial cells containing masses of rickettsiae. The disease may assume a peracute form characterized by high fever, sudden collapse, and death, or it may be mild or even abortive. In the more common acute form a rise in temperature occurs first followed by depression and loss of appetite, although some animals may continue to eat and ruminate. Nervous signs are first manifested by a high-stepping and unsteady gait followed by progressive signs of encephalitis including chewing movements, twitching of eyelids, walking in circles, aggressive and blind charges into objects, and final collapse with attendant convulsions, galloping movements, and twitching of muscles.

Animals that die with the peracute form rarely have gross lesions. Hydropericardium is not always seen in sheep with the acute form, and the absence of pericardial fluid in cattle is not uncommon. Mucous membranes are injected. Edema of the lungs is a constant finding. The peritoneal and pleural cavities contain excessive fluid with a variable amount of hemorrhage usually present on the serous membranes of the abdominal viscera and heart. The spleen and lymph nodes, particularly in cattle, are enlarged. The liver is usually enlarged and hemorrhagic, and distention of the gall bladder is common. A transparent fluid often infiltrates the mucous membrane of the abomasum. Patches of ramiform injection and diffuse hyperemia of the small intestine, particularly in cattle, produce so-called zebra markings.

The principal microscopic changes are leukostatis in all organs and perivascular infiltration in the liver and kidney and occasionally in the adrenal glands.

Immunity. Protection is usually afforded against the homologous strain, but this immunity is not complete in all animals. When animals that have recovered from natural or induced disease are challenged with other strains, only partial protection is observed as a rule. These results suggest a multiplicity of immunological strains in nature. Under field conditions animals have continuous exposure to ticks, so repeated infection produces adequate protection. These animals are protected against disease, but not infection, as they may have a rickettsemia sufficient to infect normal bont ticks feeding on them.

Calves up to 3 weeks of age are quite resistant to heartwater disease and can be rendered actively immune by infection with serum from infected animals. This procedure is practiced in certain heavily infected areas of South Africa, where the possible loss of a few young calves, through the use of live vaccine, is preferred to larger losses of older calves from natural infection (11).

Transmission. Many other kinds of ticks occur in the heartwater districts, but apparently the bont tick and other *Amblyomma* species are the only vectors. Larval ticks retain the infection through the molts to the adult form, but the parasite is not transmitted through the egg to the next generation.

The disease can be transmitted by inoculation with blood taken from sick animals during the early febrile period, but transmission is not always achieved. The route of injection is important. The preferred route is intravenous inoculation, although the subcutaneous route has been used with less success. Ingestion usually fails. It is clear that the disease is transmitted naturally solely through the activities of the *Amblyomma* ticks.

Diagnosis. Diagnosis is established by demonstration of rickettsiae in tissue smears from suspect cases or reproduction of the disease in sheep. Specimens taken 2 to 4 days after the onset of fever give the best results. After the temperature has returned to normal, blood may not be infectious. Blood should be obtained in sterile containers and inoculated intravenously into test animals as defibrinated blood immediately after withdrawal. If field material cannot be inoculated promptly into sheep, white mice inoculated intraperitoneally will preserve the organism for 90 days and permit later passage into sheep (4). The organism will infect white mice and ferrets without signs of illness. The organism is quite labile and survives in blood only for a few hours at room temperature. It is reported to survive for 2 years at −70 C. After rapid freezing at −85 C and −196 C, with or without 10 percent dimethyl sulfoxide, a Nigerian isolate remained highly virulent, killing all the goats and sheep inoculated with the frozen stabilized suspensions (8). It is also well

Figure 28.2. *Cowdria ruminantium*. In brain smear (*upper left*), stained with Giemsa. × 1,160. In choroid plexus (*lower left*) of sheep, araldite section 0.5 μm thick. × 1,160. A colony of organisms is seen in a distended endothelial cell completely obstructing the lumen of the capillary (*on right*). In adjoining capillary, at the bottom, a monocyte has organisms in a cytoplasmic vacuole. × 7,750. (Courtesy J. D. Smith.)

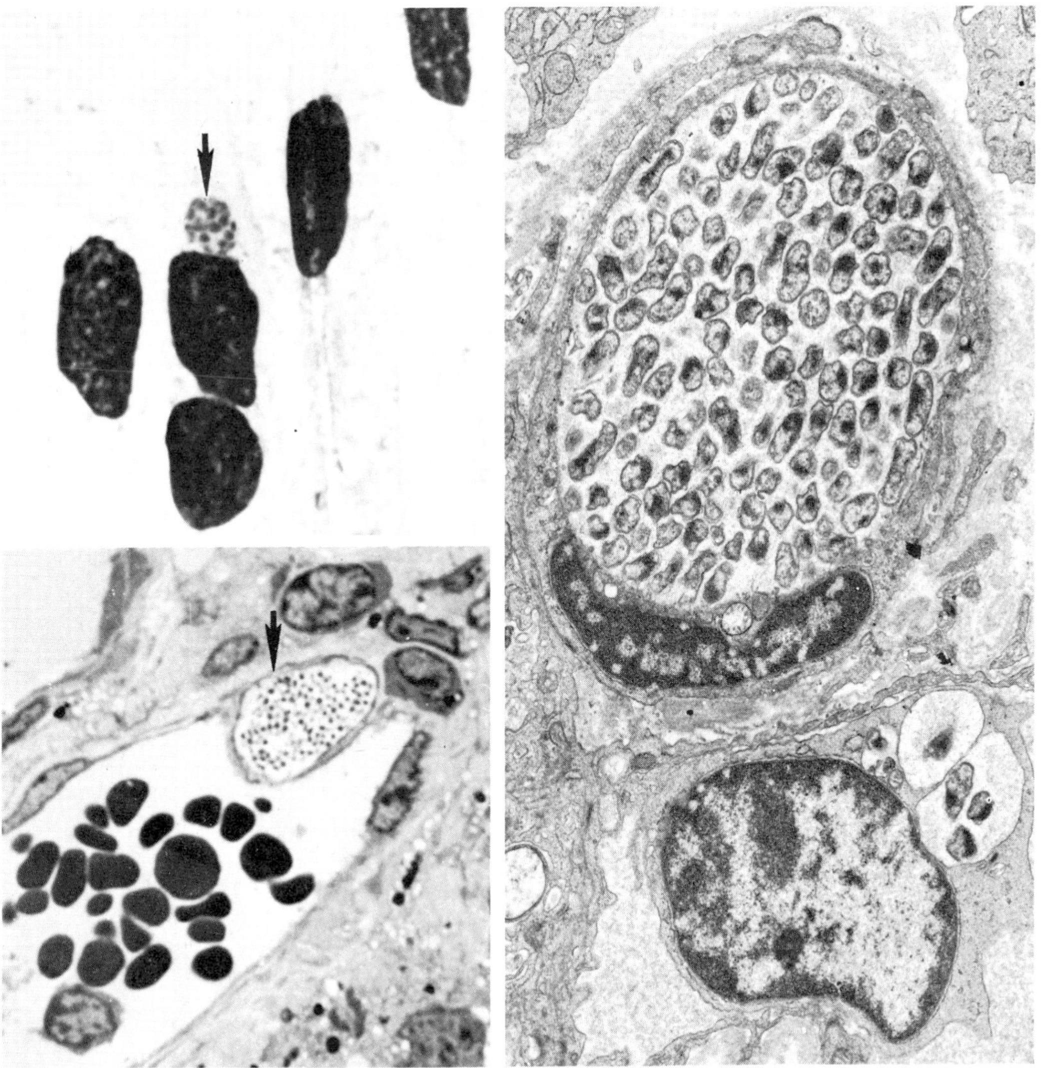

to remember that rickettsiae lose their staining properties rapidly in unfixed tissues.

Bluetongue-immune sheep should be used for the reproduction of the disease because many cattle and sheep harbor bluetongue virus which may confuse the diagnosis. There is a distinct difference in incubation period because bluetongue virus produces signs in 5 days whereas *C. ruminantium* requires 11 days. To confirm the diagnosis the rickettsial organisms should be demonstrated in endothelial cells of test animals sacrificed 2 to 4 days after onset of illness.

Although *C. ruminantium* cannot be maintained by serial passage in mice, an incubation period in this animal is required for a successful transfer to sheep. Consequently, spleens of infected mice are harvested between 14 and 21 days postinoculation and the suspension injected intravenously into susceptible sheep.

A capillary flocculation test is available to diagnose heartwater disease using antigen prepared from infective cattle or goat brain (6). Antibodies are detected 1 to 2 weeks after clinical recovery, but unfortunately persist for only 1 to 4 weeks. Consequently, the test has its limitations.

Vascular scrapings and smears from cerebral gray matter (Figure 28.2) yield equally good results after the preparations are air-dried, fixed with methyl alcohol, and stained with Giemsa. Areas rich in capillaries are sought with low power. Under high power or oil immersion the organisms appear dark blue in the cytoplasm while the nuclei of the endothelial cells are purple. The organism may be coccoid (0.3 μm diameter), bacillary (0.3 by 0.5 μm), or diplococcoid (Figure 28.2). In 1978 Ilemobade and Blotkamp (7) reported that the subcutaneous injection of brain homogenate from animals dying or dead of heartwater consistently produced the disease in susceptible goats. In attempting to diagnose heartwater brain homogenate, whole blood, and lung macrophages should be used as test materials from field cases.

According to Andreasen (2) *C. ruminantium* propagates in *Amblyomma* tick cells *in vitro*. The culture material produced heartwater in a susceptible sheep.

Treatment. Rake, Alexander, and Hamre (12) reported that this disease has proved susceptible to sulfonamide therapy, which suggests a relationship to the psittacosis group of infections, but they believe that the causative agent is neither a rickettsial nor a psittacosis agent but is related to both. Studies by Haig *et al.* (5) indicate that oxytetracycline and chlortetracycline are quite efficacious as therapeutic agents. Terramycin soluble powder (oxytetracycline) in the water has been used successfully in the treatment of sheep, goats, and cattle.

Control of ticks on sheep by dipping in benzene hexachloride helps in the prevention of the disease (10).

REFERENCES

1. Alexander. 17th Ann. Rpt., Dir. Vet. Services, Union So. Afr., 1931, p. 89.
2. Andreasen. Acta. Path. et Microbiol. Scandinavica, 1974, *82,* 455.
3. Cowdry. Jour. Exp. Med., 1925, *42,* 231 and 253.
4. Haig. Jour. So. Afr. Vet. Med. Assoc., 1952, *23,* 167.
5. Haig, Alexander, and Weiss. Jour. So. Afr. Vet. Med. Assoc., 1954, *25,* 45.
6. Ilemobade and Blotkamp. Res. Vet. Sci., 1976, *21,* 370.
7. Ilemobade and Blotkamp. Trop. An. Health and Prod., 1978, *10,* 39.
8. Ilemobade, Blotkamp, and Synge. Res. Vet. Sci., 1975, *19,* 337.
9. Lewis, Huxsoll, Ristic, and Johnson. Am. Jour. Vet. Res., 1975, *36,* 85.
10. Marsh. Adv. Vet. Sci., 1958, *4,* 164.
11. Neitz and Alexander. Onderstepoort Jour. Vet. Sci. and An. Indus., 1945, *20,* 137.
12. Rake, Alexander, and Hamre. Science, 1945, *102,* 424.

Tick-Borne Fever, Pasture Fever

Foggie (1) has described tick-borne fever in sheep and has proposed the name *Ehrlichia (Rickettsia) phagocytophilia* for the organism. Following an acute attack, the infection may persist up to 2 years in the surviving animal. The organism will infect sheep, cattle, goats, and wild ungulates. The disease has been described in Great Britain, Norway, Finland, The Netherlands, and India.

Character of the Disease. This disease is characterized by a sudden rise in temperature with the persistence of an irregular fever for 3 to 5 days in cattle and for 10 days in sheep. Dairy cattle drop in milk production and may never fully recover. Febrile relapses may occur 2 to 4 weeks after the initial attack. In some outbreaks abortions have occurred in sheep and cattle that are in the latter stages of gestation. Sometimes clinical disease is complicated by concurrent infection with *Babesia* or, virus diarrhea infection and cobalt deficiency.

The infecting agents from sheep and cattle are different strains of the same organism. They produce more severe disease in their respective natural hosts. The incubation period varies from 4 to 8 days after exposure to infected ticks and 5 to 12 days after inoculation with infective blood.

Immunity. All evidence suggests that strains of *E. phagocytophilia* are immunologically heterogenous. There is little or no apparent cross-immunity between the Scottish and Finnish strains. Experimental cattle and sheep were given successive injections with 11 Finnish strains, and some animals reacted to 6 strains. Virulent strains appear more immunogenic than mild strains. Protection appears partial and of short duration, lasting from 3 to 6 months.

In nature, repeated attacks exclusive of relapses are seldom seen. Reinfection from repeated tick bites presumably occurs and confers adequate immunity during the same tick season. The occurrence of tick-borne fever in the same animal during the following tick seasons is not rare.

Diagnosis. The ideal time to take blood specimens for demonstration or isolation of *E. phagocytophilia* is during the initial febrile period when large numbers are in the circulation. Some sheep remain carriers for 2 years, but most animals rid their tissues of demonstrable organisms within a month. Blood smears may be made directly or later from a citrated blood specimen. The organism usually remains viable for 7 days at 4 C and survives for several months at −70 C.

Either Giemsa or May-Gruenwald-Giemsa are excellent stains for demonstrating the organism in blood smears. The fluorescent antibody method can be used, but offers no advantage in ease of technique or in certainty of diagnosis. The organisms have a predilection for granulocytes, but monocytes may be infected. At the peak of infection 50 percent or more of the granulocytes may be infected with virulent strains while others may involve 6 percent. At least 100 cells should be examined before a blood smear is called negative.

The pleomorphism of *E. phagocytophilia* is apparent in stained preparations, even in the same cell (Figure 28.3). The deep-purple-staining coccoid or rod-shaped body usually situated at the periphery of the cell is about 0.5 μm in diameter. The larger homogeneously staining body more deeply situated in the cell cytoplasm is 1.3 by 2 μm and often appears to fragment into smaller irregularly shaped bodies. The rounded or oval masses, termed morulae, contain numerous distinct bodies that stain a deeper blue or purple than the surrounding matrix.

The intravenous inoculation of infective defibrinated blood into susceptible sheep or cattle constitutes another means of diagnosing the disease. To assure the diagnosis, blood smears from test animals must contain the characteristic organism in the granulocytes.

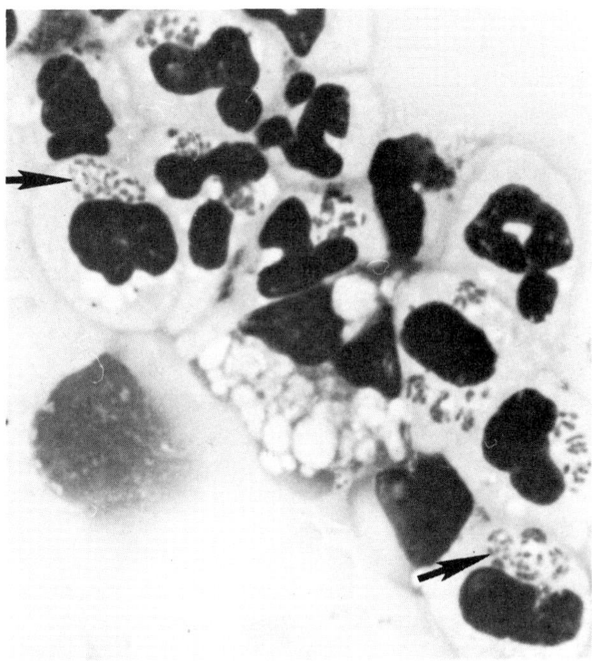

Figure 28.3. *Ehrlichia phagocytophila* in granulocytes of a leukocyte concentrate. May-Gruenwald-Giemsa stain. × 1,400. (Courtesy J. Tuomi.)

REFERENCE

1. Foggie. Jour. Path. and Bact., 1951, *63*, 1.

Bovine and Ovine Ehrlichiosis

Benign bovine and ovine ehrlichiosis is limited geographically to north and south Africa. There is only meager information about the nature of this disease in cattle and in sheep, and the immunological relationship between *Ehrlichia bovis* and *Ehrlichia ovina* has not been explored.

Character of the Disease. Cattle and sheep show an irregular fever of several weeks' duration. It is rarely a fatal disease in either species. The most significant lesion is excessive pericardial fluid similar to heartwater fever in sheep. Other consistent changes are lymphadenopathy and splenomegaly. Cattle and sheep may remain carriers for 10 months.

Immunity. Chronic infections may persist for 10 months in sheep and cattle. Recovered animals develop a solid immunity against challenge with the homologous organism, but the duration of immunity is unknown.

Transmission. *E. bovis* is transmitted to cattle by ticks of the *Hyalomma* genus whereas *E. ovina* is transmitted to sheep by the tick *Rhipicephalus bursa*. A 10 percent suspension of spleen, lung, or blood taken during the febrile stage is used to transmit the organism in its natural host. The incubation period in sheep and cattle is approximately 12 days.

Diagnosis. The organisms can be readily demonstrated in blood smears from animals in the febrile stage. Tissues from the lungs, liver, and spleen are suitable for *Ehrlichia* demonstration.

These rickettsiae are found in the cytoplasm of the circulating monocytes and monocyticlike cells in the lungs, liver, and spleen. The monocytes in the blood smear usually gather at the edge of the preparation. They frequently assemble in round colonies from 2 to 10 μm in diameter and also in closely packed granules 0.5 to 1.0 μm in diameter. With Giemsa they stain similar to *Ehrlichia phagocytophilia*. Initial bodies, 3 by 6 μm, stain a homogeneous red and later separate into elementary bodies that stain purple with May-Gruenwald-Giemsa stain. A thorough search should be made of smears as the percentage of monocytes with organisms is usually low.

Canine Ehrlichiosis

This disease has been reported in north and east Africa, India, Ceylon, Aruba, and the United States. *Ehrlichia canis* frequently occurs as a concurrent infection in dogs with *Babesia canis* because both rickettsiae are transmitted by the same tick, *Rhipicephalus sanguineus*. Wild dogs, jackals, foxes, and coyotes are also susceptible. An excellent review article on canine ehrlichiosis has been written by Ewing (2).

Character of the Disease. The onset of the disease is characterized by a high fever and depression. Icterus, vomition, progressive weakness, splenomegaly, and mucopurulent ocular discharge with photophobia are some other signs of illness. A monocytosis occurs and eosinophils almost disappear early in the disease. With disease progression a profound anemia of the normocytic normochromic type develops with depressed values for packed cell volume, hemoglobin, and total erythrocyte counts. The mortality rate among puppies is higher than in older dogs.

At necropsy the gross pathological changes include anemia, hyperactive bone marrow, enlarged spleen, liver, and lymph nodes, and petechiae of the lungs. Less commonly observed changes are hemorrhages and ulcers in the intestinal tract, hydrothorax, and pulmonary edema.

The histological lesion in the bone marrow of dogs with severe pancytopenia consisted of hypoplasia, depletion of megakaryocytes, and often loss of normal sinusoidal architecture (1). Dogs chronically infected, but without severe pancytopenia, had normocellular marrow.

Immunity. Animals that recover from an acute attack usually are immune to reinfection. Nyindo (6) suggests that the elimination of *E. canis* from a carrier dog renders it susceptible to reinfection. Others (8) suggest that there may be a correlation between a high antibody titer as determined by the indirect fluorescent antibody test and protection in the dog. Persistence of the organism in recovered dogs can be demonstrated by splenectomy with the ensuing appearance of *E. canis* in the circulating monocytes.

In experimental studies the majority of the dogs developed cell mediated responses, but they declined and disappeared in most dogs by 19 to 21 weeks after infection. Serum antibody titers as measured by the indirect fluorescent antibody test increase with time and remained at significant levels. It is interesting that lymphocytes from dogs infected with *E. canis* were shown to be toxic for autologous monocytes. Neither immune serum and complement nor anticanine globulin had any observable effect on cytotoxicity. The monocytotoxicity bore a temporal relationship to the thrombocytopenia. Kakoma *et al.* (4) suggest that T lymphocyte activation accompanying ehrlichiosis contributes to the pathogenesis of the disease and that the specific immune elimination of parasitized monocytes is antibody independent.

Transmission. *E. canis* is transmitted to the dog by the tick *R. sanguineus,* which also transmits *Babesia* to the same host.

Lung, liver, or spleen tissue as a 10 percent suspension or blood taken during the febrile stage of infective dogs produces the disease in susceptible dogs 7 to 21 days after parenteral injection.

Dogs may remain carriers for at least 29 months (3) after an acute attack and constitute a constant reservoir for the infection in nature. Unfortunately, carrier dogs may become donors of whole blood used for therapeutic purposes in veterinary hospitals. There is evidence that this has occurred despite efforts to insure that the donor was free of the disease. Puppy inoculation with donor blood is the only known means to detect carriers. Obviously, the same problem exists in other diseases where the organism persists in the blood stream after recovery from signs of illness.

E. canis may persist in adult *R. sanguineus* ticks for

155 days after detachment as engorged nymphs from a dog in the acute phase of ehrlichiosis. Infected but unfed ticks may be more important than the chroncially infected carrier dog as a natural reservoir of *E. canis* (5).

Diagnosis. This organism may be recovered from the blood of infected dogs for long periods of time. They are demonstrated most readily 2 or 3 days after the onset of fever until the end of clinical signs. If direct blood smears are negative, smears of the buffy coat of heparinized or citrated blood samples may be positive. During the febrile period *E. canis* may be demonstrated in biopsy material from the lung, liver, or spleen. As there is insufficient data on the survival of the organism, fresh test material should be injected promptly into susceptible dogs.

With the development of an indirect fluorescent antibody test for *E. canis* it is possible to detect the organism in smears of midgut tissues of *R. sanguineus* (8), and the test also is used to detect and titrate antibodies in the serum of dogs infected with *E. canis.* (7).

Stephenson and Osterman (9) developed a tissue culture system using canine peritoneal macrophages. The cultures are well established in 6 days and are maintained for at least 30 days. Infected cells were detected by 60 hours after inoculation with *E. canis,* and replication is evident by 12 to 18 days. This constitutes another test for the diagnosis of this disease.

E. canis has the same morphological and staining characteristics as *E. bovis* and *E. ovina.* Because ehrlichiae infections, particularly in the dog, are often complicated by concurrent infections with *Babesia,* a thorough search should also be made for this latter organism in the erythrocytes.

Treatment. Certain drugs, such as broad-spectrum antibiotics employed successfully in treating Rocky Mountain spotted fever and salmon poisoning disease, may alter the course of canine ehrlichiosis (and presumably *E. ovina* and *E. bovis*), but do not prevent the development of the carrier stage.

REFERENCES

1. Buhles, Huxsoll, and Hildebrandt. Jour. Comp. Path., 1975, *85,* 511.
2. Ewing. Adv. Vet. Sci., 1969, *13,* 331.
3. Ewing and Philip. Am. Jour. Vet. Res., 1966, *27,* 67.
4. Kakoma, Carson, Ristic, Huxsoll, Stephenson, and Nyindo. Am. Jour. Vet. Res., 1977, *38,* 1557.
5. Lewis, Ristic, Smith, Lincoln, and Stephenson. Am. Jour. Vet. Res., 1977, *38,* 1953.
6. Nyindo. Dissertation Abstracts International, 1976, *36B,* 4334.
7. Ristic, Huxsoll, Weisiger, Hildebrandt, and Nyindo. Inf. and Immun., 1972, *6,* 226.

8. Smith, Sells, Stephenson, Ristic, and Huxsoll. Am. Jour. Vet. Res., 1976, *37,* 119.
9. Stephenson and Osterman. Am. Jour. Vet. Res., 1977, *38,* 1815.

Equine Ehrlichiosis

This disease occurs as a distinct entity in horses located in the Sacramento Valley, California, United States. There have been five known naturally occurring cases. In 1977, Gunders and Gottlieb (2) collected ticks from burros in Israel that transmitted a granulocyte-inhabiting parasite believed to be a rickettsial organism which caused disease.

Character of the Disease. The information about the nature of this disease has been derived from the five natural cases but principally from the experimental disease produced in horses and burros (1, 5).

The disease is characterized by fever, depression, anorexia, edema of the legs, and ataxia. In experimental cases the incubation period varied from 1 to 9 days with a mean of 2.5 days with fresh blood and 6.5 days with frozen blood. Hematologic changes are thrombocytopenia, elevated plasma icterus index, decreased cell-packed volume, and marked leukopenia involving first lymphocytes and then granulocytes. Subcutaneous edema of the legs appears first at the metacarpal and metatarsal regions and may ascend to the radius and 6 to 8 inches above the hock.

At necropsy, edema and petechial and ecchymotic hemorrhage occur in the subcutaneous tissues, fascia, and epimysium of the legs distal to the elbow and stifle joints. Carcasses are frequently jaundiced, and orchitis is often seen in mature males. Some horses have excessive fluid in the peritoneal cavity and pericardial sac. Histologically, vasculitis of small arteries and veins involves swelling of endothelial and smooth muscle cells, thromboses, and perivascular infiltrations of monocytes and lymphocytes. The vessels in testes, ovaries, legs, and pampiniform plexus are principally affected.

Immunity. Present evidence suggests that one attack confers immunity. Horses recovered from experimental disease withstood challenge with infectious blood given 2.5 to 20 months later. This evaluation was based on the lack of clinical signs and of organisms in circulating granulocytes.

Transmission. No arthropod vector has been incriminated as yet in the transmission of the natural disease, except for the cases in Israel where *Ornithodoros erratius* was found on burros parasitized with a *Rickettsia*like organism in granulocytes. As the authors did not claim the organism is *E. equi,* further studies are indicated to establish the identity of the disease agent.

Infective blood produces the disease in experimental horses. Horses under 2 years of age usually do not show clinical signs other than a fever. Dogs, sheep, and goats develop a mild or inapparent infection after parenteral injection, and the organism can be demonstrated in the cytoplasm of the granulocytes.

Diagnosis. As with other *Ehrlichia* organisms blood specimens preferably are taken during the febrile period, usually 3 to 5 days after its onset. The best smears are made with fresh blood, but citrated blood samples in sterile tubes and maintained at 4 C may be used for later examination. Fresh blood is preferred for inoculation into susceptible horses, but defibrinated blood sealed in glass ampoules and stored at −70 C remains infectious although the incubation period is prolonged.

The diagnosis is based on demonstrating the presence of rickettsiae in the granulocytes contained in blood smears from natural and experimental cases that are stained with Giemsa or Wright-Leishman stains. The inclusion bodies are deep blue to pale blue-gray. They may vary from small darkly stained bodies 200 nm in diameter to large granular bodies 5 μm in diameter, which represent a cluster of smaller bodies. The percentage of parasitized granulocytes varies with the stage of the disease with mean maximum as 36 percent.

E. equi studied in equine pheripheral leukocytes has the same structure as other agents of the genus *Ehrlichia* (4). A great variation in size was observed. Lewis (3) believes *E. equi* is a different strain of the organisms of *E. canis* and *E. phagocytophilia.*

REFERENCES

1. Gribble. Jour. Am. Vet. Med. Assoc., 1969, *155,* 462.
2. Gunders and Gottlieb. Refuah Veterinarith, 1977, *34,* 5.
3. Lewis. Vet. Parasitol., 1976, *2,* 61.
4. Sells, Hildebrandt, Lewis, Nyindo, and Ristic. Inf. and Immun., 1976, *13,* 273.
5. Stannard, Gribble, and Smith. Vet. Rec., 1969, *84,* 149.

Bovine Petechial Fever, Ondiri Disease

This disease was reported in Kenya and Tanzania. It has been recognized only in the highland areas of Kenya in cattle and sheep. The involvement of an invertebrate host in the disease cycle has not been established yet. *Cytoecetes ondiri* has all the characteristics of an animal rickettsial pathogen.

Character of the Disease. Clinical bovine petechial fever develops in exotic breeds of cattle. Sahiwal crosses and Borans are susceptible while Ayrshires and Herefords were resistant to experimental inoculation with *C. ondiri. Ondiri disease* is characterized by fever, petechiae, and depression. Initially, there is a disappearance of eosinophils and a reduction in lymphocytes followed by a drop in neutrophils (2).

Latent infections may occur because the blood from some experimentally infected cattle or sheep may be infective for up to 4 weeks after the cessation of clinical signs.

Multiplication of *C. ondiri* occurs within 24 hours after inoculation into sheep or cattle, probably in the spleen because the organism could not have been demonstrated in other tissues until later (1). During the period of greatest concentration of the organism in the tissues organisms could be demonstrated in the circulating leukocytes. The spleen always had the greatest number of organisms based upon titrations in susceptible sheep.

Immunity. In his immunity studies Snodgrass (1) reported that effective immunity to challenge with homologous and heterologous strains was observed in cattle and to homologous strains in sheep. Sheep challenged with heterologous strains usually were susceptible. The duration of immunity was not ascertained.

Diagnosis. The clinical signs and necropsy findings are similar to several other diseases; so diagnosis depends on the demonstration of the organism. This usually can be done directly in blood or spleen tissue smears prepared with Giemsa stain. On occasions parasitemia may be absent when signs first appear. In these cases animal inoculations will be required to verify a presumptive diagnosis (3).

Treatment. Gloxazone is more effective in the treatment of ondiri disease in sheep than tetracycline, and it also was efficacious in infected cattle (4).

REFERENCES

1. Snodgrass. Jour. Comp. Path., 1975, *85,* 523.
2. Snodgrass. Trop. An. Health and Prod., 1975, *7,* 213.
3. Snodgrass. Vet. Rec., 1975, *96,* 132.
4. Snodgrass. Res. Vet. Sci., 1976, *20,* 108.

Contagious Ophthalmia

Colesiota conjunctivae produces conjunctivitis in sheep, cattle, goats, swine, and chickens and has been reported on all continents except Asia. Flies apparently play some role in its transmission.

The relationships between these conjunctival agents in livestock have not been well established. The strains are host-specific and not transferable among livestock. Consequently, some investigators contend that *C. conjunctivae* occurs only in sheep and the rickettsiae which infect the conjunctivae of other livestock should be given another generic name. In this respect Rizvi (2) reported a conjunctivitis in young goats caused by *Rickettsia conjunctivae*. Certain features of its morphological and staining characteristics differed from *C. conjunctivae*.

Character of the Disease. The severity of the disease varies from mild cases of purulent conjunctivitis with recovery within a week to severe cases with keratitis, vascularization, and occasionally corneal ulceration. Most severely affected eyes eventually heal without residual blemish.

The disease can be reproduced by instilling conjunctival washings into the eyes of susceptible animals of the same species. The incubation period is 2 to 4 days in the instilled eye, and the opposite eye becomes infected 3 to 4 days later.

Immunity. In sheep, immunity persists for 3 months, but after 8 months approximately 10 percent are again susceptible. The carrier stage persists in some sheep for over a year, and that fact coupled with the loss of immunity in others may account for the survival of the organism in the flock.

Immunity in animals other than sheep has not been thoroughly studied.

Diagnosis. Epithelial scrapings from the inner surface of the conjunctiva are made with a scalpel until a tinge of blood appears. The material is spread on a slide, air-dried, fixed with absolute alcohol, and stained. Saline washings from the eyes of sheep during the acute phase of the disease are an excellent source of material for transmission of the disease to experimental animals. The viability of the organism is unknown, but it should be considered labile. The organisms will not survive desiccation.

In Giemsa-stained smears several types of inclusions are observed. Many polymorpholeukocytes are observed in smear preparations taken early in the disease. Most of the organisms are found in the cytoplasm and appear as purplish-red small ovoid or short rod-shaped organisms, 0.2 by 0.5 μm. As recovery ensues, lymphocytes and monocytes replace the leukocytes. At this stage, irregular extracellular organisms, 0.8 by 1.4 μm, that stain unevenly appear as triangles, imperfect rings, and horseshoe-shaped clusters.

Treatment. In sheep, chloramphenicol reduces the severity of the disease and also the number of cases developing ulcerative keratitis. Riboflavin in 15-mg daily doses is also effective (1).

REFERENCES

1. Marsh. Adv. Vet. Sci., 1958, *4*, 164.
2. Rizvi. Jour. Am. Vet. Med. Assoc., 1950, *117*, 409.

Jembrana

A single report by Budiarso and Hardjosworo (1) described a highly fatal disease in cattle and buffaloes on Bali that killed an estimated 60,000 animals within a 3-year span. Examination of hepatic and spleen smears stained with Giemsa or Macchiavello stain revealed intracellular organisms resembling rickettsiae. Based on studies in male guinea pigs, Jembrana disease is concluded to be a rickettsiosis. Comparative studies with other bovine rickettsial organisms have not been reported.

The disease is characterized by anorexia, fever, generalized lymphadenopathy, nasal discharge, increased salivation, and anemia. At necropsy generalized vascular damage and small granulomatous nodules were observed.

REFERENCES

1. Budiarso and Hardjosworo. Austral. Vet. Jour., 1976, *52*, 97.

Salmon Poisoning

SYNONYM: Salmon disease

This disease occurs in western Oregon, northwestern California, and southwestern Washington. It is not known to occur elsewhere. It affects several members of the family Canidae. Dogs, foxes, and coyotes are known to be susceptible. House cats, mink, raccoons, and swine apparently are resistant. The disease has long been associated with the eating of salmon and trout from streams that flow into the Pacific Ocean in the region described. Although the disease has the appearance of an infection, it was long regarded as a poisoning or intoxication. Several facts about this disease indicated that it was more than a simple intestinal parasitism, and in 1954 Philip *et al.* (13, 14) proposed the name of *Neorickettsia helmin-*

thoeca for the *Rickettsia*like agent that is associated with the fluke infestation and plays an important role in the disease among mammals.

In 1973 and 1974 a series of papers (9, 11, 16) emanating from a group at Washington State University described a second agent, the Elokomin fluke fever agent, immunologically distinct from *Neorickettsia helminthoeca,* as a part of the salmon poisoning syndrome. It causes a less severe disease in dogs, with recovery ensuing in experimental dogs, whereas *N. helminthoeca* causes a high mortality.

Character of the Disease. The first sign in dogs is a slight rise in body temperature. Within 24 hours there is a complete loss of appetite and marked depression, and the temperature rises to 104 to 107 F. The animal appears very dejected and apathetic. After several days the temperature usually decreases. A slight purulent discharge may occur from the eyes during the 4th to 6th day of illness. The eyelids and adjacent tissues become edematous about this time, giving the eyes a sunken appearance. Beginning about the 4th or 5th day persistent vomiting usually occurs. This is accompanied by rapid loss of body weight. The animals become avid for water, but most of it is lost by further vomition. Diarrhea usually begins about the 5th to 7th day. In the beginning the diarrheal discharge frequently is tinged with blood, and later it is heavily impregnated with blood. After a day or two of diarrhea, many animals appear to improve, but usually this is only temporary. Finally the temperature falls to subnormal. At this time the animal is so emaciated and weak that it can hardly stand alone. Most animals die within 6 to 10 days after the appearance of signs, and from 12 to 20 days after eating the infective fish.

Autopsy examinations reveal hemorrhagic inflammation of the intestine as the most characteristic lesion. The inflammatory reaction may be observed throughout the bowel, or it may be limited to certain regions. In many cases the entire bowel is well lined with bloody exudate; in others the content is merely blood-tinged. Ulceration is unusual, but is seen in a few cases. The ulcers often are superficial and may vary in size from those barely visible to others 2 to 3 cm in diameter. Flukes and fluke eggs may be found in the intestinal content in large numbers. As many as 200,000 parasites have been recovered from a single dog. Gross changes are found in the lymphocytic tissues. Variable enlargement of the ileocecal, mesenteric, portal, and internal iliac lymph nodes are constant findings. A decrease in the number of mature lymphocytes accompanied by a proliferation of the reticuloendothelial elements in both the cortex and medulla is the predominant and most consistent microscopic finding in the lymph nodes. Similar changes are found in the tonsils, thymus, and lymphoid tissues of the spleen and intestinal tract. Coccobacillary bodies are present in the numerous reticular cells either clustered in morulalike masses or diffusely scattered in the cytoplasm. They are often numerous in the histiocytes of the intestinal villi. Some are seen as free bodies as though released by cell disintegration (3).

Follicles of the spleen rarely contain necrotic foci, but often show central hemorrhage. Flukes are found embedded in the villi or duodenal glands of the intestinal tract with no evidence of inflammatory response. Small foci of macrophages and neutrophils, often necrotic, are found frequently in the connective tissue of the lamina propria. Cellularity of the propria also may be increased, principally with plasma cells and neutrophils. Centrolobular lipidosis of the liver is common in foxes, but rare in the dog. In both foxes and dogs a moderate mononuclear infiltration of the liver interlobular connective tissue is seen. Occasionally, a few small hemorrhages beneath the bladder epithelium are observed. An accumulation of mononuclear and neutrophil leukocytes in small areas cause a slight thickening of the alveolar walls of the lungs.

A monocytic leptomeningitis is most intense over the cerebellum. Exudative and proliferative cellular changes in the sheaths of the small and medium-sized vessels in the cerebrum and focal collections of glia of mesenchymal cells (glial nodules) are commonly observed lesions.

Signs of illness usually appear on the 6th or 8th day after eating parasitized fish. In a few cases signs may be observed as early as the 5th day or as late as the 12th day.

Most untreated dogs die of the disease. Simms, Donham, and Shaw (18) observed recovery in only four dogs in a series of 102.

Simms, McCapes, and Muth (19) and Simms and Muth (20) were successful in transmitting the disease to dogs by intraperitoneal injection of blood or of ground, washed flukes from infected dogs and by the injection of metacercariae from parasitized fish, as well as by feeding fluke-infected trout and salmon. The signs produced were the same as those seen in the naturally contracted disease.

Immunity. Dogs that recover from salmon poisoning are solidly immune thereafter for long periods and perhaps for life. Simms, McCapes, and Muth (19) found it possible to immunize dogs solidly by the simultaneous injection of virulent blood and hyperimmune serum.

Shaw and Howarth (17) showed that strong immunity followed the feeding of parasitized salmon and the curing of the resultant disease with sulfanilamide.

Dogs that recover from the Elokomin fluke fever agent are fully susceptible to *N. helminthoeca* and usually succumb to infection. The reverse is also true; thus no cross-immunity develops between the two agents.

An *Ehrlichia canis*-like organism isolated in Oklahoma, USA, and termed the Oklahoma agent (OA) is pathogenic for dogs, but produces fewer deaths than *N. helminthoeca* under experimental conditions (7). Dogs convalescent from infections with either parasite (broad-spectrum antibiotics used late in the disease to permit *N. helminthoeca* infected dogs to recover) had no protection when challenged with the heterologous organism.

Transmission. In 1925 Donham (5) reported an association between the disease and an intestinal fluke, the encysted form of which occurred in fish. Chapin (1) studied this fluke and gave it the name *Nanophyetes salmincola*. It is also known as *Troglotrema salmincola*. This fluke is an essential agent in the production of the disease. The encysted form occurs in the musculature of fish of the family Salmonidae. When eaten by susceptible carnivores, the adult forms develop in the intestines. Ova escaping from these animals infect a small snail, *Goniobasis plicifera* var. *silicula*, which serves in turn to infect the fish. The limited distribution of this species of snail apparently is the factor which controls the spread of the disease.

Donham, Simms, and Miller (6) failed to produce salmon poisoning with ocean-caught salmon in which no encysted flukes could be found. The same species taken in fresh water in the salmon-poisoning area contained metacercariae and produced salmon poisoning when fed to dogs. A survey of the streams of the region showed only one species of snail occurring where fish infection existed. This was the species that was shown to be the intermediate host of the fluke. The parasitized fish included the Chinook, silverside, and chum or dog salmon, the brook or speckled trout, the cutthroat or mountain trout, the rainbow trout, and the steelhead trout. Other types of fish occurring in the region were not infected.

Until recently it was assumed that smoke-treated salmon were not dangerous to dogs, but Farrell, Dee, and Ott (8) reported signs resembling salmon poisoning in dogs after the ingestion of uncooked, smoke-treated salmon that harbored the organism.

Diagnosis. Although signs of illness are rather characteristic, the most certain method of diagnosis is the presence of fluke eggs in the feces of the patient. In most cases the eggs are so numerous that a microscopic examination of the fecal material adhering to the rectal thermometer will result in a diagnosis. These eggs appear in the feces of dogs on the 5th to 7th days after ingestion of infected fish. They are oval in shape, measuring 75 to 80 μm in length and 45 to 55 μm in breadth. There are no embryos in the eggs recovered directly from feces. When stored in cool water, embryonation occurs in 75 to 90 days.

Microscopic examination reveals intracytoplasmic, *Rickettsia*like, sometimes pleomorphic microorganisms found particularly in the reticuloendothelial cells of lymphoid tissues of infected Canidae. Suitable material for this purpose is readily obtained by aspirating cells from the mandibular lymph node with a syringe or by biopsy. Tissue smears require fixation with methyl alcohol prior to staining. Blood contains the organism during the febrile stage, but not in a sufficient number for detection by direct microscopic examination. The organisms are about 0.3 μm in diameter and Gram-negative; they stain purple with Giemsa, pale bluish with hematoxylin, red or

Figure 28.4. *Neorickettsia helminthoeca* stained by the Giemsa method in lymph node aspirations. Coccobacillary bodies (*upper left and right*) diffusely scattered in the cytoplasm of reticular cells; bacillary bodies (*lower left*) in a disintegrating macrophage; morulalike clusters (*lower right*) free and in a macrophage. × 800. (Courtesy R. K. Farrell, *Jour. Am. Vet. Med. Assoc.*)

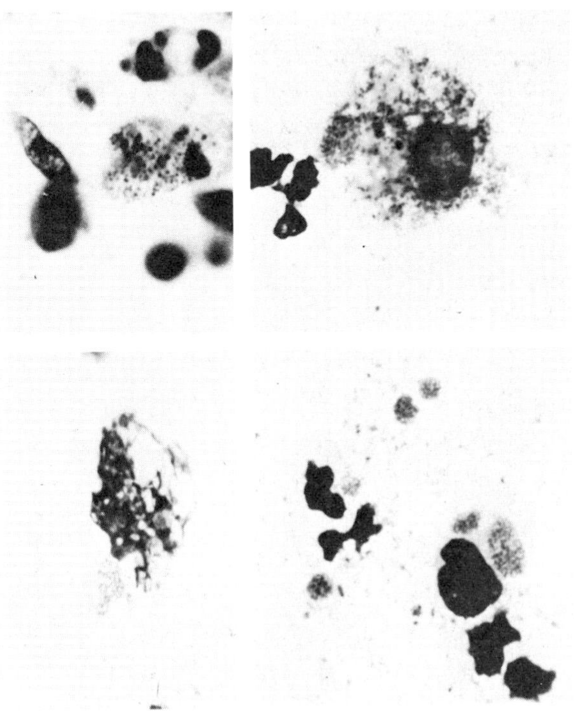

blue with Macchiavello, and dark brown or black with Levaditi. They occur in plaques or loose groups in the cells, often nearly filling the cytoplasm (Figure 28.4).

The organism can be transmitted in dogs by the inoculation of infective blood or spleen taken during the acute phase of the disease. The rickettsiae are labile, but they will survive in fresh frozen tissue stored at −70 C for at least 6 months and will withstand lyophilization. *N. helminthoeca* has been cultivated in canine monocytes (10).

Sakawa *et al.* (16) used a complement-fixation test to show a serological distinction between *N. helminthoeca* and the Elokomin fluke fever agent. A direct fluorescent-antibody test also can be applied to distinguish the same two agents (12).

Treatment. Coon *et al.* (2) showed that sulfanilamide, administered during the early febrile period of the disease in dogs, brought about rapid recovery from the disease. This was confirmed by Shaw and Howarth (17) and by Cordy and Gorham (3). The latter showed sulfamerazine and sulfamethazine to be effective. They also showed that penicillin and chlortetracycline were equally effective but streptomycin was ineffective. Philip *et al.* (15) highly recommended the use of either chlortetracycline or oxytetracycline in treating salmon poisoning.

REFERENCES

1. Chapin. North Am. Vet., 1926, *7,* 36.
2. Coon, Myers, Phelps, Ruehle, Snodgrass, Shaw, Simms, and Bolin. North Am. Vet., 1938, *19,* 57.
3. Cordy and Gorham. Am. Jour. Path., 1950, *26,* 617.
4. Cordy and Gorham. Personal communication.
5. Donham. Jour. Am. Vet. Med. Assoc., 1925, *68,* 637.
6. Donham, Simms, and Miller. Jour. Am. Vet. Med. Assoc., 1926, *68,* 701.
7. Ewing and Philip. Am. Jour. Vet. Res., 1966, *27,* 67.
8. Farrell, Dee, and Ott. Jour. Am. Vet. Med. Assoc., 1968, *152,* 370.
9. Farrell, Leader, and Johnston. Am. Jour. Vet. Res., 1973, *34,* 919.
10. Frank, McGuire, Gorham, and Davis. Jour. Inf. Dis., 1974, *129,* 257.
11. Frank, McGuire, Gorham, and Farrell. Jour. Inf. Dis., 1974, *129,* 163.
12. Kitao, Farrell, and Fukuda. Am. Jour. Vet. Res., 1973, *34,* 927.
13. Philip. Pub. Health Rpts. (U.S.), 1933, *48,* 266.
14. Philip, Hadlow, and Hughes. Exp. Parasitol., 1954, *3,* 336.
15. Philip, Hughes, Locker, and Hadlow. Proc. Soc. Exp. Biol. and Med., 1954, *87,* 397.
16. Sakawa, Farrell, and Mori. Am. Jour. Vet. Res., 1973, *34,* 923.
17. Shaw and Howarth. North Am. Vet., 1939, *20,* 67.
18. Simms, Donham, and Shaw. Am. Jour. Hyg., 1931, *13,* 363.
19. Simms, McCapes, and Muth. Jour. Am. Vet. Med. Assoc., 1932, *81,* 26.
20. Simms and Muth. Proc. 5th Pacific Sci. Congress, 1933, p. 2949.

29 The Anaplasmataceae

Members of this group are obligate parasitic organisms found within or on erythrocytes or free in the plasma of various wild and domestic vetebrates. There is no demonstrable multiplication in other tissues.

In blood smears prepared with Giemsa's strain, the organisms appear as rod-shaped, spherical, coccoid, or ring-shaped bodies staining reddish violet and measuring 0.2 to 0.4 μm in diameter. They may occur in short chains or irregular groups in blood plasma or within red blood cells. Each organism has a membrane with an internal structure resembling rickettsiae. They multiply by binary fission and have not been cultured. The organisms are Gram-negative. They are transmitted by arthropods. Any infective blood containing tissue can cause infection by parenteral inoculation. Disease may occur, but long-term persistence usually results with accompanying resistance to clinically demonstrable reinfection. Anemia is the most prominent feature. The infection occurs throughout the world. They usually respond to the tetracyclines but not to penicillin or streptomycin.

Bergey's Manual lists five genera in the family Anaplasmataceae as follows:

Genus 1. *Anaplasma*. Parasites form inclusions in erythrocytes, 0.3 to 1.0 μm in diameter. Several parasites may be found in each inclusion. No appendages to inclusions observed. The organisms infect ruminants only.

Genus 2. *Paranaplasma*. Same characteristics as anaplasma except the inclusions do have appendages and the organisms infect cattle but not deer or sheep.

Genus 3. *Aegyptianella*. They contain inclusions in erythrocytes, 0.3 to 3.9 μm in diameter, and only infect birds and some poikilothermic animals.

Genus 4. *Hemobartonella*. The parasites are within or on erythrocytes. Ring forms are rare or absent in blood preparations that stain intensely by Romanowsky methods.

Genus 5. *Eperythrozoon*. The organisms are on erythrocytes and in plasma. Ring forms are common in blood preparations stained by Romanowsky methods.

THE GENUS *ANAPLASMA*

In the course of their classical work on piroplasmosis (babesiosis), or Texas fever of cattle, Smith and Kilborne observed and described small coccuslike bodies located near the periphery of many of the red blood cells in animals suffering from the disease. They interpreted these bodies as a stage in the life cycle of the Texas fever parasite. It is clear today that these small bodies were not piroplasms and that Smith and Kilborne were dealing with animals that suffered from two diseases simultaneously, anaplasmosis and piroplasmosis. In 1910 Theiler (43) in South Africa differentiated the two diseases, but because both occurred in the same regions, there were many who disagreed with Theiler and continued to look upon the small marginal bodies either as artifacts or as piroplasms. The matter was not fully resolved until recent years when anaplasmosis was found to be prevalent in most of the southern and many of the northern states of the United States—regions that are now free of piroplasmosis (41) or, in some cases, regions that have never been known to have this disease. The parasite is widely distributed throughout the tropics, Africa, the Middle East, some parts of southern Europe, Latin America, and the Far East.

Anaplasma marginale

This name was given to the organism by Theiler. The word *Anaplasma* means "without plasma" (cytoplasm) and refers to the fact that the parasite seems to consist of nothing but a small bit of chromatic material without any evidence of cytoplasm. The specific name is derived from the fact that these bodies are located, characteristically, near the periphery of the red blood cells and thus appear, in smears, as if on the margin of cells.

Character of the Disease. Although cattle appear to be the specific host for the anaplasmas, they have been found in American deer (7) and also in water buffalo, bison, African antelopes, gnu, blesbuck, duiker, elk, and camels. Sheep and goats may develop a submicroscopic infection. The African buffalo is refractory. As in piroplasmosis, young animals are quite resistant. Cases in calves under 1 year of age are rare, although in infected territories many calves pass through the infection and become immune carriers. The natural resistance of young calves is removed by splenectomy. The marginal bodies appear in great numbers in such animals; hence they are suitable for diagnostic purposes.

In older animals the disease may be acute or chronic. In natural infections the period of incubation varies from 20 to 40 days. Experimentally, signs of illness may be produced much earlier by inoculation with large doses of acutely infected blood. Those affected with the acute form may die within 2 or 3 days after the appearance of the first signs of illness. The disease begins with a high temperature, 105 to 107 F. After a day or two, signs of anemia and icterus appear, and about this time the temperature falls to normal and even subnormal as death approaches. The mucous membranes are pale and yellowish. The yellow color is evident also in the thin-skinned parts of the body. Urination is frequent, but the urine is not blood-tinged, as it often is in piroplasmosis. The animal is usually constipated, the feces being dark, often bloodstained, and covered with mucus.

In chronic cases the animals live longer, are weak, become progressively emaciated, and show icterus and anemia. The red blood cell count may fall from a normal of about 7 million to less than 1 million per cu mm; the hemoglobin may be less than 10 percent.

The mortality is quite variable. It may be greater than 50 percent or less than 5 percent. Losses are greatest in hot weather, and in older animals.

The principal lesions are those associated with blood destruction, anemia, and icterus. The spleen is enlarged, and the pulp is dark and soft. The blood appears as if diluted with water. A catarrhal enteritis is common. There may be a few petechial hemorrhages on the heart wall and on the mucosa of the urinary bladder. The lymph nodes are swollen and edematous. The liver shows marked icterus with the bile channels engorged and the gall bladder distended with dark green, mucilaginous bile. Kreier *et al.* (17) have indicated that the anemia in *Anaplasma* infected animals is caused by intensive erythrophagocytosis initiated by parasitic damage to red blood cells and to antierythrocytic autoantibody. During the parasitemic stage of anaplasmosis serum lipids fell and gamma-globulin increased in calves (9).

Properties of the Parasite. The parasites of anaplasmosis are seen in the red blood corpuscles as minute, deeply staining points usually located near the margin of the cell. If stained with the Giemsa stain, they are deep red in color; with other stains they are apt to be so dark that color in them is not distinguished, but a one-step toluidine blue staining technique has proved useful for rapid detection of *Anaplasma* in erythrocytes in the field or laboratory (39).

With Romanowsky-type stains, this organism appears in the erythrocytes as dense, homogenous, bluish purple round structures, 0.3 to 1.0 μm in diameter. Electron microscopy reveals that these structures are inclusions separated from the cytoplasm of the erythrocyte by a limiting membrane. Each inclusion contains from one to eight subunits or initial bodies (19), which are the actual parasitic bacteria, each 0.3 to 0.4 μm in diameter that are dense aggregates of fine granular material embedded in an electronlucid plasma and all enclosed in a double membrane.

The organism (initial body) enters the erythrocyte by causing invagination of the cytoplasmic membrane and subsequent formation of a vacuole. In the vacuole the initial body multiplies by binary fusion and forms an inclusion. Thus, the formation of the inclusion body, which is most frequently encountered during the acute and convalescent phases of infection, represents only a phase in the developmental cycle of the initial body. Spores or resistant stages are not formed. The adenosine triphosphate and glutathione concentrations of erythrocytes remain essentially unchanged, regardless of the intensity of infection, and only a small quantity of methemoglobin occurs in parasitized erythrocytes. Histochemical analysis of parasites reveals DNA, RNA, protein, and organic iron. They are spherical in form, and ordinarily there is but one organism per cell, although two or more may be seen in some cells. In the early stages of the disease before the temperature rise occurs, few or no parasites can be found. When the febrile period begins, the percentage of infected cells may reach 25 percent or even more than 50 percent. If the animal recovers, the number of cells containing the marginal bodies diminishes rapidly until none can be found microscopically. The blood of recovered animals is infectious for many years and probably for life; hence it is probable that a few bodies are present indefinitely—so few as to make finding them impossible.

In 1959 Espana *et al.* (13) employed phase contrast and electron microscopy in studying hemolyzed erythrocytes from cattle infected with *A. marginale*. They found ring, match, comet, and dumbbell-like forms in natural and experimental infections. They also state that the organism is motile.

Bedell and Dimopoullos (2) claim that infectivity of *A. marginale* is destroyed by exposure to 60 C for 50 minutes and by sonic energy treatments for 90 minutes when the blood is maintained at 30 to 35 C (3). Storage of heparinized and infected *A. marginale* bovine erythrocytes in glycerol for 4.5 years at −70 C did not alter the infectivity or the virulence of the parasite (42). A concentration of 4 M dimethyl sulfoxide provides a means of preventing lysis of bovine erythrocytes when subjected to rapid freezing and thawing. This procedure also enhanced the infectivity of infected erythrocytes. (20)

Transmission. Many species of ticks have been shown to be capable of transmitting anaplasmosis. Most of these probably are mechanical rather than biological carriers, but several are biological carriers (4, 5). Among the latter are *Boophilus (Margaropus) annulatus, Dermacentor occidentalis,* and *Dermacentor andersoni,* which occur in the United States. In these species the infective agent passes through the egg into the next generation of the species. Freidhoff and Ristic (15) demonstrated *A. marginale* in the gut contents and in the Malpighian tubes of engorged *Dermacentor andersoni* nymphs by the fluorescent-antibody technique and stated that the anaplasmas multiplied in the Malpighian tubes by the process of binary fission.

In addition, at least seven species of horseflies (Tabanidae) have been shown to be mechanical carriers, and certain mosquitoes such as *Aedes* and *Anopheles* species have also been incriminated. The stable fly (*Stomoxys calcitrans*) and the horn fly (*Haematobia irritans*) apparently seldom, if ever, act as transmitters.

The fact that deer are susceptible to anaplasmosis indicates that they may constitute an important reservoir of infection in areas where they occupy the same range land as cattle (11, 22).

An important means of transmission is through the use of common surgical instruments that have not been thoroughly disinfected after being used on one animal and before being used on another. Reese (27) has shown that anaplasmosis can very easily be carried on a lancet for drawing blood if it is merely wiped after being used on an infected animal. Outbreaks have occurred in herds after dehorning operations, the drawing of blood samples, castrations, and minor operations. In areas where anaplasmosis occurs, veterinarians should be exceedingly cautious in carrying out these mass operations to avoid serious consequences resulting from the spreading of this disease to many animals from a few, or even one, carrier animal. Uterine transmission has also been reported, and Davis *et al.* (12) have demonstrated that *A. marginale* has the ability to infect via the ocular route.

Immunity. Animals that recover from anaplasmosis remain carriers for long periods and probably for life. Such animals are resistant to additional infection. Young calves are relatively resistant to the infection. Signs of illness are seldom seen in calves less than 1 year of age. Such animals can be inoculated with virulent blood, especially in the winter months when the disease is not so severe naturally as it is in the hot months, and made immune thereafter. Because they become permanent carriers and because the number of vectors is great, such animals are a source of danger to any nonimmune animals with which they come in contact at any time later in life.

In cattle infected with *A. marginale,* antibodies are found in IgG and IgM classes of immunoglobulins during the acute and convalescing phases of the infection. Erythrocytes from acutely infected cattle yield two distinct antigens, a nonsedimentable one (NS) and a sedimentable one (S). The NS antigen is active in the gel-precipitation system, and the S antigen is a suspension of initial bodies. Carson *et al.* (10) utilized the leukocyte migration-inhibition test as an index for cell-mediated immunity. The response increased greatly in cattle given virulent anaplasmas or attenuated anaplasmas.

Immunity in adult cattle persists even after the latent infection is eliminated by the use of imidocarb dehydrochloride treatment according to Roby *et al.* (35). This suggests that latency does not provide the sole means for protection.

Diagnosis. The diagnosis is made conclusive, of course, by finding the characteristic marginal bodies in the red blood cells. In this connection it is well to warn the examiner to be cautious in his identification, so as not to confuse such structures as basophilic stippling and the Jolly bodies, seen in severe anemias, with anaplasmas. Artifacts resembling these bodies also are often seen. The examinations should be made only on good films that are well stained (Figure 29.1). Ristic *et al.* (33) have detected *A. marginale* by means of fluorescein-labeled antibody.

In using splenectomized calves to diagnose anaplasmosis, Gates *et al.* (16) noted that blood obtained from cattle whose sera showed a high complement-fixation titer had a much lower degree of infectivity than that of other cattle. It should also be noted that the splenectomized cow is even more susceptible to infection than the splenectomized calf (37).

Boynton and Woods (6) have reported a simple test that seems to have some value in the diagnosis of anaplasmosis. The blood is allowed to clot, and a little clear serum is obtained. Two drops are added to 2 ml of distilled water in a tube. The serum of normal animals does not cloud the water; that of animals affected with anaplasmosis causes an immediate clouding, and after the tube stands overnight, a white precipitate covers the bottom. Animals affected with acute anaplasmosis and recently recovered carriers give this reaction. The test depends on the precipitation of euglobulin, which appears to be present in increased amount in this disease. Splenectomized, disease-free calves are suitable for use in locating carrier animals. The complement-fixation test also is used in detecting the disease. According to Price *et al.* (25), it is highly accurate. The antigen is obtained from the blood of infected splenectomized calves (14, 26).

Ristic and coworkers have employed a gel diffusion (31) and a capillary tube agglutination test (30). They claim that the latter test is as accurate as the complement-fixation test and has the advantages over gel diffusion or complement fixation of simplicity, economy, and speed of reaction in detecting anaplasmosis. A card system is used by some diagnosticians as a rapid, practical, economical, and portable procedure for the diagnosis of anaplasmosis. This modified agglutination

Figure 29.1 (*left*). *Anaplasma marginale,* a stained blood film from a cow suffering from acute anaplasmosis and showing many organisms in its blood. × 770.

Figure 29.2 (*right*). *Anaplasma centrale* in bovine blood. Two typical parasites are seen as sharply staining dots in red blood cells near the center of the illustration. Poikilocytosis and anisocytosis are present as a result of anemia. × 770.

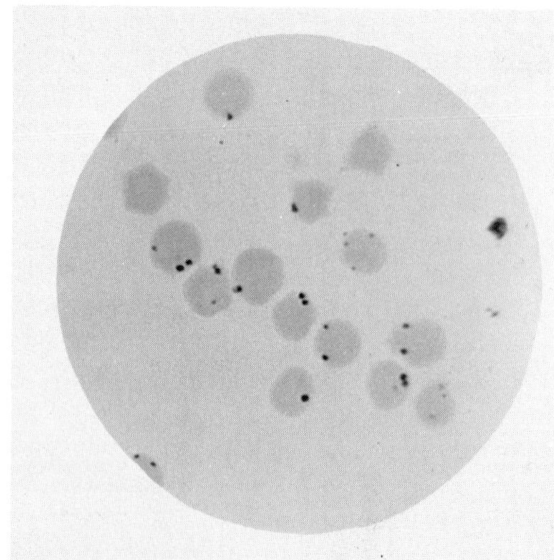

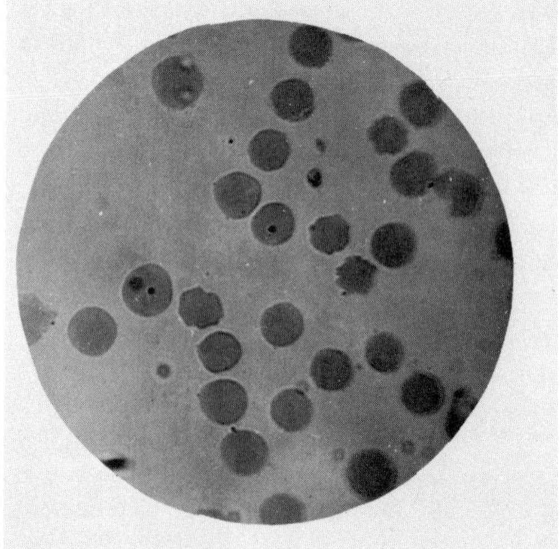

test is a direct conglutination reaction with some animals.

Prevention and Control. Various inactivated and attenuated vaccines have been developed in attempts to provide cattle with protection against natural disease with *A. marginale*. Inactivated vaccines (8, 21, 28) provide increased resistance and clearly reduce losses to the disease. Osorno *et al.* (23) used an attenuated strain produced in sheep and protected vaccinated cattle exposed to natural disease, whereas the attenuated vaccine developed by Zaraza and Kuttler (44) protected most of the immunized cattle agáinst challenge with virulent organisms. The use of either type of vaccine may complicate the control of the disease because it prevents differentiation of vaccinated and infected cattle by serologic tests (8).

The use of various chemotherapeutic agents has been under active study by numerous investigators around the world. These substances have been used to treat clinical cases and also used to eliminate the organism from carrier animals. According to Splitter and Miller (40), anaplasmosis carrier infection can be eradicated by treatment with Terramycin (5 mg per pound of animal weight per day in single or divided doses for 12 to 14 days) or by Aureomycin (15 mg per pound per day in single doses for 16 days). Pearson *et al.* (24) used intramuscular injections of tetracycline at the rate of 5 mg per pound of body weight daily for 10 consecutive days. Aralen hydrochloride, 5 percent sterile aqueous solution, has been approved for the parenteral treatment of anaplasmosis in cattle, and Roby *et al.* (36) recommend dithiosemicarbazone. Kuttler (18) combined dithiosemicarbazone with oxytetracycline to eliminate *A. marginale* in splenectomized calves that were given appropriate levels of each substance. Roby (34, 38) also has shown that imidocarb rapidly causes clearance of the organism from the blood, and it also has been used effectively in the field to treat and control the disease. Adult carrier cattle are given 5 mg per kg subcutaneously or intramuscularly at 14-day intervals to eliminate the parasite from carrier animals. Two or three doses usually suffice. Other drugs such as chloramphenicol, rolitetracycline, and dithiosemicarbazone (in combination with pytetracycline) presumably can accomplish the same objectives. Latent infections have been eliminated by feeding 1.1 mg of chlortetracycline per kg of body weight for 120 days in the ration (29).

It has been stated that the relapse which ordinarily follows splenectomy in *Anaplasma*-infected calves does not occur in those animals that have been previously treated with cortisone (32).

Eradication programs have consisted of continuing testing and stray-dipping of imported cattle, or the selection of uninfected replacement heifers from infected dams by means of the complement fixation (CF) test conducted 30 to 60 days after weaning and by placing them in CF-negative groups.

REFERENCES

1. Amerault and Roby. World An. Review, 1977, *22*, 34.
2. Bedell and Dimopoullos. Am. Jour. Vet. Res., 1962, *23*, 618.
3. Bedell and Dimopoullos. Am. Jour. Vet. Res., 1963, *24*, 278.
4. Boynton. Cornell Vet., 1928, *18*, 28.
5. Boynton. Cornell Vet., 1929, *19*, 387.
6. Boynton and Woods. Jour. Am. Vet. Med. Assoc., 1935, *87*, 59.
7. Boynton and Woods. Science, 1940, *91*, 168.
8. Brock. Proc. Am. Vet. Med. Assoc., 1963, p. 258.
9. Buening. Am. Jour. Vet. Res., 1974, *35*, 371.
10. Carson, Sells, and Ristic. Am. Jour. Vet. Res., 1977, *38*, 173.
11. Christensen, Osebold, Harrold, and Rosen. Jour. Am. Vet. Med. Assoc., 1960, *136*, 426.
12. Davis, Dimopoullos, and Roby. Res. Vet. Sci., 1970, *11*, 594.
13. Espana, Espana, and Gonzolez. Am. Jour. Vet. Res., 1959, *78*, 795.
14. Franklin, Heck, and Huff. Am. Jour. Vet. Res., 1963, *24*, 483.
15. Freidhoff and Ristic. Am. Jour. Vet. Res., 1966, *27*, 643.
16. Gates, Madden, Martin, and Roby. Am. Jour. Vet. Res., 1957, *18*, 257.
17. Kreier, Ristic, and Schroeder. Am. Jour. Vet. Res., 1964, *25*, 343.
18. Kuttler. Res. Vet. Sci., 1972, *13*, 536.
19. Lotze. Proc. Heminthol. Soc. Wash., 1946, *13*, 56.
20. Love. Am. Jour. Vet. Res., 1972, *33*, 2557.
21. McHardy and Simpson. Trop. An. Health and Prod., 1973, *5*, 166.
22. Osebold, Christensen, Longhurst, and Rosen. Cornell Vet., 1959, *49*, 97.
23. Osorno, Solana, Perez, and Lopez. Am. Jour. Vet. Res., 1975, *36*, 631.
24. Pearson, Brock, and Kliewer. Jour. Am. Vet. Med. Assoc., 1957, *130*, 290.
25. Price, Brock, and Miller. Am. Jour. Vet. Res., 1954, *15*, 511.
26. Price, Poelma, and Faber. Am. Jour. Vet. Res., 1952, *13*, 149.
27. Reese. North Am. Vet., 1930, *11*, 7.
28. Richey, Brock, Kliewer, and Jones. Am. Jour. Vet. Res., 1977, *38*, 169.
29. Richey, Borck, Kliewer, and Jones. Am. Jour. Vet. Res., 1977, *38*, 171.

30. Ristic. Jour. Am. Vet. Med. Assoc., 1962, *141*, 588.
31. Ristic and Mann. Am. Jour. Vet. Res., 1963, *24*, 478.
32. Ristic, White, Green, and Sanders. Am. Jour. Vet. Res., 1958, *19*, 37.
33. Ristic, White, and Sanders. Am. Jour. Vet. Res., 1957, *18*, 924.
34. Roby. Res. Vet. Sci., 1972, *13*, 519.
35. Roby, Amerault, Mazzola, Rose, and Ilemobade. Am. Jour. Vet. Res., 1974, *35*, 993.
36. Roby, Amerault, and Spindler. Res. Vet. Sci., 1968, *9*, 494.
37. Roby, Gates, and Mott. Am. Jour. Vet. Res., 1961, *22*, 982.
38. Roby and Mazzola. Am. Jour. Vet. Res., 1972, *33*, 1931.
39. Rogers and Wallace. Am. Jour. Vet. Res., 1966, *27*, 1127.
40. Splitter and Miller. Vet. Med., 1953, *48*, 486.
41. Stiles. U.S. Dept. Agr. Cir. 154, 1931.
42. Summers and Matsuoka. Am. Jour. Vet. Res., 1970, *31*, 1517.
43. Theiler. Transvaal Dept. of Agr., Rpt. Govt. Bact., 1908–09, p. 7.
44. Zaraza and Kuttler. Revista Instituto Colombiano Agropecuario, 1976, *11*, 363.

Anaplasma ovis

Anaplasmosis of sheep has been described by DeKock and Quinlan (1) in South Africa. In 1955 Splitter *et al.* (5) reported on a flock of sheep in Kansas. They were investigated because of an obscure debilitating condition. Routine blood examination revealed marginal bodies in the erythrocytes identical in appearance with *Anaplasma marginale,* together with extracellular forms characteristic of *Eperythrozoon ovis*. Splenectomized calves inoculated with this sheep blood did not develop evidence of *A. marginale* infection. It seems probable that they were dealing with *A. ovis*.

In 1956 an organism identified as *A. ovis* was recovered from sheep originating in the Rocky Mountain area of the United States (4). The organism produced variable degrees of subclinical anemia in sheep and goats. Cattle could not be infected with the parasite, nor did it produce any detectable immunity in these animals against *A. marginale*. This agrees with the findings of the South African workers, who have shown that cattle are not infected by *A. ovis*. In 1963 Kreier and Ristic (3) infected two Virginia white-tailed deer (*Dama virginiana*) experimentally with *A. ovis*.

Electron microscopy studies of erythrocytes infected with *A. ovis* have revealed a membrane-enclosed body, usually marginally located and filled with two initial bodies (2).

REFERENCES

1. DeKock and Quinlan. 11th and 12th Rpt. Dir. Vet. Ed. and Res., Union of So. Africa, 1926, p. 369.
2. Jatkar. Am. Jour. Vet. Res., 1969, *30*, 1891.
3. Kreier and Ristic. Am. Jour. Vet. Res., 1963, *24*, 567.
4. Splitter, Anthony, and Twiehaus. Am. Jour. Vet. Res., 1956, *17*, 487.
5. Splitter, Twiehaus, and Castro. Jour. Am. Vet. Med. Assoc., 1955, *127*, 244.

Anaplasma centrale

Theiler (2), in his studies which led to differentiation of the anaplasms from the piroplasms, distinguished two kinds of the former: the marginal bodies, which have already been described and which are the only ones found in anaplasmosis in the United States, and central bodies, which are identical in appearance with the marginal bodies, but are located characteristically in the central part of the red blood cells (Figure 29.2). The central bodies have come to be called by the name *Anaplasma centrale*.

Theiler showed that animals that had recovered from an infection with blood containing the central bodies could still be infected with blood containing the marginal bodies. He also noted that the disease caused by *A. centrale* was much milder than the other. In South Africa, according to Schmidt (1), adult cattle coming from Europe are first injected with blood containing *A. centrale* and later with *A. marginale,* the first and milder infection giving some protection against a severe second. In Australia, where immunization with *A. centrale* is practiced, it has been found that citrated calf blood infected with this parasite retains its effectiveness for 254 days when frozen in 1-ml doses and maintained at −72 to −80 C (3).

REFERENCES

1. Schmidt. Jour. Am. Vet. Med. Assoc., 1937, *90*, 723.
2. Theiler. Zeitschr. f. Infektionskr. Haustiere, 1912, *11*, 193.
3. Turner. Austral. Vet. Jour., 1944, *20*, 295.

THE GENUS *PARANAPLASMA*

In this genus there are 2 species: *P. caudatum* and *P. discoides*. The species in this genus have the same characteristics as *Anaplasma* except the inclusions have appendages. The organisms are infective for cattle but not deer or sheep. All isolations of *P. caudatum* have been from mixed infections with *A. marginale* and *P. discoides*.

REFERENCE

1. Ristic and Kreier. *In* Bergey's manual of determinative bacteriology, 8th ed., ed. Robert E. Buchanan and Norman E. Gibbons. Williams and Wilkins, Baltimore, p. 906.

THE GENUS *AEGYPTIANELLA*

Aegyptianella pullorum

This is the causative agent of aegyptianellosis in birds. Natural infections have been described in chickens, geese, ducks, turkeys, guinea fowls, pigeons, quail, and ostriches. Certain wild birds have been infected experimentally. The disease has been found in South Africa, Indochina, and the Balkans and probably exists in most subtropical and tropical countries.

Chickens are naturally infected with *A. pullorum* by the tick *Argas persicus*. Experimental infection can be achieved by parenteral injection or by scarification with infected blood. The disease is frequently associated with fowl spirochetosis. Native fowl rarely suffer an acute disease, but newly introduced stock may die within a few days with diarrhea, anorexia, a high temperature, and paralysis.

In blood smears stained with Giemsa cells, a great variety of forms, violet reddish in color with a diameter of 0.3 to 3.9 μm, appear in the infected host's erythrocytes. In larger inclusions clearly defined smaller round organisms (initial bodies) measuring up to 0.8 μm in diameter can be seen. The organisms may be found free in the plasma and in phagocytic cells. The infectivity can be preserved for 71 days by freezing in liquid nitrogen. The organism has not been cultivated *in vitro*. The organisms are sensitive to dithiosemicarbazones and tetracyclines. There are other species that eventually may be placed in this genus, but their true identity or relationship to *A. pullorum* has not been established. They are as follows: *Tunetella emydis, Sogdianella moshkovskii, Aegyptianella carpani,* and other organisms that have been reported in a number of domestic and wild birds.

REFERENCE

1. Ristic and Kreier. *In* Bergey's manual of determinative bacteriology 8th ed., ed. Robert E. Buchanan and Norman E. Gibbons. Williams and Wilkins, Baltimore, 1974, p. 909.

THE GENUS *HEMOBARTONELLA*

Most species of *Hemobartonella* are infectious, but the disease is usually not apparent except in the case of *H. felis* in cats.

Hemobartonella muris (*Bartonella muris*)

This organism was first described by Mayer (23) in Germany in 1921. It was found in laboratory rats that had been infected with trypanosomes. The organism, like the previous one, is found in and on the surface of the red blood cells. According to Peters and Wigand (29), *H. muris* when stained by Giemsa stain shows mostly coccoid forms in contrast to *Bartonella bacilliformis,* which shows mostly rod shapes. Electron microscopy studies of *H. muris* do not show structural details, cell walls like those of bacteria, or flagella. Thin sections reveal a spherical or ellipsoidal agent, 350 to 700 μm in size (43). It is nonmotile and increases by binary fission, but apparently does not multiply outside the host's blood. It is transmitted by lice and is ubiquitous in geographic distribution. It usually will not cause infection in rats unless the animals are infected with trypanosomiasis, are given certain blood-destroying poisons, or are splenectomized. Of great interest is the fact that rats in many parts of the world, including the United States, carry this organism latently. This can be demonstrated by the fact that removal of the spleen often leads to prompt development of the disease. It appears that the spleen, possibly through a protective activity of its reticuloendothelial system, is able to hold the disease in abeyance. The disease is manifested by a rapidly developing anemia and by the appearance of the organism in the blood. The animals may die, or they may recover after a few days. Other animals susceptible to infection with *H. muris* are mice, hamsters, and rabbits.

Hemobartonella canis (*Bartonella canis*)

In 1928 Kikuth (17), in Germany, described an organism similar to the other species of *Hemobartonella* which he believed to be the cause of an infectious anemia of dogs. Workers in other countries have, more recently, seen the same organism. None has succeeded in cultivating it, however; hence its relationship to the other *Hemobartonella* species has not been proved. The disease appears to be rather mild. Knutti and Hawkins (18) in the United States (1935) encountered the condition in splenectomized, bile-fistula dogs. Spontaneous periods of anemia, associated with excess bile production, were regularly associated, in some dogs, with the appearance of *Hemobartonella*like bodies in the blood (Figure 29.3). Simple splenectomy would not regularly produce the disease, but the inoculation of dog's blood containing the hemobartonellae into such animals was regularly followed by anemia and the appearance of the parasite. *H. canis* was transmitted to splenectomized dogs by all stages of *Rhipicephalus sanguineus*. There was stage-to-stage as well as transovarial transmission (33).

Hemobartonella felis

Feline infectious anemia was first described by Flint and Moss (10) in 1953. It is an acute, subacute, or chronic infectious disease of domestic cats and wild cats. When acute, it is characterized by high temperature, a marked hemolytic anemia, anorexia, depression, and rapid loss of weight. Blood smears offer the best diagnostic aid. The parasites occur as small round dots, short rods, or coccoids that sometimes are in chains. The rods are 0.2–0.5 to 0.9–1.5 μm and the coccoids are 0.1–0.8 μm in diameter. There is no rigid cell wall but it possesses a double limiting membrane. The parasites frequently occur attached to or partly embedded in erythrocyte membrane which may be eroded at point of contact. The parasites stain deep purple with Giemsa stain. Fluorescent antibody or acridine orange may reveal the organism when it cannot be seen with Giemsa stain. The organism has not been cultivated *in vitro*.

Figure 29.3. Giemsa stain of blood film from a dog showing *Hemobartonella canis*. × 1,070. (Courtesy M. M. Benjamin and W. V. Lumb, *Jour. Am. Vet. Med. Assoc.*)

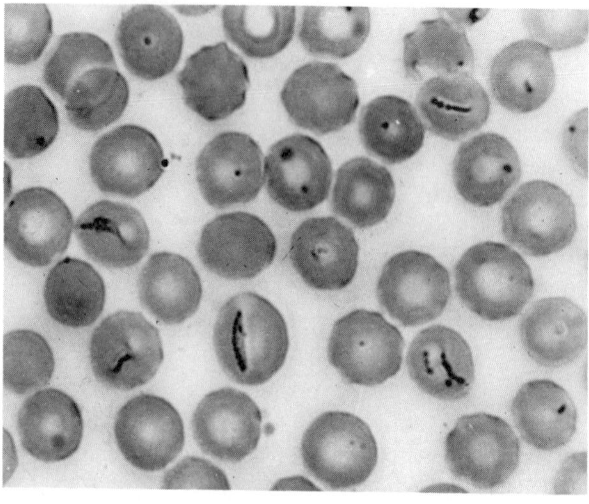

The infection can be transmitted by parenteral injection (14) or oral route. Intrauterine infection may occur, and it may be spread by biting during cat fights. Arthropod demonstration has not been established, and the organism is rather host-specific. Carriers do exist. The disease appears to be widespread in the USA.

Various chemotherapeutic agents such as chloramphenicol, tetracycline, oxytetracycline, and neoarsphenamine are effective in suppressing the disease.

Hemobartonella bovis (*Bartonella bovis*)

Donatien and Lestoquard (8) reported *Hemobartonella* in the blood of cattle in 1934. Lotze and Yiengst (22) found similar forms in American cattle in 1942. Since they were found in animals infected with anaplasmosis, the American workers were not certain that they did not represent a stage of the life cycle of *Anaplasma marginale*. Later Lotze and Bowman (20) found them in an anaplasma-free calf shortly after it had been splenectomized. It is clear, therefore, that *H. bovis* is not necessarily associated with anaplasmosis. Usually only a very few parasites are found in the blood, but they may become much more numerous during the incubation period following innoculation with anaplasms. There is no evidence, at present, that *H. bovis* is of any economic importance.

Hemobartonella are also found in goats (25), but appear to be of little economic importance.

Hemobartonella tyzzeri

This organism was found by Weinman and Pinkerton (44) in splenectomized guinea pigs from Colombia. The parasite could be transmitted to splenectomized *Hemobartonella*-free guinea pigs by intraperitoneal injection (13).

THE GENUS *EPERYTHROZOON*

Differentiation of members in this genus from *Hemobartonella* is often difficult and perhaps arbitrary in some instances. Hemobartonellae rarely occur as ring forms, while eperythyrozoa often do. Hemobartonellae

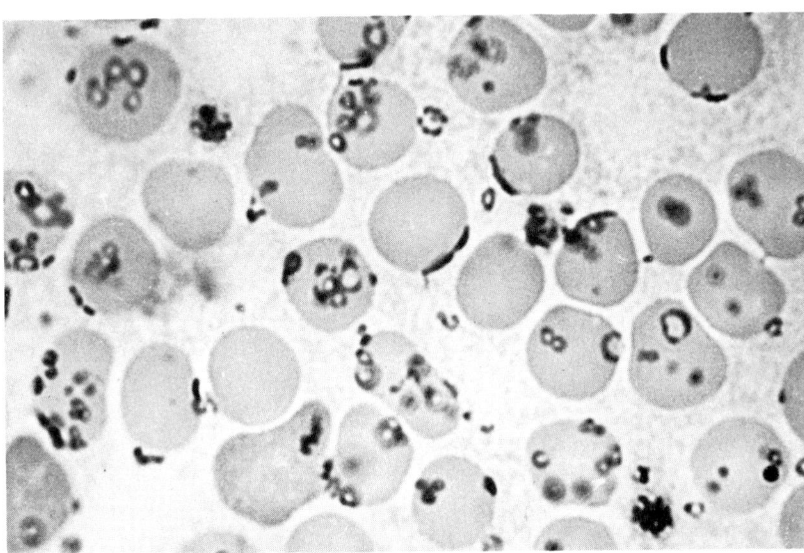

Figure 29.4. *Eperythrozoon suis* in the blood of an infected pig. × 2,225. (Courtesy A. Savage and J. M. Isa, *Cornell Vet.*)

rarely occur free in the plasma while eperythrozoa occur with equal frequency on the erythrocytes and in the plasma. Swarmlike clusters of ring-shaped eperythrozoa may occur on the surface of erythrocytes (Figure 29.4). Rod-shaped forms may occur partly or entirely circling a blood cell. In fresh preparations examined by dark-field and phase microscopy, coccoids, but no ring forms, are observed. By electron microscopy the organism appears pleomorphic surrounded by a single limiting membrane with no cell wall, nucleus, or other organelles. Typical of the family Anaplasmataceae, the organism has not been cultivated in cell-free media. Some species have been transmitted by arthropods. Infective blood readily produces the disease upon parenteral inoculation. Splenectomy activates latent infection with most species. The growth of the organism is inhibited by tetracyclines and arsenicals.

Eperythrozoon coccoides

This organism was described in 1928 by Schilling and by Dinger (7) as a blood parasite of mice. The characteristics of *H. muris* and *E. coccoides* correspond in nearly every respect, there being some trifling differences in morphology. Giemsa stains of both organisms generally show a preponderance of coccoid forms for *H. muris* and a majority of ring-shaped bodies for *E. coccoides*. Like *H. muris* this organism is nonmotile and appears not to multiply outside the host blood. It is ubiquitous in distribution and is transmitted by lice. Rats, hamsters, and rabbits are also subject to infection.

Ott and Stauber (28) observed mice that were infected with malaria and also with *E. coccoides*. In these mice the malarial infection progressed at a low-level, chronic course producing infrequent deaths. When the eperythrozoa were eliminated through treatment with oxophenarsine hydrochloride (arsenoxide), the malarial infection assumed an acute course always ending in death.

The organism inhibits the interferon response in mice during the first 3 weeks after infection (11). By 6 weeks the production of interferon in response to Newcastle disease virus returned to a normal level. Further, the clearance of parasitemia was correlated with the appearance of circulating neutralizing antibody.

Eperythrozoon suis

In 1950 Splitter and Williamson (39) found an eperythrozoon in swine associated with a clinical entity known as *anaplasmosislike disease* or *icteroanemia*. They saw the organism in three separate outbreaks. Since that time eperythrozoonosis has been found to be rather widespread in the United States (2, 4). It has also been described in western Germany associated with louse infestations (16). The causative agent has been named *E. suis*, and a second species, which apparently is a nonpathogenic blood parasite, was named *E. parvum*. The latter organism is a common parasite of swine in the Midwest. *E. suis* also shows a high incidence rate in the blood of swine in enzootic areas. The majority of young pigs acquire infection during the summer months and remain immune, latent, clinically unrecognized carriers. The clinical disease depends on the number of parasites that develop in the blood following infection. In the majority of swine, light parasitic attacks take place and cause no visible damage. Pigs heavily infected with *E. suis* show inappetence, lassitude, weakness, anemia, and often icterus. Diagnosis is made by finding small, ring-shaped bodies in or on the erythrocytes of diseased pigs. Splitter (38) has found a complement-fixation test useful in diagnosing eperythrozoonosis in swine. He employs an antigen prepared from CO_2-precipitated erythrocytes heavily parasitized with *E. suis*. Smith and Rahn (36) employed an indirect hemagglutination test for the diagnosis of *E. suis* infection in swine.

The exact mode of transmission is not known, but insect vectors such as flies and lice seem to play a role. Berrier and Gouge (3) have reported a case of *in utero* transmission.

Eperythrozoon wenyoni

Neitz (27) reported the presence of this organism in cattle in South Africa. *E. wenyoni* is observed as a mixed infection with other bovine blood organisms. Lotze and Yiengst (21) observed eperythrozoonosis in the United States in cattle experimentally infected with *Anaplasma marginale*. Mirzabekov (24) in Russia described the disease in conjunction with *Babesia bigemina*. Hinaidy (15) in Austria described the organism in a steer with severe *B. divergens* infection. In recent years the infection has also been reported in Holland (45), New Zealand (41), England (31), Columbia (1), and Ireland (30), in some instances associated with clinical signs of illness. Although the economic importance of these organisms is unknown, they are believed to be significant at times in calves. Finerty *et al.* (9) prepared an antigen by ultrasonic disruption of purified suspensions of *E. wenyoni* and claimed that it was specific when used in passive hemagglutination tests for detecting naturally occurring eperythrozoonosis in calves.

Eperythrozoon ovis

Neitz (26) reports that this organism provokes illness in sheep that are not splenectomized. It is a disease of lambs with considerable mortality and showing postmortem features of anemia, enlarged soft spleen, and an excess of pericardial fluid. More recently, Sonoda *et al.* (37) observed the disease in some adult sheep that had a fever, anemia, cardiac palpitation, tachypnea, and hemoglobinuria. In southern Australia it appears that the majority of anemic conditions of young sheep and the majority of outbreaks of ill-thrift are caused by *E. ovis* infection and that the severity of the disease may depend on complicating factors (35).

Daddow and Dunlop (6) monitored the disease in a national outbreak in Australia. The complement-fixation test (5) and blood smears were used to determine the presence of infection in the ewes and their lambs. The ewes appeared to be the main source of infection for their lambs, and the infection may have been spread by mosquitoes or sand flies. The complement-fixation test is a valuable diagnostic procedure on a herd basis.

Sutton and Jolly (42) have studied the effects of *E. ovis* in sheep under experimental conditions. Infection in lambs was characterized by a hypochromic anemia with one-half of normal hemoglobulin content. If maintained on pasture there was a retardation of growth that was not observed in housed sheep fed without restriction. The incubation period is inversely proportional to the infecting dose. Infected sheep have low venous blood glucose levels and corresponding increased blood lactic acid levels (40). The acidosis and hypoglycemia associated with infection could be potentially serious in pregnant ewes and in poorly fed sheep.

Neitz states that antimony-arsenic compounds are valuable in treating the infection. Spirotrypan forte (34) is effective but sometimes quite toxic and expensive, so it is not recommended for field use.

Eperythrozoon felis

In 1959 Seamer and Douglas (32) described a new blood parasite in cats in England and called it *E. felis*. Because the differences between *Hemobartonella* and *Eperythrozoon* are very minor, it is possible that they were dealing with feline infectious anemia.

Treatment

Organic arsenical substances, such as neoarsphenamine and arsenic-antimony compounds, are not effective in bartonellosis, but have a marked influence on hemobartonellosis and eperythrozoonosis. All three diseases are refractory to sulfa compounds. Penicillin, streptomycin, and Chloromycetin show a curative effect on bartonellosis. *H. muris* and *E. coccoides* resist penicillin and streptomycin, but are quite sensitive to Aureomycin, Terramycin, and tetracycline. Chloromycetin has little, if any, effect (29). Gledhill *et al.* (12) studied a mouse colony that had a history of long-established infection with *E. coccoides* and claimed that they were able to eliminate the organisms by regular insecticidal treatments designed to reduce infestation with lice and fleas.

REFERENCES

1. Adams, Craig, Platt, and Wyss. Revista Institutio Colombiano Agropecuario, 1976, *11*, 89.
2. Adams, Lyles, and Cockrell. Jour. Am. Vet. Med. Assoc., 1959, *135*, 226.
3. Berrier and Gouge. Jour. Am. Vet. Med. Assoc., 1954, *98*, 124.
4. Biberstein, Barr, Larrow, and Roberts. Cornell Vet., 1956, *46*, 288.
5. Daddow. Austral. Vet. Jour., 1977, *53*, 139.
6. Daddow and Dunlop. Queenland Jour. Ag. and An. Sci., 1976, *33*, 233.
7. Dinger. Zentrbl. f. Bakt., Abt. I. Orig., 1929, *113*, 503.
8. Donatien and Lestoquard. Bull. Soc. Path. Exot., 1934, *27*, 652.
9. Finerty, Hidalgo, and Dimopoullos. Am. Jour. Vet. Res., 1968, *30*, 43.
10. Flint and Moss. Jour. Am. Vet. Med. Assoc., 1953, *22*, 45.
11. Glasgow, Murrer, and Lombardi. Inf. and Immun., 1974, *9*, 266.
12. Gledhill, Niven, and Seamer. Jour. Hyg. (London), 1965, *63*, 73.
13. Groot. Proc. Soc. Exp. Biol. and Med., 1942, *51*, 279.
14. Harvey and Gaskin. Jour. Am. An. Hosp. Assoc., 1977, *13*, 28.
15. Hinaidy. Osterreich Weiner Tierärzt. Monatschr., 1973, *60*, 364.
16. Hoffman and Saalfeld. Deutsche Tierärztl. Wchnschrft., 1977, *84*, 7.
17. Kikuth. Klin. Wchnschr., 1928, *7*, 1729.
18. Knutti and Hawkins. Jour. Exp. Med., 1935, *61*, 115.
19. Kreier and Ristic. Bergey's manual of determinative bacteriology, 8th ed., ed. Robert E. Buchanan and Norman E. Gibbons, Williams and Wilkins, Baltimore, 1974, p. 912.
20. Lotze and Bowman. Proc. Helminth. Soc. Washington, 1942, *9*, 71.
21. Lotze and Yiengst. North Am. Vet., 1941, *22*, 345.
22. Lotze and Yiengst. Am. Jour. Vet. Res., 1942, *8*, 312.
23. Mayer. Arch. Schiffs-u, Trophyg., 1921, *25*, 150.
24. Mirzabekov. Veterinariya, Moscow, 1974, *6*, 68.
25. Mukherjee. Indian Vet. Jour., 1952, *28*, 343.
26. Neitz. Onderstepoort Jour. Vet. Sci. and Anim. Indus., 1937, *9*, 9.
27. Neitz. Onderstepoort Jour. Vet. Sci. and Anim. Indus., 1940, *14*, 9.
28. Ott and Stauber. Science, 1967, *155*, 1546.
29. Peters and Wigand. Bact. Rev., 1955, *19*, 150.
30. Poole, Cutler, Kelly, and Collins. Vet. Rec., 1976, *96*, 481.
31. Purnell, Brocklesby, and Young. Vet. Rec., 1976, *98*, 411.
32. Seamer and Douglas. Vet. Rec., 1959, *71*, 405.
33. Seneviratna, Weerasinghe, and Ariyadasa. Res. Vet. Sci., 1973, *14*, 112.
34. Sheriff. Vet. Rec., 1973, *93*, 288.
35. Sheriff, Clapp, and Reid. Austral. Vet. Jour., 1966, *42*, 169.
36. Smith and Rahn. Am. Jour. Vet. Res., 1975, *36*, 1319.
37. Sonoda, Takahashi, Tamura, and Koiwa. Jour. Jap. Vet. Med. Assoc., 1977, *30*, 3.
38. Splitter. Jour. Am. Vet. Med. Assoc., 1958, *132*, 47.
39. Splitter and Williamson. Jour. Am. Vet. Med. Assoc., 1950, *116*, 360.
40. Sutton. Austral. Vet. Jour., 1977, *53*, 478.
41. Sutton, Charleston, and Collins. New Zeal. Vet. Jour., 1977, *25*, 8.
42. Sutton and Jolly. New Zeal. Vet. Jour., 1973, *21*, 160.
43. Tanka, Hall, Sheffield, and Moore. Jour. Bact., 1965, *90*, 1735.
44. Weinman and Pinkerton. Ann. Trop. Med. and Parasitol., 1938, *32*, 215.
45. Wensing, Nouwens, Schotman, Vernooy, and Zwart. Tijdschr. v. Diergeneeskd., 1974, *99*, 136.

30 The Chlamydiaceae

The name that heads this chapter was suggested by Smadel (51) to designate a number of agents that have in common many characteristics not possessed by viruses. Jones, Rake, and Stearns (31) regard these agents as belonging to a higher developmental level than viruses. Some authors follow Bergey in using the generic term *Miyagawanella* for them, but most use *Chlamydia* and classify these organisms as bacteria that lack some important mechanisms for production of metabolic energy and thus lead an intracellular existence (42).

Included in this group are the agents of psittacosis, ornithosis, pneumonitis and conjunctivitis, sporadic bovine encephalomyelitis, polyarthritis, placentopathy, enteritis, cat-scratch fever, enzootic abortion of ewes, and enzootic bovine abortion. It was first suggested that the agent of salmon poisoning belonged in the family Chlamydiaceae; however, it is now generally regarded as a member of the family Rickettsiaceae.

The agents of all these diseases contain a common group antigen. All of them are susceptible to certain chemotherapeutic and antibiotic agents. Most of them are capable of producing pneumonitis in mice and are cultivable in the yolk sac of chick embryos, All of them are elementary bodies—200 to 300 nm in diameter. They have the same developmental cycle and contain RNA and DNA in relative amounts of each at different growth stages. They may vary in the specificity of cell-wall antigens, toxins, and species-differentiating biochemical properties. In studies of 4 purified strains of *Chlamydia psittaci* (1 bovine and 3 ovine) and 1 purified strain of *Chlamydia trachomatis* the number of polypeptides varied between 17 and 20 with a molecular weight range of 29,000 to 120,000 (53). Two polypeptides predominated and comprised approximately one-third of the total protein in each of the 5 strains. In another study Charton *et al.* (10) found that 2 strains of *C. psittaci* had 16 principal polypeptides, with 9 located in the envelope. Of the 5 glycopeptides one was isolated from the envelope and the others from the nucleus.

Bedson and Bland (7) studied the development of the psittacosis agent in the tissues of animals. It was observed that early in the course of infection light blue or purplish bodies appeared in the macrophages of the spleen and in the epithelial cells of the lungs, intestine, liver, and kidneys. At first these bodies appeared homogeneous, but later they became granular. Eventually they became resolved into masses of distinctly stained elementary bodies, spherical in form. These may be distinctively stained with Giemsa's stain, Macchiavello's stain, or Castaneda's stain for rickettsiae. When these bodies are fully formed, the cells that contain them rupture, discharging showers of infective elementary bodies into the tissue fluids. This developmental cycle is characteristic of all members of this group. Confirmation that the granular material in the plaques consists of psittacoid protein has been supplied by fluorescent antibody studies (17).

The bacteria that cause the psittacosis-lymphogranuloma-trachoma group diseases and that are assigned to the genus *Chlamydia* can be separated logically into two species, *C. trachomatis* and *C. psittaci,* according to Page (42). This separation is based on relatively stable morphological and chemical characteristics of the organisms rather than on their presumed natural hosts or tissue preferences or on the specific serology of their cell-wall antigens. Attempts to classify these bacteria on host specificities or serology has led to great confusion in the past.

Organisms of *C. trachomatis* that are associated with trachoma, inclusion conjunctivitis, or lymphogranuloma venereum of man or mouse pneumonitis have compact intracytoplasmic microcolonies that produce sufficient quantities of glycogen detectable by staining with iodine and that are inhibited by sodium sulfadiazine. In contrast, the members of *C. psittaci* frequently associated with psittacosis, meningopneumonitis, guinea pig conjunctivitis, bovine encephalomyelitis, feline pneumonitis, or caprine pneumonitis have diffuse microcolonies that fail to produce glycogen or to exhibit susceptibility to sodium sulfadiazine. Except for the 6BC parakeet strain which is glycogen-negative, but sulfadiazine sensitive, all strains isolated from many animal species were readily separated into one of the two species, *C. trachomatis* or *C. psittaci*. Until we obtain more concrete information regarding the epidemiology of the *Chlamydia* and develop more specific tests and information as to how they relate to the disease(s) in various hosts, the above scheme as proposed by Page (42), which as reviewed and approved by a majority of the members of the Subcommittee on the Chlamydiaceae (Taxonomy Committee, American Society of Microbiology), is logical and acceptable and will be used in this textbook. Some of the diseases caused by various strains of *C. psittaci* are given in Table 30.1, with principal emphasis on the diseases in domestic animals.

The review article (45) will provide more detailed information and additional references on chlamydial diseases in animals and in humans.

Psittacosis And Ornithosis

Psittacosis is a disease occurring in birds belonging to the parrot family (Psittacidae). Ornithosis is the same disease when it occurs in a variety of nonpsittacine birds. Formerly it was thought that ornithosis, when it affected man, was much milder than psittacosis, but this is not always the case (40). The disease contracted from pigeons generally is milder than that contracted from parrots or parakeets, but that contracted from turkeys is fully as severe as any of psittacine origin. The agent causing these diseases generates a toxin that apparently has much to do with the virulence of the strain.

Psittacosis in the United States occurs principally in green Amazon parrots and in shell parakeets. In the tropics it evidently occurs widely in many kinds of parrots and parakeets. Pinkerton and Swank (46) first reported the disease (ornithosis) in the domestic pigeon. Subsequently it has been found in this species in many American cities. Smadel, Wall, and Gregg (52) reported it in New York City; Davis and Ewing (16) in Baltimore; and Zichis, Shaughnessy, and Lemke (6) in Chicago. Meyer and Eddie (39) reported a human case of ornithosis contracted from a flock of chickens, and Wolins (59) reported a number of cases contracted from domestic ducks. Haagen and Mauer (24) identified the agent in a sea bird, the fulmar petrel, which is used for food by the inhabitants of the Faroe Islands. During the last several years a new reservoir of ornithosis infection—the domestic turkey—has come to light.

The disease has attracted wide attention from time to time because of epidemics in man. During one of these outbreaks in Paris in 1893, Nocard isolated a bacterium belonging to the *Salmonella* groups which he regarded as the causative agent. It was commonly accepted as such until the pandemic in Europe and the United States in the winter of 1929–1930, during which workers showed that Nocard's organism was not commonly present but that a psittacoid agent regularly could be isolated. The *Salmonella psittacosis* of Nocard is now known to have been *Salmonella typhimurium*, a chance contaminant.

The outbreak in man which occurred in 1929–30 was traced to green Amazon parrots imported from South America. In 1930 rigid restrictions on the importation of these birds into the United States were instituted to prevent a recurrence of the incident. In a survey made in 1932 Meyer, Eddie, and Stevens (41) discovered that the disease was well established in southern California in shell parakeets (lovebirds). It was found that more than 1,100 aviaries engaged in breeding and containing more than 100,000 birds existed as a "backyard industry" in that region, and that nearly one-half of these premises were infected. In 1933 the interstate quarantine regulations were amended to provide for the control of interstate shipment of psittacine birds in order to prevent infected birds from being shipped out of the region where the disease was enzootic. Through efforts of health authorities, the incidence of the disease has been greatly reduced in the enzootic region. In addition approximately 98 percent of psittacine birds (245,000 in 1969) are introduced into the U.S. from Public Health Service-approved treatment centers. This program

Table 30.1. Chlamydial diseases caused by *C. psittaci*

Disease manifestation	Known geographical distribution	Natural hosts	Recommended experimental hosts	Epidemiological aspects
Psittacosis (Humans)	Worldwide	Man, wild and domestic fowl	Embryonated hens' eggs, mice, guinea pigs, wild and domestic birds	Principally transmitted from birds to man, but man-to-man transmission occurs as aerosol infection. Also associated with cases of lymphogranuloma venereum and abortions in humans.
Psittacosis, ornithosis (Birds)	Worldwide	Wild and domestic fowl	Same	Endemic in psittacine and columbidine birds and probably in water fowl. Carriers exist in all fowl.
Placentopathy				
Enzootic abortion in ewes	Scotland, England, Hungary, Germany, France, United States	Sheep	Embryonated hens' eggs, guinea pigs, sheep, cattle, pigeons, and sparrows	Endemic in sheep. Arachnids and/or insects may play a role in transmission. Perhaps pigeons, sparrows, and other domestic animals as well.
Epizootic abortion in cattle	Spain, Germany, Italy, United States	Cattle	Embryonated hens' eggs, guinea pigs, sheep, and cattle	Periodically endemic in California and Oregon (USA) cattle. Arachnida and/or insects may play a role in transmission as well as sheep and other domestic animals.
Abortions in other domestic animals	United States	Pigs, goats, rabbits, mice	Embryonated hens' eggs, guinea pigs, and respective natural hosts for each *C. psittaci* isolate	Placentopathy not widely observed in these species. Interspecies disease relationships not well known.
Sporadic bovine encephalomyelitis	Australia, Canada, Germany, South Africa, United States	Cattle, dogs	Embryonated hens' eggs, guinea pigs, hamsters, cattle, and dogs	Endemic in USA cattle. Little known about the infection in dogs.
Pneumonitis				
Feline	Worldwide	Cats, man	Embryonated hens' eggs, mice, cats, hamsters, and guinea pigs	Endemic in the domestic cat. Transmitted by aerosol and infective excretions from cat to cat.
Ovine	United States	Sheep	Embryonated hens' eggs, mice, guinea pigs, sheep	Probably endemic in sheep-raising areas of USA. Sheep-to-sheep transmission.

Bovine	Czechoslovakia, Italy, Japan, United States	Cattle	Embryonated hens' eggs, mice, guinea pigs, and cattle	Endemic. Cattle-to-cattle transmission.
Caprine	Japan	Goats	Goats, embryonated hens' eggs, guinea pigs	Endemic.
Canine	United States	Dog, budgerigars, humans?	Dogs, budgerigars, embryonated hens' eggs, guinea pigs	Only one case in dog reported.
Equine	Australia, West Germany, Finland	Horse	Embryonated hens' eggs, horse	Endemic in horses.
Murine	United States	Mice	Mice, embryonated hens' eggs, guinea pigs	Endemic in certain mouse colonies.
Conjunctivitis				
Guinea pig	Worldwide	Guinea pigs	Guinea pigs, embryonated hens' eggs	Endemic as a conjunctivitis in some colonies. May be transmitted transovarially.
Hamster	Worldwide	Hamsters	Hamsters, embryonated hens' eggs, guinea pigs	Endemic as conjunctivitis in some hamster colonies.
Ovine	Worldwide	Sheep	Cell culture	Endemic in some flocks.
Polyarthritis				
Ovine	United States (principally intermountain area)	Sheep	Sheep, turkeys, guinea pigs, embryonated hens' eggs	Endemic in lambs in intermountain area of USA. Transmission from sheep to sheep, intestinal carriers may cause polyarthritic disease.
Bovine	United States	Cattle	Cattle, guinea pigs, embryonated hens' eggs	Known calf-to-calf transmission.
Equine	United States	Horses	Embryonated hens' eggs, horses	Little known.
Enteritis				
Snowshoe hare and muskrat	Canada, Wisconsin (USA)	Snowshoe hares and muskrats	Snowshoe hares, muskrats, embryonated hens' eggs	Muskrat may be principal reservoir in nature.
Bovine	Worldwide	Cattle	Cattle, guinea pigs, embryonated hens' eggs, mice.	Endemic in cattle. Many intestinal carriers.

markedly reduces transmission of bird and human psittacosis from imported psittacine birds.

From 1929 through 1942, 380 human cases of psittacosis (including ornithosis) were reported to the U.S. Public Health Service (18). Of these, 170 occurred during the epidemic of 1929–1930 and 210 later. Eighty deaths were recorded, of which 33 occurred during the epidemic. The number of cases of psittacosis in man dropped off sharply when restrictions were established by the government on the trade on psittacine birds. These restrictions were lifted in 1953 with the result that the incidence of human infections has again risen (21, 50). During 1974, 163 cases of human psittacosis were reported; during the years 1963 through 1973 the average was 46 cases per year. The majority of the reported cases in 1974 occurred in employees of turkey-processing plants (19).

From the public health viewpoint the most serious reservoir of infection in the United States is the domestic turkey. Irons, Sullivan, and Rowen (29) called attention to this in 1951 when they reported 22 human cases with 3 deaths among 78 employees in a small turkey-dressing plant in Texas. Others have since reported outbreaks in Texas, Nebraska, Oregon, California. Michigan, Wisconsin, Minnesota, Ohio, and New Jersey. It is quite obvious that the disease is widespread in turkeys in the United States and undoubtedly exists in many other areas where it has not yet been recognized. Turkey ornithosis has been identified in Canada but, according to the published literature, not in any other parts of the world.

Character of the Disease. The virulence of psittacosis and ornithosis agents varies greatly. In many outbreaks in various species, the disease was recognized only after human attendants became ill from it, and in others only by the recognition of antibodies for it. On the other hand, some outbreaks have exhibited high mortality rates among both birds and human contacts. In birds the disease generally is manifested by inappetence, great depression, the presence of nasal and eye discharges, and severe diarrhea. Recovered individuals usually continue to eliminate the agent in their discharges for long periods of time.

The mortality varies widely according to species, age, and virulence of the agent. In young psittacine birds it may be as high as 75 percent to 90 percent. In young pigeons it may be nearly as high. In turkeys it generally is much lower, but may be as high as 25 percent. Actually, the attack rate in most species is rather significant. Most infections are inapparent or undiagnosed. In man, before the advent of antibiotics, it varied between 10 percent and 30 percent, averaging about 20 percent. These cases were of parrot origin. The current mortality rate is much lower because the disease can be effectively treated with antibiotics, if diagnosed sufficiently early.

In psittacine birds. Generally speaking, psittacosis presents few or no signs of illness in the older birds. It is the younger birds that are most apt to develop acute and fatal infections, and these are the principal spreaders of the disease. The incubation period in parrots varies widely from a few days to several weeks. In young birds the course of illness is short—3 to 7 days. In older ones it is chronic as a rule. Affected birds refuse feed and are greatly depressed, their feathers become ruffled and soiled with the yellowish-green diarrheal feces, they have mucopurulent nasal discharges, and often their eyes are pasted shut with exudate. Usually they become greatly dehydrated and emaciated before death. Those that recover almost always continue to eliminate the organism in their discharges for long periods of time. It is these birds that keep the disease alive by infecting the younger birds of the flock. Parrots and parakeets that are convalescent carriers remain wholly well, or may at times suffer from transient diarrhea. The carrier state is often discovered only when the pet owners develop psittacosis.

The lesions vary in different species of birds, but the general pattern is the same. In psittacine birds swelling of the spleen is generally seen. There is an enlargement of the liver, and frequently the organ has necrotic foci. Sometimes it is covered with a layer of fibrin. Inflammation of the air sacs occurs and this lesion varies from mild clouding to the presence of caseous masses of exudate. Fibrinous pericarditis is commonly seen. In all acute cases there is a severe enteritis characterized by bloody diarrhea.

In pigeons. Adult birds may be listless, have no appetite, show nasal and eye discharges, and suffer from diarrhea. According to Coles (11), who was the first to describe ornithosis in pigeons, this disease should be suspected in any birds that are affected with conjunctivitis. The incubation period is 5 to 9 days.

Affected squabs are weak and show signs similar to those of adults. Most of these die. Many of the adult birds recover, become convalescent carriers, and serve as sources of infection to fanciers and to those who feed and fondle these birds in city parks and squares. The incidence may be very high.

The lesions are similar to those described for psittacine

birds except a swollen spleen usually does not occur in nonpsittacine birds.

In turkeys. In many outbreaks the virulence of the infection is very low (3), the losses are not serious, and the disease is likely to be undiagnosed. Graber and Pomeroy (23) have shown that strains from such outbreaks may cause human infections. On the other hand, the disease may be serious, with mortality rates of well-developed birds running as high as 25 percent. The signs of the disease often resemble those of fowl cholera or erysipelas. The birds become apathetic, do not eat well, show depression, and develop diarrhea. The diarrheal discharges are fluid, often contain blood, and generally cause matting of the feathers in the region of the vent. Many birds become greatly emaciated.

In ducks. Outbreaks in the United States have generally been inapparent. The disease has been recognized either because of human contact cases or by serological or cultural procedures.

In chickens. A few cases of ornithosis in chickens have been reported. In these instances the disease has been inapparent.

In geese. The disease in goose flocks has been of economic significance in Hungary (54). It caused between 15 and 55 percent mortality among goslings between 12 and 45 days of age in several flocks in 1972.

In other birds. Ornithosis has been recognized in geese, gray herons, and pheasants, occurring in an inapparent form. Mention has been made of the occurrence of the disease in the petrels of the Faroe Islands.

Page (44) investigated the involvement of wildlife in an epornosis of domestic turkeys and found antibodies in blackbirds, sparrows, and one of four mourning doves, but no isolations of *C. psittaci* were made.

In experimental animals. Parrots that have not previously suffered from the disease are readily infected by inoculation parenterally or orally, or by the respiratory route. Java sparrows and reed birds are readily infected by contact and by inoculation. Adult chickens are not readily infected, but young birds can easily be infected by inoculation. White mice are highly susceptible and are commonly employed for diagnostic purposes. Injection with agents of psittacine origin intraperitoneally results in infection, but injection with agents of nonpsittacine origin frequently fails. Ornithosis agents are best inoculated intracerebrally. Guinea pigs, rabbits, and monkeys can be infected by inoculation, but in these species the disease often is not fatal.

Properties of the Agent. That the disease could be produced by filtrates made from organs of diseased birds was shown, early in 1930, by Krumwiede, McGrath, and

Oldenbusch (33) in the United States and by Bedson, Western, and Simpson (8) in England, working independently.

The agent of psittacosis is filterable only through rather coarse filters. Membrane studies indicate that its particulate size is between 200 and 300 nm, a size sufficiently great that the elementary bodies are visible microscopically. The coccoid bodies found in the lesions of parrots, mice and men are of about this size. There is a general relation between the concentration of these bodies and virulence, and it is known that they are the infectious agents. These bodies were found at about the same time and were described independently in 1930 by Levinthal (35) in Germany, by Coles (11) in England, and by Lillie (36) in the United States. They are generally known as LCL bodies, the letters representing the initials of the names of these workers. Lillie at first regarded them as rickettsiae, but now they are considered to be elementary bodies of the psittacoid group. The fluorescent antibody technique has been used in recent years to prove that the LCL bodies contain RNA and DNA. The LCL bodies are Gram-negative, nonmotile organisms that multiply within the cytoplasm by a developmental cycle, unique among bacteria. Following penetration of the host cell the elementary bodies increase in size, 900 to 1,000 nm in diameter, to become initial bodies which increase to form clusters of plaques in a matrix. These thin-walled, noninfectious, larger forms multiply by fission, and daughter cells change to the smaller infectious elementary bodies, 200 to 300 μm, which contain ribosomes and a diffuse nucleus. This process takes place in a vesicle whose wall disintegrates releasing hundreds of elementary bodies into the cytoplasm. Microscopic examination of wet-cell preparations by phase microscopy or of stained preparations by regular light microscopy shows clusters of organisms of various sizes in the cytoplasm of many host cells. The small infectious form, 200 to 300 μm, stains purple with Giemsa's stain, red with Macchiavello's and Gimenez's stains, and blue with Castenada's stain. The large noninfectious form, 900 to 1,000 μm, is blue with Giemsa's and Macchiavello's stains, and purple with Castenada's stain. Phase-contrast microscopy avoids time-consuming staining procedures, and it also eliminates staining artifacts. By either method it is difficult to distinguish intracellular *Mycoplasma* organisms from chlamydiae, so diagnostic procedures other than smear preparations should be included to make a positive diagnosis.

By ultrastructural analysis of infected cell cultures and cells of the intestinal mucosa of newborn calves, four distinct morphological forms of chlamydial development were observed; elementary bodies, dispersing forms, reticulate bodies, and condensing forms which proceed to form elementary bodies (56).

Cultivation and Resistance of *Chlamydia*. The elementary bodies of members of this group may be propagated rather easily in a number of ways. Yanamura and Meyer (60) in 1941 reported successful cultivation of the agent in tissue fragments suspended in various fluids, in tissue fragments spread over the surface of serum agar slants, and in the yolk sac of developing chick embryos when the agent was introduced by a technique developed by Cox (12) for the propagation of rickettsiae. It will also develop on the chorioallantoic membrane and in the allantoic cavity of the chick embryo. Because infected cells rupture and discharge their content of elementary bodies, it is possible, in a number of ways, to obtain suspensions comparatively free from extraneous yolk-sac materials. These suspensions can be used for agglutination and complement-fixation tests. (For more information about cultivation see the section on diagnosis.)

The cell walls of chlamydiae contain considerable lipid, which makes them susceptible to lipid solvents and detergents. Consequently, a 1:1,000 dilution of quaternary compound (alkyl-dimethylbenzl-ammonium chloride) is an effective disinfectant for laboratory and hospital use. Phenol, in contrast, is a poor disinfectant. The organisms resist acid and alkali. They are rapidly destroyed by heat, but the death time is related to the amount of protective cellular material present.

Various strains produce a cytopathogenic effect in mammalian-cell cultures, but cell cultures are less commonly used than the embryonated hen's egg for research and diagnosis.

Immunity. It has been pointed out that after recovery from the active disease birds usually harbor the chlamydiae for long periods of time. During this time they possess a marked resistance to reinfection, as might be expected. The organism tends to remain in mammals also for considerable periods after clinical recovery, and it has been suggested that immunity in this disease is always due to the harboring of latent infection, but this has not been substantiated.

Neutralizing antibodies are not always demonstrable in animals immune to chlamydiae and are seldom present in great concentration. Nevertheless, animals that have received chlamydiae intramuscularly without production of disease are protected against intratracheal inoculations that produce pneumonia in nonimmunized animals.

Several workers (6, 28) have shown that mice and pigeons could be partially immunized by several injections of inactivated chlamydiae. The protection is not great enough to be useful. Turkeys vaccinated intratracheally, intramuscularly, and subcutaneously with live ornithosis agents of low virulence prepared from yolk-sac and mouse-tissue suspensions stimulated direct complement-fixing antibody titers. The presence of these titers in the vaccinated turkeys could not be equated to resistance to infection by an ornithosis isolate of high virulence (5). Adding concentrated suspensions of *Bordetella pertussis* to a bacterin of *C. psittaci* afforded significant protection to turkeys (43). Since *B. pertussis* organisms selectively stimulate T lymphocytes, cell-mediated immunity probably has an important part in the immunity to *C. psittaci*.

Transmission. These diseases apparently are transmitted in both birds and mammals largely by means of infected droplets. David, Delaplane, and Watkins (15) and others were unable to find any evidence indicating that virus was ever transmitted through the eggs of birds. A considerable number of laboratory infections in humans have occurred. In many cases these persons actually handled the infected birds and may have contracted the infection otherwise, but there have been a considerable number of persons infected without any direct contacts, and air-borne infection seems the only possible route (2, 37). In turkey-dressing establishments, it was noted that most of the infections occurred in areas where an aerosol was set up by the machinery. Rivers and Schwentker (49) found that monkeys could easily be infected by inhalation but that fully virulent material failed to infect when injected subcutaneously or intramuscularly. A number of volunteers among laboratory workers were immunized by parenteral injection of the fully virulent psittacosis agent without adverse results.

The ornithosis agent has been isolated from several species of poultry ectoparasites, suggesting that this may also be a vector-borne infection.

Diagnosis. The clinical picture may suggest psittacosis or ornithosis, but seldom can a positive diagnosis be made without confirmation by laboratory tests.

1. Animal inoculations. Experienced workers have been quite successful in isolating the agent by inoculating chick embryos into the allantoic cavity or the yolk sac (27), but the most successful way of recovering the agent is by mouse inoculation (48). Intraperitoneal injection of filtrates of human sputum or of unfiltered sputum, in case organisms are not present which kill the animals prematurely, usually kill these animals in from 5 to 14 days, occasionally as late as 30 days. If any of the mice sicken after the 4th or 5th day, they should be destroyed and examined for the characteristic focal necrosis of the liver. Films are made from the liver tissue, and a search is made for the elementary bodies of psittacosis. If the mice are still living after 30 days, it is well at that time to inject them with the known psittacosis agent to determine whether or not they may have developed immunity from an infection that did not become apparent. A 20 to 40 percent suspension of suspect tissues can be used for transfer in experimental animals.

The method described apparently is efficient for detecting the disease in man or in birds of the parrot family, but the pigeon agent usually does not kill mice or produce the liver lesions. The organism from these birds can usually be recovered, however, by inoculating the mice intracerebrally instead of intraperitoneally. The pigeon agent is more highly virulent for pigeons than that from parrots. The parrot agent will, however, usually produce inapparent infections in pigeons (39).

In using mice and guinea pigs the diagnostician and research worker should be aware that mice and guinea pig colonies may be naturally infected with chlamydiae. The murine pneumonitis strain of *C. trachomatis* has been isolated from the lungs of mice from many colonies. The organisms are demonstrated by repeated passage of homogenized lung suspensions from carrier mice into normal mice by aerosol exposure. Infected mice eventually develop a diffuse pneumonitis, and the organisms are readily demonstrated in lung-smear preparations. Guinea pigs may be naturally infected with *C. psttaci,* which manifests itself as a conjunctivitis and is readily transmitted by contact.

All strains of chlamydiae can be isolated and propagated in the yolk sac of the embryonated hen's egg. Depending on the source of inoculum, proper treatment must be performed to rid the inoculum of bacteria or *Mycoplasma,* which usually grow well in the egg. If bacterial contaminants are suspected, the test material should be ground in a phosphate-buffered saline solution (pH 7.2) containing 1 mg per ml each of streptomycin sulfate, vancomycin, and kanamycin. This markedly reduces bacterial contamination without affecting the *Chlamydia* population. Normally, a 10 percent suspension is injected into the yolk sac of 5- to 7-day-old embryonated hens' eggs with death ensuing 5 to 12 days later. The capillaries of infected eggs are not sharply outlined when candled. Infected embryos and yolk-sac membranes are congested and frequently hemorrhagic. Stained smears of yolk-sac membranes show the presence of the chlamydiae organisms (Figure 30.1). An antigen prepared from an infected yolk sac fixes complement in the presence of a positive chlamydial antiserum in the complement-fixation test. This result constitutes a positive diagnosis of chlamydiae. If no embryos die in first passage three blind passages of yolk-sac material harvested 10 to 14 days after inoculation with no specific embryo deaths are required to conclude that the avian tissue homogenate did not contain *C. psittaci*.

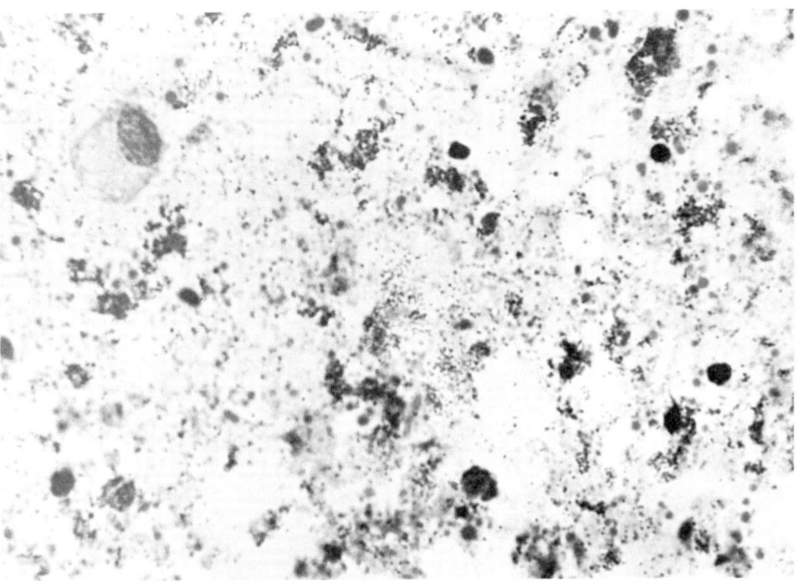

Figure 30.1. *Chlamydia psittaci.* A Gimenez-stained impression smear of a yolk-sac preparation infected with a chlamydial strain of mouse pneumonitis. × 880. (Courtesy J. Storz.)

2. Cell cultures. Most strains of *C. psittaci* propagate in cultured cells and produce sufficient cell destruction to show plaque formation (46). Intracellular microcolonies (plaques) can be seen 2 to 7 days after inoculation. Presence of chlamydiae can be demonstrated in 2 ways: (*a*) by the direct fluorescent antibody test (FAT), and (*b*) by utilization of the tissue-cultured preparation as an antigen in the complement-fixation test. The FAT is reputedly more sensitive for their identification in cell cultures, but not in smear preparations from yolk sac and other animal tissues.

Chlamydial agents multiply in cell cultures derived from various tissues of different hosts. A few such cell cultures are human embryonic skin, muscle, or lung (42), chick embryo (49), and most cells of the McCoy line (55). When a cytopathic effect occurs, it is mediated by the release of lysosomal enzymes into the host cytoplasm during the late stages of chlamydial development (54).

3. Serological tests. All members of chlamydiae contain a group-specific antigen that is a lipopolysaccharide. The antigen is resistant to phenol, heat, and various proteinases but inactivated by lecithinase and periodate. Antigens may be prepared in a variety of ways (34) to test for the group-specific antigen: in the direct complement-fixation (CF) test that is used principally for detection of CF antibodies in avian sera in which normal rooster serum is added as a test component to make the test workable; indirect CF (ICF) test; capillary tube agglutination test; gel-diffusion techniques; and hemagglutination test (4). These test procedures can be found in the textbook by Lennette and Schmidt (34).

The cell walls of chlamydiae contain a mosaic of antigens that are distinct from the group-specific antigen. The cell-wall antigens are often shared within a group of strains affecting a certain class of animals (human, mammal, and avian strains) and some antigens cross animal classes. Consequently no precise serological classification of chlamydial strains is possible at present (22).

The CF test (22) may be used to confirm the presence of the disease in flocks, but it has been shown that carrier birds of all species do not always react to this test and recent infections may not be detected. CF antibodies usually appear in birds and mammals within 7 to 10 days after infection. Some animals with intestinal infection may have no detectable CF antibodies. The height of a titer reflects the antigenic properties and recentness of infection, but it may not reflect current infection. Thus, the serologic diagnosis of infection requires demonstration of a 4-fold rise in CF antibody titer using paired sera. If 80 percent or more of individuals in a group have a demonstrable titer and half have titers of 1:64 or greater, this constitutes reasonable proof that the group of animals is currently infected with chlamydiae. The agar-gel-diffusion test has been used as an adjunct to the CF test as antibodies may be detected in serum(s) of pigeons that are negative by the CF test, thus demonstrating differing kinetics of precipitating and CF antibody formation (30).

Benedict (9) has used an intradermal test for this detection. It detects fewer chronically infected birds than the complement-fixation test. They become allergic 4 weeks after experimental infection.

4. Serum neutralization, plaque reduction, and toxin neutralization. In the neutralization test the embryo is protected from death by the neutralization of the infective particle with the specific antiserum prior to inoculation. In the toxin neutralization test the early death of mice inoculated intravenously with large numbers of organisms is prevented by the injection of specific antitoxin. The mechanism of the plaque reduction is similar to the neutralization test in the hen's egg except cell cultures are used as the indicator system for detecting *Chlamydia* activity. In these three tests high-titered antisera must be used, and results in comparative studies of chlamydiae reflect variation in cell wall antigens responsible for infectivity and provide a means to establish serotypes among some strains of *C. psittaci*.

Treatment. Unlike viruses, the psittacosis-lymphogranuloma group shows definite susceptibility to the action of some of the sulfonamides and antibiotics. Heilman and Herrell (26) in 1944 showed that large doses of penicillin would save the majority of mice inoculated with the psittacosis agent, although most of them developed inapparent infections, which made them resistant to later injections of the same strain. It has been demonstrated by several groups that the same thing is true of the disease in man. Meiklejohn, Wagner, and Beveridge (38) showed that penicillin would inhibit growth of this agent in tissues but it was ineffective in eggs. Early and Morgan (20) found that sulfadizine in food protected mice from death when the mice were inoculated with the psittacosis agent, but most of the animals became carriers. Streptomycin was not effective. The same workers found that sulfadiazine protected chick embryos from some strains but was ineffective against others.

It is apparent that many of the antibiotics exert an

influence on agents of the ornithosis group, but it appears that most are incapable of completely eliminating the chlamydiae from victims of the disease. The most successful are tetracycline compounds (13), Chloromycetin, rifampicin, nalidixic acid, and 5-fluorouracil. These must be given in rather high concentrations in the feed to accomplish sterilization. Lower doses serve to lower mortality rates, but leave many carriers. Davis and Delaplane (14) found that a concentration of chlortetracycline of 200 g per ton in an all-mash ration was required to eliminate the ornithosis agent from a group of 3-week-old poults. Experimentally infected adult turkeys, treated for 2 to 3 weeks with 200 to 400 g per ton of mash, failed to yield organisms.

In view of the initially low rate of psittacosis infection in most wild or uncrowded captive psittacines, group treatment with 0.5 percent chlortetracycline in dry pelleted feed for 45 days was practical, effective, and economically feasible, and might be considered an adequate safeguard against the hazard of psittacosis (1). More recently, Haass (25) in Southwest Germany has reported "that the widely recommended antibiotic feeding of imported psittacine birds is an inadequate control method since there is an increasing number of positive isolations of *C. psittaci* from cage birds."

Chlortetracycline is used very successfully for treating human infections, providing the diagnosis is made early and the treatment is carried on for a considerable time at a high dosage level. Too small a dosage and too short a treatment time result in relapses.

The Disease in Man. The disease in humans is characterized by fever, headache, and pneumonia. The pneumonia is an atypical, patchy, bronchopneumonia that cannot be clinically differentiated from viral-induced pneumonia. *C. psittaci* has been demonstrated in left atrial or valve biopsy specimens from 7 of 27 cases of acquired valvular heart disease (58), suggesting the organism may be cause of some cases of valvular heart disease.

The disease is seldom conveyed from person to person, although it may be unless precautions against droplet infection are taken. Ordinarily the disease in man is derived from the very considerable reservoir that exists in birds, where it often occurs as a latent disease. In recent years the majority of diagnosed human cases in the United States occurred in individuals associated with infected turkeys.

REFERENCES

1. Arnstein, Eddie, and Meyer. Am. Jour. Vet. Res., 1968, *29,* 2213.
2. Badger. Pub. Health Rpts. (U.S.), 1930, *45,* 1403.
3. Bankowski and Page. Am. Jour. Vet. Res., 1959, *20,* 935.
4. Barron, Jakay-Roness, and Bernkopf. Proc. Soc. Exp. Biol. and Med., 1965, *119,* 377.
5. Bates, Pomeroy, and Reynolds. Avian Dis., 1965, *9,* 220.
6. Bedson. Brit. Jour. Exp. Path., 1938, *19,* 353.
7. Bedson and Bland. Brit. Jour. Exp. Path. 1932, *13,* 461; 1934, *15,* 243.
8. Bedson, Western, and Simpson. Lancet, 1930, *1,* 235.
9. Benedict. Am. Jour. Hyg., 1957, *66,* 245.
10. Charton, Faye, Gueslin, Solsona, and Layee. Bull. de Acad. Vet. France, 1976, *49,* 401.
11. Coles. Lancet, 1930, *1,* 1011.
12. Cox. Pub. Health Rpts. (U.S.), 1938, *53,* 2241.
13. Cox. *In* Beaudette. Psittacosis. Diagnosis, epidemiology, and control. Rutgers Univ. Press, New Brunswick, N.J., 1955, p. 137.
14. Davis and Delaplane. Am. Jour. Vet. Res., 1958, *19,* 169.
15. Davis, Delaplane, and Watkins. Am. Jour. Vet. Res., 1957, *18,* 409.
16. Davis and Ewing. Pub. Health Rpts. (U.S.). 1947, *62,* 1484.
17. Donaldson, Davis, Watkins, and Sulkin. Am. Jour. Vet. Res., 1958, *19,* 950.
18. Dunnahoo and Hampton. Pub. Health Rpts. (U.S.), 1945, *60,* 354.
19. Durfee. Jour. Inf. Dis., 1975, *132,* 604.
20. Early and Morgan. Jour. Immunol., 1946, *53,* 151 and 251.
21. Fitz, Meiklejohn, and Baum. Am. Jour. Med. Sci., 1955, *229,* 252.
22. Fraser. *In* Analytical serology of microorganisms, vol. 1, ed. J. B. Kwapinski. Wiley, New York, 1969, pp. 257–330.
23. Graber and Pomeroy. Am. Jour. Pub. Health, 1958, *48,* 1469.
24. Haagen and Mauer. Zentrbl. f. Bakt., I Abt. Orig.. 1938, *143,* 81.
25. Haass. Tierärzt. Umschau, 1973, *28,* 625.
26. Heilman and Herrell, Proc. Mayo Clinic, 1944, *19,* 204.
27. Hudson, Bivins, Beaudette, and Tudor. Jour. Am. Vet. Med. Assoc., 1955, *126,* 111.
28. Hughes. Jour. Comp. Path. and Therap., 1947, *57,* 67.
29. Irons, Sullivan, and Rowen. Am. Jour. Pub. Health, 1951, *41,* 931.
30. Ismael, Krauss, and Geissler. Berl. und Münch. tierärztl. Wchnschr., 1975, *88,* 21.
31. Jones, Rake, Stearns. Jour. Inf. Dis., 1945, *76,* 55.
32. Kissling, Schaeffer, Fletcher, Stamm, Bucca, and Sigel. Pub. Health Rpts. (U.S.), 1956, *71,* 719.
33. Krumwiede, McGrath, and Oldenbusch. Science, 1930, *71,* 262.
34. Lennette, David A. and Nathalie J. Schmidt. Diagnostic procedures for viral and rickettsial diseases, 4th ed. Am. Public Health Assoc., New York, 1970.

35. Levinthal. Klin. Wchnschr., 1930, *9*. 654.
36. Lillie. Pub. Health Rpts. (U.S.), 1930, *45*, 773.
37. McCoy. Pub. Health Rpts. (U.S.), 1930, *45*, 843.
38. Meiklejohn, Wagner, and Beveridge. Jour. Immunol., 1946, *54*, 1 and 9.
39. Meyer and Eddie. Proc. Soc. Exp. Biol. and Med., 1932–33, *30*, 484.
40. Meyer and Eddie. Proc. Soc. Exp. Biol. and Med., 1953, *83*, 99.
41. Meyer, Eddie, and Stevens. Am. Jour. Pub. Health, 1935, *25*, 571.
42. Page. Internat. Jour. System. Bact., 1968, *18*, 51.
43. Page. Am. Jour. Vet. Res., 1975, *36*, 597.
44. Page. Jour. Am. Vet. Med. Assoc., 1976, *169*, 932.
45. Pienaar and Schutte. Onderstepoort Jour. Vet. Res., 1975, *42*, 77.
46. Pinkerton and Swank. Proc. Soc. Exp. Biol. and Med., 1940, *45*, 704.
47. Piraino. Jour. Bact., 1969, *98*, 475.
48. Rivers and Berry. Jour. Exp. Med., 1935, *61*, 205.
49. Rivers and Schwentker. Jour. Exp. Med., 1934, *60*, 211.
50. Sigel, Cole, and Hunter. Am. Jour. Pub. Health, 1953, *43*, 1418.
51. Smadel. Jour. Clin. Invest., 1943, *22*, 57.
52. Smadel, Wall, and Gregg. Jour. Exp. Med., 1943, *78*, 189.
53. Stephenson and Storz. Am. Jour. Vet. Res., 1975, *36*, 881.
54. Szemeredy and and Sztojkov. Magyar Allatorvosk Lapja, 1973, *28*, 554.
55. Tanami, Pollard, and Starr. Virol., 1961, *15*, 22.
56. Todd, Doughri, and Storz. Zentrbl. f. Bakt., 1976, *236A*, 359.
57. Todd and Storz. Inf. and Immun., 1975, *12*, 638.
58. Ward and Ward. Lancet. 1974, *2*, 734.
59. Wolins. Am. Jour. Med. Sci., 1948, *216*, 551.
60. Yanamura and Meyer. Jour. Inf. Dis., 1941, *68*, 1.
61. Zichis, Shaughnessy, and Lemke. Jour. Bact., 1946, *51*, 616.

Enzootic Abortion of Ewes

SYNONYMS: Ovine enzootic abortion, ovine virus abortion; abbreviation, EAE

This disease is caused by *C. psittaci*. It affects pregnant ewes, causing them to abort in late pregnancy. The clinical signs of the disease are indistinguishable from those of ovine vibriosis. This form of the disease is worldwide in distribution and causes marked economic losses.

Enzootic abortion of ewes was recognized as an infectious disease by Stamp *et al.* (20) in Scotland in 1950. The disease has since been diagnosed in England, Germany, France, and Hungary. In 1958 a disease which had been under observation for several years in the United States (Montana) was recognized as being caused by an agent of the psittacosis-lymphogranuloma-trachoma group (26). It was suspected to be the same as the European disease. When the agents were compared (24), they were found to be identical. *C. psittaci* can cause various disease manifestations in sheep. Schachter *et al.* (17) used the plaque reduction test to show that ovine chlamydial isolates could be separated into 2 types. Type 1 isolates usually were associated with ovine abortion and intestinal infection, whereas type 2 isolates caused polyarthritis and conjunctivitis.

Character of the Disease. Abortions occur from midgestation to late pregnancy. Retention of the placenta is frequent, and a vaginal discharge is seen for several days following lambing or abortion. The aborted fetuses may be mummified or quite normal in appearance. The cotyledons are dark red or clay-colored. The ewe is visibly ill and has fever of 2 or 3 degrees higher than normal lasting for periods up to 1 week. The genital organs quickly return to normal, and subsequent fertility is not impaired. Experimentally infected sheep react with a febrile response beginning about 3 days after inoculation. Abortions occur at least 56 days following injection or feeding the infectious agent.

The mortality rate in the ewes is virtually nil, although many lambs may be lost. In the ewe, inflammation and necrosis of the placentoma is observed. The affected fetus shows hepatopathy, occasionally edema, ascites, vascular congestion, and tracheal petechiae. Histological changes in the fetus have been described by Djurov (1).

Associated neonatal complications such as weak lambs showing nervous signs or pneumonia may occur in flocks (18). In flocks where ovine abortion occurs, epididymitis and orchitis in rams is observed. The organism has been isolated from the genital tract of 2 neonatal lambs after the clinical onset of epididymitis (11).

The Disease in Experimental Animals. Weanling white mice may be killed by intranasal inoculation of infective yolk sac material. Large doses sometimes kill adult mice when they are administered intracerebrally or intravenously. Some of these mice die as a result of intoxication from the toxin, and within a few hours following inoculation. Others die after a few days of infection. Febrile reactions may be produced in guinea pigs by intraperitoneal injections, but these animals seldom die of the infection. Animals killed during the febrile reaction show enlarged friable livers, containing minute necrotic areas, splenic enlargement, and little else (10).

Guinea pigs are the laboratory animal of choice for the isolation of ovine chlamydiae because these animals are more susceptible than chicken embryos or mice.

Strains of enzootic abortion of ewes (EAE) produce abortions in sheep under natural conditions (22). A strain of enzootic bovine abortion also has been incriminated in the production of disease and abortions of sheep (23). The goat EAE agent caused abortion in an experimental ewe and also in two experimental cows (5). The sheep EAE agent causes experimental disease in pigeons and a lethal disease in sparrows under experimental conditions (8). A sheep strain of *C. psittaci* that was isolated from a naturally occurring case of pneumonia caused abortion in experimental ewes, but the disease differed from typical EAE infection (23).

The parenteral injection of bovine or ovine chlamydial agents into rams produced seminal vesiculitis with a granulomatous response that was limited mostly to interstitial tissues (2). Excretion of *Chlamydia* in the semen continued until the experimental rams were slaughtered 8 to 22 days after inoculation. During the acute febrile stage the organism was isolated from the blood and somatic organs. Complement-fixing antibodies rose sharply 1 week after inoculation, reaching peak titers of 128 to 512. The leukocytes in semen increased in number during the experiment and the two rams receiving the calf polyarthritis strain of *C. psittaci* had pus in the semen. The frequency of secondary morphologic abnormalities of spermatozoa increased by 20 days after injection.

Properties of the Agent. The ovine abortion agent is a typical member of the psittacosis-lymphogranuloma-trachoma group. It conforms to the general characteristics of the group. Like other members of the group it is sensitive to penicillin and some of the sulfonamides, but is unaffected by streptomycin and para-aminobenzoic acid. It is highly sensitive to Chloromycetin, erythromycin, and the tetracyclines. It forms a toxin that is lethal to mice, but is is believed to play a minor role in the disease of sheep (24).

The agent causes hemagglutination of goose erythrocytes at titers varying from 1:8 to 1:128 depending on the batch of antigen and pH (4). The optimal reaction occurred at pH 6. It did not produce hemagglutination of erythrocytes of man, mouse, guinea pig, or fowl. Storz (21) showed that the fecal organism invaded the placenta and the developing fetus just as did the agent causing enzootic abortion of ewes.

Cultivation. The agent grows readily and in high concentration in the yolk sacs of embryonated hens' eggs, 5 to 7 days old. The growth of the embryos is retarded, and they succumb before hatching. Chlamydiae injected into the allantoic cavity causes death of some embryos.

Various mammalian cell cultures will support the replication of EAE strains including diploid cells from lung and myocardium of sheep embryos (9), suspension of hamster embryo cells (16), McCoy and Hela 229 cells (12). The plaque assay method in McCoy cells was highly sensitive and reproducible (12).

C. psittaci (var. *ovis*) was cultured in *Hyalomma* tick embryo cells, and the antigen was detected by direct immunofluorescence for 30 to 45 days after inoculation (19). Not all strains produce a cytopathic effect on monolayer cultures. In some instances it may be necessary to stain the cultures to enhance observation of the cytoplasmic inclusions.

Immunity. A single infection solidly immunizes ewes for their normal life expectancy (6, 7). The presence of complement-fixing antibody resulting from subclinical or clinical infection to the *Chlamydia* group antigen ameliorates the clinical response and may prevent abortion in sheep following inoculation of the epizootic bovine abortion agent. The immunity conferred by the antibody is relative because a large challenge dose may cause ewes to abort (24).

Transmission. The disease may readily be transmitted to susceptible, pregnant ewes by inoculation. Natural transmission of the disease presumably occurs by ingestion. This explains how the disease spreads in a flock of pregnant ewes. The persistence of the fecal agent may explain how the disease carries over from one lambing season to the next. The susceptibility of pigeons and sparrows to the EAE agent suggests another means of transmission to sheep and a reservoir for it in nature. It has been suggested that arachnids and/or insects may play some role in its transmission. Susceptible sheep, placed on pastures on which the disease occurs one season, seldom will show any evidence of the disease the following season (25). Venereal transmission by infected rams is probable as another means of transmission.

Diagnosis. It is difficult to make a definite clinical diagnosis, because *Chlamydia* abortion and vibriosis exhibit essentially the same signs of illness. Flocks in which vibrios cannot be found should be suspected of harboring the psittacoid agent. The diagnosis can be verified by inoculating stomach contents of aborted fetuses or placental tissues into the yolk sac of embryonated eggs or guinea pigs. The complement-fixation test will give evidence of infection with an agent of the group.

In recent years other serological tests have been recommended to reinforce the diagnosis of ovine abortion. They include the hemagglutination test (3), immunofluorescence test (13), agar-gel-precipitation test (14), and a complement-fixation micromethod (15).

The elementary bodies generally can be identified in Giemsa-stained smears of cotyledons of aborting ewes. After some experience this method may be used as a diagnostic procedure.

Control. It was found that the disease can be readily controlled by vaccinating all young ewes with a formalinized vaccine made from the infected yolk sacs of embryonated eggs. Commercial vaccine for this purpose is available. The disease has been controlled very successfully in Europe by vaccination of the young ewes prior to first breeding with the adjuvant, yolk-sac vaccine.

The Disease in Man. There is no evidence that the EAE agent has produced disease in man, but precaution and care should be exercised in handling infectious material from these cases because of the potential health hazard of the *Chlamydia* species to humans.

REFERENCES

1. Djurov. Zentrbl. fur Vet., 1972, *19B*, 578.
2. Eugster, Ball, Carroll, and Storz. 6th Internatl. Mtg. Dis. Cattle, Philadelphia, Pa., 1971.
3. Faye, Charton, Layee, Mage, and Joisel. Bull. de Acad. Vet. France, 1973, *46*, 57.
4. Faye, Charton, Mage, Bernard, and Layee. Bull. de Acad. Vet. France, 1972, *45*, 169.
5. McCauley and Tieken. Jour. Am. Vet. Med. Assoc., 1968, *152*, 1758.
6. McEwan, Dow, and Anderson. Vet. Rec., 1955, *67*, 393.
7. McEwan, and Foggie. Vet. Rec., 1956, *68*, 686.
8. Page. Am. Jour. Vet. Res., 1966, *27*, 397.
9. Pankova, Zalkind, Karavaev, Semenova, and D'yakonov. Veterinariya, Moscow, 1977, *7*, 39.
10. Parker. Am. Jour. Vet. Res., 1960, *21*, 243.
11. Rodolakis and Bernard. Bull. de Acad. Vet. France, 1977, *50*, 65.
12. Rodolakis and Chancerelle. Annales de Microbiol., 1977, *128B*, 81.
13. Russo, Vitu, Lambert, and Giauffret. Bull. de Acad. Vet. France, 1977, *50*, 415.
14. Sadowskiand Truszcynski. Bull. Vet. Inst. Pulawy, 1977, *21*, 1.
15. Saint-Aubert, Fayet, and Valette. Rev. Med. Vet., 1975, *126*, 787.
16. Saint-Aubert and Mougeot. Rev. Med. Vet., 1975, *126*, 1323.
17. Schachter, Banks, Sugg, Sung, Storz, and Meyer. Inf. and Immun., 1974, *9*, 92.
18. Schutte and Pienaar. Jour. So. Afr. Vet. Assoc., 1977, *48*, 261.
19. Shatkin, Beskina, Medvedeva, and Grokhovskaya. Med. Parazit. Parazitarnye Bolezni, 1977, *4*, 420.
20. Stamp, McEwan, Watt, and Nisbet. Vet. Rec., 1950, *62*, 251.
21. Storz. Cornell Vet., 1963, *53*, 469.
22. Storz. Jour. Comp. Path., 1966, *76*, 351.
23. Studdert and McKercher. Res. Vet. Sci., 1968, *9*, 48.
24. Studdert and McKercher. Res. Vet. Sci., 1968, *9*, 331.
25. Tunnicliff. Proc. U.S. Livestock Sanit. Assoc., 1958, *62*, 261.
26. Young, Parker, and Firehammer. Jour. Am. Vet. Med. Assoc., 1958, *133*, 374.

Placentopathy in other Domestic Animals

Placentopathy in the goat, pig, rabbit, and mouse caused by *C. psittaci* is not widely observed in the United States. The character of the disease in these species is similar to enzootic abortion in ewes. Comparative studies of the strains of *C. psittaci* that cause placentopathy in domestic animals are lacking.

A well-documented psittacosis abortion epizootic in goats appeared in the literature (1). A chlamydial organism was isolated from an aborted goat fetus in an outbreak that caused a 12 percent abortion rate during 1967 in a California flock of 216 milk goats. There was a marked decrease in incidence after penicillin therapy was given to pregnant goats. This isolate of *C. psittaci* produced abortion in two experimental pregnant cows and one experimental pregnant ewe. An accurate delayed hypersensitivity skin test has been developed for the diagnosis of chlamydiosis in goats utilizing purified *Chlamydia* from yolk sac or McCoy cells (2).

REFERENCES

1. McCauley and Tieken. Jour. Am. Vet. Med. Assoc., 1968, *152*, 1758.
2. Rodolakis, Dufrenoy, and Souriav. Annales de Recherches Veterinaires, 1977, *8*, 213.

Sporadic Bovine Encephalomyelitis

SYNONYM: Buss disease; abbreviation, SBE

This disease affects cattle, particularly those under 3 years of age, and is characterized by encephalitis, fibrinous pleuritis, and peritonitis. It occurs sporadically and is caused by an agent belonging to the psittacosis-lymphogranuloma-trachoma group. So far as is known, only cattle and buffalo are affected. It has been suspected that human infections may occur, but the evidence is inconclusive. Dogs apparently are susceptible, but little is known about the disease in this species.

The disease was first recognized and described in Iowa by McNutt (3) in 1940. It has since been diagnosed in Texas, California, South Dakota, Minnesota, and Missouri. In 1956 Schoop and Kauker (7) described a disease in Germany that was caused by a psittacoid agent that may be the same as SBE. In 1961 an outbreak was described in South Africa (8) and in Canada (1). The disease is also present in Australia. Except for a report in 1973 (5) on encephalitis in buffalo calves in which it was reported that *C. psittaci* was isolated from the brain of 2 calves, there have been no new references on this type of chlamydial disease since 1962.

It is conceivable that the organism causing SBE would fall into the serotype 2 classification of Schachter *et al.* (6).

Character of the Disease. The disease is manifested by profound depression. Fever occurs early in the course of the disease and is maintained until recovery or death approaches. Inappetence, weakness, emaciation, and prostration are characteristic. A clear mucoid discharge from the nose and eyes frequently occurs. A staggering gait is often seen, and the principal joints may be swollen and tender. Some animals develop a mild diarrhea, and some tend to walk or stagger in circles. Opisthotonos occurs occasionally. The disease appears to spread slowly, and many exposed animals seem to escape infection. This may be more apparent than real. As a rule only a few animals in a herd show illness.

By experimental inoculation the incubation period varies widely from 4 to 27 days. In the naturally transmitted disease it is not known, but apparently it is fairly long. The disease is said to have a course of from 1 to 3 weeks. Enright, Sadler, and Robinson (2) present evidence indicating that there are many mild or inapparent cases. These obviously have a much shorter course. From 40 to 60 percent of the clinically sick animals die. Many others are infected with the disease without showing detectable signs of illness; hence the mortality rate is really much lower.

The gross lesions are not conspicuous. In many cases the body cavities contain more than the usual amount of fluid, in which strings of fibrin may be found. The brain usually appears normal, but shows microscopic evidence of a severe and diffuse meningoencephalitis. The meningitis is most severe at the base of the brain.

The Disease in Experimental Animals. The disease is readily produced in young calves by intracerebral or subcutaneous inoculation. Horses, sheep, swine, and mice are not susceptible to inoculation. Guinea pigs, inoculated intraperitoneally, usually die in 4 to 5 days with a fibrinous peritonitis. Hamsters are also susceptible.

Properties of the Agent. The causative agent of SBE is a typical member of the psittacosis-lymphogranuloma-trachoma group. In morphology and growth characteristics in embryonated eggs, and by serology it is difficult to differentiate from other members of *Chlamydia*.

Cultivation. The agent reproduces readily in the yolk sac of chick embryos. We have seen no report of its cultivation in tissue cultures.

Immunity. No observations on the solidity and duration of immunity in this disease have been reported. It is probable that one experience with this disease would be sufficient to protect the animal thereafter.

Transmission. The mode of transmission of this disease is wholly unknown. The disease does not appear to be highly transmissible, but possibly this may be a misconception because many mild or inapparent cases occur. Often it appears on a single farm in a vicinity with no other recognized cases near at hand. Frequently only a small number of cases occur in a herd containing many other presumably susceptible animals. Several have shown that the disease may be transmitted to calves through the milk of infected dams (2, 4).

Diagnosis. The diagnosis is not easy, because the signs of illness often are vague. Evidence of encephalitis, combined with a stiff awkward gait, and the presence of pleuritis, peritonitis, and sometimes pericarditis are indicative. Isolation of the agent by the inoculation of yolk sacs of embryonated eggs is generally successful, and convincing.

Elementary bodies may be found by appropriate staining procedures in the cytoplasm of mononuclear cells in the exudates in the meninges and in the mononuclear cells of serosal membranes and in microglia of nodules. They are not numerous, and often embryonated hens' eggs, guinea pigs, or hamsters are inoculated where the elementary bodies are easier to demonstrate.

Control. No means of controlling this disease are known. The apparent sporadicity has not encouraged attempts to develop prophylactic immunization. Because the agent is very sensitive to most of the antibiotics except streptomycin, use of these in treatment is indicated.

The Disease in Man. Enright, Sadler, and Robinson (2) reported that 51 of 481 samples of human sera collected from persons who had had contact with cattle in California fixed complement with an antigen made from the McNutt strain of SBE. A number of these persons described clinical syndromes consisting of persisting headache and stiff necks lasting about a week, followed by complete recovery. These data provide circumstantial evidence of infection in man, but certainly not conclusive proof.

REFERENCES

1. Bannister, Boulanger, Gray, Chapman, Avery, and Corner. Can. Jour. Comp. Med. and Vet. Sci., 1962, *26,* 25.
2. Enright, Sadler, and Robinson. Proc. U.S. Livestock Sanit. Assoc., 1958, *62,* 127.
3. McNutt. Vet. Med., 1940, *35,* 228.
4. McNutt and Waller. Cornell Vet., 1940, *30,* 437.
5. Ognyanov, Panova, Pavlov, Arnaudov, and Minchev. Veterinarna Sbirka, Bulgaria, 1973, *70,* 13.
6. Schachter, Banks, Sugg, Sung, Storz, and Meyer. Inf. and Immun., 1975, *11,* 904.
7. Schoop and Kauker. Deut. tierärztl. Wchnschr., 1956, *23,* 233.
8. Tustin, Mare, and Van Herrden. Jour. So. African Vet. Med. Assoc., 1961, *32,* 117.

Enzootic Bovine Abortion

SYNONYM: Foothill abortion

This disease is caused by selective strains of *C. psittaci* that cause abortion during late gestation in pregnant domestic cows. *C. psittaci* has also been isolated from bulls with the seminal vesiculitis syndrome (13).

The abortion disease was first reported in the United States and occurs principally in California, where it is known as "foothill abortion," and in the adjoining far western states of the United States. The disease has been reported in Germany, Italy, and Spain (7). The abortion disease is endemic in California and Oregon cattle. The seminal vesiculitis syndrome in bulls is known to occur in the same areas as enzootic bovine abortion. It is now recognized as a worldwide disease of great economic importance. It is suggested that it is second only to brucellosis as a cause of abortion in the bovine species in many parts of the world.

There is evidence that a neonatal disease in calves associated with herd abortions is transmitted *in utero* and in some instances by infected colostrum (2). Prenatal and postnatal losses in 9 herds as a result of chlamydial infection were described by Ehret *et al.* (3).

Schachter *et al.* (12) serotyped chlamydial isolates of bovine origin by using the plaque reduction method. The results were similar to their studies with isolations of ovine origin. Type 1 included isolates from bovine abortion and enteric infections. Type 2 isolates were associated with polyarthritis or encephalomyelitis. Chlamydial isolates causing abortions or intestinal infections in cattle and sheep are closely related antigenically, as are those isolates producing polyarthritis, encephalomyelitis, and conjunctivitis.

Character of the Disease. The agent usually produces a febrile reaction in susceptible cows of all ages. After a latent period of a few months during which *C. psittaci* propagates in the fetus, pregnant animals abort. The disease affects pregnant heifers primarily, and the abortion losses are apt to be as high as 60 percent in these animals (5). The delivery of the aborted fetuses is uneventful, and the placenta is not retained.

Aborted fetuses in natural and experimental disease are distinctive with similar pathological changes (5). They are usually the size of a full-term fetus and die during delivery or shortly thereafter, but some premature calves may survive the disease.

The seminal vesiculitis syndrome is found in the examination of bulls for breeding soundness and is more common among younger bulls. Ball and his coworkers (1) characterized this condition as a chronic inflammation of the seminal vesicles, accessory sex glands, epididymides, and testicles. Affected bulls have inferior semen quality, and some testicles were atrophic. The incidence in a herd may reach 10 percent.

The gross lesions of the abortion disease are limited to the aborted fetus and the fetal membranes (5). The latter are usually thick and edematous. Pale and anemic fetuses usually show petechial hemorrhages of the skin and mucuous membranes. Subcutaneous tissues are wet and edematous. Straw-colored peritoneal and pleural fluid is present. A swollen nodular liver caused by chronic passive congestion may sometimes occur. Petechial hemorrhages are often seen in trachea, tongues, thymus, and lymph nodes. Lymphoid tissues are enlarged with associated lymph stasis. Tiny gray foci that are most difficult to see without proper lighting are irregularly scattered in all tissues. Granulomatous lesions may be present in any organ. Histologically, the disease in the fetus is characterized by a diffuse or focal reticuloendothelial hyperplasia which may involve all organs, but the spleen, thymus, and lymph nodes are most apt to be severely affected.

The Disease in Experimental Animals. Guinea pigs are the laboratory animal of choice for isolation and study of enzootic bovine abortion agents. The embryonated hen's egg and mice are also susceptible. These hosts show the same general signs as described for the EAE (enzootic abortion of ewes) agent.

The injection of pregnant cows with either enzootic bovine abortion or EAE agent produces an abortion disease comparable to natural disease. Signs of impending abortion, consisting of a thin, yellowish vaginal discharge, occurred in 6 of 12 heifers that aborted (6). The elementary bodies were frequently demonstrated in stained smears of this vaginal discharge. It was further observed that pathologic changes of extragenital organs occurred only in internal iliac lymph nodes of infected heifers. Because these nodes drain the genital organs, the lesions are probably the result of the inflammatory process in the gravid uterus where the EBA agent localizes after a short initial blood infectious stage. Omuri *et al.* (10) have induced endometritis by intrauterine inoculation of nonpregnant cows with a *C. psittaci* strain.

A strain of *C. psittaci* isolated from a bull with seminal vesiculitis produced interstitial orchitis and epididymitis, testicular degeneration, and granulomas adherent to the tunica vaginalis propria in inoculated male guinea pigs (13). In contrast, uninoculated male control-guinea pigs failed to show genital lesions.

Properties of the Agent. The enzootic bovine abortion agent shares the properties of all members of *C. psittaci*. The strain of Storz *et al.* isolated from seminal vesiculitis was indistinguishable from a California enzootic bovine abortion strain in the neutralization test (13).

A bull injected intravenously with a strain of *C. psittaci,* which had been recovered from the joint of a calf with polyarthritis, developed a seminal vesiculitis similar to the disease described in rams in the previous section on enzootic abortion in ewes (4). The organism persisted in the semen after recovery from acute disease.

Cultivation. The enzootic bovine abortion strains of *C. psittaci* have the same cultivation characteristics as the EAE strains.

Immunity. All field strains of enzootic bovine abortion that have been compared by neutralization tests are immunologically identical. This information helps us to explain, in part, the field experience of various investigators and clinicians, which indicates that a single exposure to enzootic bovine abortion affords protection against this disease for the normal lifetime of the animal. In experimental studies Lincoln *et al.* (6) indicated the presence of CF antibodies and intestinal *Chlamydia* infection, seemingly had no influence on the experimental production of enzootic bovine abortion disease in pregnant heifers.

The seminal vesiculitis syndrome is observed most frequently in young bulls. After recovery it is possible that they are solidly immune, but there is no experimental evidence to support this concept.

Transmission. The abortion disease may be readily produced in susceptible pregnant cows. Natural disease may spread by ingestion of infected tissues. Another likely route is venereal transmission (8) because the bull may harbor the organism in the semen. There is some suggestion that *Archnida* and/or insects may play a role in the transmission of enzootic bovine abortion and EAE in a herd. Reindeer may be another source of infection for cattle as Neuvonen (9) reported an incidence of 21 percent (63 of 291) in a group that had CF antibody titers of 1:16 or greater.

The persistence of fecal agent results in carriers, and may also explain how the disease persists in a herd.

Diagnosis. To make a positive diagnosis requires isolation and identification of *C. psittaci*. In making a clinical and pathological diagnosis, differentiation from *Brucella abortus* is one principal concern. Granulomatous lesions may be present in any organ of enzootic bovine abortion fetuses, and those in the kidney are similar to *Brucella* infection, but the bronchopneumonia characteristics of fetal *Brucella* infection is lacking (5). Cultural examinations for *Brucella* and *Campylobacter* are indicated in herds troubled with abortions. The cultural smear and serological procedures previously described in this chapter should be utilized for the isolation or identification of *C. psittaci*.

Control. No vaccine is currently recommended for the control of this disease.

The Disease in Man. There is no evidence that the enzootic bovine abortion strains have caused disease in man, but the possibility certainly exists. Page and Smith (11) experimentally produced abortion in a pregnant cow with a strain of *C. psittaci* isolated from aborted human placental tissue.

REFERENCES

1. Ball, Griner, and Carroll. Am. Jour. Vet. Res., 1964, *25,* 291.
2. Blanco-Loizelier and Page. Abst. Ann. Meet. Am. Soc. Microbiol., 1974, *74,* 73.
3. Ehret, Schutte, Pienaar, and Henton. Jour. So. Afr. Vet. Assoc., 1973, *46,* 171.
4. Eugster, Ball, Carroll, and Storz. 6th Internatl. Mtg. Dis. Cattle, Philadelphia, Pa., 1971.
5. Jubb, K. V. and P. C. Kennedy. Pathology of domestic animals, 2nd ed. Academic Press, New York, 1970.
6. Lincoln, Rivapien, Reed, Whiteman, and Chow. Am. Jour. Vet. Res., 1969, *30,* 2105.
7. McKercher. Jour. Am. Vet. Med. Assoc., 1969, *154,* 1192.
8. McKercher, Wada, Robinson, and Howarth. Cornell Vet., 1966, *56,* 433.
9. Neuvonen. Acta Vet. Scandinavica, 1976, *17,* 362.

10. Omuri, Ishii and Matumoto. Am. Jour. Vet. Res., 1960, *21*, 564.
11. Page and Smith. Proc. Soc. Exp. Biol. and Med., 1974, *146*, 269.
12. Schachter, Banks, Sugg, Sung, Storz, and Meyer. Inf. and Immun., 1975, *11*, 904.
13. Storz, Carroll, Ball, and Faulkner. Am. Jour. Vet. Res., 1968, *29*, 549.

Feline Pneumonitis

SYNONYMS: Feline distemper, feline influenza

This is an infection of the respiratory tract and conjunctiva of domesticated cats caused by *C. psittaci*. In 1944 Baker (1) showed that it was caused by an agent which could be transmitted from cat to cat and, experimentally, from cats to white mice. Later in the same year Hamre and Rake (6) showed that the agent belonged to the psittacosis-lymphogranuloma-trachoma group. The disease is worldwide in distribution.

Character of the Disease. The disease is contagious. Affected animals usually do not die, but they become greatly debilitated, and recovery is slow. In the beginning the disease is manifested by fever and inappetence. A mucopurulent discharge appears in the eyes and nose, and the animal coughs and sneezes a great deal. In most cases signs of pneumonia are not detected. The period of incubation varies from 6 to 10 days, and the illness usually continues for about 2 weeks, after which there is gradual improvement. Much weight is lost during the time when signs are most obvious. It is usually at least a month before the affected animals regain their original body weight. Unless complicated by other factors, the mortality is very slight.

Lesions are confined principally to the upper respiratory tract and the conjunctival membranes. The mucosa of these regions are reddened, swollen, and covered with exudate. Pneumonic lesions may be found when the animal is destroyed during the period of acute signs. These lung lesions disappear promptly as recovery begins. The consolidated portions are of a pinkish-gray color. The bronchial nodes are not noticeably enlarged. Histologic sections of the pneumonic areas show that alveoli to be filled with exudate consisting largely of monocytic and polymorphonuclear leukocytes. Occasional areas of necrosis are found, but in general the epithelium of the air passages is intact. Elementary bodies are found in the cytoplasm of the monocytic cells. Cello (4) states that significant involvement of the lung is a rare occurrence in the cat.

The Disease in Experimental Animals. It is possible to transmit the chlamydiae of this disease to white mice, hamsters, guinea pigs, and rabbits by inoculating them with infective material intranasally while they are under light anesthesia, a technique that has been used successfully in work with the influenza viruses. Using doses 10 to 50 times greater than were needed to infect by the nasal route, Baker (1) was unable to infect mice by parenteral injection. Hamre and Rake (6), however, using much larger doses of yolk sac material, were successful in producing infections by intracerebral and intraperitoneal injection. The disease in adult guinea pigs and in rabbits is manifested by fever and pneumonia, but the animals do not die. Young guinea pigs, hamsters, and mice exhibit the same signs of illness, but the disease usually is fatal, mice dying on the 2nd or 3rd day, hamsters on the 3rd or 4th day, and the young guinea pigs on the 5th to 7th day.

Properties of the Agent. The agent of feline pneumonitis usually failed to pass Berkefled N filters (1). Lung tissue contains bodies similar to those of *C. psittaci,* and large numbers could be produced in the yolk-sac membrane of developing chick embryos by inoculating virus into the sac. In the lungs of mice and hamsters, dense structures or plaques were recognized, which suggested that the agent was undergoing a developmental cycle, now recognized as characteristic of this group of chlamydial agents. Centrifugation at 10,000 rpm for 30 minutes caused sedimentation of large numbers of elementary bodies from suspensions derived from yolk sac membranes. The supernatant fluid lost most of its pathogenicity for mice, but this was regained when these suspensions were shaken and the elementary bodies were resuspended.

Hamre and Rake (6) have shown that the elementary bodies of feline pneumonitis, like those of several other diseases of this group, produce an endotoxin which in large doses ($>10^8$ ID_{50}) kills mice within 12 to 24 hours after intravenous injection.

The organism is destroyed when heated at 50 C for 30 minutes and at 60 C for 10 minutes. It is not completely inactivated, but its pathogenicity is reduced, by heating at 45 C for 30 minutes or 50 C for 10 minutes. Lung suspensions in 50 percent glycerol lose most of their disease-producing power in 30 days. Suspensions of yolk-sac material retain their activity for at least a week at room temperature, and for at least a month at 4 C. In the lyophilized state the agent retains its activity for 6 months or longer, but there is a significant loss in titer. Storage at −70 C preserves infectivity in most instances.

The group and specific antigens of the feline pneumonitis agent are located in the cell wall. When the cell walls of the feline agent are isolated by treatment of the elementary bodies with deoxycholate and trypsin, the group antigen is found in the deoxycholate extract and the specific antigens remained in the cell wall (7).

The feline pneumonitis agent hemagglutinates mouse erythrocytes only. Differential centrifugation shows that the activity is found in particles distinct from the elementary bodies.

Yerasimides described a strain isolated from a feline case of acute catarrhal conjunctivitis (11). Neutralization tests showed a one-sided relationship because antiserum to Baker's virus did not neutralize Yerasimides's isolate, but equal cross-neutralization occurred with antiserum produced by the Yerasimides isolate. These antiserums were specially prepared for these tests, and these data demonstrate a close, but not complete, antigenic relationship.

Cats convalescent from feline pneumonitis infection do not always have demonstrable serum-neutralizing antibodies. Some cats do not have complement-fixing antibodies in their convalescent serum.

Cultivation. The agent is readily propagated in the yolk sac of developing chick embryos (1). Using eggs that had been incubated for 5 days, embryonic deaths were found to occur on the 2nd or 3rd day, and large numbers of elementary bodies were present in the cytoplasm of the cells from the yolk-sac membrane. Development of the organism also occurs when infective material is dropped on the chorioallantoic membrane of 10-day embryos. The membranes become thickened, but the embryos are not affected by this method of inoculation.

Immunity. The degree and duration of immunity to the feline pneumonitis agent in the domestic cat has not been clearly established (2, 3, 4). The study of immunity in pathogen-free cats with various strains of the feline pneumonitis agent is needed to clarify the degree and duration of immunity in the domestic cat.

Based on our limited knowledge of feline pneumonitis immunity in cats and of immunity to psittacoid agents, it is reasonable to assume that the resistance of cats to the feline pneumonitis agent may be partial and transitory. Apparent remissions and exacerbations of the disease in an individual animal may represent recovery and reinfection rather than activation of a latent infection (4). Then, too, some presumed recurrent infections of *C. psittaci* may be caused by a feline respiratory viral pathogen. We know that carriers of *C. psittaci* exist as well as viral carriers, such as feline calicivirus and feline rhinotracheitis virus, and this obviously leads to considerable confusion in diagnosis. Cello (4) has found that *Mycoplasma* infection of the conjunctival sac, nasal passages, and sinuses often develops in cats that have had chlamydial infections. This also could lead to the erroneous impression that the original infection had developed into a chronic state or that it had recurred unless agent isolation attempts were performed in a complete and precise manner.

In experimental trials McKercher (8) felt that inactivated elementary body suspensions of the feline pneumonitis agent were relatively ineffective in producing immunity in kittens and in mice. Mitzel and Strating (9) tested a commercially available modified live chlamydial vaccine and found that the vaccine afforded some degree of protection, although not complete, and *C. psittaci* could be isolated from tissues of 34 percent of the vaccinated cats 3 days after challenge by the aerosol route.

In 1971 at an American Veterinary Medical Association Colloquium on Selected Feline Infectious Diseases, a panel of experts evaluated the only modified hen's-egg-propagated vaccine for immunization of domestic cats against feline pneumonitis. The vaccine stimulated CF antibodies. The duration of immunity and the degree of protection were unknown. The more recent studies by Mitzel and Strating suggest some degree of protection with this type of vaccine. The panel recommended yearly vaccination until the duration of immunity is known and the most reasonable time for the first immunization is weaning time. Care should be exercised in its use because ocular contamination may cause inflammation. Its use in pregnant cats was not recommended because the data on its use in pregnant cats was limited. The panel recognized that *C. psittaci* of cats is only one of many feline respiratory pathogens. Consequently, vaccine efficacy in a respiratory outbreak may be questioned at times.

Transmission. The natural disease in cats evidently is transmitted by direct contact with infected secretions and by droplet infection. The disease in mice and guinea pigs will not transmit naturally from animal to animal.

Diagnosis. The clinical diagnosis is exceedingly difficult because many viruses have been isolated from respiratory cases with signs of illness similar to those described for feline pneumonitis. Only by isolation and identification is it possible to differentiate *C. psittaci* from other respiratory and conjunctival pathogens in the cat such as feline viral rhinotracheitis, feline calicivirus, and feline reoviruses. Of course, concurrent infections with one or more of these pathogens can and do occur.

According to Cello (4) the large microcolonies (2 to 12 μm in diameter) with elementary bodies (Figure 30.2) in various stages of development may be seen in Giemsa-stained conjunctival cells from cats infected with feline pneumonitis and represent a reliable and accurate diagnostic feature of infection.

Control. This can be best achieved by taking advantage of the feline pneumonitis agents' susceptibility to certain antibiotics. Tetracyclines will free diseased animals of infection, but the problem is to keep them free (4).

The Disease in Man. Schachter, Ostler, and Meyer (10) isolated a *Bedsonia* organism from conjunctival scrapings of a man with acute follicular keratoconjunctivitis. The patient owned two cats, one of which had clinical manifestations of feline pneumonitis. *Bedsonia* isolates from the two cats and their owners had the same characteristics as *C. psittaci*. The human isolate produced typical, acute, inclusion-positive conjunctivitis in experimental cats. This suggests that certain strains of feline and human *C. psittaci* with an affinity for the conjunctiva may produce disease in both humans and domestic cats.

REFERENCES

1. Baker. Jour. Exp. Med., 1944, *79,* 159.
2. Baker. Jour. Am. Vet. Med. Assoc., Colloquium (Cornell Univ.), 1971, *158, 941.*
3. Bittle. Jour. Am. Vet. Med. Assoc., Colloquium (Cornell Univ.), 1971, *158,* 942.
4. Cello. Jour. Am. Vet. Med. Assoc., Colloquium (Cornell Univ.), 1971, *158,* 932.
5. Expert Panel. Jour. Am. Vet. Med. Assoc., Colloquium (Cornell Univ.), 1971, *158,* 835.
6. Hamre and Rake. Jour. Inf. Dis., 1944, *74,* 206.
7. Jenkin, Ross, and Moulder. Jour. Immunol., 1961. *86,* 123.
8. McKercher. Cornell Univ. thesis, 1949.
9. Mitzel and Strating. Am. Jour. Vet. Res., 1977, *38,* 1361.
10. Schachter, Ostler, and Meyer. Lancet, 1969, *1,* 1063.
11. Yerasimides. Jour. Inf. Dis., 1960, *106,* 290.

Pneumonitis and Conjunctivitis in Other Animals

In general, the diseases in sheep, cattle, goats, dogs, and mice are characterized by a conjunctival and nasal discharge, lethargy, anorexia, labored breathing, signs of pneumonia, and hyperthermia. Diarrhea may occur. The diseases are rarely fatal, and their severity is largely determined by secondary bacterial infections, but in some instances by other viral or *Mycoplasma* pathogens

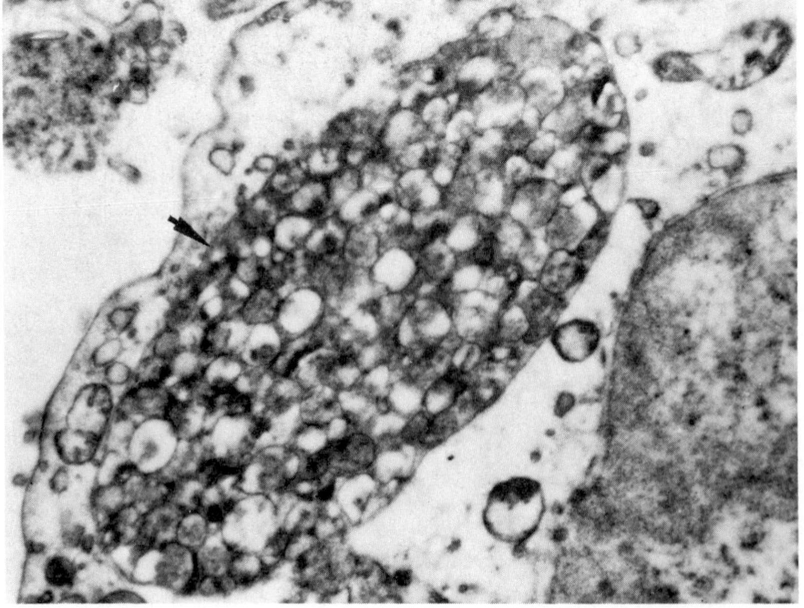

Figure 30.2. Feline pneumonitis, showing elementary bodies. Electron micrograph of metallic-shadowed preparation. × 17,600. (Courtesy J. A. Baker.)

of the respiratory tract. A lethal pneumonia in animals as in mice can be produced by serial passage in young animals by the intranasal route.

The pulmonary lesions of experimental psittacoid infections are characterized by an intense neutrophilic response, whereas viral infections are proliferative (6). Copious mucoid exudates of tracheobronchitis may be present with red, lobular consolidation in the anterior lobes. The histological lesion is an exudative bronchopneumonia of the bronchioles with extension into adjacent alveoli. Demonstration of elementary bodies in smears or in histological sections is difficult. Diagnosis should emphasize demonstration of elementary bodies in smears of yolk sac, of mouse lung, or of guinea pig peritoneal exudate of experimentally inoculated hosts; or of a rising serum titer utilizing paired serum samples.

The strains isolated from pneumonitis of a given animal species can produce experimental pneumonia by intratracheal inoculation in the homologous species. In some instances these strains can produce disease in another body system such as the genital tract of the homologous animal species. Occasionally, a strain that produces a characteristic disease in one species can do likewise in another mammal. One can only conclude that *C. psittaci* organisms contain a specific antigen(s) in their structure that has a selective cell-tropism for one or more animal hosts and this dictates the nature of the disease. The carrier state persists in many animals and serves as a source of infection for susceptible animals.

Various colonies of guinea pigs are chronically infected with *C. psittaci* that produce conjunctivitis. The guinea pig organisms also are transmitted transovarially (17). *C. psittaci* has been isolated from diseases conjunctiva of hamsters (11). Because guinea pigs and hamsters are used for diagnostic and research studies of *C. psittaci,* the worker must be aware of possible latent psittacoid infections in colonies of these species.

Presumably, the strains of *C. psittaci* that cause pneumonia and conjunctivitis are serotype 2.

In sheep. An agent was described by McKercher (8) that causes pneumonia in sheep. A sheep pneumonic strain of *C. psittaci* studied by Studdert and McKercher (19) produces abortion in ewes, but the disease differed from typical enzootic abortion of ewes. Dungworth (3) has produced experimental pneumonitis in lambs with an ovine abortion strain, while experimental abortions in ewes with an ovine pneumonitis strain was reported by Page (14). Abortion and pneumonia in sheep are caused by similar chlamydial agents, although some serotypic differences exist between ovine pneumonic and abortion strains. A pneumonic condition of goats in Japan may be caused by *C. psittaci*. The agent was transmissible to many other domestic animals.

Follicular conjunctivitis, sometimes with complicating eye lesions, occurs commonly in sheep. Storz *et al.* (18) have isolated *C. psittaci* from sheep with follicular conjunctivitis in 3 different herds. (Figure 30.3) The isolates were specifically related to strains of *C. psittaci* causing

Figure 30.3. Early (*upper*) and mature (*lower*) chlamydial inclusions in conjunctival cells of infected sheep. Giemsa stain. × 1,300. (Courtesy J. Storz.)

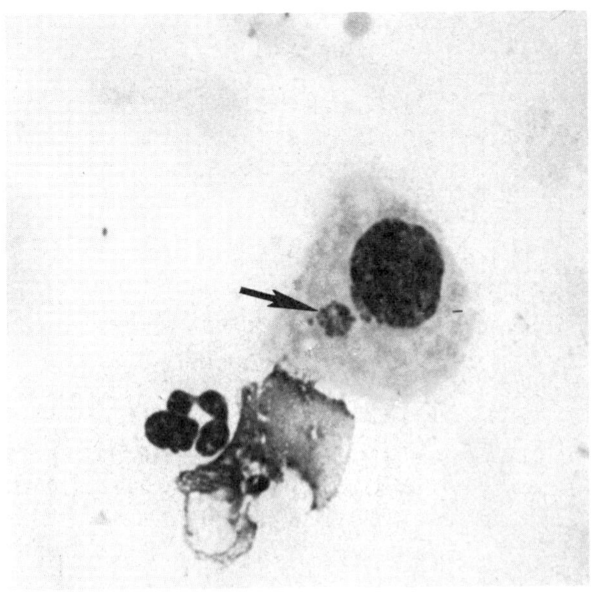

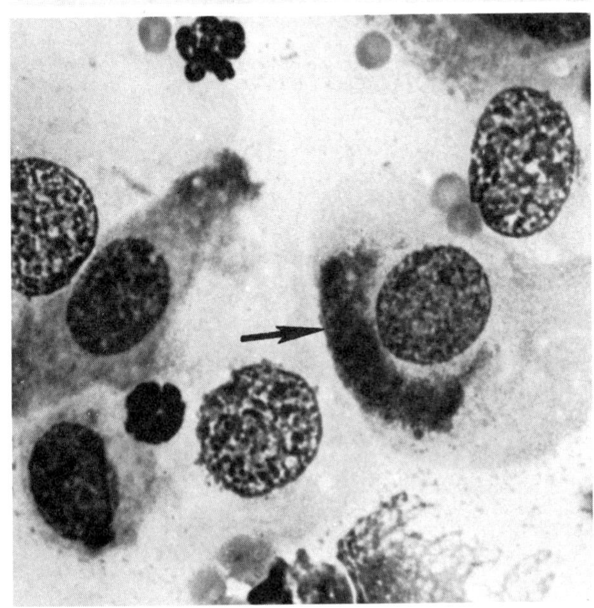

polyarthritis. Some of the sheep with follicular conjunctivitis also had polyarthritic signs. Parenteral injection of conjunctival *C. psittaci* resulted in follicular conjunctivitis and polyarthritis in lambs. Cooper (2) described the transmission of *C. psittaci* isolated from conjunctivokeratitis of New Zealand sheep.

In Cattle. Bovine strains of *C. psittaci* are responsible for pneumonitis in cattle of Czechoslovakia (5) and for pneumoenteritis in cattle of Italy (9) and Japan (13). The disease also has been described in the United States.

Werdin (21) in the USA. and German investigators (1, 16) have been studying the etiology of calf pneumonia. Particular emphasis is placed on the effects of *C. psittaci* in experimental calves. The isolates from natural cases produced respiratory signs and pathological changes of varying intensities with the reisolation of the organism from the respiratory tract in all cases and from the intestinal tract of some animals.

In Dogs. At a local dog pound (Fort Collins, Colorado) more than 50 percent of 119 dogs contained group-specific chlamydial antibodies, with greatest incidence in older male dogs. In a serological survey for chlamydial antibodies in laboratory dogs 7.6 percent (77 of 1,007 random samples) had CF titers between 1:5 and 1:40 (20). Ten of the 15 colonies under test had dogs with antibodies.

Fraser *et al.* (4) have described respiratory signs of illness in a dog that had access to an aviary in which psittacosis occurred. There is strong evidence that the dog as well as three human beings associated with the aviary had psittacosis. *C. psittaci* may also cause nervous manifestations in conjunction with pneumonic signs, or chronic keratitis as a single entity.

Maierhofer and Storz (7) described clinical and serological responses in dogs inoculated parenterally with a chlamydial strain isolated from a case of ovine polyarthritis. The affected dogs had fever, anorexia, signs of depression, pneumonia, incoordination, muscle and joint pain, and diarrhea. The chlamydial agent was isolated from somatic organs, including brain and portions of intestinal tract, and also from joints. CF group-specific antibodies were produced with maximum titers 21 to 28 days after inoculation and were still detectable 1 year later.

In Horses. In serological survey of horse populations in Finland (12) and Western Germany (15) CF antibodies were found in a sufficient percentage of animals to indicate that *C. psittaci* is a common infection. Its importance as a disease entity still has not been established. *C. psittaci* has been isolated from the nasal tract of 2 horses with acute respiratory disease (10), but transmission trials in horses were not performed with these isolates.

REFERENCES

1. Baumann. Arch. Exp. Vet.-Med. 1974. *28,* 847.
2. Cooper. New Zealand Vet. Jour., 1974, *22,* 181.
3. Dungworth. Jour. Comp. Path. and Therap., 1963, *73,* 68.
4. Fraser, Norval, Withers, and Gregor. Vet. Rec., 1969, *85,* 54.
5. Gmitter. Sborn. Ces. Akad. Ved. Vet. Med., 1960, *5,* 475.
6. Jubb, K. V. and P. C. Kennedy. Pathology of domestic animals, 2nd ed. Academic Press, New York, 1970.
7. Maierhofer and Storz. Am. Jour. Vet. Res., 1969, *30,* 1961.
8. McKercher. Science, 1953, *115,* 543.
9. Messieri. Atti. Soc. Ital. Sci. Vet., 1959, *8,* 702.
10. Moorthy and Spradbrow. Equine Vet. Jour., 1978, *10,* 38.
11. Murray. Jour. Inf. Dis., 1964. *114,* 1.
12. Neuvonen and Estola. Acta Vet. Scandinavica, 1974, *15,* 256.
13. Omuri, Ishii, and Matumoto. Am. Jour. Vet. Res., 1960, *21,* 564.
14. Page. Am. Jour. Vet. Res., 1966, *27,* 397.
15. Schmatz, Schmatz, Weber, and Sailer. Berl. und Münch tierärztl. Wchnschr., 1977, *90,* 74.
16. Stellmacher, Baumann, and Ilchmann. Monatshefte fur Vet., 1974, *29,* 539.
17. Storz. Jour. Inf. Dis., 1961, *109,* 129.
18. Storz, Pierson, Marriott, and Chow. Proc. Soc. Exp. Biol. and Med., 1967, *125,* 857.
19. Studdert and McKercher. Res. Vet. Sci., 1968, *9,* 48.
20. Weber, Krauss, and Schmatz. Zeitschr. fur Versuchstierkunde, 1977, *19,* 270.
21. Werdin. Dissertation Abst. Internatl., 1973, *33B,* 5569.

Ovine Polyarthritis

Polyarthritis in sheep was first observed in Wisconsin by Mendlowski and Segre in 1957 (1) and further described as an arthritic disease caused by a chlamydial agent (2). The disease was found also by Storz *et al.* (5) to be widespread in the intermountain area of the United States.

Character of the Disease. The main habitat for the polyarthritic agents of sheep may be the intestinal tract. Infections producing polyarthritis are systemic, and *Chlamydia* can be isolated from many tissues.

The disease affects lambs up to 6 months of age. The principal feature of the disease is lameness, and a few animals become permanently lame. There is also depression, reluctance to move, and a conjunctivitis. Tetanus-like spasms may be seen occasionally. The morbidity is high and the mortality 3 to 7 percent as a rule.

At necropsy, a constant finding is a serous to serofibrinous or fibrinous synovitis. The subcutaneous and adjacent periarticular tissues are edematous with clear fluid with extension around tendon sheaths. Surrounding muscles are hyperemic and edematous with petechial hemorrhages in the fascia. The viscera may show change associated with systemic infection with histologic changes of inflammation of soft tissues, including the central nervous system.

The Disease in Experimental Animals. The experimental disease in 5- to 6-month-old lambs is similar to the naturally occurring disease (6).

The sheep polyarthritis agent produced a severe polyarthritis in the leg joints of sheep and in the hock joint of turkeys (3). The sheep polyarthritic agent failed to affect mice inoculated intraperitoneally or pigeons inoculated intracerebrally, but caused disease in guinea pigs inoculated intraperitoneally. Both the pigeon ornithosis and sheep polyarthritic agents produced aerosacculitis in intraperitoneally inoculated turkeys. These observations may be important to our understanding of natural interspecies transfer.

Properties of the Agent. The isolates of *C. psittaci* from the intestinal tract and affected joints of polyarthritic lambs are antigenically identical, but differed from EAE isolates from the same flock or other flocks with EAE (4). All strains of ovine polyarthritis Chlamydiae seem to be antigenically identical (4).

The organism is readily cultivated in the embryonated hen's egg (2). The guinea pig, turkeys, and lambs readily grow the ovine polyarthritis psittacoid agents (3).

Immunity. Convalescent sheep that are injected with ovine polyarthritis strains of *C. psittaci* do not develop polyarthritis, although they harbor the organism 21 days after challenge (6).

The natural disease is limited to lambs, so it is a self-limiting disease in this respect. Whether this is an age factor or a very common disease with ensuing protection after recovery is unknown, but it is probably the latter.

Diagnosis. Microscopic examination of wet mounts of joint exudates with a phase-contrast microscope often reveal numerous mononuclear cells whose cytoplasm contains elementary bodies. As this is a systemic infection, the organism can be isolated in the hen's egg, guinea pig, or turkeys from visceral tissues, feces, or from joint exudate.

The psittacoid organisms are principally responsible for polyarthritis in lambs, although *Mycoplasma* have been incriminated.

Control. Procedures for control are still being sought.

The Disease in Man. Caution must be exercised especially because the turkey can be readily infected with the ovine polyarthritis agent and many human cases are derived from infected turkeys.

REFERENCES

1. Mendlowski and Segre. Am. Jour. Vet. Res., 1960, *21*, 68.
2. Mendlowski, Kraybill, and Segre. Am. Jour. Vet. Res., 1960, *21*, 74.
3. Page. Am. Jour. Vet. Res., 1966, *27*, 397.
4. Storz. Jour. Comp. Path., 1966, *76*, 351.
5. Storz, McKercher, Howarth, and Staub. Jour. Am. Vet. Med. Assoc., 1960, *137*, 509.
6. Storz, Shupe, Marriott, and Thornley. Jour. Inf. Dis., 1965, *115*, 9.

Bovine Polyarthritis

Polyarthritis in calves has been recognized for years. In this species it is caused by certain bacteria, *Mycoplasma,* and *Chlamydia*. Bovine psittacoid polyarthritis occurs in the United States.

Character of the Disease. Chlamydial infection in calves is severe, causing a high mortality. Some affected calves are weak at birth implying intrauterine infection. The infant calves have a fever and develop anorexia, reluctance to move or stand, and swelling of the joints in 2 to 3 days, and death ensues 2 to 12 days after appearance of signs of illness. The limb joints are most severely affected with the synovial structures distended with a turbid yellowish fluid and strands of fibrin adhering to the synovium. The surrounding subcutaneous and adjacent periarticular tissues are edematous with an extension around the tendon sheaths. Muscles around the joints are edematous and hyperemic with petechial hemorrhages in the fascia. The visceral organs may show changes attributable to systemic infection.

The natural and experimental disease in calves is similar (1). In the experimental disease of calves, chlamydiae are recovered from the blood within 18 hours after intra-articular inoculation. The *C psittaci* organisms persist in the blood for 6 days. The organism also is readily isolated from the joint fluids in the embryonated hen's egg by the yolk-sac route.

Properties of the Agent. The bovine polyarthritic psittacoid strains are antigenically related to each other and to the ovine polyarthritic psittacoid strains, but apparently are different from epizootic bovine-abortion psittacoid strains (1). There is also a close relationship between one bovine polyarthritis psittacoid strain and one guinea pig psittacoid strain that causes inclusion conjunctivitis and systemic infection.

The guinea pig and embryonated hens' eggs are excellent experimental hosts.

Immunity. Little is known about the immunity, but one probably expects protection aginst this systemic disease if the calf recovers from polyarthritic psittacoid infection.

Diagnosis. The same diagnostic procedures apply for ovine and bovine psittacoid polyarthritis. In bovine polyarthritis other infectious agents must be sought as well. Certain bacterial organisms such as *Escherichia coli* and streptococci cause polyarthritis in calves, and occasionally the former may be present together with *C. psittaci* in the joint exudate. *Mycoplasma* frequently cause polyarthritis in calves, but cytopathogenic viruses have not been isolated (2).

Control. No effective measures presently exist.

The Disease in Man. There are no reports of this agent causing disease in humans, but caution should be exercised in handling cases of polyarthritis in calves.

REFERENCES

1. Storz, Shupe, Smart, and Thornley. Am. Jour. Vet. Res., 1966, *27*, 987.
2. Storz, Smart, Marriott, and Davis. Am. Jour. Vet. Res., 1966, *27*, 633.

Equine Polyarthritis

Chlamydial polyarthritis was diagnosed in a newborn foal (1). The disease was characterized by fever, leukocytosis, conjunctivitis, depression, and polyarthritis. Most joints in all four limbs were swollen, contained large amounts of fluid, and were sensitive to pressure. Clinical recovery was complete after treatment with penicillin and tetracycline.

The diagnosis was confirmed in the laboratory by the isolation of *C. psittaci* by the demonstration of the organism after yolk-sac inoculation with infective joint fluid.

REFERENCE

1. McChesney, Becerra, and England. Jour. Am. Vet. Med. Assoc., 1974, *165*, 259.

Bovine Enteritis

Pneumoenteritis of dairy calves is a very important disease and one of the limiting factors in a successful vealing operation. In all likelihood there is no single pathogenic organism responsible for this disease. Certain respiratory viruses may be responsible, and pneumoenteritis reputedly also occurs as a psittacoid disease in cattle of Italy (2) and of Japan (3).

In 1951 York and Baker (4) described an agent isolated from the intestinal tract of calves, which they named *Miyagawanella bovis,* and later suggested it may produce enteritis in colostrum-deprived calves. *C. psittaci* is commonly present in the feces of a large proportion of animals in infected herds, and a high percentage of herds in New York State harbor this fecal organism and also have antibodies to this agent. In all likelihood a comparable herd situation exists in other states of the United States and also in other countries of the world. Because there is a close antigenic relationship between many intestinal strains of *C. psittaci* and many strains that cause EAE, epizootic bovine abortion, or ovine and bovine and psittacoid polyarthritis, the intestinal-carrier strains may explain, in part, the epidemiology of psittacoid disease in domestic ruminants.

In experimental studies in newborn colostrum-deprived or colostrum-treated Hereford calves infected orally with a bovine chlamydial strain, Doughri *et al.* (1) described clinical and pathological changes associated with the disease (Figure 30.4). The gross lesions were found in the abomasum and the intestinal tract with terminal portion of the ileum most severely affected. There is edema, petechial hemorrhage, and epithelial erosion and ulceration. Histological features included desquamation of surface epithelium, central lacteal dilatation, occlusion, and dilatation of Lieberkühn's glands, and infiltration of the lamina propria by neutrophils and mononuclear cells.

REFERENCES

1. Doughri, Young, and Storz. Am. Jour. Vet. Res., 1974, *35*, 939.
2. Messieri. Atti. Soc. Ital. Sci. Vet., 1959, *8*, 702.
3. Omuri, Ishii, and Matumoto. Am. Jour. Vet. Res., 1960, *21*, 564.
4. York and Baker. Jour. Exp. Med., 1951, *93*, 587.

Cat-Scratch Disease in Man

SYNONYMS: Cat-scratch fever, nonbacterial regional lymphadenitis

This is an ulceroglandular disease of man. It does not produce disease in any animals, so far as is known. It is

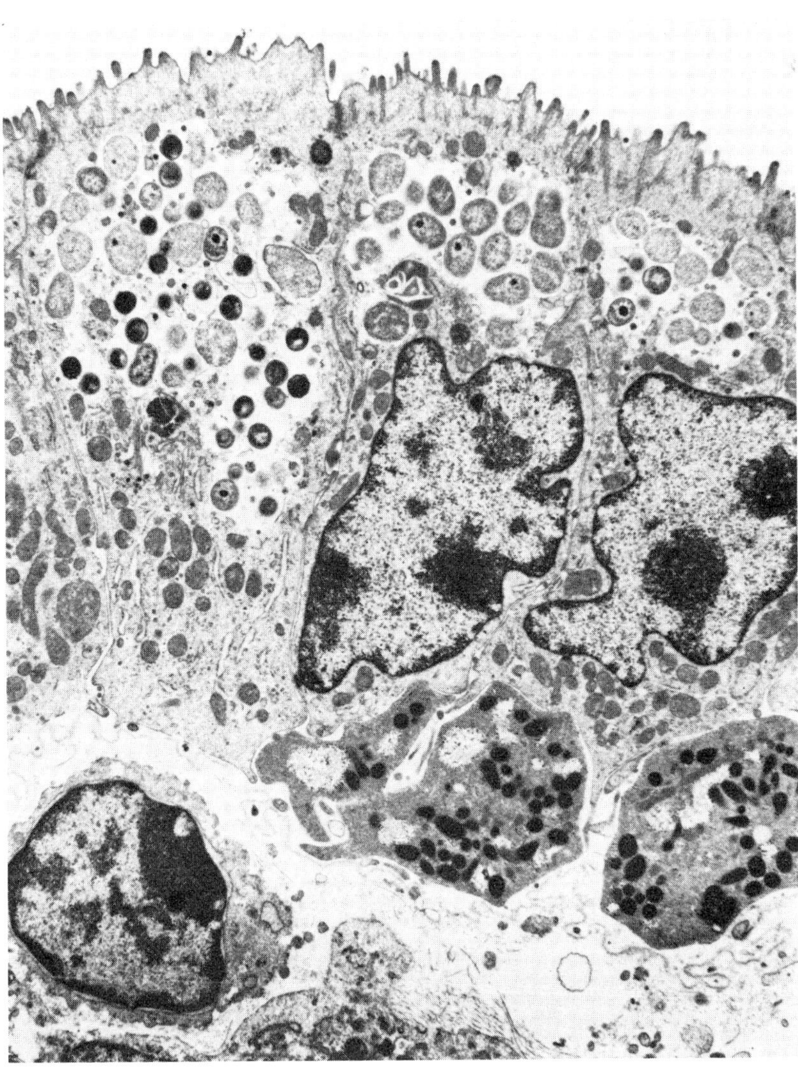

Figure 30.4. *Chlamydia*-infected enterocytes of a calf with dense-centered, infectious forms; intermediate and reticulated developmental forms. Microvilli and terminal web of enterocytes are altered. × 13,650 (Courtesy Doughri, Altera, and Storz.)

included here because many infections of man appear to be associated with *C. psittaci,* although the etiology is unclear. Frequently, the disease in man is concerned with scratches from the household cat, but not always. The cat may be a mechanical carrier of the infecting agent, or perhaps the injury by a cat scratch may incite a latent agent of humans such as a herpeslike virus or *C. psittaci*. Possibly rodents, or other natural prey of the cat, are the original source of the infection.

The disease affects human males and females alike, and all age groups may be involved. Young people appear to be infected more often than older, but this may be because of greater exposure.

In its typical form the disease in man presents an initial skin lesion at the site of the scratch, bite, or abrasions caused by other experiences. Initially this seems to be an ordinary wound infection that occurs within a few days after the infliction of the wound. The local lesion heals slowly, assuming the form of a local ulcer. Two or 3 weeks after the local wound develops, the regional lymph glands swell and become painful. Fever and constitutional symptoms usually appear at this time. The nodes may eventually become reduced in size and heal, but in most instances they remain enlarged for a long time. Suppuration occurs, and the nodes have to be lanced, or they will rupture and discharge a thick pus. In rare circumstances, the patient has nervous manifestations characterized by a rapid recovery from encephalitis (8).

Clinical diagnosis of the disease presents some difficulties. Of assistance has been the use of an intradermal test, utilizing aspirated, heat-treated pus as antigen (1). McGovern and his group (5) found that of 120 persons tested with such an antigen, two out of three reacted when there was a history of an attack of disease sometime in the past. Among 99 persons who had no history of an attack there were 10 reactors. Four of these were members of families in which there had been cases of the disease. A group of the personnel of the hospital were studied. Of the animal house personnel 22 percent gave positive reactions, whereas of the general personnel the percentage was 4.5. It was concluded that there probably were appreciable numbers of undiagnosed, or perhaps inapparent, cases and that the disease probably was much more common than had been supposed.

McGovern *et al.* (5) made a comprehensive study of the disease in patients and animal house attendants. Neither his group nor many others who have worked with this disease were able to isolate any disease-producing agent, but McGovern *et al.* transmitted the infection to human volunteers and monkeys by inoculation with pus from the abscessed nodes. Support for the viral nature of the causative agent was supplied by Dodd and coworkers (2), Manning and Reid (6), and Kalter *et al.* (4). Dodd *et al.* showed that the pus from cases of this disease had the property of agglutinating the red blood cells of rabbits, and that this property was neutralized by the serum of a human case and also by the serum of rabbits prepared by several injections of cat scratch fever pus. The hemagglutinating agent was described in a later paper as a herpeslike virus that lacked cytopathogenicity (9). Kalter, Kim, and Heberling (4) described the presence of numerous herpeslike virus particles in electron microscope photographs of biopsied lymph node material from 8 persons with the clinical diagnosis of cat-scratch disease. Attempts to isolate a herpesviruslike agent from this material have not succeeded (3). Manning and Reid conducted studies on patients suffering from this disease, using the complement-fixation test with a psittacosis antigen. Sixty percent of 10 cases with a histologic diagnosis of cat-scratch fever, and 23 percent of 35 persons having positive skin tests fixed complement. No positives were found among 44 persons who were negative to the skin test. These results support previous findings by Mollaret (7) indicating that the causative agent probably belongs to the *Chlamydia* group. Most individuals think in the terms of a single etiology for this disease, but it is possible that more than one pathogenic organism may be responsible for the entity that we call *cat-scratch disease*.

REFERENCES

1. Daniels and MacMurray. Ann. Int. Med., 1952, *37*, 697.
2. Dodd, Graber, and Anderson. Proc. Soc. Exp. Biol. and Med., 1959, *102*, 556.
3. Kalter. Personal communication, 1970.
4. Kalter, Kim, and Heberling. Nature, 1969, *224*, 190.
5. McGovern, Kunz, and Blodgett. New Eng. Jour. Med., 1955, *252*, 166.
6. Manning and Reid. Am. Jour. Clin. Path., 1958, *29*, 430.
7. Mollaret. Comp. rend. Soc. Biol. (Paris), 1950, *144*, 1493.
8. Pollen. Neurology, 1968, *18*, 644.
9. Turner, Bigley, Dodd, and Anderson. Jour. Bact., 1960, *80*, 430.

PART V

THE PATHOGENIC FUNGI

31 Classification of the Fungi

The fungi comprise kingdom III of the current five-kingdom classification of living organisms (1). They are filamentous or unicellular organisms with chitin, chitosan, glucan, and mannan in their cell walls. They do not produce flagella, are either haploid or dikaryotic, and exhibit meiotic division and propagation by haploid spores.

Nutrition is absorptive. Both carbohydrate and nitrogen sources must be supplied. The nitrogen source may be inorganic. Fungi are autotrophic in respect of vitamin requirements, with the exception of some species of *Trichophyton* that are unable to synthesize certain B vitamins—a defect which can be helpful in their identification.

The fungi are either saprophytes, symbionts, or parasites. Some have become highly adapted parasites of animals and cause a variety of diseases of the skin and internal organs.

Fungal classification is based on the mode of conidial and sexual spore production and on the morphologic characteristics of these structures, the colonies, and their constituent hyphae. Identification of some fungi such as yeasts requires study of certain biochemical and physiologic characteristics. The following explanations of the more commonly used terms in veterinary mycology may prove useful in the chapters that follow.

Hypha — A single vegetative filament that may contain a number of cells joined end to end.

Mycelium — A mass of hyphae

Septate — Divided by cross-walls, or septations

Coenocytic — Having few or no septations

Yeast — A unicellular growth form of a fungus

Conidium — A cell that is the product of asexual multiplication

Spore — A cell that is usually the product of sexual multiplication

There are at least seven kinds of conidia, each of which is named according to its mode of production. These names will be mentioned separately as each fungus is discussed. Also, it should be mentioned that sporangiospores formed by the Zygomycota are an *asexual* form of reproduction and thus are an exception to the rule that spores are the product of sexual reproduction.

The kingdom Fungi contains six phyla. These are the Chytridomycota, the Zygomycota, the Ascomycota, the Basidiomycota, the Deuteromycota (Fungi Imperfecti), and the Mycophycophyta. Only the Zygomycota, Ascomycota, and Deuteromycota contain genera of veterinary importance.

The Zygomycota are characterized by the formation of zoospores and/or sporangia during asexual reproduction. Sexual reproduction results in zygospores. The hyphae are coenocytic. Examples of genera in this phylum are *Mucor* and *Rhizopus*.

The Ascomycota reproduce asexually by conidia. Sexual reproduction occurs in an ascus, a sacklike structure that eventually contains 8 ascospores. The hyphae are septate. *Arthroderma, Nannizzia, Aspergillus* (*Eurotium*), and *Penicillium* (Talaromyces) are examples of genera in this phylum. The genera *Arthroderma* and *Nannizzia* have been established for *Trichophyton* sp. and *Microsporum* sp. where a sexual stage (perfect state) in the life cycle has been observed.

The Deuteromycota are often called *Fungi Imperfecti* because their life cycle is as yet incompletely worked out. A sexual stage has not been observed. The hyphae are septate. Most of the Deuteromycota probably belong to the Ascomycota. Examples of genera in this phylum are *Candida, Cryptococcus, Microsporum,* and *Trichophyton*.

The fungi that cause disease in animals are organized in the following chapters into general categories:

(*a*) Specific fungi that cause *superficial mycoses* in which the lesions involve the skin and mucous membranes (Chapters 32 and 33).

(*b*) Specific fungi that cause *internal mycoses* in which the lesions predominantly involve the deep structures and organs of the body (Chapter 34).

(*c*) Various unrelated fungi that cause specific diseases such as abortion, mastitis, rumenitis, and keratitis (Chapter 35).

Chapters 32, 33, and 34 are arranged according to genera of fungi, and Chapter 35 is arranged according to diseases caused by the unrelated fungi. These categories, although convenient, are quite arbitrary. Some of the internal mycoses, for instance, are frequently present in a form that includes skin lesions.

Many fungal diseases such as ringworm, mycotic abortion, or mycotic mastitis can be caused by a variety of fungi, some of which are common contaminants of the animal's environment and its skin. Thus mere isolation of such fungi from a specimen would not be proof of its role in the etiology of the lesion. Such proof should include the presence of fungal elements in the lesion, repeated isolation of the same fungus, and the presence of many colonies of the same fungal species on the isolation medium. However, even a few fungal colonies from normally sterile specimens such as brain or bone marrow would be regarded as significant. Some fungal pathogens such as *Blastomyces dermatitidis* or *Coccidioides immitis* are very unlikely to be found as contaminants.

REFERENCE

1. Whitaker. Science, 1969, *163,* 150.

32 The Fungi That Cause Superficial Mycoses, I

The most frequent causes of superficial mycoses in the domestic animals are members of the genera *Microsporum* and *Trichophyton*. These fungi are often referred to as *dermatophytes* because of their association with the skin. They are unique among the pathogenic fungi both in causing contagious infections and in their dependence on keratin as a nutrient source—they are among the very few microorganisms that can hydrolyze this substance.

The dermatophytes have considerable zoonotic importance because man has been known to contract infection by all the common species found on animals. Their growth on feathers, hair, nails, and skin elicits host responses manifested in a variety of diseases. These diseases are commonly referred to as *ringworm* (from the circular nature of the lesion) or *tinea* (from the Latin word for the clothes moth, whose feeding on woollen cloth results in circular holes).

GENERAL CHARACTERISTICS OF THE GENERA *MICROSPORUM* AND *TRICHOPHYTON*

Morphologic Features. Both *Microsporum* sp. and *Trichophyton* sp. produce colonies that have a variety of textures, pigments, and rates of growth—characteristics that are valuable in identification. Both genera produce fine, branching, septate hyphae and varying numbers of macroconidia and microconidia. The macroconidia are large and multilocular (Figure 32.1) with either rough (*Microsporum*), or smooth (*Trichophyton*) walls.

The macroconidia in *Microsporum* are concentrated toward the center of the colony and in *Trichophyton* are found on the periphery. Other microscopic features such as chlamydoconidia or spiral hyphae may be present and are of value in identification.

Culture. Good growth occurs on media (such as Sabouraud's) that contain glucose, neopeptone, and agar. Chloramphenicol and cycloheximide may be added to inhibit bacterial contaminants and saprophytic fungi, as in Mycobiotic or Mycosel agars. A selective and differential medium (dermatophyte test medium) that changes from yellow to red when dermatophytes are growing and producing alkali on it is also available. Potato dextrose agar that contains potato extract is useful for identification studies since it promotes sporulation, in contrast to dermatophyte test medium, which tends to inhibit it.

Incubation of *Microsporum* sp. and *Trichophyton* sp. is performed at 30 C, with the exception of bovine samples suspected to contain *T. verrucosum;* these should be incubated at 37 C. A humid environment must be provided and the incubation time may be as long as 3 or 4 weeks because of the slow growth of some dermatophytes.

A series of seven media (*Trichophyton* media) that contain different B vitamins and other growth factors is used for identification of some of the *Trichophyton* species. *T. verrucosum,* the common cause of bovine ringworm, requires inositol and thiamine, and *T. equinum,* a cause of ringworm in the horse, requires nicotinic acid for growth.

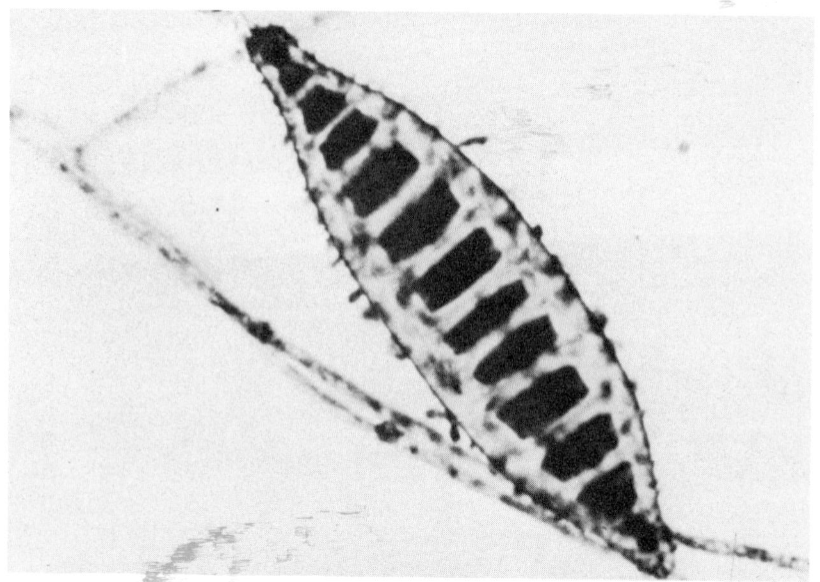

Figure 32.1. A multilocular macroconidium of *Microsporum canis* showing the rough surface typical of the genus. × 880.

At least 15 species of *Microsporum* and 21 species of *Trichophyton* have been described (1), but only a small number of these are commonly involved in cases of animal ringworm, and some, although keratinophilic, are not known to cause disease. Table 32.1 lists the *Microsporum* and *Trichophyton* species that commonly affect domestic animals.

Epidemiology and Pathogenesis. *Microsporum* and *Trichophyton* sp. are classified either as geophilic, zoophilic, or anthroprophilic dermatophytes on the basis of their natural habitat. Geophilic dermatophytes live in the soil and resist the degrading effects of soil bacteria by means of antibacterial substances in their cell walls (*M. gypseum, M. nanum*). Zoophilic dermatophytes are specialized parasites of the skin of animals and are not known to live in soil as saprophytes (*M. canis, M. distortum, T. gallinae; T. verrucosum, T. equinum*). Several of these are readily transmitted from animals to man. Anthropophilic dermatophytes are parasites of human skin and can survive briefly in the soil (*T. mentagrophytes* var. *interdigitale, T. tonsurans, M. audouini*).

Animal infections by geophilic dermatophytes are contracted by exposure to infected soil. These infections are sporadic and do not spread readily between animals. An important factor in the infectivity of soil is the presence of hair. For instance, soil-derived infections of dogs by *M. gypseum* occurred only in situations where hair and macroconidia were present together in the soil (22). The infections were observed in autumn after a period of fungus multiplication on the hair during the summer. In Australia, moist atmospheric conditions and the activi-

Table 32.1. The common dermatophyte species affecting animals

Host animal	Dermatophyte
Horse	*T. equinum**
	T. mentagrophytes
	T. verrucosum
	M. gypseum
	M. canis
Ox	*T. verrucosum**
	T. mentagrophytes
	T. equinum
Sheep†	*M. canis*
	T. mentagrophytes
Pig	*M. nanum**
	M. gypseum
Poultry	*T. gallinae** (M. gallinae)
	T. simiae
Dog	*M. canis**
	M. gypseum
	T. mentagrophytes
	M. audouini
Cat	*M. canis**
	M. gypseum
	T. mentagrophytes

*The most common dermatophyte species.
†Rarely infected by dermatophytes.
Note: A more exhaustive list of species of dermatophytes found in animals is given in Ainsworth and Austwick, Fungal diseases of animals (Commonwealth Agricultural Bureaux, Farnham Royal, England, 1959).

ties of biting insects were factors in outbreaks of *M. gypseum* infection in horses (29).

Infections by zoophilic dermatophytes are seen mostly in young, sexually immature animals that are kept in close contact. High humidity and environmental temperature, traumatization of the neck and shoulder areas by collars or chains, and poor nutrition are other important predisposing factors (18). Causes of friction such as harness straps, brushes, and self-grooming activities are other important influences on the occurrence and transmission of zoophilic dermatophyte infections. Thus lesions in cats and dogs are common on the head and paws.

Survival of the conidia (arthrospores) of zoophilic dermatophytes on the interior surfaces of buildings depends on the availability of moisture. The conidia are highly resistant to freezing but extremely susceptible to desiccation and also to temperatures greater than 50 C (13). Conidia of *T. verrucosum* that contaminate buildings are probably the most important means by which the infection is maintained from one season to the next. In the case of *M. canis,* carrier cats and dogs are a very important source of infection for other animals. The conidia of *T. equinum* have been observed to remain infective for 3 years (20).

Both *Microsporum* spp. and *Trichophyton* spp. enter the skin via abrasions. The conidium germinates and hyphae appear within the stratum corneum and invade the walls of the hair follicles. They then emerge into the follicular canal and grow downward between the hair cuticle and the wall of the follicle. The hyphal tip penetrates into the hair cortex by dissolving the keratin and by mechanical pressure. Massive hyphal and conidial (arthrospore) formation then occurs in the peripilar space, and to a lesser extent in the cortex (14). As the hair grows, the fungal elements are carried out of and above the surface of the skin. Many of these hairs fall out or are broken off.

In the case of endothrix infections, the hyphae and conidia are located within the hair, whereas in ectothrix infections the conidia are located to the outside of the hair (Figure 32.2). All of the common dermatophyte infections of animals are ectothrix. The conidia of *Microsporum* spp. generally form a mosaic pattern while those of *Trichophyton* spp. form linear chains on the hair.

Extensive hyphal growth and spore formation also occurs in the stratum corneum of the epidermis and a hyperkeratosis soon develops. The fungus invasion spreads centrifugally from the point of initial invasion, resulting in a ring-shaped lesion. Since the greatest inflammatory response is at the zone of recent fungal invasion, the circular nature of the lesion is emphasized. The

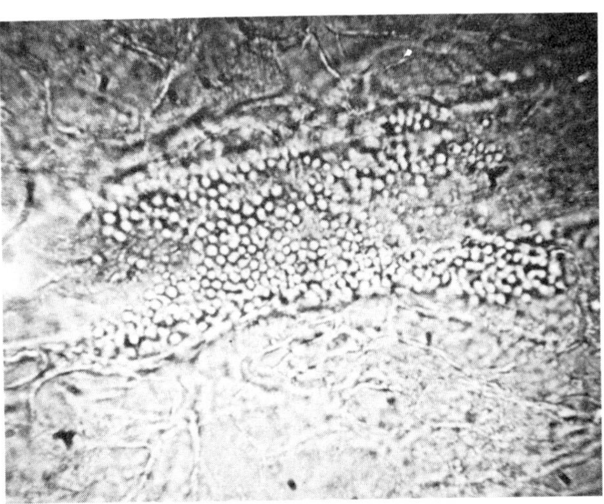

Figure 32.2. Ectothrix conidia (arthrospores) of *Trichophyton mentagrophytes* on the exterior of a hair from an infected rat. × 400.

dermatophytic fungi do not invade the living areas of the skin, although their presence in the dead layers does provoke an active inflammatory response beneath the *stratum Malpighii*. They show a preference for the hairy body surfaces. The hairs become brittle and appear dry and lusterless. The skin of affected areas becomes scaly and harsh, and crusts are formed. In cats and dogs the lesions are most common on the head, elbows, and paws (Figure 32.3). In cattle, the lesions involve principally

Figure 32.3. Ringworm in a dog. (Courtesy H. J. Milks and H. C. Stephenson.)

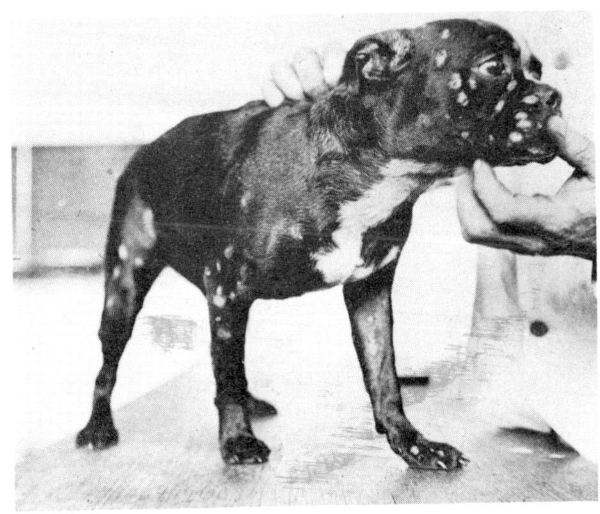

the head and neck. In horses, friction areas such as the saddle girth are usually affected. The lesions in cats may be difficult to detect and may be present as a faint scurfiness in the fur resembling cigarette ashes.

Generally speaking, ringworm thrives best in young animals and in older ones that have been devitalized by disease or malnutrition. It is seen more often in stabled animals than in those on pasture, and more often in winter than in summer. Ringworm infection that has become widespread in groups of calves will often clear up spontaneously in the spring several weeks after the animals have been turned out into the sunshine. This may be a result of better nutrition or it may be caused by the direct influence of the light. Ultraviolet light has proved useful in treating many forms of ringworm.

Immunity. *Microsporum* spp. and *Trichophyton* spp. possess both group- and species-specific antigens which are highly allergenic and cause a state of delayed hypersensitivity (15). Precipitins and complement-fixing antibodies appear about 30 to 80 days after infection in some animals but are usually present in low titer. In addition most animal sera contain a nonantibody antifungal factor which restricts the growth of dermatophytes to the stratum corneum (10).

Dermatophyte infection may result in the development of a resistance to reinfection. This resistance may be local and such that reinfection of the original infection site is of restricted duration and severity. *T. verrucosum* antigen apparently persists at the site of original infection in cattle and/or stimulates formation of persisting sensitized immunocytes which give rise to an immediate skin reaction at this site when an extract of the fungus is injected intravenously (24). Immunity is always associated with the development of delayed hypersensitivity which appears in cattle 14 days after infection with *T. verrucosum* (24). It disappears on healing of the lesions but is recalled within 2 days after reinfection. This memory persists for at least a year.

In horses, *T. equinum* infection produces a strong stable immunity lasting at least 3 to 4 years (28). The strength of the immunity depends on the length and severity of clinical disease (31).

Vaccines prepared from the mycelium of *T. verrucosum* have been successfully used in cattle (7, 17). Sarkisov *et al.* (32) showed that a *T. verrucosum* vaccine gave protection for 3 to 5 years. This was confirmed by Krdzalic *et al.* (19), who used LTF-130 vaccine to produce similar effects. These workers found that this vaccine was also effective when used therapeutically and produced remissions within a few weeks of administration.

Diagnosis. Direct microscopic examination and culture of skin scrapings and hairs from the periphery of suspect lesions is necessary to confirm a clinical diagnosis of dermatophyte infection. The steps involved in the laboratory diagnosis of ringworm are shown in Figure 32.4. Detection of lesions in cats and dogs may be greatly enhanced by preliminary screening with ultraviolet light from a Wood's lamp. An apple-green

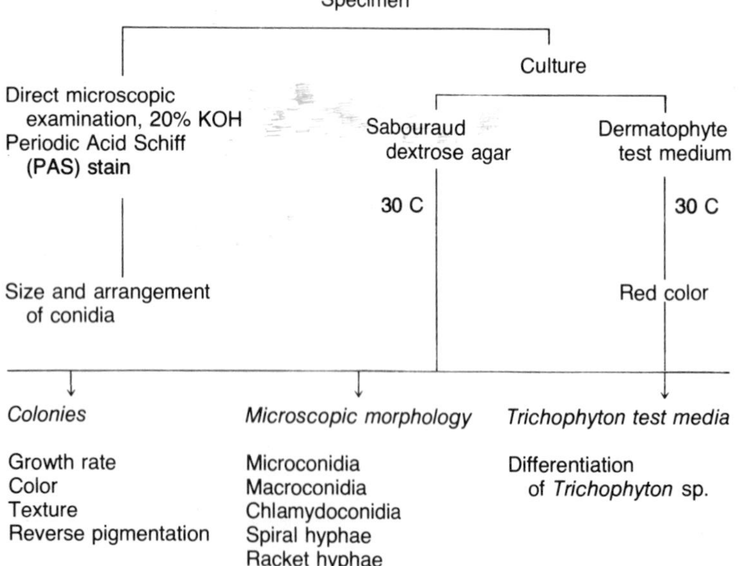

Figure 32.4. Laboratory diagnosis of ringworm.

fluorescence is produced by hairs invaded by *M. canis*, *M. distortum*, or *M. audouini*. Fluorescent hairs may be removed with a forceps and examined microscopically. A toothbrush may also be used to check the coats of animals for dermatophytes. Skin scrapings are placed in a drop of 20 percent KOH solution, gently warmed, and examined under the microscope with reduced lighting. Preparations stained with Periodic Acid Schiff (PAS) are more reliable and easier to interpret than KOH preparations as the fungal elements stain a deep red. However the latter is simpler and more suited to the practice laboratory. Hyphae and conidia may be present both in infected skin scales and on hairs.

Specimens for culture should be transported in an envelope or petri dish. Sealed glass containers are unsuitable because moisture may permit growth of contaminating bacteria and fungi. The specimens should be placed on dermatophyte test medium, on Mycobiotic (Mycosel) agar, and on Sabouraud dextrose agar. Plates should be incubated at 30 C. If *T. verrucosum* is suspected, the incubation temperature should be 37 C. A moist atmosphere must be maintained during incubation, which may, if necessary, be continued for 1 to 4 weeks.

Culture of specimens is necessary not only to confirm direct microscopic diagnoses but also to allow identification of the dermatophyte. The elements present in skin scrapings are usually not characteristic enough to permit definitive identification.

Immunologic methods are not used for detection of dermatophyte infections of animals.

Chemotherapy. Griseofulvin, an antibiotic produced by *Penicillium griseofulvum*, is highly effective in treatment of dermatophyte infections in cats (16), chinchillas (3) and cattle (6, 23). The antibiotic is administered orally for up to 6 weeks and becomes incorporated into keratin in the skin and hair. Treated animals are therefore refractory to reinfection for a number of weeks after treatment is discontinued (12). Griseofulvin binds to intracellular lipids and interferes with the function of the mitotic spindle so that fungal cells are unable to divide normally. Thus it has a fungistatic effect. Teratogenic effects in pregnant cats (33) have also been observed.

Preparations that contain oils, iodine, sulfur, salicylic acid, and other drugs are used in treating ringworm. Lies (25) recommends spraying cattle with 20 percent sodium caprylate. Hayes (11) used iodochlorohydroxyquinoline as an economical and successful treatment of ringworm in chinchillas. In horses Batte and Miller (2) found that successful healing followed the application of N-trichloromethylthio-tetrahydrophthalimide. Dermatomycosis in man responds to treatment with salts of undecylenic acid, to derivatives of salicyl anilide, and to racemic 2-dihydroemetine.

Natomycin has been successfully used in a topical application for treatment of horses with *T. equinum* infection (27). Thiabendazole has also been shown to inhibit *T. verrucosum* infection in cattle when applied topically (20).

THE GENUS *MICROSPORUM*

Microsporum canis

PERFECT STATE: *Nannizzia otae*

M. canis is distributed throughout the world and causes almost all ringworm cases in the cat and about 70 percent of cases in the dog. The natural host of this dermatophyte is probably the cat, but a wide variety of animals as well as man may be infected. Siamese and Persian cats appear to be more susceptible than other breeds.

The disease appears as small scabby areas on any part of the body but is seen most frequently on the ears, face, neck, and tail. These areas do not appear to cause much irritation, nor do they have any appreciable effect upon the general health of the animal as a rule. The hair is not shed; in cats especially, if the disease affects the long-haired breeds and occurs on parts that are especially well covered with fur, the lesions may be overlooked until the disease has spread over a considerable part of the body. Such cases are stubborn to treat, and such animals readily infect other cats, dogs, and often human beings with whom they come in contact. Rebell *et al.* (30) have found that kittens react to experimental infection with *M. canis* by producing only a minimal inflammatory response, which reaches a peak in about 28 days and then regresses. In man the disease may appear on the scalp, or circinate lesions may appear on the relatively hairless parts of the body. There are records of the disease being transmitted from one cat to another through the agency of an intermediate human being.

Microsporum gypseum

PERFECT STATES: *Nannizzia gypsea* and *Nannizzia incurvata*

This dermatophyte commonly occurs in the soil in all parts of the world and causes sporadic infections in many different animal hosts. The typical colonial appearance and macroconidia are shown in Figure 32.5. Macroconidia may contaminate the skin and hair from soil contact in the absence of any disease. *M. gypseum* causes about a quarter of all canine ringworm cases in the United States and about 1 percent of cases in the cat. It causes the majority of equine ringworm cases in the southern United States.

There are at least two perfect states of *M. gypseum* where a sexual phase in the life cycle has been seen—*Nannizzia gypsea* and *N. incurvata*. The epidemiologic significance of these two species in relation to animal disease is not known.

Figure 32.5. *Microsporum gypseum*. (*Upper*) Cultural appearance on Sabouraud's glucose agar. (*Lower*) Macroconidia. × 315. (Courtesy R. W. Menges, *Cornell Vet.*)

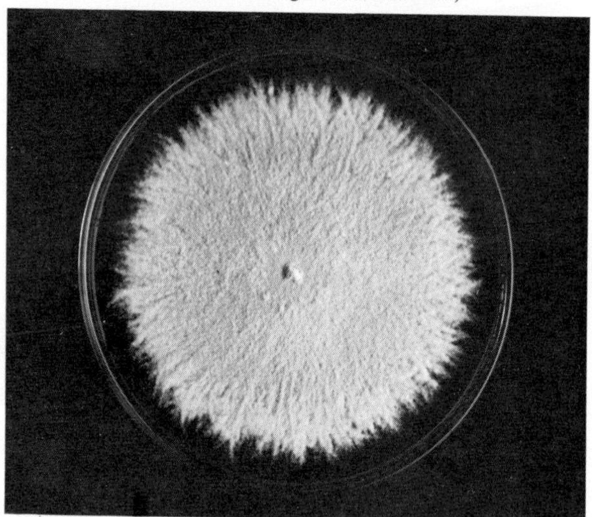

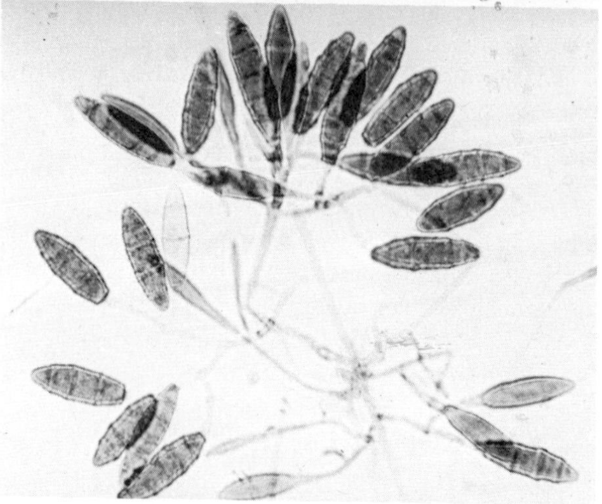

Microsporum nanum

PERFECT STATE: *Nannizzia obtusa*

M. nanum has been reported on swine in the United States (5), Australia, New Zealand, Kenya, and Cuba (1). Although the infection was not reported until 1964, it must have been present before this in the United States since the fungus is common in soil in many regions. Lesions begin as small circular areas which gradually enlarge in a circular fashion until they may cover much of the animal's body. Most have a somewhat roughened, though not obviously raised, surface that is covered with thin, easily removed brown crusts. The crusts may cover the area uniformly or they may be more prominent at the periphery, making a band that clearly outlines the infected area. Other lesions have few brown crusts, but have a red cast or a brown speckled appearance. There is no alopecia, pruritus, or general involvement, and lesions may be hidden by dirt and easily overlooked. Hyphae are the only fungal elements usually found in lesions.

This organism has been isolated from cases of ringworm in human beings.

Microsporum distortum

M. distortum has been reported only in Australia, New Zealand, and the United States (1). Infections in cats and dogs have occasionally been reported, but the

Figure 32.6. Macroconidia of *Microsporum distortum* showing their characteristic bizarre shapes. × 400.

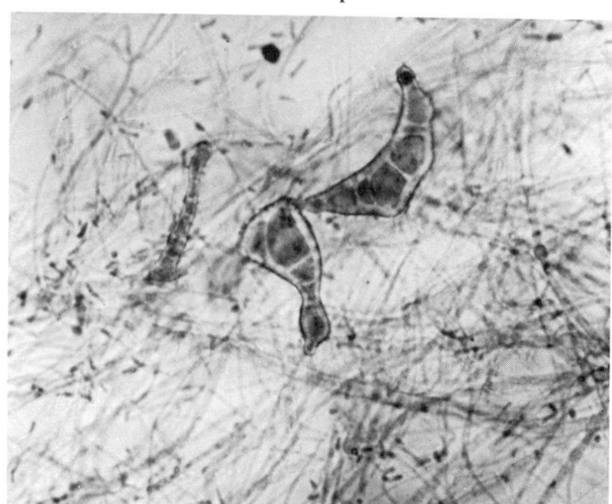

most important host appears to be primates in laboratory colonies. The macroconidia have bizarre shapes that are highly characteristic (Figure 32.6).

Microsporum audouini

M. audouini is the most common of the anthropophilic *Microsporum* sp. and is the primary agent of tinea capitis among children. Puppies and monkeys may be infected from human cases and may therefore serve as sentinels of infection in human communities. These infections are usually seen in animals from economically depressed urban areas. The circular lesions have been single or scattered, with loss of hair, scaling and some erythema.

THE GENUS *TRICHOPHYTON*

Trichophyton verrucosum

SYNONYMS: *Trichophyton faviforme, Trichophyton ochraceum, Trichophyton album, Trichophyton discoides*

Ringworm of cattle is a very common disease, especially in young animals kept indoors during winter months. The causative agent is easily demonstrated, but the lesions are so characteristic that demonstration of the fungus is unnecessary for diagnosis. Hairs plucked from the margins of the lesions and examined microscopically have large, ectothrix conidia (arthrospores). The fungus grows slowly and is often overgrown by contaminants. It requires thiamine and inositol for growth.

It survives for years in farm buildings; Muende and Webb (26) found colonies of the calf ringworm fungus growing on semidried fecal material in a stable in England. The fungus produced colonies large enough to be macroscopically visible. Blank (4) states that animal dermatophytes may persist and keep their virulence outside the body on such material as soil, straw, and wood, especially if mixed with keratinaceous material shed from infected animals.

The lesions are usually found on the face, particularly around the eyes, and also occur on the neck and shoulders. They consist of raised, dry, crusty, grayish white masses from which a few broken hairs protrude. The disease spreads rapidly among calves kept under crowded conditions in damp, dark housing.

Infections are frequent in humans who have contact with infected stock.

Trichophyton equinum

Ringworm of horses occasionally causes a great deal of trouble in large stables. The disease spreads readily, principally through the use of common grooming tools, harnesses, and blankets. Outbreaks can be controlled only by treatment of the affected animals and by thorough disinfection of all stable equipment.

The disease is seen on parts of the body where harness or blanket straps rub the skin. The face, breast, croup, flanks, and back where the saddle and saddle girth rub are the areas most often involved. The hair on these areas breaks off and much of it comes out, leaving semibald patches. The skin becomes progressively thickened and overlaid with flaky crusts. The underlying skin is dry and has a dull luster. Infections often complicate the picture, making the areas moist and reddened. The disease is transmissible to man, although apparently its contagiousness is not so great as that caused by *Microsporum*. These infections seem to cause little inconvenience to the animal. The principal damage is the temporary disfigurement of its coat. If untreated the disease may spread over large areas. A case of infection by this species has been recorded in the dog (9).

Trichophyton mentagrophytes

SYNONYMS: *Trichophyton gypseum, Trichophyton granulosum, Trichophyton quinckeanum*

PERFECT STATES: *Arthroderma benhamiae, Arthroderma vanbreuseghemii*

T. mentagrophytes commonly infects mice, rats, dogs, cats, rabbits, chinchillas, and guinea pigs in laboratory colonies (Figure 32.7). It is seen occasionally in horses, cows, muskrats, opossums, squirrels, and foxes, and rarely in swine (8). Mice infected with this species have transmitted it to cats, in which the lesions most commonly occur around the paws and on the ears. Wild rodents appear to be the natural reservoir of the zoophilic variant *T. mentagrophytes* var. *mentagrophytes*. The zoophilic variant has granular and red pigmented colonies whereas the variant found in man (*T. mentagrophytes* var. *interdigitalis*) produces white downy colonies. The latter, with *T. rubrum*, is the prime cause of athlete's foot in man in the United States (1).

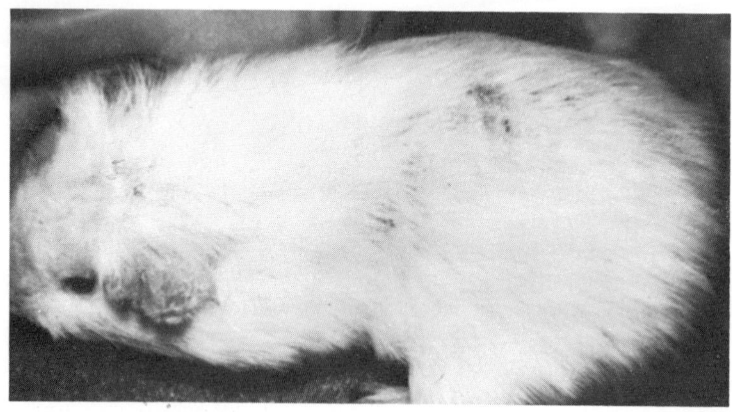

Figure 32.7. *Trichophyton mentagrophytes* infection in a laboratory guinea pig.

It should be mentioned that the zoophilic strains isolated from animals frequently change to the white downy form upon prolonged subcultivation. Humans directly infected by the zoophilic form from contact with animals develop typical ringworm.

Trichophyton gallinae

SYNONYMS: *Achorion gallinae, Microsporum gallinae*

Favus or *white comb* of fowls, particularly of chickens and turkeys, is now a disease of minor importance in Europe and the United States. It occurs in wild birds, although it has been reported in man and dog. It appears as small white patches on the comb, usually of male birds (Figure 32.8). These enlarge and coalesce, so that finally the comb may be covered with a dull white, moldy layer several mm thick. The disease usually is self-limiting, healing after several months if untreated. Scutula are not found on the comb lesions, but occasionally the disease extends into the feathered parts, in which case typical shields are formed. So long as the disease is limited to the comb, there is little effect upon the health of the bird. When the feathered portions are involved, however, the bird becomes emaciated and may die. There is evidence that *T. gallinae* is incorrectly classified and should instead be placed in the genus *Microsporum*.

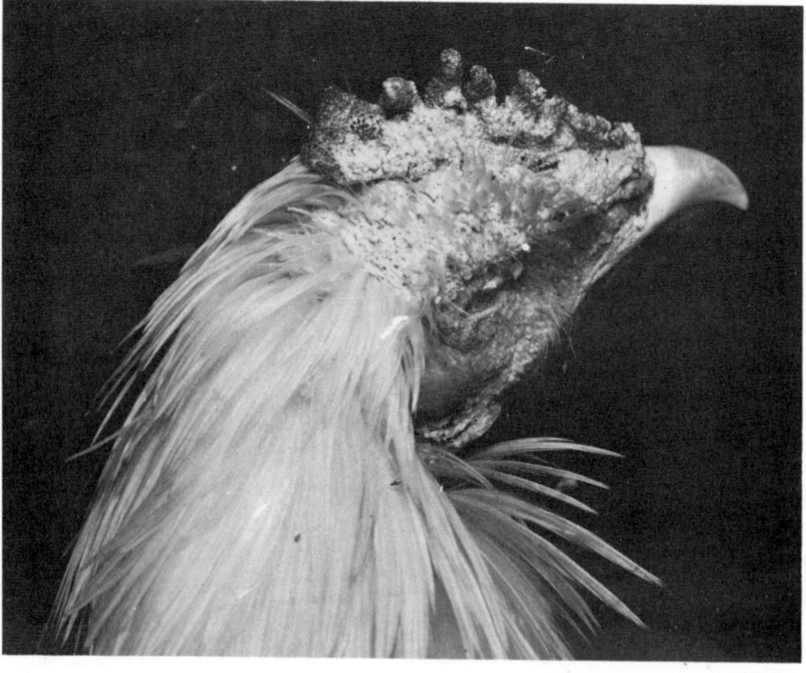

Figure 32.8. Lesions of favus in a chicken. This condition is caused by *Trichophyton* (*Microsporum*) *gallinae*.

REFERENCES

1. Ajello. Mycopath. et Mycolog. appl., 1974, *53,* 93.
2. Batte and Miller. Jour. Am. Vet. Med. Assoc., 1953, *123,* 111.
3. Belloff. Vet. Med., 1967, *62,* 438.
4. Blank. Am. Jour. Med. Sci., 1955, *299,* 252.
5. Bubash, Ginther, and Ajello. Science, 1964, *143,* 366.
6. Edgson. Vet. Rec., 1970, *86,* 58.
7. Florion, Nemeseri, and Lovas. Magy. Allatorv. Lapja, 1964, *19,* 529.
8. Ginther and Ajello. Jour. Am. Vet. Med. Assoc., 1965, *146,* 361.
9. Goldberg. Jour. Am. Vet. Med. Assoc., 1965, *147,* 845.
10. Grappel, Bishop, and Blank. Bacteriol. Rev., 1974, *38,* 222.
11. Hayes. Jour. Am. Vet. Med. Assoc., 1956, *128,* 193.
12. Hiddleston. Vet. Rec., 1973, *92,* 123.
13. Hoshimoto and Blumenthal. Appl. and Envir. Microbiol., 1978, *35,* 274.
14. Hutton, Kerbs, and Yee. Inf. and Immun., 1978, *21,* 247.
15. Jodassohn, Schoaf, and Laetsch. Arch. Dermatol. Syph., 1935, *31,* 461.
16. Kaplan and Ajello. Jour. Am. Vet. Med. Assoc., 1959, *135,* 253.
17. Kielstein and Richter. Monatsh. f. Vet.-Med., 1970, *25,* 334.
18. Klofusicky and Buckvald. Arch. f. Exp. Vetmed., 1974, *28,* 409.
19. Krdzalic, Stojicevic, and Brezjonac. Vet. Glasnik., 1978, *32,* 343.
20. Krivanec, Dvorak, and Hanak. Zentrbl. Vet.-Med., 1978, *25B,* 356.
21. Kriz, Jagos, and Marjonkova. Acta Vet. (Brno), 1971, *40,* 199.
22. Kushida. Jap. Jour. Vet. Sci., 1978, *40,* 1.
23. Lauder and O'Sullivan. Vet. Rec., 1958, *70,* 949.
24. Lepper. Res. Vet. Sci., 1972, *13,* 105.
25. Lies. Jour. Am. Vet. Med. Assoc., 1949, *115,* 458.
26. Muende and Webb. Arch. Dermatol. and Syph., 1937, *36,* 987.
27. Oldenkamp. Eq. Vet. Jour., 1979, *11,* 36.
28. Pascoe. Austral. Vet. Jour., 1976, *52,* 419.
29. Pascoe and Connole. Austral. Vet. Jour., 1974, *50,* 380.
30. Rebell, Timmons, Lamb, Hicks, Groves, and Coalson. Am. Jour. Vet. Res., 1956, *27,* 74.
31. Sarkisov and Petrovich. Vet. Moscow, USSR, 1976, no. 11, 39.
32. Sarkisov, Petrovich, Nikiforov, Yablochnik, and Korolov. Vet. Moscow, USSR, 1971, *47,* 54.
33. Scott, de Lahunta, Schultz, Bistner, and Riis. Teratology, 1975, *11,* 79.

33 The Fungi That Cause Superficial Mycoses, II

THE GENUS *CANDIDA*

This genus belongs to the class Blastomycetes of the phylum Deuteromycota (Fungi Imperfecti). The Blastomycetes are yeastlike fungi, with or without pseudohyphae, that produce blastoconidia and rarely produce a true mycelium.

Candida spp. are a frequent component of the normal flora of the skin and digestive tract of domestic animals. Candidiasis (moniliasis) is a general term applied to disease caused by *Candida* spp., usually *C. albicans*. Mucosal invasion by *Candida* spp. is frequently seen in animals stressed by poor nutrition, immunosuppression, or prolonged antibiotic therapy.

Candida albicans

SYNONYM: *Monilia albicans*

This is the species that causes thrush in human infants. Members of this genus are also found in animals and in birds.

Morphology and Cultural Features. Young cultures consist of oval, budding, yeastlike cells that measure 3.5 by 5.5 μm. *C. albicans* produces chlamydoconidia when grown on corn meal agar. Most other species of *Candida* do not. In lesions, the yeastlike cells in process of budding, as well as fragments of mycelium, can be seen. Pseudohyphae formed from blastoconidia buds that continue to elongate are frequently seen in culture (Figure 33.1).

On Sabouraud's agar, soft creamy colonies that are very convex appear in 24 to 48 hours when incubated at 30 C. In gelatin stabs, short villus streaks extend out from the main spike of growth. The medium is not liquefied. Acid and gas are formed from glucose, levulose, maltose, and mannose. A little acid but no gas is formed from sucrose and galactose. Lactose, raffinose, and inulin are not attacked.

Reliable techniques for the identification of *C. albicans* have been published (14, 15). Eosin–methylene blue agar, infused corn meal, and rapid fermentation tests are employed in identification procedures.

Pathogenicity. Thrushlike lesions in birds—chickens, pigeons, turkeys, pheasants, and grouse—are quite common and often very serious. They involve the mouth, the crop, the proventriculus, and the gizzard. The lesions consist of whitish circular areas or of elongated patches along the crests of folds in the mucosa. The areas may become confluent and finally involve large parts of the linings of these organs. The invaded tissues finally slough off, leaving superficial ulcers. Epizootics in very young birds may cause heavy mortality. The infections also occur in older birds, but recovery is the rule. Venereal disease has also been reported in geese (2).

A systemic disease of cattle has been reported to be candidiasis (8), and *Candida* spp. have also been found in bovine mastitis (Chapter 35) and have been associated with chronic pneumonias, vaginal discharges, aborted fetuses, and specific inflammations of the esophagus. In calves following prolonged antibiotic therapy the liver, lungs, brain, kidneys, and forestomachs have been in-

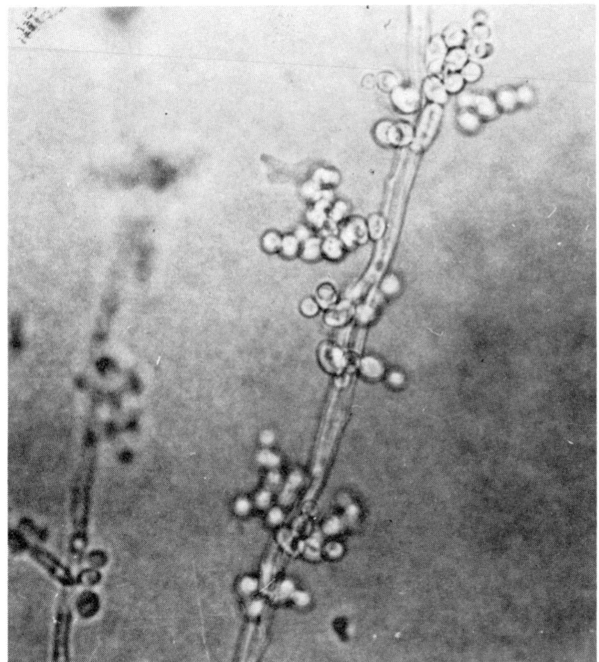

Figure 33.1. *Candida* sp., an unstained preparation from a deep colony in agar showing pseudohyphae and the yeastlike blastoconidia that arise at the ends of filaments and at mycelial nodes. Surface colonies of *Candida* consist largely of yeastlike cells. Pseudomycelium is produced only under conditions of reduced oxygen tension. Both pseudomycelium and yeastlike blastoconidia are found in lesions. × 500.

fected. Candidial rumenitis in young calves has been reported in Europe and in Connecticut (4). Thrush has been described in a small pig being reared artificially (9) and in pigs in Wisconsin (1), where the organism appeared to have a predilection for the esophageal region of the gastric mucosa and the lower portion of the esophagus. It has also caused cutaneous candidiasis in swine (12). It has produced cutaneous candidiasis (mycotic dermatosis) in dogs and cats (6, 7).

Immunity. According to Comaish *et al.* (3), a clear relation between *Candida* infection and the level of serum agglutinins has been found. Vaccinated mice show a significant degree of resistance to challenge (11). Rabbits respond by producing antibodies of the IgG and IgM classes when injected intravenously with heat-killed *C. albicans* (10). Beemer *et al.* (2) have successfully controlled endemic venereal disease caused by *C. albicans* in geese following vaccination.

Inherited defects in cell-mediated immunity in humans predispose to candidiasis and indicate that this phase of the immune response is most important in normal protection against the disease.

Diagnosis. Mere culture and isolation of a *Candida* sp. from a specimen is not evidence for diagnosis of candidiasis. The organism must be demonstrated in sections, scrapings, and squash mounts of lesion material. In tissue, the organism has the form of round or oval budding cells and pseudomycelia.

C. albicans may be identified by the production of chlamydoconidia on corn meal agar containing 1 percent Tween 80 (Dalmau plate). The inoculated area of the plate should be protected by a coverslip during the incubation period. Another presumptive test for the identification of *C. albicans* is its ability to form a germ tube when incubated for 3 hours in serum at 37 C (13).

Chemotherapy. *Candida* spp. are sensitive to nystatin and amphotericin B, but these drugs have restricted application in veterinary practice because of toxicity and cost. Haloprogin has been used successfully in treating topical infections (5), candicidin has been used in curing mycotic dermatoses in dogs and cats (7), and formic acid has been sprayed on food to reduce the severity of lesions in partridge chicks (16).

REFERENCES

1. Baker and Cadman. Jour. Am. Vet. Med. Assoc., 1963, *142,* 763.
2. Beemer, Kuttin, and Katz. Avian Dis., 1973, *17,* 629.
3. Comaish, Gibson, and Green. Jour. Invest. Dermatol., 1963, *40,* 139.
4. Cross, Moorhead, and Jones. Jour. Am. Vet. Med. Assoc., 1970, *157,* 1325.
5. Harrison, Zwadyk, Bequett, Hamlow, Tavormina, and Zygmunt. Appl. Microbiol., 1970, *19,* 746.
6. Kral and Uscavage. Jour. Am. Vet. Med. Assoc., 1960, *136,* 612.
7. Litwack. Jour. Am. Vet. Med. Assoc., 1966, *148,* 23.
8. McCarty. Vet. Med., 1956, *51,* 562.
9. McCrea and Osborne. Jour. Comp. Path. and Therap., 1957, *67,* 342.
10. Matthews and Inman. Proc. Soc. Exp. Biol. and Med., 1968, *128,* 387.
11. Mourad and Friedman. Proc. Soc. Exp. Biol and Med., 1961, *106,* 570.
12. Reynolds, Miner, and Smith. Jour. Am. Vet. Med. Assoc., 1968, *152,* 182.
13. Taschdjian, Burchall, and Kozinn. Jour. Dis. Child., 1960, *99,* 212.
14. Walker and Huppert. Am. Jour. Clin. Path., 1959, *31,* 551.
15. Widra. Jour. Inf. Dis., 1957, *100,* 70.
16. Wood. Vet. Rec., 1970, *87,* 656.

THE GENUS *RHINOSPORIDIUM*

This genus contains one species, *R. seeberi,* which causes a chronic infection of the nasal and ocular mucosa and is characterized by polypoid growth. The disease is seen mainly in man, horses (2, 5, 6), mules, cattle (4), and to a lesser extent in goats, dogs (3), and waterfowl (1).

The fungus can be demonstrated microscopically in tissues or in exudates from polyps, in which it is seen as white specks. These specks are the sporangia, are about 300 to 400 μm in diameter, and are filled with thousands of endospores. The latter are about 5 μm in diameter and leave the ripe sporangia by means of an exit pore.

R. seeberi has not been cultured, and its ecology and mode of transmission are not understood. The infection is endemic in India and Ceylon but occurs only sporadically in the southern United States, South Africa, South America, Japan, and parts of Europe. There appears to be positive correlation between the amount of water contact and the frequency of occurrence of the infection.

The polypoid lesions may be pedunculated or sessile; they are less than 3 cm in diameter and pinkish in color. They consist of fibromyxomatous tissue that is heavily vascular and bleeds easily. Affected animals may have a unilateral mucopurulent nasal discharge. Lesions have also been found in the conjunctival sac, ears, vagina, and other external parts of the body.

Diagnosis is made by finding the giant sporangia in the polyps. Treatment consists of surgical removal and cautery of the base of the polyp.

REFERENCES

1. Farn and Herm. Mycopathologia, 1957, *8,* 54.
2. Myers, Simon, and Case. Jour. Am. Vet. Med. Assoc., 1964, *145,* 345.
3. Nino and Freine. Mycopath. and Mycol. Appl., 1964, *24,* 92.
4. Saunders. Cornell Vet., 1948, *38,* 213.
5. Smith and Frankson. Southwest. Vet., 1961, *15,* 22.
6. Zschokke. Schweiz. Arch. f. Tierheilk., 1913, *55,* 641.

THE GENUS *SPOROTHRIX*

This genus belongs to the Ascomycota, the generic name *Ceratocystis* being applied to the perfect state of the fungus. *Sporothrix schenckii* is the only pathogenic species in animals.

Sporothrix schenckii

SYNONYMS: *Sporotrichum schenckii, Sporotrichum beurmonsis*

PERFECT STATE: *Ceratocystis stenoceras*

S. schenckii was first described in the United States in man. It is now known to be widely distributed geographically, and to affect both man and animals. It has been observed in horses, donkeys, mules, cattle, a pig, dogs, cats, fowl, camels, rats, and mice. Records of sporotrichosis in animals far outnumber those in man (1).

Morphology and Staining Reactions. *S. schenckii* is a dimorphic fungus, growing in a yeast form in tissue and in culture at 37 C, but as a filamentous fungus at 30 C. At 30 C it forms fine, septate, branching hyphae which carry ovoid sympoduloconidia either on short support hyphae or directly on the sides of the main hyphae. In pus, the organism is difficult to demonstrate microscopically. The characteristic form in tissue are cells resembling elongated yeasts, sometimes described as "cigar-shaped" (4). The vary in length from 2 to 10 μm and in breadth from 1 to 3 μm.

Cultural Features. Growth occurs on all the ordinary laboratory media, but solid media are more productive than fluid. Maltose favors growth. Good growths are obtained on potato dextrose agar where the characteristic brownish black pigment is best seen.

Small whitish filamentous colonies appear on potato slants on the second day of incubation at 30 C. These gradually enlarge and darken until finally the color is almost black. The surface is woolly because of the short aerial hyphae. Old cultures develop convoluted, wrinkled surfaces.

On mycobiotic agar the growth is similar to that on potato but the colonies remain whitish in color. They adhere because the mycelium penetrates the medium. Gelatin is slowly liquefied. Most of the growth is near the surface, but spikelike growth occurs along stabs. There may be some blackening of the surface growth. Loeffler's blood serum shows a slight depression under the colonies, but general liquefaction does not occur.

Epidemiology and Pathogenesis. *S. schenckii* is a common saprophyte on dead plant material such as sphagnum moss. Thus most cases in humans are found in forestry workers, gardeners, and miners who handle timber props left under damp conditions underground. The conidia are also common in the soil. The organism enters via skin wounds, the usual sites being the hands,

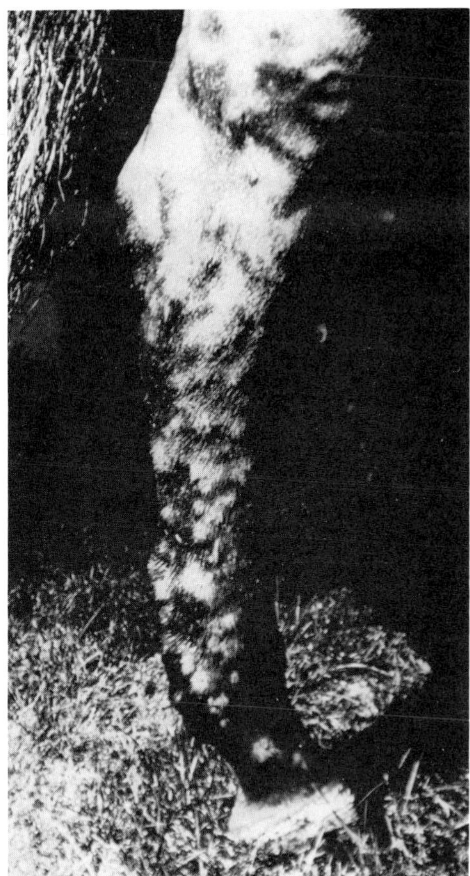

Figure 33.2. Sporotrichosis of the right hind limb of a horse. Note the extensive nodule formation and thickening of the fetlock area because of subcutaneous fibrosis and lymph stasis.

feet, and head. Horses (Figure 33.2) and dogs are much more commonly infected than other animals. A lesion begins as a small reddish nodule which may exude a thin seropurulent fluid. Infection then spreads via the lymphatic channels. Nodules form along these channels and ulcerate to the surface, discharging a thick, pale yellow pus. The lymph nodes are also enlarged. The subcutaneous tissues of the limb may become thickened because of accumulated lymph fluid, return of which to the general lymphatic circulation is restricted by lesions in the lymph channels. Dissemination to other tissues is rare in the horse but sometimes occurs in the dog.

The organism is sparse in lesions and is usually found intracellularly in macrophages. It is pleomorphic and exhibits multiple budding.

Immunity. There is both a humoral and cell-mediated response to infection. Agglutinins to the yeast form rise during infection. Complement-fixing antibodies are present in about 50 percent of cases. A rapid rise in antibody titer suggests a favorable prognosis. Filtrates of old fluid cultures (sporotrichin) will give specific delayed type hypersensitivity reactions in infected animals.

Diagnosis. The tiny spherical and cigar-shaped yeast bodies of *S. schenckii* in tissues and pus are best observed by the fluorescent-antibody technique (3) and by the Periodic Acid Schiff staining procedure. These procedures are rapid but must be supported by culture of specimens on brain-heart infusion or mycobiotic agar slants at 37 C and at 30 C or room temperature. The typical colonies are seen after about 1 week—initially white and glabrous and becoming brown-pigmented as they age. The yeast phase is produced at 37 C and differentiates *S. schenckii* from infections by other *Sporotrichum* spp. and *Sporothrix* spp., which occasionally have caused lesions in the subcutaneous tissues of man.

Diagnosis may also be confirmed by intraperitoneal inoculation of mice with tissue macerates or exudates. Mice develop peritonitis, and the cigar-shaped and pleomorphic budding yeast forms are abundant in the peritoneal exudate a week after inoculation.

Chemotherapy. Intravenous or oral potassium iodide is recommended for treatment of horses, but treatment failures are frequent. Griseofulvin has also been recommended in treating horses (2). Amphotericin B is effective in treatment of cases in man.

REFERENCES

1. Ainsworth and Austwick. Fungal diseases of animals. Commonwealth Agricultural Bureaux, Farnham Royal, England, 1959, p. 26.
2. Davis and Worthington. Jour. Am. Vet. Med. Assoc., 1964, *145*, 692.
3. Kaplan and Gonzalez. Jour. Lab. and Clin. Med., 1963, *62*, 835.
4. Young and Ulrich. Arch. Dermatol. Syph., 1963, *67*, 44.

34 The Fungi That Cause Internal Mycoses

THE GENUS *ASPERGILLUS*

This genus belongs to the phylum Ascomycota and contains a large number of saprophytic species that are very common in the air and soil and in animal feed. Some of these species can opportunistically cause disease in animals under conditions of stress, excessive exposure to fungal contamination, or prolonged antibiotic and/or corticosteroid therapy. *Aspergillus flavus* and *A. parasiticus* produce aflatoxins in moldy feed, which, when ingested, cause acute or chronic aflatoxicosis (17) in swine, cattle, and poultry. In cattle, various species have been found to be associated with abortions. Cases of pulmonary and cutaneous aspergillosis have also been reported in cattle, (3, 4, 11), generalized infection has been recorded in lambs (5), and aspergilli have been associated with abortion in mares (6) and persistent diarrhea in foals (9). Aspergilli have been isolated from frontal sinus infection in the dog (12) and from pulmonary disease in the cat (13). Bovine abortion, rumenitis and gastritis, mastitis, and equine guttural pouch mycosis caused by fungi including *Aspergillus* sp. are described in detail in Chapter 35 and will not be mentioned further here.

One of the most important disease-producing *Aspergillus* spp. is *Aspergillus fumigatus,* a common cause of respiratory disease of poultry and of penguins in captivity.

Aspergillus fumigatus

The most characteristic feature of the aspergilli is the structure of the expansions of the tips of certain of the aerial hyphae which bear the conidia (Figure 34.1). These expansions carry small papillae on which the conidia are borne externally. Colonies are woolly, dense, and quite unlike the loose mycelium of *Mucor*. Most of the aspergilli have pigmented conidia, and these give color to the entire colony. *A. fumigatus* has dark-green conidia; hence colonies have a dusty, dark-green color.

Culture of the causative organism is very easily accomplished on plain agar or Sabouraud's agar. The organism grows best at about 30 C, although it will grow at body temperature. Fine woolly colonies appear. After a day or so these enlarge, and greenish yellow specks appear in the aerial hyphae. These are the fruiting bodies (Figure 34.2). Later the entire surface is covered with a thick, matted, mycelial growth, yellowish green in color and dusty.

A. fumigatus apparently is introduced into flocks principally in moldy grain feeds and in moldy litter. The species seems to be widely scattered in nature and can readily multiply in feeds that become wet or are stored in a damp room. Outbreaks seem to be produced by the inhalation of conidia from such sources. The disease is not contagious, but *A. fumigatus* is an airborne fungus that can penetrate sound and cracked eggs in the incubator (18). The disease has been reported in chickens,

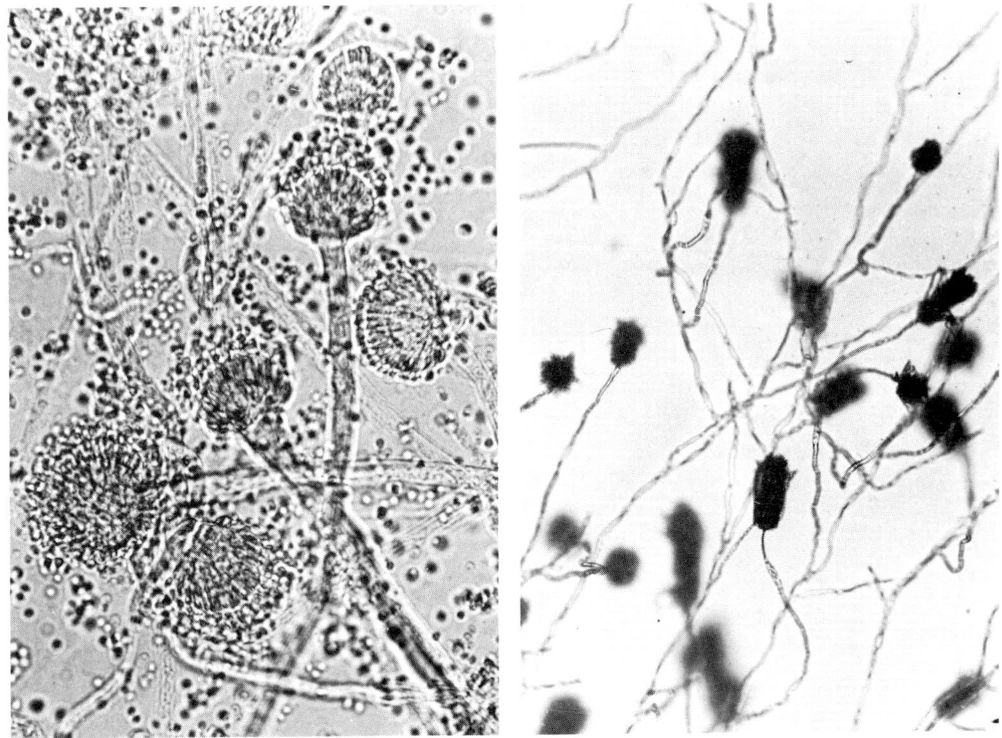

Figure 34.1 (*left*). *Aspergillus fumigatus,* an unstained preparation showing mycelium, fruiting bodies, and free conidia. The straight, stiff stalks are aerial hyphae. The bulbous expansions at their free tips contain papillalike processes (phialides) which bear long chains of highly refractile conidia of a yellowish-green color. The photograph was made from a bit of culture removed from a solid medium and immersed in a clearing solution. The majority of the conidia have broken loose from their attachments. × 550.

Figure 34.2 (*right*). *Aspergillus fumigatus,* a photograph of the aerial hyphae and the fruiting bodies in a Henrici slide preparation. × 55.

pigeons, turkeys, ducks, geese, canaries, mynah birds, and many kinds of wild birds. So far as is known all birds are susceptible.

For birds this organism is very dangerous, producing a disease known as *brooder pneumonia,* or *aspergillosis.* This infection sometimes occurs in epizootic form, in which case large losses may be sustained. Unlike most of the other fungi that produce deep-seated diseases, this one infects young birds more often than older ones. Hatchery-borne outbreaks have been seen in day-old chicks, although usually the classical disease does not appear before the birds are 5 days of age (2).

The infection is limited to the upper air passages and sometimes the mouth, the lungs, and the air sacs. In these locations the mold has access to air and vegetates readily. Tuberclelike bodies containing giant cells and lymphocytes usually form, and these quickly go on to caseation. The lungs, therefore, may show caseous areas, and the air sac walls may be thickened. Sometimes the air sacs are lined with greenish areas because of the presence of large numbers of conidia of the organism. In other cases the air sacs are not uniformly thickened, but many small, whitish bodies of dense composition are present. The mold hyphae in many of these lesions may be recognized by crushing them with a little caustic potash. In the green areas the conidia are readily found. In some of the denser lesions it is difficult or impossible to find evidence of the mold except by cultural means.

Encephalitic aspergillosis has been described in very young poults. It appears that the fungus invaded the eggs during incubation and infected the embryos (15).

Austwick *et al.* (1) have described seven cases of pulmonary aspergillosis in lambs, one of them subclinical. *A. fumigatus* was recovered from all lung lesions. It has been recovered from amniotic fluid of ewes and from the skin and lungs of fetal sheep (8). Jasmin *et al.* (7) have isolated the organism from pneumonic lesions in captive alligators (*Alligator mississippiensis*). It has also been found in calves and horses. In man, *A. fumigatus* is found infrequently in pulmonary infections, where it produces aspergillomas which may develop into lobar pneumonia (14, 19).

Chemotherapy. Experimentally amphotericin B has shown strong antifungal action against *A. fumigatus* (4). However, Utz (16) states that most strains from clinical cases are resistant.

REFERENCES

1. Austwick, Gitter, and Watkins. Vet. Rec., 1960. *72,* 19.
2. Clark, Jones, Crowl, and Ross. Jour. Am. Vet. Med. Assoc., 1954, *124,* 116.
3. Davis and Schaefer. Jour. Am. Vet. Med. Assoc., 1962, *141,* 1339.
4. Evans and Baker. Antibiotics and Chemother., 1959, *9,* 209.
5. Gracey and Baxter. Brit. Vet. Jour., 1961, *117,* 11.
6. Hensel, Bisping, and Schimmelpfennig. Jour. Am. Vet. Med. Assoc., 1961, *139,* 883.
7. Jasmin, Carroll, and Baucom. Am. Jour. Vet. Clin. Path., 1968, *2,* 93.
8. Leash, Sachs, Abrams, and Limbert. Lab. Animal Care, 1968, *18,* 407.
9. Lundvall and Romberg. Jour. Am. Vet. Med. Assoc., 1960, *137,* 481.
10. Molello and Busey. Jour. Am. Vet. Med. Assoc., 1963, *142,* 632.
11. Nag and Malik. Can. Vet. Jour., 1960, *2,* 30.
12. Otto. Jour. Am. Vet. Med. Assoc., 1970, *156,* 1903.
13. Pakes, New, and Benbrook. Jour. Am. Vet. Med. Assoc., 1967, *151,* 950.
14. Parker, Sarosi, Doto, and Tosh. Am. Rev. Resp. Dis., 1970, *101,* 551.
15. Raines, Kuzdas, Winkel, and Johnson. Jour. Am. Vet. Med. Assoc., 1956, *129,* 435.
16. Utz. *In* Host-parasite relationships in systemic mycoses, Part II, ed. A. M. Beemer, A. Ben-David, M. A. Klingberg, and E. S. Kuttin. Karger, Basel, London, New York, 1977.
17. Wilson, Campbell, Hayes, and Hanlin. Appl. Microbiol., 1968, *16,* 819.
18. Wright, Anderson, and Epps. Avian Dis., 1960, *4,* 369.
19. Young, Vogel, and DeVita. Jour. Am. Med. Assoc., 1969, *208,* 1156.

THE GENUS *BLASTOMYCES (AJELLOMYCES)*

This genus is included in the phylum Ascomycota. Although the generic name *Ajellomyces* has been applied to the perfect state of *Blastomyces dermatitidis,* we will describe this fungus by its older name.

Blastomyces dermatitidis

PERFECT STATE: *Ajellomyces dermatitidis*

This organism causes *North American blastomycosis,* a chronic granulomatous and suppurative mycotic infection that occurs occasionally in man and animals. The lesions may be confined to the skin and subcutaneous tissue or the disease may be generalized. The organisms appear as yeastlike bodies in infected tissues, but in cultures they produce a mycelial growth.

B. dermatitidis seems to be confined to the United States, Canada, and Africa, but the reported incidence of blastomycosis in any area is related to interest in the disease. Blastomycosis was recognized in 1912 in dogs by Meyer (13). Since that time the organism has been reported in a number of instances in dogs (14, 15, 16), in a horse (3), in Siamese cats (8), in a sea lion (21), and in man.

Morphology and Cultivation. The organism is a spherical, thick-walled, budding, yeastlike fungus in tissue or exudates and in culture at 37 C. In culture at room temperature it develops slowly as a typical, moldlike, filamentous fungus. It grows well on common laboratory media, where it becomes wrinkled, waxy, and yeastlike in appearance. The yeastlike phase is composed of cells (7 to 15 μm) with single buds resembling those found in exudates or tissues. Occasionally pseudohyphae or incomplete hyphae are present.

Pathogenicity. The organism causes a chronic granulomatous infection of the skin and internal organs. In dogs it can be characterized as a chronic, debilitating pulmonary condition often accompanied by some degree of lameness. Palpable cutaneous or subcutaneous swellings are frequent. Infection may start as a cutaneous lesion in the form of a papulopustule. In systemic blastomycosis the lungs are most frequently infected and show the most extensive lesions. Most cases reported in animals have been of the systemic type. A case in a dog, studied by Lacroix *et al.* (11), showed no cutaneous involvement. Lesions were confined to the lungs, which were dotted with miliary nodules of the type found in infectious granulomas. Saunders (17), however, reported a case of cutaneous blastomycosis in the dog which was a primary skin infection, and Foshay and Madden (6) described another case in a dog in which lesions appeared in the subcutaneous tissues, lymph nodes, spleen, liver, kidneys, lungs, and intestines. Ocular involvement has been diagnosed in dogs (19), and also secondary amyloidosis of the kidneys, liver, and spleen (18).

Systemic blastomycosis has been described in Siamese cats (8) and because most reported cases in the cat have occurred in this breed there may be a breed susceptibility.

Blastomycotic mange has been reported in mice (7).

In man the disease may occur as the cutaneous form with the initial lesion appearing on the exposed skin surface following trauma. In these cases healing usually occurs with scar formation of the keloid type.

The systemic infection in man is usually pulmonary in origin but may result from metastasis of a cutaneous lesion. The disease extends mainly by hematogenous routes.

Transmission. Blastomycosis is more prevalent in the middle Atlantic, south central, and St. Lawrence and Ohio-Mississippi River Valley states. There is no evidence that the disease is contagious and no proof that it is transmitted from man to man or from animals to man. There has been much speculation over the role of soil as a source of infection, and in 1961 Denton *et al.* (5) isolated *B. dermatitidis* from a Lexington, Kentucky, soil sample that came from a tobacco-stripping barn that had sheltered a dog that died of blastomycosis 2 years previously. In 1964 it was recovered from 10 of 356 soil samples collected in an endemic area at Augusta, Georgia (4). The organism appears to be a self-sufficient saprophyte, capable of surviving and thriving in nature, but the yeast phase of the organism seems to be the important agent in promoting infection, and this phase survives for only a short time in soil (12). Ajello (1) has stated that *B. dermatitidis* presents one of the greatest ecological challenges. As yet, its natural habitat remains unknown. It is difficult to imagine the precise conditions required to permit its existence in such diverse regions as the Americas and Africa.

Immunity. Complement-fixing antibodies can be demonstrated in the serum of human patients with extensive or progressive infection but not in patients with localized cutaneous lesions. A delayed hypersensitivity reaction can be demonstrated in infected individuals by injecting extracts of the organism.

Diagnosis. The characteristic spherical thick-walled budding yeast 8 to 20 μm in diameter in tissues, exudates, or tracheal aspirates is easily recognised. However, spherules may be difficult to find in some specimens. On Sabouraud dextrose agar at room temperature, *B. dermatidis* grows as a white to tan mold that produces round to oval conidia ranging in size from 3 to 5 μm. Such cultures can be confused with unusual isolates of *Histoplasma capsulatum* and with some *Chrysosporium* spp. that bear small conidia (10). Definitive identification in this situation requires conversion to the typical tissue (yeast) form, which may be difficult for some strains. Alternatively, the antigen produced by the mycelial form can be identified by immunodiffusion using standard antisera prepared against the A precipitin (9).

Chemotherapy. In an outbreak of North American blastomycosis Smith *et al.* (20) treated nine patients with stilbamidine or 2-hydroxystilbamidine and reported that eight responded rapidly and without toxic manifestations to the therapy. A 7-month-old infant died. In 1959, Baum and Schwarz (2) reported that North American blastomycosis is an almost-conquered disease due to the effectiveness of amphotericin B and stilbamidine and its derivatives.

REFERENCES

1. Ajello. Bact. Rev., 1967, *31*, 6.
2. Baum and Schwarz. Am. Jour. Med. Sci., 1959, *238*, 661.
3. Benbrook, Bryant, and Saunders. Jour. Am. Vet. Med. Assoc., 1948, *112*, 475.
4. Denton and DiSalvo. Am. Jour. Trop. Med. and Hyg., 1964, *13*, 716.
5. Denton, McDonough, Ajello, and Aushermann. Science, 1961, *133*, 1126.
6. Foshay and Madden. Am. Jour. Trop. Med., 1942, *22*, 565.
7. Galton. Am. Jour. Path., 1963, *43*, 855.
8. Jasmin, Carroll, Baucom, and Beusse. Vet. Med., 1969, *64*, 33.
9. Kaufman, McLoughlin, Clark, and Blumer. Appl. Microbiol., 1973, *26*, 244.
10. Kaufman and Standard. Current Microbiol., 1978, *1*, 135.
11. Lacroix, Riser, and Karlson. North Am. Vet., 1947, *28*, 603.
12. McDonough, Prooien, and Lewis. Am. Jour. Epidemiol., 1965, *81*, 86.
13. Meyer. Proc. Path. Soc. Philadelphia, 1912, *15*, 10.
14. Newberne, Neal, and Heath. Jour. Am. Vet. Med. Assoc., 1955, *127*, 220.
15. Ramsey and Carter. Jour. Am. Vet. Med. Assoc., 1952, *120*, 93.
16. Saunders. Cornell Vet., 1948, *38*, 213.
17. Saunders. North Am. Vet., 1948, *29*, 650.
18. Sherwood, LeMay, and Castellanos. Jour. Am. Vet. Med. Assoc., 1967, *150*, 1377.
19. Simon and Helper. Jour. Am. Vet. Med. Assoc., 1970, *157*, 922.

20. Smith, Harris, Conant, and Smith. Jour. Am. Med. Assoc., 1955, *158,* 641.
21. Williamson, Lombard, and Getty. Jour. Am. Vet. Med. Assoc., 1959, *135,* 513.

THE GENUS *COCCIDIOIDES*

Coccidioides immitis

This organism was originally thought to be a protozoon. The form that occurs in the lesions resembles an oocyst of a coccidium, and it is from this resemblance that the generic name was derived.

The fungus is the causative agent of a human disease of considerable importance, especially in the valleys of central and southern California. It also occurs in Argentina, Paraguay, Bolivia, Guatemala, Honduras, Venezuela, Colombia, and Mexico.

Most of the early cases of human infection originated in the valley of the San Joaquin River, and the disease became well known as the *San Joaquin Valley disease.* For years only the chronic cases, characterized by the formation of granulomas in the internal organs and especially in the lungs and by a mortality rate in excess of 50 percent, were recognized. In 1938, Dickson (10) showed that the disease occurred in another much more prevalent form. This is the *valley fever* or *desert fever,* an influenzalike disease that had long been known in the valleys of central California without its real nature being suspected. It is now known that large numbers of residents and transient workers in these valleys become infected. Most cases recover in 3 to 6 weeks. Only a few lapse into the chronic form characterized by granulomatous lesions (*coccidioidal granuloma*).

In 1918, Giltner (14) identified this organism in an infection of a cow that had lived in the San Joaquin Valley. The disease has now been recognized in many cattle, dogs, burros, swine, sheep, horses, a monkey, a gorilla, a chinchilla, a llama, a tapir, and several species of wild rodents (23).

Morphology and Staining Reactions. As it occurs in the purulent material and the granulation tissue of lesions, the fungus appears as spherical bodies (spherules or sporangia) that vary greatly in size from 10 to 80 μm in diameter. The wall is double-contoured and highly refractile (Figure 34.3). The protoplasm is finely granular. In many of the larger spherules a number of endospores may be seen as spherical bodies varying from 2 to 5 μm in diameter. Mycelium is rarely seen in the tissues, although Puckett (27) claims that mycelial growth of *C. immitis* may develop in focalized and stabilized lesions in the human host in the same manner that it develops in cultures. He states that hyphae are more common in cavities (73 percent) than in granulomatous lesions (30 percent).

When tissues are planted on suitable culture media, protoplasmic shoots appear from the spherules. These develop into hyphae, and soon a well-developed mycelium is formed. The hyphae branch extensively and exhibit well-marked septa (Figure 34.4). In time aerial hyphae appear and a white woolly colony is formed (Figure 34.5). Microscopically, numerous chlamydoconidia may be seen and some arthroconidia. The spherical structures found in tissues are never present in cultures unless they are incubated under special conditions semianaerobically (3) or in special media (4, 6, 24). It is also claimed that *C. immitis* can be identified readily by the use of specialized media (7). It appears that the yolk sac of the embryonated chicken egg is a good medium for growing the tissue phase of *C. immitis* (33).

All forms of this parasite can be stained, but for most purposes fresh material unstained is preferable for study.

Cultural Features. *C. immitis* will grow on all the common media of the bacteriological laboratory. When cultures on solid media are incubated at 20 C, growth does not appear for 3 or 4 days, but at 37 C it is usually evident within 24 hours. The colonies are circular in outline, or a silvery gray color, and slightly raised. The mycelium penetrates deeply into the medium, so that the colonies cannot be removed except by digging out the medium. After a few days the cultures develop a whitish, moldy appearance because of the development of short aerial hyphae. In some tubes these are abundant and from 2 to 3 mm long; in others they may be scarce and short. In old cultures the medium develops a brownish discoloration but the growth remains white. Gelatin and coagulated bovine serum are slowly liquefied. Milk is gradually digested. Broth cultures produce fluffy masses in the bottoms of the tubes, and some tubes show rather tough pellicles. Sugars are not fermented.

Epidemiology and Pathogenesis. The endemic region in the United States is the desert country of the southwest and the San Joaquin Valley of California (1). These areas are in the lower Sonoran Life Zone, an ecologically distinctive area characterized by low rainfall, high ambient temperature, and vegetation comprised to a great extent of cacti and creosote bushes.

Desert rodents infected with *C. immitis* inhabit the

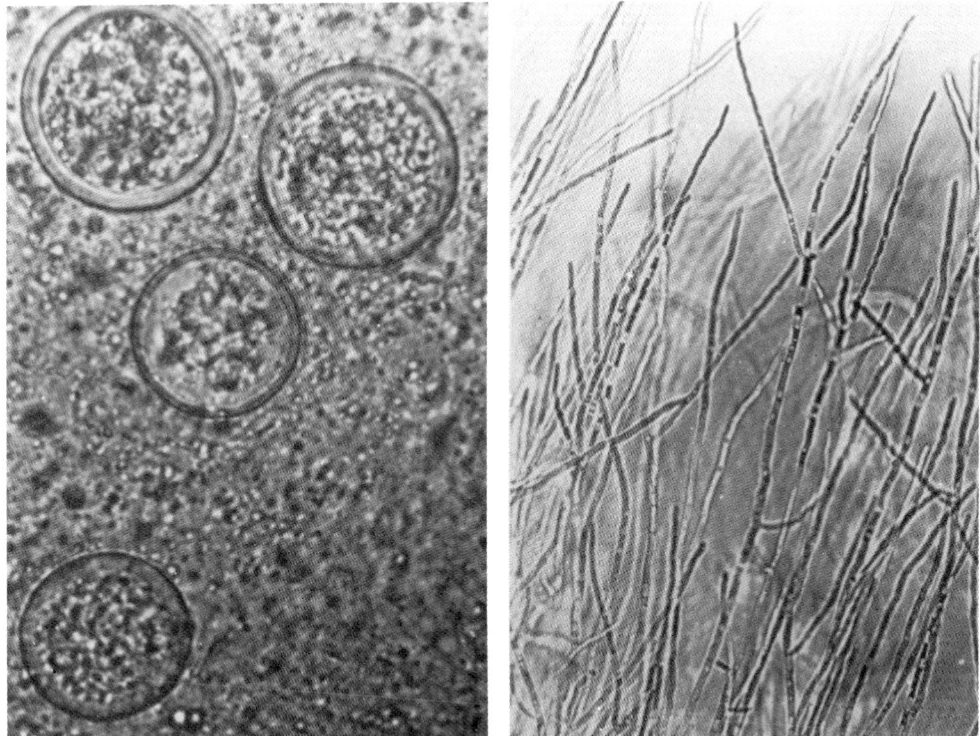

Figure 34.3 (*left*). *Coccidioides immitis,* showing several of the spherules contained in pus expressed from a lesion in a lymph node. × 550. (Courtesy Stiles and Davis, *Jour. Am. Med. Assoc.*)

Figure 34.4 (*right*). *Coccidioides immitis,* a hanging drop preparation from a culture showing mycelium of the organism. × 210. (Courtesy Stiles and Davis, *Jour. Am. Med. Assoc.*)

ground beneath these plants and may excrete large numbers of spherules in their feces which germinate and multiply vegetatively in nearby soil after rain (12). When the ground dries, large numbers of arthroconidia are produced and released. These are readily spread to surrounding areas by the wind. Animals grazing these areas or dogs that sniff in the area of rodent burrows may inhale large numbers of arthroconidia. Most animals that live in the endemic zone are exposed and infected during their lifetimes, but few develop serious disease.

The disease is not transmitted from animal to animal. Maddy (22) made a 2-year study of a site in Arizona

Figure 34.5. (*Left*) *Coccidioides immitis.* A single colony of the organism growing on a solid medium. Note the cottonlike appearance. × 2. (*Right*) Coccidioidal granuloma. Lesions in a bovine lymph node which strikingly resemble those of tuberculosis. The lesions vary in size. They are caseous in their centers. Note the hemorrhages and the encapsulation. About × 2. (Courtesy Stiles and Davis, *Jour. Am. Med. Assoc.*)

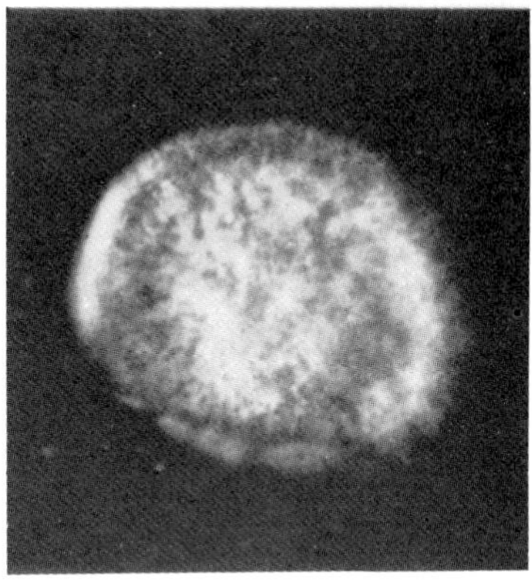

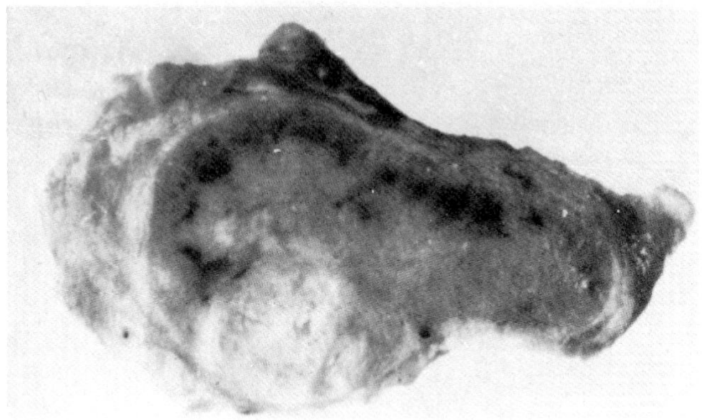

where a dog had acquired *C. immitis* infection. Soil samples collected from areas not near rodent burrows were negative for this fungus. Some positive results were obtained when soil was taken directly from the burrows. Most of the samples that yielded *C. immitis* were collected during the months of September through December, when the fall rains may have supplied the moisture needed for the growth of the fungus. In 1961 the organism was recovered from an ancient Indian camp site in San Diego County, California (34). Although direct transmission is unlikely, bedside interhuman transmission of coccidioidomycosis via growth on fomites has been reported in a hospital epidemic that involved six persons (11). Fifty dogs (29) were exposed in an area where coccidioidomycosis was known to exist and 29 (58 percent) became infected. Most cases developed in the cool months of the year, in contrast to the warm-season pattern of infection reported for man.

Cattle. Coccidioidomycosis in cattle (2, 8, 14, 32) is a benign disease which ordinarily involves only the lymph nodes of the chest—the posterior mediastinal and the bronchial. In a few cases small granulomatous lesions have been found in the lungs and in the submaxillary, retropharyngeal, and mesenteric lymph nodes. The affected glands are enlarged and contain a yellowish, glutinous pus, similar to that of tuberculosis (Figure 34.5). The abscess wall consists of granulation tissue (Figure 34.6). According to Maddy (2), some degree of calcification is shown by 15 percent of the lesions. Symptoms are not elicited.

With but few exceptions all cases have originated in the inland valleys of California, where the human infection occurs. The diseases in the human and bovine species have no direct relationship to each other because the infection is not transmitted from man to animals or vice versa. Both species contract the disease from the same source, that is, from dust infected with chlamydoconidia. As several cases have been found in cattle that were raised in Colorado and in Arizona, it is evident that the infection is not restricted to California.

Horses. In 1958, Zontine (35) reported a case of generalized coccidioidomycosis in a horse. The main clinical features of the disease were a course of 4 months, severe progressive emaciation, variable temperature, moderate anemia, pronounced leukocytosis, edema of the lower parts of the legs, and a peculiar attitude of the front feet. At necropsy it was found that the animal had died from recent abdominal hemorrhage resulting from a ruptured liver. Granular abcesses of various sizes were seen scattered throughout the lungs (Figure 34.7), spleen, and liver. Other cases have been observed in horses and in a pony (9).

Sheep. Coccidioidomycosis in a sheep was described in 1931 by Beck *et al.* (2). Since then a number of reports have appeared. The lesions are like those in cattle.

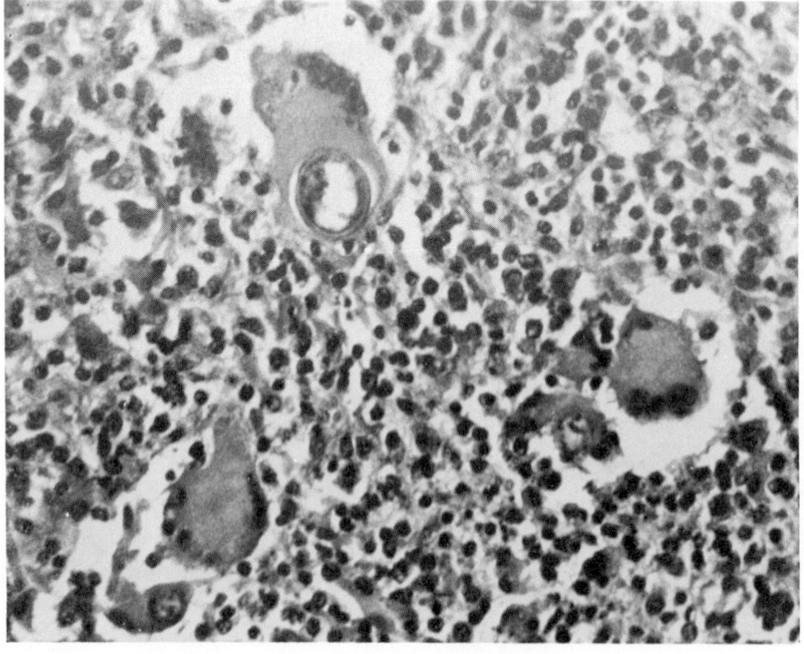

Figure 34.6. Coccidioidal granuloma section of a bovine lymph node showing granulation tissue and several giant cells, one of which contains a spherule of the causative agent. × 400. (Courtesy Stiles and Davis, *Jour. Am. Med. Assoc.*)

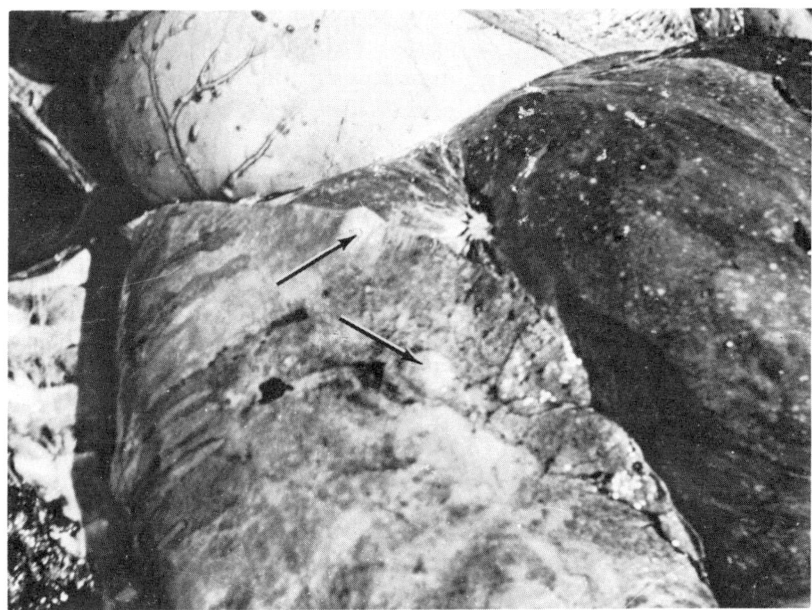

Figure 34.7. Coccidioidomycosis in a horse. Note raised nodules of coccidioidal granuloma (arrows) on surface of the lung. The largest nodule measured 3 cm in diameter. (Courtesy J. A. Rehkemper, *Cornell Vet.*)

Swine. In 1966, Prchal and Crecelius (26) described an infection in pigs raised in the area of Tucson, Arizona. Lesions occured as granulomas in the bronchial lymph nodes and were found to contain the fungus *C. immitis*.

Dogs. More cases of coccidioidomycosis have been described in the dog than in any other domestic animal (13, 15, 25, 28). Boxers and Doberman pinschers appear to be more susceptible than other breeds. Cases have been reported from Arizona, California, Iowa, Kansas, Texas, and Quebec. In general, granulomatous lesions involve the lungs as the primary site, but they are also seen in the pleura, liver (Figure 34.8), spleen, kidneys, and bones (Figure 34.9). The picture grossly resembles tuberculosis. In affected animals partial anorexia, vomition, and distress or collapse after eating are frequent. The disseminated form occurs frequently in this animal and usually produces a hopeless invalid if it does not

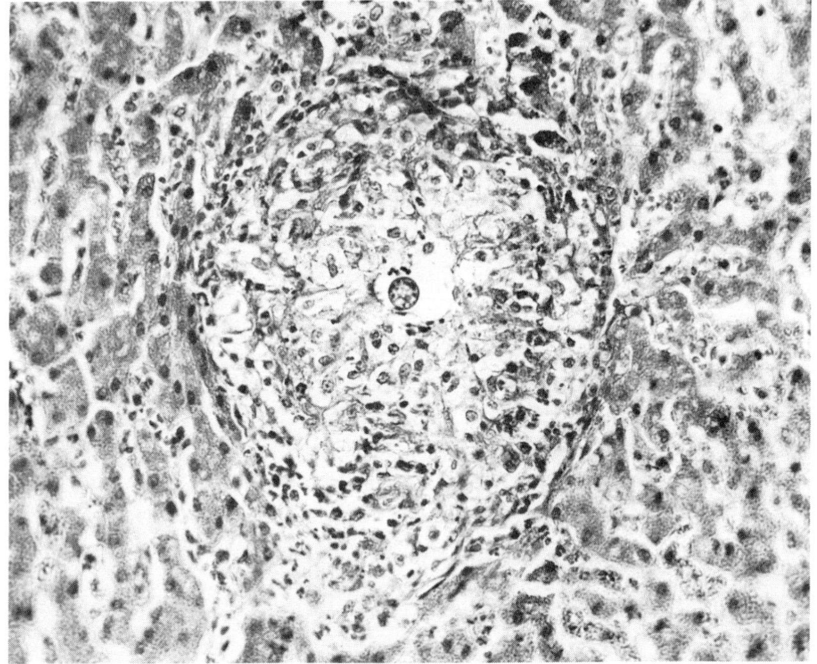

Figure 34.8. Coccidioidal granuloma in the liver of a dog showing central spherule and surrounding epithelioid cells. (Courtesy T. J. Hage, *Cornell Vet.*)

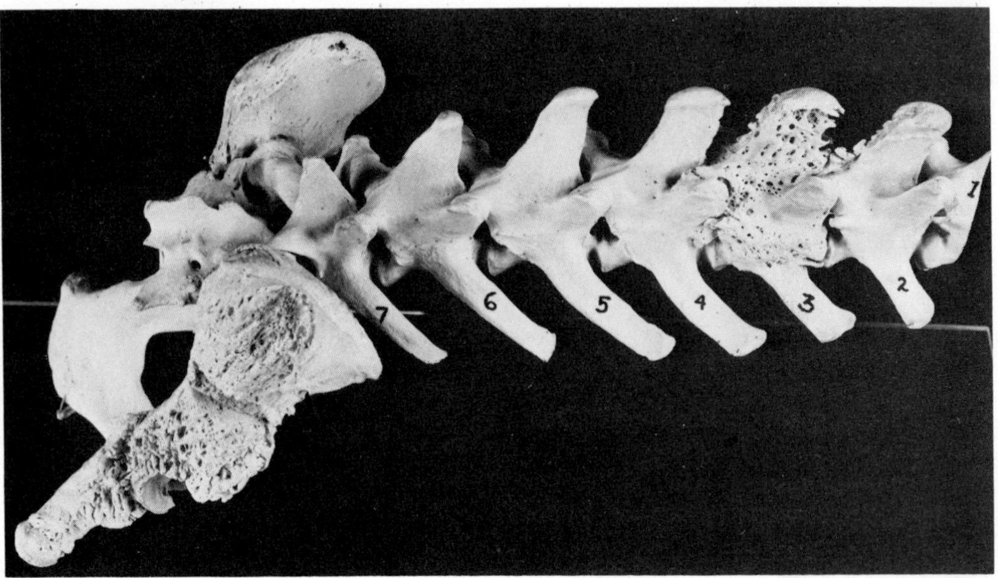

Figure 34.9. Lumbar vertebra and pelvis of dog showing coccidioidal lesions. (Courtesy T. J. Hage, *Cornell Vet.*)

result in death. This illness is common in the dog in the Southwest.

Cats. Coccidioidomycosis has been diagnosed in two cats in Arizona (30). One animal developed an abscess on the hip, and histologic sections of the subcutaneous tissue, lungs, and thoracic lymph nodes all showed *C. immitis*. In the second cat granulomas were found in the liver and kidneys in addition to the sites listed for the first victim.

Chinchillas. A case of coccidioidomycosis in a chinchilla has been described by Jasper (16). The disease was similar to that in the dog.

Man. Primary pulmonary coccidioidomycosis in man may be subclinical or clinical. The subclinical type occurs with minimal manifestations and is often overlooked. More severe cases show low-grade fever and other symptoms of pulmonary disease. Some patients may develop a hypersensitivity, indicated by erythema several weeks later. The coccidioidin skin test becomes positive within about 3 weeks after exposure or within days after symptoms appear. The longer this test remains positive the better the prognosis. A positive complement-fixation (CF) test is indicative of active or progressive infection.

Rarely the disease is primary in the skin or subcutaneous tissues with or without a history of trauma. Ulcerating painless nodules are produced.

Diagnosis. Coccidioidin, a product made from filtrates of broth cultures, is used for diagnostic purposes. The CF test also is useful, especially in indicating the progress of the disease. The fluorescent-antibody (FA) technique applied with absorbed conjugates has been useful in detecting *C. immitis* in clinical materials (17). The agar-gel-diffusion test with soluble spherule antigens is recommended in detecting *C. immitis* antibody in sera from suspect patients (20). Demonstration of the fungus either in the lesions or by cultural means provides a definitive diagnosis.

An exoantigen test developed by Kaufman and Standard (18) can be used for rapid identification of suspect cultures. This test is based on the reaction in agar gel of extracts from the fungal mycelium with specific precipitating antiserum to the TP and F antigens of *C. immitis*.

Immunity. Recovered animals are immune to reinfection. Infection results in development of cell-mediated immunity and a delayed hypersensitivity response. Vaccines have not been used in the field, although Castleberry *et al.* (5) have successfully vaccinated dogs with a killed arthroconidia (arthrospore) preparation.

Chemotherapy. Amphotericin B has been successfully used for therapy in humans (19).

REFERENCES

1. Ajello. Bact. Rev., 1967, *31*, 6.
2. Beck, Traum, and Harrington. Jour. Am. Vet. Med. Assoc., 1931, *78*, 490.
3. Breslau and Kubota. Jour. Bact., 1964, *87*, 468.
4. Burke. Proc. Soc. Exp. Biol. and Med., 1951, *76*, 332.

5. Castleberry, Converse, Sinski, Lowe, Pakes, and Favero. Jour. Inf. Dis., 1965, *115,* 41.
6. Converse. Proc. Soc. Exp. Biol. and Med., 1955, *90,* 709.
7. Creitz and Puckett. Am. Jour. Clin. Path., 1954, *24,* 1318.
8. Davis, Stiles, and McGregor. Jour. Am. Vet. Med. Assoc., 1938, *92,* 562.
9. DeMartini and Riddle. Jour. Am. Vet. Med. Assoc., 1969, *155,* 149.
10. Dickson. Jour. Am. Med. Assoc., 1938, *111,* 1362.
11. Eckmann, Schaefer, and Huppert. Am. Rev. Resp. Dis., 1964, *89,* 175.
12. Emmons. Pub. Health Rpts. (U.S.), 1942, *57,* 109.
13. Farness. Jour. Am. Vet. Med. Assoc., 1940, *97,* 263.
14. Giltner. Jour. Agr. Res., 1918, *14,* 533.
15. Hage and Moulton. Cornell Vet., 1954, *44,* 489.
16. Jasper. North Am. Vet., 1953, *34,* 570.
17. Kaplan and Clifford. Am. Rev. Resp. Dis., 1964, *89,* 651.
18. Kaufman and Standard. Current Microbiol., 1978, *1,* 135.
19. Klapper, Smith, and Conant. Jour. Am. Med. Assoc., 1958, *167,* 463.
20. Landay, Pash, and Millar. Jour. Lab. and Clin. Med., 1970, *75,* 197.
21. Maddy. Jour. Am. Vet. Med. Assoc., 1954, *124,* 456.
22. Maddy. Am. Jour. Vet. Res., 1959, *20,* 642.
23. Maddy. Vet. Med., 1959, *54,* 233.
24. Northey and Brooks. Jour. Bact., 1962, *84,* 742.
25. Plummer. Can. Jour. Comp. Med. and Vet. Sci., 1941, *5,* 146.
26. Prchal and Crecelius. Jour. Am. Vet. Med. Assoc., 1966, *148,* 1168.
27. Puckett. Am. Rev. Tuberc., 1954, *70,* 320.
28. Reed. Jour. Am. Vet. Med. Assoc., 1956, *128,* 196.
29. Reed and Converse. Am. Jour. Vet. Res., 1966, *27,* 1027.
30. Reed, Hoge, and Trautman. Jour. Am. Vet. Med. Assoc., 1963, *143,* 953.
31. Short, Schleicher, and Rice. Jour. Am. Vet. Med. Assoc., 1955, *127,* 352.
32. Stiles, Shahan, and Davis. Jour. Am. Vet. Med. Assoc., 1933, *82,* 928.
33. Vogel, Peace, and Koger. Am. Jour. Path., 1957, *33,* 1023.
34. Walch, Pribnow, Wyborney, and Walch. Am. Rev. Resp. Dis., 1961, *84,* 359.
35. Zontine. Jour. Am. Vet. Med. Assoc., 1958, *132,* 490.

THE GENUS *CRYPTOCOCCUS*

Cryptococcus neoformans

SYNONYMS: *Torula histolytica, Cryptococcus hominis*

PERFECT STATE: *Filobasidiella neoformans*

European blastomycosis is a subacute or chronic mycotic infection of animals and man caused by *C. neoformans*. The organism frequently attacks the tissues of the nervous system, but lesions may also be found in the lungs, skin, lymph glands, and other tissues. The disease has been reported from all parts of the world (17). In the United States cryptococcosis has been reported in horses, cattle, sheep, goats, a pig, dogs, cats, foxes, mink, ferrets, koala bears, cheetahs, a civet cat, guinea pigs, monkeys, and man (2, 8, 14, 18).

Morphology and Cultivation. *C. neoformans* grows rapidly on Sabouraud's glucose agar. The colony is flat or slightly heaped, shiny, moist or mucoid, with smooth edges. The color is cream at first, later becoming brown. The organism grows as a yeast at room temperature and at 37 C. It is spherical or ovoid in shape, thick-walled, single or budding, and refractile and measures from 3 to 8 μm in diameter (Figure 34.10). It develops capsules, but no mycelium. Variants that have lost their capsules are avirulent. The genus is characterized by inositol assimilation and urease production. Incubation at 40 C destroys the organisms (11). Shields and Ajello (19) have developed a selective medium that permits recovery of *C. neoformans* from heavily contaminated materials. It contains creatinine as a nitrogen source, diphenyl ($C_6H_5C_6H_5$) and chloramphenicol as mold and bacterial inhibitors, and *Guizotia abyssinica* seed extract as a specific color marker.

Epidemiology and Pathogenesis. *C. neoformans* has been isolated from soil (4), which appears to be its natural habitat. Emmons (5) examined pigeon nests and pigeon droppings from 19 premises by mouse inoculation for the presence of pathogenic fungi. *C. neoformans* was isolated from 63 of 111 specimens that came from 16 of these 19 premises. Ajello (1) has indicated that habitats that favor growth of *C. neoformans* occur throughout the world. It flourishes in bird manures, especially that of pigeons. This association may be governed by the presence of creatinine, which is utilizable as a nitrogen source by *C. neoformans* but not by competing microorganisms. Most cases of cryptococcosis result from inhalation of the fungus, but direct implantation of the skin or entry through the teat meatus in the cow and goat also frequently occur.

The disease is slow in development and predominantly involves the central nervous system. The organism's tropism for nervous tissue is probably related to its ability to metabolize nitrogen-containing substances of low molecular weight such as urea, uric acid, and creatine, which are relatively plentiful in the cerebrospinal fluid. Capsule formation prevents phagocytosis, and,

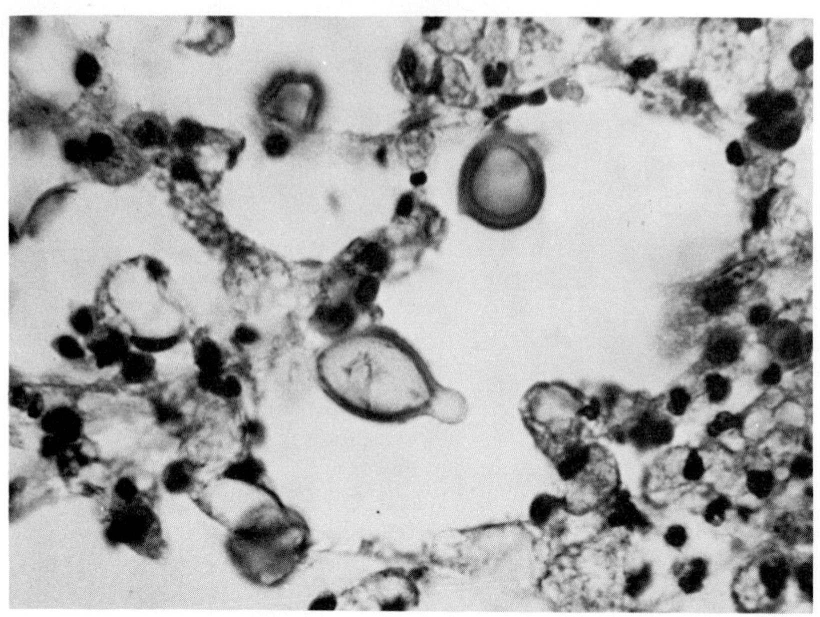

Figure 34.10. Photomicrograph showing a round cell of *Cryptococcus neoformans* with thick capsule in the upper part of the field. Below is an oval cell in the process of budding. × 790. (Courtesy Jean Holzworth, *Cornell Vet.*)

since capsular material is nonantigenic, there is no opsonic antibody response. The organism continues to grow extracellularly in the tissue and causes pressure atrophy of surrounding areas. The great mass of capsular material may give affected tissue a gelatinous appearance. There is little inflammatory response.

Dogs. Encephalitis or a chronic respiratory condition may herald the disease. Cases have been accompanied by pulmonary, generalized and intraocular involvement. The usual pathologic findings reported in dogs are those of a granulomatous destructive process involving nasal mucosa and turbinates, facial sinuses, adjacent osseous structures, and meningitis. Primary pulmonary lesions with secondary meningitis may also occur (15).

Cats. Cryptococcosis in cats (6, 8) has also been characterized by lesions in the central nervous system and granulomas involving the eye, sinuses, and nasal septum. There may be a chronic ocular and nasal discharge. Lesions involving the skin of the head have also been observed (Figure 34.11).

Sheep. Laws and Simmons (12) have reported a case of cryptococcosis in a sheep in which organisms were present in the leptomeninges, brain, mucosa of the nose and maxillary sinuses, and in the lungs. Clinically the sheep presented with swollen maxillary sinuses, mucoid nasal discharge, dyspnea, coughing, and anorexia.

Other animals. In cattle, outbreaks of cryptococcic mastitis with regional lymph node involvement have occurred (2, 9). See Chapter 35.

In horses, respiratory disease accompanied by nasal obstructive growths and lesions on the lip have been caused by *C. neoformans.*

The disease has been reported in monkeys (7). Although it was not suspected clinically, it was diagnosed on histologic examination by finding typical cryptococcic granulomas in the lungs and deep in the brain parenchyma.

Man. In man, *C. neoformans* may produce a cutaneous form of disease in which healing sometimes occurs spontaneously after several weeks; a pulmonary disease with unilateral or bilateral lesions and a low-grade pneumonia; or a central nervous disease in which symptoms suggestive of a subacute or chronic meningitis, abscess, or brain tumor appear. Meningitis may follow the cutaneous form or it may occur as a primary condition. A case of cryptococcal hepatitis was reported in 1965 (16).

Diagnosis. Spinal fluid and material from lesions should be spread in a drop of India ink and examined microscopically. *C. neoformans* appears as a large transparent halo surrounding a cell which may carry a single bud. No other similar capsulated organism is known to invade the nervous system in animals (13).

On culture, a moist, creamy, spreading growth appears in a few days at 30 C. Capsule development is slow and is not optimal for some days more. Chloramphenicol or other broad-spectrum antibiotics should be included in the medium to inhibit bacterial contaminants. Nonpathogenic *Cryptococcus* spp. cannot be differentiated by physiological tests from pathogenic species.

Pigeons and mice are very susceptible to experimentally induced infections. Intracerebral or intraperitoneal inoculation of specimens containing *C. neoformans* will cause death in 3 to 18 days. Pigeons and mice both show signs of CNS disturbance before death.

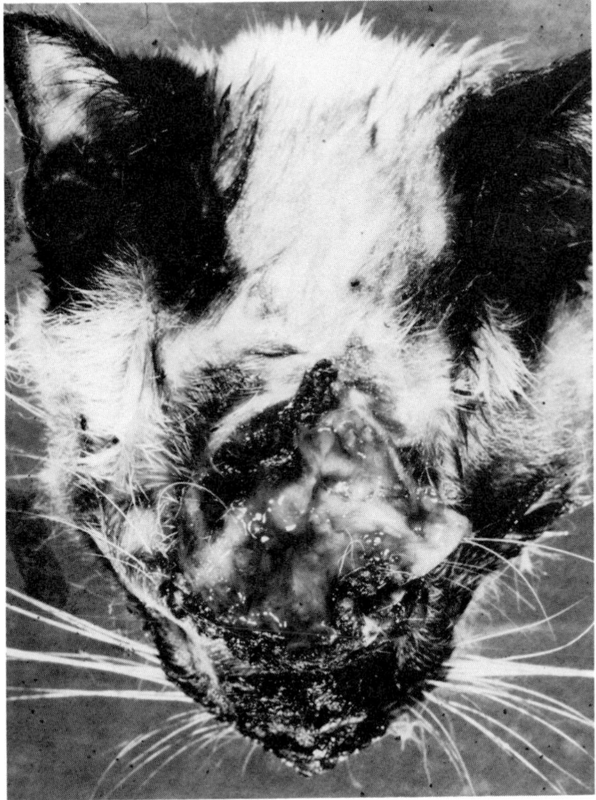

Figure 34.11. Lesion caused by *Cryptococcus neoformans* on the head of a cat. (Courtesy Joseph Kowalski).

Immunologic methods are of little value in diagnosis. However, a sensitized latex particle test is available for detection of capsular antigen in cerebrospinal and other fluids.

Chemotherapy. *In vitro* tests have shown that the thiosemicarbazones, cycloheximide (actidione), polymyxin B, ethyl vanillate, prophylparaben, methylparaben, and neomycin sulfate are inhibitory for this organism (3, 10, 20). Amphotericin B has been used with varying success. The application of an aqueous solution of hydrated lime and sodium hydroxide has been used to eliminate *C. neoformans* from contaminated pigeon coops (21).

REFERENCES

1. Ajello. Bact. Rev., 1967, *31,* 6.
2. Barron. Jour. Am. Vet. Med. Assoc., 1955, *127,* 125.
3. Eisen, Shapiro, and Fischer. Can. Med. Assoc. Jour., 1955, *72,* 33.
4. Emmons. Jour. Bact., 1951, *62,* 685.
5. Emmons. Am. Jour. Hyg., 1955, *62,* 227.
6. Fischer. Jour. Am. Vet. Med. Assoc., 1971, *158,* 191.
7. Garner, Ford, and Ross. Jour. Am. Vet. Med. Assoc., 1969, *155,* 1163.
8. Holzworth. Cornell Vet., 1952, *42,* 12.
9. Innes, Seibold, and Arentzen. Am. Jour. Vet. Res., 1952, *13,* 469.
10. Johnson, Joyner, and Perry. Antibiotics and Chemother., 1952, *2,* 636.
11. Kligman, Crane, and Norris. Am. Jour. Med. Sci., 1951, *221,* 273.
12. Laws and Simmons. Austral. Vet. Jour., 1966, *42,* 321.
13. Littman, Borok, and Dalton. Am. Jour. Epidemiol., 1965, *82,* 197.
14. Pounden, Amberson, and Jaeger. Am. Jour. Vet. Res., 1952, *13,* 121.
15. Price and Powers. Jour. Am. Vet. Med. Assoc., 1967, *150,* 988.
16. Procknow, Benfield, Rippon, Diener, and Archer. Jour. Am. Med. Assoc., 1965, *191,* 269.
17. Saunders. Cornell Vet., 1948, *38,* 213.
18. Seibold, Roberts, and Jordan. Jour. Am. Vet. Med. Assoc., 1953, *122,* 213.
19. Shields and Ajello. Science, 1966, *151,* 208.
20. Simon. Am. Jour. Vet. Res., 1955, *16,* 394.
21. Walter and Coffee. Am. Jour. Epidemiol., 1968, *87,* 173.

THE GENUS *HISTOPLASMA*

This genus belongs to the phylum Ascomycota. There are two species of importance as causes of disease in man and animals, *Histoplasma capsulatum* and *H. farciminosum*.

Histoplasma capsulatum

PERFECT STATE: *Ajellomyces capsulatus*

This intracellular organism was first described by Darling (6) in the tissues of natives in the Canal Zone in 1906. Its fungal nature was demonstrated by De-Monbreun (7) in 1934, who cultured the fungus from a human case. Since then, histoplasmosis has been described in a wide variety of species in many parts of the world. The majority of cases are subclinical, inapparent infections.

Morphology and Cultivation. The organism is a small (about 1 to 3 μm in diameter), oval, yeastlike fungus in tissues (Figure 34.12) and in media incubated at 37 C and can be stained by Giemsa, Periodic Acid Schiff, or hematoxylin and eosin methods. Cultures are made on Sabhi, Sabouraud, or Mycobiotic agars at 30 C and should be held for up to 10 weeks as some strains are very slow growing. In culture at room temperature, the organism is a typical moldlike, filamentous fungus. In fact, it is sometimes difficult to distinguish it from cultures of *Blastomyces*. In old cultures or under adverse

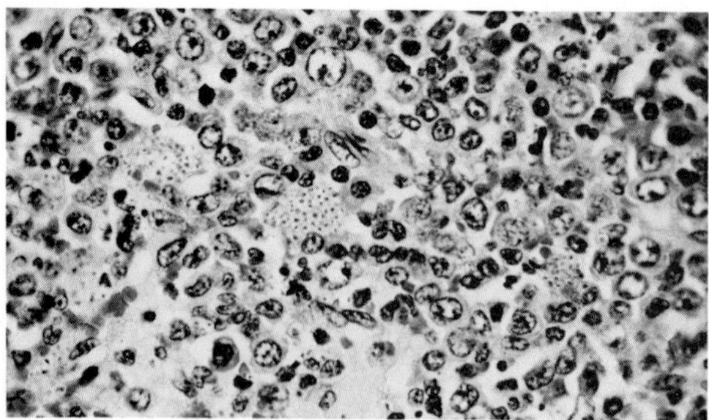

Figure 34.12. Hypercellular bone marrow of a horse containing many *Histoplasma capsulatum*. H and E stain. × 390. (Courtesy Roger J. Panciera, *Cornell Vet.*)

conditions, *H. capsulatum* produces diagnostic chlamydoconidia—round, thick-walled structures 7 to 15 μm in diameter.

Small, pear-shaped microconidia are also produced in cultures at 30 C. The yeast phase is produced on brain-heart infusion agar with glutamine 37 C. Tissue culture has also been used to convert *H. capsulatum* to the yeastlike phase (20). Smith and Furcolow (28) studied 3 techniques for isolating *H. capsulatum* from soil and recommend a modified oil flotation method. By employing FA techniques, Kaufman and Blumer (16) have demonstrated the existence of five *H. capsulatum* serotypes.

Epidemiology and Pathogenesis. Endemic areas in the United States include the Mississippi, Ohio, and St. Lawrence river valleys. The natural reservoir of the fungus is soil (19), which does not appear to be generally contaminated but which supports concentrations of *H. capsulatum* in particular areas where certain organic matter is found. For instance, the soil of chicken houses and yards located in endemic regions frequently carries high concentrations of this organism (14, 31, 32). Investigations indicate that chickens are not a reservoir of histoplasmosis, and their association with the fungus remains unexplained. Data suggest that urban starling-blackbird roosts may harbor *H. capsulatum* and contribute significantly to the prevalence of cutaneous sensitivity to histoplasmin among children residing or attending school near the roosts (30).

Emmons (10) reported that dung from bats was the factor responsible for the constant saprophytic infestation of soil in certain premises that he investigated, and Shacklette *et al.* (26) recovered the organism from the liver and spleen of bats. Subsequent investigations (1, 2, 8, 11) concerning the role of bats in the spread of histoplasmosis have shown that they harbor *H. capsulatum,* that their feces contain the organism, and that caves inhabited by bats have been shown to be heavily contaminated with the fungus (27). It seems likely that bats seed the soil with infected feces and that *H. capsulatum* may then be transmitted by air from these foci.

In tap water the yeast phase will change to the mycelial phase and grow (24).

Man has acquired histoplasmosis in the laboratory (23), and feathers from a pillow yielded the fungus in an epidemiologic study of the disease in an infant (3).

Entry into the body is via airborne conidia into the lung, where phagocytosis occurs. Infection then spreads throughout the reticuloendothelial system by means of migrating mononuclear cells that contain the parasite. The infection may be inapparent (19) or may cause acute, subacute, chronic, localized, or disseminated disease. Primary lesions often are located in the lungs. Severe systemic infections are associated with splenomegaly, hepatomegaly, leukopenia, anemia, and emaciation. Ulcerations of the intestine may occur and produce diarrhea. The central nervous system, kidneys, bone marrow, and skin are frequently involved in clinical cases. The organism is packed within mononuclear phagocytic cells in great numbers (Figure 34.13).

The dog is the most commonly infected domestic animal. The disease is characterized by a chronic, debilitating digestive disturbance with enlarged abdomen, heptomegaly, lymphadenopathy, and ascites. A chronic cough, irregular pyrexia, and dyspnea are frequent (25).

The communicability of *H. capsulatum* from dog to dog has been established, and although there is at present no proof of a relationship between the disease in dogs and that in man, the infected dog must be considered a potentially dangerous source because it can disseminate the organism by saliva, vomitus, feces, and urine (4).

Spontaneous infections have also been found in cats, cattle, a horse, a pig, a woodchuck, a skunk, an opossum, a gray fox, a ferret, and a monkey, but the incidence of the disease in these animals is low. Sheep, a pig, and fowl have been recorded as histoplasmin-positive. According to Furcolow and Ruhe (12), histoplasmin sensitivity can be demonstrated in cattle, and it is probable that cattle and human beings are infected from the same source, but it appears that cattle are not an important animal reservoir.

Naturally infected bats have been located in the United States (Alabama, 1; Arizona, 8; Maryland, 11; Oklahoma, 2; and Texas 11) and in the Canal Zone. The

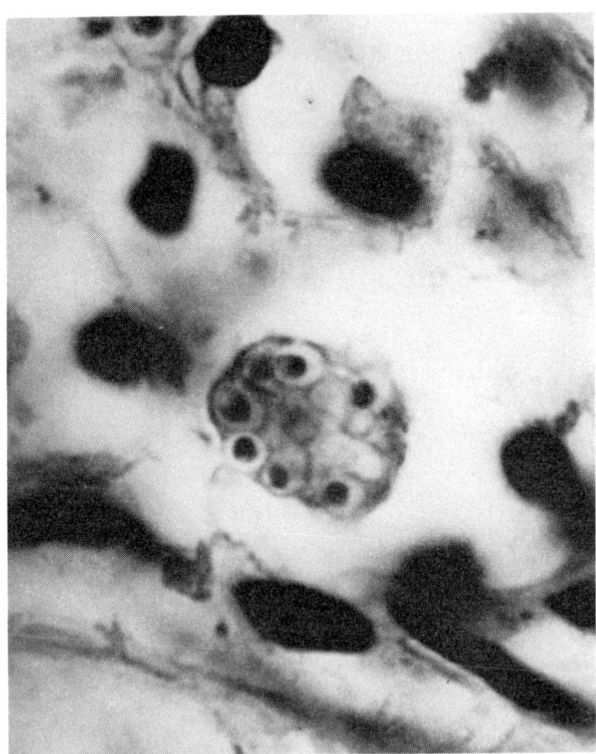

Figure 34.13. *Histoplasma capsulatum,* parasites in macrophage of a dog; natural infection. × 2800. (Courtesy Oreg. Agr. Exp. Sta., J. W. Osebold.)

fungus has been isolated from the liver, lungs, spleen, intestines, and feces of this mammal.

A spontaneous outbreak of histoplasmosis has been described in guinea pigs (5). Adult animals showed a chronic disease with progressive emaciation and lameness of the hind legs. The young below 3 months of age died in 2 to 4 weeks, presenting ruffled fur, great dorsal curvature, and sometimes closed eyelids and catarrhal conjunctivitis. At necropsy the principal lesions were ulcerative gastritis, hemorrhagic and catarrhal enteritis, and enlarged spleen and mesenteric lymph nodes.

Immunity. Recoveries from localized infections are common and are associated with the development of cell-mediated and humoral immunity. With recovery, antibody titers tend to wane, but the delayed hypersensitivity reaction persists and so the skin test with histoplasmin remains positive (21). Hemagglutination, complement-fixation, agar-gel precipitin (15), and sensitized latex particle tests are available for measuring antibody titers.

H. capsulatum shares H or H and M precipitinogens with *H. capsulatum* var. *duboisii* and *H. farciminosum* (18). This cross-reactivity limits the value of the exoantigen test (18) for identification of *Histoplasma* isolates in areas such as Africa where all 3 strains occur.

Diagnosis. Stained smears and cultures on Sabouraud agar of lesions, peritoneal fluid, cerebrospinal fluid, tracheal aspirates, bone marrow, and other materials are prepared. The organism is frequently difficult to culture from specimens. Smears may also be examined by the fluorescent-antibody technique (17).

Complement-fixation tests with the yeast and mycelial antigens, and immunodiffusion tests are used for serologic diagnosis. Skin testing with histoplasmin is not useful diagnostically because of cross-reactions with other fungi.

Isolation of a hyphomycete that bears tuberculate macroconidia is suggestive of *H. capsulatum.* However, a number of saprophytic *Arthroderma, Chrysosporium,* and *Sepedonium* spp. grossly and microscopically resemble the mycelial form of *H. capsulatum.* They can be distinguished by the exoantigen test (18).

Chemotherapy. *In vitro* studies have shown *H. capsulatum* to be sensitive to ethyl vanillate (13) and nystatin. According to Drauhet *et al.* (9), the treatment with nystatin of fulminating, moderately acute, or chronic disease in hamsters and mice has decreased mortality, inhibited dissemination of the disease in many animals, and sterilized the tissues in selected animals. Administration of sulfonamides, admixed in the diet, has also proved highly effective in treating mice infected with lethal doses of the organism (22). There is evidence that amphotericin B is effective in treating chronic pulmonary histoplasmosis where there are active lesions and positive sputum cultures (29). Amphotericin B is not recommended for the treatment of acute histoplasmosis.

REFERENCES

1. Ajello, Hosty and Palmer. Am. Jour. Trop. Med. and Hyg., 1967, *16,* 329.
2. Bryles, Cozad, and Robinson. Am. Jour. Trop. Med. and Hyg., 1969, *18,* 399.
3. Campbell, Hill, and Falgout. Science, 1962, *136,* 1050.
4. Cole, Farrell, Chamberlain, Prior, and Saslaw. Jour. Am. Vet. Med. Assoc., 1963, *122,* 471.
5. Correa and Pacheco. Can. Jour. Comp. Med. and Vet. Sci., 1967, *31,* 203.
6. Darling. Jour. Am. Med. Assoc., 1906, *46,* 1283.
7. DeMonbreun. Am. Jour. Trop. Med., 1934, *14,* 93.
8. DiSalvo, Ajello, Palmer, and Winkler. Am. Jour. Epidemiol., 1969, *89,* 606.
9. Drauhet, Schwarz, and Bingham. Antibiotic and Chemother., 1956, *6,* 23.

10. Emmons. Pub. Health Rpts. (U.S.), 1958, *73,* 590.
11. Emmons, Klite, Baer, and Hill. Am. Jour. Epidemiol., 1966, *84,* 103.
12. Furcolow and Ruhe. Am. Jour. Pub. Health, 1949, *39,* 719.
13. Hansen and Beene. Proc. Soc. Exp. Biol. and Med., 1951, *77,* 365.
14. Ibach, Larsh, and Furcolow. Science, 1954, *119,* 71.
15. Kaufman, Leo. Serodiagnosis of fungal disease. Manual of clinical immunology. Am. Soc. Microbiol., Washington, D.C., 1976, p. 363.
16. Kaufman and Blumer. Jour. Bact., 1968, *95,* 1243.
17. Kaufman and Kaplan. Jour. Bact., 1963, *85,* 986.
18. Kaufman and Standard. Current Microbiol., 1978, *1,* 135.
19. Larsh, Hinton, and Cozad. Am. Jour. Hyg., 1956, *63,* 18.
20. Larsh, Hinton, and Silberg. Proc. Soc. Exp. Biol. and Med., 1956, *93,* 612.
21. Loosli, Procknow, Tanzi, Grayston, Combs, and Lowell. Jour. Lab. and Clin. Med., 1954, *43,* 669.
22. Mayer, Eisman, Geftic, Konopka, and Tanzola. Antibiotics and Chemother., 1956, *6,* 215.
23. Murray and Howard. Am. Rev. Resp. Dis., 1964, *89,* 631.
24. Ritter. Am. Jour. Pub. Health, 1954, *44,* 199.
25. Schwabe. Vet. Med., 1954, *49,* 479.
26. Shacklette, Diercks, and Gale. Science, 1962, *135,* 1135.
27. Shacklette, Hasenclever and Miranda. Am. Jour. Epidemiol., 1967, *86,* 246.
28. Smith and Furcolow. Jour. Lab. and Clin. Med., 1964, *64,* 342.
29. Sutliff. Veterans Administrations - Armed Forces cooperative study on histoplasmosis. Am. Rev. Resp. Dis., 1964, *89,* 641.
30. Tosh, Doto, Beecher, and Chin. Am. Rev. Resp. Dis., 1970, *101,* 283.
31. Zeidberg and Ajello. Jour. Bact., 1954, *68,* 156.
32. Zeidberg, Ajello, Dillon, and Runyon. Am. Jour. Pub. Health, 1952, *42,* 930.

Histoplasma farciminosum

SYNONYMS: *Cryptococcus farciminosus, Saccharomyces farciminosus, Endomyces farciminosa, Histoplasma farciminosa, Saccharomyces equi, Blastomyces farciminosa*

H. farciminosum (2) is the causative agent of *epizootic lymphangitis* or *pseudofarcy* of horses and mules. A few cases have been reported in cattle, but the latter are not highly susceptible. The infection is endemic in countries bordering the Mediterranean, particularly in Italy and North Africa. It is also found in central and southern Africa, and in parts of Asia and Russia. The disease caused a great deal of trouble during the Boer War, and cases were brought back to England after its conclusion. It also was of much concern during World War I. Some doubtful cases have been reported in the United States. Most of these, possibly all, were cases of sporotrichosis.

The organism was first demonstrated in pus by Rivolta in 1873. It was not successfully cultivated until 1896. The first pure cultures were obtained by Tokishiga (5) in Japan.

Morphology and Staining Reactions. In pus the organism appears as a double-contoured oval or ovoid body, measuring 2.5 to 3.5 by 3 to 4 μm. The cells resemble those of yeasts very closely. The cytoplasm is granular, and here and there bits of cytoplasm may be seen extruding from a break in the cell wall, forming buds from which daughter cells are formed. In cultures the organism produces both hyphae and ascospores (3).

The fungus cells can be stained, though not very satisfactorily. Structural details are best seen in fresh, unstained preparations. The Gram stain usually is retained.

Cultural Features. *H. farciminosum* is strongly aerobic. It has been successfully cultivated on a variety of media, but growth is slow and uncertain. When incubated under the most favorable cultural conditions now known, growth usually is not evident for 1 to 3 weeks or longer, and of many tubes inoculated similarly a considerable part may fail to exhibit growth. Growth may be obtained on plain agar and broth and on potato, coagulated egg medium, coagulated serum medium, and various other special media. On solid media, growth appears in the form of small grayish white granules that have a dry appearance and may become leatherlike in structure. In liquid media, growth generally occurs in the form of scanty, granular sediment. Sugar media are not fermented.

H. farciminosum is characteristically sterile in its mycelial form. These cultures can be identified by the type of exoantigen produced (4).

Pathogenicity. Epizootic lymphangitis of horses is characterized by inflammation of the superficial lymphatic vessels and nodes, principally of the legs, the chest, and the neck. Infection is believed to occur through wounds. In severe cases lesions may be found on any part of the body and even on the mucous membranes.

The lymph channels become enlarged and appear as tortuous cords beneath the skin, connecting the swollen lymph nodes. The nodes soften and rupture, forming craterlike ulcers from which a thick pus exudes. The yeastlike organism can easily be demonstrated in such pus. When mucosal lesions occur, they are most likely to be found in the nasal passages, but there are records of their occurrence on the genitalia and of the transmission of the disease from stallions to mares by copulation.

Bennett (1) described a type of equine pneumonia that was believed to be caused by *H. farciminosum*. It was of an interstitial type beginning with infiltrations of lymphocytes and then monocytes. Syncytia and giant cells next appeared and in these the *Histoplasma* could be seen. The organisms then multiplied profusely, leading to extensive destructive changes and fatality. The condition was not associated with skin manifestations. The organism was not cultivated and therefore was not certainly identified.

Treatment. The disease is chronic as a rule, though some cases heal spontaneously after a few weeks. The chronic cases usually are incurable. Sodium iodide given intravenously has some effect in treating the infection.

REFERENCES

1. Bennett. Jour. Comp. Path. and Therap., 1931, *44,* 85.
2. Dodge. Medical mycology. C. V. Mosby, St. Louis, Mo., 1935.
3. Eberbeck. Arch. f. Tierheilk., 1926, *54,* 1.
4. Kaufman and Standard. Current Microbiol., 1978, *1,* 135.
5. Tokishiga. Zentrbl. f. Bakt., I. Abt., 1896, *19,* 105.

35 Mycotic Diseases Associated with a Variety of Fungal Genera

In this chapter, we shall describe a number of important fungal diseases that can be caused by any of a number of different and unrelated fungi. Most of these infections are examples of opportunism where fungal contamination is introduced either iatrogenically as in mastitis or through damaged epithelia or mucous membranes as in mycotic rumenitis or keratitis. In the case of mycotic abortion heavy fungal contamination of the animal's immediate environment is an important factor in the infective process.

Mycotic Abortion

Fungal infections of the placenta are a well-known and important cause of abortion in the bovine. One survey found that fungal infection accounted for 13.4 to 24.9 percent of all abortions investigated annually in a large area of southern England between 1959 and 1966 (17). In the United States about 5 percent of bovine abortions are caused by fungi (16). Fungal abortions have also been reported in the horse (15) and sheep (19, 20).

Etiology. The primary species known to cause mycotic abortion are:

Aspergillus fumigatus
Other *Aspergillus* spp.
Absidia ramosa
Mucor pusillus
Mortierella wolfii
Cephalosporium spp.
Candida tropicalis
Allescheria boydii (Petriellidium boydii)
Torulopsis glabrata.

Mortierella wolfii is the most important cause of bovine mycotic abortion in New Zealand (7). This fungus has also been found in aborted bovine fetuses in the United States (35), and may be more important than hitherto realized because it is relatively difficult to culture and isolate from specimens.

Epidemiology and Pathogenesis. The majority of fungal abortions in cattle occur in winter and spring during the time when hay, silage, and other conserved feeds are fed (1, 34). Part of the high incidence in winter, however, may be explained by the greater number of calves born at this time. In the northeastern United States and in England mycotic abortions peak in January and February, and the majority occur during the last trimester of pregnancy. The abortion rate for English cattle fed hay in cowsheds was much higher than that for animals kept in loose housing systems (34). Thus there is circumstantial evidence that close, prolonged exposure to sources of spores in feed such as hay is important in the infectious process. According to Bendixen and Plum (5), infection takes place by the respiratory or alimentary route. Subsequent hematogenous spread leads to placental infection. The ability of blood-borne spores to produce placental infection has been demonstrated experimentally (10, 26). Mycotic pneumonia associated with mycotic abortion occurs frequently (9, 11) and suggests that infection initially enters the respiratory tract—a conclusion supported by the much higher incidence of mycotic abortion in cattle tied close to their feed in cowsheds and so

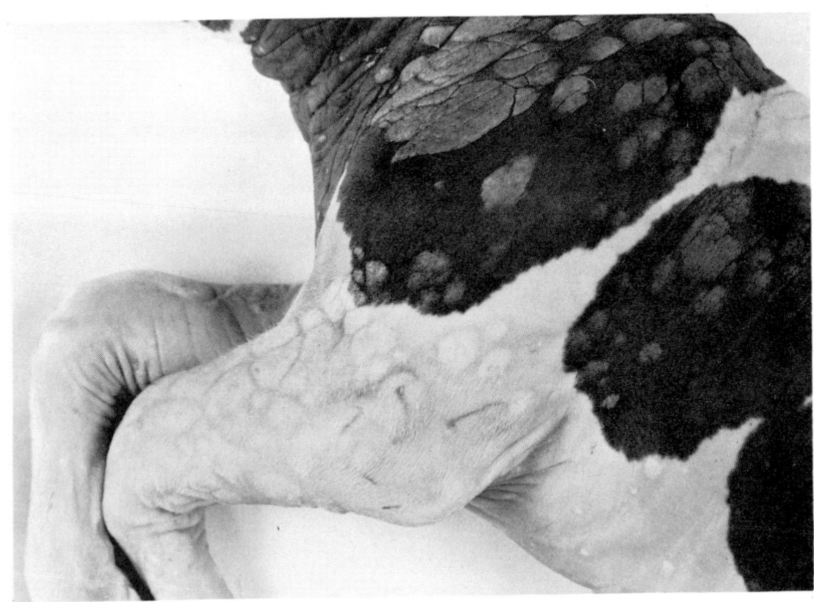

Figure 35.1. Lesions on skin of fetus aborted because of *Aspergillus* spp. infection. (Courtesy Kenneth McEntee.)

continuously exposed to potentially high local concentrations of fungal spores in the air they inspire. However, spores in the feed may also enter the bloodstream from the intestine (3).

Initial germination of spores in the bovine placenta is stimulated by a carbohydrate-containing substance of low molecular weight in the placental tissue (8, 33). Fungal growth in the placenta leads to areas of infarction in the caruncles. The fetal membranes become infiltrated with gelatinous lemon-yellow masses. Hyphae proliferate in the arterial walls of the cotyledons and also in the skin of the fetus, where necrotic plaques are produced (Figure 35.1).

Serous fluid accumulates in the fetal peritoneum and pericardium. Abortion apparently occurs because the fetus dies due to impaired placental circulation.

There is evidence (34) that not all placental fungal infections result in abortion and that a viable fetus may be born of infected dams. The amount of placental damage is probably critical in determining whether abortion of a dead fetus occurs.

The cotyledons are usually necrotic and dry (Figure 35.2), and portions of the maternal caruncles may remain adherent to the fetal villi. Although endometritis is present in mycotic abortion, the subsequent reproductive performance of the cows is frequently unaffected, and

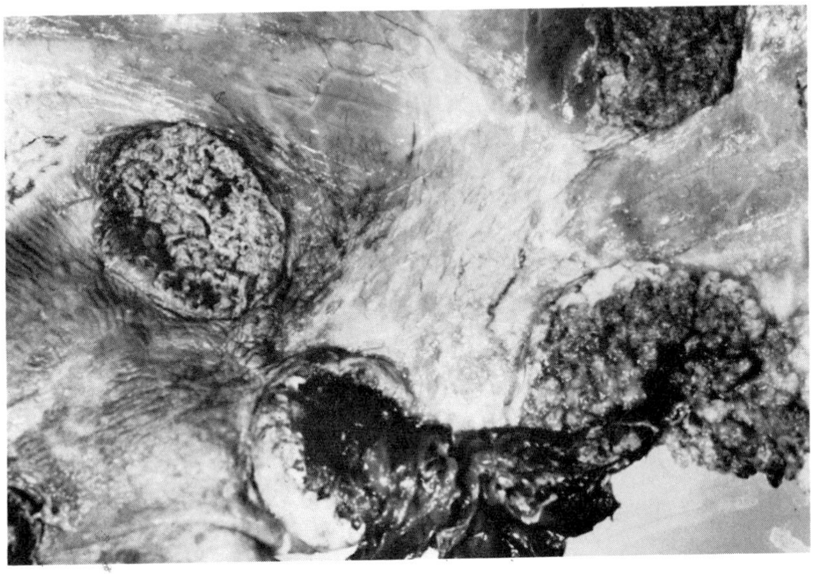

Figure 35.2. Placenta aborted because of *Aspergillus* spp. infection. The fetal cotyledons on the right have areas of necrosis and adherent tissue from the maternal caruncle. (Courtesy John King.)

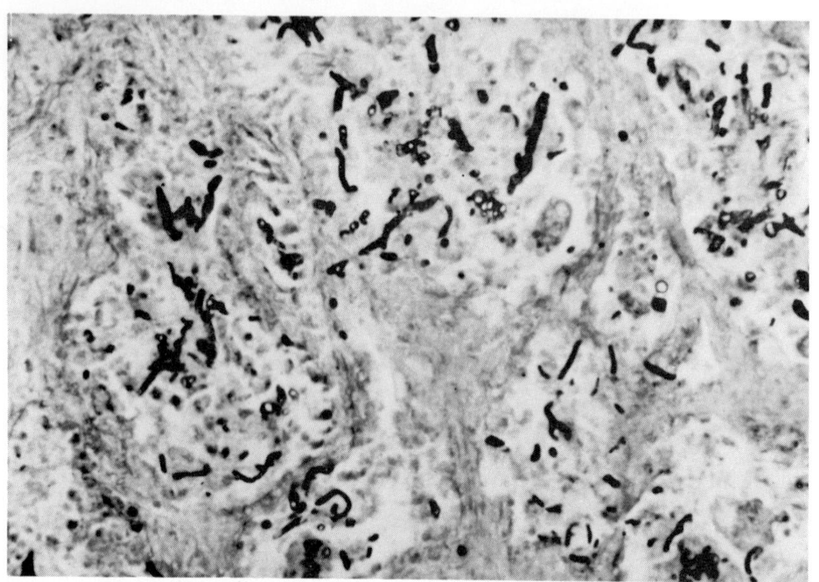

Figure 35.3. A section of placenta from a case of mycotic abortion showing many hyphal segments. × 400. (Courtesy Clyde Boyer.)

cows apparently do not continue to carry the infection in their reproductive tracts.

Diagnosis. Fungal elements in fetal stomach contents and in the placenta (Figure 35.3) are diagnostic and can be demonstrated by direct microscopic examination and by culture on Sabouraud's medium. Mycotic placentitis is usually accompanied by hyphae in the fetal stomach contents (34). There is no available method of diagnosing mycotic placentitis before abortion occurs.

Mycotic Mastitis

Fungal mastitis is usually caused by yeastlike fungi and its incidence has greatly increased with the advent of intramammary antibiotic therapy during the 1950s and 1960s. The disease is fairly common in dairy-cow and goat herds.

Etiology. The majority of isolations from cases of fungal mastitis in the United States belong to the genera *Candida, Trichosporon,* and *Cryptococcus* (12). In other parts of the world other genera such as *Pichia* and *Torulopsis* may be important. The following are the more common genera and species that have been reported:

Candida krusei, parakrusei, guilliermundi, tropicalis, pseudotropicalis, albicans, parapsilosis, norvegensis, albidus, and *stellatoidea*
Trichosporon cutaneum
Torulopsis spp.
Rhodotorula spp.
Allescheria boydii (Petriellidium boydii)
Pichia spp.
Cryptococcus neoformans
Aspergillus fumigatus
Geotrichum candidum

Epidemiology and Pathogenesis. Epizootics of yeast mastitis have been traced to the use of intramammary antibiotic preparations that were contaminated with yeasts (4, 22). Thus the disease may be iatrogenic. The disease has often occurred 4 to 5 days after treatment of a herd infected with *Streptococcus agalactiae* (13). Many of the yeast infections were associated with the administration of home-produced infusions or the use of the same cannula or syringe to infuse a number of quarters. The use of single-dose antibiotic preparations from disposable tubes is much less likely to be associated with fungal mastitis (12). Thus there is good circumstantial evidence that the organisms causing yeast mastitis frequently enter the teat via contaminated infusions.

However, the disease also occasionally occurs in cows with no history of antibiotic administration (30). This suggests that other unknown factors may be involved in the pathogenesis of mycotic mastitis. Yeasts may occasionally colonize the teat canal and/or the teat and gland cysterns without causing disease. If a bacterial mastitis should occur, these yeasts may multiply and invade the damaged parenchyma, causing a secondary fungal mastitis. It is probable that commensal bacteria on and in the udder inhibit yeast multiplication and that their removal by antibiotics is an important factor in multiplication of the yeast.

The wide variety of genera and species implicated in

this disease certainly emphasizes the importance of the primary contaminative aspect of its epidemiology. Consistent with this is the fact that infection does not secondarily spread from quarter to quarter or from cow to cow. Mastitis due to *Cryptococcus neoformans* is often associated with soiling of the barn by pigeon feces, resulting in heavy local environmental contamination. This fungus has infected cows udders by way of contaminated distilled water used to prepare intramammary infusions for dry cow therapy (28).

The severity of mycotic mastitis is related to the number of organisms that enter the gland, the genus of fungus involved, and its ability to grow at 40 C (31). *Candida, Trichosporon,* and other similar yeasts in sufficient numbers cause severe local inflammation, swelling, fever, loss of milk production, and a greatly increased leukocyte count in the milk. Most of these infections are cleared in 1 to 2 weeks and udder function returns to normal.

Infection by *Cryptococcus neoformans* is more severe, and milk production is often permanently lost when the secretory parenchyma is replaced by granulation tissue (18). Many affected cows must eventually be culled for economic reasons (28).

Cows that have clinically recovered from mastitis caused by *Candida* spp. may continue to shed the organism for many months.

Diagnosis. Farnsworth and Sorensen (13) have reported that 2.0 percent of Minnesota dairy cattle with clinically normal udders shed yeast organisms in their milk. Thus mere isolation of yeast organisms is not proof of their etiologic significance in cases of mastitis. The presence of large numbers of a single yeast species that grows well at 37 C in conjunction with a history of previous antibiotic infusion are helpful criteria in diagnosing fungal mastitis. Milk samples should be cultured on both blood and Sabouraud's agars at 37 C. The latter should contain antibiotics such as penicillin and streptomycin to inhibit bacteria which grow faster than and tend to obscure yeast colonies. Subsequent identification of yeast isolates is based on characteristics such as colony color, sugar assimilation, and formation of chlamydoconidia, blastoconidia, and arthroconidia (2).

Treatment. Most yeast species are sensitive to nystatin, to amphotericin B, and 5-fluorocytosine. However, treatment of yeast-induced mastitis is frequently unsuccessful. All of the abovementioned antifungal agents are toxic both locally in the mammary gland and also systemically and may cause as much or more damage as the yeast infection itself, which often clears up spontaneously in a few days (32). Other less toxic antifungal

agents such as undecylenic acid (6), pimaricin, and miconazole may be more satisfactory in therapy.

Mycotic Rumenitis (Mycotic Gastritis)

Mycotic infections of the bovine stomach are caused mainly by fungi of the class Phycomycetes (phylum Zygomycota) and by the yeast *Candida albicans*. These fungal diseases have increased greatly with the increased use of antibiotics for prophylaxis and therapy and with the advent of systems of husbandry that include concentrate feeding.

Etiology. The following have been identified in cases of mycotic rumenitis and gastritis:

Absidia spp.
Mucor spp.
Rhizopus spp.
Aspergillus spp.
Candida albicans

Epidemiology and Pathogenesis. The fungi involved in lesions of bovine rumenitis or gastritis are common contaminants of the animals' feed and of the normal gastrointestinal contents. They are opportunistic invaders of the stomach mucosa given the appropriate predisposing conditions. Prolonged antibiotic treatment, for example, because it reduces the normal bacterial flora, diminishes the controlling effect of the latter on fungal multiplication; stimulation of epithelial renewal is also reduced and so the mucosa is more susceptible to fungal invasion. Furthermore, it has even been suggested that antibiotics stimulate the growth of some fungi, including *Candida* spp. (23, 27).

Mycotic gastritis associated with antibiotic administration is seen most often in calves, whereas the disease in older bovines is more often associated with rumenitis caused by excess acid from consumption of unaccustomed large quantities of grain or concentrates. In these animals the pH of the rumen contents drops as low as 3.5 and so the normal protozoal fauna and bacterial flora are destroyed. The rumenal mucosa, particularly in the ventral sacs, becomes ulcerated and is then invaded by fungi from the gastric contents.

The fungal hyphae penetrate the mucosa, infiltrate the walls of blood vessels, and obstruct blood flow by formation of thrombi. This may lead to ischemic infarction and necrosis of neighboring tissue. Gross lesions in the rumen, omasum, or abomasum consist of circumscribed

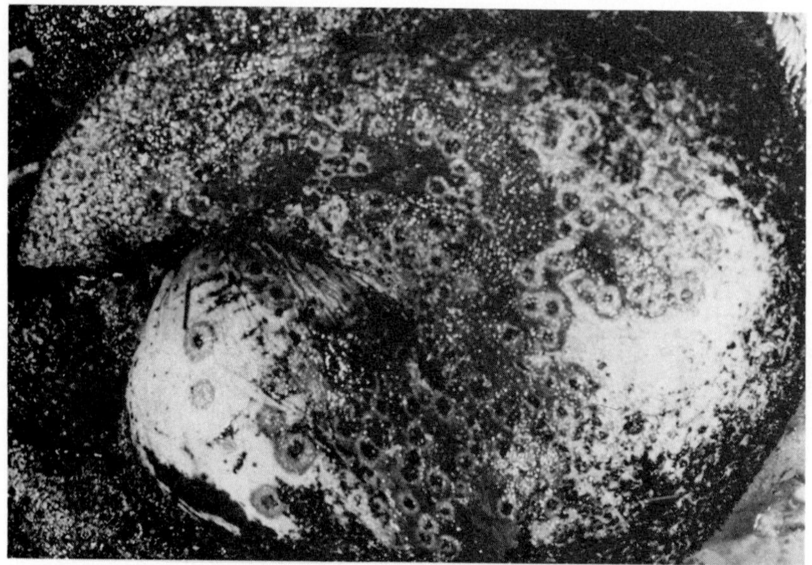

Figure 35.4. Lesions of mycotic rumenitis in a cow. (Courtesy John King.)

areas of necrosis surrounded by a zone of congestion (Figures 35.4 and 35.5). The stomach may also adhere to other organs such as the liver and diaphragm. Histologically, lesions are characterized by necrosis, congestion, and occlusion of blood vessels by thrombi and fungal hyphae. Hyphae and other fungal elements are present also in the necrotic tissue (24).

Affected animals exhibit rumen atony, anorexia, depression, and foul-smelling feces (21). There is no effective treatment.

Diagnosis. Microscopic evidence of fungal elements in lesions provides good support for a diagnosis of mycotic rumenitis-gastritis. Phycomycetes in lesions of calves are not readily cultured (14). The constant presence of fungi in the digesta and on the mucosal surface also complicates the interpretation of cultural findings.

Guttural Pouch Mycosis

Infection of the guttural pouch by *Aspergillus fumigatus,* other *Aspergillus* spp., and *Mucor* spp. is occasionally found in stabled horses and may be associated with damage to the internal carotid artery or nerves that pass close to the guttural pouch. Infections are found most often on the left side but can occur bilaterally. They apparently originate in moldy feed, the spores being inhaled.

Affected horses may have a unilateral nasal discharge,

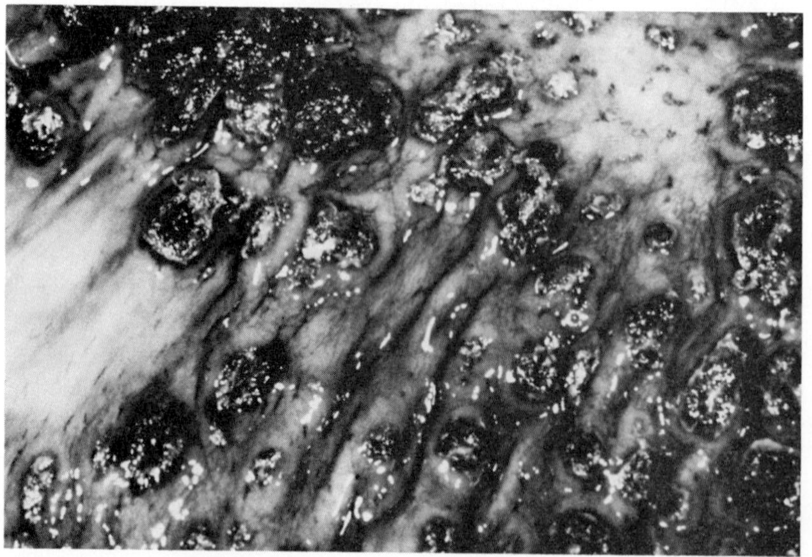

Figure 35.5. Lesions of mycotic abomasitis in a cow. Note the raised circular lesions with depressed necrotic centers. (Courtesy John King.)

epistaxis, and dysphagia caused by involvement of the pharyngeal branch of the vagus or the glossopharyngeal nerves. Treatment involves ligation of the internal carotid artery to prevent epistaxis, surgical removal of mycelium, and intravenous administration of sodium iodide (25).

Diagnosis is based on detection of hyphal elements in tissue and exudates.

REFERENCES

1. Ainsworth and Austwick. Vet. Rec., 1955, *67,* 88.
2. Ajello, Georg, Kaplan, and Kaufman. *In* Laboratory manual for medical mycology. Pub. Health Serv. Pub. No. 994, U.S. Govt. Printing Office, Washington, D.C., 1963.
3. Angus, Gilmour, and Dawson. Jour. Med. Microbiol., 1973, *6,* 207.
4. Beck. Michigan State Univ. Vet., 1957, *17,* 82.
5. Bendixen and Plum. Acta. Pathet. Microbiol. Scand., 1929, *6,* 252.
6. Biancardi, Binaghi, Georgi, Milani, Morgenti, and Bandini. Atti. delle Soc. Ital. Buiatria, 1976, *8,* 158.
7. Carter, Cordes, Menna, and Hunter. Res. Vet. Sci., 1973, *14,* 201.
8. Corbel and Eades. Brit. Vet. Jour., 1973, *129,* 75.
9. Cordes, Dodd, and O'Hara. New Zeal. Vet. Jour., 1964, *12,* 95.
10. Cordes, Menna, and Carter. Vet. Path. 1972, *9,* 131.
11. Donnelly. Vet. Jour., 1967, *21,* 82.
12. Farnsworth. Jour. Amer. Vet. Med. Assoc. 1977, *170,* 1173.
13. Farnsworth and Sorensen. Can. Jour. Comp. Med., 1972, *36,* 329.
14. Gitter and Austwick. Vet. Rec., 1957, *69,* 924.
15. Hensel, Bisping, and Schimmelpfennig. Jour. Am. Vet. Med. Assoc., 1961, *139,* 883.
16. Hubbert, Booth, Bolton, Dunne, McEntee, Smith, and Tourtellotte. Cornell Vet., 1973, *63,* 291.
17. Hugh-Jones and Austwick. Vet. Rec., 1967, *81,* 273.
18. Innes, Siebold, and Arentzen. Am. Jour. Vet. Res., 1952, *13,* 469.
19. Korotchenko, Gavdye, and Saposkinsky. Problemy Vet. Sanitarii, 1974, *49,* 62.
20. Leach, Sachs, Abrams, and Limbert. Lab. Animal Care, 1968, *18,* 407.
21. Lock. Vet. Med./Small Animal Clin., 1975, *70,* 197.
22. Loken, Thompson, Hoyt, and Ball. Jour. Am. Vet. Med. Assoc., 1959, *134,* 401.
23. Mills. Jour. Am. Vet. Med. Assoc., 1967, *150,* 862.
24. Neitzke and Schiefer. Can. Vet. Jour., 1974, *15,* 139.
25. Owen and McKelvey. Vet. Rec., 1979, *104,* 100.
26. Pier, Cysewzki and Richard. Am. Jour. Vet. Res., 1972, *33,* 349.
27. Seelig. Am. Jour. Med., 1966, *40,* 887.
28. Sipka and Petrovic. Zentrbl. Vet.-Med., 1975, *22B,* 353.
29. Smith and Tourtellotte. Cornell Vet., 1973, *63,* 291.
30. Stuart. Vet. Rec., 1951, *63,* 314.
31. Topolko. Vet. Archiv., 1968, *38,* 242.
32. Weight. Habilitationschrift, tier. Hoch. (Hannover) 1973. 160 pp.
33. White and Smith. Proc. Soc. Gen. Microbiol., 1973, *1,* 27.
34. Williams, Shreeve, Hebert, and Swire. Vet. Rec., 1977, *100,* 382.
35. Wohlgemuth and Knudfson. Jour. Am. Vet. Med. Assoc., 1977, *171,* 437.

Mycetomas (Maduromycosis and Chromomycosis)

Mycetomas are localized chronic fungal infections, usually involving the cutaneous and subcutaneous tissues of the legs and feet, and characterized by formation of excessive granulation tissue that contains abscesses. The causative fungi are present in the lesions in the form of granules.

The term *maduromycosis* is derived from the Indian province of Madura, where mycetomas were first described in man. The term *chromomycosis* has been specifically applied to mycetomas caused by darkly pigmented (dematiaceous) fungi.

Etiology. The following species are most often involved in mycetomas:

Cladosporium spp.
Allescheria boydii (*Petriellidium boydii*)
Curvularia geniculata
Helminthosporium spp.
Fonsecaea pedrosoi
Phialophora spp.

Epidemiology and Pathogenesis. The fungi that cause mycetomas are saprophytes of the soil and decaying vegetation and enter the skin via small wounds. Bridges (1) has stated that most cases of maduromycotic mycetomas seen in the United States have appeared in the southern regions. He reported three cases in dogs and one in a horse and identified *Curvularia geniculata* as the etiological agent affecting the feet of one of the dogs. This genus is closely related taxonomically to *Helminthosporium,* another genus that has been associated with the disease. In 1967, Brodey *et al.* (4) described a case of eumycotic (maduromycotic) mycetoma in a Coonhound that had been used for hunting in Virginia and Pennsylvania. Clinically the dog had intermittent lameness and a progressively enlarged swelling in the right shoulder. *C. geniculata* was determined to be the causative agent. In 1970, two cases of eumycotic mycetoma in dogs were reported (5, 6). In one case the lesion was in

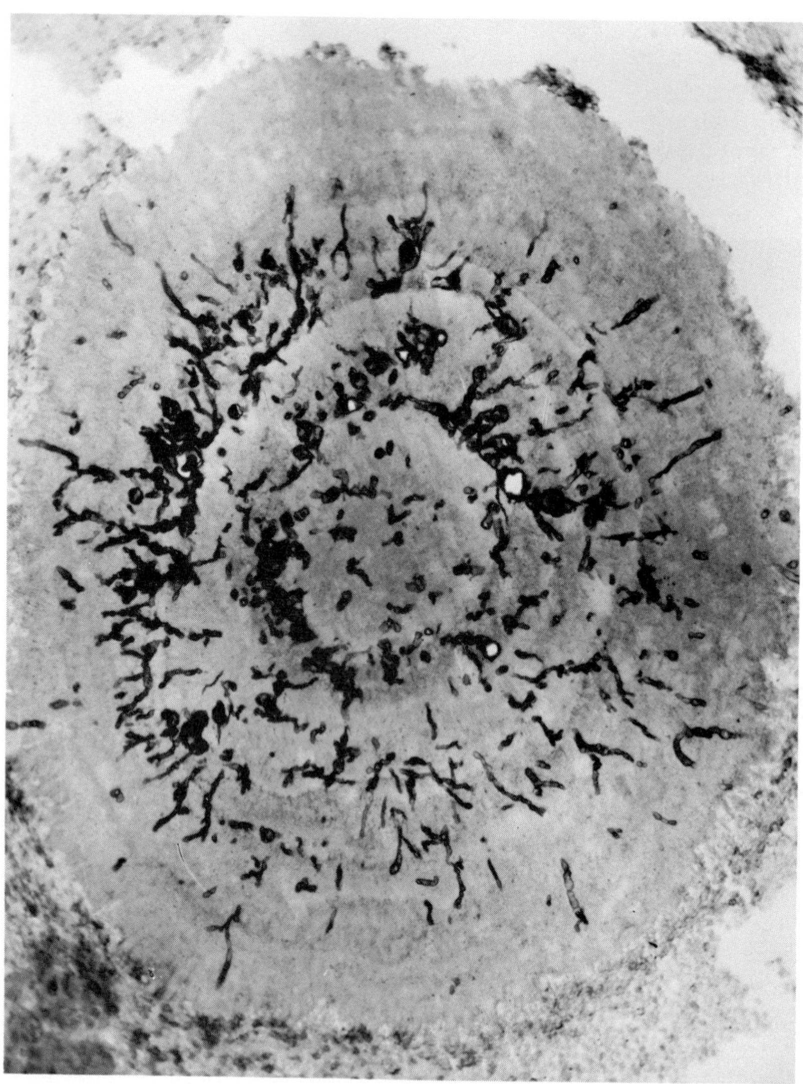

Figure 35.6. A large laminated acidophilic body from a case of bovine maduromycosis containing many chlamydoconidia and hyphae. The white holes represent microchlamydoconidia which extend to both surfaces of the section. Gridley fungus stain. × 190. (Courtesy Charles H. Bridges, *Cornell Vet.*)

the abdominal region and in the other one-half of the spleen and portions of the gastric and duodenal walls were involved. In both cases, *Allescheria boydii,* an ascomycete, was found to be the inciting agent. Mycetomas are most common in tropical and subtropical areas.

In 1960, Bridges and Beasley (3) stated that he had diagnosed maduromycotic mycetomas in a cat, a horse, and a dog. *Brachycladium spiciferum* was identified as a causative agent in the cat and the horse. Generally, the clinical signs were manifested by chronic inflammation with formation of nodular granulomatous masses in the foot of the cat, skin of the head and body of the horse, and in a prescapular lymph node of the dog. Pigmented colonies of fungus could be seen as brown to black specks in the lesions from the dog and the horse. Colonies of fungus were easily found in stained smears of pus taken from draining sinuses of the cat's foot. According to Mahaffey and Rossdale (7), *A. boydii* has caused abortion in the horse. They found lesions in the fetal membrances and in the lungs of the fetus.

Bridges (2) in 1960 and Roberts *et al.* (9) in 1963 recorded the finding of maduromycosis (maduromycotic mycetoma) of the bovine nasal mucosa. It appears that nasal granuloma in American cattle was first described in Louisiana in 1933. Since then cases have been seen in Texas and Colorado.

The disease is similar to the so-called *snoring disease* of cattle in India. Growth appears on the turbinate bones, causing the animals to sneeze and rub their nostrils on any available object. After several months a thick mucous discharge may block the nasal passages to the point where breathing is difficult. Microscopically there is an eosinophilic granulomatous proliferation of the nasal mucosa and submucosa accompanied by the appearance of deep epithelial crypts. Langhans' giant cells, and thin-walled chlamydoconidia. In some areas, segmented hyphal elements also can be seen.

A *Helminthosporium* sp. is believed to be the cause of the disease in American cattle.

Chromomycosis is rare in animals. Natural infection in a horse and a dog has been described by Simpson (10). The mycetomas in this condition contain small (6 to 12 μm) dark single or clustered bodies. The causative fungi—*Fonsecaea* sp., *Curvularia* sp., and *Phialophora* sp.—are slow growing.

Diagnosis. Maduromycotic mycetomas are recognized by the presence of granules (100 to 300 μm) composed of compact masses of hyphae, chlamydoconidia in pus, and granulation tissue (Figure 35.6). The granules of chromomycotic mycetomas are much smaller (6 to 12 μm) and do not contain hyphae. Identification of the causative fungi may be performed following culture and isolation on Sabouraud agar containing a broad-spectrum antibiotic to inhibit bacterial contaminants. Incubation must be continued for 2 to 3 weeks because most of the fungi that cause mycetomas are very slow growing.

Treatment. Small lesions may be eradicated by surgical excision. Larger lesions are difficult to remove completely and recur. Amphotericin B may have application in therapy (8), but there are no clinical reports of its use in animals.

REFERENCES

1. Bridges. Am. Jour. Path., 1957, *33*, 411.
2. Bridges. Cornell Vet., 1960, *50*, 468.
3. Bridges and Beasley. Jour. Am. Vet. Med. Assoc., 1960, *137*, 192.
4. Brodey, Schryver, Deubler, Kaplan, and Ajello. Jour. Am. Vet. Med. Assoc., 1967, *151*, 442.
5. Jang and Popp. Jour. Am. Vet. Med. Assoc., 1970, *157*, 1071.
6. Kurtz, Finco, and Perman. Jour. Am. Vet. Med. Assoc., 1970, *157*, 917.
7. Mahaffey and Rossdale. Vet. Rec., 1965, *77*, 541.
8. Moss, Emma S. and Albert C. McQuown. Atlas of medical mycology, 2nd ed. Williams & Wilkins, Baltimore, 1960, p. 163.
9. Roberts, McDaniel, and Carbrey. Jour. Am. Vet. Med. Assoc., 1963, *142*, 42.
10. Simpson. Vet. Med., 1966, *61*, 1207.

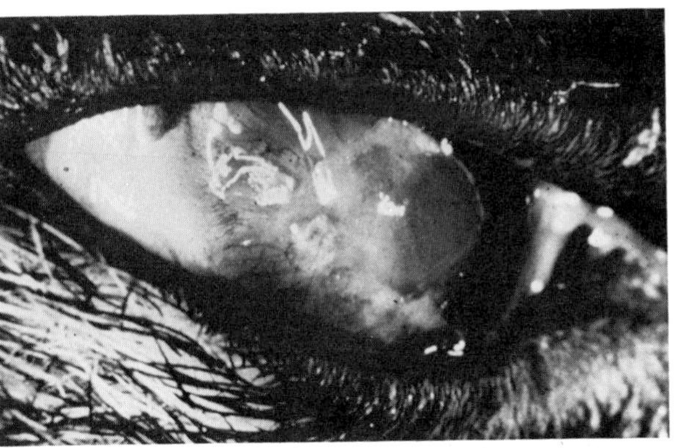

Figure 35.7. Mycotic keratitis in a horse. Note the extensive opacity and formation of scar tissue.

Mycotic Keratitis

A variety of saprophytic, commensal, and pathogenic fungi have been isolated from ocular lesions in animals and man. They include *Aspergillus* spp., *Blastomyces dermatidis, Candida* spp., *Cryptococcus neoformans, Drechslera* spp., *Fusarium* spp., and *Penicillium* spp.

Mycotic keratitis usually results from corneal injury, which allows opportunistic entry of fungal cells into the corneal stroma. It may also result from dissemination of a systemic infection by *B. dermatidis* or *C. neoformans*. Both of these fungi, in a minority of cases, invade the eye during a systemic infection (3).

Opportunistic fungal invasion may be suspected if a primary bacterial infection does not respond to prolonged antibiotic therapy. Combined antibiotic-corticosteroid medication is particularly likely to be associated with secondary fungal invasion of the cornea. As the cornea undergoes fungal invasion it slowly becomes opaque and ulcerates (Figure 35.7). The ulcer is often accompanied by characteristic endothelial plaques in the center of the cornea. If hypopyon is present it is generally sterile.

Diagnosis. Mycotic keratitis may be misdiagnosed as bacterial infection or as squamous cell carcinoma. Material is scraped from the edge of the ulcer on the anesthetized cornea and is stained by Gram, Giemsa, and Periodic Acid Schiff. Hyphae, blastoconidia, and/or pseudohyphae may be observed in this material. Fungal identification requires culture of specimens and isolation of the causative fungus.

Treatment. The most effective chemical or physical agents in the management of mycotic keratitis include amphotericin B, nystatin, pimaricin, and potassium iodide. The condition may be treated by cryotherapy, laser beam, and surgical debridement (1, 2).

REFERENCES

1. Bistner and Riis. Cornell Vet., 1979, *69,* 364.
2. De Voe. Am. Jour. Opthal., 1971, *71,* 406.
3. Wold, Schwartzman, and Sautter. Vet. Med., 1958, *53,* 595.

Phaeohyphomycosis

Phaeohyphomycosis is a name applied to diseases caused by various species of dematiaceous fungi whose tissue form consists of septate, dark-walled hyphae. Unlike mycetomas, granules are not present.

The disease is rare in animals (1). *Drechslera spicifera, Cladosporium* spp., and *Curvularia* spp. are the most frequent causative agents.

Isolates of *Drechslera* have been erroneously identified as *Helminthosporium*. The former produce sympoduloconidia whereas the conidia of *Helminthosporium* are borne on straight conidiophores of a definite length.

In the horse, lesions consisting of multiple cutaneous plaques 1 to 3 cm in diameter have been observed on various parts of the body. The lesions were black, denuded, and covered with small pustules and papules. The fungus in these lesions was in the form of individual and small groups of darkly pigmented septate hyphae (1).

Both in the horse and the cat the lesions are localized in the subcutaneous tissues (2).

Treatment. Kaplan *et al.* (1) reported that iodovet detergent applied frequently to the lesions resulted in clinical improvement.

REFERENCES

1. Kaplan, Chandler, Ajello, Ganthier, Higgins, and Cayonette. Can. Vet. Jour., 1975, *16,* 205.
2. Muller, Kaplan, Ajello, and Padhye. Jour. Am. Vet. Med. Assoc., 1975, *166,* 150.

PART VI

THE VIRALES

36 The Viruses

Quite understandably the early bacteriologists held the belief that all contagious and infectious diseases were caused by bacteria, except for a few which were known to be caused by higher fungi and protozoa. But time showed that bacteria and other known disease-producing agents could not be identified with many diseases. Eventually it was learned that some of these infective fluids retained their ability to produce disease after they had been forced through fine-pored clay filters that retained all ordinary bacteria. This indicated that agents smaller than bacteria were capable of causing infectious diseases. For more than 40 years (1892 to 1935) this was about all that was known of such agents, which became known as filter-passing or filterable viruses. The adjective *filterable* is not used now because it is known that not all viruses are small enough to be filterable and some well-known bacteria can be made to pass through the so-called bacteria-proof filters. The word virus now connotes a series of characteristics among which filter passing is only one probable feature.

The first known virus was that of the tobacco mosaic disease (Figure 36.1). It was demonstrated by a Russian, Iwanowski (22), in 1892. In 1898 Loeffler and Frosch (23), in Germany, demonstrated that foot-and-mouth disease of cattle was caused by an agent that readily passed bacteria-proof filters and could not be seen with the microscope. It was the first animal virus discovered. In the same year Sanarelli (31) proved that a highly contagious rabbit tumor (myxomatosis) was caused by a virus. In the years that have elapsed since these early discoveries, many viruses and virus diseases have been found or differentiated.

In 1920 D'Herelle (17) described the first of a series of viruses which he named *bacteriophages* because they parasitized bacterial cells, causing them to swell and burst. The ease with which these agents could be studied greatly stimulated the study of viruses, and many of the observations on bacteriophages have been applicable to the viruses that infect plant and animal cells. An even greater stimulus to the study of viruses was the announcement by Stanley (34) in 1935 that he had been successful in extracting a crystalline nucleoprotein that

Figure 36.1. A model of tobacco mosaic virus showing 2,130 elongated capsomeres, consisting of protein molecules, arranged around a hollow core. The helical coil embedded in the capsomeres represents the viral nucleic acid. (Courtesy Franklin, Klug, Caspar, and Holmes, *17th Ann. Symposium, Fundamental Cancer Res.*, Williams and Wilkins, 1963.)

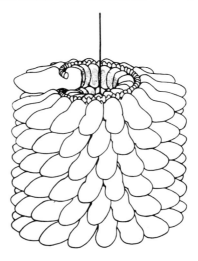

had all the properties of the virus from tobacco plants affected with mosaic disease. The virus research field has been very active and productive in recent years because of the introduction of a number of new techniques. A new science of virology has been formed, staffed by individuals who have training in biochemistry, genetics, microbiology, biophysics, statistics, and/or pathology.

TERMS COMMONLY USED BY VIROLOGISTS

Virion: The complete infective virus particle; may be identical to nucleocapsid; more complex virions include the nucleocapsid plus the surrounding envelope.

Capsid: The protein shell that encloses the nucleic acid core (genome).

Nucleocapsid: The capsid together with the enclosed nucleic acid.

Structure units: The basic units of similar structure in the capsid; may be individual polypeptides.

Capsomeres: Morphologic units seen on the surfaces of isometric virus particles. They represent clusters of structure units.

Primary nucleic acid structure: The sequence of bases in the nucleic acid chain.

Secondary nucleic acid structure: The spatial arrangement of the complete nucleic acid chain. For example, is the nucleic acid single- or double-stranded, circular or linear in conformation, or branched or unidirectional?

Tertiary nucleic acid structure: Refers to fine spatial detail in the helix such as super-coiling, breakage points, deletions, gaps, catenation, and regions of strand separation.

Envelope: The outer coat some viruses acquire as they penetrate or are budded from the nuclear or cytoplasmic membrane. Envelopes always contain altered host-cell membrane components.

Peplomers: Morphological units composed of structure units that are embedded in the envelope.

Complementation: A general term to describe situations where mixed infections result in enhanced yields of one or both viruses in the mixture.

Translation: The mechanism by a particular base sequence in messenger RNA results in the production of a specific amino acid sequence in a protein.

Transcription: The means by which specific information encoded in a nucleic acid chain is transferred to messenger RNA.

Transcapsidation: A form of complementation where two viruses ''hybridize''; for example, adenovirus capsid is spontaneously transferred to SV40 nucleoids (or DNA).

Helper virus: Certain viruses are defective and require a closely related ''helper'' virus to complete their replication.

Defective virus: Functionally deficient particles in some aspect of replication. May interfere with replication of normal virus.

Pseudovirions: The capsid sometimes erroneously encloses host nucleic acid and the virions appear as normal particles under an electron microscope. As such they do not replicate.

THE BIOLOGIC NATURE OF VIRUSES

From the time that viruses were discovered until Stanley initiated a new series of research attacks on their nature, little had been learned. They were known for what they could do, not for what they were. The only criterion for their recognition was their ability to produce recognizable signs of disease in plants or animals and, in some cases, to form certain foreign bodies (inclusion bodies) within parasitized cells. Many speculated about the possibility that a whole host of living beings, too small to be seen with the microscope and many perhaps leading a wholly saprophytic existence, might eventually be found to exist. There were no ways by which such a hypothesis could be proved or disproved. Gradually it became generally accepted that viruses could not be propagated like most bacteria in artificial culture media which was devoid of living cells—that growth and multiplication occurred only in living cells. Whether viruses are living or nonliving entities was a subject of considerable controversy until 2 decades or so ago. Some virologists still speak of *live* and *killed* viruses. A Dutchman, Beijerinck (9), started the controversy in 1899 with his idea of a *contagium vivum fluidum,* a form of life which, if it existed, would certainly be different from anything known since it would be a noncellular form of life. A still more unorthodox idea appeared—that viruses might be nonliving autocatalytic chemical agents that had the property of instigating abnormal metabolic activities in the cells that they attacked, one of the products of such abnormal activity being more of the instigating substance, which then became available in increased quantity for repeating the process in other cells of the same individual or, if it could escape to another host, of causing in it the same chain of events.

Life in the higher plants and animals generally is easily detectable by a series of well-known criteria. When it comes to determining life in very primitive beings, which probably are at a subcellular level, the usual distinctions fail. Unless new distinctions are made, we must regard viruses as nonliving agents. The basic structure of a virus is shown in Figure 36.2. It is perfectly clear that a strand of nucleic acid, which forms the core of a virus, is a macromolecule with a somewhat simple and definable chemical structure that can perform essential functions of living things in a suitable environment. This macromolecule can replicate itself and also direct the synthesis of proteins. The newly formed nucleic acid and proteins are then assembled to consitute a complete virus particle. While the controversy was still raging in 1945, Burnet suggested that the epidemiologist and public health workers think of viruses as microorganisms. In 1966 Lwoff and Tournier (24) made it clear that viruses differ from other living things including microorganisms by five characters: (*a*) mature virus particles (virions) have only one type of nucleic acid, either DNA or RNA, whereas microorganisms possess both types; (*b*) virions are unable to grow or undergo binary fission; (*c*) virions make use of the ribosomes of their host cell; (*d*) virions are reproduced solely from their nucleic acid; other agents grow from the integrated sum of their constituents and reproduce by division; and (*e*) viruses lack genetic information for the synthesis of essential cellular systems such as that responsible for the production of energy with high potential. As our knowledge of viruses increases, it is unlikely that Lwoff's concepts will encompass all discoveries; for example, the satellite viruses (24) cannot reproduce from their own nucleic acid, and neither the nucleic acid nor the virions are infectious. Even some bacteria such as chlamydiae with some ribosomes also are dependent on host-cell ribosomes (2).

Figure 36.2. A diagram of a complete virus particle or virion. The core is either ribonucleic acid or deoxyribonucleic acid. (Courtesy R. W. Horne, *Sci. Am.*)

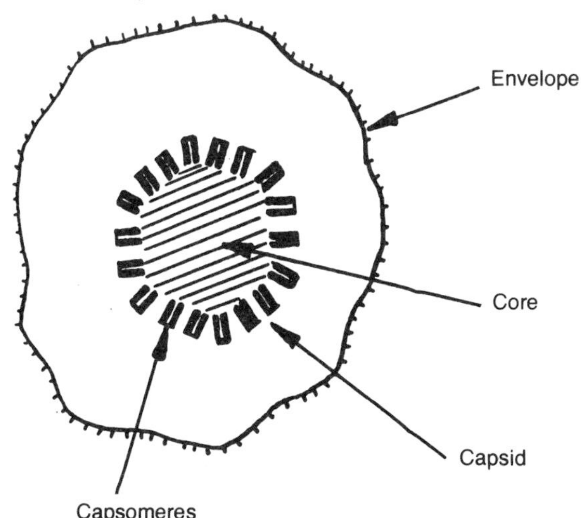

The contagious living fluid concept is no longer tenable. Although there are many differences among virologists on other points, all now agree that viruses are particulate in nature; that is, they may be filtered out of suspensions with appropriate filters, and they may be centrifuged out of suspensions with ultracentrifuges. Many virus particles have been photographed with the electron microscope and their morphology and size accurately determined.

Animal and bacterial viruses contain either RNA or DNA, but not both, while plant viruses have RNA. To release the nucleic acid from its protein outer coat involves lysis of the capsid by a detergent such as sodium dodecyl sulfate and further treatment of the nucleic acid with Pronase and phenol. Viruses from various groups, such as the enterovirus, yield infectious RNA by such treatment, and members of Papovaviridae and bacteriophage have yielded infectious DNA. Infectious RNA and infectious DNA are inactivated by their respective enzymes (ribonuclease or deoxyribonuclease) whereas the infectivity of intact particles is not affected by such treatment. On the other hand, antiserum produced for intact particles readily neutralizes the virion as the antibodies react with the antigens of the protein coat, but fail to inactivate free viral infectious nucleic acid. It is known that purified DNA is not immunogenic, but DNA complexes containing appreciable protein not readily dissociated from DNA are antigenic producing precipitating and C^1-fixing antibodies in rabbits.

Some viruses are toxic as evidenced by the peracute death of mice within a few hours after parenteral injection of concentrated suspensions of influenza virus. At necropsy these animals show no pathological lesions except marked vascular congestion. In most viral diseases the inflammatory response is characterized by an infiltration of mononuclear cells and lymphocytes whereas polymorphonuclear leukocytes predominate in the lesions of acute bacterial diseases. In many viral diseases pathogenic bacteria play a significant role as secondary invaders in the disease process of ectodermal tissues, so polymorphonuclear leukocytes invade the infected tissues after the mononuclear-type cells.

CLASSIFICATION AND NOMENCLATURE OF VIRUSES

With the rapid advances in virology during the last two decades, virologists are producing a reasonable classification and nomenclature of viruses including vertebrate, invertebrate, plant, and bacterial viruses. The responsibility for this task lies in the hands of an International Committee on the Taxonomy of Viruses (ICTV), which was established at the IXth International Congress of Microbiology. The Commission approved a number of rules with the purpose of establishing uniformity and standardized terminology. Many virologists other than the Commission were involved in the task, so the final product represents a consensus but by no means unanimity.

Many virus groups were proposed for consideration at the International Congress of Virology in Hungary, 1971. As taxonomy is a dynamic, ever changing scheme, Figures 36.3 and 36.4 represent the latest changes (1979) established by the ICTV on recommendation of its Vertebrate Virus Subcommittee, presently chaired by Dr. Fred Murphy. Detailed characterization data of virus groups usually are published in *Intervirology,* the official journal of the Virology Section of the International Association of Microbiological Societies. Viruses have been separated into families based on their physical, chemical, and biological characteristics. For all virus groups family names now have been established, and these end in *idae*. Names of genera end with the word *virus,* and members of each genus share certain common characteristics. In general an effort has been made to provide for a latinized binomial nomenclature, and existing latinized names are to be retained if possible. Each virus-group description must include a designated type species, its taxonomic position (genus or family), its main characteristics, a list of viruses in the group, and a file of probable or possible members belonging in the group. The description should also include cyrptograms for the groups and its individual viruses. Each cryptogram should contain: (*a*) the type of nucleic acid/strandedness of nucleic acid, (*b*) molecular weight of the nucleic acid in millions/percentage of nucleic acid in virus particle, (*c*) outline of virus particle/outline of nucleocapsid, and (*d*) kinds of host infected/kinds of vector. A proposed classification for viruses should be based on the features just cited in the cryptogram and, in addition: (*a*) the presence or absence of an envelope; (*b*) certain measurements for helical viruses such as the diameter of the nucleocapsid, and for cubical viruses including the triangulation number and the number of capsomeres; (*c*) the symmetry of the nucleocapsid (helical, cubical, or binal), and (*d*) certain characteristic biological and biophysical features. Ultimately, the classification undoubtedly will include comparisons of the nucleotide sequences of the viral nucleic acids and presently could also include nucleic acid homology (genetic relatedness) and nearest neighbor analyses.

Figure 36.5 is a diagram illustrating the shapes and relative sizes of animal viruses of the major families except the proposed family Caliciviridae.

DNA Viruses

Parvoviridae. The members of the family presently are the only known viruses with single-stranded DNA. The type species is *Parvovirus* n-1. These small DNA viruses, 18 to 22 nm in diameter, are divided into 2 genera. The *Parvovirus* genus includes the Kilham rat virus, the X14 virus of rats, hamster osteolytic H viruses, minute virus of mice, porcine parvovirus, human parvovirus, and infectious feline panleukopenia virus and its closely related mink enteritis virus. Other members in the genus are avian parvovirus, canine parvovirus, minute virus of canines, hemorrhagic encephalopathy virus, and bovine parvovirus. The adeno-associated viruses 1, 2, 3, and 4 comprise the *Adeno-associated virus* genus. The DNA liberated from adeno-satellites by conventional procedures acts like double-stranded nucleic acid, but the DNA within the virion stains with acridine orange and reacts with formaldehyde as single-stranded. The single-stranded DNA within the satellite particles exists as positive and negative complementary strands in separate particles. Upon extraction of DNA the positive and negative strands unite to form double-stranded DNA helix. The adenovirus satellites are defective and require an adenovirus "helper" to complete its replication. Members of the *Parvovirus* genus are nondefective and replicate without assistance from another virus. Their DNA is single-stranded inside and outside of all particles indicating the strands have a similar polarity. The icosahedral particles probably have 32 capsomeres, 2 to 4 nm in diameter, with a buoyant density in cesium chloride of 1.4 g per cm^3 and with a molecular weight of 1.4×10^6 daltons. The nonenveloped particles are acid-

Figure 36.3. Taxonomy of DNA Animal Viruses

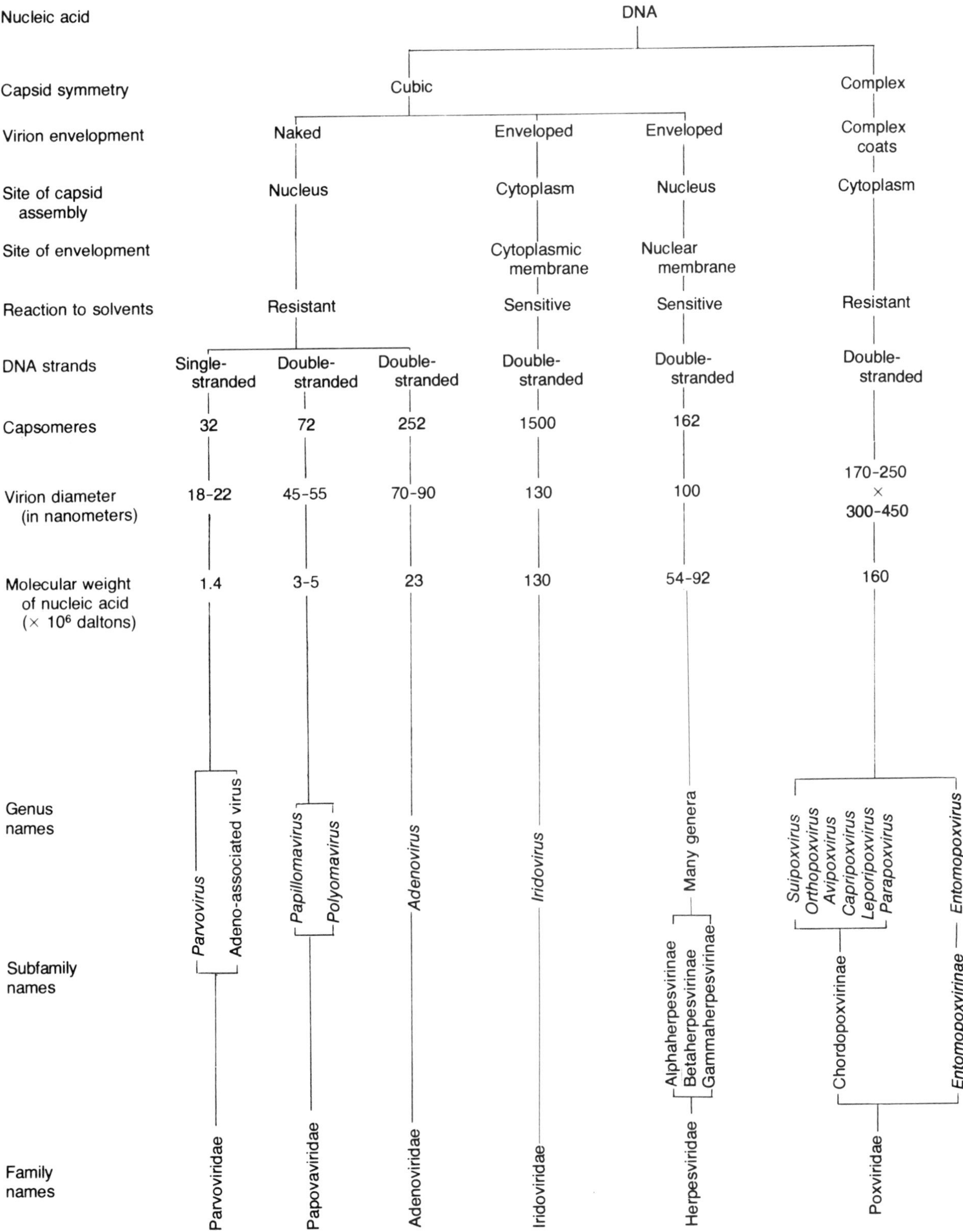

Information for this figure courtesy Fred Murphy, Chairman, Vetebrate Virus Committee, International Committee on Taxonomy of Viruses.

Figure 36.4. Taxonomy of RNA animal viruses

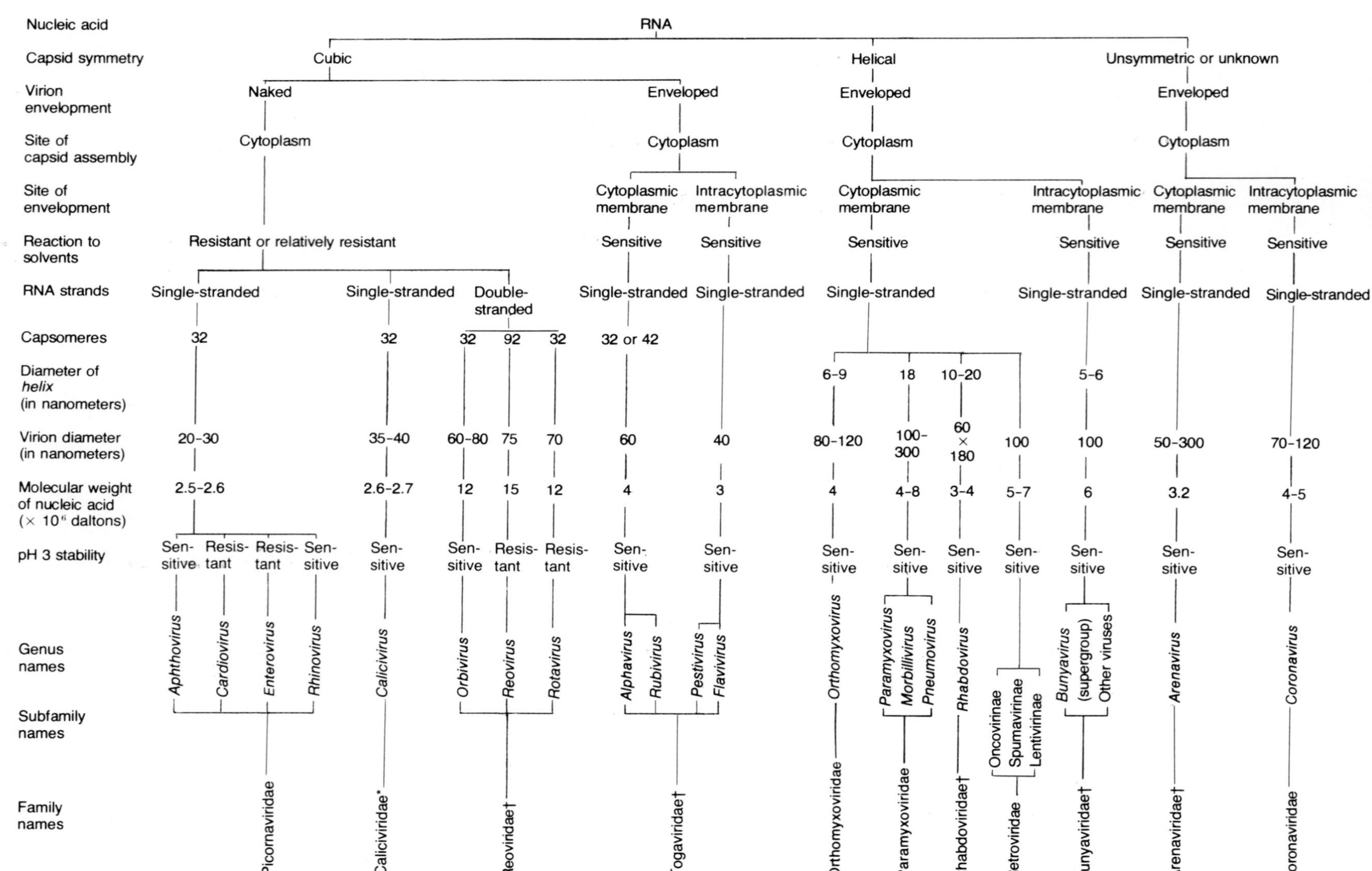

*Not yet approved by the International Committee on Taxonomy of Viruses.
†Arboviruses included; cytoplasmic polyhedrosis viruses included in Reoviridae.
Information for this figure courtesy Fred Murphy, Chairman, Vertebrate Virus Committee, International Committee on Taxonomy of Viruses.

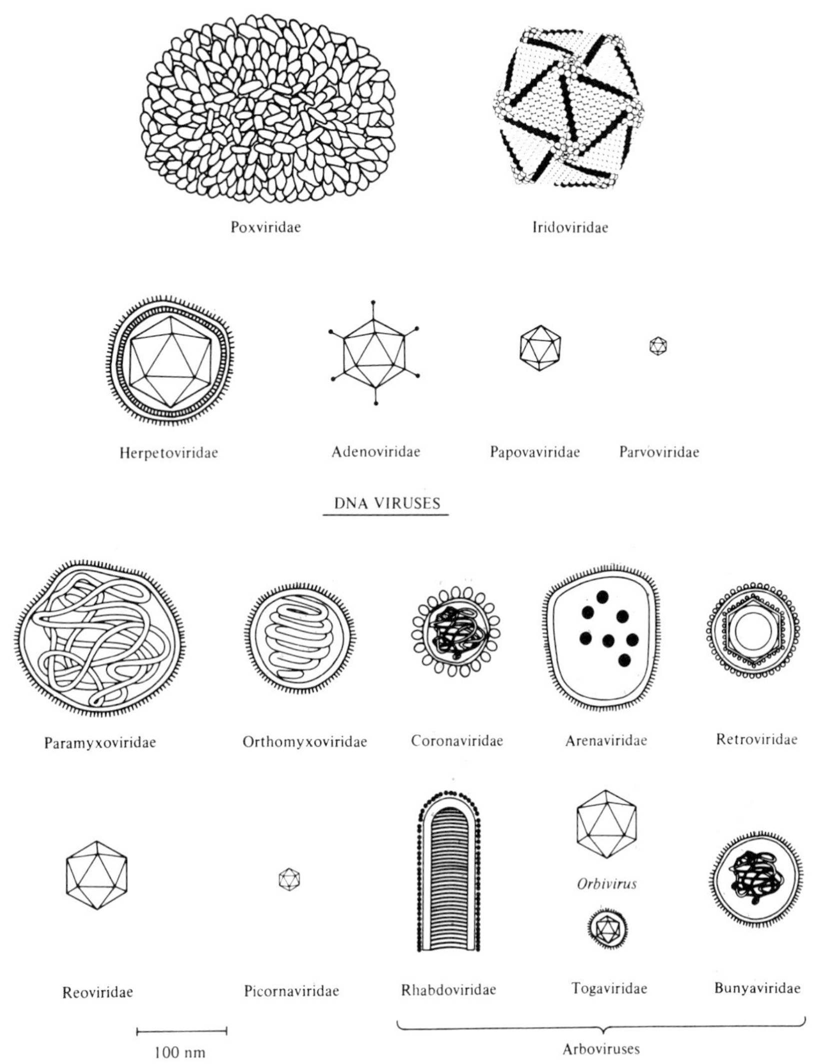

Figure 36.5. Diagram illustrating the shapes and relative sizes of animal viruses of the major families (bar = 100 nm). (From Frank Fenner and David O. White, *Medical Virology*, 2nd ed., Academic Press, New York, 1976.)

and heat-stable and ether-resistant. The guanine-cytosine (GC) content is 39 percent.

Viral replication occurs in the nucleus and intranuclear inclusion bodies are formed.

Papovaviridae. The family has two genera: *Polyomavirus* and *Papillomavirus*. The type species for the genus *Polyomavirus* is *Polyomavirus* m-1 (murine). Other viruses in the genus are simian vacuolating virus (SV40), rabbit-vacuolating virus, and K virus, and also the virus associated with leukoencephalopathy in man. The viruses contain double-stranded, cyclic DNA (Figure 36.6) with a GC ratio of 41 to 49 percent. The icosahedral particles, 45 nm in diameter and with 5-3-2 symmetry, have a buoyant density in cesium chloride of 1.34 g per cm^3, a molecular weight of 3×10^6 daltons, and a sedimentation rate of 240 S. The nonenveloped capsid has 72 capsomeres in a skew arrangement. The particles are acid- and heat-stable and ether-resistant. The viruses are assembled in the nucleus with the formation of intranuclear inclusion bodies. Some are oncogenic under certain conditions but inapparent infections are the rule in most hosts. Several viruses hemagglutinate by reacting with neuraminidase sensitive receptors.

The *Papillomavirus* S-1 (Shope papillomavirus) is the type species for the genus *Papillomavirus*. Other members of the genus are rabbit oral papilloma, human papilloma, canine papilloma, canine oral papilloma, and bovine papillomaviruses. Probable members include papillomata of horses, monkeys, sheep, goats and other

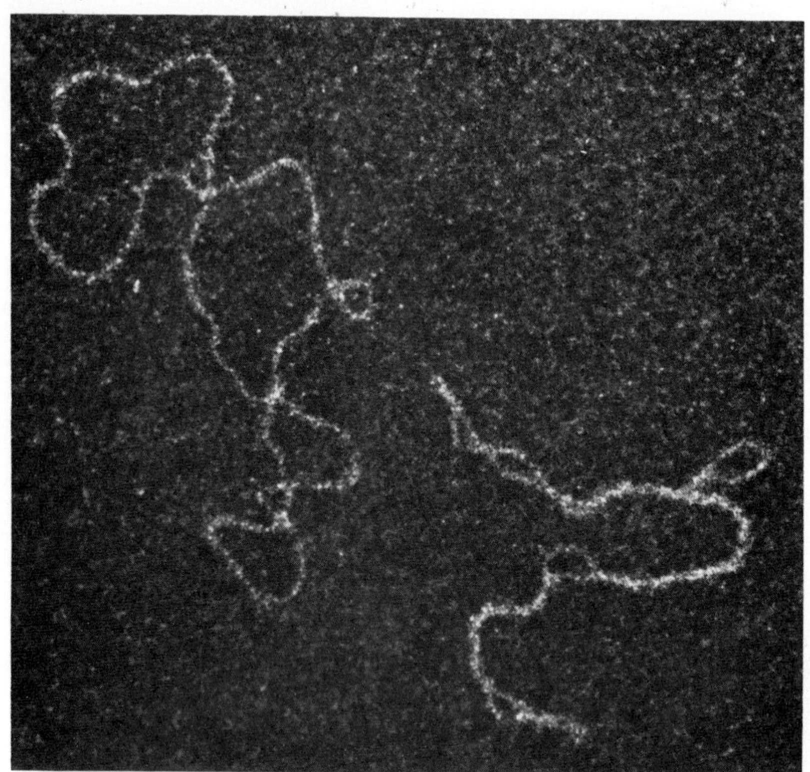

Figure 36.6. Electron micrograph of SV40 DNA circular molecules. DNA molecules were picked up on 20 Å thick carbon-aluminum film and spread by the aqueous technique. The DNA samples were imaged by titled beam dark field electron microscopy. Final magnification was 230,600. The length of both the relaxed form II SV40 DNA (*left-hand side*) and that of the superhelical form I SV40 DNA (*right-hand side*) was 1.5 μm. (Courtesy George Ruben and Ray Wu, Section of Biochemistry, Molecular and Cell Biology, Cornell University, Ithaca, N.Y. Reprinted with permission from *Biochemistry,* 1976, *15,* 738. Copyright by the American Chemical Society.)

species. Members of this genus contain double-stranded, cyclic DNA with a GC ratio of 49 percent. The nonenveloped icosahedral particles, 55 nm in diameter and with 5–3–2 symmetry, have a molecular weight of 5×10^6 daltons, a buoyant density in cesium chloride of 1.34 g per cm^3, a sedimentation rate of 280 to 300 S, and 72 capsomeres in a skew arrangement. The virions are ether-resistant and heat- and acid-stable.

The viruses replicate in the nucleus and cause papillomata in many animal hosts. Several viruses hemagglutinate by reacting with neuraminidase-sensitive receptors.

Adenoviridae. The genus *Adenovirus* includes a rather large number of viruses represented by the type species, *Adenovirus* h-1 (human). Other members of the genus include human types 2 to 35, 25 simian, 2 canine, 9 bovine, porcine, murine, avian, and other mammalian adenoviruses from sheep, horse, opossum, and cat. These double-stranded DNA viruses, 70 to 90 nm in diameter, have a GC content of 48 to 57 percent. Isometric nonenveloped particles with icosahedral symmetry have 252 capsomeres, 7 nm in diameter, arranged in a 5–3–2 axial symmetry. The vertex capsomeres carry a filamentous projection which are antigenically distinct from other capsomeres of the particle. The virions have a molecular weight of 23×10^6 daltons, a buoyant density in rubidium chloride of 1.34 g per cm^3, and a sedimentation rate of 795 S. The particles are ether-resistant and heat- and acid-stable.

The virus replicates in the nucleus where it causes intranuclear inclusion bodies. Some viruses hemagglutinate red blood cells of various species. Some adenoviruses are ocogenic in hamsters. A common antigen shared by all mammalian adenoviruses differs from a corresponding antigen of avian strains.

Iridoviridae. The type species to the single genus in this family is *Iridovirus* t-1 (tipula iridescent virus). Other members are *Sericesthis iridescent* virus and *Chilo iridescent* virus; probable members are *Aedes iridescent* virus and other iridescent viruses of the mosquito. Other members include *Lymphocystis* virus of fish, African swine-fever virus, *Amphibian cytoplasmic* virus, and Gecko virus. The viruses contain approximately 15 percent double-stranded DNA (a single molecule) with a molecular weight of 130×10^6 daltons and with a guanine-cytosine content of 29 to 32 percent. The icosahedral particles, 130 nm in diameter, have an icosahedral edge length of approximately 85 nm and a sedimentation rate of 2,200 S. The complex particle contains several proteins, and the outer icosahedral shell contains approximately 1,500 capsomeres. Members in the genus have an envelope and are sensitive to solvents.

The site of capsid assembly and envelopment is in the cytoplasm.

Herpesviridae. This family provisionally is divided into three subfamilies: Alphaherpesvirinae (prototype virus—human herpes simplex), Betaherpesvirinae (prototype virus—human cytomegalovirus), and Gammaherpesvirinae (prototype virus—Epstein-Barr virus). The family contains an exceedingly large number of viruses involved in the production of disease. The type species is *Herpesvirus* h-1 (herpes simplex virus). Other members are *Herpesvirus simiae* (B virus), *Herpesvirus T* (of marmosets), perhaps two herpesviruses of *Cercopithecus,* herpesvirus of patos monkeys, herpesvirus of saimiri, *Herpesvirus cuniculi* (virus III of rabbits), pseudorabies virus, infectious bovine rhinotracheitis virus, varicella virus, equine rhinopneumonitis and other related equine herpesviruses, malignant catarrhal fever virus of cattle, bovine ulcerative mammillitis (Allerton) virus, feline rhinotracheitis virus, canine herpesvirus, Epstein-Barr virus (associated with infectious mononucleosis and Burkitt lymphoma), Marek's disease virus, avian infectious laryngotracheitis, avian herpesviruses of pigeons, parrots, owls, and cormorants, herpesvirus associated with lymphosarcoma in the African clawed frog, snake herpesvirus, cytomegaloviruses affecting various species including man, porcine inclusion body rhinitis virus, sheep pulmonary adenomatosis (jaagziekte) virus, duck plague virus, and fish viruses.

The herpesviruses contain linear double-stranded DNA with terminal reiterations and internal repetition of terminal sequences. The viruses have a molecular weight of 54 to 92 $\times$ 10^6 daltons and a guanine-cytosine content of 57 to 74 percent. The nucleocapsid, 100 nm in diameter, shows cubic and icosahedral symmetry with 162 hollow and elongated capsomeres that usually are hexagonal, but some are pentagonal in cross section. Lipid membrane surrounding the capsid is 150 nm in diameter. The particles are sensitive to lipid solvents and also are acid-labile. The particle DNA content is approximately 7 percent of its weight, and it has a buoyant density in cesium chloride of 1.27 to 1.29 g per cm^3. The development begins in the nucleus, and the particle is completely formed by the addition of protein membranes as the virus passes into the cellular cytoplasm.

Intranuclear inclusion bodies are formed by these viruses. A few contain hemagglutinins. Viruses in this group cause a broad variety of infectious diseases ranging in character from acute catarrhal disease to chronic and even oncogenic disease.

Poxviridae. This family has two subfamilies: Chordopoxvirinae, which contains six genera of mammalian viruses, and Entomopoxvirinae, consisting of one genus of insect viruses.

Member viruses in the genera of the subfamily Chordopoxvirinae are as follows. *Orthopoxvirus* includes vaccinia, variola, alastrim, cowpox, horsepox, ectromelia, rabbitpox, monkeypox, buffalopox, and camelpox. *Avipoxvirus* includes turkeypox, canarypox, fowlpox, quailpox, lovebirdpox, sparrowpox, starlingpox, and pigeonpox. *Capripoxvirus* includes sheeppox, goatpox, and lumpy skin disease virus. *Leporipoxvirus* includes myxoma viruses, rabbit fibroma, hare fibroma, and squirrel fibroma. *Parapoxvirus* includes contagious pustular dermatitis of sheep (orf), sealionpox virus, bovine papular stomatitis, and pseudocowpox viruses. *Suipoxvirus* includes swinepox. It is interesting to note that no poxvirus has been described in the dog or domestic cat. There are many important animal pathogens in this group that cause fatal disease and serious economic losses.

The symmetry of the capsid of these largest vertebrate viruses is unknown. The poxviruses contain 5 to 7.5 percent double-stranded DNA in linear form with a molecular weight of 160 $\times$ 10^6 daltons. The guanine-cytosine content of the nucleic acid is 35 to 40 percent. Brick-shaped or ovoid complex particles, 170 to 250 by 300 to 450 nm have a buoyant density in cesium chloride varying from 1.1 to 1.33 g per cm^3. The particles have characteristic surface patterns and lateral bodies and some poxviruses have an envelope. Some poxviruses are known to contain RNA polymerase. There is an NP antigen common to all members, and members of Chordopoxvirinae also have other antigens in common and can recombine genetically. All poxviruses exhibit nongenetic reactivation and replicate in cytoplasmic foci.

RNA Viruses

There is a group of more than 350 viruses, called the arbovirus group, that have interesting ecological cycles involving vertebrate hosts and arthropods which serve as vectors in the transmission of the viruses to humans and domestic and wild animals. Many arboviruses are pathogenic in vertebrate hosts. As our knowledge of these viruses has advanced and our system of viral classification improved, it has been possible to place many arboviruses into one of five RNA virus families: Reoviridae, Togaviridae, Bunyaviridae, Rhabdoviridae, and Arenaviridae.

Picornaviridae. This family now has four genera: *Aphthovirus, Cardiovirus, Enterovirus,* and *Rhinovirus.* Member viruses in the genus *Enterovirus* are the three poliovirus serotypes; Coxsackie A and B viruses; human ECHO viruses; bovine, porcine, murine, and simian enteroviruses; Nodamura virus; avian encephalomyelitis; duck hepatitis virus; and human hepatitis A virus. The *Rhinovirus* genus includes human (> 90 serotypes), bovine, and equine rhinoviruses. *Aphthovirus* genus contains seven foot-and-mouth disease serotypes. The *Cardiovirus* genus only has one virus, encephalomyocarditis (rarely infects man).

Member viruses contain single-stranded RNA in linear form. The molecular weight of RNA is 2.5 to 2.6 × 10^6 daltons. G and C content of virus is 40 to 54 percent. Virions are isometric, nonenveloped, and 20 to 30 nm in diameter, with icosahedral symmetry (T = 3, 32 capsomeres probably). Virions are assembled in cytoplasm. Buoyant density in cesium chloride is 1.34 to 1.35 g per cm^3 (enteroviruses) or 1.38 to 1.45 g per cm^3 (rhinoviruses). Infectivity is ether-resistant. Enteroviruses and encephalomyocarditis virus are acid-stable, and rhinoviruses and foot-and-mouth disease virus are acid-labile. Enteroviruses and some rhinoviruses are stabilized against heat inactivation by magnesium chloride. Many viruses hemagglutinate. Replication involves functional protein formation by posttranslational cleavage or an unpunctuated precursor. There are very important human and animal pathogens in this family.

Caliciviridae. This is a provisional family with a single genus, *Calicivirus,* which includes vesicular exanthema viruses of swine, sea lions, and fur seals and also feline caliciviruses. These viruses cause disease in their respective hosts.

Member viruses contain single-stranded RNA. The molecular weight of RNA is about 2.6 to 2.7 × 10^6 daltons. The G and C content is about 46%. Virions are isometric, nonenveloped, and 35 to 40 nm in diameter, with icosahedral symmetry (probably T = 3). Virions are assembled in cytoplasm. Buoyant density in cesium chloride is 1.36 to 1.39 g per cm^3. Virions contain only one structural polypeptide. Infectivity is ether-resistant, and stability at acid pH is variable (generally labile at pH 3). The capsomeres are cup-shaped and 32 in number.

Reoviridae. This family has been expanded considerably in the last few years and now includes many important animal pathogens, particularly in the genera *Orbivirus* and *Rotavirus*. The three mammalian serotypes in the genus *Reovirus* have been associated with respiratory and enteric diseases of animals, but most frequently as inapparent infections.

The viruses in this family contain double-stranded RNA in ten linear segments. It is the only family with double-stranded RNA animal viruses. Molecular weight of RNA segments varies from 0.3 to 3.0 × 10^6 daltons, and total genome is 15 × 10^6 (reovirus) or 12 × 10^6 daltons (orbivirus and rotavirus). The G and C content is 42 to 44 percent. Virions are isometric, nonenveloped and 75 nm (reovirus), 60 to 80 nm (orbivirus), or 70 nm (rotavirus) in diameter. Virions have a double capsid shell, and the structure of outer capsid layer is indistinct. Structure of inner capsids of orbiviruses and rotaviruses have icosahedral symmetry (T = 3 plus complex secondary symmetry). Virions are assembled in cytoplasm. Buoyant density in cesium chloride is 1.36 g per cm^3. Infectivity is resistant (reoviruses) or partly resistant (orbiviruses) to ether treatment; infectivity is resistant (reoviruses and rotaviruses) or sensitive (orbiviruses) to acid conditions. Intracytoplasmic inclusion bodies are formed by many viruses. Reoviruses and rotaviruses hemagglutinate.

Important diseases in the genus *Orbivirus* are African horse sickness, bluetongue in sheep and cattle, Colorado tick fever, and epizootic hemorrhagic disease of deer. The genus *Rotavirus* includes such diseases as human infantile diarrhea disease, rotavirus diarrheal disease of neonatal cattle, neonatal horses, swine, and dogs, and epizootic diarrhea of infant mice virus. Infectious pancreatic necrosis virus of trout and infectious bursal disease virus of chickens are placed in this family.

Togaviridae. There are four genera in this family: *Alphavirus, Rubivirus, Pestivirus* and *Flavivirus*. Member viruses contain single-stranded RNA in linear form. The molecular weight of RNA is 3 or 4 × 10^6 daltons. The G and C content is 48 to 51 percent. Virions are either isometric and enveloped, 60 nm (alphaviruses and rubiviruses), or 40 nm (flaviviruses and pestiviruses), in diameter including envelope and surface projections. Icosahedral symmetry has been proven for capsid of alphaviruses only (T = 3 or T = 4). Virions are assembled in cytoplasm by budding from host cell membranes. Buoyant density in cesium chloride is 1.25 g per cm^3. Infectivity is ether-sensitive and variably sensitive to acid conditions. Alphaviruses and flaviviruses replicate in vertebrate and arthropod hosts; rubiviruses and pestiviruses have no invertebrate host. Virions act as hemagglutinin. There are a large number of viruses assigned to this family. Only those members that are significant pathogens in humans and/or animals will be listed.

In the genus *Alphavirus,* eastern, western, and Venezuelan equine encephalitides; and Sindbis virus are worthy of mention. Yellow fever; dengue 1–4; Japanese B, Murray Valley, Russian spring-summer, and St. Louis encephalitides; louping ill; Israel turkey meningoencephalitis; and West Nile fever are important pathogens in the genus *Flavivirus.* In the genus *Rubivirus* rubella and possibly equine arteritis are assigned to this group. *Pestivirus* includes two important viral diseases in domestic animals: bovine virus diarrhea and hog cholera.

Orthomyxoviridae. The well-characterized viruses in this group compromise one genus *Orthomyxovirus.* The member viruses contain single-stranded RNA in eight segments. The molecular weight of RNA segments varies from 1.1×10^5 to 1×10^6 daltons, and total genome is 4×10^6 daltons. The G and C content is 41 to 43 percent. Virions are spherical, elongated, or filamentous, and 80 to 120 nm in diameter, and filaments may reach several nm in length. Virions consist of a unit-membrane envelope modified with viral M protein that has two types of precise projections, hemagglutinin and neuraminidase, and helically symmetric ribonucleocapsid, 6 to 9 nm. Viral ribonucleocapsid accumulates in the nucleus, and virions are formed by budding from plasma membrane. Buoyant density in sucrose is 1.19 to 1.21 g per cm^3. Infectivity is sensitive to ether, acid, and heat. Viruses hemagglutinate by attachment to neuraminidase-sensitive receptors except for influenza C, which does not have demonstrable neuraminidase. Recombination is common between influenza A viruses. Antigenic variation is frequent as drifts and shifts occur. An RNA-dependent RNA polymerase is associated with purified virions.

This well-characterized group includes viruses of types A, B, and C. Type A viruses include human influenza, porcine influenza, equine influenza, and avian influenza. Types B (B/Lee/40) and C (C/Taylor/1233/47) are human-influenza serotypes. Inflenza A viruses have fifteen hemagglutinin variant types, and nine neuraminidase types are recognized. Strains from different species may share these antigens. Hemagglutinin and neuraminidase differences in influenza B virus distinguish antigenic variants, but no types are specified. Influenza C strains show hemagglutinin variations, but no types have been specified. Influenza A viruses cause respiratory infections of pigs, horses, and birds. The orthomyxoviruses are sensitive to dactinomycin.

Paramyxoviridae. This family consists of three genera: *Paramyxovirus, Morbillivirus,* and *Pneumovirus.* Viruses in this family contain single-stranded RNA in unsegmented linear form. The molecular weight of RNA is 4 to 8×10^6 daltons. The G and C content is 48 to 52 percent. Virions are spherical or pleomorphic and 100 to 300 nm in diameter. Virions consist of a unit-membrane envelope with surface projections containing a single, helically symmetric ribonucleocapsid, 18 nm in diameter. Virions are formed in the cytoplasm by budding from the cytoplasmic membrane. The buoyant density in cesium chloride is 1.23 g per cm^3. Virions are sensitive to acid, ether, and heat. Viruses in the genus *Paramyxovirus* hemagglutinate by attachment to neuraminidase-sensitive receptors, whereas members of the genus *Morbillivirus* do not contain neuraminidase. The paramyoxviruses are resistant to dactinomycin.

Viruses in the genus *Paramyxovirus* include Newcastle disease virus, mumps virus, parainfluenza viruses 1–4, turkey paramyxovirus, and Yucaipa virus. There are four important pathogens in the genus *Morbillivirus:* measles virus, canine distemper virus, rinderpest virus, and peste de petite ruminant virus. The respiratory syncytial virus and pneumonia virus of mice are members of the genus *Pneumovirus.*

Rhabdoviridae. Members of this family contain 2 percent single-stranded RNA with a molecular weight of 3 to 4×10^6 daltons and with a guanine-cytosine content of approximately 42 percent. The helical nucleocapsid, 10 to 20 nm in diameter is surrounded by a shell to which is closely applied an envelope with 10 nm spikes. The whole particle is bullet-shaped measuring 60 by 180 nm and has a buoyant density in cesium chloride of 1.2 g per cm^3. Infectivity is destroyed by ether and by acid. Some viruses hemagglutinate, and antigenic relationships exist between some members. The particles maturate at the cytoplasmic membrane. Most members multiply in arthropods as well as vertebrates.

The type species is *Rhabdovirus* b-1 (vesicular stomatitis virus). Other members are cocal, Hart Park, Kern Canyon, Flanders, and rabies viruses, and also viruses of fish, bats, flies, and plants.

Retroviridae. This family has been divided into three subfamilies: Oncovirinae, Spumavirinae, and Lentivirinae. The viruses contain single-stranded RNA in linear form. The molecular weight of RNA is 5 to 7×10^6 daltons consisting of two subunits of equal size. The G and C content is 47 to 57 percent. Virions are complex, enveloped, and about 100 nm in diameter. Virions consist of a unit-membrance envelope with surface projections (knobs), an inner shell with icosahedral symmetry, and a central core or nucleocapsid probably with helical symmetry. Virions are assembled by budding through cytoplasmic and plasma membranes after the formation of inner structures in the cytoplasm. Buoyant density in cesium chloride is 1.18 g per cm^3. Infectivity is destroyed by ether, acid, and heat. All viruses contain antigenically specific RNA-dependent DNA polymerase (reverse transcriptase), and replication of viral RNA involves a DNA provirus which is integrated into host DNA. Many viruses cause neoplastic diseases, especially leukemias, sarcomas, mammary carcinomas, and degenerative diseases.

Members of Oncovirinae include many murine leukemia and sarcoma viruses, feline leukemia and sarcoma viruses, and tumor pathogens from many other species including rats, guinea pigs, cattle, pigs, monkeys, baboons, chickens, and reptiles. Visna and maedi viruses of sheep comprise the subfamily Lentivirinae. In the subfamily Spumavirinae are the foamy viruses of primates, cats, hamsters, cattle, and man.

Bunyaviridae. All viruses in this family are arboviruses that contain single-stranded RNA in three or four linear segments. The total genome has a molecular weight of 6×10^6 daltons. Virions are spherical, enveloped, and 100 nm in diameter. Virions consist of a unit-membrane envelope with surface projections, which may be randomly placed or clustered in arrays with icosahedral symmetry, containing helically wound symmetric ribonucleocapsids with circular configuration, 5 to 6 nm in diameter. Virions are formed by budding from intracytoplasmic (primarily Golgi) membranes. Buoyant density in potassium tartrate is 1.20 (g per cm^3). Infectivity is destroyed by ether, acid, and heat. Virus particles hemagglutinate.

Important diseases in this family are Nairobi sheep disease, sandfly fever, Rift Valley fever, and Crimean hemorrhagic fever.

Arenaviridae. Members of the only genus, *Arenavirus,* in this family contain single-stranded RNA in linear segments. Molecular weight of four large RNA segments varies from 2.1, 1.7, 1.1, and 0.7×10^6 daltons; one to three small RNA segments are about 0.03×10^6 daltons. Virions are spherical or pleomorphic and 50 to 300 nm in diameter. Virions consist of unit-membrane envelope with surface projections containing varying numbers of ribosome particles (20 to 25 nm) either free in interior or, less commonly, connected by a linear structure. Virions are formed by budding from plasma membrane. Buoyant density in cesium chloride is 1.19 to 1.20 g per cm^3. Infectivity is sensitive to ether, acid, and heat. Most viruses have a limited rodent host range in nature in which maintenance is by persistent infection with viruria. All viruses share a group-specific antigen determined by the immunofluorescence test and in some instances by the complement-fixation test.

Important diseases caused by viruses in this family include lymphocytic choriomeningitis, Bolivian and Argentinian hemorrhagic fever, and Lassa fever.

Coronaviridae. Member viruses contain single-stranded RNA. The molecular weight of RNA is 4 to 5×10^6 daltons. Virions are spherical or pleomorphic and 70 to 120 nm in diameter. Virions consist of a unit-membrane envelope with unique, definitive, bulbous projections; the interior structure is not fully resolved, but probably is a loosely wound, helically symmetric nucleocapsid. Virions are formed by budding from intracytoplasmic membranes. Buoyant density in sucrose is 1.18 g per cm^3. Infectivity is sensitive to ether. acid, and heat.

Viruses in this family cause a variety of illnesses. Infectious bronchitis virus causes a respiratory disease in chickens. Coronaviruses have been implicated in gastrointestinal disease in cattle, pigs, dogs, humans, and possibly the horse. One member causes bluecomb disease in turkeys. Hemagglutinating encephalomyelitis virus causes encephalitis in pigs.

Viroids. A new class of infectious agents, viroids are smaller than viruses. Viroids exhibit the characteristics of nucleic acids in crude extracts. They are insensitive to heat and organic solvents but sensitive to nucleases and do not appear to possess a protein coat. Viroids consist solely of a short strain of RNA with a molecular weight of 75,000 to 100,000 daltons. These agents cause five separate plant diseases and may cause disease in humans and animals, although this is only speculative at present.

VIRAL SIZE AND MORPHOLOGY

Electron Microscopy. Electron micrographs are photomicrographs made with an instrument known as an electron microscope (Figure 36.7). This is an instrument of magnification that uses beams of electrons, instead of light rays, and electromagnetic fields instead of lenses of glass or quartz. Because the beams of electrons cannot be seen with the eye, the images are projected on a fluorescent plate, which renders them visible just as x-rays can be visualized on a fluoroscope. The micrographs are the images secured on photographic plates.

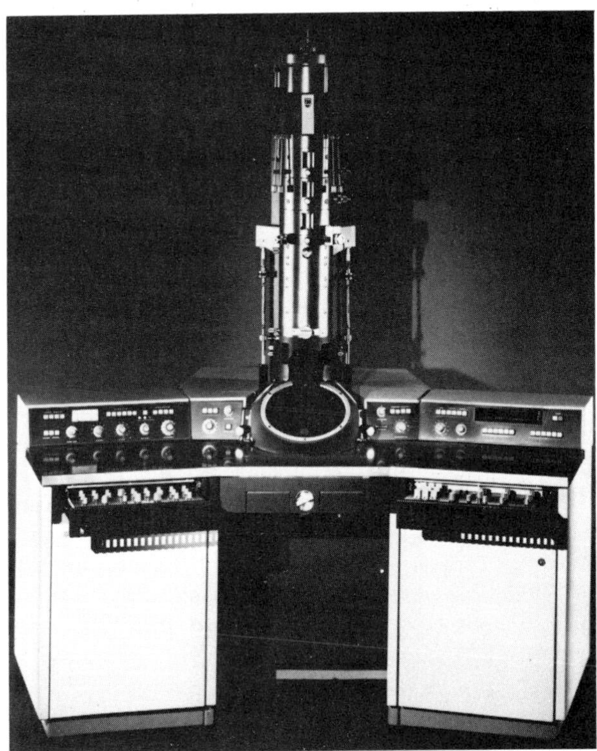

Figure 36.7. Electron microscope. Philips Model 302. (Courtesy Philips Electronic Instruments, Inc., Mahwah, N.J.)

With an electron microscope, images with sharp definition can be secured at magnifications as high as 1 : 1,000,000 by enlarging electron photomicrographs. The advantages can be appreciated when it is pointed out that, with the best optical equipment, resolution is difficult to obtain with magnifications greater than 1,200 diameters.

The objects from which electron micrographs are made usually are mounted on very thin collodion films supported on fine metallic screens. Because the density of many of the very small particles is not great, the early micrographs were not clear. This was remedied by the work of Williams (37), who introduced metallic shadowing into the process (Figure 36.8). This not only provided the needed contrast, but also made possible the introduction of a third dimension into the photographs. The prepared films are dried and then introduced into a small chamber, which is evacuated. They are carefully oriented with reference to a focal point where a small particle of the shadowing metal (silver, gold, chromium, etc.) is placed. The metal is then raised in temperature by an electric current until it is vaporized. In the vacuum the vaporized metal molecules are dispersed in every direction, lodging upon the first surfaces encountered. Because the films on the collodion membranes are deliber-

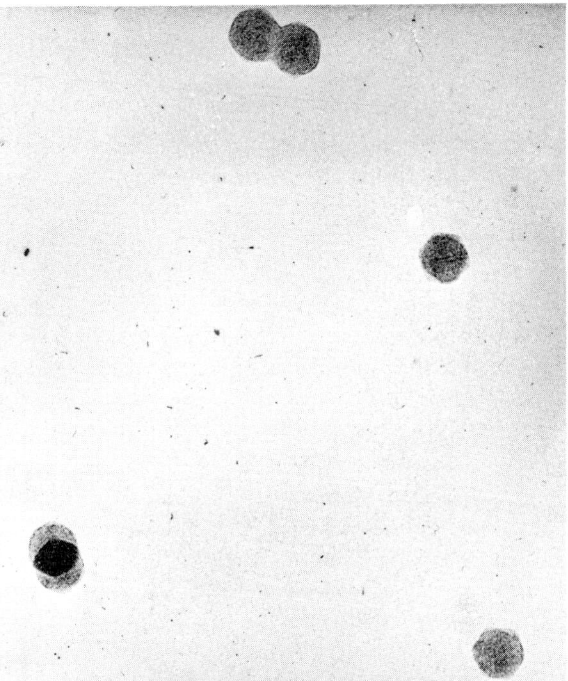

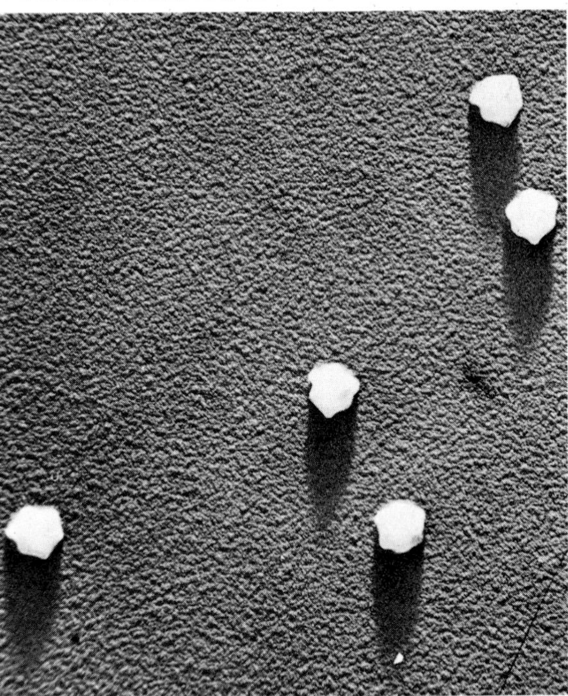

Figure 36.8. Electron micrographs of air-dried particles of the *Tipula* (crane fly) virus. × 52,000. (*Upper*) Unshadowed particles. (*Lower*) Metallic shadowed particles. (Courtesy Robley C. Williams and Kenneth M. Smith, *Biochem. Biophys. Acta.*)

ately oriented at an angle to the source of the metallic dispersion, the metal film will be deposited on any particles in this film, and there will be "shadows" on the side of the particles where the metallic molecules are prevented from reaching the surface by the height of the particles. These shadows give a realistic idea of the third dimension of the particles.

The negative staining technique that employs the use of phosphotungstic acid is excellent for studying structures of viruses with the electron microscope. The phosphotungstate permeates the virus particle as a cloud and clearly shows the surface structure of viruses by the virtue of negative staining. It also enters the core of particles without nucleic acid that the noninfectious. Thus, it is possible to study the development of viral particles at different stages of replication.

Thin stains of infected animal tissues or pellets of centrifuged cells from infected cell culutres have also advanced our knowledge of viral structure. Unless special precautions are taken, electron photomicrographs may overestimate the diameter of viruses.

The size of some animal viruses, in comparison with some other microorganisms and protein molecules, is indicated in Table 36.1. It is customary in measuring such small objects to use the *nanometer* (nm) as the unit of measure, this unit being 0.001 of a micrometer (μm). By such a scale the elementary bodies of chlamydiae measure about 0.3 μm or 300 nm. In the table micrometers are used as the unit to avoid confusion. Particles with a 2-fold difference in diameter have an 8-fold difference in volume.

Ultrafiltration. Because it is known that the pore size of silica filters (Pasteur, Berkefeld) is not the sole factor that determines whether or not particles in suspension will be passed, such filters have been discarded as a means of determining the approximate size of virus elements.

To avoid the absorbing properties of silica filters, Bechhold (8) as early as 1907 introduced the use of collodion membranes as filters for virus suspensions. Many years later, Elford (14) and Bauer and Hughes (6) standardized such filters (gradocol membranes) so that they might be used for determining the approximate size of virus particles. By the use of membranes of differing pore sizes, it was possible to determine the approximate diameter of the elements of many viruses. The size of the limiting APD (average pore diameter), multiplied by 0.64, yields the diameter of the virus particle. Later, when other methods of determining particle size were discovered, it was found that the membrane filters had given reasonably accurate results. Early studies for estimation of size by filtration often underestimated the size.

Ultracentrifugation. The ordinary laboratory centrifuges, operating at full speed, rarely spin faster than 4,000 revolutions per minute. At this rate most bacteria and larger particles with a specific gravity heavier than the fluids in which they are suspended gravitate rapidly to the bottoms of the tubes that contain them. Most virus particles, being much more minute, are thrown down at a very much slower rate—so slow, in fact, that it is not practicable to remove most of them from suspensions in this way. More successful are the angle centrifuges in which the tubes are held at an angle while spinning; here sedimenting particles have to travel only a short distance before they come in contact with the fluid-glass interface. For sedimenting the smaller virus particles, ultracentrifuges are needed. These are instruments of several types which can be operated at speeds of 60,000 rpm and more with centrifugal forces up to 200,000 times the force of gravity. One of them is described by Bauer and Pickels (7). These instruments have been used to determine physical characteristics of virus elements, as well as of other minute bodies such as albumin molecules. The approximate size can be calculated from data yielded by the sedimentation constants. The agreement between these calculations and the data derived from filtration studies is very good. It was known before the electron

Table 36.1. The approximate size of virus units in comparison with other well-known molecules and other microorganisms

	Micrometers		Micrometers
Staphylococcus aureus	0.8 to 1.0	St. Louis encephalitis	0.025
Psittacosis	0.3	Louping ill	0.015–0.020
Vaccinia	0.20	Foot-and-mouth disease	0.023
Pseudorabies	0.12	Poliomyelitis	0.025
Vesicular stomatitis	0.176 by 0.069	Serum globulin	0.0063
Fowl plague	0.080	Serum albumin	0.0056
Rift Valley fever	0.030	Egg albumin	0.004

microscope was developed that different viruses varied in size, some being only a little larger than protein molecules and others as large as some of the smaller bacteria.

Ionizing Radiation. A beam of charged particles such as high-energy electrons, alpha particles, or deuterons passing through a virus causes a loss in primary ionization. The release of these ions within the virion inactivates particle infectivity, antigenicity, and hemagglutinins.

By ascertaining the number of ionizations per unit volume or area required to inactivate 63 percent of the infectivity of the viral preparation, the average sensitive volume or area per ionization can be determined. This is the point at which there has been an average of one hit per sensitive target, according to the Poisson distribution, so the volume or area per ionization is equivalent to volume or area of the sensitive unit measured. Thus, knowledge of the volume or area permits calculation of the diameter or area of the infective unit in the virus particle. In the same way it is possible to measure the sizes of complement-fixing antigens and hemagglutinins.

Ultraviolet and rays and x-rays inactivate viruses. The inactivating dose varies for different viruses.

Viral Morphology. The morphology of viruses is determined principally by the use of the electron microscope and x-ray diffraction.

The capsids of animal viruses are arranged in two forms of symmetry, cubic and helical. All cubic symmetry in animal viruses is characteristic of an icosahedron with its 5:3:2 pattern of rotational symmetry. The arrangement of capsomeres to comply with icosahedral symmetry is limited. This limitation in its simplest form can be expressed by the formula $N = 10\ (n-1)^2 + 2$, where N represents the number of capsomeres and n signifies the number of capsomeres on one side of each equilateral triangle. The icosahedron has 20 equilateral triangular faces with 12 vertices (see Figure 41.1 of an adenovirus, in chapter 41), although the face (30 in number) of the Picornaviridae members may be a rhombus thus changing the formula to $N = 30\ (n-1)^2 + 2$.

The triangulation number can also be used to group viruses with icosahedral symmetry. The number of capsomeres (morphologic units) is expressed by the formula $M = 10T + 2$. One class has values of 1, 4, 9, 16, and 25; a second class, values of 3 and 12; and a third class, values of 7, 13, 19, and 21.

Properties of Viral Components

Viral Nucleic Acid. The viral nucleic acid carries the genetic information for the replication of the virus. The type of nucleic acid can be determined by various means using the intact virus particle or the free nucleic acid. The enzyme digestion tests with free virus nucleic acid constitute a method reliable for determining the nucleic acid type. The type of nucleic acid and its strandedness can be determined by fixing smears of purified virus with an alcohol fixation followed by staining with acridine orange (pH 4.0, dye concentration 0.01 percent). Double-stranded viruses, either RNA or DNA, stain yellow, and single-stranded DNA and RNA viruses stain red in the fluorescent microscope. Uranyl acetate is a specific stain for DNA while having no affinity for RNA. This stain is often used in electron microscope preparations for this purpose. Density-gradient centrifugation in cesium salts also is used to differentiate RNA from DNA.

The viral nucleic acids are physically fragile once removed from their capsid protection. This made it difficult to study their structure. It is possible now to examine many nucleic acid molecules in the electron microscope without disrupting them. The molecules are spread in a special inert protein monofilm so their complete contour lengths can be measured with accuracy. In most viruses the nucleic acids are linear, but in some the molecule takes the form of a circle. In the case of the Papovaviridae the viruses have a double-stranded circle,

Figure 36.9. Forms of DNA of *Papovavirus* SV40 and sedimentation coefficients in neutral sucrose gradients: supercoiled (I), nicked (II), linear (III), and replicative intermediate (RI). Linear DNA is formed by restriction endonucleases, which cleave both strands of the DNA at a single site. The RI shows 2 forks, 3 branches, and no ends, as seen in electron microscopy. (From E. Jawetz, J. L. Melnick, and E. A. Adelberg, *Review of Medical Microbiology*, 13th ed. Copyright 1978 by Lange Medical Publications, Los Altos, Calif.)

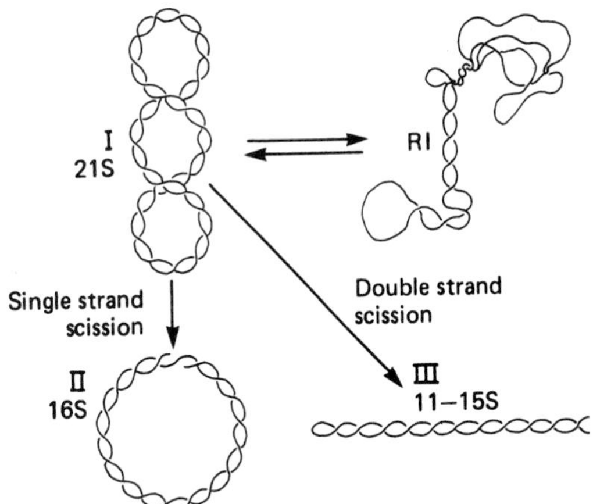

often hypercoiled (Figure 36.9). By using linear densities of approximately 2 by 10^6 daltons (1 dalton equals the mass of one hydrogen atom) per micrometer for double-stranded forms and one-half that amount for single-stranded forms the molecular weights of viral genomes can be calculated from direct measurements.

A finding of great interest and significance cited the presence of a DNA polymerase in RNA viruses that synthesizes DNA from an RNA template. Thus, it has been demonstrated that an RNA virus can make DNA.

Viral Protein. Viral proteins have several important functions. These proteins determine the antigenicity of the virus and are very much involved in the immunogenic process. Thus the viral structural proteins are of great interest to individuals concerned in the production of vaccines. In addition, these proteins determine the relatedness of viruses and thus are important to the diagnostician. The proteins also protect the viral genome against inactivation by nucleases present in tissues, participate in the adsorption of the virus particle to a susceptible cell, and serve as the structural units providing structural symmetry to the virus. Viral protein as such is not pathogenic.

The structural proteins of a few viruses have been extensively studied, including those of poliovirus. Despite some knowledge of the structural arrangement and chemical composition from poliovirus protein, there is little known about the binding of its RNA to the protein. Using polyacrylamide gel electrophoresis, the polypeptides of purified poliovirus particles obtained by treatment with detergents were analyzed. Four polypeptides were found to exist in poliovirus. Other analyses suggested that these polypeptides exist as precursors of the infectious virus in cells and in some unknown fashion become assembled with the viral RNA to form the virion.

In addition to the structural proteins, other virus specific proteins are formed in an infected cell such as the virus specific enzyme, thymidine kinase, in herpes- and vaccinia-infected cells.

Viral Lipids. Lipids are found in those viruses that have an envelope. Those viruses containing essential lipids are ether-sensitive and chloroform-sensitive. It has been observed that certain poxviruses are ether-resistant and chloroform-sensitive, but this is the only viral family showing this distinction among certain of its members.

The study of viral lipids presents real problems because their distinction from contaminating host cell lipids associated with viral particles is difficult. In general the lipids are added to the viral particle as it matures or buds through the cell or nuclear membrane. In the process the host membranes are incorporated into the complete virus particle. The host membrane of the viral-infected cell differs from a noninfected cell. For example, the limiting membrane of orthomyxoviruses contains neuraminidase, an enzyme not found in normal cell membranes. Another RNA virus whose lipid envelopes have been studied with interesting results is the SV5, a simian parainfluenza virus. The lipid content of its envelope is related to the nature of its host substrate. The SV5 virions grown in monkey cells or in baby hamster kidney cells have a lipid composition that is closely similar to the plasma membrane composition of the particular cell in which the virus replicated. The proposed structure of the envelope of Sindbis virus, an arbovirus in the family Togaviridae, is depicted in Figure 36.10. In the case of a DNA virus, such as a *Herpesvirus* which is assembled as a nucleocapsid within the nucleus, the nucleocapsid contacts the nuclear membrane whose inner membrane thickens and becomes electron-dense. The nucleocapsid is progressively enveloped by the thickened membrane and finally "buds" off as an enveloped virion in the perinuclear cisterna of the cell. Nucleocapsids can also bud off into nuclear vacuoles which seem to be continuous with the cisterna. The enveloped nucleocapsid is released from the cell by (*a*) the incorporation of some virions within cytoplasmic vacuole formed by the outer lamella of the nuclear envelope and sequestration of it from the cytoplasma to the outside of the cell and (*b*) movement through the cisternae of the endoplasmic reticulum to the cell exterior. In the late stages of infection unenveloped virions appear as breaks in the nuclear membrane occur.

Figure 36.10. Proposed structure of Sindbis virus, an arbovirus. (After Harrison and others. From E. Jawetz, J. L. Melnick, and E. A. Adelberg, *Review of Medical Microbiology*, 13th ed. Copyright 1978 by Lange Medical Publications, Los Altos, Calif.)

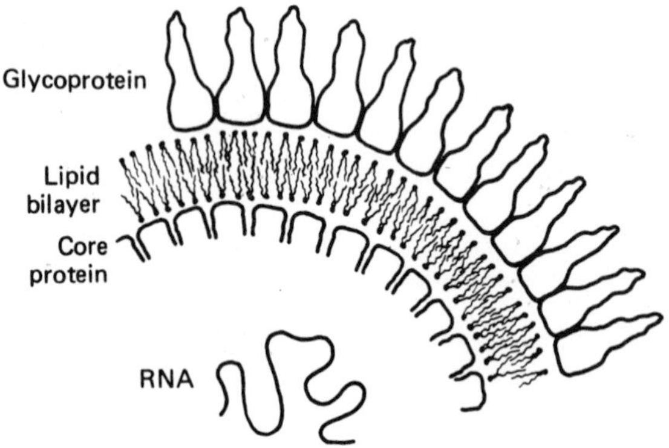

Viral Carbohydrates. The viral envelope contains carbohydrates as well as lipids, principally as glycoproteins. The glycoproteins are important parts of viral antigenic determinants. Their synthesis is controlled by the viral and host cell genome.

Hemagglutination. The hemagglutination phenomenon was described independently in 1941 by Hirst (18) and McClelland and Hare (25) as a property of human influenza virus. A wide variety of animal viruses are capable of agglutinating red blood cells of various animals and under a variety of conditions. The hemagglutination and hemadsorption techniques are now widely used in both the diagnostic and experimental laboratory to assay for virus and antibody. This test also serves as a model for host-virus interactions. It is a viral property useful in classifying viruses. The same can be said for the hemadsorption test, which is a useful manifestation of the hemagglutination phenomenon. This method has been used to demonstrate the presence of some viruses in tissue culture systems. The erythrocytes added to such a culture form red cell clumping at the cell sites of viral activity.

Certain Physical and Chemical Characteristics of Viruses

Effects of Heat and Cold. Most viruses are inactivated by heating at 56 C for 30 minutes, although some resist this treatment.

The ideal way to preserve viruses in the laboratory is storage at low temperatures, perferably −60 C or lower. All viral preparations stored under dry ice refrigeration must be tightly stoppered as the liberated CO_2 will cause a drop of pH of poorly buffered viral suspensions and inactivate those viruses that are sensitive to acid conditions. Lyophilization is another means by which many viruses can be preserved in the dry state for long periods of time at 4 C. Heat-resistant viruses withstand the lyophilization process reasonably well, but there usually is some loss in viral titer during lyophilization.

Enveloped viruses are less stable than viruses without an envelope, even at −90 C, and do not withstand repeated freezing and thawing. The addition of dimethyl sulfoxide (DMSO) in concentrations above 5 percent provides enveloped viruses with greater stability when maintained at very low temperatures.

Inactivation by Vital Dyes. Vital dyes such as toluidine blue, neutral red, and acridine orange penetrate many viruses to varying degrees. The dyes combine with the viral nucleic acid, and when exposed to light, inactivation results. These dyes do not penetrate some viruses, such as polio; thus, inactivation does not occur. Others are moderately susceptible such as adenoviruses and reoviruses, while still others such as *Herpesvirus* and vaccinia are readily suceptible. When poliovirus is grown in the presence of a vital dye in the absence of light, dye penetrates the nucleic acid and is then susceptible to photodynamic inactivation. The protein-coat antigen is not affected by this process.

Effect of pH. Practically all viruses are stable between pH 5 and pH 9. A notable exception is foot-and-mouth disease virus, which is readily inactivated at pH 6.

Electrostatic forces play an important role in hemagglutination reactions. Sometimes a variation of a few tenths of a pH Unit may determine a negative or positive reaction.

Virus Stabilization by Salts. Many viruses, such as poliovirus, can be stabilized by molar concentrations of salts. The mechanism is unknown. Viruses are preferentially stabilized by certain salts. Certain members of the Picornaviridae family and reoviruses are stabilized by 1 M magnesium chloride. The orthomyxoviruses and paramyxoviruses stabilize in the presence of 1 M magnesium sulfate, while 1 M sodium sulfate stabilizes herpes simplex virus.

This phenomenon can be utilized to rid certain polio preparations of viral adventitious agents such as SV40, foamy virus, and herpes B virus which are susceptible to heating in 1 M magnesium chloride, whereas this treatment has no adverse effects on the infectivity of poliovirus.

Antibiotic Sensitivity. With one exception, antibiotics and the sulfonamides, which are used so successfully in the treatment of bacteria, have no effects on viruses. The antibiotic rifampin readily inactivates bacterial RNA but not animal RNA polymerase. It also is active against poxviruses, presumably acting against the RNA polymerase of the particle, which is essential to poxvirus replication.

Metabolic analogues or antibiotics that interfere with DNA or RNA synthesis will inhibit viral replication. They also adversely affect RNA and DNA synthesis of the host cell. Consequently most are too toxic for use as viral chemotherapeutic agents.

Chemical Inactivants. Several classes of organic compounds are reactive with viruses. Aldehydes and ethylene oxide or imine react with primary valence bonds while others such as urea, phenol, detergents, guanidine, and lipid solvents affect mainly salt linkages or secondary valence bonds. Organic solvents such as ether and chloroform readily inactivate viruses with an envelope.

Phenol and hexylresorcinol are excellent protein denaturants that strip protein from some viruses releasing the infectious nucleic acid, which usually contains sufficient RNase to slowly inactivate the acid.

Formaldehyde, ethylene oxide, acetylethyleneimine, and glycidaldehyde are alkylating agents used for viral inactivation. Formaldehyde has been commonly employed to inactivate viruses for vaccine use. It reacts with amino, guanidyl, and amide groups of the viral protein and with nonhydrogen-bonded amino groups of the purine and pyrimidine bases of the nucleic acid. Ethylene oxide in a humid atmosphere is an effective virucide. Acetylethyleneimine appears to have great promise as an inactivant for foot-and-mouth disease virus vaccine because its kinetic curve for inactivation is essentially first-order, without tailing, and inactivation takes place in 24 to 48 hours without destruction of the viral immunizing properties; any excess can be neutralized with sodium thiosulfate. Organic iodine compounds are relatively ineffective against viruses because small amounts of organic matter rapidly deplete the active iodine.

Recently, Scott (32) reported on the activity of selected virucides against certain feline viruses that include a feline *Parvovirus,* feline *Calicivirus,* and feline *Herpesvirus* which can be considered as representative of their respective virus families. The former two viruses are known to be quite resistant because they do not contain an envelope. The information is given in Table 36.2.

Replication of Viruses

Viruses are highly parasitic and require living cells to furnish the energy, the enzymes for metabolic activity, and the low molecular weight precursors for viral protein and nucleic acid. Viruses do contain the essential genetic material for their replication in the host cell. The number of enzymes and structural antigens produced in the cell is a function of the size of the viral genome.

Successful replication studies were first accomplished with the T series of bacteriophages. The bacterial system is relatively easy to prepare and manipulate, and the growth cycle is short, being measured in minutes, whereas animal viruses take many hours to complete their growth cycle. Lastly, the assay of bacteriophages is more accurate and simple.

With the advent of improved methods of *in vitro* cultivation of animal cells, in assay for viral content and for study of biophysical, biochemical, and biological characteristics of viruses, some of the steps of interaction between animal viruses and tissue cells have been elucidated. The principal studies involving the adsorption of viruses to specific receptor sites has been done with the orthomyxoviruses. The receptor sites for these viruses are mucopolysaccharides on the cell surface. Viral adsorption can be prevented by the pretreatment of the host cells with an enzyme (receptor destroying enzyme, RDE) from *Vibrio cholerae* which destroys the mucopolysaccharide receptors involved in the hemagglutination reaction. This test procedure has been extensively used in the study of cell receptor sites. Viruses that contain lipid in their structure are released continuously from the cells. In contrast, viruses without lipid are released in large numbers at the time of cell lysis (burst process) similar to bacteriophages.

The replication of RNA and DNA viruses, in general, is similar, but differences do exist. The following two sections cite a replication of an RNA and a DNA virus.

RNA Viral Replication. The replication of foot-and-mouth disease virus (FMDV), which contains a single-stranded RNA genome, has been studied in great detail, beginning with the process of infection and ending with the release of viral progeny. Moreover, the stage of the cycle dealing with the replication of viral RNA has been accomplished in a cell-free system. The complete growth cycle takes place in the cytoplasm, a known characteristic of all RNA viruses whose replication has been studied in any detail. Further, all steps of the cycle apparently are independent of the cellular DNA genome.

Infection of pig kidney cell cultures by FMDV is a two-step process involving adsorption and penetration. Adsorption of virus requires calcium ions and is temperature-dependent with an activation energy of 6,000 calories per mole. The cells appear to possess between 30 and 100 receptor sites for virus. At low temperatures (2 to 4 C) the virus remains attached without penetration and can be released by certain chemicals. At higher temperatures (37 C) the attached virus penetrates the cell by a first-order reaction with an activation energy of 24,000 calories per mole. The half-time of penetration at 37 C of 30 seconds allows infection of 90 percent of the cells within 3 minutes. Virus attaches itself to dead cells, but does not penetrate them. Following engulfment by the cell, fragmentation of the virion into infectious RNA and viral protein subunits occurs within the cytoplasm. Because the host range of the disease is not widened by infection with free FMDV-RNA, this is further proof that cellular engulfment of the virion occurs.

Table 36.2. Activity of virucides against feline viruses

Virucide	Manufacturer's recommended dilution	Dilution of virucide tested*	Percent of viral activity†		
			Feline panleukopenia virus (*Parvovirus*)	Feline *Calicivirus*	Feline viral rhinotracheitis virus (*Herpesvirus*)
I. *Alcohols*					
Methyl alcohol	78%	35%	–	–	+++
Ethyl alcohol	70%	50%	–	+	NT
Isopropyl alcohol	70%	50%	–	±	NT
Lysol spray	U	1/2	–	±	+++
Pentacresol	U	1/2	–	±	+++
II. *Coal and Wood Tars*					
Creolin	1/21	1/16	–	+++	+++
Hexachlorophene	3%	1/2 (1.5%)	NT	–	NT
Pine oil	1/180	1/180	NT	–	NT
III. *Iodines*					
Betadine	U	1/2	±	++	+++
GSI	1/64	1/64	–	–	+++
Hi-Sine	1/256	1/256	–	–	+++
Iodophor	1/640	1/640	–	–	+++
IV. *Phenolics*					
Amerse	1/32	1/32	–	+++	+++
Lysol solution	1/32	1/32	–	+++	+++
Lysol spray	U	1/2	–	±	+++
Matar	1/256	1/256	–	+++	+++
1-Stroke Environ	1/256	1/256	±	+++	+++
O-Syl	1/32	1/32	–	+++	NT
V. *Quaternary Ammonium Compounds (Cationic Detergents)*					
A-33	1/64	1/64	–	–	+++
Hi-TOR	1/256	1/256	–	–	+++
Omega	1/256	1/256	–	–	NT
Roccal-D	1/200	1/200	–	–	+++
VI. *Soaps (Anionic Detergents)*					
Klomine	5%	5%	NT	±	NT
Silk Floss	U	1/2	–	+++	+++
Super Green	1/42	1/42	NT	–	+++
VII. *Miscellaneous*					
Clorox	1/32	1/32	+++	+++	+++
Formaldehyde	4%	4%	+++	+++	+++
Gluteraldehyde	2%	1%	+++	+++	+++
Hydrogen peroxide	3%	1/2 (1.5%)	+	+	NT
Nolvasan	1/128	1/128	–	–	+++

–, No infective virus detected at lowest virus test dilution (1/10).
±, 10 to 99 percent virus remaining.
+, 99 to 99.9 percent virus remaining.
++, 99.9 to 99.99 percent virus remaining.
+++, > 99.99 percent virus remaining.
NT, No test.
U, Undiluted.
*Exposed to virus dilutions for 10 minutes at room temperature.
†After treatment with virucide.
Courtesy F. W. Scott.

Within 30 minutes after infection, cellular protein synthesis is decreased by 50 percent and followed by bursts of virus-specific protein as a result of translation by viral RNA. The first burst occurs at 60 minutes postinfection. It can be inhibited by guanidine and has a temporal correspondence with the expected synthesis of FMD-specific RNA polymerase. Appreciable amounts of polymerase can be extracted from the cell after 2 hours with a peak activity of 3.5 hours after infection. The VIA (virus infection associated antigen) appears to be enzymatically inactive FMDV-specific RNA polymerase because its antibody inhibits polymerase activity. The VIA-RNA polymerase antigen is formed prior to virions and only when virus replicates in cells indicating that it is translated from noncapsid cistrons of the viral genome.

The nature of the second burst is unknown, but the third one coincides with viral maturation. In the interim between the first and third burst of virus-specific protein, single-stranded viral RNA molecules (+ strands) presumably are synthesized from the viral RNA in replicate form. More recently it has been demonstrated that C-type particle RNA tumor viruses contain an enzyme, DNA polymerase, that synthesizes DNA from the viral RNA template thus representing an early event in the replication of RNA tumor viruses and that the newly formed DNA serves as the template for viral RNA synthesis or more likely for a complementary DNA strand. The latter transcribes for viral RNA. It is known that actinomycin D inhibits DNA-dependent RNA synthesis and thus inhibits the multiplication of DNA viruses, and also a few RNA viruses such as Rous sacoma virus and RNA myxoviruses. The exact mechanism for this inhibition of RNA viruses is unclear, but perhaps the answer lies in the above explanation for the C-type particle RNA viruses.

The synthesis of viral capsid proteins apparently occurs at the same time. At a subsequent time the proteins then form procapsids or empty protein shells. In some unknown manner the viral genome is incorporated in the procapsids to form the virion that represents maturation. The FMD viral particles are released when the cell undergoes lysis.

DNA Viral Replication. The replication of adenoviruses has been thoroughly studied. Adsorption, penetration, and uncoating of a DNA virus such as an *Adenovirus* is similar to that described for FMDV, an RNA virus. After uncoating, the viral DNA migrates to the nucleus where a viral DNA strand is transcribed into specific messenger RNA that is translated to synthesize virus-specific proteins (such as tumor antigen) and to synthesize enzymes necessary for the biosynthesis of viral DNA. Host-cell DNA synthesis is initially elevated, but becomes suppressed as the cell manufactures viral DNA. Messenger RNA transcribed during the late stage of cellular infection migrates to the cytoplasm where translation into viral capsid protein occurs. The capsid protein is transported to the nucleus where it incorporates the viral DNA to form a mature virus particle. The virions are released after cell lysis.

Infectious viral DNA also has been synthesized *in vitro* by the use of a DNA template molecule from the bacterial virus ΦX-174 which can occur as a single- or double-stranded particle. In the presence of a monomer mixture used for polymerization this covalently closed circular viral DNA template (+) is copied by purified DNA polymerase with the formation of linear (−) strand complementary to the (+) circle that the joining enzyme converts into a covalent duplex circle similar to that which occurs *in vivo*.

Genetics of Animal Viruses

A vast amount of knowledge about genetics has been derived from studies of bacterial viruses. Within the last two decades two major advances in the animal virology field have made possible meaningful studies of animal viruses. The development of accurate and sensitive plaque assay procedures in cell culture systems permitted the quantitation of virus infectivity. Through the study of biophysical, biochemical, and biological characteristics of many animal viruses many stable genetic markers were observed that were amenable to experimental manipulation, easy to recognize, and resulting from single mutations. Some markers that are used include plaque size, pathogenicity, specific viral induced antigens, drug resistance, and inability to grow at a higher temperature. These mutations may occur spontaneously or arise after treatment with a mutagen.

Conditional-lethal mutants are noninfective under a set of conditions termed nonpermissive but which yield normal infectious progeny under conditions termed permissive. These mutants may be either host range (hr) mutants or temperature-sensitive (ts) mutants. Ts mutants have been isolated from nearly all animal viruses. These mutants grow at low temperatures (permissive) but not at high temperatures (nonpermissive). At a nonpermissive temperature the particles are defective because an altered amino acid sequence in some essential virus-specified protein renders that protein incapable of functioning. Hr mutants replicate and form plaques in one kind of cell (permissive) whereas abortive infection occurs in another cell type (nonpermissive). With hr bacterial virus mutants the permissible cell carries a transfer RNA that recognizes the altered nucleic acid base sequence as a codon and inserts an amino acid resulting in the formation of a functional polypeptide. It is conceivable such a mechanism is also operative in the host range mutants of animal viruses.

When more than one virus particle infects the same cell, they may act in various ways. These types of interactions are given in Table 36.3. In genetic interaction some progeny emerge that are genetically different from either parent. Several types of viral interaction can occur simultaneously under the proper conditions. The true viral genetic reactions are recombination, cross-reactivation, and multiplicity reaction as their progeny are genetically stable and some differ from their parents.

Cross-reactivation takes place between the genome of an infectious particle and the genome of an inactivated virus particle. Certain markers of the inactivated parent are rescued in viable progeny as a result of combination between a portion of the inactivated particle genome with the genome of the active particle. None of the progeny has the same characteristics as the inactivated parent. This phenomenon can be used to produce desirable vaccine strains as was done with influenza virus.

Recombination occurs when some progeny are produced that carry traits not found together in either parent. It is thought that nucleic acid strands break, resulting in the recombination of a part of the genome from one parent with part of the genome of the second parent. Recombinant progeny are stable and yield like progeny upon replication. Recombination has been demonstrated with polio and influenza viruses.

Multiplicity reactivation involves the combination between the genomes of two inactive particles in the same cell that results in the production of a viable genome that can replicate. None of the progeny produced is identical with either parent. This phenomenon has been demonstrated with vaccinia virus.

Phenotypic mixing has been demonstrated with some of the viruses in the *Enterovirus* group. It involves random incorporation of the genome of one virus such as poliovirus into the capsid of another heterologous virus

Table 36.3. Types and characteristics of interactions between animal viruses

Type of interaction	Viability of parental viruses	Some progeny different from parental virus	Progeny genetically stable	Example
I. Genetic				
A. Recombination	Active + active	Yes	Yes	Influenza, herpesvirus
B. Cross-reactivation	Active + inactive	Yes	Yes	Influenza
C. Multiplicity reactivation	Inactive + inactive	Yes	Yes	Vaccinia
II. Nongenetic				
A. Phenotypic mixing	Active + active	Yes	No	Picornaviruses
B. Genotypic mixing	Active + active	Yes	No	Paramyoxiviruses
C. Interference	Active + active	No	Yes	Coxsackieviruses
	Defective + active	No	Yes	Satellite + adenovirus
D. Enhancement	Active + active	No	Yes	NDV + parainfluenza
E. Complementation	Active + inactive	No	Yes	Poxviruses
	Active + defective	No*	Yes	(a) Rous-associated virus + Rous sarcoma virus† (b) Murine leukemia + sarcoma† (c) SV40 + adenovirus (d) Adenovirus + satellite
	Defective + defective	No*	Yes	PARA (SV40-adeno) + adenovirus

*In those cases in which the helper virus is supplying the coat (RSV-RAV, MSV-MLV, PARA-adenovirus), the progeny defective virus will be antigenically different if a heterologous helper virus is present and transcapsidation or pseudotype formation occurs.

†Shares certain similarities with an extreme form of phenotypic mixing.

Slightly modified from E. Jawetz, J. L. Melnick, and E. A. Adelberg, *Review of Medical Microbiology*, 13th ed., Lange Medical Publications, Los Altos, Calif., 1978.

such as Coxsackie virus. A stable genetic change does not occur as the phenotypically mixed parent will produce progeny with a capsid homologous to the genotype because protein synthesis is controlled by the viral genome. In this instance the phenotypically mixed parent would have a Coxsackie virus capsid, but its progeny would have a poliovirus capsid.

Genotypic mixing is characterized by a single virus particle that produces progeny of two distinct parental types. This is probably an accidental incorporation of two genomes in a single capsid. This unstable genetic change has been seen in the study of the orthomyxoviruses.

Complementation is the interaction between two viruses (one or both may be defective or inactive) that permits replication of either one or both of them. Neither the phenotype nor the genotype of the virus changes, and the progeny are like the parents. Different types of complementation between viruses are indicated by the following examples: (*a*) active fibroma virus provides the stimulation for an uncoating enzyme necessary for the genomal release of inactive myxoma virus; (*b*) active *Adenovirus* provides the production of the coat protein that is required by defective SV40 (PARA) virus.(*c*) active *Adenovirus* may provide some essential gene product that induces replication of the defective adeno satellite virus; and (*d*) viable Rous-associated virus probably supplies genetic material for the replication of defective Rous sarcoma virus particles (21) and murine leukemia virus likewise serves as a "helper" for its defective murine sarcoma virus particles.

Interference. In the course of investigational studies it has been noted that simultaneous injection of two viruses into a host may result in interference of one of the two viruses. This phenomenon may occur, wholly or in part, between two viruses of different antigenicity, between two strains of the same virus with differences in virulence, or between inactivated and virulent particles of the same virus. The phenomenon is discussed in detail by Vilches and Hirst (36) who cite many examples. It is known that monkeys infected with lymphocytic choriomeningitis fail to become paralyzed when given polio virus. Distemperoid (ferret distemper virus) or egg-adapted distemper virus interferes with the multiplication of virulent distemper virus in dogs. Inactivated influenza virus interferes with virulent influenza virus. The protective action in these cases cannot be due to antibodies because ample time had not elapsed for antibody formation. One plausible mechanism is the finding by Isaacs and Lindenmann in 1957 (21). These investigators described a macromolecular substance which they named *interferon*. In other instances of interference, interferon is not demonstrated. It is believed that the initial virus may alter either the host-cell surface, its metabolic pathways, or possibly the production of defective particles (DI) may cause interference of the superimposing virus. Many investigators have reported that continued passage of animal viruses in cell culture produced a cyclic variation in viral titers. Huang (20) showed that this variation is due to defective particles (Figure 36.11). There is an intracellular accumulation of nucleocapsids in cells when the largest amount of defective particles are synthesized by the cells. There also may be other unknown factors that affect the relative proportions of defective and standard particles during continuous passages. In this cyclic viral production it is noted that the DI particles lag slightly behind those representing standard virions. It is interesting to speculate on how these observations would relate to pathogenesis and the appearance and disappearance of clinical signs during certain diseases. In any instances of viral interference the process is generally short-lived as cell susceptibility recurs soon after the disappearance of interfering virus or interferon.

The discovery of interferon and its potential use in the treatment and prevention of viral diseases has created much excitement and considerable study. This viral inhibitor can be produced by cells in animals or in culture after infection with viruses. It appears in appreciable

Figure 36.11. Many investigators have reported that continued passage of animal viruses in cell culture produced a cyclic variation in viral titers. Huang showed that this variation is due to defective particles (DI). (Courtesy Alice S. Huang. Reproduced, with permission, from the *Annual Review of Microbiology*, Volume 27. © 1973 by Annual Reviews, Inc.)

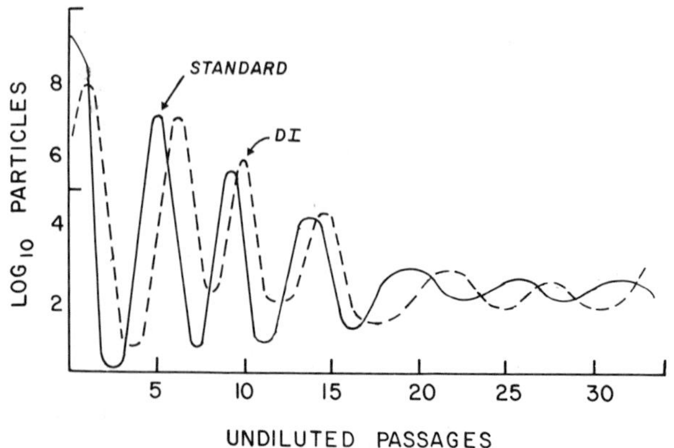

quantities after maximum virus production in the host animal but before circulating antibodies appear, suggesting an important role for interferon in the body defenses against viral infection. The cells of the reticuloendothelial system seem to provide most of the interferon, although most cells of the body are believed to contribute to its production.

Interferon is a protein which is heat-labile, acid-stable at pH 2, nondialyzable, trypsin-sensitive, nonneutralizable by virus, and weakly antigenic. It is effective as an antiviral substance on cells from the host species from which it was produced; thus, it is species-specific. It is not viral-specific. As a matter of fact, interferon can be produced *in vitro* in cultures of cells when stimulated with viruses (particularly double-stranded RNA is produced during replication) or synthetic double-stranded polynucleotides; and also by cells in the intact animal (*in vivo*) with viruses, rickettsiae, bacterial endotoxins, synthetic anionic polymers, or polynucleotides. After stimulation of animals with various interferon inducers, different classes of interferon are demonstrable, as evidenced by molecular weight differences. One class with a molecular weight of 8.5×10^4 daltons appears 2 hours after induction whereas one with a molecular weight of 3.4×10^4 daltons appears at 18 hours. The cellular events of the induction and action of interferon are presented in schematic summary in Figure 36.12.

The use of interferon and interferon inducers in the prevention and treatment of disease has tremendous potential, but many important problems must be recognized and solved prior to general use in man and animals. It has been possible to demonstrate the effectiveness of exogenous interferon in preventing disease or reducing its severity, if given early enough in the disease. Exogenous interferon is very costly to produce, and al-

Figure 36.12. Cellular events of the induction and action of interferon (IF). Virus comes in contact with the cell (1) and penetrates the cell membrane. The virus then releases its genetic material, and replication of the virus occurs (2). The new virus leaves the cell (3), enters the fluid around the first cell, and some of the replicated virus infects a second cell (4), where the release of the genetic material again takes place (5). During the early stages of infection of the first cell, some event (viral nucleic acid?) stimulates a gene in the DNA which contains the stored genetic information for interferon (A). This leads to the production of a messenger RNA for interferon, which leaves (B) the nucleus, and is translated by the cell's ribosomes (C), into the interferon protein.

Several events now occur more or less simultaneously. Some interferon is secreted by the first cell (D), enters the surrounding fluid, where it comes into contact with and stimulates the second cell (E). The second cell is thereby induced to produce a new messenger RNA (F) which is translated to a new protein(s) (G), the antiviral protein (AVP). This in turn modifies the cell's protein synthesizing machinery, such that cell messenger RNA is translated into protein, but viral RNA is poorly bound or translated or both. In the first cell processes E, F, and G may, in some instances, also operate to form AVP and thereby reduce the virus yield in the first cell. Shortly after interferon is synthesized in the first cell, another messenger RNA (H) is believed to be synthesized from the cell's DNA and is translated (I) into a regulatory protein (RP) (hypothesized). This regulatory protein combines with the messenger RNA for interferon, thereby preventing the further synthesis of more interferon (J). There is recent evidence that the antiviral state may be directly transferred between adjacent cells (from second to third cell at right) by the passage of an unknown (?) inducer of the antiviral protein. (Courtesy Samuel Baron and Ferdinando Dianzani.)

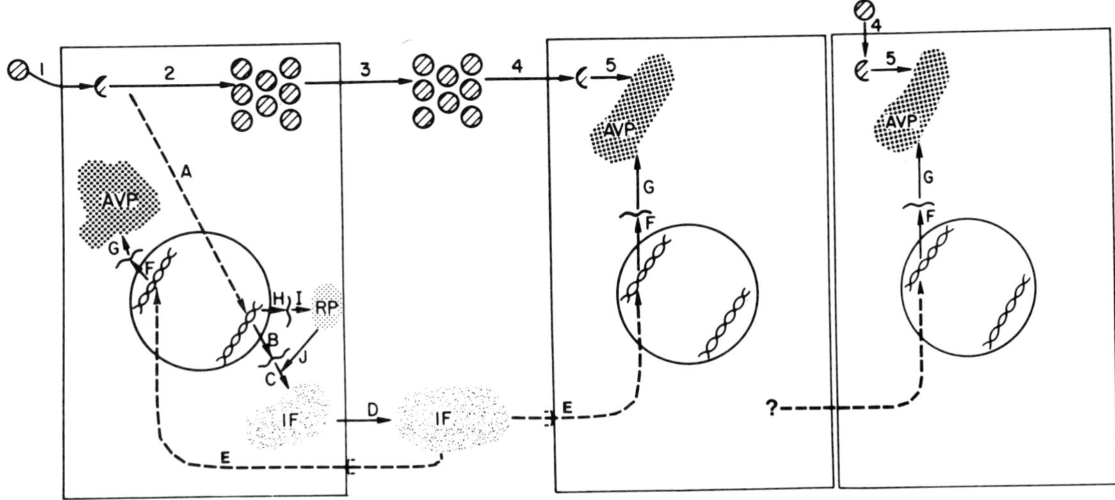

though interferon-inducers offer the greatest hope in controlling certain virus infections, they often are toxic in therapeutic doses, and nontoxic antilogues must be developed that are efficacious and reasonable in cost. The half-life of exogenous interferon is very short, and frequent injections are required to maintain effective prophylactic levels.

Enhancement, or dual infection, is the antithesis of interference. The demonstration of dual infection of single cells with viruses producing intranuclear (herpes simplex) and cytoplasmic (vaccinia) inclusions was reported by Syverton and Berry (35). This suggests that interference may not take place between viruses that require different pathways for their replication. Another mechanism may be concerned with the activity of one virus that inhibits the formation of interferon. It is known that parainfluenza virus reduces autoinhibition by Newcastle disease virus, a very potent interferon producer. Often coinfection enhances the production of one of the two viruses involved with the emergence of progeny similar to the parents.

Exaltation of disease may result when dual infection occurs in a host. For example when dogs are given distemper and infectious canine hepatitis viruses simultaneously, a more severe disease results than in dogs given either virus alone (17).

CHEMOTHERAPY OF VIRAL INFECTIONS

The control of disease is based on health measures, immunization, and treatment. The first two criteria have proved to be successful against many viruses and are responsible for the reduced incidence of serious diseases such as canine distemper, hog cholera, rinderpest, feline panleukopenia, and many other infectious viral diseases of domestic animals. With very few exceptions at present, treatment of viral diseases consists of amelioration of signs rather than reduced replication of the virus.

There are two major deterrents to the effective treatment of viral disease. The first, and perhaps the most important, is the strict parasitic relationship of virus and its host cell. It is quite clear that a virus depends on the metabolism of the host cell for its replication, and the majority of viral inhibitors act against cellular processes. A useful viral inhibitor must prevent completion of the viral growth cycle in the infected cell without causing lethal damage of the uninfected cells. This desirable effect can be achieved by a compound that acts directly on a component of the virus or on a viral product such as a virus-specific enzyme that is essential for successful replication. With the finding of virus-specific enzymes, the outlook for viral chemotherapy has brightened considerably. Inhibitors that prevent adsorption or penetration of the cell without damaging it are also being sought. The second problem involves the nature and pathogensis of viral diseases and the attendant problem of an early and accurate diagnosis. Many viral diseases may be recognized too late for effective treatment with a viral inhibitor. In other instances success depends on the availability of safe and effective viral inhibitors.

Amantadine, a symmetrical amine, inhibits certain members of the *Orthomyxovirus* and *Paramyxovirus* groups, pseudorabies virus (a *Herpesvirus*) and Rous sarcoma virus by blocking the penetration of the virus. It has no effect on adsorption of the virus. When administered prophylactically it is very effective in protecting experimental animals and man against influenza A strains. Therapeutic treatment has little or no effect on the course of the disease.

Many viruses of the Picornaviridae family are inhibited *in vitro* (tissue cultures) by guanidine and hydroxybenzylbenzimidazole (HBB). These compounds interfere with the synthesis of viral RNA polymerase, thus preventing the formation of viral protein and viral RNA. After the RNA polymerase is formed, neither drug can prevent viral replication. The inhibitory effect can also be overcome by dilution with fresh tissue culture medium. The therapeutic action of the two drugs with marked structural difference presumably is similar but not identical as some viruses can be inhibited by one drug but not the other. In some instances HBB and guanidine have a synergistic effect. Unfortunately there is no protection by either drug in experimental animal infections. This may be due, wholly or in part, to the rapid production of drug-resistant mutants.

Thiosemicarbazones were shown to inhibit the growth of poxviruses. Later isatin B-thiosemicarbozone (methisazone) and its N-methyl derivative were shown to have greater protective capacity in experimental animals. These compounds are also an effective prophylactic for smallpox in man if given within 24 to 48 hours after exposure. The drug is virus-specific without any effect on normal cell metabolism. There is normal synthesis of viral DNA and of the two enzymes (thymidine kinase and DNA polymerase) concerned in DNA synthesis. The synthesis of many, but not all, of the 20 or more soluble viral antigens that are formed during normal viral growth is inhibited, resulting in the formation of immature, noninfectious particles. Mutants resistant to this drug have been isolated.

Actinomycin D (dactinomycin) inhibits the replication of DNA viruses and some RNA viruses such as Rous sarcoma virus and some orthomyxoviruses. The drug inhibits DNA-dependent RNA synthesis by a mechanism that is not clear.

The antibiotic rifampin shows a preferential inhibition of bacterial RNA polymerase. Poxviruses carry their own RNA polymerase for synthesizing viral messenger RNA, and this antibiotic was very effective against smallpox virus in tissue-culture studies by inhibiting the viral polymerase but not materially affecting cellular polymerase.

Analogues of purine and pyrimidine bases may inhibit both RNA and DNA synthesis. Iododeoxyuridine (IUDR) has been used topically with success in the treatment of corneal lesions caused by herpes simplex, a DNA virus. It cannot be used routinely for systemic infections because it is too toxic. Under heroic circumstances, massive near-lethal doses have been administered in cases of *Herpesvirus* encephalitis with complete recovery ensuing. In tissue-culture studies of Papovaviridae-infected or *Herpesvirus*-infected cells, IUDR arrests the synthesis of the virion but not the viral components, because large amounts of viral antigen have been found in the cells. Electron-microscopic examination reveals the presence of immature virus particles in large numbers. Other halogenated deoxyuridines such as 5-fluoro-2′-deoxyuridine (FUDR), and 5-bromo-2′-deoxyuridine (BUDR), as well as IUDR, inhibit replication of members of the major DNA virus groups by the production of an improperly functioning nucleic acid. Drug-resistant mutants of some viruses have emerged by growth in the presence of IUDR or BUDR.

The activity of a purine or pyrimidine analogue can be enhanced by incorporation of ribose or deoxyribose into its molecule. The action of riboside or deoxyribose can be directed preferentially toward the inhibition of RNA or DNA. It has been found that ribosides of halogenated benzimidazoles are more selective inhibitors of influenza virus replication than the free benzimidazoles or their deoxyribosides.

The size of the halogen atom of the halogenated pyrimidine analogue determines the nature of its viral inhibitory action. The size and shape of 5-bromouracil (BU) is very similar to thymine, and 5-fluorouracil (FU) is similar to uracil. Thus, BU has been shown to inhibit DNA bacteriophage, but has no effect on the RNA tobacco mosaic virus. FU inhibits RNA virus, and its action is reversed by the addition of uridine but not by the thymidine. In the study of specific viral inhibitors this reversion technique involving the addition of analogous normal metabolic compounds is essential to the proof of drug-specificity, rather than inhibition caused by drug-toxicity.

Certain protein inhibitors have been useful in the study of viral replication. Cycloheximide, p-fluorophenylalanine, and puromycin inhibit synthesis of viral and cell protein. Consequently, they can interrupt the cycle of viral replication at various stages. Because they also inhibit cell-protein synthesis, these drugs are not viral chemotherapeutic candidates.

Virazole is a synthetic nucleoside which appears to inhibit an early step in viral replication involving the synthesis of viral nucleic acid, either DNA or RNA. As such it has a broad spectrum of possibilities as an antiviral drug. Although not completely free of toxic reactions, it is sufficiently nontoxic to be used by the aerosol or parenteral routes. It has been licensed in several European countries but not in the USA. It is contraindicated during pregnancy.

Disodium phosphoroacetate is a promising, stable, nontoxic antiviral drug that selectively inhibits DNA-dependent DNA polymerase essential to DNA replication. The inhibition appears to be specific for the viral enzyme of several herpesviruses with little effect on cellular DNA synthesis.

HOST RESPONSE

Viruses are completely dependent on the living cell for their survival and replication. The alterations caused by viruses in cells are regulated by the cell-virus relationships. Some viruses produce little or no alteration in the biochemical mechanisms of the cell. This represents the ultimate in parasitism, because the virus and cell perform their physiological functions for survival with no adverse structural effects on each other. Others have a severe effect, resulting in pathological changes.

As a result of their marked dependence on cell functions for replication, many newly developed and refined techniques and procedures are used for the study of the host-virus relationships. With advances in electron-microscope techniques, this methodology permits the study of many ultrastructural features of cell tissue invaded by virus. Immunofluorescence procedures have

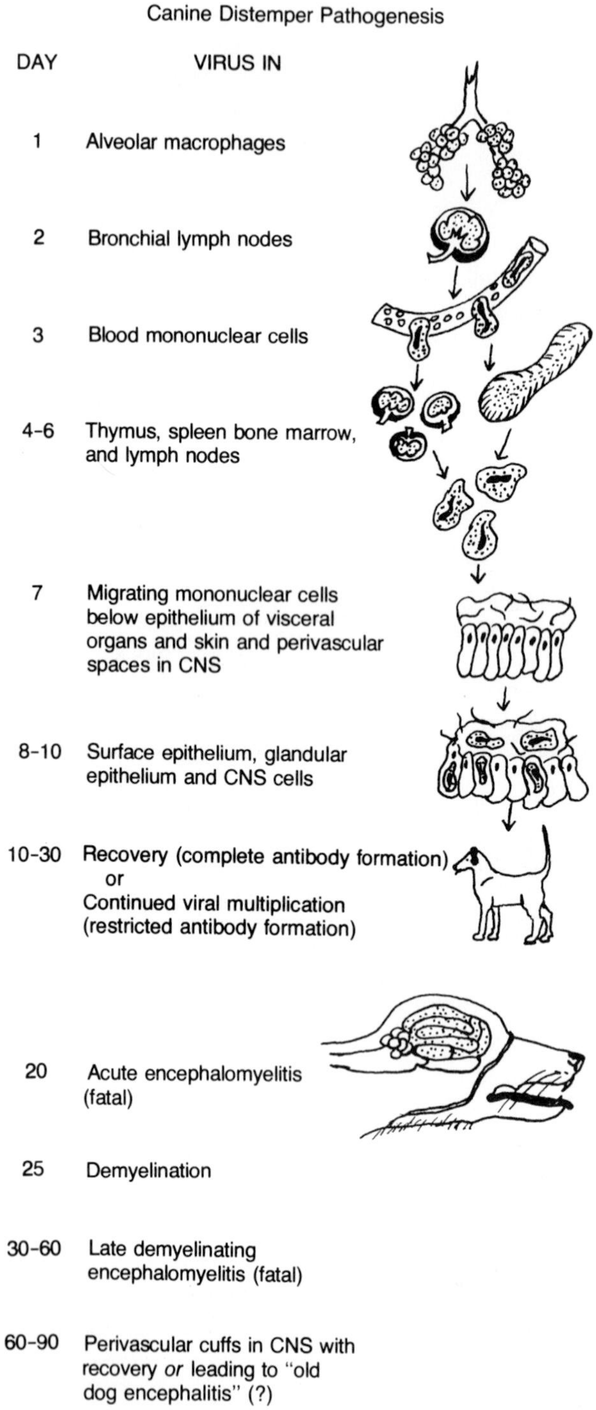

Canine Distemper Pathogenesis

DAY	VIRUS IN
1	Alveolar macrophages
2	Bronchial lymph nodes
3	Blood mononuclear cells
4-6	Thymus, spleen bone marrow, and lymph nodes
7	Migrating mononuclear cells below epithelium of visceral organs and skin and perivascular spaces in CNS
8-10	Surface epithelium, glandular epithelium and CNS cells
10-30	Recovery (complete antibody formation) or Continued viral multiplication (restricted antibody formation)
20	Acute encephalomyelitis (fatal)
25	Demyelination
30-60	Late demyelinating encephalomyelitis (fatal)
60-90	Perivascular cuffs in CNS with recovery *or* leading to "old dog encephalitis" (?)

Figure 36.13. Schematic illustration of canine distemper pathogenesis. (Drawing by Cynthia J. Holmes. Modeled from similar schemata by E. Jawetz, J. L. Melnick, and E. A. Adelberg, with modifications by M. Appel.)

enhanced pathogenesis studies, permitting investigators to study the pattern of viral infections in various hosts and in tissue and organ cultures. Improved tissue-culture methods also are used to excellent advantage in assaying virus for pathogenesis studies. Histochemistry and radioautography also are being used for studies of this nature. Both standard and phase microscopy provide the means for correlating the gross lesions of viral disease with the molecular level processes.

Pathogenesis

The induction of infection by viruses varies markedly depending on the viral tropism, cell susceptibility, the means of transmission, and the site of body contact.

As a rule, the initial site of contact occurs in cells that line the superficial tissues of exposed surfaces of various body systems including the reproductive, digestive, and respiratory tracts and also the skin. In some instances, but not in all, initial replication of a virus will occur in these primary sites of contact and adsorption. In some instances viral replication will be limited to these superficial tissues. After a sufficient concentration of virus has been attained, its spread involves other cells in neighboring tissues. Prime examples of this type would be parainfluenza in dogs and in cattle, and influenza infection in pigs. This localized process also operates in the case of certain viral skin diseases such as molluscum contagiosum and papilloma. Dissemination of some viruses may extend to other remote areas in the body from initial sites through transport in the lymph and blood streams where replication occurs and pathological lesions are formed. Herpes infection in man and animals constitutes a good example of this type of pathogenesis.

In other instances the virus gains entrance into the body through superficial tissues without viral replication and invades the macrophages, leukocytes, and other cellular elements in the blood stream and is then transported to various tissues throughout the body with adsorption and replication of virus occurring in other fixed, susceptible cells. Canine distemper is an excellent example. (Figure 36.13). In neurotropic canine cases of distemper, virus also penetrates the blood-brain barrier with virus antigen appearing first in meningeal macrophages, long after viremia occurs, and then in perivascular cells, ependymal cells, and later in glial and neuronal cells (3).

In the case of arthropod-borne viruses, transmission of the disease is dependent on insect vectors, which inject the virus through a bite. The virus invades the blood stream and replicates in cells of the endothelial lining of lymph and blood vessels.

A variety of mechanisms operate in the successful adsorption of viruses to cells. Proper receptor sites on cell surfaces are essential to viral adsorption. Certain orthomyxoviruses contain a surface enzyme necessary for union with specific receptors at definite loci on the cell surface. Specific receptor sites also are involved in cell-enterovirus union. Phagocytosis of attached virus by the cell occurs at a time when the viral nucleic acid is released from its protein coat, permitting viral nucleic acid to direct the cellular activity essential to its successful replication (described in the section called "Replication of Viruses" in this chapter).

Cells in an animal host at different ages may vary in their susceptibility to viruses producing diverse disease pictures. Infectious bovine rhinotracheitis virus in neonatal calves causes a generalized disease with the most dramatic lesions occurring in the anterior portion of the digestive tract, but with generalized pustular lesions in most body systems. In contrast, lesions in the anterior portion of the digestive tract in older calves or young adults do not occur, and lesions are likely to be confined to one body system (5). Less dramatic differences are observed with experimental foot-and-mouth disease in the avian host, but prominent heart lesions and the highest virus titers in this organ occur in the 14-day-old chicken embryo, whereas lesions and the higher virus titers occur in the gizzard muscle of the 1-day-old chick (15). This demonstrates a remarkable difference in cell susceptibility of the developing avian host to FMDV within a period of 8 days.

The effective transmission of viruses from one host to another is essential in the pathogenesis of any viral disease. This subject is covered in Chaper 37, Epidemiology of Viral Infections.

Pathology

The various routes of viral transport within the body serve as a means to establish infection in these cells for which each virus has an affinity or tropism. The nature of the infection (and disease) is determined by the degree of parasitism, the number and type of cells involved in the viral-host relationship, and the nature of viral replication within the cell.

The intracellular processes leading to degeneration and necrosis manifest themselves in many different pathological changes in cells. Viral infections are usually characterized by vacuolation, ballooning degeneration, syncytium formations, hypertrophy, and hyperplasia. Nucleolar displacement, margination of nuclear chromatin, and the production of cytoplasmic or intranuclear inclusions are changes at the cellular level. The degree, nature, and type of cellular involvement determine the severity and nature of the disease. In some instances no clinical signs or lesions are associated with the infection, while in others severe disease with resulting death ensues. In most viral infections the initial stages of the pathogenesis are clinically inapparent, and in some diseases signs of illness do not occur until late in acute stages of the disease, often when antibodies are first demonstrable.

Inclusion Bodies. In many virus diseases round or oval bodies may be found in the cytoplasm or within the nuclei of affected cells. These have long been known to pathologists as *inclusion bodies*. They are indicative of the presence of virus in the cell. Some are so characteristic in appearance and staining qualities that they are of diagnostic importance. They are not used so often as formerly for diagnosis because better methods are available in most cases. The Negri body, found in certain nerve cells of animals suffering from rabies, is an inclusion body still commonly sought as a means of quick diagnosis of that disease.

Inclusion bodies have not been detected in some virus diseases, and in others their presence is not constant. The majority of inclusion bodies stain with acid dyes. A few are basophilic, and others are basophilic and Feulgen positive in their early stages and acidophilic later. The inclusion bodies of trachoma of man, of psittacosis in man and animals, and of some related diseases of the psittacosis-lymphogranuloma-trachoma group are quite different from those of virus infections. They have been described in Chapter 30.

The eosinophilic cytoplasmic inclusions vary in size in different diseases, and in variant cases of the same disease, up to 20 or more micrometers in diameter. There may be only one, or several, bodies with a single cell. Some of these may be large and others much smaller. Some appear to be quite hyaline, but most are granular, and some contain distinctly stained "inside" bodies.

Two types of intranuclear inclusions may be distinguished. Cowdry (13) refers to them as A- and B-types. The *Type A inclusions* are found in nuclei in which there is evidence of severe disruption of the chromatic structure. The chromatin fragments are crowded around the nuclear membrane (margination). The inclusion body, or bodies, usually lie near the center of the nucleus and appear as amorphous or granular, generally acid-staining material. The affected tissue often shows cells with bodies in different stages of development; that is, fully developed bodies may be seen in some cells and much smaller ones in neighboring cells. The *Type B inclusions* may vary in size, but they are better circumscribed, there is no margination of chromatin, and the nucleus presents a less disorganized appearance than in the other type. Type A bodies are found in such diseases as canine hepatitis, canine distemper, infectious enteritis, and pseudorabies. A good example of the Type B inclusion is the Joest body found in Borna disease.

Some of the earlier workers regarded inclusion bodies as the infective agent; some regarded them in protozoa; others thought them to be aggregates of minute parasites embedded in capsular or other hyaline material. When filtration experiments demonstrated that the viruses of many diseases obviously were much smaller than the inclusion bodies seen in those diseases, there was a tendency to regard them as specific degeneration products of the cell substance. More recently, however, evidence has accumulated that some of the bodies contain aggregates of virus elementary bodies.

Borrel (11) studied the inclusions, known as *Bollinger bodies*, found in pox of fowls. These are rather large structures that occur in the cytoplasm of diseased epithelial cells. Microscopically, minute spherical corpuscles were detected within the larger body, which, when crushed, released smaller bodies. These are now known as *Borrel bodies*. Borrel bodies may be separated from affected tissues by crushing, by tryptic digestion, and by differential centrifugation. After many washings these bodies are capable of inducing fowlpox; that is, they contain virus. Borrel bodies may be specifically agglutinated by the serum of animals that have recovered from the disease or have been immunized against it. They are regarded as the virus particles, or *elementary bodies*. A similar condition can be demonstrated in several other virus diseases.

It has now been established that the intranuclear inclusion bodies may contain virus. It has not been proved that all inclusion bodies are virus carriers. It is possible, of course, that some are specific degenerative structures and others are essentially virus aggregates.

Inflammatory Response. The inflammation that accompanies viral infections is usually secondary to the primary cellular alterations. There is little to distinguish viral infections based on the character of the inflammatory response. Edema is often observed as an early and persistent feature, but the reason for its occurrence is unknown. The early cellular response to most viral infections is mononuclear and lymphocytic.

Polymorphonuclear leukocytes are commonly found in bacterial infections, but the initial and, in many instances, the whole reaction to viruses depends on mononuclear cells, including macrophages, lymphocytes, and plasma cells. Inflammation is found in most viral diseases but not in all of them. In louping ill, Purkinje cells undergo complete necrosis before any infiltration is observed. In rabies, neuronal cells are completely destroyed, and yet there is often no inflammatory response.

When secondary bacterial infection does occur in viral diseases, infiltration of polymorphonuclear leukocytes is presumably a response to cell necrosis and degeneration. The leukocytes predominate in the lesions of infectious bovine rhinotracheitis infection where massive necrosis is observed. Perivascular infiltration with lymphocytes is especially characteristic of various types of viral encephalitis such as the equine encephalomyelides. The lymphocytic pleocytosis in the cerebrospinal fluid usually distinguishes aseptic meningitis from purulent meningitis.

Secondary bacterial infection often complicates viral diseases. This is especially true in viral respiratory and skin diseases, particularly the former. Many potential bacterial pathogens reside on the skin and in the respiratory tract. The initial damage to the superficial cells of these organs by the virus provides the necessary conditions for the rapid invasion and multiplication of the bacterial pathogens, whose influence changes the nature and character of the disease to an acute pyogenic inflammatory infection that is often responsible for the high morbidity and mortality rates encountered in many viral epidemics. This sequence of events is characteristic for most viral respiratory diseases of domestic animals.

Virus infections of cells cause chromosome damage with derangement of the karyotype. Most changes are random in nature. Most frequently breakage, fragmentation, and rearrangement of the chromosomes occur. Abnormal chromosomes and changes in their number also are observed. Cell cultures infected with or transformed to malignancy by certain adenoviruses, such as infectious canine hepatitis virus, exhibit such changes as well as random chromosomal abnormalities in addition to fragmentation. Certain viruses, such as herpes simplex virus in the Chinese hamster cell, cause chromosome breaks that are not random in distribution. Replication of the virus is necessary for induction of the chromosome aberrations. As yet, chromosome alterations cannot assist in the identification of virus-infected or virus-transformed cells.

Constitutional Effects. Each viral infection is recognized by a number of nonspecific constitutional disturbances including fever, myalgias, anorexia, malaise, and headaches. These signs are attributed to a number of factors such as absorption of degradation products from injured cells, viral toxicity, vascular abnormalities producing circulatory disturbances, degree of viremia, and other less specific factors. Usually the mechanism that leads to the production of signs of disease, and certainly death, in viral diseases is unknown. Vascular shock, viral toxicity, and functional faiure of one or more vital organs are believed to account for death.

Immunopathic Viral Diseases

Certain viruses cause chronic diseases. The presently accepted hypothesis holds that the immunologic response of the host to persisting viruses in these diseases causes the formation of circulating virus-antibody complexes which results in cellular alterations with the production of disease. This mechanism apparently exists in lymphocytic choriomeningitis in mice. If adults are rendered immunologically incompetent by immunosuppressive drugs, irradiation, or antiserum produced against the lymphoid elements of the mouse, no illness is produced after inoculation with the virus. The virus replicates and persists until immunocompetence is reestablished, at which time the mouse becomes ill. Infection of newborn mice before they become immunocompetent results in a lifetime viral infection without illness. Age plays a definite role in the persistence of certain viruses. This may be related to the development of immunocompetence. Other notable examples that may have a similar basic mechanism include Aleutian disease of mink and equine infectious anemia. These are characterized by persisting virus and by pathologic alterations of blood vessels and kidneys not unlike those seen in certain connective-tissue disorders of man.

Latent Virus Infections

A few decades ago only a limited number of viruses were believed to persist in the host. Now the vast majority of viruses are known to persist, and this has been determined through new and refined techniques for the detection of incomplete and complete virus. In some viral diseases the agent is transmitted vertically from mother to progeny and horizontal transmission is not necessary—an ideal situation for the perpetuation of the parasite.

Many viral diseases occur as inapparent (or silent) infections in the human or animal populations. Such infections are important in the epidemiology and immunity of a given population. In many instances these inapparent viral infections end with the elimination of the parasite from the host. In others, especially in subclinical infections, this does not occur, but results in the phenomenon known as latent infection. With some diseases such as lymphocytic choriomeningitis in mice and Rous sarcoma infection in chickens, the virus persists, but antibody does not develop, and the animal remains a virus carrier for an indefinite period. In other diseases caused by herpesviruses, adenoviruses, and varicella-zoster virus, virus persists after the initial infection despite the production of antibody. The basic nature of latent infection with these viruses is poorly understood *in vivo*. For example, *Herpesvirus* is known to survive within certain cells of the buccal mucous membranes, lymph nodes, or local sensory ganglia. It is not known if the virus persists as a complete virion or as "occult" virus, or if latent infection is established in all individuals after a primary experience with the virus. It is known that reactivation follows stimulation by a physical, nutritional, or endocrine alteration or during a fever or cold. An interesting observation has been made in a tissue culture system which may explain the pathogenesis of the reactivated latent disease (19). Certain variants of *Herpesvirus* induce the formation of syncytia by which adjacent cells can be invaded by virus through interconnecting cytoplasmic channel ways. By this route virus avoids contact with antibody.

Occult (or masked) virus may account for the long duration of immunity attributed to such diseases as canine distemper, but presently there is no adequate way to detect this type of virus. In the case of certain tumor viruses such as Shope papilloma virus, the course of the infection is long, and eventually the virus becomes occult. The phenomenon of masked virus occurs with other DNA viruses such as polyoma, SV40, and human adenoviruses 12 and 18. With polyoma, the antigenic components for the virus become undetectable, and there is no evidence of virus or viral genome in the transformed cells. It has been postulated that SV40 induced transformed cells carry the viral genome in a noninfec-

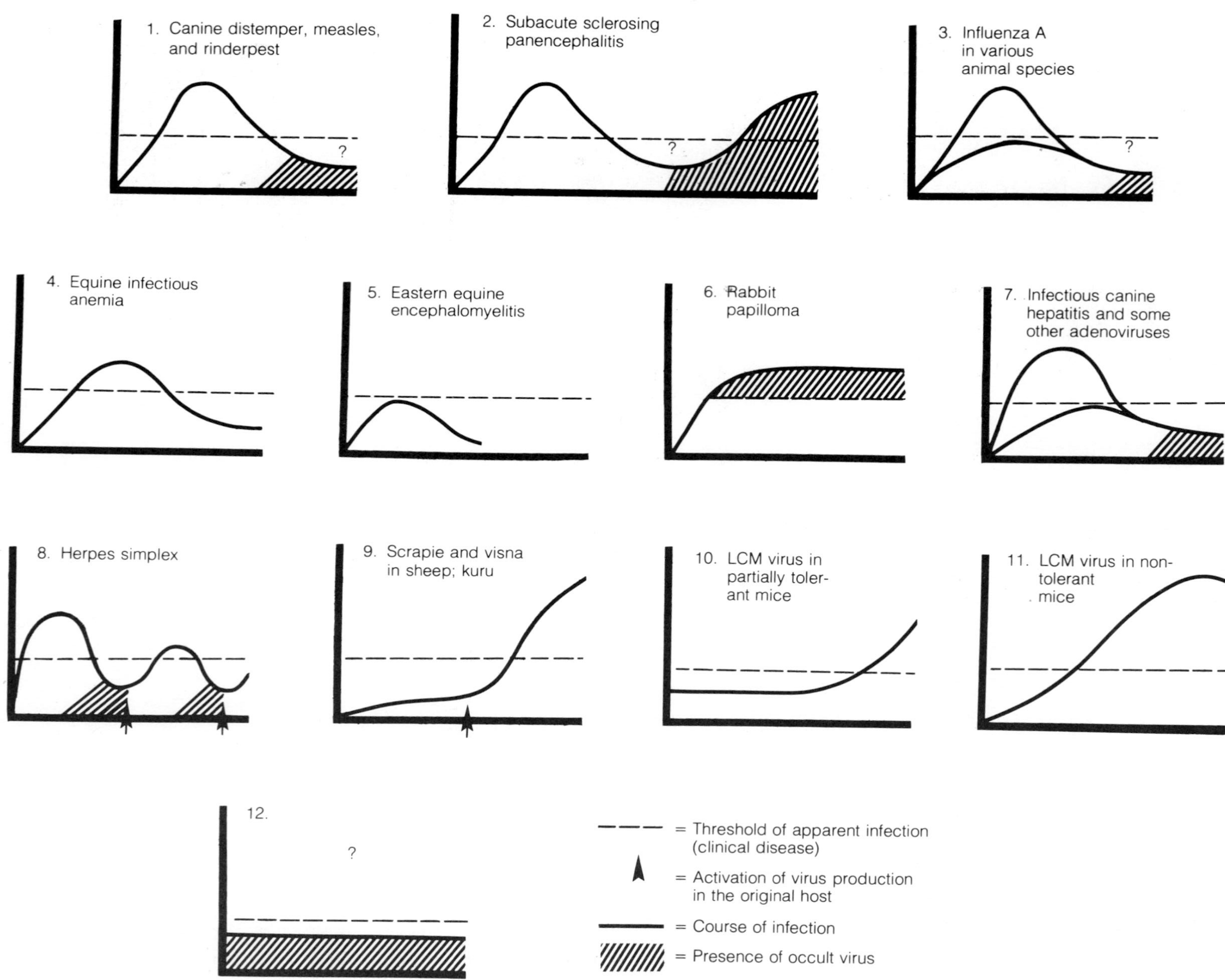

1. Canine distemper, measles, and rinderpest
?
2. Subacute sclerosing panencephalitis
?
3. Influenza A in various animal species
?
4. Equine infectious anemia
5. Eastern equine encephalomyelitis
6. Rabbit papilloma
7. Infectious canine hepatitis and some other adenoviruses
8. Herpes simplex
9. Scrapie and visna in sheep; kuru
10. LCM virus in partially toler- ant mice
11. LCM virus in non- tolerant mice
12.
?
= Threshold of apparent infection (clinical disease)
= Activation of virus production in the original host
= Course of infection
= Presence of occult virus

tious state and on the rare occasions a parasitized cell produces infectious virus. On the other hand, certain RNA tumor viruses such as Rous virus and feline leukemia viruses persist in transformed cells. Defective Rous virus can produce transformed cells in culture. For example, cells may grow in culture for many generations despite replication of a virus. Usually, only a small proportion of the cells is infected with virus. This may be likened to slow virus infections in a natural host that are characterized by a prolonged incubation period lasting months or years during which time the virus replicates with progressive destruction of tissue as occurs in diseases like visna, maedi, Aleutian disease, and equine infectious anemia. In some viral cell-culture systems the cell continues to survive despite viral replication in that cell, thus resembling a moderate virus infection. In these virus-carrier cultures the virus seems to be under some control; perhaps inferferon is responsible in some instances. By various means, the virus can be released in these cultures by cell crowding, lowering the temperature, or medium exhaustion. Although cell cultures have helped to increase our knowledge of viral latency, the results must be viewed with caution as they may apply to the natural host where defense mechanisms are in operation that are lacking in an *in vitro* system.

Figure 36.14 provides various examples of apparent, inapparent, latent, and occult viral infections in graphic form.

Figure 36.14. Apparent, inapparent, latent, and occult virus infections. (1) CD, measles, and rinderpest run an acute, almost clinically apparent course resulting in long-lasting immunity. (2) Measles may also be associated with persistence of latent infection in sclerosing panencephalitis. (3) Influenza A may be more often subclinical than clinical. (4) In equine infectious anemia, recovery from clinical disease may be associated with latent infection in which fully active virus persists in the blood. (5) Some infections are, in a particular species, always subclinical, such as equine encephalomyelitis in some species of birds that act as reservoirs of the virus. (6) In rabbit papilloma, the course of infection is chronic, and chronicity is associated with the virus becoming occult. (7) Infection of animals with certain adenoviruses may be clinical or subclinical. There may be a long latent infection during which virus is present in small quantity in urine after recovery from disease (infectious canine hepatitis). (8) The periodic activation of latent herpes simplex virus, which may recur throughout life in humans, often follows an initial acute episode of stomatitis in childhood. (9) In many instances, infection is wholly latent for long periods of time before disease occurs. Examples of such "slow" virus infections characterized by long incubation periods are scrapie and visna virus in sheep, and kuru in humans. (10) Lymphocytic choriomeningitis (LCM) virus may be established in mice by *in utero* infection. A form of modified immunologic tolerance develops in which only low levels of antibody are produced. This antibody and circulating LCM virus form antigen-antibody complexes that ultimately produce immune complex disease in the partially tolerant host. The presence of LCM virus in this latent infection (circulating virus with little or no apparent disease) may be readily revealed by transmission to an indicator host, e.g., nontolerant adult mice from a virus-free stock. All nontolerant mice develop classic acute symptoms of LCM and die (11). The possibility is shown of latent infection with an occult virus that is not readily activated (12). Proof of the presence of such a virus remains a difficult task which, however, is attracting the attention of cancer investigators. (Modified from E. Jawetz, J. L. Melnick, and E. A. Adelberg, *Review of Medical Microbiology*, 13th ed., Lange Medical Publications, Los Altos, Calif., 1978.)

Natural and Acquired Resistance in Virus Diseases

Natural Resistance. It is quite clear now that mechanisms for resistance to viral infections involve more than the production of circulating antibodies. This became apparent as a result of viral and bacterial resistance studies with hypogammaglobulinemia patients, absence of an antibody response in certain congenital viral infections, and the role of antibodies in the protection of animals against the production of tumors by oncogenic viruses.

Innate susceptibility or resistance are terms commonly used in discussing so-called natural resistance (or susceptibility) of a given species to a particular viral infection. This may also apply to the marked variation in resistance of individuals to a given virus within a species. The mechanisms involved in innate resistance are poorly understood. but they may operate at the level of the cell or organism (host). The route of viral entry also is a factor.

At the cellular level, adsorption of the virus to the cell receptors is the first and perhaps most important factor in cellular resistance or susceptibility. In some instances, such as poliovirus, other human enteroviruses, and phage-resistant strains of *Escherichia coli,* cellular insusceptibility is caused by the failure of adsorption and not the ability of the nucleic acid to replicate in cells. Actually, little is known about intracellular factors affecting the susceptibility of cells to viral infection, but such things as pH, temperature, interferon, and genetics can play a role.

Two known forces operating at the organism level that are generally recognized are the blood-brain barrier and the role of the reticuloendothelial system.

At present, the only effective experimental approach

to the study of the mechanisms of innate resistance to virus infections can be made in "inbred" mouse colonies or perhaps in chicken flocks. These animal lines may differ markedly in their resistance to certain viral diseases. The mechanism of resistance in these "inbred" lines to various viruses may differ. Susceptibility by mouse lines to St. Louis encephalitis and louping ill viruses was correlated with the level of viral multiplication in the mouse brain. The Princeton Rockefeller Institute mice are highly resistant to 17D strain of yellow fever virus, and this observation (30) extended to the other group B arboviruses but not the group A arboviruses. In the intact animal it is sometimes possible to produce resistance by transfer of macrophages from resistant to susceptible animals. Macrophages also play the same role in infectious hepatitis of mice. Unfortunately, this does not seem to be the case with mousepox where macrophages apparently had no influence on the susceptibility of mice to this disease. It is well to note that selective breeding to one viral disease does not insure resistance to others.

Natural selection in a population plays an important role in the history (ecology) of a viral disease. Most diseases as we know them represent such a situation where adjustment of the host and virus occur over a long period of time. An excellent opportunity for the study of innate resistance occurred in Australia two decades ago when virulent myxoma virus was introduced into a previously unexposed, highly susceptible wild rabbit population. Initially the case-mortality rate was 90 percent, but within 7 years fell to 25 percent under standardized conditions.

Other environmental factors known to operate in disease resistance include age, ambient temperature, and a poorly developed thermal regulating mechanism of most species at time of birth. Neonatal animals are often highly susceptible to viruses during the first weeks of life. Consequently, neonatal animals are often used for study of viruses. Certainly, dogs are more susceptible to canine distemper and canine *Herpesvirus* during the first 1 to 2 weeks of life. Fortunately, maternal antibodies are conferred to the progeny counteracting this highly susceptible period. Temperature also may have an effect on the viral multiplication, antibody response, and interferon production of the organism. The aged often are more susceptible to virus infections—for reasons unknown.

Acquired Resistance. Acquired resistance (or immunity) is obtained by contact with the antigens of infectious agents, and specific antibodies to these substances play an important role in the resistance of the host organism. There are two main segments in the immune response, namely, (*a*) the production and effects of humoral antibodies, and (*b*) cell-mediated immunity generated by cells of the reticuloendothelial system.

Immunity in a considerable proportion of all virus diseases is absolute and relatively long-lasting. This is quite different from that which is found in bacterial diseases where immunity is relative and usually short-lived. Such solid and lasting immunities do not occur in all virus diseases; in fact in many, especially those which affect superficial structures such as herpes infections and foot-and-mouth disease, it is solid but not long lasting.

The prolonged solid immunity found in many virus diseases cannot be explained with certainty. When antigens come in contact with tissues, antibodies are produced, and these usually may be recognized by a variety of established methods. If the antigen is contained in a parasitic or pathogenic organism that multiplies and retains its position in the body for a considerable period of time, antibodies will be stimulated as long as the stimulus remains. If it is a nonviable antigen that is quickly eliminated from the body, antibody formation quickly ceases and the blood titer is soon lost. The same thing ordinarily happens when an animal recovers from an infection. How then can continued virus-neutralizing power be maintained, as it is in many virus diseases, long after all evidence of the disease has disappeared?

No definite answer can be given to this question at present. The fact that viruses develop only intracellularly whereas bacteria usually develop in the body fluids may be responsible for the difference. In these cases viruses may find it possible to continue to exist in certain cells of the recovered host as latent or occult virus in spite of the fact that the body fluids contain virus-neutralizing antibodies. Such an individual may have little or no ability to infect others because the neutralizing antibodies bathing the infected cells would prevent the escape of virus into any of the secretions or excretions of the body under most circumstances, but might not prevent the passage of virus through intercellular bridges to other susceptible cells of the same individual. In virus diseases it is at least theoretically possible that many individuals will continue to harbor the virus as long as they live. Such individuals would be expected to show continuous production of antibodies especially if the virus persisted in cells involved in antibody production and maintain a solid immunity to reinfection. This theory is supported by Poppensiek and Baker (28), who showed that virus in the urine and immunity persisted in dogs that recovered from infectious canine hepatitis.

Rivers, Haagen, and Muckenfuss (29) inoculated rabbit cornea with vaccinia virus and then maintained the viability of the corneal cells by submerging them in antivaccinal plasma. They found that corneal lesions developed in spite of the virus-neutralizing antibodies in the plasma. When the vaccinia virus was first mixed with the plasma before the addition of the corneal tissue, the tissue did not become infected. These experiments prove that viruses may develop in cells that are bathed with antiviral substances. Such experiments serve to explain the frequent clinical experiences indicating that viral antisera may be useful as preventive agents but are usually useless in treating already existing disease.

Another interesting possibility was pointed up by the findings of van Bekkum and colleagues (10) with animals that have recovered from foot-and-mouth disease. This is a disease in which immunity is relatively short-lived and in which it has always been believed that virus disappears rather quickly after recovery. The Dutch workers discovered that FMD virus could be recovered from the saliva of a considerable portion of recovered cattle for several months after all evidence of the disease had disappeared even though these animals did not transmit the disease to susceptible cattle which were kept in close contact with them. Convalescing animals apparently continued to produce a small amount of virus for a long period, the amount being too small to cause infection by ordinary contacts.

Passive Immunity. Specific hyperimmune sera are useful against a number of animal virus diseases. When these sera are administered before infection occurs, or perhaps very early in the course of the infection before the virus has been widely disseminated, they are fairly effective. The protection given by such sera usually is complete and solid, but it is of short duration. It is not safe to depend on passive immunity lasting for more than 1 to 2 weeks. Additional doses can be given to prolong this period. Antiserum is often used to protect susceptible animals during critical periods. If the passively immunized animal comes in contact with virus during the period of protection, active immunization often occurs.

In general, it is useless to administer antisera to animals that exhibit well-marked signs of virus infections. The virus, in these cases, has already reached the susceptible cells, where it is beyond the reach of the antibodies.

Hyperimmune antisera are used effectively in combating hog cholera of swine and feline panleukopenia. It may be used in many more virus diseases, but in some either it is impracticable, ineffective, or better methods of protection are known.

In *maternal immunity* the temporary immunity is conferred by the mother to her progeny. This is very important in many virus diseases, as neonatal infections are often fatal. Certainly this is true for many human and animal viruses. In general, there is a quantitative relationship between the serum titer of the dam at birth and the duration of the passive protection for the progeny. For example, the duration of maternal protection for puppies against distemper and infectious canine hepatitis viruses, in general. persists from 4 to 15 weeks. Obviously, dams with the highest serum antibody titers confer protection to their progeny for the longest period of time. Most domestic animals receive the major portion of their maternal antibody through the colostrum; thus it is important for them to nurse well in the first 24 to 48 hours of life. For more information about maternal immunity, see the section on canine distemper under "Pathogenesis" earlier in this chapter.

Active Immunization. The methods of actively immunizing against virus infections fall into four categories: (*a*) the use of fully virulent virus alone, (*b*) the use of virulent virus and antiserum simultaneously, (*c*) the use of vaccines made from attenuated virus, and (*d*) the use of inactivated virus. A list of viral vaccines licensed by the United States Department of Agriculture for animal use in the USA is provided in Tables 36.4 and 36.5.

Fully virulent virus. When fully virulent virus is used, it is introduced by a route different from natural transmission. This is a relatively dangerous method because the virulent material does not always behave in a predictable manner, and at best it is undesirable to spread virulent material to premises where it did not formerly exist. When it is used, *all susceptible stock* on the same premises should be treated; otherwise there is danger of producing an epizootic among the unprotected animals. This method is seldom used now, but it formerly was employed for the control of some animal diseases in the USA including contagious ecthyma of sheep and infectious laryngotracheitis and infectious bronchitis of chickens.

Virus and antiserum stimultaneously. The best-known example of the use of virus and antiserum simultaneously

Table 36.4. Inactivated (killed) virus vaccines* licensed in the United States for immunization of animals in 1979

Disease	For use in	Preparation method
Avian encephalomyelitis	Chickens	Chicken embryo
Bovine rhinotracheitis	Cattle	Cell culture
Parainfluenza 3 infection	Cattle	Cell culture
Bursal (Gumboro) disease	Chickens	Chicken embryo
Eastern, Western, and Venezuelan encephalomyelitis	Horses	Cell culture
Equine influenza	Horses	Chicken embryo or cell culture
Feline panleukopenia	Cats	Cell culture or infected tissue
Feline rhinotracheitis	Cats	Cell culture
Feline calicivirus infection	Cats	Cell culture
Fox encephalitis	Fox	Cell culture
Mink enteritis	Mink	Cell culture
Newcastle disease	Chickens	Chicken embryo
Pseudorabies (Aujeszky's disease)	Swine	Cell culture
Rabies	Dogs and cats	Cell culture or infected tissue
Sendai virus infection	Mice	Chicken embryo
Bovine warts	Cattle	Infected tissue

*There are many licensed veterinary biological products containing more than one immunizing component. Complete directions for use and appropriate cautions are provided on the label for each product.

This table was compiled from information provided by Biologics Licensing and Standards Staff, Veterinary Services, Animal and Plant Health Inspection Service, U.S. Department of Agriculture. (Courtesy D. Long.)

is in hog cholera. In this method of immunization, the antiserum is depended upon to lessen the virus effect so the animal suffers only a mild or inapparent infection.

Attenuated virus. Attenuated viruses for immunization purposes are generally made by adapting them to hosts other than the one on which the vaccine is to be used. In many cases this increases the virulence for the new host but reduces it for others. The first virus vaccine, the rabies vaccine of Pasteur (26), was of this type. This was produced by passing virulent virus through a series of rabbits. Finally when the virus had developed great virulence for the rabbit, it was found that it had lost most of its pathogenicity for other animals and man. This attenuated virus thus could be used to stimulate antibodies that would protect against the more virulent strains. Other examples of such attenuated virus vaccines are the ferret-adapted virus vaccine for canine distemper, the mouse-brain vaccines for yellow fever of man and the horsesickness of Africa, and the vaccines for rinderpest, distemper, and rabies made by cultivating the viruses in fertile hens' eggs. Viruses adapted to rabbits, to hens' eggs, or to tissue-cultured cells are called *lapinized, avianized,* or *tissue cultured* vaccines respectively.

The propagation of viruses in cell cultures from tissues of the same or alien hosts usually results in their attenuation for the natural host by the simple procedure of numerous transfers in cultures. More recently the selection of temperature-sensitive mutants and their repeated transfer through a susceptible cell system at 32 C has resulted in sufficient attenuation to use the altered virus as a safe and efficacious virus vaccine. Another genetic manipulation now being used experimentally to produce attenuated virus is recombination. Cell-cultured attenuated virus vaccines now are used to protect individuals against many diseases, and they are rapidly replacing attenuated virus vaccines produced *in vivo.* Tissue-cultured vaccines are usually simpler and cheaper to produce and also easier to assay for viral content because

Table 36.5. Attenuated virus vaccines* licensed in the United States for immunization of animals in 1979

Disease	For use in	Preparation method
Avian encephalomyelitis	Chickens	Chicken embryo
Bluetongue	Sheep	Cell culture
Bovine rhinotracheitis	Cattle	Cell culture
Parainfluenza 3 infection	Cattle	Cell culture
Virus diarrhea	Cattle	Cell culture
Infectious bronchitis	Chickens	Chicken embryo
Bursal (Gumboro) disease	Chickens	Chicken embryo
Canine adenovirus Type 2 infection	Dogs	Cell culture
Canine hepatitis	Dogs	Cell culture
Canine parainfluenza virus infection	Dogs	Cell culture
Mink distemper	Mink	Cell culture
Canine distemper	Dogs	Cell culture
Duck virus enteritis (plague)	Ducks	Chicken embryo
Duck virus hepatitis Type 1	Ducks	Chicken embryo
Venezuelan equine encephalomyelitis	Horses	Cell culture
Equine rhinopneumonitis	Horses	Cell culture
Feline panleukopenia	Cats	Cell culture
Feline rhinotracheitis	Cats	Cell culture
Feline calicivirus infection	Cats	Cell culture
Fowl laryngotracheitis	Chickens	Chicken embryo or cell culture
Fowlpox	Chickens, turkeys, and pigeons	Chicken embryo or cell culture
Marek's disease	Chickens	Cell culture
Newcastle disease	Chickens	Chicken embryo
Ovine ecthyma	Sheep	Cell culture or infected tissue
Pseudorabies (Aujeszky's disease)	Swine	Cell culture
Rabies	Dogs, cats, horses, cattle, sheep, and goats	Cell culture or chicken embryo
Bovine rotavirus infection	Cattle	Cell culture
Bovine coronavirus infection	Cattle	Cell culture
Tenosynovitis (viral arthritis)	Chickens	Chicken embryo
Transmissible gastroenteritis	Swine	Cell culture

*There are many licensed veterinary biological products containing more than one immunizing component. Complete directions for use and appropriate cautions are provided on the label for each product.

This table was compiled from information provided by Biologics Licensing and Standards Staff, Veterinary Services, Animal and Plant Health Inspection Service, U.S. Department of Agriculture. (Courtesy D. Long.)

most viruses cause a cytopathogenic effect in cell cultures or provide some other indicator of their viral concentration. They are only approved after the produce is determined to be safe and efficacious.

The major concern in the production of attenuated virus vaccines *in vivo* and *in vitro* is the problem of latent viruses and *Mycoplasma* contamination. The latter seems to be easier to detect, but it is quite difficult to control. Latent viruses in both systems confront our medical professions with major problems. There is a slow but gradual shift from primary or secondary cell cultures to the use of diploid- or stable-line cell cultures for the production of veterinary and human viral vaccines. These lines are carefully monitored for all known viruses, particularly the respective hosts from which the cell cultures were derived, and also for *Mycoplasma*. In addition, critical cytological studies including karyography, possible reversion to virulence, and oncogenic capabilities are made before approval is given for the production of viral vaccines in these cell lines.

The duration of the immunity conferred by vaccines containing active virus depends on the pecularities of the virus itself. When the natural disease confers a solid and permanent immunity, attenuated virus vaccines generally will do the same.

Inactivated virus. The word "inactivation" is used in viral terminology to avoid the use of the word "killed," which is commonly used in bacteriology. The implications with respect to life are thus avoided. Viruses may be inactivated with heat, chemicals, ultraviolet rays, ultrasonic vibration, and other processes that commonly destroy life in higher forms. Care must be exercised to be certain that complete inactivation results (14).

There are those who do not believe that fully inactivated virus vaccines can induce useful immunity in animals. These people have felt, and more recent knowledge of the nature of viruses lends plausibility to their beliefs, that the so-called inactivated viruses generally contain some active elements. It is possible that inactivation may prove to be a reversible phenomenon, that inactivated agents may be reactivated in some degree by contact with susceptible cells. It has been conclusively demonstrated many times that so-called inactivated viruses really have contained a very small fraction of active virus, a portion which has much greater resistance to the inactivating agent than most of the virus particles (4, 14).

Today most virologists accept the concept that it is possible to induce serviceable immunity with wholly inactivated viruses. To be effective such vaccines must contain relatively large amounts of virus protein, because there can be no increase of protein in the body such as occurs when active virus is used. It is often difficult to produce vaccines with sufficient protein to provide satisfactory antigenic stimulus, and it is believed that this has been the reason for many failures. Moreover, inactivated virus cannot supply continuing stimulation; hence the induced immunity may be initially solid but cannot last, unless repeated immunizations are made leading to two concerns: (*a*) reaching the patients a sufficient number of times and (*b*) possible hypersensitivity reaction to repeated administration of foreign proteins. Further, it is known that some inactivated virus vaccines have induced hypersensitivity to subsequent infection. The inactivated virus vaccines for eastern and western equine encephalomyelitis and for feline panleukopenia are examples of excellent biologics.

Replication of foot-and-mouth disease virus produces an enzyme (VIA) detectable in the agar-gel diffusion test (12). Sera from animals given inactivated FMD virus fail to show this enzyme antibody. It is possible that this phenomenon may be used to test other inactivated virus vaccines for infectious virions.

Other Procedures for Improving Vaccines and Their Use. Manufacturers are using chemical and physical means such as zonal centrifugation to eliminate nonviral proteins in an effort to reduce adverse reactions. There also is great activity by virologists to produce subunit vaccines that include only those fractions necessary to stimulate antibody production essential to protection. These viral surface components, usually protein in nature, are not infectious or involved in the coding mechanism of the virion. As a consequence they are completely safe and promise to be the vaccines of the future.

More attention is being paid to the type of immunoglobulins involved in protection and their location in the body to make the best use of a biological product for host protection. For example, it may make more sense to administer a vaccine by the aerosol route to protect against respiratory viral diseases; by the oral route for enteric diseases. In essence, we are making use of our knowledge of immunology and pathogenesis to enhance the effectiveness of a biological product.

Cross Immunity in Viral Infections

It has been pointed out that antigenicity is a property of the protein fraction of the virus moiety, the innocuous portion which serves to protect the nucleic acid.

As known for a long time with bacteria, there are antigenic relationships and similarities among viruses. These do not necessarily mean that common pathogenic factors exist, or that the agents are biologically related. The literature contains a number of examples. One of the most intriguing of these is the relationship that exists between measles in man, distemper in dogs, and rinderpest in cattle (1, 27). The protection conferred by measles virus in dogs against virulent distemper virus is based on the anamnestic response (16). The protection conferred by bovine virus diarrhea virus in pigs against virulent hog cholera virus is based upon a similar phenomenon (33).

Viral Resistance

In general, viruses seem to possess about the same degree of resistance to heat, drying, and many chemical agents as the vegetative forms of most bacteria. Moist heat at 55 to 60 C for 30 minutes serves all practical purposes of disinfection; yet is has been shown that a very small residuum of active FMD virus remains after exposure at these temperatures for several times as long. This same situation exists for some other viruses. Drying is destructive to most viruses; yet there are some that survive very long periods of ordinary drying. Freeze drying, or lyophilization, is one of the best methods of preserving viruses for long periods of time. Another method is the storage of viruses at −60 C or lower.

To chemical disinfectants, viruses respond in the same way as vegetative forms of bacteria, but there are important differences. Most viruses are wholly unaffected by concentrations of most antibiotics that will inhibit and destroy bacteria. In most tissue culture work it is standard practice to incorporate such substances as penicillin, streptomycin, or mycostatin in the culture media to restrain the growth of bacteria and molds and allow unrestricted growth of viruses.

Viruses, it should be remembered, are usually present in necrotic tissue fragments and mixed with coagulable proteins that may serve as effective protective coatings, delaying access of chemicals to the active agents. Because strongly alkaline solutions are effective tissue solvents, it has been believed that they were particularly effective agents in chemical disinfection. Two percent lye solution has been used for many years in disinfection following outbreaks of FMD, apparently with complete success. Recently it has been found in laboratory experiments that this solution is not very effective with this virus, and with the virus of vesicular stomatitis. It is probable that the virtue of the lye has resided not so much in its virucidal properties as in its solvent and detergent properties, because these have resulted in exposing the virus particles, diluting them, and removing them from the environment. (See the section on chemical inactivants earlier in this chapter.)

Most viruses are well preserved in strong solutions of glycerol (50 to 100 percent). Such concentrations cause dehydration of the cells containing virus and tend to prevent their autolysis.

REFERENCES

1. Adams and Imagawa. Proc. Soc. Exp. Biol. and Med., 1957, *96,* 240.
2. Anderson, Hopps, Barile, and Bernheim. Jour. Bact., 1965, *60,* 1387.
3. Appel. M. J. G. Am. Jour. Vet. Res., 1969, *30,* 1167.
4. Bachrach, Breese, Callis, Hess, and Patty. Proc. Soc. Exp. Biol. and Med., 1957, *95,* 147.
5. Baker, McEntee, and Gillespie. Cornell Vet., 1960, *50,* 156.
6. Bauer and Hughes. Jour. Gen. Physiol., 1934–35, *18,* 143.
7. Bauer and Pickels. Jour. Exp. Med., 1936, *64,* 503.
8. Bechhold. Zeitschr. phys. Chem., 1907, *60,* 257.
9. Beijerinck. Zentrbl. f. Bakt., II, Abt., 1899, *5,* 27.
10. Van Bekkum, Frenkel, Fredericks, and Frenkel. Tijdschr. Diergeneeskd., 1959, *84,* 1159.
11. Borrel. Comp. rend Soc. Biol. (Paris), 1904, *57,* 642.
12. Cowan and Graves. Virol. 1966, *30,* 528.
13. Cowdry. Arch. Path., 1934, *18,* 527.
14. Elford. Jour. Path. and Bact., 1931, *34,* 505.
15. Gillespie, Cornell Vet., 1955, *45,* 170.
16. Gillespie and Karzon. Proc. Soc. Exp. Biol. and Med., 1961, *105,* 547.
17. D'Herelle. The bacteriophage: Its role in immunity. Eng. trans., Williams and Wilkins Co., Baltimore, 1922.
18. Hirst. Science, 1941, *94,* 22.
19. Hoggan, Roizman, and Roane. Am. Jour. Hyg., 1961, *173,* 114.
20. Huang. Ann. Rev. Microbiol., 1973, *27,* 101.
21. Isaacs and Lindenmann. Proc. Roy. Soc., 1957, *147,* 258.
22. Iwanowski. Bull. Acad. Imp. Science, St. Petersburg, 3rd ser., 1892–94, *35,* 67.
23. Loeffler and Frosch. Zentrbl. f. Bakt., I Abt., 1898, *23,* 371.
24. Lwoff and Tournier. Ann. Rev. Microbiol., 1966, *20.* 45.
25. McClelland and Hare. Can. Pub. Health Jour., 1941, *32,* 530.
26. Pasteur. Comp. rend. Acad. Sci., 1885. *101,* 765.
27. Polding, Simpson, and Scott. Vet. Rec., 1959, *71,* 643.
28. Poppensiek and Baker. Proc. Soc. Exp. Biol. and Med., 1951, *77,* 279.
29. Rivers, Haagen, and Muckenfuss. Jour. Exp. Med., 1929, *50,* 673.

30. Sabin. Proc. Natl. Acad. Sci., 1952, *38*, 540.
31. Sanarelli. Zentrbl. f. Bakt., I Abt., 1898, *23*, 865.
32. Scott. Proc. Am. An. Hosp. Assoc., 1979, *46*, 105.
33. Sheffy, Coggins, and Baker. Proc. Soc. Exp. Biol. and Med., 1962, *109*, 349.
34. Stanley. Science, 1935, *81*, 644.
35. Syverton and Berry. Jour. Exp. Med., 1947, *86*, 145.
36. Vilches and Hirst. Jour. Immunol., 1947, *57*, 125.
37. Williams and Wyckoff. Science, 1945, *101*, 594.

37 Epidemiology of Viral Infections

The epidemiology of viral diseases is an exceedingly fascinating area of microbiology because of the unique biochemical, biophysical, and biological characteristics of viruses. With their highly parasitic nature and small size, certain problems arise that make the viruses more difficult to recognize in nature than other microorganisms. With the advent of modern tissue-culture techniques, as well as improved methods of purification, concentration, and visualization, the detection of viruses in our environment is more easily accomplished now than two decades ago. Our increased knowledge of the host spectrum of viruses has also aided in their detection as we still rely heavily on the effects that viruses produce in various animal species for their recognition. Thus, our knowledge of the epidemiology and ecology of viral diseases has grown at a rate commensurate with our technological advancements in animal virology. Consequently, it is obvious that a meaningful program in viral epidemiology requires competent laboratory support utilizing various viral isolation and serological procedures.

According to Shope (9) periodicity and seasonal prevalence are two characteristic features of most viral diseases, but these are incompletely understood. The terms "distemper years," "hog cholera years," "foot-and-mouth disease years," and so on, are expressions used for our recognition of the periodicity of viral diseases. These years of significant disease caused by various animal viruses are explained on the basis of increased virulence or invasiveness of the virus or on the fluctuating ratio of immune and susceptible animals in a population. Thus, the virus and the host both play a major role in the periodicity of disease. Certain viral diseases do have a seasonal prevalence, such as canine distemper, which occurs more frequently in the fall and winter. Where arthropod vectors are involved in disease transmission, such as the arboviruses, the disease occurs during the summer season in temperate zones.

For many years epidemiologists limited their studies of an outbreak from the time it appeared as a disease in a single host species until it disappeared from that population, treating each experience as an episode. More recently, epidemiologists have broadened their interests by concerning themselves with the ecology and natural history of viral disease(s), seeking more information about the location and survival of the virus during the interepidemic phase. The epidemiology of animal viral diseases, generally speaking, is less complex and less difficult to study than human viral diseases. Farm and pet animals usually are confined to limited areas of travel, and contact with large numbers of animals from outside sources is the exception rather than the rule. Our greatest disease problems in veterinary medicine are usually associated with the movement of animals from one location to another where assembly of animals from many sources occurs. Even wild animals, except certain species of birds and bats, tend to reside within a limited geographic area; thus exposure to various disease agents is restricted. This situation does produce a more susceptible population which leads to more explosive outbreaks when an agent is introduced into a virgin population. For example, rather severe outbreaks of canine distemper with a high morbidity and mortality rate in dogs of all ages have been reported in isolated arctic communities. Obviously, it is simpler to study the natural history of disease under these circumstances than a population in various stages of immunity; thus, animal models are often applied to enhance one's knowledge of the epidemiology of certain human viral diseases. There are many notable examples, but the earliest and perhaps in many ways the most important was the finding, by Smith and Kilbourne (11), of the arthropod transmission of Texas fever in cattle. Of course, many viruses produce infection and disease in animals and man under natural conditions, and these particular infections are of great interest to human and veterinary medicine.

Persistence of Virus in Nature

In an account of viral persistence in nature two major factors are taken into consideration: (*a*) the biophysical and biochemical characteristics of a virus that permit it to retain its infectious nature in the environment outside of its natural host(s), and (*b*) its biological characteristics that facilitate persistence in one or more hosts for varying periods of time. If failure occurs on both counts, the virus passes into oblivion.

Most viruses cannot withstand severe environmental conditions. The majority are destroyed in a strong alkali or acid solution, or even in strong salt solutions. In the presence of fat solvents, viruses with a lipid coat are quickly inactivated. High temperatures for relatively short periods of time destroy viral infectivity. Certain viruses are quickly inactivated in direct sunlight. On the other hand many viruses in well-buffered media or in tissue are maintained for long periods of time at exceedingly low temperatures (−60 C and lower) and also in a dried state at regular refrigeration temperature for a long time. In a study of viral ecology it is well to know the biophysical and biochemical characteristics in an assessment of their ability to survive in an environment outside of the body of their natural host(s). It soon becomes apparent that the chances for viral survival outside of the host(s) in most instances are rather meager.

The successful spread and the perpetration of virus in the host are the principal mechanisms by which a viral species is maintained in nature. There exist several known epidemiological models which explain the successful spread and maintenance of certain viral diseases. These models will be considered in some depth in subsequent sections of this chapter.

According to Shope (9) the epidemiology of clinically apparent viral illnesses may be classified as intermittent and nonintermittent. The intermittent diseases have no good evidence for the existence of a continuous chain of animal-to-animal infection either by contact or by a vector or intermediate host. The nonintermittent viral diseases apparently are maintained by contact infections either as clinical or subclinical infections. In addition, indigenous viral infections occur in nature and serve as a source of disease in more susceptible hosts. As our knowledge of animal viral diseases has improved, it has become apparent that viruses can readily exist in the host as persisting or occult virus, or even as a virogene, representing a potential source of virus in nature, not necessarily requiring a broad host spectrum to enhance its perpetuity.

Direct Species-to-Species Transmission

The infections transferred by direct contact from an animal of one species to another animal of the same species are usually spread by salivary contamination, aerosal, or fecal contamination. Examples of this type of situation in the animal kingdom are not uncommon—the most notable examples are vesicular exanthema, transmissible gastroenteritis, and hog cholera in swine; virus diarrhea-mucosal disease (VD-MD) of cattle; avian bronchitis of chickens; and murine hepatitis. We know little about these diseases in our wildlife, but in reality some viruses, such as VD-MD in deer, likely appear in very closely related species and are not limited to a single animal species. Subclinical infections often play an important role in maintaining the chain of infection.

Most of the diseases in this epidemiological group have a long-lasting immunity. Earlier, it was believed that these viruses did not persist, but it is known now that some of them do remain under certain conditions serving as probable links in any subsequent chain of infection.

Virus Transmission by Virus Carriers

A large number of animal virus infections are transmitted by virus carriers. After initial infection of an individual, the virus persists in a superficial tissue of the body that readily permits elimination of the agent in various body excretions. This includes viruses in various families such as Adenoviridae, Herpesviridae, Picornaviridae, and Poxviridae to mention a few. The virus carriers are a source of potential infection to all susceptible species.

Some of the diseases in this group such as herpes simplex of man are characterized by clinical relapses that usually occur after some stress such as another infection. The coexistence of immunity and infection are in delicate balance in these persisting viral infections. In an interesting experiment Good and Campbell (3) precipitated latent herpes simplex encephalitis in rabbits by anaphylactic shock, a severe form of stress.

Arthropod-Borne Virus Transmission

Four principal cycles are involved in the transmission of the arboviruses: (*a*) arthropod to man (urban yellow fever is an example); (*b*) arthropod-lower vertebrate cycle with tangential infection of man (Examples are jungle yellow fever and equine encephalomyelitis); (*c*) arthropod cycle with occasional infection of lower vertebrates and man (an example is Colorado tick fever); and (*d*) lower vertebrate-arthropod (African horsesickness is a prime example—another probable one is turkey meningoencephalitis, although essential insect transmission has not been completely proved).

In the arthropod-anthropod transmission the virus may be transmitted from the adult arthropod to its offspring by transovarian passage not involving a vertebrate host in its successful transmission. Often the virus produces little or no disease in the arthropod host, and the agent persists in an infective form in the insect host which serves for its complete life-span as the reservoir for the infection. In contrast, the arboviruses produce a severe disease of short duration in most vertebrate hosts. The disease terminates quickly in survival or death. Survival results in the formation of an excellent immunity that persists for a long period of time. In some arbovirus infections the presence of the virus in the vertebrate is temporary and short, and it therefore plays a minor role in perpetrating the agent in nature.

Transmission of Viral Diseases by Accidental Bite Infection

There are two well-known viral diseases transmitted by a bite. Rabies is a disease of considerable historical importance. This virus has a broad host spectrum, and the main means of transmission is a bite by an infected carnivorous animal or by an infected bat. Its epidemiology will be discussed at length in the section on rabies in Chapter 51. Another disease is monkey B-virus infection in man, caused by a bite from an infected monkey that shows no evidence of illness. The clinically apparent disease in man occurs as encephalitis and is often fatal.

Certain diseases can readily be produced by the accidental infection of a viral contaminant or by blood transfusion from viral carriers to susceptible individuals. These diseases are obviously produced by man, and some simple procedures can correct some of these situations by observation of sterile techniques in the vaccination of animals and by strict control in the production and testing of biologics. When fresh animal tissues (including blood) are used in therapy, certain hazards such as the occurrence of persisting microbes must be weighed in their usage. Certain blood protozoan agents and equine infectious anemia virus are readily transmitted by these means.

Indigenous Viral Infections

Some notable examples include lymphocytic choriomeningitis in mice, viral encephalitides in birds and rodents, bovine malignant catarrhal fever, and East African swine fever. In these situations healthy carriers exist in a given species that have never shown disease and yet serve as the means of perpetuating and transmitting the viruses that they may carry. Indigenous viral infections have three main features, namely, (*a*) inapparent infection, (*b*) persisting virus, and (*c*) infection at an early age.

Immunological tolerance may be an important characteristic of lymphocytic choriomeningitis, an indigenous infection in mice. In this infection, mice are infected *in utero* and as sucklings from their clinically well mothers. Through the excreta of the latently infected mouse, humans may contract clinical disease. Indigenous viral encephalitis infections in birds and in rodents may play important roles in the epidemiology of these important viruses in which frank disease develops in other hosts, such as the horse and man, through the medium of the arthropod that has contact with indigenous viral hosts.

In bovine malignant catarrhal fever, cattle are the disease (indicator) host of a virus carried as a silent infection in the wildebeests and possibly by sheep. African swine-fever virus is an indigenous viral infection in the wart hog. In contrast, it is a highly acute and fatal disease in domestic swine as a rule.

Parasite Reservoir Hosts for Viral Diseases

There are three animal diseases in whose epidemiology a worm may play a role. Swine influenza and hog cholera are virus diseases of swine, and salmon poisoning of dogs is caused by a rickettsial agent. There are no known human viral or rickettsial agent counterparts.

The causative agent of salmon poisoning in dogs is carried by the trematode, *Troglotrema salmincola*. The complete life cycle of this fatal disease of dogs has been established by Simms, McCapes, and Muth (10) and Cordy and Gorham (2). The details of the cycle are given in the chapter on rickettsiae.

Shope's studies with influenza and hog cholera viruses incriminated the swine lungworm and its intermediate host, the common earthworm (9). The transmission of these viruses is complicated by the occult (masked) form that the virus assumes in lungworm intermediate host, and once within the swine, the virus must be provoked to the infective state by a stress induced in the infected swine. In nature stress is associated with the onset of cold and wet weather.

The Case for the Virogene and the Oncogene

Lysogeny (prophage) is a state in bacteriophage replication known for a long period of time. Bacteria in the prophage stage may lose the prophage for reasons presently unknown, retain that state, or develop from prophage to vegetative form with phage maturation and eventual lysis. It is believed that there is a comparable prophage stage for animal viruses which has been called by Luria (7) "parasitism at the genetic level." Shope (9) has called it "masked" virus, while the terms "occult" or "virogene" have also been suggested. This viral stage is most difficult to prove, especially when it cannot be reactivated into an infective form. There are a number of viruses capable of causing tumors in animals in which the agent presumably becomes integrated into the genetic apparatus of the parasitized cell. Although the virus may lose its infectivity under these circumstances, it retains the capacity to elicit the formation of specific antiviral antibodies. The first notable example of this phenomenon involved the Shope papilloma rabbit virus. In cottontail rabbits that are naturally infected with this virus, active virus could usually be demonstrated in the papillomas. In contrast, no infective virus could be demonstrated in the papillomas induced by the cottontail virus in domestic rabbits. Viral antigen was demonstrated in these noninfective domestic rabbit papillomas (8) and also in the carcinomas arising from them (6). This noninfectious antigenic virus was called "masked virus" by Shope. Other oncogenic DNA viruses such as the polyoma and certain adenoviruses behave in a similar manner. Infective virus often is not demonstrable in polyoma-induced tumors in hamsters (4). Similarly, Huebner *et al.* (5) failed to isolate infective virus from tumors in hamsters induced by adenovirus types 12 and 18 or in rats by adenovirus 12, although antigens that produce antibodies capable of reacting with type-specific viral antigens of a given serotype were demonstrated in the tumor mass. The studies of Black *et al.* (1) with simian virus (SV40), hamster tumors, or with cells transformed in culture gave similar results, causing the investigators to conclude that the noninfective antigen is synthesized by information from the SV40 viral genome integrated in the tumor and *in vitro*-transformed cells. Thus, we have four examples of DNA oncogenic viruses that are usually free of infective virus in the tumor tissue but contain viral antigen(s).

The Epidemiology of Tumor Viruses

There are a number of viral-induced tumors in mammals and birds. Many of these tumors are similar in structure to certain tumors in man. Although no virus has been proved to cause a tumor in man, certain human tumors may eventually be found to be viral-induced.

In general, our limited knowledge of viral-induced tumors suggests that these diseases sometimes are vertically transmitted, thus limiting the means by which they may ultimately be controlled from an epidemiological standpoint. The principal method would appear to be the use of drug therapy aimed at the replication of specific viral enzymes.

The Bittner mouse virus that causes mammary carcinoma is an interesting epidemiological model. Virus is present in the milk and other tissues of certain strains of mice. The virus is transmitted to the offspring through the milk at nursing. The agent may remain dormant for the lifetime of the infected mouse without manifesting itself as a disease, but may readily be transmitted to its offspring. In most instances, the infected adults develop mammary carcinoma at a certain stage of hormonal function and subsequently die.

Certain tumor viruses such as the murine leukemia,

avian leukemia, and feline leukemia viruses may be transmitted directly from the dam to the progeny *in utero*. Much must be done to determine the precise pathogenesis. There has been speculation that the virus is transferred in the germ cell of the female and perhaps even in the male germ cell. These viruses may persist within the cells for the lifetime of an individual without disease manifestation. Why some individuals harboring the agent develop leukemia and/or sarcomas and others do not is unknown. This close association of the virus with the genetic apparatus of the cell and its ability to persist for long periods of time assures the viral parasite of perpetuation as long as its natural hosts do not become extinct.

Certain superficial surface tumors such as rabbit fibroma and papillomas of rabbits and some domestic animals can be transmitted surgically and presumably by certain insects as well. For example, there is definite field evidence that the rabbit fibroma is transmitted in nature by a flying biting insect (9). The rabbit papilloma also appears to be insect transmitted in cottontail rabbits.

The epidemiological study of animal tumors has been rather limited. There is considerable interest now in these diseases, particularly those for which good viral assay and serological methods exist. Until the etiology of human tumors is determined, the measure of success in epidemiology in this area will be rather limited. Consequently most of our basic knowledge of tumor epidemiology will be developed with animal tumor models of known viral etiology.

The Epidemiology of Chronic and Degenerative Diseases

This includes a group of diseases caused by agents called slow viruses. The incubation period of the disease manifestation is as a rule extremely long in the natural host, and virus can be isolated from the tissues of these infected animals for long periods of time. There is strong evidence that some of these diseases are autoimmune conditions with lesions resulting from the combined action of antigen, antibody, and complement.

Little is known about the transmission of these diseases. Is vertical or horizontal transmission the main mechanism for its spread from one individual to another? Are vectors required for their transmission? Do they have a narrow or broad host spectrum? How long do these disease agents persist in the host? These are some of the questions still unanswered about the nature of these diseases which are essential to an understanding of their ecology.

Eradication of Viral Diseases

In veterinary medicine slaughter has been the principal method used to eradicate certain viral diseases. Foot-and-mouth disease is the prime example, and success has been achieved in certain countries where the infection was limited to a single country bordered by others free of the disease or by navigable waters. It is quite remarkable that this success has been achieved in many instances by slaughtering the afflicted ruminant species and pigs in infected herds with no particular effort pursued in the direction of other domesticated animals or wildlife species that are susceptible to some degree to FMD virus. In Great Britain, where the disease has occurred frequently in the past, the reinfection of the population usually has been traced to the introduction of the virus in an animal product from a country where the disease is epizootic. Yet the virus does persist in recovered animals, in animals given attenuated virus vaccine, or in animals vaccinated with inactivated virus vaccine and subsequently exposed to infective virus. Consequently the slaughter method seems the only reasonable approach to eradication with this virus disease. Where latency and vertical transmission are features of a viral disease, the slaughter method is probably the only means by which it can be eradicated.

Hog cholera has been eradicated from Canada by the slaughter method. A similar effort achieved this goal in the USA. This disease affects only domestic and wild pigs with no positive proof that the virus affects other hosts naturally, so it was reasonable on the basis of the Canadian experience to expect that the USA program also be successful. This proved to be the case despite the complex pig-industry system, which involves frequent and rapid movement of hogs over long distances. The latency of the virus presents a problem that is overcome by the slaughter technique. Inactivated virus vaccine is not a very good biologic and has never completely controlled the disease. Attenuated virus vaccine helped to control the disease, but led to latency and chronicity in certain animals, so this procedure was terminated as a method of eradication. Vaccination was helpful in preventing and controlling the disease, but not in its eradication.

In certain arbovirus diseases, insects are true biological vectors and are essential to disease perpetuation in man and animals. If these vectors are removed from the environment where susceptible animals or humans reside, the disease is eliminated. Of course the eradication of insects also poses a formidable task that it is not usually feasible or practical to execute.

The elimination of viral disease from a country by vaccination has not been too successful. The notable exception is rinderpest of cattle. Inactivated virus vaccines generally provide insufficient immunity to prevent the replication of virus in a vaccinated animal even though disease may not occur. Attenuated virus vaccines provide greater immunity and usually prevent the residence of virulent (street) virus in the animal, but often the attenuated virus may be transmitted to susceptible animals. After repeated transfer of attenuated vaccine virus in nature it may revert to virulence with the production of acute or chronic disease depending on its nature. With properly attenuated rinderpest vaccines the virus does not produce disease or transmit to susceptible hosts and constitutes a blind-ended infection in the vaccinated animal. This is an ideal vaccine, which leads to disease eradication when a large percentage of the population are vaccinated in a unified, country-wide campaign. Theoretically, this should be possible to accomplish with canine distemper in dogs because excellent biologics that do not spread the disease also are available. It would require a well-organized nationwide campaign to eliminate a virulent agent that spreads as readily in a susceptible population as does the distemper virus. This may not be a desirable situation unless very strict quarantine and vaccination procedures were enforced. At best it would be difficult to control in pets while international travel is so common and there is a close companionship between man and dog.

REFERENCES

1. Black, Rowe, Turner, and Huebner. Proc. Natl. Acad. Sci., 1963, *50,* 1148.
2. Cordy and Gorham. Am. Jour. Path., 1950, *26,* 617.
3. Good and Campbell. Proc. Soc. Exp. Biol. and Med., 1948, *68,* 82.
4. Habel and Atanasiu. Proc. Soc. Exp. Biol. and Med., 1959, *102,* 99.
5. Huebner, Rowe, Turner, and Lane. Proc. Natl. Acad. Sci., 1963, *50,* 379.
6. Kidd, Beard, and Rous. Jour. Exp. Med., 1936, *64,* 76.
7. Luria. Science, 1950, *111,* 507.
8. Shope. Jour. Exp. Med., 1937, *65,* 219.
9. Shope. *In* Viral and rickettsial infections of man, 4th ed., ed. Frank L. Horsfall and Igor Tamm. J. P. Lippincott, Philadelphia, 1965, pp. 385–404.
10. Simms, McCapes, and Muth. Jour. Am. Vet. Med. Assoc., 1932, *81,* 26.
11. Smith and Kilbourne. Investigation into the nature, causation, and prevention of Texas or southern cattle fever. Bull. 1, B.A.I., USDA, Govt. Printing Office, Washington, D.C., 1893.

38 Laboratory Diagnosis of Viral Infections

Ideally, disease is diagnosed at the clinical level, using anamnesis, physical examination, and the signs of illness of a single patient or herd for this purpose. The veterinarian, especially the small-animal practitioner, often resorts to fluoroscopic x-ray, surgical, and other specialized procedures to facilitate a proper diagnosis. Most cases can be adequately diagnosed in this manner. With the availability of more specialized equipment and increased knowledge, more veterinary practitioners are requiring laboratory examinations involving such disciplines as pathology, microbiology, physiology, and biochemistry. Many laboratory procedures today are simple, rapid, accurate, and inexpensive to conduct, and constitute ideal diagnostic tests. A small laboratory for such tests is maintained and operated in conjunction with many veterinary practices. An occasional case demands more sophisticated equipment and a specialized approach to diagnosis that requires the services of a state or university veterinary diagnostic laboratory. Biological specimens for this purpose must be properly prepared, stored, and sent to the laboratory. These latter points cannot be overemphasized because a poor specimen often receives (and deserves) a poor answer.

Many viral diseases have rather characteristic features that permit identification at the clinical and pathological level. In other instances it may be deemed essential to establish a diagnosis either by isolation of the virus or by serological methods. Isolation of the virus often entails techniques that require a few days or weeks for identification. Most serological tests require the use of paired sera taken 2 to 3 weeks apart for a proper diagnosis of viral disease. It is apparent that most viral diagnostic test results become available after the patient has recovered or passed away. A notable exception is immunofluorescence (fluorescent antibody) testing, which is being rapidly developed for the diagnosis of many viral diseases. Some viral diseases, notably rabies, presently are diagnosed by this method.

Isolation of Viruses from Infected Animals

The effort and cost involved in a viral etiological diagnosis requires careful selection of case material as well as the proper collection and handling of the right type of specimen. As a rule, a virus isolation is desirable for the following reasons: (*a*) to identify a virus concerned in a herd health program; (*b*) to point out a public health problem that may be involved, such as rabies; (*c*) to establish the viral etiology of a disease not previously encountered in a practice; (*d*) to determine the immunological type of a given virus when epidemics such as foot-and-mouth disease occur; and (*e*) to pinpoint the exact agent when serological test methods fail because it shares common antigens with other viruses.

The isolation of a virus from a diseased animal does not necessarily mean that the isolate is the cause of the diseased state. Many viruses, including pathogens, persist in animals for long periods of time and their presence would tend to confuse the diagnosis. Some of these viruses, such as bovine enteroviruses, will be of the orphan type in that they are not proved pathogens. A knowledge of clinical and epidemiological patterns for the various viruses is useful in assessing the significance of a viral isolate from a diseased animal. On occasion more than one virus is isolated from a patient. This can be a difficult problem if both isolates are known pathogens. In a given patient at a particular time, one virus may be causing an inapparent infection while the other is responsible for the observed clinical signs of illness. A knowledge of the clinical signs produced by each virus is important as this may help to establish the primary disease agent in that situation. If both viruses produce comparable signs the etiological diagnosis becomes academic unless it is known that the patient may have had previous experience with one or both agents. It may then be possible to evaluate the facts and decide on the real culprit in a given situation. It also becomes apparent that the right diagnosis would be missed if antibody (serological) studies were made only for the virus causing the inapparent infection.

There are a number of excellent textbooks, papers, and monographs devoted to the laboratory diagnosis of viral diseases. The most desirable sources, which give an excellent, authoritative, and up-to-date coverage, are the multiauthored books edited by Lennette and Schmidt (5) and by Cottral (2). The latter book deals with standarized methods for veterinary microbiology.

Collection of Clinical Material for Viral Diagnosis

The ideal time to collect biological material for viral isolation is during the acute stage of illness prior to the formation of antibodies.

Various materials such as blood, nasal swabs, nasopharyngeal swabs, feces, urine, pus, vesicular fluid, skin lesions, spinal fluid, and biopsy material as well as tissues obtained at autopsy are used for the isolation of viruses. The biological specimens required for each specific disease can be obtained by referring to the description of the disease in this textbook, particularly the section of each disease dealing with diagnosis.

Some general rules can be stated that apply to the proper selection of tissues for viral isolation. Respiratory illnesses in their acute stage usually are associated with the excretion of virus in the nasal or pharyngeal secretions. Virus can be demonstrated in the fluid of vesicular lesions or in the scabs from pox lesions. Many generalized catarrhal diseases have a viremic state, and the virus can be readily isolated from the blood; virtually all body excretions contain virus during the acute stage of illness. Diseases referable to the central nervous system often present a problem, but it is reasonable to attempt isolation from the blood and also from the brain of animals that succumb to the disease. It is most important to obtain tissue specimens from deceased animals immediately after death—in some instances an owner may agree to sacrifice a moribund animal, which further enhances viral isolation. Often a blood sample is taken from an animal for serologic tests at the same time. It is important that the serum be harvested from the whole blood prior to freezing because lysis of red blood cells often renders a sample useless for certain serologic tests.

The biophysical and biochemical properties of viruses vary markedly. Many viruses are heat-sensitive and acid-sensitive, and great care must be exercised in handling such materials. In particular, fresh tissues must be used and then frozen to −60 to −70 C immediately after harvesting. Furthermore, a minimum of time is desirable in attempted isolations with these tissues in cell cultures or test animals. If there is no alternative, the tissue specimens may be placed in a deep freeze maintained at −20 C until dry ice is obtained for storage and shipment to the laboratory. A wide-mouthed thermos jug or a styrofoam-insulated carton, filled with dry ice after the specimens are inserted, is used for this purpose. If dry ice is not available, 50 percent glycerol can be used recognizing that certain viruses remain viable longer than others in this solution. Small pieces of tissue, fecal material, or mucus are placed in a vial, and the vial is completely filled with 50 percent glycerol and stored at 6 C.

Most laboratories do not operate over a weekend, so it is wise to ship the biological material during the early part of the week unless other arrangements are made.

Naturally, the tissue specimens should be taken with sterile instruments in a sterile manner. If an individual is concerned with the viral distribution in the tissues, separate sterile instruments must be used for procuring each tissue. Tight, sterile screw-cap vials often are used for storage of suspect tissues and fluids. If the fluid specimens are stored in dry ice, the vials should be air-tight as the gaseous phase of dry ice is CO_2, which changes the pH of fluids—resulting in inactivation of acid pH-labile viruses. When vials are not air-tight, they can be placed in a sealed, air-tight plastic bag, which accomplishes the same purpose.

Isolation of Virus

Susceptible animals, cell cultures, and embryonated hens' eggs are used for viral isolation. Fluid specimens that are bacteria-free can be inoculated directly or after dilution with a buffered solution (pH 7.2 to 7.6).

Solid tissues are prepared as 10 to 20 percent suspensions using a buffered solution (pH 7.2 to 7.6) as diluent. This suspension is given a light centrifugation to remove the coarse particles which tend to plug the inoculating equipment and often are toxic to cells in the test system. The supernatant fluid is used as the inoculum after centrifugation at 2,000 rpm for 10 minutes.

Certain test inocula such as feces, oral and nasal swabs, insects, and some infected tissues contain bacteria, and these should be eliminated prior to inoculation. Various procedures are used for this purpose, but for various reasons they do not always succeed. Ether is bactericidal, but may not be harmful to the virus under consideration. In such instances 10 to 15 percent ether can be added to the test suspension. Antibiotics are used and a mixture of penicillin (1,000 units per ml) and streptomycin (100 mg per ml) is most commonly employed. The dye proflavine is often used to photodynamically inactivate microbes in stool and throat specimens as it has little or no effect on enteroviruses or rhinoviruses. The specimen is treated with 10^{-4} M proflavine for 1 hour at pH 9 at 37 C after which the dye is removed by cation resins. The photosensitized bacterial and fungal contaminants are inactivated by exposure to light. Microbes also can be removed by mechanical means such as ultrafiltration and differential centrifugation. Earthenware, porcelain, and asbestos filters are used for this purpose, but viral concentration is reduced by adsorption to these materials. Differential centrifugation is a convenient and excellent method to remove many bacteria from a heavily contaminated specimen of the smaller viruses. For viruses smaller than 100 nm in size a run in the centrifugation at 18,000 rpm for 20 minutes in a 6-inch rotor will sediment the bacteria but not the virus. With specimens containing a minimal amount of virus, centrifugation at 40,000 rpm for 60 minutes in a 6-inch rotor will concentrate most viruses in a small gelatinous pellet at the bottom of the tubes. The supernatant of such runs contains less than 1 percent of the original virus. The pellet is then resuspended in a small volume of buffered solution.

Isolation of Viruses in Embryonated Hens' Eggs

Marked progress made in the field of virology during the past 30 years has been due, in part, to the use of the chicken embryo as a medium for the propagation of viral agents. Most viruses under natural conditions are relatively host-specific. Moreover, they show a marked predilection for groups of highly specialized tissue cells of the host, for example, those comprising nerve tissue, epithelial tissue, etc. Although growing readily in these tissues, they fail to grow in all or most others of the body. This tissue affinity, which is one of the unique properties of viruses, is known as tropism. While a number of viruses show marked host-specificity or tissue tropism, the great majority can be adapted by various procedures to foreign hosts. Inasmuch as the cells and the extraembryonic membrances of the developing chicken embryo, like most embryonic tissues, lack a high degree of specialization, these provide a general substrate containing some constituents conducive to the growth of all or most viruses. By virtue of the ability to alter their tropism and to adapt to new host species, many viruses become fully capable of growing in chicken embryo tissues wherein they frequently attain a much higher concentration than in the tissues of the natural host species.

Inoculation Procedures

The methods described below for the inoculation of the chicken embryo do not comprise a complete list, but represent rather those that are practiced most commonly. Likewise, while there are a number of techniques for inoculating by each of the routes listed, the one most widely used is described herein (Figure 38.1).

Yolk Sac. The large elementary-body viruses and the rickettsiae grow readily in the yolk-sac membranes. Although many of the smaller viruses also are inoculated by the yolk-sac route, they invade the embryo proper and multiply in the body tissues of the embryo rather than in the yolk-sac tissues.

1. *Age and preparation.* Fertile eggs that have been incubated for 5 to 7 days are suitable because the yolk sac is relatively large at this time. The eggs are candled and the boundary of the air sac pencilled in. The shell over the air space, which is referred to as the shell cap, is disinfected by an application of iodine to one small area. When the iodine is dried, a hole is made through the shell over the center of the natural air space by means of a drill.

2. *Inoculation and incubation.* By means of a syringe fitted with a 1-inch, 23-gauge needle, the inoculum is deposited in the yolk sac by passing the needle through the hole in the shell cap and directing it downward to its full length, parallel to the long axis of the egg. From 0.2

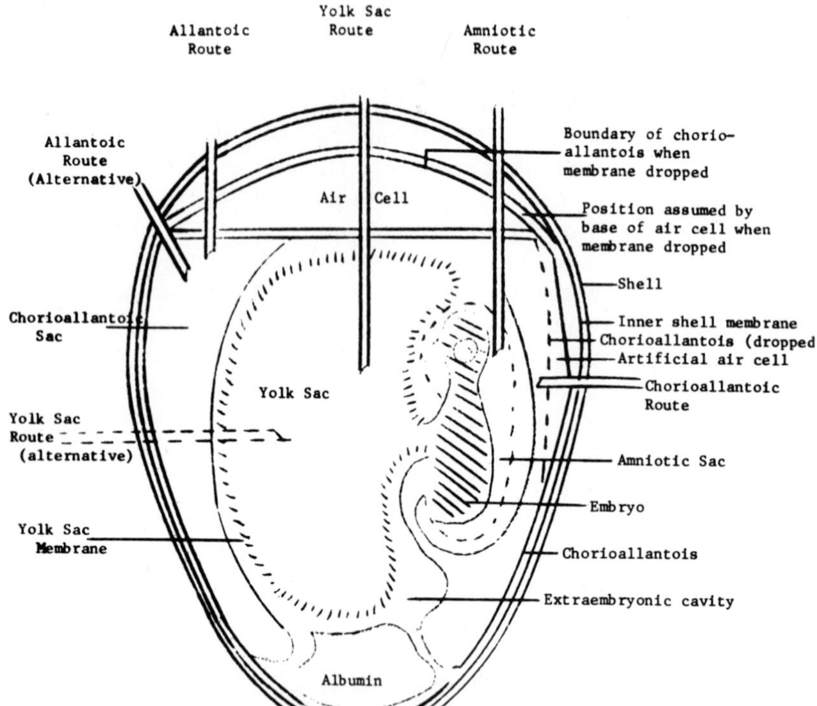

Figure 38.1. Various routes of inoculation into embryonating hens' eggs for the propagation of viruses.

to 0.5 ml is usually inoculated. The hole in the shell is then sealed with hot vaspar (paraffin-vaseline mixture), and the eggs are incubated at 37 C.

3. *Harvesting procedure.* The egg is placed in a container that maintains it in the upright position during the harvesting procedure. The shell is cracked with sterile forceps and the cap lifted off. The exposed membranes are torn away, and the yolk-sac contents may be removed with a special sterile 10-ml pipette with the tip removed. If the yolk-sac membrances are to be harvested, the contents of the egg are quickly emptied into a sterile petri dish. The yolk sac is usually ruptured in the process. The yolk-sac membranes, which are easily recognized by their deep yellow color, are detached from the embryo, separated from the chorioallantois with sterile forceps, and quickly transferred to a sterile petri dish. When the embryo is to be harvested, it is withdrawn by hooking the curved end of a dental probe around the neck. It is then separated from the adherent membranes with sterile scissors and transferred to a sterile petri dish.

Allantoic Cavity. The influenza and the Newcastle disease viruses, and most other viral agents that cause respiratory infections, grow readily in the entodermal cells of the allantoic sac wall and are liberated into the allantoic fluid. The encephalomyelitis viruses and the mumps virus also multiply readily when inoculated by this route.

1. *Age and preparation.* Embryonating eggs that have received a preliminary incubation of from 8 to 11 days are candled and the boundary of the air space pencilled in. The eggs are held in the upright position with the air sac uppermost. A point is selected several millimeters above the floor of the air space on the side of the egg where the chorioallantois is well developed but free of large vessels. Iodine is applied to the area around the site. A hole is then drilled or punched through the shell.

2. *Inoculation and incubation.* A 0.5-inch, 24-gauge needle, fitted to a small syringe containing the inoculum, is inserted into the allantoic cavity by passing it through the hole in the shell parallel to the long axis of the egg or at an angle directed towards the apical extremity. From 0.2 to 0.5 ml of inoculum is injected into each egg. The hole in the shell is then sealed with hot vaspar, and the eggs are incubated at 37 C.

3. *Harvesting of allantoic fluid.* To avoid hemorrhage into the allantoic fluid while harvesting, the eggs are chilled by holding in the refrigerator from 4 to 6 hours prior to the harvesting procedure. They are held in an upright position, and the shell over the air sac is removed with sterile forceps. The floor of the air space is exposed. The floor consists of the inner shell membrane overlaying the chorioallantois. With a pair of small, sterile, curved forceps these membranes are torn away. To facili-

tate the harvesting of the allantoic fluid, the embryo is displaced to one side by placing the forceps against the embryo with the tips toward the shell wall. The allantoic fluid then can readily be aspirated with a 5- or 10-ml sterile pipette.

The Chorioallantoic Membrane. 1. *Age and preparation*. Nine- to eleven-day-old embryonating eggs are candled, and an area about 1 centimeter square is outlined with a pencil on the shell over the most vascular underlying portion. The surrounding shell is treated by applying 5 percent phenol, which is permitted to dry. Iodine is not used to sterilize the shell because the alcoholic solution is absorbed through the shell and causes lesions on the chorioallantois which could be mistakenly attributed to the virus. With a drill, the shell is cut along the pencilled lines, great care being exercised to avoid cutting the inner shell membrane. A hole is then drilled or punched through the shell and inner shell membranes into the natural air space, as for yolk-sac inoculation. The egg is now placed on its side in a holder with the drilled side uppermost. With a pair of sharp pointed forceps or a dental probe the excised piece of shell is gently removed, exposing the white inner shell membrane, to the underside of which is attached the chorioallantois. A small drop of sterile saline is placed on the center of this area to soften the membrane. The bevelled surface of a 27-gauge, 0.25-inch needle (depending on the preference of the operator) fitted to a 1-ml syringe is applied at a 45-degree angle to this area with gentle downward pressure and, by traction, a slit is made in the membrane. Care must be exercised to avoid damage to the underlying chorioallantois. Because the fibers of the inner shell membrane run obliquely, the syringe should be held at a 45-degree angle to the long axis of the egg so that the pressure exerted will tend to separate rather than to tear the fibers. Suction is then applied with a rubber bulb to the hole in the natural air space. If preferred, a drop of sterile saline may be dropped on the slit before suction is applied. The saline, as it is drawn in, aids in separating the chorioallantois from the inner shell membrane. The former then drops as part of the egg contents is displaced into the space occupied originally by the natural air space. This is indicated by a clearing of the inner shell membrane as the chorioallantois separates from it.

2. *Inoculation and incubation*. By carefully passing the needle through the inner shell membrane from 0.1 to 0.2 ml of inoculum is dropped on the chorioallantois with a 1-ml syringe fitted with a 22- or 23-gauge needle. In very critical studies the egg should be candled during this procedure to insure that the inoculum is deposited on, rather than through, the membrane. After inoculation the egg is gently rocked in order to spread the inoculum uniformly over the surface of the chorioallantois. The opening in the shell is covered with a small square of scotch tape, and the inoculated eggs are incubated with the shell window uppermost.

An alternative method for inoculating by this route, which eliminates much of the tedium connected with window cutting, is carried out as follows: At a selected point a hole is drilled through the sterilized shell to the inner shell membrane. Using a 19-gauge needle with the bevel held downward, the inner shell membrane is carefully separated from the shell around the margin of the hole by exerting a slight downward pressure on the needle. The egg is then placed on a candler and suction applied to the hole that has previously been made into the air space. The dropping of the chorioallantois can then be readily observed.

3. *Harvesting of the membrane tissues*. The egg is placed in the horizontal position with the window uppermost. Iodine is applied to the area around the window with a cotton swab and the tape then peeled off. The surrounding shell is broken away with sterile forceps and the chorioallantois exposed. The membrane is grasped with forceps, detached with scissors, and quickly transferred to a sterile petri dish.

Inasmuch as the chorioallantois of eggs that have been incubated for 9 or 10 days adhere firmly to the inner shell membrane, a common practice is to drop these membranes at 7 or 8 days and to hold the eggs in the incubator until they are ready to be inoculated. They are candled during the inoculation procedure in order to insure that the chorioallantois has not risen in the meantime, and that the inoculum is deposited on the membrane rather than in the allantoic sac. The hole in the shell is then sealed with vaspar or scotch tape. Incubation and harvesting is the same as described for the first method.

Amniotic. This method is used principally for the isolation of the influenza virus from throat washings. The embryo during the course of its development swallows the amniotic fluid, thereby bringing the inoculated virus it contains into contact with the tissues of the respiratory and intestinal tracts where multiplication presumably occurs. The amniotic route of inoculation is used also for the isolation of the encephalomyelitis viruses.

1. *Age and preparation*. Embryos from 7 to 15 days of age are used. The position of the embryo is determined by candling, and then a point is marked on the shell over the air space on the side of the egg in which the embryo

is situated. The site is prepared in the usual manner, and a hole is drilled or punched as for yolk-sac inoculation.

2. *Inoculation and incubation.* A 1-ml syringe fitted with a 0.75-inch, 24-gauge needle is used for the inoculation. The egg is placed horizontally on the candler, and the needle is introduced and gently stabbed in the direction of the embryo. Penetration of the amniotic sac is indicated by a sudden movement of the embryo. The needle is then withdrawn slightly and from 0.1 to 0.2 ml of the inoculum injected. The hole in the shell is sealed with vaspar, and the eggs are incubated in the vertical position.

3. *Harvesting of amniotic fluid.* The shell is removed as for the allantoic and yolk-sac routes of inoculation. A few drops of saline are placed on the floor of the air space to render the membrane transparent. Using the eyes of the embryo as a reference point, the amniotic fluid is aspirated by means of a syringe fitted with a short 23-gauge needle.

Miscellaneous. 1. *Intravenous.* This method of inoculating chicken embryos is not practiced to any extent. In carrying it out, 12- to 14-day-old chicken embryos are used. A large vein is located by candling and marked. A rectangular piece of shell directly over the vein is removed in the manner already described, and a droplet of sterile mineral oil is placed on the inner shell membrane to render it transparent. A 27-gauge needle fitted to a small syringe is introduced through the membrane into the vein in the direction of blood flow. From 0.1 to 0.5 ml of inoculum is then injected. Incubation and harvesting of the embryo is carried out as already described.

2. *Intracerebral.* This method was occasionally used for the cultivation of the rabies virus.

Isolation of Viruses in Tissue Culture

Advances in the methods of cell culture have provided the virologist with a highly valuable tool for isolation and propagation of viruses. Certain knowledge of the techniques of cell cultivation and maintenance is, therefore, a prerequisite to the study of viruses. Tissue cultures are the most widely used methods for isolation of viruses from clinical material. Replication of viruses in cell cultures can be recognized in various ways, such as cytopathic effects, viral interference, hemadsorption and hemagglutination, fluorescent antigen, and complement-fixing antigen.

The usage of the following terms has been recommended by the Committee on Terminology of the Tissue Culture Association. Dependent on whether cells, tissues, or organs are to be maintained or grown, two methodological approaches—cell culture, and tissue or organ culture—have been developed in the field of tissue culture. The cell culture denotes the growing of cells *in vitro,* including the culture of single cells. In these, the cells are no longer organized into tissues. In tissue or organ cultures, tissues, or a whole organ or parts of an organ, are grown or maintained *in vitro* in a way that may allow differentiation and preservation of the architecture and/or function. A single layer of cells growing on a surface is called a monolayer. Suspension culture denotes a type of culture in which cells multiply while suspended in medium. A primary culture may be regarded as such until it is subcultured for the first time. It then becomes a cell line. A cell line may be said to have become established when it demonstrates the potential to be subcultured indefinitely *in vitro*. Diploid cell line denotes a cell line in which, arbitrarily, at least 75 percent of the cells have the same karyotype as the normal cells of the species from which the cells were originally obtained. A diploid chromosome number is not necessarily equivalent to the diploid karyotype because there are situations in which a cell may lose one type of chromosome and acquire another type. Thus the karyotype of the cell has changed, but the diploid number of chromosomes remains the same. Such cells should be referred to as pseudodiploid.

Primary cultures are prepared from a variety of tissues of human and animal origin and are routinely employed in the cultivation of a large number of viruses. Primary cultures are preferred in many instances for their increased susceptibility to viruses. On the other hand, lack of uniformity in susceptibility in different batches of cells and the possible presence of occult viruses are some of the inherent dangers involved in their use. Certain viruses such as some human coronaviruses will replicate only in organ cultures.

Only under special circumstances can cell lines be grown continuously without changes in karyotype. Usually the conditions of culture select out variants in the cell population. These may differ radically from the predominant cell type in a primary culture. Most established cell lines used today are of this selected type, although increasing use is made of diploid or pseudodiploid cell lines. By preserving large batches of these cells in the frozen state it is possible to work with cells of constant characteristics. In addition, cell lines offer advantages for their availability and rapid growth. At the same time, more attention is required to maintain them free of contaminants.

Viruses do not propagate outside living, actively

metabolizing cells. For this reason it is necessary to consider the cell, its nutritional requirements, and its susceptibility to viruses, as well as the virus itself when working with tissue-culture systems. While the body of the natural or experimental animal host species provides the necessary conditions for virus multiplication, it becomes necessary to manipulate the tissue-culture system in such a way that optimal virus-growth conditions are satisfied in the test tube. This has been accomplished to a considerable degree by providing the cells with media designed to assure satisfactory growth and maintenance. The conditions necessary for virus multiplication are intimately associated with and dependent on the maintenance of viable cells. To this end a formidable formulary of media has been devised to suit the requirements for growth of various cell types. In general, all media contain the following general substances in varying combinations and amounts: (*a*) balanced salt solutions—Earle's, Hanks', and Tyrode's solutions, to mention only a few media; (*b*) "fortification substances"—lactalbumin hydrolysate, embryo extracts, amniotic fluid, vitamins, hormones, amino acids, minerals, and yeast extract; (*c*) serum—human, horse, dog, calf, rabbit, sheep, and other species free of inhibitors and antibodies to the virus under study; and (*d*) antibiotics—penicillin, streptomycin, Mycostatin, tetracyclines, and many others used in dosage levels not toxic to cells.

Cell-culture work was plagued with contamination by unwanted bacteria and molds until the introduction of antibiotics, which allowed a much wider group of workers to do satisfactory tissue culture in mass quantity. Contamination is still, however, one of the major hazards; for this reason strict asceptic technique is necessary.

The many techniques of tissue culture applied to virus cultivation are modifications of 5 basic methods:

1. *The suspended-cell method*. This is an old and still employed method used for the production of virus for foot-and-mouth disease.

2. *Plasma-clot method*. Tissue fragments (explants) are made to adhere to the wall of a glass slide or test tube with the aid of clotted plasma, often chicken plasma. A film of plasma is layered onto a glass surface and induced to clot by the addition of embryo extract. Into this matrix are placed tissue fragments which adhere and proliferate. By this method one can observe the cellular proliferation and measure growth of the explants. Growth of viruses in such cultures can be determined by several methods: (*a*) sampling the virus in the liquid or cellular phase of the culture and inoculating susceptible laboratory hosts which are known to become infected; (*b*) noting the effect on cellular metabolism (i.e., inhibition of certain metabolic pathways); (*c*) observing cell-death (necrosis); (*d*) testing for presence of hemagglutinins; and (*e*) using electron microscopy of cells and purified fluids.

3. *Monolayer cell cultures*. Stationary-tube cultures are by far the most widely used in virology. These cultures are prepared from trypsin-dispersed tissues and consist of small clumps of cells and single cells derived from the particular source suited for use: kidney, testicle, skin, tumors, and other tissues. Tissues to be used are finely minced with scissors, washed with saline to remove blood cells and tissue debris, and placed in a trypsin solution that is kept constantly stirred with a magnetic stirring device. When the cells are dispersed (the time depending on the temperature of trypsinization and the type of tissue being prepared), they are lightly centrifuged, washed with media two or three times to remove the trypsin, filtered through several layers of cheesecloth, diluted to contain sufficient cells per ml to insure good growth (the amount of cells depends upon the type), and inoculated into test tubes. The cell suspensions prepared from kidney fragments produce luxuriant monolayer cultures on any clean glass surface, petri dish or test tube, or bottle held in a stationary position. Tube cultures prepared in this way are used for virus isolations, titrations, neutralization tests, and studying the growth of viruses in cells.

4. *Direct cultures*. The procedure is the same as described for monolayer cell cultures. In this situation, tissues are taken at autopsy or by biopsy from the diseased animal for the production of monolayer cell cultures to enhance the opportunity for viral isolation where little virus is likely to be present or virus may be rendered inactive by antibodies present in the tissues. As little trypsin as possible should be used because some viruses are inactivated by trypsin.

5. *Organ cultures*. These cultures, used for the inoculation of suspect viral material or organ cultures, can be made directly from diseased tissues as indicated in the previous section. Organ cultures contain the differentiated tissues characteristic of a given organ. In some cases a virus—such as certain human coronaviruses—requires a specialized cell essential for its replication that is not present in a monolayer cell culture from the same organ. Organ cultures are used principally in research studies, for the technique is time-consuming and tedious in its present technology. Most viral studies in organ cultures involve the use of respiratory viruses in organ cultures derived from respiratory

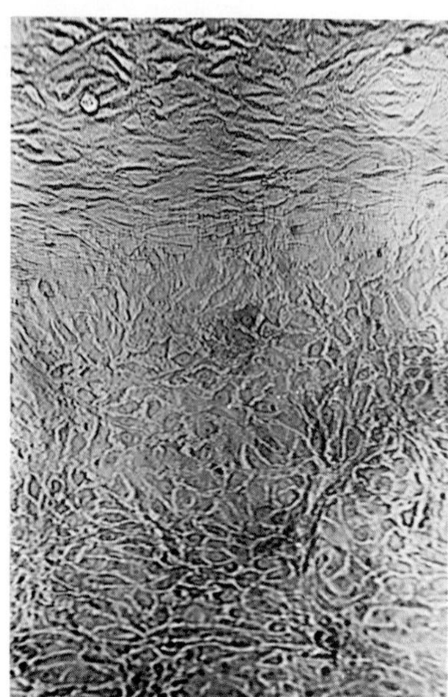

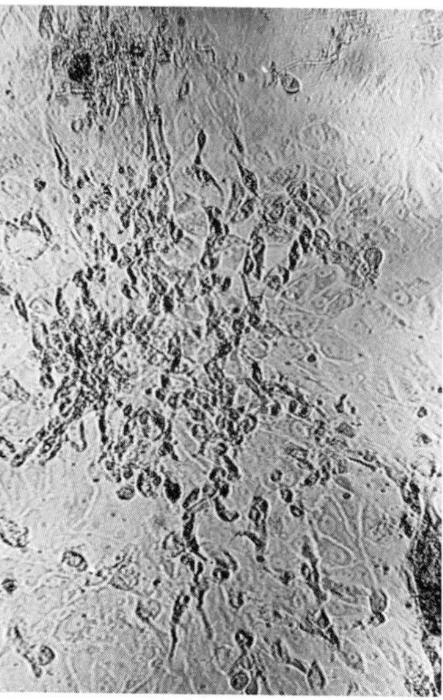

Figure 38.2. (*Left*) Uninoculated feline kidney cell culture. (*Right*) Cytopathic effect (CPE) induced by a virus in feline kidney cell culture. × 82. (Courtesy F. Scott, C. Csiza, and J. Gillespie, *Am. Jour. Vet. Res.*)

embryonic tissues with emphasis on viral propagation and its cytomorphological effects in the *in vitro* differentiated tissues. Investigators interested in the pathogenesis and immunity of viral diseases will continue to apply this method in future studies.

The most characteristic change in virus-infected cultures is a degenerative or necrotic change in the cellular elements of the culture (Figure 38.2). These cytopathic changes (cytopathic effect or CPE) are microscopically visible with a light microscope, and first involve individual cells and then spread to all susceptible cells in a culture. The effect of the virus on the cells depends on the type of virus and cell. With certain viruses such as infectious bovine rhinotracheitis, infectious canine hepatitis, human adenoviruses, poliovirus, vesicular stomatitis virus, and foot-and-mouth-disease virus, the cells become granular, round up into clumps of degenerated cells, and finally drop from the glass surface, leaving islands of clear spaces. Eventually all the cells of a culture may become infected. In some infections the cells tend to clump together in aggregates to form "giant cells," which are syncytial formations of multinucleate cells. These are characteristic of distemper, mumps, measles virus, parainfluenza viruses, and syncytium-forming viruses of monkeys, humans, cattle, and cats (Figure 38.3). In such infected cultures there is a liberation of virus into the fluids bathing the cells, although with certain viruses the concentration of virus at any time in the growth cycle may be higher within the cell (cell-associated virus) than in the tissue culture fluid. Certain tumor viruses cause a loss-of-contact inhibition, and the cells tend to pile upon each other forming a plaque. The characteristic cytopathic effect produced by some viruses along with their clinical history permits a rapid presumptive diagnosis. Because some viruses replicate without producing a cytopathic effect other means are used for their identification in cell cultures.

Such viruses as feline infectious panleukopenia virus produce intranuclear inclusion bodies, which can be readily observed after May-Gruenwald staining, without a significant destruction of the cell layer, so staining

Figure 38.3. Cytopathic effects by a bovine syncytium-forming virus characterized by syncytium formation with marked vacuolation and numerous cytoplasmic inclusion bodies clearly demonstrated by staining a cover-slip preparation(s) with May-Gruenwald-Giemsa stain. × 1,250. (Courtesy F. Scott.)

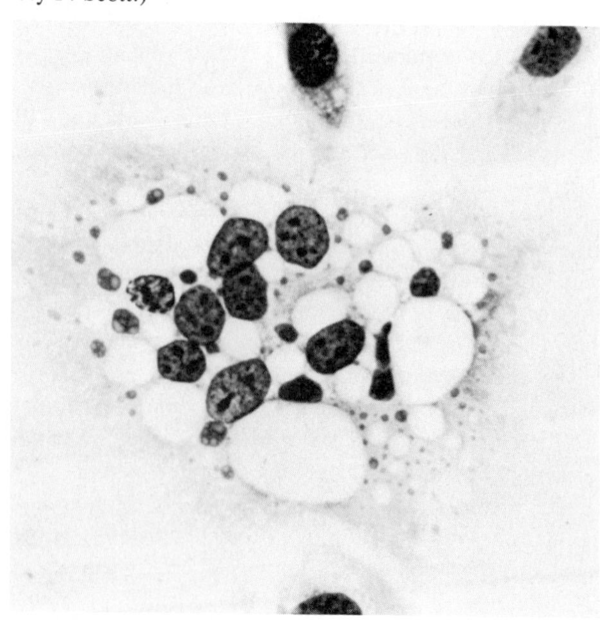

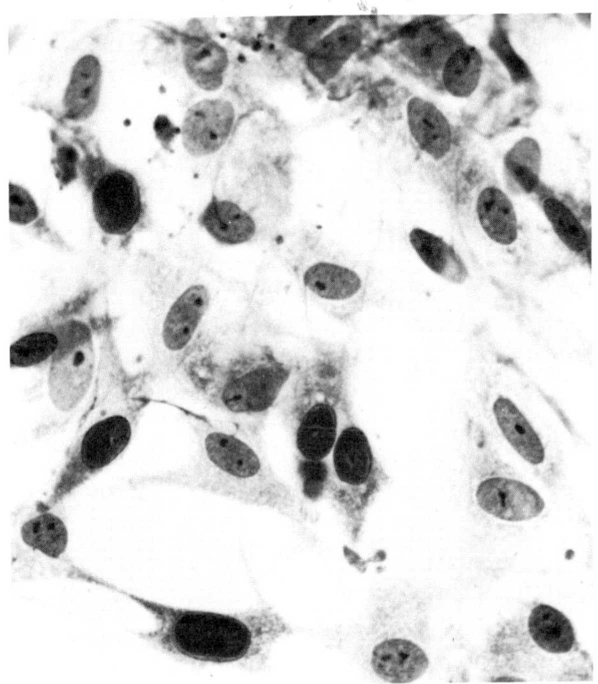

Figure 38.4. Note Cowdry type A intranuclear inclusion bodies produced by feline panleukopenia virus in tissue-cultured feline kidney cells. May-Gruenwald stain. × 370. (Courtesy C. Geissinger, E. Tompkins, and F. Scott.)

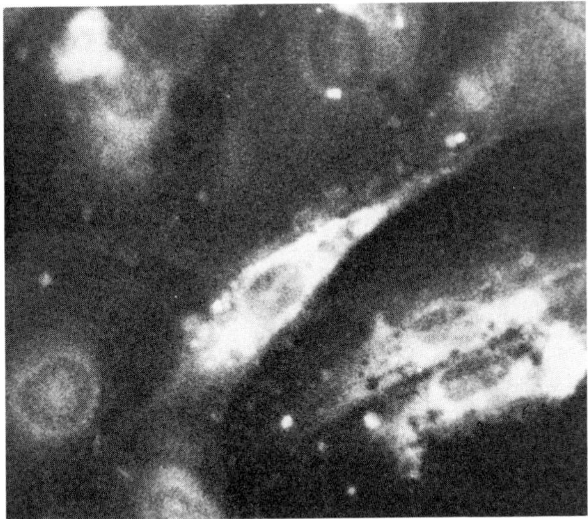

Figure 38.5. Immunofluorescence test (FAT). Specific cytoplasmic fluorescence (white area) in a cell culture infected with mucosal disease-virus diarrhea virus stained with MD-VD antiglobulin conjugate. × 1060. (Courtesy R. Schultz.)

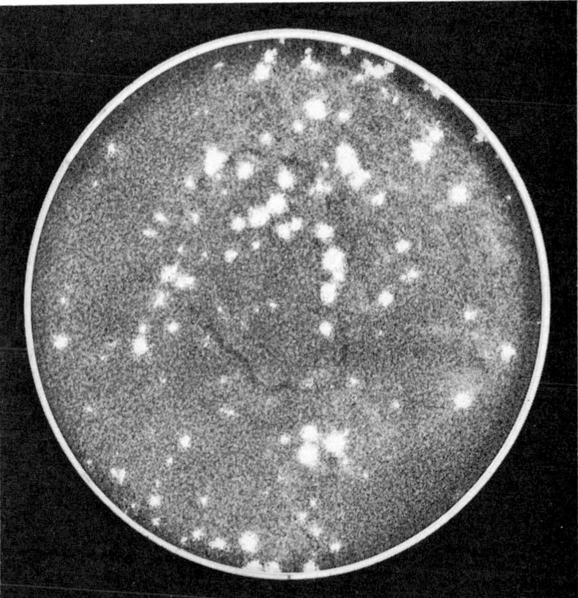

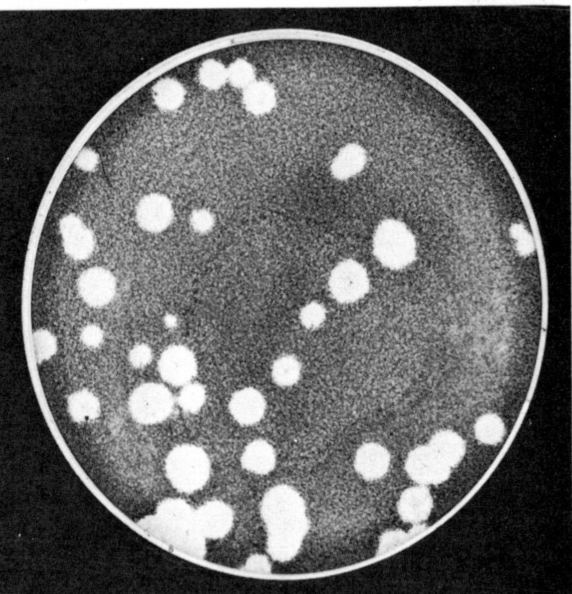

Figure 38.6. (*Upper*) Plaques produced in NL-111 rabbit kidney cells by a field isolate of equine herpesvirus 1. (*Lower*) Plaques produced in NL-111 rabbit kidney cells by a modified live virus vaccine strain of equine herpesvirus 1. (Courtesy D. Holmes and M. Kemen.)

procedures of cover-slip cell cultures offer a better means for diagnosis (Figure 38.4). The diagnostician can use immunofluorescent staining with a specific conjugate (Figure 38.5) or a vital stain such as May-Gruenwald for identification. When a virus such as a noncytopathic strain of virus diarrhea-mucosal disease virus produces absolutely no cell alterations, a fluorescent antibody conjugate or the viral interference test with a cytopathic strain of virus diarrhea-mucosal disease virus can be used to assist in identification. In the interference test the noncytopathic strain interferes with a precalculated amount of cytopathic virus (usually 100 $TCID_{50}$ per 0.1 ml) and

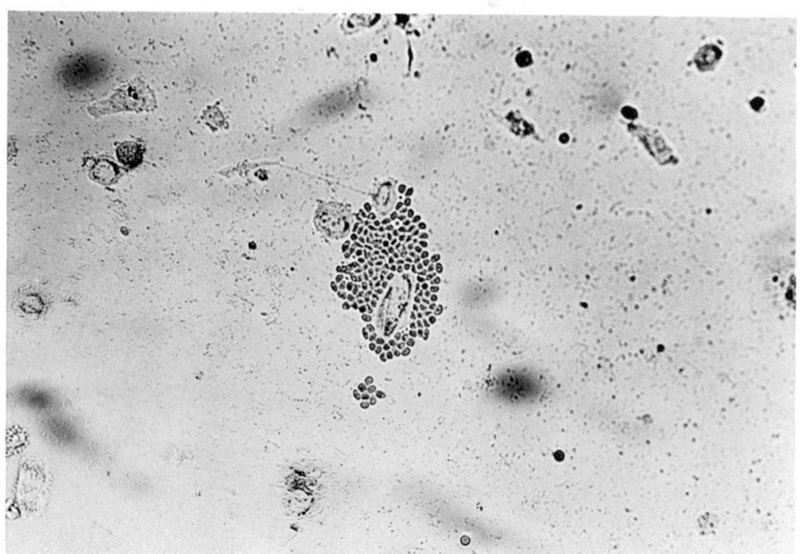

Figure 38.7. Mumps virus causing hemadsorption (clumping) of chicken red blood cells in a cell culture of Vero cells. × 260. (Courtesy R. Schultz and F. Scott.)

prevents the production of a cytopathic effect, often manifested as a plaque (Figure 38.6).

Some viruses, such as members of the Orthomyxoviridae and Paramyxoviridae cause hemagglutination and/or hemadsorption. The hemadsorption phenomenon can be used for viral detection by adding 0.15 ml of a 0.25 percent suspension of red blood cells directly to washed tube cell cultures and incubating at 37 C for 48 to 72 hours. In cultures containing virus the red blood cells are adsorbed to the infected cell sheets (Figure 38.7).

Production of virus in large quantities, as required for production of vaccines or complement-fixing antigens, is possible then using sheets of cells grown in bottles. By using protein-free media (such as Parker-Morgan media 199) virus can be harvested in large quantities by withdrawing the fluid at a time when the maximum yield is expected. Once the immunizing dose is established, the fluid can be harvested and either inactivated with formalin or phenol to produce a killed vaccine or, if the agent has been adequately attenuated, diluted properly to contain sufficient virus to immunize.

Isolation of Viruses in Animals

The selection of a susceptible host for the isolation of a virus is essential to a diagnosis by this means. In certain instances age is important; suckling animals are more likely to develop recognizable infection than older animals. It is not a wise idea to use an animal more than once for viral isolation as subclinical infections do occur, and this would cause a false negative result. In studying a new viral agent the best chance for its successful propagation is in the natural host. In veterinary medicine we have this distinct advantage for the isolation of a virus in an animal. Often the natural host is a large animal, a fact that reduces its usefulness in achieving quick and easy solutions. The researcher then studies the effects of the virus in many other hosts, particularly in caged laboratory animals such as mice, hamsters, guinea pigs, rats, cats, and rabbits. In some instances adaptation to an unnatural host requires the use of a special virus strain, or by alteration of viral transfers between natural host and unnatural host it is possible to select viral particles which can be maintained in serial passage in the new host. The laboratory animal of choice for the various viruses, if one is available, is given under each virus infection discussed in this book. The route of inoculation of the virus in a laboratory host is critical with certain viruses. In unknown situations the most successful route is directly into the body system, where the virus produces lesions in the natural host; for example, suspect brain material from encephalitic cases would be inoculated intracerebrally into suckling and older mice.

The source of animals is exceedingly important as latent viruses occur in many animal colonies. To counteract this problem in part, animal colonies have been established by using caesarian-derived animals as the breeding stock. It is important to maintain these colonies as pathogen-free stocks by the use of isolation procedures. In some instances germ-free colonies are established for selected types of biological research problems. The caesarian-derived animal gives reasonable assurance that it is not harboring a viral agent which is transmitted horizontally. In the case of vertically transmitted viruses, such as the RNA (type C) endogenous viruses, this procedure does not eliminate the viral agent. Consequently, there is little chance of establishing a colony which is free of all viruses or their viral genomes. Of course the problem of latent viruses also applies to the chick embryo and tissue culture as well. *Mycoplasma* and other microbes constitute a similar problem for all three systems often used for virus isolations. At best one can only hope to achieve a colony which is well defined and can be monitored for diseases for which adequate and specific tests exist for their identification.

With the introduction of the chick embryo technique, and particularly tissue culture techniques, animal inoculations are seldom used for diagnosis of viral infections. They are still essential for viral research studies, so the student should have some knowledge of their use and the problems associated with their use.

Intracerebral Inoculation. The intracerebral route of inoculation in mice is used for the isolation of neurotropic viruses. Either suckling mice or recently weaned mice (3 to 4 weeks old) are used for this purpose. On occasion, guinea pigs and rabbits are used. The inoculum should be virtually free of bacteria because the brain has little resistance to bacterial agents. Mice are lightly anesthetized with anesthetic ether before inoculation of 0.03 ml of test inoculum with a sharp needle, 27-gauge, 0.25-inch long, and syringe, above the orbital ridge directly into the brain. Similarly, control mice are given a comparable amount of buffered physiological salt solution in a test to activate a latent brain virus such as lymphocytic choriomeningitis virus if it should exist in the test mice.

After inoculation all mice should be observed daily for signs of illness for approximately 30 days. Any mice that die during this period should be autopsied using sterile techniques in an attempt to isolate microbes from the brain and heart blood. Negative cultures rule out contamination with bacteria, fungi, and *Mycoplasma*, assuming the proper type of media were used to isolate these agents. Brain tissue should also be retained for additional viral tests if required to establish the diagnosis. Careful observation is made for macroscopic lesions followed by the study of stained sections of various tissues, particularly the brain, for the microscopic lesions. In viral encephalitides macroscopic brain lesions usually are lacking, but microscopic lesions are quite pronounced. If the control mice given sterile buffered physiological salt solution (PSS) develop nervous manifestations, the test is declared void and another source of test mice sought if the infection is viral in nature. If all mice appear healthy at 30 days, they are sacrificed and examined carefully for lesions.

Intranasal Inoculation. As a rule the mouse is the animal of choice for the isolation of pneumotropic viruses. Occasionally ferrets are used, but they are generally avoided if possible because the ferret is a difficult animal to handle.

The mice are anesthetized in a covered jar containing cotton soaked with ether and 0.05 ml of test material applied to the nares with a fine pipette. If properly anesthetized the mouse will inhale the fluid preparation with no difficulty; otherwise it will discharge the fluid. Conversely, too much anesthesia or fluid inoculum causes death of the mouse.

Most respiratory diseases have a short incubation period, so a 14-day observation period for signs of illness is usually adequate time. Mice that die are examined carefully at autopsy for lesions, especially of the respiratory tract. If the test mice show signs of respiratory illness, some are sacrificed. Some lungs are harvested for future virus studies. Others are used for macroscopic and microscopic study of the lesions. Surviving mice are examined at autopsy at the end of the observation period. Although virus may have replicated in the mouse lung, no pneumonic lesions are produced in first passage. Depending on the virus, it may be possible to detect it by various means such as the hemagglutination phenomenon. Subsequent passages of infective mouse lungs in mice may select a viral population which does cause pneumonia. The number of mouse transfers required will vary with the virus and also with the strain of virus.

Intraperitoneal Inoculation. This route of inoculation is commonly used for isolation of agents in guinea pigs, particularly the psittacoid and rickettsial organisms. Mice are also used but less frequently. The peritoneal cavity of the guinea pig is particularly effective in the destruction of most nonpathogenic bacterial organisms present in feces of various domestic animals; consequently, it serves as an effective filter to eliminate most bacteria from fecal specimens not treated with antibiotics and being tested for psittacoid and rickettsial agents.

The guinea pigs are inoculated directly into the peritoneal cavity with a sharp needle, 24- to 25-gauge and 0.5-inch long, and syringe with 0.5 ml of the lightly centrifuged test suspension. Daily temperatures and observations are made of the guinea pigs maintained in a temperature-controlled environment. The guinea pig's thermal-regulating mechanism is sensitive to a marked rise in room temperature, and its normal temperature range is exceeded at 38 to 39.5 C. This becomes especially important when a rise in temperature may be the only indication of infection. If the guinea pigs sicken, the appropriate tests from spleen, blood, and peritoneal cavity are made for possible baterial contamination. Tissues also are selected for further study of the pathogenic agent, usually the spleen. Quite often guinea pigs recover from active infection, which is a distinct advantage for serological studies.

Serological Diagnosis of Viral Diseases

The immunological response of an animal to natural or planned viral infection can be detected and measured by a large number of serological procedures. There are two indispensable elements in any serological test: the antigen and the antibody. The viral antigen(s) may be detected, identified, and quantified by testing it against a number of specific antibody preparations. Conversely, the antibody in the serum of a recovered or vaccinated animal can be identified and quantitated by testing against a number of prepared viral antigens.

At present the greatest number of diagnostic tests performed in a microbiological laboratory are serological tests. The most widely used tests are the serum-neutralization, complement-fixation, and hemagglutination-inhibition. Other methods include the hemadsorption, hemadsorption-inhibition, precipitation, agglutination, immunodiffusion radioimmunoassay, indirect hemagglutination, enzyme-linked immunoabsorbent assay (ELISA), and flocculation tests. The procedures with the greatest potential as quick and accurate diagnostic tests for viral diseases are the direct and indirect fluorescent antibody techniques (FAT) involving immunofluorescence and the ELISA test. A fluorescent virus precipitin test (FVPT) for the serologic identification of small particulate antigens such as virus has been described and probably is as sensitive as any serologic test (3). It is rapid and reliable, and only a single fluorescent conjugate is needed to permit the detection of many viruses. Cottral (2) and Lennette and Schmidt (5) cover most of these tests in detail.

In 1955 Takatsy (8) described the use of spiral loops in serological and virological micromethods and Sever (7) utilized the microtechnique for viral and serological investigations in the United States (Figure 38.8). With the availability of accurately calibrated equipment for measuring small volumes from a commercial source,* microserological techniques have been developed for the diagnosis of viral diseases in the United States and elsewhere. At present microtests for the hemagglutination-inhibition, complement-fixation, gel-diffusion, and neutralization tests (Figure 38.9), and more recently the ELISA test, are in usage (1) in viral serological diagnosis, and they give comparable results to the macromethods. The microtests are preferred because they contribute to an economy in time, space, and reagents.

*Cooke Engineering Company, Medical Research Division, Alexandria, Virginia, 22314, USA.

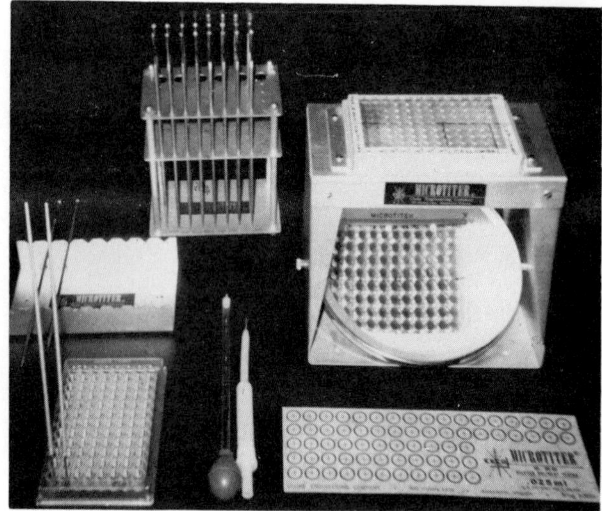

Figure 38.8. A photograph depicting most of the equipment (produced by Cooke Engineering Co., Alexandria, Va.) essential for the performance of viral and serological microtiter plate tests. (Courtesy R. Schultz and D. Holmes.)

The ELISA test (Figure 38.10) is exceedingly sensitive in detecting antigen and antibody. The test procedure has been automated with appropriate equipment to provide minimal operator involvement, increased productivity, and precise answers. Its accuracy, simplicity, and low cost provides the diagnostician and epidemiologist with a procedure to test large numbers of serum samples for antibody within a short time. As a consequence, it promises to become the test of choice in diagnostic laboratories for antigen-antibody systems that can be adapted to the automated procedure. In addition to the direct system an indirect ELISA microplate test has been devised as a diagnostic and surveillance tool to aid in the control of animal disease (6).

With most serological methods antibody titers are expressed as the reciprocal of the highest serum dilution causing a positive observable antigen-antibody reaction. In such tests as the neutralization test, which is based on the inhibition of viral replication by specific antibody the level (titer) can be expressed as the neutralization index (alpha test procedure) or as the highest dilution which protests 50 percent of the test host against a precalculated virus dosage (beta test procedure). The 50 percent end

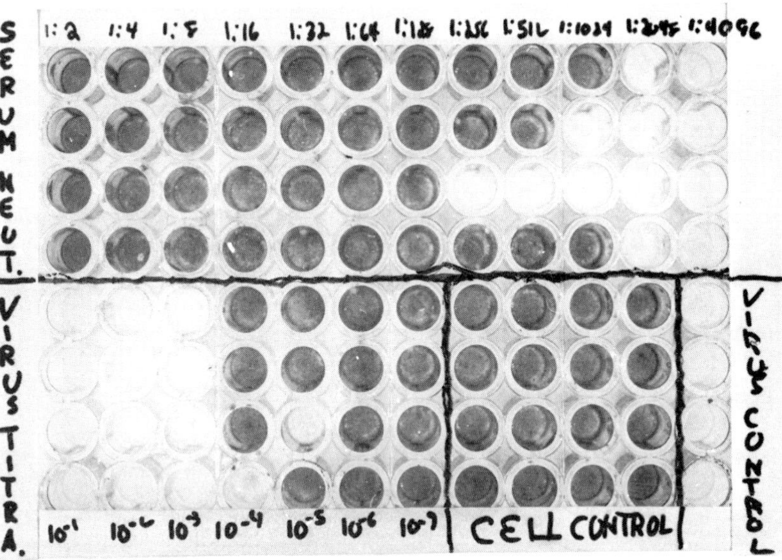

Figure 38.9. Test results of a microtiter serum neutralization test with an accompanying virus titration using a feline herpesvirus antigen-antibody system. In the SN test 100 $TCID_{50}$ of virus was used against varying 2-fold dilutions of serum. After appropriate incubation at 37 C the nutrient fluid is discarded and cell layers in the plate are rinsed with saline, fixed with methanol, and stained with Giemsa. The stained wells (dark) indicate lack of viral cytopathic effect; the clear wells lack cells as a result of viral cytopathic activity. (Courtesy D. Holmes and R. Schultz.)

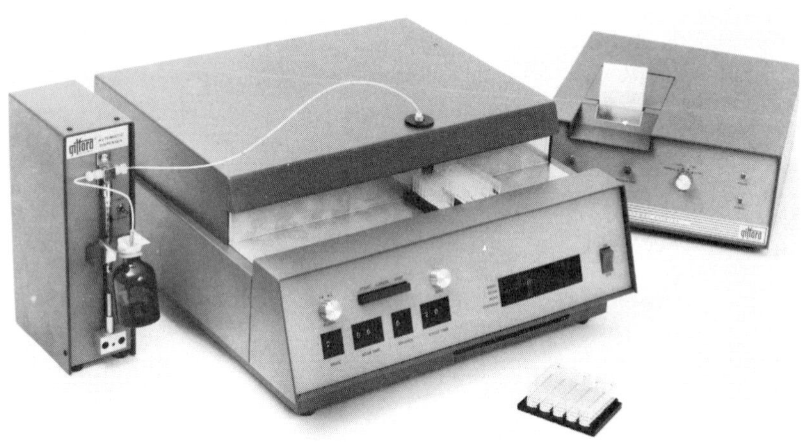

Figure 38.10. An automated system for performing the enzyme-linked immunoabsorbent assay procedure. (Courtesy Gilford Instrument Laboratories, Inc., Oberlin, Ohio.)

points for the beta test procedure can be calculated by the methods of Kärber (4).

To perform satisfactory serological tests blood samples should be collected in sterile sealed units. The recommended unit is the B-D Vacutainer* (without additive). The specimens should be allowed to clot at room temperature for a few hours before overnight refrigeration. The following day the serum is decanted from the clot into a sterile centrifuge tube. Centrifuge the sample at 2,500 rpm for 20 to 30 minutes and remove the serum into a sterile vial without disturbing the red cells. The nonhemolyzed serum sample can be frozen at −10 to −20 C and shipped immediately, under refrigeration, or sent later with a second sample drawn from the same animal. Under no circumstances should the blood sample be frozen before the serum is harvested from the collected specimen. Proper labeling of each sample identified with a given animal and with proper date is essential to a correct diagnosis.

*Becton-Dickinson Company, Rutherford, New Jersey, USA.

REFERENCES

1. Casey. Health Lab. Sci., 1970, *7,* 233.
2. Cottral, George E. (ed.). Manual of standardized methods for veterinary microbiology, Cornell University Press, Ithaca, N.Y., 1978.
3. Foster, Peterson, and Spendlove. Proc. Soc. Exp. Biol. Med., 1975, *150,* 155.
4. Kärber. Arch Exp. Path. Pharmokol., 1931, *162,* 480.
5. Lennette, David A., and Nathalie J. Schmidt. Diagnostic procedures for viral and rickettsial infections, 4th ed. Am. Pub. Health Assoc., New York, 1969.
6. Saunders, Clinard, Bartlett, and Sanders. Jour. Inf. Dis., 1977, *136,* 258.
7. Sever. Jour. Immunol., 1960, *88,* 320.
8. Takatsy. Acta Microbiol. Acad. Sci., 1955, *3,* 1955.

Diagnosis of Viral Diseases by Electron Microscopy

With improvements in the performance of the electron microscope and new techniques such as negative-staining with phosphotungstic acid in the preparation of specimens diagnosis of some viral diseases has become possible, particularly those agents involved in the production of enteric viral diseases.

This method was used by Mebus (1969), who found viral particles about 65 nm in the feces of calves with acute diarrhea. About 4 years later medical virologists described the presence of similar particles in infants and young children with acute diarrhea. Now the examination of excretions, secretions, and solid tissues for viral particles has become a routine procedure in some diagnostic laboratories and especially in research laboratories in a search for viral particles as a possible etiology of an animal disease epidemic.

The method of preparing specimens for electron microscopy allows for some concentration of the virus so that virus at 10^5 particles per ml is just detectable, 10^6 particles provides a greater degree of detection, and 10^8 particles provides a rapid diagnosis (1). The diagnosis is possible if the particles have a characteristic morphology. This is the case for the most important viruses causing acute diarrhea in any species (Figures 38.11, 38.12, and 38.13). The sensitivity and accuracy of the diagnosis can be enhanced by mixing known viral antisera with the suspect viral specimen. This procedure is known as the immune electron microscopy technique. In a positive reaction there is a clumping of viral particles bound together by antibody (Figure 38.14). This latter technique provided the breakthrough on hepatitis A infection in humans that defied the efforts of many talented and experienced investigators for many years.

The procedure for preparing fecal specimens for examination is easy but time-consuming (1). An experienced worker can check at most 40 fecal specimens in one day. As a consequence, with the development of other procedures for diagnosis such as tissue culture, ELISA test, crossed-electrophoresis, or complement fixation in which 400 specimens can be processed in the same time, electron microscopy is being superseded, yet it is still used to verify a diagnosis in doubtful cases, and particularly where mixed viral infection may be responsible for enteric disease. Various viruses have been demonstrated in stool specimens such as rotaviruses, parvoviruses, coronaviruses, caliciviruses, adenoviruses, astroviruses, and enteroviruses (such as hepatitis A). Some are definitely responsible for disease in domestic animals—rotaviruses, parvoviruses, coronaviruses (Figures 38.11, 38.12, and 38.13), caliciviruses, and adenoviruses.

The electron microscope definitely plays an important role in the modern and well-equipped diagnostic laboratory. It clearly has its limitations and never serves as a sensitive method for detecting small concentrations of virus and obviously can never supplant viral isolation in cell culture or in animals.

REFERENCES

1. Flewett. Jour. Am. Vet. Med. Assoc., 1978, *173,* 538.

The Differential Diagnosis of Viral Respiratory Diseases of Domestic Animals

The differential diagnosis of infectious diseases of domestic animals offers the student and veterinary practitioner one of his greatest challenges yet also contributes to their frustrations. This is especially true of the respiratory diseases, principally those of viral origin. Their disease manifestations are so similar that differential diagnosis is possible only through laboratory procedures ranging from simple cytologic examination to the isolation of the agent(s). Some viral respiratory diseases are further complicated by secondary infections with opportunist bacterial pathogens or even another virus. A clinical diagnosis can be no more than a calculated guess as the problem in domestic animals is similar in complexity to the "common cold" in humans.

To assist the practitioner in the proper selection of biological materials for diagnosis of respiratory infections, tables depicting the major characteristics of the principal respiratory viral infections of domesticated animals are given below. In the preparation of Tables 38.1 (1) and 38.2 (2) some of the information was extracted from information developed by the respective panels of the American Veterinary Medical Association Symposia. The practitioners on these panels felt that this type of table would be quite useful to the student and veterinarian in their understanding of respiratory complexes and as an aid in arriving at a differential diagnosis.

REFERENCES

1. American Veterinary Medical Association. Panel, Bovine Respiratory Disease Supplement. Jour. Am. Vet. Med. Assoc., 1968, *152,* 713.
2. American Veterinary Medical Association. Panel, Feline Infect. Diseases Report. Jour. Am. Vet. Med. Assoc., 1971, *158,* 835.

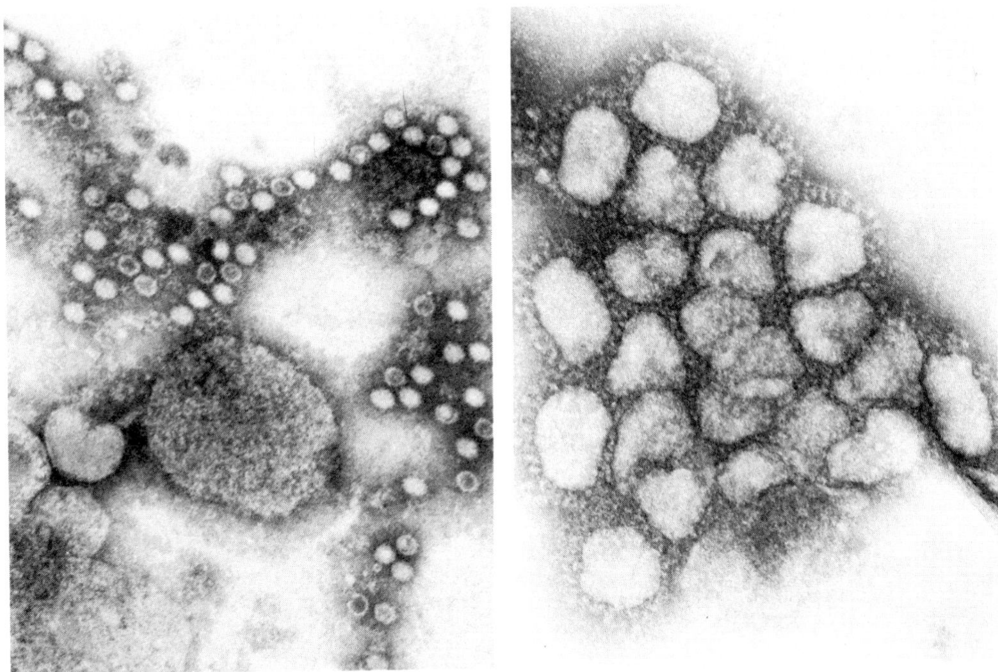

Figure 38.11 (*left*). Canine parvovirus. Viral particles in feces of a dog with a natural case of acute diarrhea. × 127,000. (Courtesy Helen Greisen.)

Figure 38.12 (*right*). Canine coronavirus. Particles in the feces of a dog with a natural case of acute diarrhea. × 122,000. (Courtesy Helen Greisen.)

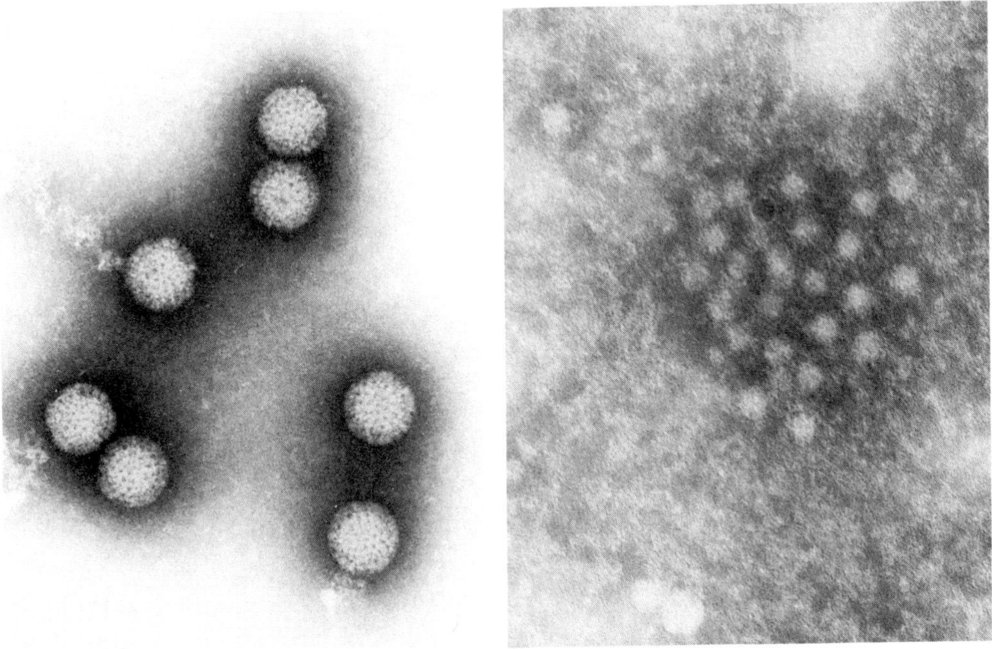

Figure 38.13 (*left*). Canine rotavirus isolated in Vero cells from a dog with acute diarrhea. × 127,000. (Courtesy Helen Greisen.)

Figure 38.14 (*right*). Human hepatitis A virus (enterovirus). Particles in infective spleen demonstrated by immune electron microscopy. Note the fuzzy outline of the particles caused by the antigen-antibody interaction. × 154,000. (Courtesy M. Frey and J. Gillespie.)

Table 38.1. Characteristics of chlamydial* and viral respiratory infections of cattle†

	Infectious bovine rhinotracheitis (IBR) (respiratory form only)	Parainfluenza 3 Infection (PI-3)‡	Bovine rhinovirus (BRH)
Agent	Infectious bovine rhinotracheitis virus, a bovine herpesvirus	Bovine parainfluenza 3 virus	Bovine rhinovirus, 2 sero-types
Known geographic distribution	Worldwide	Worldwide	Germany, USA, England
Incubation, natural infection	4 to 5 days	5 to 10 days	2 to 4 days
Age	Any, usually in young stock	Any	Any
Signs	Respiratory form only—varies markedly in severity as a herd infection. Characterized by high fever, depression, inappetence, and copious mucopurulent exudate initially followed by nasal ulcers, necrosis of muzzle and nostril wings, dyspnea, mouth breathing, conjunctivitis, coughing, and sometimes bloody feces. WBC mostly normal	Seldom occurs in calves. In adult cattle respiratory signs encompass those associated with a fibrinous pneumonia such as coughing, difficult breathing, extended neck, foamy saliva	Serous nasal discharge, temperature, coughing, depression, dyspnea
Course of disease	In respiratory form some cattle may die acutely, but most of them run a disease course for a few days	4 to 7 days, occasionally longer	Approximately 1 week
Morbidity	In USA varies from 10 to 35 percent in cattle population	High in infected herds	Probably high
Mortality	Varies but in U.S. feedlots the average mortality is 10 percent	Varies markedly, but can be moderate in cattle shipped during cold weather	Little or none
Pathologic findings	Highly inflamed mucous membranes of upper respiratory tract with shallow erosions with a glary, fetid mucopurulent exudate. These lesions may be found in the pharynx, larynx, trachea, and larger bronchi. Sometimes patchy purulent pneumonia. Ulceration and inflammation of the abomasal mucosa is found, and catarrhal enteritis may occur	Lesions confined principally to respiratory tract. White fibrinous mass on lung surface. Lungs may be solid and heavy, filling the thoracic cavity. Cut sections show deep red and grayish lobules separated by interlobular tissue, greatly thickened by infiltration of coagulated exudate on serous surface	Principal lesions occur in nasal passages. A pneumonia in calves can occur after experimental intratracheal inoculation
Inclusions	Intranuclear inclusion bodies occur in epithelial cells of respiratory tract	Intracytoplasmic inclusion bodies in nasal and bronchial epithelial and alveolar macrophages that show marked fluorescence with specific antibody conjugate	None reported in cattle or in cell culture

Bovine adenovirus (BA)	Bovine virus diarrhea-mucosal disease (BVD-MD)	Malignant catarrhal fever (MCF)	Bovine reoviruses (BRE)
Eight serotypes	BVD-MD virus	A bovine herpesvirus	Bovine reovirus—3 serotypes
USA, England, Hungary, Japan	Worldwide	Africa, most countries of south and central Africa, North America	Probably worldwide
Several days	6 to 9 days	Unknown. Exp. infection in cattle 10 to 44 days	Few days
Usually in calves	Any	Any	Any
Signs associated with a pneumoenteritis	In clinical cases, diphasic temperature reaction, usually a dry, harsh, nonproductive cough, and a watery conjunctivitis, no dyspnea, excessive salivation with erosions in oral cavity, mucoid and sometimes blood-tinged diarrhea, and bluish discoloration of muzzle. Abortions. Leukopenia often followed by leukocytosis	Initially, a fever lasting 1 to 2 days coinciding with inappetence and depression. Then inflammation of nasal passages, oral cavity, and eyes occurs. Difficult breathing follows and fibrinopurulent pneumonia may occur. Nervous signs develop early in most cases with either stupor or excitement	Usually inapparent infection. Presently recognized as a mild respiratory infection
Weeks in some instances	Usually subclinical, few days as a rule, occasionally chronic, persisting for months	Varies markedly. Sometimes death in 24 hours; usually 5 to 14 days	Unknown
High in infected herds	Moderate to high	Low; usually only 1 to 2 cattle in herd will show signs	Believed high
Low to moderate in infected herds	Low to high	Extremely high	Little or none
Varying degrees of pneumonia with proliferative bronchiolitis with necrosis and bronchiolar occlusion causing alveolar collapse. Lesions may persist for weeks	The lesions are not confined to the respiratory tract; in fact the principal lesions are found in the oral cavity, digestive tract, and lymphatic system	Dark, swollen glassy membranes of turbinates and nasal sinuses covered with fibrin shreds and purulent excretion with shallow ulcers under this mass. Similar lesions seen in larynx, trachea, bronchi, and sometimes bronchopneumonia. Swollen head and lymph nodes. Inflammation and erosion of abomasum and small intestine sometimes occurs. Meninges congested and hemorrhagic. Nonpurulent encephalitis	Interstitial pneumonia and lymphadenitis of regional nodes
Intranuclear inclusion bodies in bronchiolar epithelium, septal cells, and bronchial lymph nodes	None	Inconclusive. Some investigators report nerve-cell intranuclear inclusion bodies; others cytoplasmic inclusion bodies in epithelial cells	Unknown but should be present in bronchiolar epithelium

Table 38.1.—*continued*

	Infectious bovine rhinotracheitis (IBR) (respiratory form only)	Parainfluenza 3 infection (PI-3)‡	Bovine rhinovirus (BRH)
Other natural hosts	None known; goats can be experimentally infected	PI-3 virus has been isolated from man, water buffalo, horses, and monkeys	None reported
Propagation	Tissue culture; cytopathic effects in kidney cells from cattle, pig, dog, sheep, goat, and horse	Replicates in many types of cell cultures from many species, causing CPE and hemadsorption. Causes syncytia and cytoplasmic and intranuclear inclusion bodies	CPE produced in bovine kidney cell cultures at 33 C
Carrier state	Virus may persist for weeks	Known to persist in lungs for at least 18 days	Unknown
Diagnosis	Sometimes possible on basis of history and character of the disease. Viral isolation from exudate of nasal passage in tissue culture. SN, FA, CF, gel-diffusion tests	Virus readily isolated from nasal exudate in cell culture. HI, HA-I, FA, and SN tests	Difficult clinically. Virus isolation in cell culture. SN test
Immunity	Long-term serviceable immunity	Maternal immunity apparently confers protection. The degree and duration of active immunity is yet to be determined with certainty	Status vague, immunity may be incomplete
Prophylaxis	Inactivated and attenuated virus vaccines	Inactivated vaccines, one incorporating PI-3 virus and *Pasteurella* organism, appear to be effective in controlling field disease	No vaccine available
Treatment	Antibiotic therapy and supportive measures	Antibiotic therapy is useful, as bacteria play an important role in the pathogenesis of the disease. Warm and dry quarters and supportive measures are important	Antibiotic therapy may be useful; supportive treatment

*Chlamydial respiratory disease in cattle is similar to that described for sheep and goats in Table 38.6, and it is sometimes called pneumoenteritis in calves.

†See Table 38.6 for description of Rift Valley fever in sheep and cattle; the disease is less severe in cattle.

‡*Pasteurella* organisms are usually involved in this disease.

Bovine adenovirus (BA)	Bovine virus diarrhea-mucosal disease (BVD-MD)	Malignant catarrhal fever (MCF)	Bovine reoviruses (BRE)
Not determined	Perhaps sheep, goats, and also white-tailed and mule deer	Possibly sheep and African wildebeests	May infect man and other animals; not known for certainty
Tissue culture; calf kidney and testes	Tissue culture; cell cultures derived from bovine tissues. Some strains produce CPE, others do not	Tissue culture; thyroid or adrenal gland cultures	Tissue culture—produces CPE in bovine kidney, pig kidney, and monkey kidney
21 days known but probably longer	Possibly, but little known	Unknown	At least 1 month
Isolation in calf testes cell cultures from exudate of nasal passages or from feces; SN, HI, and agar gel tests	Clinical signs, but more specifically upon lesions in severe cases; may be confused with rinderpest, malignant catarrhal fever, and certain respiratory diseases. Isolation of virus from blood or excretions and selected tissues in cell culture. Noncytopathic strains are identified in culture by exaltation or interference tests. SN and agar gel tests	Clinical diagnosis is possible when sporadic cases with nervous and eye manifestations occur in a herd	Virus is isolated from nasal passages and conjunctiva in tissue culture. SN, HI tests
Duration of immunity presently unknown	Complete and long-lasting immunity	Uncertain	No evidence of maternal immunity. Degree and duration of active immunity unknown
None	Attenuated virus vaccine available; do not use in pregnant cows	None. Keep sheep away from cattle	None at present
Antibiotics to assist in control of bacterial invaders; supportive measures	Supportive measures	None	Antibiotics may be useful in controlling secondary bacterial infections such as *Pasteurella* organisms

Table 38.2. Characteristics of chlamydial and viral respiratory infections of cats

	Rhinotracheitis (FVR)	Calicivirus infection (FPI)	Reovirus infection (FRI)	Pneumonitis (FPN)
Agent	Herpesvirus serotype 1	Calicivirus; 1 serotype and 1 serological variant (picornavirus)	Reovirus serotypes 1 and 3	*Chlamydia psittaci (Miyagawanella felis; Bedsonia felis)*
Known geographic distribution	USA, Europe, New Zealand	USA, Europe, Australia, New Zealand, Japan	USA	USA, Europe
Incubation, natural infection	Several days	Usually 1 to 3 days shorter than for FVR	4 to 19 days	6 to 10 days
Age	Any	Any	Any	Any
Signs	Sneezing and coughing, sometimes paroxysmal; salivation, ocular and nasal exudation, oral breathing, fever, inappetence, weight loss; pregnant females occasionally abort; some fatal generalized infection in newborn kittens; sinusitis, ulcerative keratitis, panophthalmitis in chronic infections. Leukocytosis when accompanied by bacterial infection	Asymptomatic to severe, depending on virus strain. Conjunctivitis, ocular discharge often unilateral, rhinitis, sneezing, depression, inappetence, dyspnea, rales, other abnormal lung sounds, and pneumonia; fever, often diphasic; ulcers on tongue and hard palate, preceded by salivation; mortality in newborn cats. Early transient lymphopenia in some cases. May be involved in urolithiasis	Generally mild, with lacrimation, photophobia, serous conjunctivitis, gingivitis, and depression; nasal discharge and fever rarely. WBC mostly normal; no leukopenia	Sneezing, drooling, lacrimation, ocular and nasal discharge, occasional cough, fever, and inappetence. A related strain thought to cause unilateral purulent conjunctivitis often affects other eye in 5 to 7 days. May be enzootic in catteries. May infect newborn or newly introduced cats. Occasional sneezing and nasal discharge; fever uncommon. Leukocytosis inconsistently
Course of disease	Usually 2 to 4 weeks	Average of 7 to 10 days	1 to 26 days	A few days to several weeks
Morbidity	High	High	About 50% among contact controls	Variable
Mortality	Low in adults	Variable; up to 30% in experimental infections	Low	Low in adults

Pathologic findings	Necrotizing conjunctivitis, rhinitis, and tracheitis associated with intranuclear inclusions; sinusitis, resorption of turbinates in chronic infections; in some cases, patchy or general consolidation in anterior lung lobes characterized by necrotizing bronchiolitis and proliferation of alveolar septal cells; secondary bacterial or mycotic infections may occur*	Conjunctivitis, rhinitis, ulcers of the tongue and palate, patchy bronchopneumonia. Alternately dark and pale red banding of spleen associated with calicivirus infection in some cats	Conjunctivitis	Conjunctivitis, rhinitis, laryngitis, pharyngitis, patchy pneumonic consolidation in anterior lung lobes
Inclusions	Intranuclear inclusions in respiratory epithelial cells, nictitating membrane, tongue, and tonsils	None	Paranuclear cytoplasmic inclusions	Intracytoplasmic elementary bodies in respiratory and conjunctival epithelial cells
Other natural hosts	None known	None known	Reovirus 1 and 3 isolated from many mammals	None
Propagation	Tissue culture; cells of feline origin	Tissue culture; cells of feline origin	Tissue culture, feline and bovine kidney cells	Chicken embryo or cell culture
Carrier state	Yes	Yes	Not determined	Yes
Diagnosis	Demonstration of intranuclear inclusions early in course of infection, tissue culture isolation, SN, HA, HI, FA tests	Tissue culture isolation, SN, FA tests	Tissue culture isolation, SN, HA tests	Demonstration of elementary bodies in Giemsa-stained material, animal inoculation, CF test
Immunity	Weak, transient	Many serotypes; homologous protection likely	Not determined, but likely	Weak, transient
Prophylaxis	Attenuated virus vaccine	Attenuated virus vaccine (1 serotype)	None	Vaccine is available
Treatment	Antibiotics indicated for secondary invaders, supportive measures	Antibiotics indicated for secondary invaders, supportive measures	Symptomatic	Tetracyclines systemically and in ophthalmic ointment; supportive measures occasionally needed

*Experimental intravenous inoculation results in necrosis in growth regions of all bones, focal necrosis in adrenal glands and liver, and, in pregnant females, placental necrosis, fetal death, and abortion.

Table 38.3. Characteristics of viral respiratory infections of horses

	Equine herpesvirus infection (EHI)	Equine influenza (EI)
Agent	Equine herpesvirus 1 (equine rhino-pneumonitis virus); equine cytomegaloviruses under investigation	Equine influenza virus. Two types designated A/Equi-1/Praha/56 and A/Equi-2/Miami/63
Known geographic distribution	USA, Europe	Worldwide
Incubation, natural infection	*Weanling disease*—a few days *Abortion disease*—3 to 4 weeks	1 to 3 days
Age	Any	Any
Signs	*Weanling disease*—mild febrile reaction accompanied by rhinitis or nasal catarrh; usually in fall of year *Abortion disease*—infection in mares causes abortion (usually between 6 and 10 months of pregnancy) with no other signs. Rare cases of nervous disease. Sometimes a leukopenia in weanlings	Coughing is most common sign of illness. High temperature, inappetence, mental depression, photophobia, lacrimation, cloudy cornea, nasal catarrh, swollen lymph nodes of head. If pneumonia develops, horse usually dies from bacterial infection
Course of disease	Foals usually recover in 8 to 10 days	1 to 3 weeks, sometimes longer
Morbidity	Very high in foals in infected herds; varies from 10 to 90 percent on stud farms	Highly contagious with high morbidity
Mortality	No mortality in weanlings. Only rarely in mares, but loss of foals through abortions may be high	Usually does not exceed 5 percent
Pathologic findings	*Weanlings*—Reddening of mucous membranes of upper air passages with a collective mucopurulent exudate *Aborting mares*—No lesions *Aborted fetuses*—Multiple focal liver necrosis, petechial hemorrhages in heart muscle and in capsules of spleen and liver; lung edema	Principal lesions in fatal cases are extensive edema of lungs or a bronchopneumonia with pleurisy; hydrothorax; gelatinous infiltrations around larynx and in the legs; swollen lymph nodes
Inclusions	Intranuclear inclusion bodies are found in hepatic cells, and also in epithelial cells and endothelial cells of various organs of aborted fetuses	None
Other natural hosts	None known	Only members of equine family

Equine rhinovirus infection (ERI)	Equine parainfluenza infection (EPI)	African horsesickness (AHS)
2 Equine rhinovirus serotypes; possibly a third serotype	Parainfluenza virus. Limited information about virus and the disease	Equine orbivirus (Reoviridae). Nine distinct immunological types
North America, South America, Africa	USA and Canada	Africa, Middle East, parts of Asia
3 to 7 days	Few days	Probably 7 to 9 days
Any, mostly young animals	Any. Usually occurs in young horses.	Any
Fever, anorexia, serous, followed by mucopurulent nasal discharge, cough	Mucopurulent discharge and other signs referable to respiratory tract, fever	Acute form characterized by respiratory signs with death resulting from severe edema in the lungs. There is fever, labored breathing, coughing, severe dyspnea, and copious foamy nasal discharge. Chronic cases also include heart distress coupled with edema of head and neck tissues
About 1 week	4 to 7 days, sometimes longer	3 to 5 days average; may be longer
Infected stables—high morbidity	Moderate to high in limited surveys	Usually high; spreads very rapidly
Low	Low	25 to 95 percent
Marked pharyngitis, lymphadenitis, abscesses in submaxillary lymph nodes	Insufficient information	Depends upon severity of case. *In acute type* thoracic cavity contains liters of fluid and lungs are distended. A yellowish fluid separates interlobular tissue from alveolar portions. The lung surfaces are wet and fluid runs from cut surface. Pericardial sac may have excess fluid and subendocardial hemorrhages usually are present. Some fluid is present in abdominal cavity, the liver is swollen and intestines reddened. *In chronic form,* edema of head and neck; hydropericardium and hydropic degeneration of myocardium. Lungs and thoracic cavity have moderate edema
None	Unknown	Unknown—should be present in bronchiolar epithelium
None known	Unknown	Zebras, dogs, angora goats, mules, donkeys

Table 38.3.—*continued*

	Equine herpesvirus infection (EHI)	Equine influenza (EI)
Propagation	It has been adapted to hens' eggs. Replicates and produces CPE in cell cultures of fetal horse kidney, lamb kidney, and rabbit kidney	Embryonated hen's egg is best. Tissue cultures of monkey kidney more susceptible than bovine, equine, or human kidney cells
Carrier state	Not studied	Suggested that some horses remain carriers for months
Diagnosis	Clinical diagnosis of respiratory disease is difficult; aborting disease less complicated. Intranuclear inclusion bodies help establish diagnosis. Virus can be isolated from affected tissues in cell culture. SN, CF, precipitation tests	Usually can be diagnosed in an outbreak on basis of history, clinical signs and lesions. virus isolation from nasal exudate in hens' eggs or tissue culture. SN and HI tests
Immunity	Probably transitory immunity, lasting few years	Solid immunity to natural disease for 1 year
Prophylaxis	In USA an attenuated virus vaccine is recommended	Two types of inactivated vaccine available. Yearly vaccination required
Treatment	None	Antibiotic therapy indicated to control bacterial infection. Supportive measures

Equine rhinovirus infection (ERI)	Equine parainfluenza infection (EPI)	African horsesickness (AHS)
Rabbits, guinea pigs, monkeys and man susceptible to intranasal instillation. Tissue culture: cells of many animal species	Tissue culture	Tissue culture: cell cultures derived from baby hamster, bovine kidney and others with production of CPE and cytoplasmic inclusion bodies; suckling mice
At least 1 month	Unknown	*Culicoides* (midges) are probable vectors. Direct transmission does not occur
Isolation of virus in cell culture from nasal excretions. SN test	Isolation of virus in cell culture. SN, HA-I, HA, HI, CF tests	May be confused with other diseases, especially when first occurring in virgin territory. Laboratory diagnosis required by virus isolation from infective blood or tissues inoculated intracerebrally into suckling mice. SN, CF, agar gel, FA, HI tests, HI used for viral serotyping
Limited knowledge. Evidence of maternal immunity and active immunity protection	Unknown	Apparent excellent immunity to homotypic serotype
No vaccine available although one is needed	No vaccine available	Multiple mouse-brain virus vaccine available. Given annually. Stable nonvaccinated horses at night
Antibiotic therapy to help control bacterial invaders	Antibiotic therapy may be useful. Supportive measures and good nursing in warm, dry quarters	No treatment is effective

Table 38.4. Characteristics of chlamydial* and viral respiratory infections of dogs

	Canine distemper (CD)	Infectious canine hepatitis (ICH)
Agent	Canine distemper virus	Canine adenoviruses 1 & 2; canine 2 causes its major effects in the respiratory tract
Known geographic distribution	Worldwide	Worldwide
Incubation, natural infections	4 to 6 days	5 to 9 days
Age	Any	Any
Signs	Some infections are inapparent; principal signs in others may be respiratory, enteric, or nervous or a combination of them. Respiratory signs include watery discharge from eyes and nose, which may become mucoid in 24 hours; diphasic temperature; and pneumonia may develop as a result of bacterial infection. Leukopenia followed sometimes by leukocytosis	*Classic hepatic form* characterized by fever, intense thirst, sometimes edema of extremities, diarrhea, vomiting, intense pain, serous nasal discharge. *Respiratory form* characterized by 1- to 3-day fever, harsh and dry hacking cough, serous nasal discharge sometimes becoming purulent, muscular trembling, depression, dyspnea. In hepatic form there is a leukopenia, but in respiratory form total WBC are variable
Course of disease	Usually 2 to 3 weeks; may last longer in few cases	*Hepatic form*—5 to 10 days *Respiratory form*—5 to 28 days
Morbidity	High	High
Mortality	Varies markedly in outbreaks, usually related to brain involvement. Probably averages 20 percent in clinical cases	10 to 25 percent overall; especially high in puppies
Pathologic findings	Viremic disease with affinity for epithelial cells thus capable of producing a wide variety of lesions. There is a viral-induced giant cell pneumonia which may be complicated by bacterial infection causing a purulent bronchopneumonia. There may be enteritis, encephalitis, vesicular and pustular skin lesions, atrophied and gelatinous thymus gland, eye lesions, urinary and reproductive system lesions	*Hepatic form*—characterized by edema and hemorrhage. Fibrinous peritonitis with blood-tinged fluid in cavity; hydrothorax; marked thickening of gall bladder; swollen liver; lung edema; uveitis. *Respiratory form*—moderate to severe pneumonic changes. Proliferative, adenomatous changes are seen in lungs of dogs with infection for 10 days
Inclusions	Cytoplasmic and/or intranuclear inclusion bodies in many epithelial cells; particularly seen in bronchi, bladder, renal pelvis, and glial cells	*Hepatic form*—intranuclear inclusion bodies in hepatic and endothelial cells. *Respiratory form*—intranuclear inclusion bodies in bronchial epithelium, alveolar septal cells, and turbinate epithelium
Other natural hosts	Principally members of canine family	Foxes (often show nervous disease), wolves, coyotes, bears, raccoons?

Canine parainfluenza (SV-5)	Canine reovirus infection (CRI)	Canine herpesvirus (CH)
Parainfluenza II virus (SV-5)	Canine reovirus 1	Canine herpesvirus
USA	USA	USA, Great Britain, and Europe
2 to 3 days	Uncertain	3 to 8 days in puppies
Any	Any	Any
Sudden onset, copious nasal discharge, fever, and coughing. If *Bordetella bronchiseptica* and *Mycoplasma* are involved, a dry cough persists for weeks	Experimental dogs from conventional sources showed elevated temperature and respiratory signs and pneumonia. Sometimes causes enteritis. Germ-free dogs became infected without signs of illness	*Puppies*—labored breathing, abdominal pain, yellowish green stool, anorexia, and acute death. *Older dogs*—vaginitis and mild rhinitis
1 to 7 days; weeks in cases with complications	Not well studied	In 1- to 2-week-old puppies 1 to 2 days; older dogs—unknown
Low to moderate	Low to moderate	Low to moderate
Low	Low	High in 1- to 2-week-old puppies; negligible in older dogs
Usually no gross lesions except petechial hemorrhages in respiratory tract. Microscopic catarrhal changes are present in lower and upper respiratory tract and also in regional lymph nodes	Pneumonia and enteritis	*Puppies*—disseminated focal necrosis and hemorrhages found in virtually all internal organs, especially kidney. Lungs are diffusely pneumonic. Meningoencephalitic lesions frequently seen but without nervous signs
Unknown	Unknown	Intranuclear inclusion bodies in cells in areas of necrosis are found
Monkeys, man, dogs, perhaps others	Unknown, may infect man and other animals	Not known

Table 38.4.—*continued*

	Canine distemper (CD)	Infectious canine hepatitis (ICH)
Propagation	Tissue culture—primary and cell lines from various dog tissues support the replication and show CPE. Embryonated hens' eggs with adapted strains. Suckling mice, suckling hamsters, ferrets and many other species are susceptible	Tissue culture; canine, ferret, and swine-kidney monolayer cultures
Carrier state	Footpads—4 to 6 weeks. Brain—at least 49 days in some nervous cases of dogs	Urine—39 weeks Kidney—unknown Tonsils—unknown
Diagnosis	Demonstration of inclusion bodies constitutes a presumptive diagnosis. Isolation of virus constitutes a positive diagnosis—this can be done in dog macrophage cultures. FA and SN tests are excellent methods	Demonstration of intranuclear inclusion bodies. Isolation of virus from pathological lesions in tissue culture; SN, FA, and CF tests
Immunity	Long-term durable immunity to natural disease. Maternal protection may persist for 15 weeks	Solid and long lasting, perhaps life
Prophylaxis	Excellent vaccines are available; for maximum protection yearly vaccination is advised	Inactivated and attenuated virus vaccines
Treatment	Antibiotic therapy recommended for control of bacterial disease; supportive measures	Antibiotics indicated for bacterial invaders, especially respiratory form; supportive measures

*The disease in dogs is similar to that described for sheep and goats in Table 38.6 except dogs have muscle and joint involvement in addition to respiratory signs.

Canine parainfluenza (SV-5)	Canine reovirus infection (CRI)	Canine herpesvirus (CH)
Replicates with CPE and cytoplasmic inclusion bodies in kidney cultures of dog, rhesus monkey, and human embryos. Replicates in amniotic cavity of hens' eggs without death	Produces CPE in dog kidney cell culture	Tissue culture; dog kidney cells
Unknown	Spleen—3.5 weeks	Turbinates—3 weeks Kidney—unknown Nasal—3 weeks
Clinically difficult. Virus isolation with respiratory exudates in cell cultures; HA, HA-I, HI, SN, FA tests	Isolation of virus from nasal exudate or feces in cell culture	Focal renal hemorrhages not seen in CD and ICH. Intranuclear bodies must be differentiated from ICH intranuclear inclusions. Virus can be isolated from many tissues of dead puppies in dog kidney cell cultures. SN, CF tests
Dogs infected naturally or by intranasal route are completely protected. Duration of immunity is low so it has little significance in natural protection	Unknown	Duration of immunity unknown, but puppies from immune mothers are temporarily resistant
No vaccine available although there is a need for one	None	No vaccine available
Antibiotic therapy is indicated to control secondary invaders; supportive measures and good nursing	Antibiotics may be indicated; supportive measures	Supportive measures and especially warm environment for puppies

Table 38.5. Characteristics of viral respiratory infections of swine

	Swine influenza (SI)	Porcine inclusion body rhinitis (PIBR)	Pseudorabies (PR)
Agent	Swine influenza A virus	Type B herpesvirus of pigs	Pseudorabies virus, a herpesvirus
Known geographic distribution	Worldwide	Worldwide	Worldwide
Incubation, natural infection	1 to 3 days	5 to 10 days	4 to 7 days, occasionally longer
Age	Any	Any	Any
Signs	Whole herds seem ill at once. Disease begins with fever, extreme weakness, prostration. Swine exibit muscular stiffness and pain. Some show lung edema and bronchopneumonia and usually die. Coughing also is observed	Severe disease in piglets as acute infection. In pigs over 2 weeks a subacute disease. Signs include sneezing, nasal exudate, inappetence, rapid loss of weight, paralysis, and death in 5 days. Subacute infections limited to respiratory tract. Severe anemia	Pruritis does not occur. Signs in sows usually are mild. Characterized by fever, depression, vomition, respiratory signs, and abortions. In suckling and recently weaned pigs the above signs are more severe
Course of disease	2 to 6 days	Several days	4 to 8 days
Morbidity	High	1- to 2-week-old piglets—probably high. Older pigs—low	May be high
Mortality	Usually less than 4 percent, but may go to 10 percent	1- to 2-week-old piglets—high, Older pigs—low	Young pigs—high Older pigs—very low
Pathologic findings	Principal lesions are in the lungs. Thick, mucilaginous exudate in the bronchioles and bronchi cause atelectasis while remainder is usually pale because of interstitial emphysema. In some cases pneumonia develops and involves the areas in which atelectasis first occurred. Regional nodes are swollen and wet. Spleen is enlarged, and there is hyperemia of stomach mucosa	Mucopurulent rhinitis, sinusitis, and sometimes turbinate atrophy, petechial hemorrhages in kidneys and myocardium	The gross lesions are not extensive; in fatal cases cellular infiltrations and necrosis occur in various parts of nervous system as seen in microscopic sections. Animals may die before virus reaches and causes lesions in anterior part of cord and brain

Inclusions	None	Intranuclear inclusion bodies in enlarged cells of many organs, including brain and particularly tubuloalveolar glands of nasal mucosa	Intranuclear inclusion bodies are not found in swine
Other natural hosts	Man	None known	Cattle, cats, dogs, sheep, rats; horses?
Propagation	Intra-amniotic and intra-allantoic inoculation of 10- to 12-day-old embryonated hens' eggs. Various tissue cultures useful for cultivation and assay	Primary porcine lung-cell cultures—produces CPE and intranuclear inclusion bodies	Chick embryos. Tissue culture; chick, rabbit, guinea pig, dog, and monkey tissues
Carrier state	Complex epizootiology involving earthworms, lung worms, and pigs not completely understood or accepted by all investigators	Unknown	Animals that exhibit no visible signs can transmit the virus
Diagnosis	Embryonated hens' eggs with respiratory exudates. SN, FA, HI, CF, HA-I tests	Herd history, signs, and lesions allow good field diagnosis. Virus from lesions can be isolated in cell culture	More difficult in swine than other animals unless nervous signs occur. Virus can be isolated from lesions by inoculating into brain of rabbits; SN test
Immunity	Believed to be immune after disease but not all investigators agree. Maternal immunity lasts for as long as 13 to 18 weeks	Piglets derive maternal protection from immune dams	Long lasting, perhaps life
Prophylaxis	No vaccine available now: previous one not effective	None	Inactivated and attenuated virus vaccines available. Keep swine separated from cattle. Rat control
Treatment	Antibiotic therapy. Dry, warm quarters beneficial	None	None

Table 38.6. Characteristics of chlamydial and viral respiratory infections of sheep and goats

	Adenomatosis (sheep)	Psittacosis (sheep and goats)	Parainfluenza virus (PIV) infection (sheep)	Rift Valley fever (RVF) (sheep)
Agent	Herpesvirus	*Chlamydia psittaci*	Parainfluenza virus 3. Closely related to bovine and human PI-3 viruses, but not identical	Rift Valley fever virus, arbovirus (Bunyaviridae)
Known geographic distribution	Europe, Peru, Iceland, South Africa, India, Israel, USA	Probably worldwide	USA, Australia	Africa only
Incubation, natural infection	Very long	Usually 6 to 10 days	Unknown	1 to 3 days
Age	Any	Any	Any	Any
Signs	Signs are seen only in sheep over 4 years of age. As air spaces in lungs become obliterated the animals become dyspneic and emaciated	Conjunctival and nasal discharge, lethargy, labored breathing, pneumonia, and hyperthermia. Sometimes diarrhea	Signs referrable to respiratory tract with production of pneumonia	Fever, prostration, rapid course, some vomiting, also show purulent nasal discharge and bloody stools. Ewes abort sometimes without other signs. Severe leukopenia
Course of disease	When sheep become dyspneic, they die in a few days to several weeks from anoxia	Varies, but generally 2 weeks	Usually 1 week; longer in some cases	2 weeks
Morbidity	Low	High in affected flocks	Common and widespread in USA	High
Mortality	High	Rarely fatal; severity determined by secondary bacterial, viral, or *Mycoplasma* infections	Low	*Lambs*—high, often 95 to 100 percent; *Ewes*—probably less than 20 percent; *Cattle*—less than 10 percent
Pathologic findings	Proliferation of cells in lung-supporting tissues with gradual filling of alveoli causing lung consolidation. Recognized as primary lung carcinoma which may metastasize	Intense neutrophilic response; copious mucoid exudates may be found with red lobular consolidation in anterior lobes of lungs. Histologically, it is a typical exudative bronchopneumonia of bronchioles with extension into alveoli	A fibrinous type of pneumonia	Most characteristic lesion is focal necrosis of the liver Other lesions are principally hemorrhages in lymph nodes, gastric and intestinal mucosa, endocardium, and epicardium

Inclusions	Unknown	Elementary bodies are found in cytoplasm of infected cells	Unknown	Intranuclear inclusion bodies in liver
Other natural hosts	None known	Not thoroughly studied. Some strains of *C. psittaci* may cause similar disease in other mammals	Unknown	Cattle and humans
Propagation	Unknown except in sheep	*C. psittaci* grows well in yolk sac of embryonated egg. Also in certain tissue cultures. Mice and guinea pigs are best laboratory animals for propagation	Sheep kidney cell cultures	Cell cultures of chick, rat, mouse, human, lamb, and hamster. Replicates in embryonated hens' eggs. In white mice
Carrier state	Unknown	Carriers do exist	Unknown	Unknown
Diagnosis	Typical lesions at autopsy	Demonstration of elementary bodies are difficult in smears or histological sections of lesions. Principal means is by isolation of exudates in hen's egg, in mouse lung, or guinea pig peritoneal cavity. CF, SN, and other serological tests	Isolation of virus from respiratory exudates in cell culture. SN, HA, HA-I, HI tests	Clinical signs and history highly suggestive. Massive liver focal necrosis characteristic. Inoculation of white mice causes prompt fatal infection with liver and other infective tissues. CF, agar gel, HI tests
Immunity	Animals with signs of illness do not recover	Immune status is unclear	Maternal immune protection exists. Little known about active immunity	Long-term, durable immunity in animals and humans that recover
Prophylaxis	Remove affected sheep from flock	No vaccines are available	No vaccine available	Live-virus vaccines are available but not safe in young lambs or pregnant cattle and ewes. Inactivated vaccines also avaliable. Move animals into mountains away from mosquito vectors if possible
Treatment	None	Chemotherapy is useful—various antibiotics are effective	Antibiotic therapy, but it may not be feasible or practical	No effective treatment

Table 38.7. Characteristics of respiratory viral infections of chickens

	Newcastle disease (ND)	Avian infectious bronchitis (AIB)
Agent	Paramyxovirus	Coronavirus
Known geographic distribution	Worldwide	North America, Japan, England, Europe
Incubation, natural infection	4 to 14 days	2 to 4 days
Age	Any	Any
Signs	Outbreaks vary in intensity—older birds may have inapparent infection, but chicks usually show marked respiratory distress and nervous manifestations appear in a varying percentage a few days later. When nervous signs occur, the death rate is high. In laying birds respiratory signs occur accompanied by a complete cessation in egg production	Severity of respiratory signs is age-dependent, with chicks showing greatest effects, including listlessness, depression, rales, gasping. In laying flocks egg production drops dramatically, and full production is not usually achieved until next laying period
Course of disease	6 to 8 days with respiratory disease; with CNS involvement usually longer	6 to 18 days
Morbidity	High	High
Mortality	Low to high depending on incidence of birds with nervous manifestations	Chicks—25 to 90 percent Older birds—none to low
Pathologic findings	Gross lesions not particularly striking. Fluid or mucous in the trachea, cloudy air-sac membranes. Spleen may be enlarged. Typical viral encephalitic lesions in birds with nervous signs	Mucoid or caseous plugs overlying highly inflamed bronchi and sometimes in nasal passages. Chicks that die usually have fibrinopurulent exudate in lower trachea and larger bronchi
Inclusions	None seen	None

Laryngotracheitis (LT)	Fowlpox virus	Fowl plague (FP)
Laryngotracheitis virus, an avian herpesvirus	Fowlpox virus	Avian influenza A virus
Worldwide	Worldwide	USA, Canada, Europe, South America
2 days	Several days	3 to 5 days
Any	Any	Any
High contagious. Respiratory signs include mouth breathing, gurgling and rattling sounds, nasal exudate in some birds	As a rule, the pox lesions are confined to head; occasionally they are limited to oral cavity and trachea causing a respiratory like disease	Mucoid nasal discharge, fever, edema of head and neck, lethargy, bluish black discoloration of combs and wattles; rapid deaths
5 to 6 days in individual 3 to 4 weeks as a flock	Most birds recover in 3 to 4 weeks	1 to 3 days
Approaches 100 percent in susceptible flocks	High in affected flocks	High
Depends on time of year and stage of production. Young birds in warm weather have low mortality. In heavy layers during winter months may be high	Low to moderate	As a rule, high in chickens
Lesions confined to larynx, trachea, and bronchi and characterized by a reddened petechiated, slimy exudate containing blood. Sometimes exudate is caseous forming a plug which occludes trachea causing suffocation and death	In respiratory form, the infraorbital sinus is involved and greatly distended as a result of a yellowish or brownish caseous exudate. In mouth and trachea there are whitish cankerlike lesions that tend to ulcerate	Usually not numerous. Petechial hemorrhages in heart, gizzard, proventriculus and body cavity serosa. Principal organs may show cloudy swelling and petechial hemorrhages. By microscopic examination, there is a diffuse encephalitis
Intranuclear inclusion bodies in epithelial cells of tracheal lesions	Cytoplasmic inclusions in swollen epithelial cells are termed Bollinger bodies	None

Table 38.7.—*continued*

	Newcastle disease (ND)	Avian infectious bronchitis (AIB)
Other natural hosts	Turkeys, pheasants, ducks, geese, and many other species are naturally infected	None
Propagation	Readily propagated in embryonated hens' eggs and produces a CPE and also replicates in cell cultures of chick origin. Cytoplasmic and intranuclear inclusions occur in cell cultures	Causes dwarfing and curling of chick embryos. Cytopathic effect in chicken embryo kidney cultures
Carrier state	Perhaps as long as 1 month	At least 49 days
Diagnosis	Chicks with respiratory and nervous signs suggest the disease is Newcastle disease; in this instance it must be distinguished from fowl plague. Virus isolation from nasal exudate or tissues with lesions. Can be isolated in hens' eggs. SN, HI tests useful in diagnosis	Difficult to distinguish from Newcastle unless nervous signs are observed, then it can be diagnosed as Newcastle. In older birds must be distinguished from other respiratory infections requiring cultural tests for virus and bacteria. SN, FA, agar gel tests
Immunity	Immunity persists for years	Immune for at least 8 months after infection
Prophylaxis	Vaccines are available. Caution should be exercised in their use in laying flocks	Complicated by multiple serotypes, although attenuated virus vaccines are available and apparently useful
Treatment	Replacement of laying flock at appropriate time may be required to prevent infection of susceptible young stock	Often flocks are disposed of after disease if vaccination is not feasible or desirable

Laryngotracheitis (LT)	Fowlpox virus	Fowl plague (FP)
Occasionally pheasants	Turkeys, pheasants, canaries, and some wild birds	Turkeys (main host in USA and Canada), pheasants, and certain wild birds
Chicken embryos	Chorioallantoic membrane of hens' embryonated eggs. Tissue-culture cells derived from chick embryo tissues	Embryonated hans' eggs and in certain tissue cultures
Yes, for months after infection and serve as source for future infections	Some recovered birds are carriers	Unknown
As flock becomes diseased, diagnosis can be made by signs and lesions. Inoculation of 2 susceptible and 2 resistant birds with trachea exudate provides positive diagnosis	Typical skin pox lesions—or by demonstration of Bollinger bodies in wet preparations. Virus isolation in hens' eggs or tissue culture. SN, HI, CF, agar gel tests	Exceedingly high mortality accompanied by peracute deaths highly suggestive. Confirmation by viral isolation and serology. HI test best
Long-term and complete	Permanent	Solidly immune for several months at least
Conjunctivally administered vaccine strain 146 provides durable immunity after production of conjunctivitis without permanent damage, but carriers may exist	Attenuated fowlpox vaccines available	No vaccine available in USA
Flock disposal may be indicated	In some instances flock disposal may be desirable	Flock disposal may be indicated

SECTION II DNA VIRUS FAMILIES

Viruses are divided into two major groups by the International Committee on Taxonomy of Viruses depending on whether they contain ribonucleic acid (RNA) or deoxyribonucleic acid (DNA). The viruses that contain DNA comprise six families: Parvoviridae, Papovaviridae, Adenoviridae, Iridoviridae, Poxviridae, and Herpesviridae.

39 The Parvoviridae

The family Parvoviridae consists of two genera: *Parvovirus* and *Adeno-associated virus*. The parvoviruses contain single-stranded DNA with a molecular weight of 1.4×10^6 daltons. In members of the *Adeno-associated virus* genus the single strands are complementary and band together *in vitro* to form a double strand. The isometric nonenveloped particles, 18 to 22 nm in diameter with icosahedral symmetry, probably have 32 capsomeres, 2 to 4 nm in diameter. The buoyant density in cesium chloride is 1.4 g per cm^3. The particles are heat-stable and ether- and acid-resistant. Members of the adeno-associated viruses replicate only in the presence of an adenovirus which serves as the "helper" virus (Figure 39.1). All members multiply in the nucleus of the dividing cell.

The type species for the genus *Parvovirus* is *Parvovirus* n-1 (Kilham rat virus). Other members of the genus are the H viruses (H1 and X14), minute mouse-viruses, porcine parvovirus, bovine parvovirus, canine parvovirus, feline panleukopenia (feline parvovirus), minute virus of canines, avian parvovirus, and goose parvovirus. The *Adeno-associated virus* genus includes types 1, 2, 3, and 4. Mink enteritis virus is considered a biological variant of feline panleukopenia virus. Many investigators feel that canine parvovirus is a biotype of feline panleukopenia virus. The inclusion of Aleutian mink virus in the genus *Parvovirus* is done with some reservation, but Porter *et al.* (2) suggest that it is a member of this group; others feel it is a picornavirus (4).

The most significant pathogens of domesticated animals are feline panleukopenia virus, canine parvovirus, mink enteritis virus, and Aleutian disease virus of mink. Other pathogens include the porcine parvovirus and bovine parvovirus (Table 39.1). For information about members of the genus *Parvovirus* that are not discussed in this chapter the reader is referred to articles by Kilham (1) and Toolan (3).

Table 39.1. Diseases in domestic animals caused by viruses in the Parvoviridae family, genus *Parvovirus*

Common name of virus	Natural hosts	Type of disease produced
Feline panleukopenia virus (FPL in cats, enteritis in mink)	Cats, mink	Leukopenia, enteritis, cerebellar hypoplasia (cats)
Bovine parvovirus	Cattle	Fetal death, enteritis, (myocarditis?)
Canine parvovirus (closely related to FPL)	Dogs	Leukopenia, enteritis, myocarditis
Minute virus of canines	Dogs	Diarrhea
Porcine parvovirus	Swine	Fetal death, abortions, infertility
Aleutian disease virus	Mink	Chronic progressive disease. Anorexia, polydipsia, and hemorrages

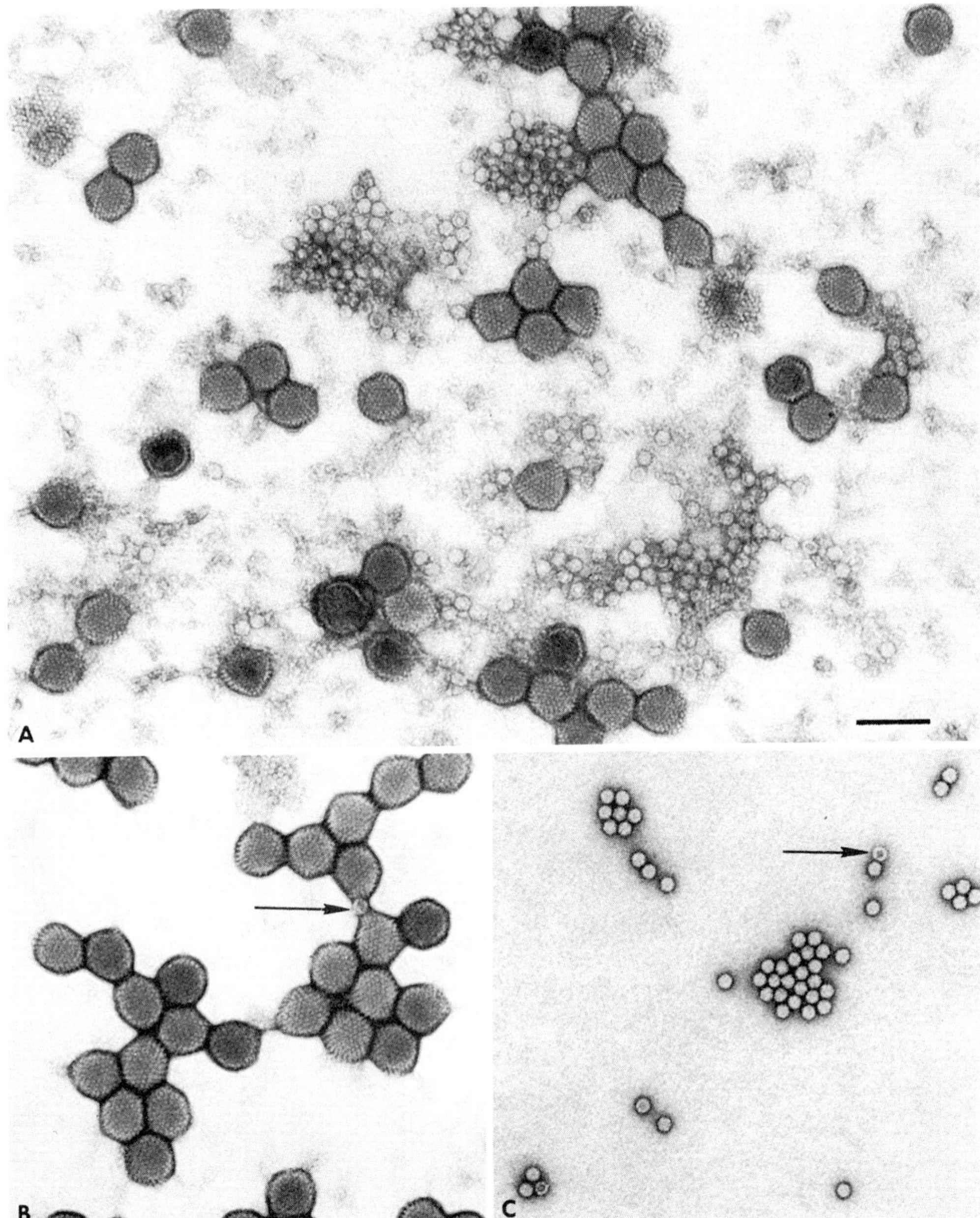

Figure 39.1. (*A*) Crude tissue culture harvest showing many empty and full 22-nm adeno-associated virus (AAV) particles as well as many 80-nm infectious canine hepatitis (ICH) virions. (*B*) ICH virions from the adenovirus band after 48 hours of centrifugation in an isopycnic CsCl gradient; *arrow* shows a single empty 22-nm particle. (*C*) Micrograph showing 22-nm AAV virions in AAV band of 48-hour-old isopycnic CsCl gradient; *arrow* again points out empty AAV capsid. Each preparation stained with 1 percent uranyl acetate. × 102,500. (Courtesy M. David Hoggan and Gunter F. Thomas, NIH.)

REFERENCES

1. Kilham. Viruses of laboratory rodents. Natl. Cancer Inst. Monograph no. 20, 1966, p. 117.
2. Porter, Larsen, Cox, Porter, and Suffin. Intervirol., 1977, *8*, 129.
3. Toolan. Int. Rev. Exp. Path., 1968, *6*, 135.
4. Yoon, Dunker, and Kenyon. Virol., 1975, *64*, 575.

THE GENUS *PARVOVIRUS*

Feline Panleukopenia

SYNONYMS: Feline distemper, feline agranulocytosis, cat plague, cat fever, feline infectious enteritis, feline ataxia; abbreviation, FPL

This disease is highly contagious, and often the mortality rate is high. It undoubtedly occurs in all parts of the world and has been described in France, England, India, Brazil, Canada, and the United States. A disease which may be the same but which is manifested a little differently was described by Seifried and Krembs (36) in Germany. The disease destroys many pet animals and formerly was a scourge in catteries and in animals that had been exposed in cat shows. In the past the disease has been ascribed by various authors to different bacterial agents. The true cause, a virus, was first identified by Verge and Cristoforoni (38) in 1928. The findings of the French workers were confirmed by Hindle and Finlay (14) in England in 1933 and by Leasure, Lienhardt, and Taberner (26) in the United States in 1934. In 1938 Lawrence and Syverton (24) studied a disease that occurred spontaneously in cats kept for laboratory purposes. The disease was manifested by signs that will be described below, but the most striking characteristic was the rapid disappearance of white blood cells from the blood during the early stages of the illness. It was shown to be caused by a virus. The following year Hammon and Enders (13) described the disease independently. They gave it the name *panleukopenia,* because of the almost total disappearance of leukocytes from the blood. There is no doubt that these workers were dealing with the disease known in veterinary circles at that time as *infectious enteritis.* The panleukopenia had not been previously recognized.

Character of the Disease. The disease is seen most often in domestic cats, usually during August, September, and October. Cockburn (4) reports deaths in the London zoo in tigers, leopards, lynxes, servals, ocelots, cheetahs, and some others. He believed the majority of wild Felidae to be susceptible, excepting lions, civets, and genets. Torres (37) found this virus in a fatal disease of caged wild cats. Hyslop (15) transmitted the virus from a domestic cat to two lynxes, then to a cheetah, and then back to a domestic cat in which the typical disease was produced. The signs in the wild cats were very similar to those seen in the house cat.

Schofield (31) in 1949 described a highly fatal disease of mink in Canada which could be readily transmitted with bacteria-free filtrates. In 1952 Wills (39) studied this disease more fully and came to the conclusion that its causative agent was the same as that of feline enteritis. This was confirmed by Gorham and Hartsough (12) in 1955, although Burger *et al.* have some reservations about it (2). Thus, all members of the cat family (Felidae) are susceptible as well as the raccoon, coatimundi, and ringtail in the family Procyonidae and also mink.

The disease infects young cats especially, although older ones are susceptible if they have had no previous contact with it. The affected animal develops lassitude, inappetence, and fever. In animals that are closely watched following natural exposure, a diphasic fever curve usually occurs. The first febrile reaction may reach a peak of 104 to 105 F within a few hours and remain at this level for about 24 hours. It then usually falls to normal, or near-normal, for 36 to 48 hours, at the end of which time it again rises. By the time of the second rise the cat is very ill. It is depressed, has a rough, unkempt coat, lies on its abdomen with its head on its front paws, and is indifferent to its owner or surroundings. Death usually occurs shortly after the peak of the second temperature curve is reached, or the temperature will fall precipitously and the animal recover. Animals lose weight rapidly because of dehydration. Retinal dysplasia has been observed. Vomiting is common. Many of the cases develop a profuse watery diarrhea which is often blood-tinged. Most of them exhibit mucopurulent discharges from the eyes and nose. Gochenour (11) has seen cases in which there was no temperature rise.

Intrauterine infection with FPL virus may result in abortions, stillbirths, early neonatal deaths, or cerebellar hypoplasia (Figure 39.2) manifested by ataxia first seen at 2 to 3 weeks when the kittens become ambulatory (6, 7, 22, 23). The type of teratogenic effects depend on the stage of gestation at the time of infection.

In artificially inoculated animals the incubation period may be as short as 48 hours, but it usually is about 4 days. By natural contact it is generally longer—sometimes as long as 9 days but usually not more than 6 days. The disease progresses to its crisis very rapidly in most instances. According to Riser (29), the average duration is about 5 days, but some animals may die within 3 days and others may last more than a week. Animals that survive as long as 9 days practically always recover.

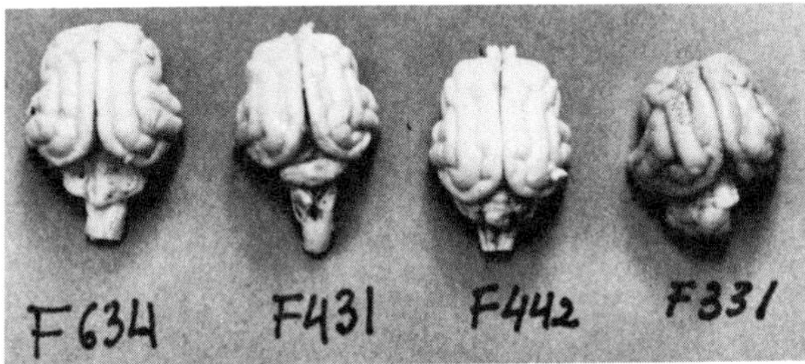

Figure 39.2. Cerebellar hypoplasia caused by feline infectious panleukopenia virus. Infected neonatal kittens F634, F431, and F442 show varying degrees of hypoplasia. The brain labeled F331 has a normal-sized cerebellum removed from an uninfected kitten. (Courtesy C. Csiza.)

The incidence, morbidity, and mortality may vary considerably under field conditions. The morbidity is usually high, but the mortality may run from low to high, in some instances 90 percent. Subclinical infections must occur, as most unvaccinated adult cats have antibody and many cats have never exhibited clinical disease.

Lesions of enteritis are found, usually in the terminal portion of the ileum, where the mucosa may be only slightly inflamed or there may be severe pseudomembranous inflammation. In some cases the inflammation may be more extensive, involving much of the small intestine. The mesenteric lymph nodes may be swollen and hemorrhagic. The red marrow of the long bones is greasy and gelatinous. Microscopically, the principal changes are found in the intestine, bone marrow, and lymphoid organs of natural cases (8). Intestinal lesions were characterized by degenerative changes accompanied by the appearance of intranuclear inclusion bodies in the epithelial cells of the crypts. In contrast to the crypts, the villi were seldom involved (Figure 39.3). Hypoplasia, parenchymal degeneration, and activation of the reticuloendothelial system were observed in the bone marrow and lymphoid organs. Intranuclear inclusion bodies were found occasionally also in the reticular and parenchymal cells of the bone marrow, lymphoid organs, liver, adrenals, and pancreas. Most of the inclusion bodies were amphophilic when stained with hematoxylin and eosin and occupied the whole area of the nucleus without producing any zone of clear halo. While cells bearing inclusion bodies underwent degenerative changes constantly in the intestinal crypts, the formation of inclusion bodies was not accompanied by the degeneration of corresponding cells in any other organ. Pathological changes as mentioned above were considered to be closely related to the systemic infection of feline panleukopenia virus.

The blood reaction in this disease is exceedingly interesting. Lawrence, Syverton, Shaw, and Smith (25) divided their cases into two classes according to the manner in which the leukocytes disappeared from the peripheral circulation under the influence of the virus. In the first group the leukocytes gradually diminished from the time of exposure until the time of the temperature peak. In the other there was little change in the leukocyte count for 5 to 6 days; then during the febrile reaction there was a precipitous drop. From a normal of about 15,000 leukocytes per cu mm the count usually dropped

Figure 39.3. Feline infectious panleukopenia. Intranuclear inclusion bodies in epithelial cells of the small intestine. × 985. (Courtesy C. Csiza.)

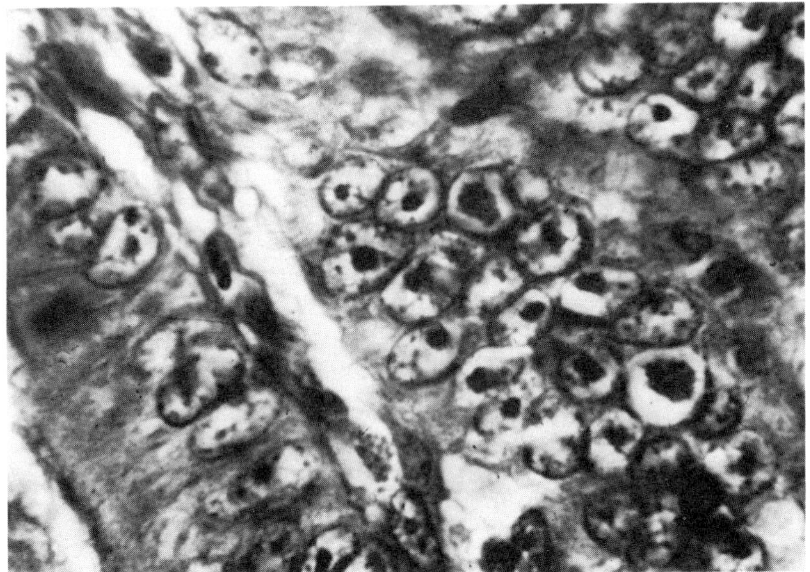

to 2,000 or less, and not infrequently to zero. In about 20 percent of their cases the count varied from 0 to 200 cells per cu mm. During this time there was only a slight decrease in the red cell count and the percentage of hemoglobin. The virus obviously has a severely distructive effect upon the hemopoietic centers.

Mink affected with mink enteritis virus are anoretic and have abnormal enteric mucoid discharges often with blood streaks and intestinal casts. The mortality varies between 10 and 80 percent (9, 31).

The Disease in Experimental Cats. Subclinical or mild infections occur in gnotobiotic cats given virulent virus (30). More recently a study of the infection was made by Carlson and Scott (3) in germ-free and specific-pathogen-free (SPF) kittens. Clinical illness was observed only in the SPF kittens. They had anorexia and slight diarrhea with no deaths. Both groups had thymic involution—the only gross lesion observed. There were more virus-infected cells and lesions in the intestine of SPF kittens. The incidence of infected cells was greater in the proximal jejunum and decreased along the small intestine.

In a pathogenesis study of newborn kittens, every tissue in the body contained virus following intranasal or oral inoculation (6, 7). It appears that the virus first establishes itself in the oral pharynx at 18 hours and then a viremia develops. At 48 hours every tissue has significant amounts of virus, and high titers persist through day 7. As serum antibody appears, virus titers drop precipitously with little or no virus by day 14 in most tissues. Small quantities of virus may persist for 1 year in some tissues such as the kidney (5).

The pathogenesis in the cat is dependent largely on the mitotic activity of various tissues within the body. In the newborn cat the thymus and external granular layer of the cerebellum are undergoing rapid development, and these tissues are severely affected at this stage. In older kittens the infection occurs primarily in the lymphoid tissues of the oropharynx, epithelium of the intestinal crypts, and bone marrow.

The neonatal ferret inoculated intracerebrally is the only animal known to be susceptible other than those previously mentioned (22).

Properties of the Virus. The virus has the principal characteristics of the type species for the genus *Parvovirus*. This DNA virus, which is probably double-stranded, (18, 20, 38) resists ether, chloroform, heat (56 C for 30 minutes), acid, phenol, and trypsin, but can be inactivated by 0.2 percent formalin (16). Its size by electron microscopy is 20 to 25 nm, and the specific gravity is 1.33 g per cm^3 (18, 21). At low temperatures or in 50 percent glycerol the virus is infective for long periods of time.

Reciprocal serum neutralization tests with many isolates and their antisera resulted in equivalent titers in all cases (32). The same results were obtained with mink enteritis, feline ataxia, and feline panleukopenia isolates (17, 19). This is rather good evidence that FPL virus is a single antigenic serotype, and the recently isolated canine parvoviruses are biological variants of FPL virus.

The complement-fixation test has been used by employing a purified mink enteritis virus antigen (21). There is no evidence that FPL virus contains a hemagglutinin (28).

There is no evidence of cross-reaction between FPL virus and other members of the genus, but complete cross testing has not been done. The Kilham rat virus inoculated into neonatal kittens produces degeneration of the cerebellum similar to FPL virus (28).

Cultivation. Cell cultures of feline kidney origin are preferred for the isolation and cultivation of FPL virus. The virus has a selective affinity for the mitotic cell so the best results are obtained when cultures are inoculated with virus 2 to 3 hours after cell seeding. The maximum cytopathic effects are observed after 4 to 5 days at 37 C. Unless the cultures are inoculated with a high viral content the use of May-Gruenwald-Giemsa stain, hematoxylin-eosin stain, or specific fluorescein isothiocyanate conjugate is required to identify the virus in culture as the cytopathic effect (CPE) in unstained cultures is negligible. With the dye stains Cowdry type A intranuclear inclusion bodies can be detected (Figure 39.4). The virus also replicates in cell cultures of a feline-tongue diploid line, of a feline-thymus diploid line, and of a cell line of feline kidney (Crandell), lion kidney, and a feline neurofibrosarcoma (27).

No multiplication of virus occurs in the embryonated hen's egg (10).

Immunity. Neutralizing antibodies appear in the circulation of cats about 3 days after the onset of illness. The titers develop rapidly to reach 1,000 to 10,000 about 10 to 11 days after onset of illness (33). Neutralizing antibody presumably persists in the cat for years, and such cats are protected against a subsequent exposure to virulent challenge virus by various routes of inoculation or by contact exposure to cats acutely ill with FPL infection.

Maternal antibody conferred from the immune dam to its progeny interferes with vaccination and also protects

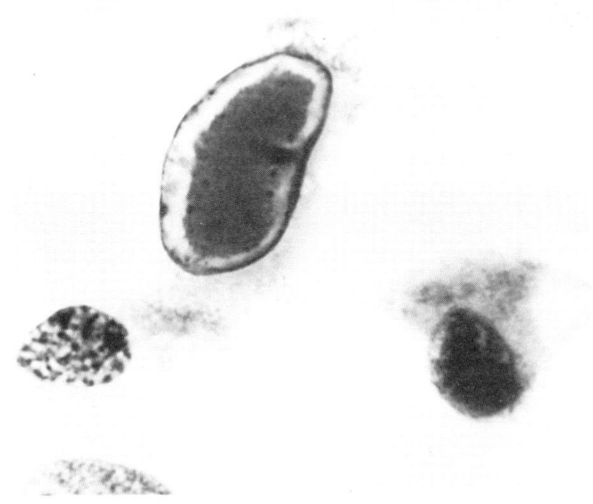

Figure 39.4. Feline infectious panleukopenia. Cowdry type A inclusion bodies in feline kidney cell culture. May-Gruenwald-Giemsa stain. × 880. (Courtesy F. Scott.)

against virulent virus (34). The serum-neutralizing antibody titer of the progeny is equivalent to the dam's 24 to 48 hours after birth, then gradually declines with an antibody half-life of approximately 9.5 days (Figure 39.5). Maternity titers of 30 or greater (tested against 100 $TCID_{50}$ of virus) usually protect kittens against challenge with 1,000 to 3,000 $TCID_{50}$ of virulent challenge virus, and seroconversion does not occur. Attenuated

Figure 39.5. The mean maternal immunity to feline panleukopenia in a group of kittens born to immune queens. (Courtesy F. Scott, C. Csiza, and J. Gillespie, *Jour. Am. Vet. Med. Assoc.*)

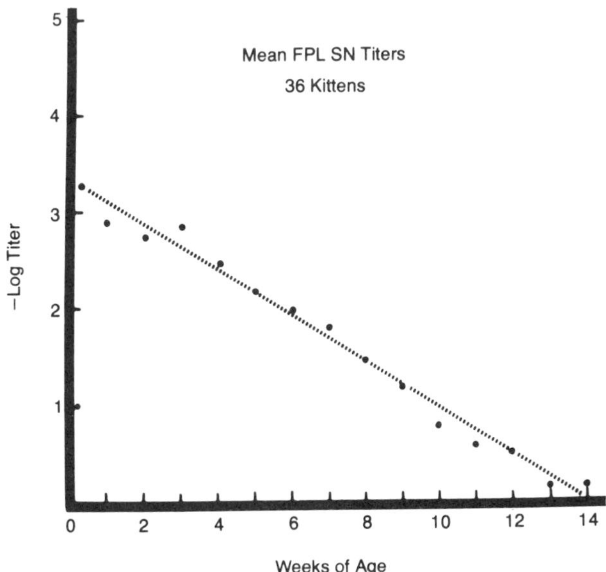

virus vaccines will replicate in kittens with titers of 10 or less and produce an active immunue titer at a high level; any demonstrable maternal antibody interferes with inactivated virus vaccines.

Most field strains produce frank disease in experimental kittens purchased from farms. Subclinical or mild infections occur frequently in susceptible cats with some strains, so the investigator must be selective in his choice of test strain used for challenge (32).

Transmission. Viral transmission usually occurs by direct contact of susceptible cats with infected cats in the acute stage of illness when the virus is excreted in the feces, urine, saliva, and vomitus. It may also occur mechanically by contact with contaminated food dishes, bedding, infected cages, or by humans. Recovered cats may shed the virus in their feces or urine for considerable periods of time with virus known to persist for several weeks in the kidneys of recovered cats and for at least 1 year in the kidneys of neonatally infected cats (5). Recovered mink may shed the virus in their feces for at least 1 year (1).

During acute stage of illness fleas may transmit the disease (18), and it seems likely that biting insects may do likewise.

The virus is extremely stable and probably survives for a considerable period of time in the environment of infected premises.

The facts cited above readily explain how this virus maintains itself in nature.

Diagnosis. A presumptive diagnosis of FPL can be made on basis of the clinical signs and the presence of leukopenia. The diagnosis can be confirmed by pathological lesions, viral isolation, demonstration of immunofluorescence of infected tissues with a specific FPL conjugate, or demonstration of a rising serum titer. The direct immunofluorescent test can be used for detection of virus in cell culture or in tissues.

The serum-neutralization test is generally used to detect antibody (34). Serum dilutions are mixed with an equal volume of virus (100 to 300 $TCID_{50}$ per 0.1 ml). Aliquots of the serum-virus mixtures are incubated at room temperature for 1 hour, and 0.2 ml of each is inoculated into secondary feline kidney cells in Leighton tube coverslip cultures 2 to 3 hours after transfer. After 4 days at 37 C the coverslips are stained and examined for intranuclear inclusion bodies as outlined in the section on cultivation. The metabolic inhibition test or direct examination of unstained cultures can be used if the cultures are good and the proper amount of virus is used in the respective tests. Nonspecific degeneration of cultures often makes the end point difficult to ascertain with these latter methods.

Prevention. There are several excellent biologics for the prevention of feline panleukopenia. Inactivated and attenuated virus vaccines produced an immunity that presumably persists for years, although there is no definite information on this point. Because the disease can be prevented by immunization, clinicians should emphasize the importance of proper vaccination. An evaluation of the types of biologics was made, and various guidelines for their use were recommended by the Panel of the American Veterinary Medical Association Colloquium on Selected Feline Infectious Diseases (9). The Panel made the following recommendations for vaccination based upon information presented at the colloquium.

> The Panel recommends the use of tissue culture origin (TCO), inactivated or modified live-virus (MLV) vaccines, although tissue-type vaccines have been known to be efficacious for years. However, The Panel notes that, according to the information provided at the colloquium, TCO vaccines appear to have a slight advantage for the following reasons: These vaccines tend to break through a low level of maternally derived immunity and hence may be effective in cats of a slightly younger age. They contain less organic material and cause less discomfort at the time of administration. The antigenic content of TCO vaccines is easier to monitor.
>
> Due to varying degrees of maternal antibody in kittens, the Panel recommends administration of two doses of vaccine starting at 9 to 10 weeks of age. For the MLV vaccines, the second vaccination should be given at 14 to 16 weeks of age. If the kittens are older than 12 weeks at the time of the first vaccination with MLV vaccines, a second vaccination is not necessary.
>
> For the inactivated vaccines, the second dose should be given 2 weeks later. For maximum protection, a third vaccination should be given when the cat is 16 weeks old.
>
> Annual revaccination is recommended for maximum protection. Unvaccinated kittens should not be admitted to an area of possible exposure to FPL without immediate vaccination or administration of antiserum. Colostrum-deprived kittens should be given antiserum for immediate protection followed by repeated doses of vaccine as indicated.

The Panel's recommendations for the use of antiserum are as follows: "There are two specific indications for the use of antiserum (or normal serum). First, susceptible cats that have been exposed to FPL should be given antiserum immediately at the rate of 1 ml per pound of body weight. Second, colostrum-deprived kittens should be given antiserum as soon after birth as possible. Vaccines should be given later at appropriate intervals."

Aerosal exposure with modified live-virus vaccine is an effective and practical method for immunization of large numbers of cats against FPL (35).

Control. The disease is difficult to control in a group of cats once the infection starts. Antiserum is quite effective in outbreaks where certain cats have not shown signs of illness at the time of its administration. After signs are observed, the antiserum has little or no benefit.

The stability of this virus dictates thorough cleansing and disinfection of infected premises before the introduction of infected cats. Unless several months have passed, new cats should be vaccinated approximately 2 weeks before introduction into infected premises.

The Disease in Man. There is no evidence that FPL virus causes disease in humans.

REFERENCES

1. Bouillant and Hanson. Can. Jour. Comp. Med. and Vet. Sci., 1965, *29,* 183.
2. Burger, Farrell, and Gorham. West. Vet., 1958, *5,* 68.
3. Carlson and Scott. Vet. Path., 1977, *14,* 79.
4. Cockburn. Vet. Jour., 1947, *103,* 261.
5. Csiza, Scott, de Lahunta, and Gillespie. Am. Jour. Vet. Res., 1971, *32,* 419.
6. Csiza, Scott, de Lahunta, and Gillespie. Jour. Inf. and Immunity, 1971, *3,* 838.
7. de Lahunta. Jour. Am. Vet. Med. Assoc., 1971, *158,* 901.
8. Doi, Okawa, Sokuma, and Okaniwa. Natl. Inst. An. Health Q., 1975, *15,* 76.
9. Feline Infectious Diseases Colloquium. Jour. Am. Vet. Med. Assoc., 1971, *158,* 835.
10. Gillespie. Unpublished observations, 1971.
11. Gochenour. North Am. Vet., 1943, *24,* 104.
12. Gorham and Hartsough. Am. Fur Breed., 1955 (Apr). (Abstract in Jour. Am. Vet. Med. Assoc., 1955, *126,* 467.)
13. Hammon and Enders. Jour. Exp. Med., 1939, *69,* 327.
14. Hindle and Finlay. Jour. Comp. Path. and Therap., 1932, *45,* 11.
15. Hyslop. Brit. Vet. Jour., 1955, *111,* 373.
16. Johnson. Res. Vet. Sci., 1966, *7,* 112.
17. Johnson. Jour. Small Anim. Pract., 1967, *8,* 319.
18. Johnson and Cruickshank. Nature, 1966, *212,* 622.
19. Johnson, Margolis and Kilham. Nature, 1967, *214,* 175.
20. Judkins and Gillespie. Unpublished observations, 1968.
21. Kääriäinen, Kangas, Keränen, Sirkka, Nyholm, and Weckström. Arch. f. die gesam. Virusforsch, 1966, *19,* 197.
22. Kilham, Margolis, and Colby. Lab. Invest., 1967, *17,* 465.
23. Kilham, Margolis, and Colby. Jour. Am. Vet. Med. Assoc., 1971, *158,* 888.

24. Lawrence and Syverton. Proc. Soc. Exp. Biol. and Med., 1938, *38,* 914.
25. Lawrence, Syverton, Shaw, and Smith. Am. Jour. Path., 1940, *16,* 333.
26. Leasure, Lienhardt, and Taberner. North Am. Vet., 1934, *15,* 30.
27. Lee, Kniazeff, Fabricant, and Gillespie. Cornell Vet., 1969, *59,* 539.
28. Margolis and Kilham. Internatl. Acad. Path. Monograph no. 9. Williams and Wilkins, Baltimore, 1968, ch. 8.
29. Riser. North Am. Vet., 1943, *24,* 293.
30. Rohovsky and Griesemer. Path. Vet., 1967, *4,* 391.
31. Schofield. North Am. Vet., 1949, *30,* 651.
32. Scott. Feline panleukopenia. Cornell Univ. thesis, 1968.
33. Scott, Csiza, and Gillespie. Cornell Vet., 1970, *60,* 183.
34. Scott, Csiza, and Gillespie. Jour. Am. Vet. Med. Assoc., 1970, *156,* 439.
35. Scott and Glauberg. Jour. Am. Vet. Med. Assoc., 1975, *166,* 147.
36. Seifried and Krembs. Arch. f. Tierheilk., 1940, *75,* 252.
37. Torres. North Am. Vet., 1941, *22,* 297.
38. Verge and Cristoforoni. Comp. rend. Soc. Biol. (Paris), 1928, *99,* 312.
39. Wills. Can. Jour. Comp. Med., 1952, *16,* 419.

Bovine *Parvovirus*

A hemadsorbing enteric virus (HADEN) was isolated from the gastrointestinal tract of normal calves by Abinanti and Warfield (1) and later classified as a parvovirus by Storz and Warren (9). Other isolates later were made in the USA (3), Algeria (10), and Japan (4). Parvoviruses sometimes were found in naturally occurring mixed infections with bovine enteroviruses, coronaviruses, adenoviruses, and adeno-associated viruses (8).

In limited serological surveys the incidence of the disease in the USA ranged from 65 to 86 percent (1, 7) and 70 percent in Algeria (10).

Character of the Disease. Diarrhea is the principal sign of illness in calves. Calves that recover from the disease may be stunted. Parvoviruses have been isolated from calves with serous conjunctivitis (5). On occasion it causes a fever and respiratory and enteric signs (4). In Japan it has been associated with abortion (4). Virus can be isolated intermittently from the feces of recovered calves.

In experimental studies with colostrum-deprived and newborn calves the virus produced illness 24 to 48 hours after oral or intravenous inoculation (8). Initially, the feces were watery then became mucoid. Body temperature reached 41 C 2 days after inoculation. The calves were listless, but they usually drank milk.

Storz *et al.* (8) found that virus could be demonstrated by the fluorescent antibody technique rather consistently in cells of the jejunum, ileum, and cecum. Fluorescing cells were found in the intestinal epithelium of the crypts, in the transition and intervillous zones of villi, central lacteals, and in cells of the laminae propria mucosae. Epithelial cells in crypts of Lieberkühn, regional lymph nodes, thymus gland, nodular areas of spleen, adrenal glands, and heart muscle also had fluorescing cells. There were recognizable nuclear changes in cells of infected adrenal glands. Cowdry type A inclusions are produced by this virus.

Properties of the Virus. The HADEN strain has all the characteristics of a parvovirus (2, 9). Its size is approximately 23 nm, and it is resistant to ether and sodium deoxycholate (6). It is stable over a pH range of 3 to 9. Intranuclear inclusion bodies of the Cowdry type A are produced in bovine embryonic kidney cells. The virus produces hemagglutination and hemadsorption of human, dog, and guinea pig red blood cells, but elution of virus does not occur (1, 2). Actinomycin D, and also bromo- and 5-fluoro-2′-deoxyuridine (BUDU and FUDR) inhibited the replication of virus in cell culture.

Comparative HI serological test investigations revealed no relationship between the bovine parvovirus and other parvoviruses (2). All bovine parvovirus isolates are antigenically related or identical to the original HADEN strain, but one strain isolated in Japan may be different (4).

Cultivation. Virus can be isolated readily by using parasynchronous bovine fetal spleen cell cultures and employing a technique of partial cell removal (1/4 to 1/2 of a culture) and cell growth stimulation with fresh medium through 2 to 5 subpassages until a cytopathic effect is observed (8). These results correlate quite favorably with viral detection in tissues by fluorescent antibody technique (FAT). Sera used to stimulate cell growth must be screened for inhibitory factors.

Immunity. This aspect of the disease has not been studied. It is safe to predict that recovered animals will have a solid and long-lasting immunity as this is a characteristic of members of the genus. Likewise, maternal immunity should have an impact on the incidence and epidemiology of this disease in calves because limited surveys show it is a common infection in cattle in the USA.

Transmission. Because recovered cattle intermittently shed the virus in the feces, this is the most likely mechanism for its spread to susceptible animals. Likewise, viruses in this family are stable and exceedingly resistant, so they likely can persist on the premises for an appreciable period of time.

Diagnosis. The importance of bovine parvovirus as a natural cause of diarrhea has not been ascertained, but should be considered when diarrhea in calves, abortions, stillbirths, and congenital anomalies occur in cattle.

Diarrhea in calves can be caused by other pathogens such as rotaviruses, conoraviruses, *Salmonella* species, and pathogenic *Escherichia coli*. A precise clinical diagnosis of bovine parvovirus disease is virtually impossible without assistance from a diagnostic laboratory equipped to provide a complete microbiological service. As mixed enteric infections often occur, this clearly complicates the diagnosis. Under these conditions it is difficult to determine the precise agent causing the disease in question. Then, too, synergistic effects by pathogens must be weighed in evaluating the problem.

A definitive diagnosis can be made by isolating the virus from infected feces or other selected tissues described in the section under disease characteristics. In some instances the electron microscope could be used to identify the agent in feces.

The hemagglutination test also can be used to render a diagnosis, but only if acute and convalescent paired serum samples from a given animal are available to the laboratory so that a rising titer can be demonstrated. Sometimes test sera contain inhibitory HA substances, but these can be eliminated or materially reduced by treatment with kaolin.

Control. Until we ascertain the true significance of this viral agent in the population, it is unlikely that a vaccine will be developed for its prevention and control.

It has been observed that some herds are free of the infection, but once it is introduced on a premises, control is difficult because some animals are viral carriers and the virus itself persists in the environment.

REFERENCES

1. Abinanti and Warfield. Virol., 1961, *14*, 288.
2. Bachmann. Zentrbl. Vet.-Med., 1971, *18B*, 80.
3. Bates, Storz and Reed. Jour. Inf. Dis., 1972, *126*, 531.
4. Inaba, Kurogi, Takahashi, *et al.*, Arch. f. die gesam. Virusforsch., 1973, *42*, 54.
5. Matteson. Quoted from Storz *et al.*, Jour. Am. Vet. Med. Assoc., 1978, *173*, 624.
6. Spahn, Mohanty, and Hetrick. Can. Jour. Microbiol., 1966, *12*, 653.
7. Storz, Bates, Warren, *et al.*, Am. Jour. Vet. Res., 1972, *33*, 269.
8. Storz, Leary, Carlson, and Bates. Jour. Am. Vet. Med. Assoc., 1978, *173*, 624.
9. Storz and Warren. Arch. f. die gesam. Virusforsch., 1970, *30*, 271.
10. Vincent. Ann. Inst. Pasteur (Paris), 1972, *126*, 531.

Canine *Parvovirus*

A canine virus was isolated from the feces of four adult dogs. The recovered isolates had many of the properties of the *Parvovirus* genus, so it was proposed that this canine virus be designated a member of the genus and called the minute virus of canines (MVC) (5). Based on limited serological studies, it appears that this virus infection may occur frequently in canine populations.

In 1978, outbreaks of acute diarrheal disease in dogs from many parts of the United States occurred and caused severe illness and mortality of dogs of all ages (7). A parvovirus was isolated from the feces of these dogs and called canine parvovirus (CPV); occasionally a fecal specimen also contained a coronavirus. MCV isolated by Binn *et al.* (5) appears to be unrelated to CPV isolates made from diseased dogs in the United States (including Alaska), Europe, and Australia since 1978. There is evidence to suggest that it is a new disease in the United States (1).

CPV is closely related antigenically to feline panleukopenia virus, which also is indistinguishable serologically from mink enteritis virus. The parvolike virus disease outbreaks in dogs resemble closely the outbreaks of mink enteritis observed by Gorham before vaccine for that disease was available (8).

Character of the Disease. Clinical signs associated with CPV are vomiting, often severe and protracted, anorexia, diarrhea, and rapid dehydration, especially in pups. The feces are generally a light grayish or yellow gray color at the onset of disease; however, fluid stools either streaked with blood or frankly hemorrhagic may be present as the initial sign and may persist until recovery or death.

Some animals vomit at frequent intervals and have diarrhea, sometimes projectile and hemorrhagic, until they die; others have only a loose stool and recover uneventfully. Temperatures ranging from 104 to 106 F are observed in some animals, especially pups; however, there may be little if any elevation of temperature in older dogs. Sudden "shocklike" death may occur in some puppies as early as 2 days after the onset of illness.

A common feature of the CPV disease is leukopenia, especially during the first 4 to 5 days of illness. White cell counts less than 100 cells per cu mm have been recorded; however, counts of 500 per cu mm through

2,000 per cu mm seem more common at the peak of illness. The data cited was obtained principally from field cases where hemograms were not done on a daily basis. Leukopenia is often accompanied by fever.

Another syndrome that might be related to parvovirus infection is sudden heart failure in young pups, sometimes after they have recovered from enteritis. Dogs may die suddenly after a brief and inconspicuous illness. Respiratory signs caused by congestive heart failure, crying, or unproductive vomiting may occur. Invasion of the heart muscle by inflammatory cells was found, and parvovirus has been demonstrated by electron microscopy in heart muscle cells by workers at the Angell Memorial Hospital in Boston, Massachusetts.

When freshly isolated virus is inoculated into laboratory-reared dogs, fever and low lymphocyte counts were the only signs, and intestinal lesions were mild. This is not surprising because disease in specific pathogen-free animals is often milder than that observed naturally. It is likely that several factors are necessary to produce severe disease.

CPV causes necrosis of the crypt epithelium in the small intestine (6). There is often extensive loss of epithelium cells with dilatation of remaining crypts. In advanced cases there is regeneration of epithelium, and the lamina propria may be infiltrated by inflammatory cells. Intranuclear inclusion bodies in epithelial cells may be present, but only rarely. There often is necrosis or depletion of lymphoid tissue. The lesions are remarkably similar to the intestinal changes caused by feline panleukopenia virus.

The original isolates of MVC were associated with cases of diarrhea in dogs. More information is required to establish its importance as a pathogen in canines, although most investigators now view it as a major infectious disease.

Properties of the Virus. There is evidence that two serotypes of canine parvovirus exist. It has been shown that dog antiserum to MVC does not neutralize CPV. Likewise, dog antiserum to CPV does not neutralize MVC (4). CPV isolates are closely related antigenically to feline panleukopenia virus. It has been noted (2) that living attenuated as well as inactivated feline panleukopenia (FPL) virus vaccines protect dogs against virulent CPV. Further, this close relationship between CPV and FPL virus is clearly revealed by serum-neutralization, hemagglutination-inhibition, and immunofluorescence tests. MVC agglutinates simian erythrocytes but not guinea pig, human O, rat, or pig red blood cells. CPV has a greater spectrum of hemagglutinating activity than the MVC. CPV isolates strongly hemagglutinate swine and rhesus monkey erythrocytes under restrictive conditions of pH and temperature. CPV has all the biophysical and biochemical characteristics of other parvoviruses. It is extremely resistant, but can be inactivated by using a 1:30 dilution of Clorox in water.

Cultivation. The MVC produces a cytopathic effect in a continuous cell line, WRcc, characterized by infected cells becoming rounded, developing distinct cell membranes and cytoplasmic strands, and, finally, detaching from the glass. Viral titers of $TCID_{50}$ 10^7 per ml usually were achieved. The isolates failed to induce CPE in cell cultures of primary dog kidney, of human embryonic kidney, of African green monkey kidney, of feline kidney, and of kidneys from many other animal species. Attempts to produce overt signs of illness in newborn and weanling mice, hamsters, and guinea pigs failed.

CPV produces a cytopathic effect in dog kidney cell cultures, and unlike other parvoviruses that are highly host-specific, the CPV replicates in cells of noncanine origin.

Immunity. Very little is known about CPV except that dogs that recover from the disease are immune to challenge with homologous virulent virus. Dogs immunized with homotypic formalin-inactivated virus, formalin-inactivated feline panleukopenia virus (2 doses given 1 to 2 weeks apart), or attenuated feline panleukopenia virus are also protected against CPV (3).

It is reasonable to anticipate that recovered or vaccinated dogs will have a long and durable immunity characteristic of other well-studied viruses in this family. Maternal immunity can be expected to interfere with active immunization.

Transmission. Dog-to-dog contact is probably the most common means of viral spread. Fecal material also contains large amounts of virus that is extremely resistant to heat, acid, and many disinfectants. The virus may survive in the environment for long periods and be carried by individuals from kennel to kennel.

Diagnosis. A presumptive diagnosis of CPV is based on clinical signs and necropsy where there is a history of contagious enteritis. Other diseases cause vomiting and diarrhea in the dog such as coronavirus infection, so-called atypical distemper, bacterial and parasitic diseases, acute pancreatitis, poisonings, and tryptic enteritis. When several dogs are involved, viral enteritis should be given special consideration. A rapid diagnosis can be made by electron microscopy when fresh fecal material is available by applying the conventional negative staining technique. With fatal cases the immunofluorescent (IF) antibody technique using feline panleukopenia IF conjugate can be used to examine tissues from the mesenteric lymph node, ileum, or spleen for CPV antigen. Cell cultures can be used for isolating virus or conducting the serum-neutralization test for detecting antibody. The hemagglutination inhibition test also provides an excellent way to demonstrate antibody.

Control. As a temporary measure until a licensed product for CPV becomes available, inactivated FPLV vaccination of young puppies should be safe. Licensed attenuated FPLV vaccines for cats have proved effective and safe in dogs to immunize against CPV (1980).

The Disease in Man. There is no evidence that CPV produces infection in humans.

REFERENCES

1. Appel. Personal communication, 1979.
2. Appel, Cooper, Greisen, Scott, and Carmichael. Cornell Vet., 1979, *69,* 123.
3. Appel, Scott, and Carmichael. Vet. Rec., 1979, *105,* 156.
4. Binn. Quoted by Appel *et al.* in Cornell Vet., 1979, *69,* 123.
5. Binn, Lazar, Eddy, and Kajima. Inf. and Immun., 1970, *1,* 503.
6. Cooper, Carmichael, Appel, and Greisen. Cornell Vet., 1979, *69,* 134.
7. Eugester and Nairn. Southwest Vet., 1977, *30,* 59.
8. Gorham. Personal communication, 1978.

Porcine *Parvovirus*

SYNONYM: Porcine picodnavirus;
abbreviation, PPV

Originally, pathologic changes generally were not attributed to the porcine parvovirus, although a small DNA virus was described in England (3) that was believed to be responsible for abortions, stillbirths, and infertility in swine. This English isolate had properties similar to PPV described earlier by Mayr and Mahnel (8). Since 1975 reports from investigators in many countries provided positive evidence that under natural conditions PPV can cause abortions, stillbirths, and infertility in susceptible pregnant gilts or sows that become infected during the early stages of gestation (5, 6, 11–14). Evidence that PPV could cause similar effects in pregnant sows under experimental conditions was reported about the same time (2, 9, 10). A large percentage of pigs in New York State (15) and Germany (1) have antibodies. The pig is the only species known to be susceptible to PPV.

Neonatal and older pigs develop antibodies without the production of clinical disease or pathological lesions (1, 4). Fetuses from sows experimentally infected at 72, 99, and 105 days of gestation survived (2), but developed high-antibody titers. In dead fetuses or stillborn piglets, histological brain lesions usually were found. The lesions were typical of a meningoencephalitis consisting of perivascular cuffing of proliferating adventitial cells and a few plasma cells. Lesions were localized in a few plasma cells. Lesions also were localized in the cerebral gray and white matter and leptomeninges (12).

This virus was isolated from several stocks of tissue-cultured hog cholera virus (1, 7) and from primary monolayer cultures of kidneys from healthy piglets (7). The virus produced a cytopathic effect characterized by a diffuse granulation and by rounding and detachment of cells from the glass of primary and cell line pig kidney cell cultures. Intranuclear inclusion bodies occur. Maximum virus yields of $TCID_{50}$ 10^4 to 10^5 per 0.1 ml are attained by inoculating cultures before they become confluent and harvesting the fluid at 72 to 108 hours later (7).

The virus contains a hemagglutinin. The HA test is performed at 4 C using erythrocytes of the guinea pig, mouse, rat, cat, chicken, or human type O, but not hamster, pig, rabbit, dog, sheep, mouse, or goose (7). Its virus particles are 20 to 22 nm in diameter with a morphology comparable to other parvoviruses (7). It has a buoyant density of 1.38 g per cm^3 (7). No pathological changes are produced in newborn hamsters or rats by PPV (7).

Immune sows or gilts that are exposed to virus during gestation have normal piglets. It is anticipated that the immunity is solid and long lasting. The hemagglutination-inhibition and serum-neutralization tests can be used to test for antibodies. Pig serums used in the hemagglutination-inhibition (HI) test first must be treated with kaolin. Transmission of the infection moves rapidly through a herd once it is introduced.

Diagnosis can be verified by isolation of virus from many tissues of infected fetuses in cell culture. Lesser amounts of virus are present in tissue from macerated and mummified fetuses collected in the late stages of fetal disease. Direct tissue examination by immunofluorescence examination reveals large masses of viral antigen in all stages of fetal disease (9).

The true eonomic significance of this disease has not been ascertained; consequently, a vaccine has not been developed, but it certainly is within the realm of possibility to produce one.

REFERENCES

1. Bachmann. Zentrbl. Vet.-Med., 1969, *16B*, 341.
2. Bachmann, Sheffy, and Vaughn. Inf. and Immun., 1975, *12*, 455.
3. Cartwright and Huck. Vet. Rec., 1967, *81*, 196.
4. Cutlip and Mengeling. Am. Jour. Vet. Res., 1975, *36*, 1179.
5. Donaldson-Wood, Joo, and Johnson. Vet. Rec., 1977, *100*, 237.
6. Foreman, Lenghaus, Hogg, and Hale. Austral. Vet. Jour., 1977, *53*, 326.
7. Mayr, Bachmann, Siegl, Mahnel, and Sheffy. Arch. f. die gesam. Virusforsch., 1968, *25*, 38.
8. Mayr and Mahnel. Zentrbl. f. Bakt., I Abt. Orig., 1966, *199*, 389.
9. Mengeling and Cutlip. Am. Jour. Vet. Res., 1975, *36*, 1173.
10. Mengeling and Cutlip. Am. Jour. Vet. Res., 1976, *37*, 1393.
11. Mengeling, Cutlip, Wilson, Parks, and Marshall. Jour. Am. Vet. Med. Assoc., 1975, *166*, 993.
12. Narita, Invi, Kawakami, Kitamura, and Maeda. Natl. Inst. An. Health Q. (Tokyo), 1975, *15*, 24.
13. Pini. Jour. So. Afr. Vet. Assoc., 1975, *46*, 241.
14. Rodeffer, Leman, Dunne, Cropper, and Sprecher. Jour. Am. Vet. Med. Assoc., 1975, *166*, 991.
15. Sheffy. Personal communication, 1969.

Aleutian Disease in Mink

SYNONYMS: Plasmacytosis, hypergammaglobulinemia; abbreviation, AD

Aleutian disease (AD) in mink is characterized by genetic predisposition, presistent blood-borne infection, pronounced plasmacytosis, hypergammaglobulinemia, progressive immune complexes, and other signs consistent with slow virus infections. The increased susceptibility of genetically defined types of mink appears to be associated with inheritance of a dysfunction of the protective mechanism, comparable to the Chediak-Higasi syndrome seen in man and in cattle.

The disease was first described by Hartsough and Gorham (14), and it has been reported in the United States, Canada, and Denmark. It is suggested that this disease may be an excellent natural model for the study of collagen diseases of man (7).

Character of the Disease. It is a chronic progressive disease of high mortality and morbidity characterized by anorexia, loss of weight, lethargy, polydipsia, and hemorrhages. It has a long incubation period, and death usually occurs in a few to many months. According to Bazeley (3), there is strong evidence for vertical transmission occurring at the rate of 100 percent in infected herds. The well-being of an animal consists of periodic low-level hypergammaglobulinemia accompanied by minute vascular occlusions. The spontaneous lethal change in an individual arises during one of the hypergammaglobulinemia episodes representing a failure of the immune system to control an inherent virus-induced mononucleosis.

At necropsy the kidneys are enlarged, pale yellow, and mottled, and the liver is slightly enlarged. Histological alterations are characterized by marked plasmacytosis of the lymph nodes, spleen, liver, and kidneys; marked rise in serum gamma globulin; hepatic degeneration with bile duct proliferation; and smudging of glomerular basement membranes (15). The severity of lesions is related to the degree of hypergammaglobulinemia. In one quarter of natural cases there are vascular lesions consisting of segmental periarteritis and fibrinoid degeneration of small and medium-sized arteries. There are many points of histochemical similarity to human connective tissue diseases, but also differences (20). The serum protein alterations and pathologic changes are similar to those seen in certain human connective tissue disorders such as disseminated lupus erythematosus, rheumatoid arthritis, and plasma cell hepatitis. The intercapillary nodular lesions are similar to those found in diabetes mellitus. The presence of a monoclonal type of gamma globulin late in the disease is comparable to changes seen in multiple myeloma or monoclonal gamma globulin production in man.

The Disease in Experimental Animals. The disease is readily produced in genetically susceptible mink. Although the Aleutian type of mink develop lesions more quickly and die sooner after injection, other genotypes are also susceptible (22, 25). The virus can be serially transferred in mink (12).

Overt signs of Aleutian disease are not seen in naturally or experimentally infected ferrets (19). The infection produced a systemic proliferation of lymphoid elements in association with a hypergammaglobulinemia and vasculitis. Most ferret sera examined electrophoretically had gamma globulin levels about 20 percent, considered to be the upper normal limit for most domestic animals (1). A monoclonal type of hypergammaglobulinemia was frequently found in ferrets; usually observed only in mink that survive early AD. Natural subclinical infection also occurs in ferrets maintained on ranches where AD is found in mink.

Properties of the Virus. In 1962 Russell (23), Karstad and Pridham (17), and Trautwein and Helmboldt (25)

independently reported that Aleutian disease is caused by a virus. The disease is reproducible with filtrates of infected tissues or with pellets after ultracentrifugation. Fluorocarbon extraction fails to reduce appreciably its infectivity (6). The virus is present in blood, serum, bone marrow, spleen, feces, urine, and saliva of infected mink (12).

The size of Aleutian disease virus particles ranges from 23 to 25 nm (8, 26). In a cesium density gradient of a highly purified and concentrated suspension derived from early infected mink tissues using fluorocarbon extraction procedures, 3 distinct bands of buoyant densities were observed. The more dense Aleutian disease virions (1.4 g per cm^3) had a higher infectivity rate than the virions with a density of 1.3 g per cm^3 (8). ADV is resistant to detergents and lipid solvents. Its titer was reduced by 700-fold by proteolytic enzymes, but not by DNase or RNase (13). The virus is inactivated slowly at 56 C; the initial half-life is 90 minutes. There is a suggestion that it is a DNA virus, and extracted DNA from spleens of mink with viral plasmacytosis is infective for mink (5). This may account for the unusual heat resistance of the infective agent. At present we are including the virus in the family Parvoviridae but with considerable reservation as it has certain characteristics that are atypical for the family.

Cultivation. Specific morphological alterations are produced by the agent in cultures of mink testis and mink kidney cells (4) or of feline kidney cells (Crandell cell line).

Immunity. Although plasmacytosis and hypergammaglobulinemia are characteristic of the disease, there is no evidence of natural or acquired immunity. Gamma globulin from infected mink fails to neutralize virus. This indicates that virus and gamma globulin can exist together in a cell-free environment (11) and also in the serum of infected mink. Circulating infectious antigen-antibody complexes have been detected, and it is probable that these complexes deposited in blood-vessel walls cause the hyaline degeneration associated with disease (16). These same lesions are seen during late stages of lymphocytic choriomeningitis of mice. It appears that antiglobulin antibodies (positive Coombs' test) are produced as a result of AD infection (24). Counter-electrophoresis and complement-fixation were reliably specific for AD antibody whereas immunofluorescence was less reproducible (10). Immunofluorescence complement fixation was 4- to 8-fold more sensitive than regular or modified counter-electrophoresis, but limited by background staining and anticomplementary activity when used to detect small amounts of antibody in undiluted sera.

Karstad *et al.* (18) produced an inactivated vaccine by treating tissues of infected mink with 0.3 percent of formalin at 37 C. Vaccinated mink maintained in contact with infected mink failed to develop the disease, but they succumbed to injection with infective tissue suspension—even after vaccination with three doses.

Transmission. Horizontal and vertical transmission undoubtedly occur. In horizontal, 2 routes are possible: (*a*) fecal-oral and (*b*) saliva-aerosol-respiratory circuits. Indeed, mink were infected experimentally by both routes (12). Often only certain individuals in litters show signs of illness. The isolation of virus in the saliva of mink 4 months after exposure suggests an extended infectious period (12). Mink with inapparent infection are capable of transmitting the disease, but the risk is less than with mink with progressive Aleutian disease (2). Vertical transmission of infection from the dam to its progeny does occur. Although the agent was isolated with equal facility from both susceptible and resistant breeds of pregnant females, the fetal mortality was greater in the genetically susceptible mink (21).

Diagnosis. This can be established by three means: (*a*) a series of positive iodine agglutination tests of increasing activity (*b*) clinical signs, and (*c*) typical lesions at necropsy. The iodine test reveals an increase in gamma globulin, a decrease in albumin, an increase in total serum proteins, and a change in the A:G ratio (12). The cytoplasmic inclusion bodies of Aleutian disease stain strongly by the periodic acid-Schiff (PAS) method differentiating them from distemper inclusions.

Control. Mink that have AD antibody also harbor the virus. By eliminating mink with AD antibody from a ranch it is possible to eliminate the infection; the counter-immunoelectrophoresis test (Figure 39.6) is extremely useful in achieving this objective (9).

The Disease in Man. This agent is not known to cause infection in man. It has been compared with periarteritis nodosa in humans.

REFERENCES

1. Abinanti. Ann. Rev. Microbiol., 1967, *21,* 467.
2. An and Ingram. Am. Jour. Vet. Res., 1978, *39,* 309.
3. Bazeley. Jour. Inf. Dis., 1976, *134,* 252.
4. Bosrur, Gray, and Karstad. Can. Jour. Comp. Med. and Vet. Sci., 1963, *27,* 301.
5. Bosrur and Karstad. Can. Jour. Comp. Med. and Vet. Sci., 1966, *30,* 295.

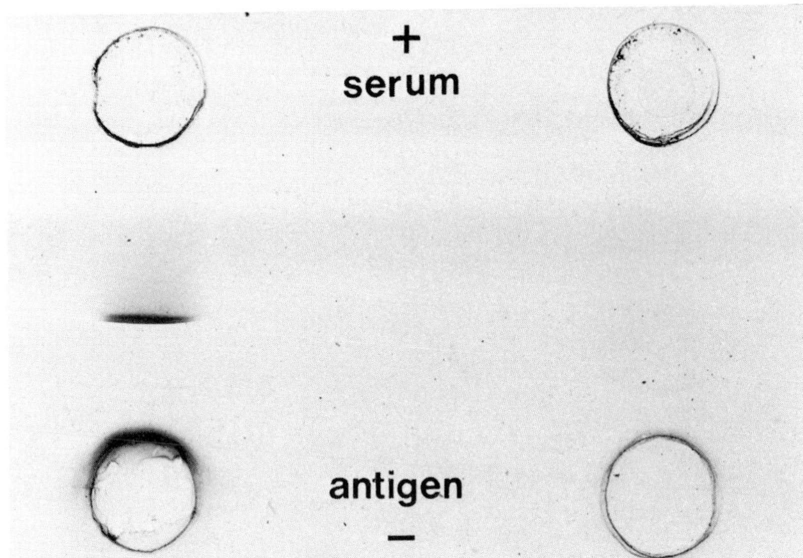

Figure 39.6. The counter-immunoelectrophoresis test for Aleutian disease. The positive antigen-antibody system is on the left as indicated by the line of identity between the two wells, while the negative one is on the right side. The positive (+) and the negative (−) signs indicate the presence of an electrical system. (From Ian R. Tizard, *An Introduction to Veterinary Immunology*, Saunders, Philadelphia, 1977.)

6. Burger, Gorham, and Leader. Quoted by Leader in Arch. Path., 1964, *78,* 390.
7. Cabasso. Vet. Rec., 1975, *96,* 563.
8. Cho. Can. Jour. Comp. Med., 1977, *41,* 215.
9. Cho and Greenfield. Jour. Clin. Microbiol., 1978, *7,* 18.
10. Crawford, McGuire, Porter, and Cho. Jour Immunol., 1977, *118,* 1249.
11. Gorham, Leader, and Henson. Fed. Proc., 1963, *22,* abstract 627.
12. Gorham, Leader, and Henson. Jour. Inf. Dis., 1964, *114,* 341.
13. Hahn, Ramos, and Kenyon. Arch. Virol., 1977, *55,* 315.
14. Hartsough and Gorham. Natl. Fur News, 1956, *28,* 10.
15. Helmboldt and Jungherr. Am. Jour. Vet. Res., 1958, *19,* 212.
16. Karstad. Can. Vet. Jour., 1970, *11,* 36.
17. Karstad and Pridham. Can. Jour. Comp. Med. and Vet Sci., 1962, *26,* 97.
18. Karstad, Pridham, and Gray. Can. Jour. Comp. Med. and Vet. Sci., 1963, *27,* 124.
19. Kenyon, Williams, and Howard. Proc. Soc. Exp. Biol. and Med., 1966, *123,* 510.
20. Leader. Arch. Path., 1964, *78,* 390.
21. Padgett, Gorham, and Henson. Jour. Inf. Dis., 1967, *117,* 35.
22. Padgett, Leader, and Gorham. Quoted by Leader in Arch. Path., 1964, *78,* 390.
23. Russell. Natl. Fur News, 1962, *34,* 8.
24. Saison, Karstad, and Pridham. Can. Jour. Comp. Med. and Vet Sci., 1966, *30,* 151.
25. Trautwein and Helmboldt. Am. Jour. Vet. Res., 1962, *23,* 1280.
26. Yoon, Dunker, and Kenyon. Virol., 1975, *64,* 575.

40 The Papovaviridae

In the family Papovaviridae there are two genera: *Papillomavirus* and *Polyomavirus*. The division is based on the size of their genomes and the diameter of their capsids. Because the viruses in the genus *Polyomavirus* do not include diseases of domestic animals, this chapter will cover only the diseases in the genus *Papillomavirus*.

THE GENUS *PAPILLOMAVIRUS*

The type species for the genus *Papillomavirus* is *Papillomavirus* S-1 (Sylvilagus), commonly known as the Shope papillomavirus. Other members of the genus are the rabbit oral papillomavirus, human papillomavirus, canine papillomavirus, canine oral papillomavirus, and bovine papillomavirus. Additional members include the viruses causing papillomata of horses, sheep, goats, hamsters, monkeys, and other species.

The particles of viruses studied in this genus are 53 nm in diameter. They contain double-stranded cyclic DNA with a GC ratio of 49 percent and a molecular weight of approximately 5×10^6 daltons. The capsid is composed of 72 capsomeres in a skew arrangement. The buoyant density in cesium chloride is 1.34 g per cm^3. Particles are assembled in the nucleus. They are ether-resistant, acid-stable, and heat-stable. Several papillomata viruses hemagglutinate by reacting with neuriminidase-sensitive receptors. Each papovavirus is antigenically distinct, and all those that have been studied differ in their base composition of their nucleic acid.

The principal viruses in the genus are oncogenic, especially in young or new born animals. Nucleic acid extracted from these viruses is oncogenic. Subacute, latent, and chronic infections are commonly produced by these viruses. Papillomas, or common warts, occur in many species of animals. They seem to be most frequent in man, cattle, dogs, and rabbits. All of these tumors contain filterable agents with which the tumors may be induced in other individuals. They appear to have a high degree of host specificity, and some of them even have specificities for particular kinds of epithelium within a single host. Warts occur in epizootic form in herds of cattle and in kennels of dogs. All varieties are most prevalent in the young of the species.

Bovine Papillomatosis

Character of the Disease. Warts frequently occur in calves and young stock less than 2 years old. They appear most often in the winter months when the animals are closely housed. The head, especially the region about the eyes (Figure 40.1), is most frequently involved, but they may appear on the sides of the neck and less commonly on other parts of the body. They usually do not occur on the legs. They appear first as small nodular growths, which develop slowly for a time and then often grow rapidly into dry, horny, whitish, cauliflowerlike masses, which finally fall off as a result of dry necrosis of their bases. Sometimes hundreds of these masses occur on a calf at the same time. The size varies from small ones no larger than a pea to confluent masses sev-

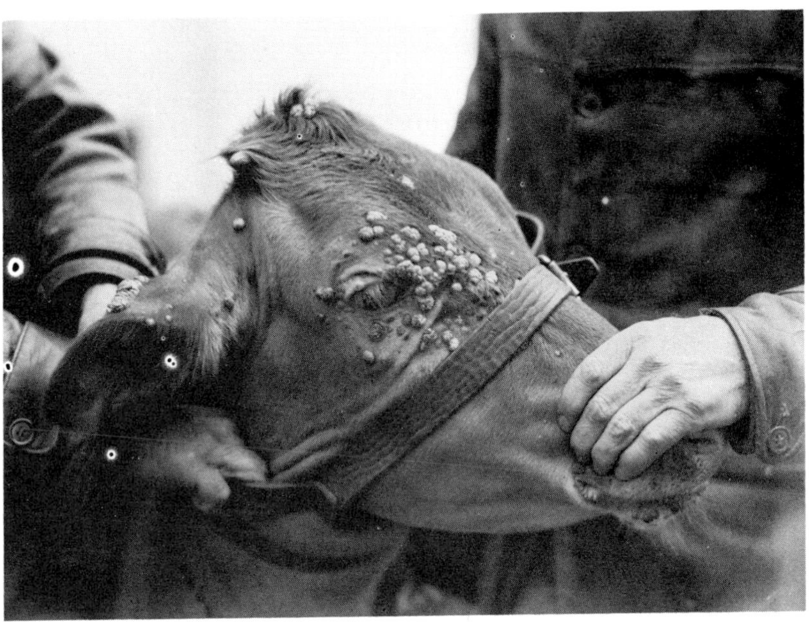

Figure 40.1. Bovine papillomatosis (warts).

eral inches in diameter. Such warts have been seen along the sides of the neck beginning at points where blood samples have been drawn from the jugular vein, an indication that an infected bleeding needle has been the transmitting agent. Warts have also been found in the nasal openings of many animals in the same herd, apparently transmitted by the fingers of persons who have held the animal or by a bull lead that has been used as a means of restraint.

Occasionally infectious papillomas occur in dairy herds, the tumors appearing only on the teats. These cause difficulty in milking, and evidently are spread in the milking process. Whether they are caused by the same virus that causes general skin warts is not known. Another rather common papilloma of cattle is seen on the end of the penis of bulls and in the vagina of cows. Clinical evidence of transmissibility exists, but experimental evidence is lacking (7). There also is an atypical cutaneous form recognized as different from the typical cutaneous fibropapilloma by the lack of the fibromatous dermal component (3). Transmission and immunization characterization of this virus have failed.

The losses from warts are considerable. In young animals affected with many of these tumors, the general growth rate may be retarded. The greatest losses are in damages to the hides of slaughtered animals. Frequently the owner is most concerned by the reduction in the sales value of warty animals, especially in purebred stock.

Properties of the Virus. The virus is typical of members in this genus. According to Favre and Breitburd, "Purified preparations of bovine papillomavirus (BPV) agglutinate mouse erythrocytes. Maximal hemagglutination (HA) activity occurs at 4°[C], between pH 6.8 and 8.4. The adsorbed virus is readily eluted at 37°[C]. The BPV receptors on mouse erythrocytes show a high resistance to receptor-destroying enzyme or Influenza A2 neuraminidase. The BPV hemagglutinin is associated to both full and empty viral particles. Sera of animals infected with BPV contain antibodies inhibiting the HA reaction" (6).

Creech (5) inoculated 11 calves with ground unfiltered wart material and 11 additional with filtrates of the same materials from Berkefeld N filters. The filtrates were bacteriologically sterile. Eight "takes" were secured with the unfiltered material and 7 with the filtered. The inoculations were made by scarification and intradermal injections.

Cultivation. The virus of bovine papillomatosis can readily be cultivated on the chorioallantoic membrane of developing chick embryos. The presence of virus is indicated by marked epithelial thickenings that are rich in virus. It is the only member of the genus that grows in the embryonated hen's egg.

Newborn Afghan pikas, an Asian lagomorph similar to the rabbit, are susceptible to bovine papilloma virus. After subcutaneous inoculation, cutaneous or subcutaneous fibromas and fibrosarcomas were observed approximately 9 months later (13).

Immunity. Although warts affecting animals always clear up spontaneously after a time, varying from 1 to several months, owners often demand curative treatment. Surgical removal of a few warts often leads to rapid regression and disappearance of the others. This has been interpreted as meaning that wart virus, escaping from the tumors during the operative procedures and absorbed in the wounds produced, has resulted in immunization. This explanation has not been confirmed by experimental proof, and it should always be kept in mind that warts retrogress spontaneously. All methods of treatment should be accepted with caution for this reason.

Artificial immunization of cattle with finely ground wart tissue suspended in a 0.4 percent formalin solution has been used for many years to combat wart outbreaks. In recent years, since it has been possible to propagate the virus on the membranes of embryonated eggs, most commercial companies have used the artificially produced virus for vaccine manufacture. In many instances the results have appeared to be excellent; in others they were poor.

Experimentally, Bagdonas and Olson (2) and Olson and Skidmore (11) found that vaccines were of limited value. They agree that autogenous vaccines were more effective than stock vaccines. Olson, Segre, and Skidmore (9) found that inactivated bovine tissue vaccine did not produce complete immunity to all bovine virus strains and that vaccine produced by cultivation of the virus in eggs is worthless (10). On the other hand, Pearson *et al.* (12), working in the British Isles, found that autogenous vaccines made from bovine tissues gave protection to 87 percent of a large group of cattle, and nonautogenous bovine tissue vaccines protected 76 percent. These were general body surface tumors. Teat wart vaccines were successful only in 4 out of 12 cases. Unvaccinated control cattle were kept on each of the farms where autogenous vaccines were used. These animals showed little change in their wart load while the vaccinated were showing wart regression.

Bagdonas and Olson found that animals that had been vaccinated with autogenous vaccines responded to inoculation with wart virus by connective tissue rather than epithelial growths. This was interpreted to mean that the vaccine had protected only against the epithelial elements of the warts.

Cattle given 3 injections of formalin-inactivated bovine papillomavirus vaccine produced significant levels of precipitating antibody similar to that produced to infective papillomavirus (4), but the titer decreased markedly within 24 months after the last vaccination. Multiple, repeated vaccination provided the best serologic response.

Transmission. The mode of natural transmission of warts is unknown. It has been pointed out above that there are indications that transmission may occur through the handling of animals by people and by needles used for breeding. Presumably they may be transmitted by friction between warty and normal animals. Often, in the same pens, animals may be found with extensive crops of warts and others of about the same age with few or none. Bagdonas and Olson (1) studied an extensive wart epizootic in a large herd of beef cattle in a feed lot. They discuss possible alternative routes of transmission of the disease. The use of a tattoo instrument for placing an identification number in the ears of cattle causes a high incidence at this site in herds infected with this virus. This does not occur when metal ear tags are used.

Schultz (15) claims to have succeeded in transmitting bovine warts to man. Under natural exposure this seldom or never occurs. Olson and Cook (8) succeeded in producing connective tissue tumors, resembling sarcoids, in horses by inoculation with bovine wart material. In studies by Ragland and Spencer (14), there was no evidence that the equine sarcoid and bovine papilloma agents were similar. Serums from horses with equine sarcoid failed to neutralize bovine papillomavirus. Furthermore, the response in horses with equine sarcoid to bovine papillomavirus was indistinguishable from that produced in normal horses.

REFERENCES

1. Bagdonas and Olson. Jour. Am. Vet. Med. Assoc., 1953, *122*, 393.
2. Bagdonas and Olson. Am. Jour. Vet. Res., 1954, *15*, 240.
3. Barthold, Koller, Olson, Studer, and Holtan. Jour. Am. Vet. Med. Assoc., 1974, *165*, 276.
4. Barthold, Olson, and Larson. Am. Jour. Vet. Res., 1976, *37*, 449.
5. Creech. Jour. Agr. Res., 1929, *39*, 723.
6. Favre and Breitburd. Virol., 1974, *60*, 572.
7. McEntee. Cornell Vet., 1950, *40*, 304.
8. Olson and Cook. Proc. Soc. Exp. Biol. and Med., 1951, *77*, 281.
9. Olson, Segre, and Skidmore. Jour. Am. Vet. Med. Assoc., 1959, *135*, 499.
10. Olson, Segre, and Skidmore. Am. Jour. Vet. Res., 1960, *21*, 233.
11. Olson and Skidmore. Jour. Am. Vet. Med. Assoc., 1959, *135*, 339.
12. Pearson, Kerr, McCartney, and Steele. Vet. Rec., 1958, *70*, 971.
13. Puget, Favre, and Orth. Comptes Rendus Acad. Sci. D. (Paris), 1975, *280*, 2813.
14. Ragland and Spencer, Am. Jour. Vet. Res., 1968, *29*, 1363.
15. Schultz. Deut. med. Wchnschr., 1908, *34*, 423.

Equine Papillomatosis

Skin warts in horses and mules (Figure 40.2) have long been recognized, although they do not appear to be as common as those affecting cattle. They develop most commonly on the nose and around the lips, appearing as small, elevated, horny masses that vary in number from a few to several hundred. Usually they remain quite small, but occasionally they may be large, especially when they are few in number. Generally they are not larger than 1 cm in diameter.

Cook and Olson (1) studied the transmissibility of equine warts and also some of the characteritics of the virus. They had no difficulty in infecting horses, but they did not succeed in infecting calves, lambs, dogs, rabbits, and guinea pigs. Some degree of immunity was produced by experimental infections. Natural infections produced solid immunity. The agent remained alive for 75 days when stored in 50 percent glycerol at 4 C, but was inactive after 112 days. It remained viable in a frozen suspension at −35 C for 185 days but not for 224 days.

REFERENCE

1. Cook and Olson. Am. Jour. Path., 1951, *27*, 1087.

Caprine and Ovine Papillomatosis

Warts in goats are not common; however, one outbreak in a herd was reported by Davis and Kemper (1). The tumors were located in various parts of the skin. They closely resembled those which occur in cattle. Although no transmission experiments were attempted, it is clear that they were infectious because the disease spread to many animals in the same herd. The herd was not in contact with cattle or other species of animals. It was believed that the disease had been introduced into the herd by purchased animals.

There is a report in the literature of the identification and transmission of a papillomavirus in sheep (2).

REFERENCES

1. Davis and Kemper. Jour. Am. Vet. Med. Assoc., 1936, *88*, 175.
2. Gibbs, Smale, and Lawman. Jour. Comp. Path., 1975, *85*, 327.

Canine Papillomatosis

Benign epithelial growths, commonly called *warts*, are not uncommon in young dogs. The tumors usually are found around the lips and in the mouths of the animals, where they may cause serious inconvenience. The condition is highly contagious, often spreading through all the dogs in a kennel, according to Penberthy (3).

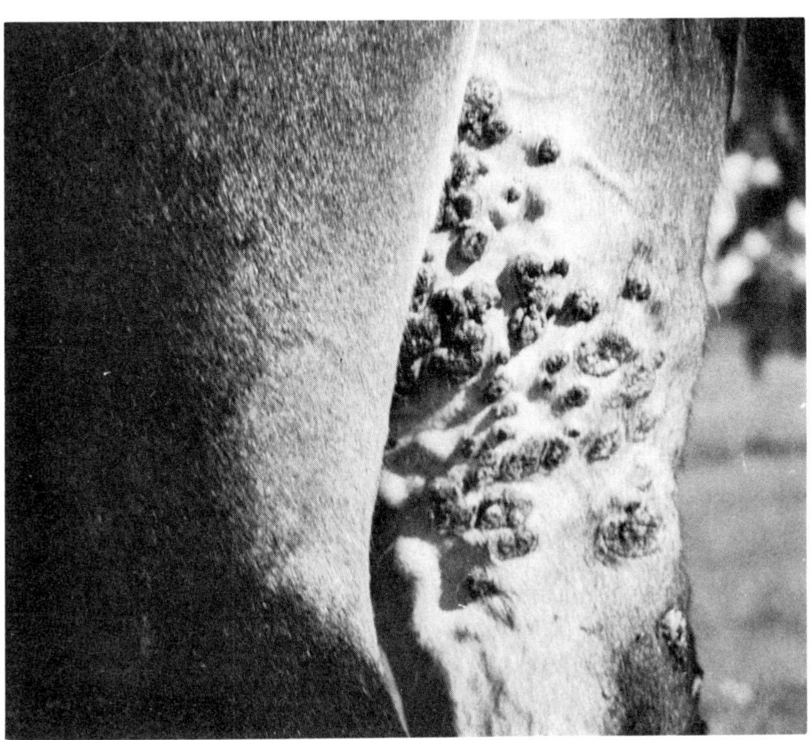

Figure 40.2. Papillomas on leg of mule. (Courtesy W. Cameron and C. Milton.)

Character of the Disease. The warts begin around the lips, as a rule, as smooth whitish elevations, which later develop a roughened surface and appear as typical papillomas (Figure 40.3). Usually following the first one or two tumors, a secondary crop appears on the insides of the cheeks, the hard palate, the tongue, and even on the walls of the pharynx. The tumors have the appearance of cauliflowers. They may interfere considerably with mastication. After several months without any sort of treatment they disappear spontaneously.

Properties of the Virus. McFadyean and Hobday (2) showed that the warts were infectious by rubbing pieces of the tumors on the scarified mucous membranes of other dogs. DeMonbreun and Goodpasture (1) likewise found it easy to propagate the tumors in this way. McFadyean and Hobday state that the incubation period is from 4 to 6 weeks. DeMonbreun and Goodpasture found that it was about 30 to 32 days as a rule, but it was somewhat longer in malnourished dogs. The latter workers passed tumor suspensions through Berkefeld N and W filters and found that the virus was present in abundance in the filtrates. Wart material was dried while frozen and kept in this state for 64 days. At the end of this time it readily produced tumors, the incubation period being 32 days, an indication that there had not been appreciable attenuation of the virus. Wart tissue kept in glycerol for the same period likewise kept its virulence relatively unimpaired. Wart tissue that had been heated at 45 C for 1 hour retained its virulence, but that heated at 58 C and 80 C proved inactive.

The attempts of DeMonbreun and Goodpasture to produce warts on the vaginal mucous membrane, on the mucous membrane of the conjunctiva, and on the skin of the abdomen proved unsuccessful, both with filtrates and with fresh unfiltered wart tissue. They also failed to infect the mouths of cats, rabbits, guinea pigs, and rats.

Immunity. Clinical experience indicates that dogs that recover from an attack of warts seldom or never are infected again. McFadyean and Hobday, and also DeMonbreun and Goodpasture, found it impossible to reinfect, experimentally, dogs that had recovered.

Vaccines are sometimes used for treatment. These are made like those of cattle. Some veterinarians have re-

Figure 40.3. Canine oral papillomatosis. (*Left*) Puppy's mouth showing the warts as they appeared 66 days after injection of a Berkefeld filtrate of tumor emulsion. In this case the incubation period was 33 days. (*Right*) A transverse section of a papilla of an actively growing wart. The inner core of Malpighian cells is approximately normal in size. They are surrounded by the enlarged, vacuolated wart cells. × 132. (Courtesy DeMonbreun and Goodpasture, *Am. Jour. Path.*)

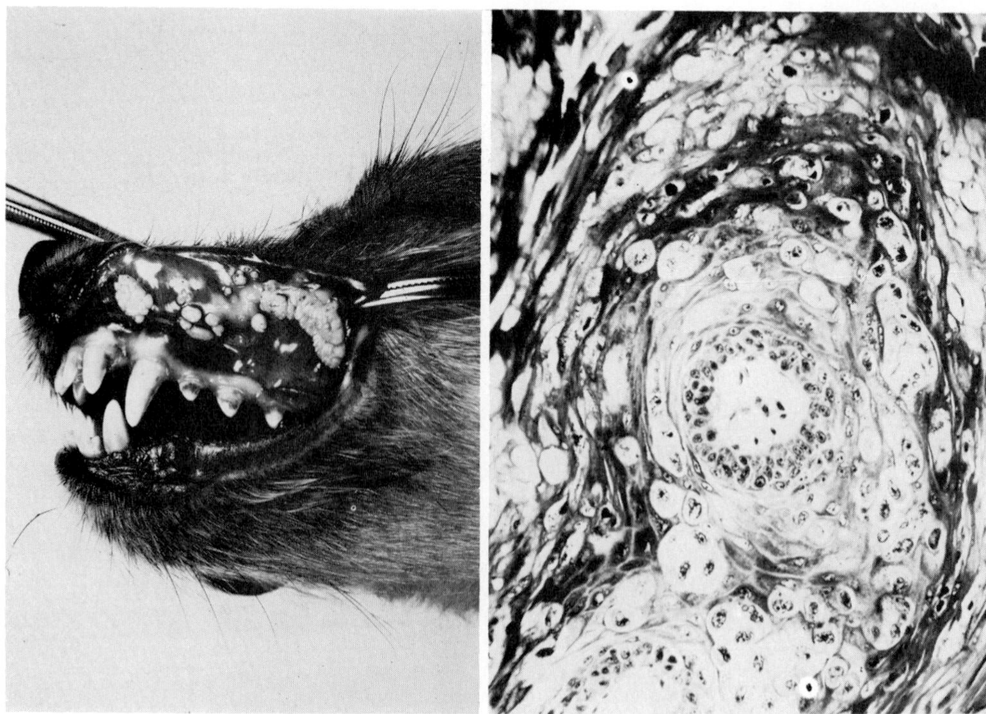

ported good results from the use of these vaccines. Since the disease is self-curing, the results of the use of vaccines must be accepted with caution.

REFERENCES

1. DeMonbreun and Goodpasture. Am. Jour. Path., 1932, *8*, 43.
2. McFadyean and Hobday. Jour. Comp. Path. and Therap., 1898, *11*, 341.
3. Penberthy. Jour. Comp. Path. and Therap., 1898, *11*, 363.

Papillomatosis of Rabbits

Two kinds of virus-induced papillomas occur in rabbits. One, commonly known as the *Shope papilloma,* occurs on the skin and is never found on the mucous membranes of the mouth. The other occurs on the oral mucosa and is never found on the skin. The viruses of these tumors are not related to each other serologically, and neither immunizes against the other.

The Shope Papilloma of Rabbits

In 1933 Shope (9) showed that the common wart of the western wild cottontail rabbit was infectious and that the infectious agent was a virus. These warty growths are not uncommon among wild rabbits of the midwestern part of the United States. Usually there are from 1 to 10 of these tumors on the infected animal, but occasionally there may be hundreds of small tumors covering almost the entire body surface. Even when the tumors are numerous, they have little effect on the general health of the rabbit.

Character of the Disease. The naturally occurring tumors appear as tall, thin, horny structures, usually grayish or even black in color. Hunters sometimes refer to such animals as "horned" rabbits, especially when the warts occur on the head. The sides of the neck, the shoulders, the abdomen (Figure 40.4), and the inside of the thighs are the sites of predilection.

Experimentally the disease may be transmitted easily by inoculating scarified skin areas with filtered or unfiltered tumor tissue. These tumors can be transmitted in series in the cottontail rabbit, but those produced in domestic rabbits by such inoculations are not transmissible although otherwise typical. Rous and Beard (8) showed that if the tumor-bearing domesticated rabbits are kept for long periods (200 days or longer), a considerable number of the benign papillomas become transformed into malignant carcinomas. Kidd and Rous (5), studying the matter further, showed that the same thing was true of such tumors produced by inoculation in jackrabbits and snowshoe rabbits. In rabbit species in which the virus is foreign, there apparently is virus variation which leads to malignancy. By gradual change in character, the malignant tumors arise from cells which are already neoplastic as a result of virus action.

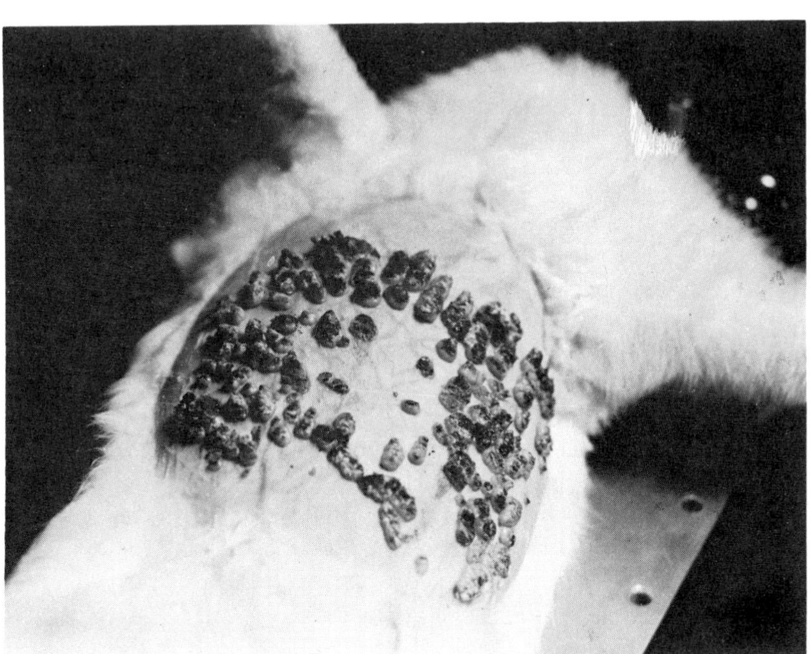

Figure 40.4. Rabbit papillomatosis. Warts on the scarified skin of the abdomen of a rabbit were produced experimentally. The inoculation had been carried out about 1 month previously. (Courtesy R. E. Shope, *Jour. Exp. Med.*)

Properties of the Virus. This is a double-stranded DNA virus (12) whose particles are icosahedral and 53 nm in diameter. The virus starts its development in the nucleolus and shortly involves the rest of the nucleus.

It is quite heat-resistant, requiring a temperature of 70 C for 30 minutes for inactivation. It survives for many years in glycerol and at low temperatures and is quite resistant to x-radiation and entirely resistant to ether. Purification can be accomplished with fluorocarbon or by precipitation with methanol (4). Analysis of rabbit papillomavirus on strained gels revealed 5 bands with a major polypeptide molecular weight of 60,000 daltons comprising 48 percent of the virion protein (11), while iodinated preparations of the same virus yielded 7 polypeptides. Isoelectrofocusing of iodinated virions had an isoelectric point of pH 4.0.

The fluorescent antibody technique has shown that the viral antigen is located in the keratohyaline and keratinized layers of the skin (7). Rabbit red blood cells absorb the virus, but the cells are agglutinated (2). Complement-fixing antigen is extractable from warts of cottontail rabbits, to a lesser degree from warts of domestic rabbits. No cross-neutralization or cross-immunity is demonstrable between the Shope papilloma and the papillomas of cattle and dogs or the rabbit oral papilloma (1).

Cultivation. Proliferation of epidermal cells was observed in skin organ cultures of newborn rabbits, but propagation of virus was not proved (6).

Immunity. Shope (9, 10) has shown that rabbits carrying experimentally produced papillomas are partially or wholly immune to reinfection, and also that the sera of such animals are capable of partially or completely neutralizing the virus *in vitro*. Even though the tumors produced in domesticated rabbits contain no demonstrable virus, injections or suspensions of such tumors will actively immunize susceptible animals. Shope concluded that in the tumors of the domestic rabbit the virus is present, but is masked in some unknown way. Bernheim and coworkers (3) claimed to have obtained the virus from cottontail rabbit tumors in the form of a homogeneous protein, but they were unable to find this protein in domesticated rabbit tumors. They did find in the latter, however, a noninfectious, antigenic protein that immunizes animals to the virus. They suggest that a factor exists, possibly enzymic in nature, in the domesticated rabbit which destroys the virus. They also speculate about the chance of the existence of such agents in other mammalian tumors and the possibility that this may explain why viruses have not been recognized in many of them.

Transmission. In view of the fact that animals can easily be infected through superficial scarifications of the skin, it is presumed that natural infections occur through direct contacts between infected and susceptible animals.

REFERENCES

1. Andrewes, Christopher. Viruses of vertebrates. Williams and Wilkins, Baltimore, 1964.
2. Barbadze. Virol., 1960, *5,* 103.
3. Bernheim, Bernheim, Taylor, Beard, Sharp, and Beard. Science, 1942, *95,* 230.
4. Fischer. Proc. Soc. Exp. Biol. and Med., 1949, *72,* 323.
5. Kidd and Rous. Jour. Exp. Med., 1940, *71,* 469.
6. deMaeyer. Science, 1962, *136,* 985.
7. Noyes and Mellors. Jour. Exp. Med., 1957, *106,* 555.
8. Rous and Beard. Jour. Exp. Med., 1935, *62,* 523.
9. Shope. Jour. Exp. Med., 1933, *58,* 607.
10. Shope. Jour. Exp. Med., 1937, *65,* 219.
11. Spira, Estes, Dreesman, Butel, and Rawls. Intervirol., 1974, *3,* 220.
12. Watson and Littlefield. Jour. Mole. Biol., 1960, *2,* 161.

The Oral Papilloma of Rabbits

Parsons and Kidd (1) described oral papillomatosis of the rabbit in 1943. These are benign growths which were found in a rather high percentage of "normal" domestic rabbits in the New York City area. They are readily transmitted by filtrates to other domestic rabbits, to the cottontail rabbit and the jackrabbit of the midwestern states, and to the snowshoe rabbit of the north, although they apparently do not occur naturally in any but the domestic species. They are not transmissible to other species of animals.

Character of the Disease. The tumors consist of small, gray white, sessile or pedunculated nodules found usually on the under surface of the tongue, occasionally on the gums, and rarely on the floor of the mouth. They often are multiple and sometimes quite numerous. The larger ones have cauliflowerlike surfaces and may be as large as 5 mm in diameter and 4 mm in height. The smaller ones usually are smooth and domelike.

Microscopically they are typical papillomas, the epithelial cells being swollen and vacuolated. In the cells near the surface, intranuclear inclusion bodies are found in about 10 percent of the lesions in the domestic rabbit. They are never found in lesions in other species.

The tumors are benign and cause little inconvenience to the host. Usually they are not noticed unless the oral mucosa is closely scrutinized.

Intranuclear inclusions were found by Parsons and Kidd in about 10 percent of the tumors in domestic rabbits, but none was found in the induced tumors in other species of rabbits. When present they were located in the outer 6 to 10 layers of epithelial cells. They varied greatly in size and shape. Some were hyaline, and others showed a stippled structure. They were basophilic and located near the center of the nucleus, the chromatin being marginated. Such bodies were not found in normal oral epithelium of domestic rabbits.

The disease is transmissible by scarification to rabbits that have not previously been infected. The lesions in experimental animals do not differ in appearance from those occurring naturally.

Properties of the Virus. The virus readily passes Berkefeld V and N candle filters. The average incubation period of unfiltered virus is 15 days; of Berkefeld V filtrates, 19 days; and of Berkefeld N filtrates, 23 days. The virus is a very stable one. Tissues stored in 50 percent glycerol at 4 C retain their pathogenicity relatively undiminished for 2 years and more. Those stored while frozen remain potent for long periods, and material dried while frozen remains potent many months. The resistance to heat is rather remarkable. Heating at 65 C for 30 minutes appears to do little injury. Some tumors were produced by materials heated at 70 C.

Cultivation. Reports of attempts to cultivate the virus of rabbit oral papillomatosis have not been found.

Immunity. After recovery from oral papillomatosis animals are solidly immune to reinfection for at least several months. There is no immunological relationship with the Shope papilloma. Animals affected with one type of tumor can readily be infected with the other, and animals solidly immune to one type as a result of regression are fully susceptible to the other.

Transmission. The disease does not appear to be particularly contagious because Parsons and Kidd observed no general spread among stock in animal quarters. It was noticed, however, that the tumor incidence of the litters from females that had papillomas was much higher (11.8 percent) than those from females free of tumors (1.3 percent). Virus was recovered in several instances from mouth washings of animals that had no papillomas. The authors believed that the virus is present in a dormant state in the mouths of many animals and that tumors are induced only when the mucous membrane is injured by rough feed or other agents. Several experiments in which coal tar was smeared on the skin of rabbits without tumors led to a higher incidence of tumors than in animals not so treated. Since the tar is licked off by the animals, it was thought that the tar was the precipitating factor. Abundant quantities of virus were recovered from the tar-induced tumors. The same tar did not induce tumors in wild rabbits, which do not carry this virus, but are fully susceptible to it by inoculation. It was thought, too, that the virus might be transmitted from doe to offspring in the process of suckling.

REFERENCE

1. Parsons and Kidd. Jour. Exp. Med., 1943, *77*, 233.

Genital Papilloma of Pigs

This condition was described by Parish in 1961 (1). He observed the natural occurrence of papillomas in the genital region of boars. The papilloma was transmissible by scarification or injection into the genital skin of adults. The warts appeared 8 weeks after injection. Cytoplasmic inclusion bodies were observed in the lesions.

This agent is inactivated readily by heat, and survival at 4 C and −20 C is poor. It is resistant to ether. Neutralizing antibodies can be detected in the sera of hyperimmunized pigs and rabbits, but not in convalescent pig sera. Pigs that recover from the infection are resistant to challenge. Antigen can be demonstrated by the use of the gel-diffusion or conglutination complement-absorption tests (2).

REFERENCES

1. Parish. Jour. Path. and Bact., 1961, *81*, 331.
2. Parish. Jour. Path. and Bact., 1962, *83*, 429.

41 The Adenoviridae

The type species for the single genus *Adenovirus* in the family Adenoviridae is *Adenovirus* h-1 of man; 35 serotypes of man are at present recognized. These are divided into 4 subgroups on the basis of their ability to agglutinate rhesus monkey and rat red blood cells. There is some correlation between this method of grouping and immunological groupings based on cross-reactions with sera from volunteers inoculated with various members of the group. Hemagglutination-inhibition and neutralization tests have also demonstrated antigenic relationships among members of the 4 respective hemagglutinating groups, although cross-reactions are generally of low level and vary with the virus strain and the method employed. Other members of the genus include 2 canine, 25 simian, 9 bovine, 4 porcine, 5 ovine, 11 fowl, 4 turkey, and 3 goose serotypes. Adenoviruses also have been isolated from the horse, mouse, and opossum.

In general, the members of this family have been well characterized, especially the human adenoviruses, and excellent reviews are available (1–4). The virions contain double-stranded DNA with a molecular weight of 23 $\times$ 10^6 daltons. Isometric nonenveloped particles have icosahedral symmetry, 70 to 90 nm in diameter, with 252 capsomeres, each 7 nm in diameter (Figure 41.1). Twelve vertex capsomeres are antigenically distinct from the other capsomeres and carry a filamentous projection. The particles are ether-resistant. They have a buoyant density in rubidium chloride of 1.34 g per cm^3 and a sedimentation coefficient of 795 S. Viral assembly takes place in the nucleus of the cell where inclusion bodies are seen. A common antigen shared by all mammalian strains differs from the corresponding antigen of avian strains. Some viruses hemagglutinate cells of various species.

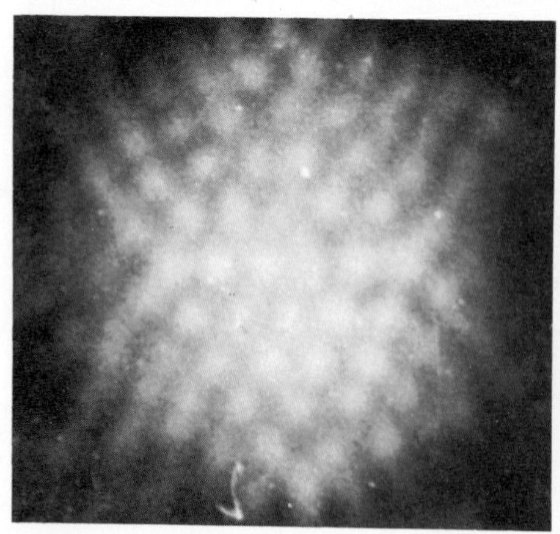

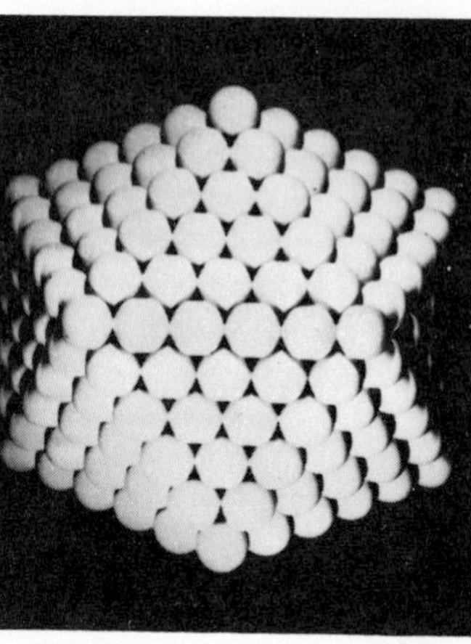

Figure 41.1. (*Left*) Electron micrograph of an adenovirus, an icosahedral virus. It is embedded in phosphotungstate, magnified about 1 million diameters. (*Right*) A model of the figure on the left showing how the particles, 252 surface subunits or capsomeres, are arranged with icosahedral symmetry. (Courtesy R. W. Horne, S. Brenner, P. Wildy, and A. P. Waterson, *Jour. Mole. Biol.*)

Table 41.1. Diseases in domestic animals caused by viruses in the Adenoviridae family, genus *Adenovirus*

Common name of virus	Natural hosts	Type of disease produced
Infectious canine hepatitis (canine adenovirus type 1)	Dogs	Hemorrhagic and hepatitic
Canine adenovirus, type 2	Dogs	Respiratory
Bovine adenoviruses, types 1-9	Cattle	Variety of clinical syndromes—conjunctivitis, pneumonia, pneumoenteritis, diarrhea, polyarthritis (weak calf syndrome)
Porcine adenoviruses, types 1-4	Swine	Type 4 usually is the only pathogen causing diarrhea and/or meningoencephalitis
Ovine adenoviruses, types 1-5	Sheep	Respiratory and enteritic, usually mild or inapparent unless complications arise
Equine adenovirus infection, type 1	Horses	Pneumonia; Arabian foals seem most susceptible
Turkey adenoviruses, types 1-4	Turkeys	Respiratory disease and occasionally enteritis in poults; marble spleen disease
Avian adenoviruses, types 1-11	Chickens (domestic)	Respiratory illness, enteric disease, egg-drop syndrome, aplastic anemia, atrophy of bursa of Fabricius

Under certain conditions some viruses are oncogenic. They produce a rather characteristic cytopathology in monolayer cell cultures with marked rounding of cells that form aggregates in grapelike clusters. The host specificity is relatively narrow, and persistence of the virus in the natural host is quite common.

The important diseases in this family are respiratory and ocular disease in humans and other species and infectious canine hepatitis (Table 41.1).

REFERENCES

1. Cabasso and Wilner. Adv. Vet. Sci. and Comp. Med., 1969, *13*, 159.
2. Huebner. Modern Med. (Minneapolis), 1958, *26*, 103.
3. Pereira. Brit. Med. Bull., 1959, *15*, 225.
4. Sohier, Chardonnet, and Prunieras. Prog. Med. Virol., 1965, *7*, 253.

Canine Adenoviruses (Infectious Canine Hepatitis)

SYNONYMS: Hepatitis contagiosa canis, Rubarth's disease, fox encephalitis; abbreviation, ICH

This disease has long been confused with canine distemper. It affects foxes as well as dogs, and according to Chaddock (10), it also occurs in timber wolves, coyotes, and bears. Bolin, Jarnevic, and Austin (5) found neutralizing antibodies in the blood of a wild raccoon. Green (23) first described the disease in foxes, at which time it was thought to be a form of salmonellosis, but in 1930 Green, Ziegler, Green, and Dewey (25) published evidence that indicated the causative agent was a virus. As early as 1927 Green and coworkers showed that the disease could be readily transmitted to dogs. The experimental disease in the dog was described in detail by Green and Shillinger (24) in 1934, and by Beckman and Torrey (4) in 1940. That the disease occurred naturally in dogs was soon recognized. DeMonbreun (16) in 1937 described the histological lesions accurately, but assumed that the disease was canine distemper. Rubarth (36) in Sweden published a detailed account of the disease in 1947, and it was he who supplied the name *infectious canine hepatitis,* by which it is now generally known. Rubarth recognized that the disease was the same as that which American authors had been discussing for some years under the name of fox encephalitis infection of dogs.

Canine adenovirus type 1 (strain Utrecht) was the first canine adenovirus officially recognized. The canine virus Toronto A26/21 of Ditchfield *et al.* (17) is now regarded as type 2 because biophysical data and also differences in complement-fixing, hemagglutinating, and neutralizing antigens suggest a significant variation from type 1 and it has a marked predilection for respiratory tissue.

Character of the Disease. *Hepatic form in dogs.* This classical form is very widespread and probably occurs wherever dogs are numerous. Rubarth diagnosed 190 cases in Stockholm between 1928 and 1946, this number being 3.4 percent of all canine fatalities coming under his observation. The disease is very common in the British Isles, Denmark, Norway, Australia, and North America. Natural infections have been recognized in the United States by many; Storm and Riser (37), Riser (35), Coffin (13), and Chapman (12) were among the early reporters. It is now known that ICH is a common and destructive disease of dogs in the United States. Mixed infections with canine distemper (CD) may occur, and such cases have an unusually high death rate.

The disease occurs at all times of the year. It is most frequent in young dogs, but has been seen in all age groups. Young puppies, shortly after weaning, seem most susceptible, and in them the mortality rate is highest.

The affected animal becomes apathetic and loses its appetite, but frequently shows an intense thirst. At this time the temperature is likely to be as high as 105 F or higher; later it may fall and become subnormal. Some cases exhibit edema of the head, neck, and lower portion of the abdomen. Vomiting and diarrhea are common. Many animals manifest pain by moaning, especially when pressure is brought to bear on the abdominal wall.

During the early temperature reaction, a blood count will disclose a leukopenia, the leukocytes usually falling to 2,500 per cu mm or less. Nervous signs usually are absent, and only rarely does icterus appear. A common sign is a transient opacity of the cornea (uveitis), which may appear in one or both eyes from 7 to 10 days after the disappearance of the acute signs (1, Figure 41.2).

The mucous membranes are usually pale, and sometimes petechiae appear on the gums. The tonsils frequently are acutely inflamed and enlarged. The heart action is often accelerated, and the respiratory rate increased. Albuminuria occurs in many cases.

The incubation period is short. Baker *et al.* (2) report that after intravenous inoculation dogs showed signs on the 2nd or 3rd day; after subcutaneous inoculation, in 3 to 4 days; after being fed virus, in 4 to 6 days; and when susceptible dogs were allowed natural contact with infected ones, the susceptible usually developed signs in 6 to 9 days.

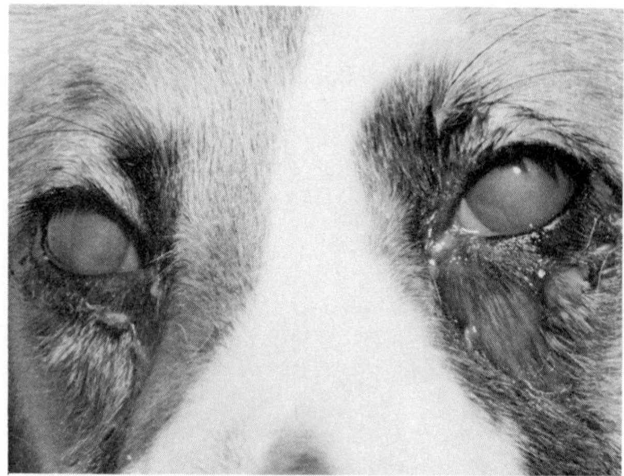

Figure 41.2. Corneal opacity of both eyes of an experimental dog following intravenous inoculation of an attenuated canine adenovirus serotype 1 strain, classical ICH virus. (Courtesy L. Carmichael.)

The progress of this disease is much more rapid than that of distemper. Most dogs have recovered or are dead within 2 weeks, and many succumb within a few days.

The mortality varies according to the age of the dog. Chaddock and Carlson (11) report about 25 percent mortality for artificially infected dogs. Baker *et al.* experienced only about 10 percent.

The autopsy findings of the hepatic form are rather characteristic. Because of the rapid progress of the disease, there is no evidence of emaciation. Edema of the subcutaneous tissues frequently occurs, and fluid is found in the peritoneal cavity in half or more of the cases. This fluid may be clear, but more often it is blood-tinged, and usually it appears to consist almost wholly of pure blood. Upon exposure to the air this bloody exudate often coagulates. A fibrinous exudate is usually found among the intestinal loops even when no fluid is present in the cavity. Hydrothorax occurs only occasionally. Sometimes subserous hemorrhages are seen on the stomach, intestines, gall bladder, and diaphragm.

The liver may not be greatly changed in appearance, but usually it is somewhat swollen and light in color. The capsule is tense, and the lobules appear more prominent than normal. The gall bladder generally shows a marked edema of its wall. The thickened wall may be hemorrhagic, in which case the whole sac may appear black or reddish black. The mucosa of the gall bladder is not changed in appearance, but fibrinous deposits are usually found in the vicinity of the organ. The spleen seems normal or slightly enlarged. The intestines may appear normal, but the contents are often mixed with blood. Edema of the lungs may occur, but pneumonia is absent.

The principal histological changes are found in the liver and endothelial cells (Figure 41.3). The blood content is increased, and the larger vessels are greatly dilated. The distended sinusoids cause pressure on the liver cells. The endothelial cells of the sinusoids and Kupffer cells are greatly swollen and undergoing degeneration. Nuclear inclusions occur to a varying degree in the liver cells, as well as in the lining cells of the sinusoids and the Kupffer cells and in the endothelial cells of the veins. Rubarth considers the primary damage to be in the endothelial cells and the circulatory disturbances to be secondary. In the brain, serous effusions frequently occur under the pia mater, and there are cellular infiltrations around the blood vessels. The endothelial cells of the blood vessels often are swollen and undergoing degeneration, and many of the smaller veins are filled with such cells. Inclusion bodies are usually found in these cells. The picture is that of a nonpurulent encephalitis.

Inclusion bodies can be found readily in most cases, but sometimes they are not numerous. They occur in the endothelial cells of the sinusoids of the liver, of the spleen, of the lymph nodes, of the vascular system of the brain, and less commonly elsewhere in the hepatic form. They may be found in detached endothelial cells in the small blood vessels, especially in the brain and in the glomeruli of the kidneys. They are always intranuclear and acidophilic. The chromatic material of the affected nuclei breaks down and marginates, leaving a clear central area in which the inclusion bodies may be found. Usually there is but one inclusion body in each nucleus, but multiples are occasionally seen. They may be round or oval. The inclusion bodies may be found in tissue sections, or they may be demonstrated in touch preparations of fresh liver tissue (15).

Figure 41.3. Canine adenovirus serotype 1 (ICH) virus in vascular endothelial cells. FA. × 125. (Courtesy L. Carmichael and M. Appel.)

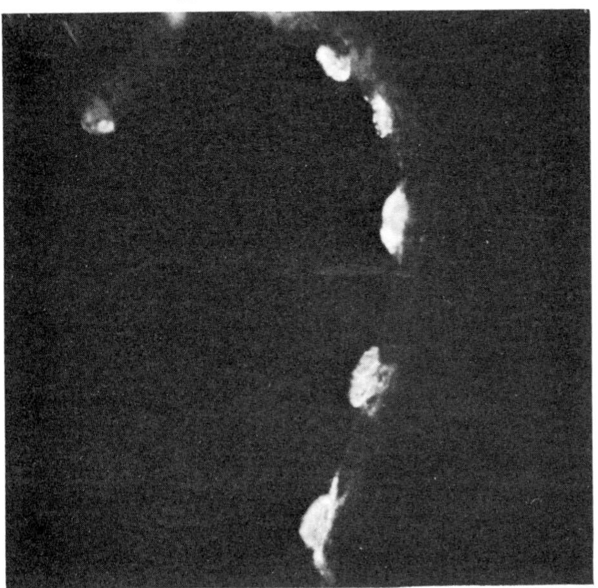

The disease can be reproduced in dogs and foxes by inoculation. It is innocuous for ferrets, a fact used in differentiating this virus from that of canine distemper. It does not affect mink or the ordinary small laboratory mammals. Dogs, raccoons, and ferrets do develop interstitial keratitis following injection of virus into the anterior chamber of the eye. Carmichael *et al.* (8) reported that canine adenotype 1 antibody complexes caused severe anterior uveitis with corneal edema when the virus was injected into the anterior chamber of normal dogs' eyes (Figure 41.4). The response to such immune complexes was similar to the spontaneously occurring disease. Similar immune complexes have been found in the serum of experimental dogs during the acute stage of the disease when serum antibody titers were low (30).

Respiratory form in dogs. The Toronto A26/21 strain of canine adenovirus was isolated from a dog with a respiratory illness (17). These original observations have been extended by others, so it is accepted now that certain strains of canine adenovirus have a strict affinity for the epithelial cells lining the respiratory tract (Figure 41.5) and fail to produce hepatitis in dogs (39). Virus persisted in organ cultures from nasal nucosa for at least 12 weeks after oronasal exposure with A26/61 respiratory-type strain, whereas cultures from dogs given hepatic-type virus were negative for virus (28). Conversely, virus was isolated from cell cultures derived from kidneys of these dogs, but kidney cultures from dogs given A26/61 virus were negative.

The infection produced by the A26/61 was inapparent or quite mild (1, 20). In contrast, more severe respiratory signs of illness in dogs were described by Swango *et al.* (39) with their C955L strain, which is serologically identical to A26/61. Certain bacteria, either pathogens or potential pathogens, were isolated singly or in various combinations from the lungs of dogs at necropsy. They probably contributed a great deal to the severity of the disease. The signs were observed in their contact dogs as well as the dogs infected by the aerosol method.

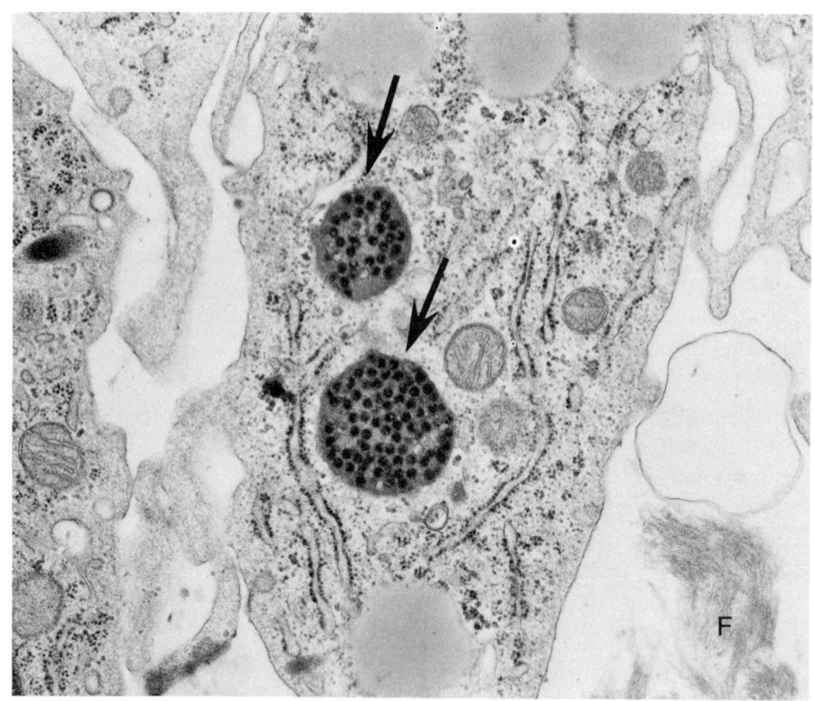

Figure 41.4. Double membrane body aggregates (immune complexes) in the cytoplasm of a macrophage comprising portion of the keratic precipitate. Note fibrin *(F)*. × 13,000. (From Carmichael, *Cornell Vet.*, 1975, *65*, 331.)

A fever usually persists for 1 to 3 days after an incubation period of 5 to 6 days for contact dogs. The disease may vary in severity from a harsh, dry hacking cough of 6 to 7 days duration to a fatal pneumonia. Other signs include depression, anorexia, dyspnea, muscular trembling, and serous nasal discharge. In some dogs the nasal discharge became mucopurulent. Vomition occurs in some animals, and some have soft, mucoid feces. Dogs with a harsh and dry cough had less lung involvment than those dogs with a soft, moist, pulsating cough. The leukocyte counts were variable and inconclusive.

The gross lesions apparently are confined to the respiratory tract. There is atelectasis and congestion of the lungs with varying degrees of consolidation sharply demarcated from normal tissue. Congestion and hemorrhages of the bronchial lymph nodes and congestion of

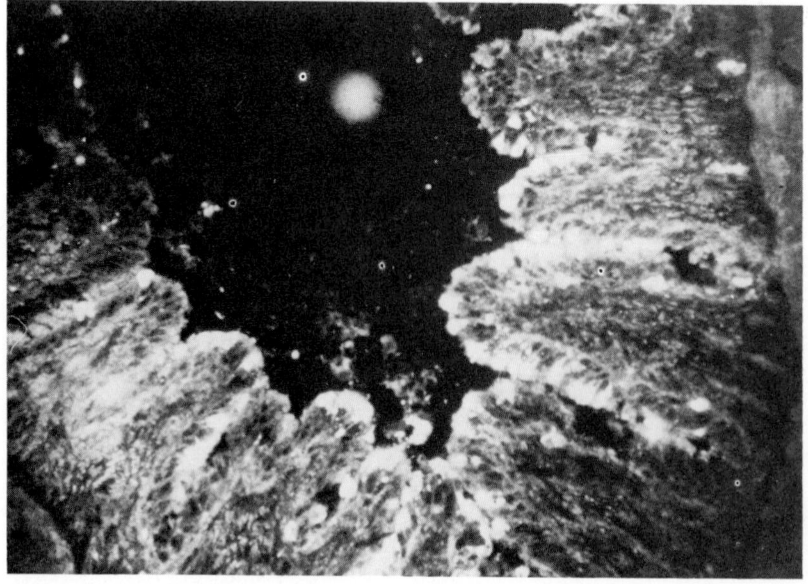

Figure 41.5. Canine adenovirus serotype 2 virus (respiratory form) in bronchial epithelial cells of a dog, 6 days after aerosol exposure. FA. × 120. (Courtesy M. Appel and I. Parkinson.)

mesenteric lymph nodes is seen in most dogs. There were no gross lesions in the liver or gall bladder as is characteristic of the hepatic form in dogs.

In histological studies moderate to severe pneumonic changes were observed in dogs infected with A26/21 type virus. Cowdry type A intranuclear inclusion bodies may occur in the bronchial epithelium, alveolar septal cells, and turbinate epithelium. Proliferative, adenomatous changes are seen in the lungs of dogs 10 days after infection ensues. The bronchial lymph nodes are congested and edematous. Similar but more severe histologic changes are seen in the lungs than in dogs infected with hepatic form, but centrilobular necrosis and intranuclear inclusion bodies in the liver and marked edema and hemorrhage in the gall bladder were lacking in A26/21-type infections.

In studies with Toronto A26/61 strain, corneal opacities were not seen in 24 experimental dogs after infection (1). Corneal opacities are known to occur in a small percentage of dogs given attenuated vaccine produced with hepatic-type virus strains, or after natural disease with canine adenovirus type 1.

Encephalitic form in foxes. The disease occurs among wild animals, but the losses are seen principally on fur ranches. They may amount to 15 or 20 percent of the population of the ranch. The disease appears suddenly, and the course in affected animals is very short. Loss of appetite may be noted for a day or two before other signs appear. In many cases animals are found dead without signs having been observed. Violent convulsions often initiate the signs. These are followed by a lethargic state in which the animal wanders about aimlessly and blindly. This may be interrupted by other convulsions. Usually the affected animal dies within 24 hours of the time when the first sign is seen. Toward the end various paralytic signs may be noted: paralysis of one leg, of the hind quarters, or of the entire body. A terminal coma may last for periods up to 24 hours. At the onset of the disease a watery nasal discharge is common, and sometimes there is a similar discharge from the eyes. The feces become soft and filled with mucus; sometimes there is a profuse diarrhea in which blood streaks are common.

Chaddock (10) says that the incubation period in artificially inoculated animals varies from 2 to 6 days depending on the virulence of the strain.

The disease runs a very rapid course in foxes. It may be as short as 1 hour, and it usually is less than 24 hours, but a few cases may last as long as 3 days. Foxes that succumb to this disease generally have lost little weight because of the rapidity of its course.

Nearly all animals that show signs die. The spread of the disease in breeding pens is rather slow, and usually not more than 5 percent of the animals contract it. The disease persists for many years on fox farms, reappearing annually. The losses over a period of years may be great.

Gross lesions consist of hemorrhages in various parts of the body. These occur as rather large extravasations in some cases, and are small or absent in others. Large hemorrhages into the brain or into the cord serve to explain the paralytic signs often seen in this disease. Large hemorrhages into the lungs sometimes occur.

Although the name of this disease suggests that it is caused by a neurotropic virus, this is not the case. The disease in foxes is generalized, involving primarily the endothelial system, especially the endothelial linings of the smaller blood vessels. Injuries to these cells result in hemorrhages and in cellular degenerations. As the nervous system is very susceptible to this form of damage, the signs are largely referable to it.

Nuclear inclusion bodies may be readily demonstrated in endothelial cells of various organs and in epithelial cells of the liver. These are identical in appearance with those found in dogs.

Properties of the Virus. The negative staining technique has shown in electron photomicrographs that the virus particles are rigid icosahedra with 252 protein subunits (capsomeres) that comprise the overcoat (capsid) (14). The diameter is estimated at 75 to 80 nm. Some strains produce intranuclear virus crystals (27).

It survives well when frozen or dried. It is inactivated in 24 hours by 0.2 percent formalin, but survives for days in 0.5 percent phenol (38). It is inactivated at 50 C after 150 minutes, or at 60 C in 3 to 5 minutes. It is ether- and chloroform-resistant and survives between pH 3 and 9 at room temperature.

The virus hemagglutinates chicken red blood cells at 4 C and pH 7.5 to 8 (21). It also hemagglutinates rat and human O cells at pH 6.5 to 7.5 (19). Viral hemagglutination is inhibited by antibody.

A group complement-fixing antigen is shared by ICH virus and other adenoviruses (7, 26). Complement-fixation and precipitin reactions are unilateral between ICH virus and human adenovirus types, since human adenovirus antiserums react with both human and canine virus types, but ICH antiserum fails to react with the human adenovirus antigens. No cross neutralization occurs between ICH virus and certain other adenovirus types (26). Interferon is not produced by ICH virus in dog kidney tissue cultured cells, nor is the virus sensitive to interferon.

Cultivation. Up to the present little success has been realized in attempts to cultivate this virus in embryonated eggs. Miles *et al.* (29), in England, claim to have secured propagation in serial passage, but these studies have not been confirmed. Cabasso and coworkers (6) reported successful cultivation of this virus in roller-tube tissue cultures of dog kidney cells, in which specific cytopathogenic effects are produced (Figure 41.6). The virus can be carried indefinitely in such cultures. Independently and at about the same time, Müller and Thordal-Christensen (31), in Norway, also succeeded in propagating the ICH virus and demonstrating cytopathogenic effects in tissue cultures of canine kidney monolayer cells. Fieldsteel and Yoshihara (22) were the first to report success in propagating the ICH virus in tissue cultures consisting of cells other than those of dogs. They were successful with ferret kidney and swine kidney cells. Emery and York (18) likewise succeeded with swine kidney cell tissue cultures. They reported that the virus lost a substantial part of its virulence for dogs as a result of replication in swine cells.

Immunity. Canine adenovirus type 1 protects dogs against itself and against Toronto A26/61 type virus, and A26/21 type virus protects dogs against itself and against canine adenovirus type 1 (1). Consequently, presently available vaccines for ICH protect dogs against both types of canine adenovirus.

One attack of this disease confers a solid and permanent immunity. It has already been pointed out that immune animals may, nevertheless, shed virus in their urine for long periods of time. There is no cross immunization between infectious hepatitis and canine distemper. Rubarth, in Sweden, and several workers in the United

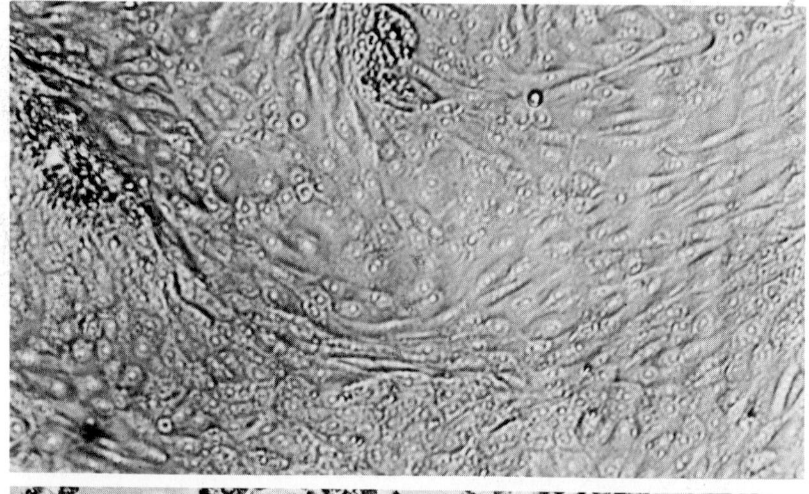

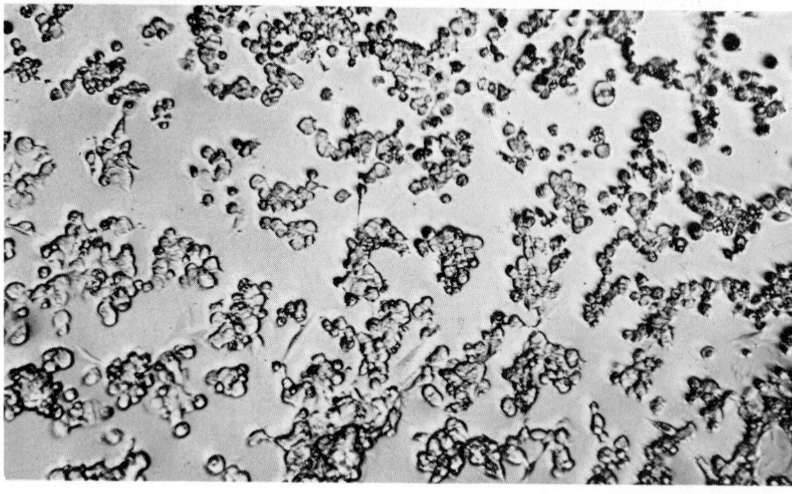

Figure 41.6. Roller-tube cultures of canine renal cortex. (*Upper*) Uninoculated control showing solid sheet of epithelial cells. (*Lower*) Epithelial cells 3 days after inoculation with 10^4 tissue culture inoculation doses of infectious canine hepatitis virus. × 90. (Courtesy Fieldsteel, *Am. Jour. Vet. Res.*)

States have found that a considerable number of puppies having no history of the disease are, nevertheless, resistant to infectious hepatitis by virtue of neutralizing antibodies which they carry. This indicates that the virus is considerably more prevalent in our dog population than the recognized number of cases would indicate.

Poppensiek (32) showed that it was possible to protect susceptible puppies by passively immunizing them with homologous hyperimmune serum, and that solid, active immunization could be accomplished with serum and virus administered simultaneously. These dogs quite generally proved to shed virus in their urine as in the natural disease; hence they were hazardous to nonprotected puppies with which they came in contact.

As with canine distemper the virus-neutralization test is the only serological test that has been shown to indicate immunity. Other tests may be used for diagnosis, but CF antibodies do not persist long after initial infection whereas neutralizing antibodies remain for a long period of time. Most dogs possess high levels of neutralizing antibodies at least 3.5 years after vaccination and at least 5.5 years after experimental infection.

The results obtained by Carmichael, Robson, and Barnes (9) with maternal immunity to ICH in puppies are remarkably but predictably similar to those obtained in distemper because the antibody half-life for both viruses is 8.5 days. Appel *et al.* (1) suggested a practical way to overcome maternal immune interference. In their experiments, 4-week-old puppies with ICH maternal antibody titers ranging from 10^2 to $10^{2.4}$ were inoculated with their respiratory strain DK_{12} (closely related to Toronto A26/61) by the oronasal route. Virus was found in pharyngeal swabs 4 to 7 days after exposure, but serum antibody titers continued to decline at a half-life rate of 8.5 days. When antibody titers of 10^1 were reached, a sudden increase in antibody occurred suggesting the production of an active immunity presumably due to persisting virus replication. These antibody levels remained, and when some puppies were challenged at 14 weeks of age with canine adenovirus type 1 and the homotypic virus, the puppies showed no signs of illness, nor could virus be isolated from pharyngeal swabs or blood.

Immunization. Inactivated and attenuated virus vaccines, alone or in combination with the distemper and other components, are manufactured in the United States and abroad. The ICH virus has been attenuated by transfer in dog, ferret, or pig kidney culture. The dual vaccine containing attenuated distemper and attenuated ICH viruses is used most commonly in the United States. On rare occasions the attenuated virus vaccine causes a corneal opacity, but this is the only sign of disease that ever occurs. The lesion disappears without treatment. Certainly cortisone therapy is contraindicated.

More recently attenuated canine adenovirus type 2 was approved to replace canine adenovirus type 1 in vaccines so postvaccination corneal opacity should no longer constitute a problem.

If the dual attenuated virus vaccine (or the triple vaccine) is given to puppies with an unknown maternal immunity for ICH or CD, it should be administered preferably at 9 weeks of age or whenever they are first presented, and then again at 15 weeks of age. This will cover the period of maternal insusceptibility for both diseases. Immunity acquired from the mother is likely to vary among litters of puppies because the mother will probably have a different antibody level of protection for each disease.

It is known that attenuated ICH virus is eliminated from the urine of vaccinated dogs. Susceptible dogs that come in contact with the attenuated virus will be immunized without signs of illness.

Foxes that recover from the natural infection are permanently immune thereafter, and it is possible to immunize with hyperimmune homologous serum and with vaccine (10). Hyperimmune serum is used principally to stop outbreaks. Green, Ziegler, Green, and Dewey (25) failed in their attempts to immunize foxes with serum and virus used simultaneously. Animals treated in this manner did not sicken and die immediately as did the control animals, but most of them died about 5 weeks after treatment. It appeared that virus had persisted and produced disease only after the serum immunity had worn off.

Formalinized-tissue vaccines have been used successfully in foxes. Some of the commercial companies that make vaccine for canine use also recommend the vaccine for use on this animal.

Transmission. Baker and coworkers (2) have shown that this disease, unlike canine distemper, is not transmitted by droplet infection, but requires more or less direct contact. Susceptible dogs, kept in cages separated from those of infected dogs by no more than 6 inches, remained uninfected. On the other hand, it was easy to infect through the mouth with infective materials. Transfer of saliva on the fingertips usually succeeded. More recently other investigators (39) suggested that the respiratory form of ICH, in contrast to the classical form, may be conveyed by aerosol transmission. Poppensiek and Baker (33) showed that canine adenovirus type 1 virus is liberated in the urine during the acute phases and for many months afterwards in some dogs; this undoubtedly is the usual source of infection.

Diagnosis. Clinically, ICH is difficult to distinguish from other infectious diseases of the dog, principally canine distemper (CD) and others that cause respiratory signs of illness. Because CD is the most serious malady of the dog, the differentiation of ICH and other canine respiratory diseases from CD constitutes a major problem for the practitioner. ICH and CD vary in their signs of illness, but there is sufficient overlapping in the signs that a positive diagnosis is difficult. One major difference was cited by Poppensiek (32), who stated that the coagulation time of the blood is much increased in clinical cases of hepatic ICH while it is unchanged in CD.

At necropsy the hepatic form of ICH in dogs can be readily distinguished from CD. The characteristic liver and gall bladder lesions and the effusions that occur in the body cavities of hepatic ICH distinguish it from CD. Intranuclear inclusion bodies are found in tissues infected with ICH, whereas CD has intracytoplasmic inclusion bodies—this readily differentiates the two viral diseases regardless of the disease form of ICH. ICH can be transmitted to susceptible dogs and foxes like CD, but unlike CD the virus of ICH is not transmissible to ferrets.

The methods that are used in dogs are applicable to the disease in foxes. In general, the acute course and the pronounced nervous signs make the clinical diagnosis easier in this species than in dogs.

Rubarth found that the complement-fixation test could be used successfully for diagnosing ICH. Extracts of the liver may be used as antigen, these being set up against a specific antiserum produced for the purpose. With such a test he reported that he was able to make specific diagnoses on dogs in which postmortem decomposition had made any other method of diagnosis impossible. The test was used in a survey of 100 dogs in the clinic at Stockholm which, at the time, were not suffering from hepatitis. Seventy percent of the animals were positive to the test, the incidence of reactors increasing with age. This would have to be taken into consideration when using the test for diagnostic purposes. In endeavoring to find a practical means of determining whether dogs of unknown history had or had not previously suffered from ICH, Prier and Kalter (34) compared the complement-fixation test with an intradermal test, using as antigen formalinized lymph node tissues from a dog acutely ill with ICH. They found the intradermal test much more accurate than the CF test.

Field strains of ICH virus readily produce a cytopathic effect in monolayer cultures of primary or secondary dog-kidney cells. This offers a convenient and excellent way of diagnosing the disease as the tissue-cultured virus can be readily recognized by its characteristic adenovirus type of cytopathic effect, by its ability to hemagglutinate erythrocytes from several animal species, by its production of intranuclear inclusion bodies in tissue-cultured cells, and by its neutralization with immune and convalescent ICH serum. The demonstration of a rising antibody titer utilized with paired sera from an active case is another means of diagnosing the disease.

Control. Because it appears that a high percentage of dogs harbor the virus of infectious hepatitis, it follows that most animals will come in contact with it sooner or later, unless they live an isolated and sheltered life. Apparently most cases are mild and result in permanent immunity. The greatest mortality apparently occurs when hepatitis and distemper infections occur simultaneously. Because the distemper mortality is much greater than that from hepatitis, it is most important to protect dogs against the former, but it is possible to vaccinate against both, and this probably is the best course.

The Disease in Man. The virus of canine hepatitis is not infective for man. The agent of a viral-induced infectious hepatitis of man was compared by Bech (3) with the ICH virus in many ways, and no antigenic relationship between them could be detected.

REFERENCES

1. Appel, Pickerill, Menegus, Percy, Parsonson, and Sheffy. Gaines Symposium, 1971.
2. Baker, Richards, Brown, and Rickard. Proc. Am. Vet. Med. Assoc., 1950, p. 242.
3. Bech. Proc. Soc. Exp. Biol. and Med., 1959, *100,* 135.
4. Beckman and Torrey. North Am. Vet., 1940, *21,* 232.
5. Bolin, Jarnevic, and Austin. Proc. Soc. Exp. Biol. and Med., 1958, *98,* 414.
6. Cabasso, Stebbins, Norton, and Cox. Proc. Soc. Exp. Biol. and Med., 1954, *85,* 239.
7. Carmichael and Barnes. Proc. Soc. Exp. Biol. and Med., 1961, *107,* 214.
8. Carmichael, Medic, Bistner, and Aquirre. Cornell Vet., 1975, *65,* 331.
9. Carmichael, Robson, and Barnes. Proc. Soc. Exp. Biol. and Med., 1962, *109,* 677.
10. Chaddock. Auburn Vet., 1948, *5,* 11.
11. Chaddock and Carlson. North Am. Vet., 1950, *31,* 35.
12. Chapman. North Am. Vet., 1948, *29,* 162.
13. Coffin. Jour. Am. Vet. Med. Assoc., 1948, *112,* 355.

14. Davies, Englert, Stebbins, and Cabasso. Virol., 1961, *15,* 87.
15. Davis and Anderson. Vet. Med., 1950, *45,* 435.
16. DeMonbreun. Am. Jour. Path., 1937, *13,* 187.
17. Ditchfield, MacPherson, and Zbitnew. Can. Vet. Jour., 1962, *3,* 238.
18. Emery and York. Science, 1958, *127,* 148.
19. Espmark and Salenstedt. Arch. f. die gesam. Virusforsch., 1961, *11,* 61.
20. Fairchild, Medway, and Cohen. Am. Jour. Vet. Res., 1969, *130,* 1187.
21. Fastier. Jour. Immunol., 1957, *78,* 413.
22. Fieldsteel and Yoshihara. Proc. Soc. Exp. Biol. and Med., 1957, *95,* 683.
23. Green. Proc. Soc. Exp. Biol. and Med., 1925, *22,* 546.
24. Green and Shillinger. Am. Jour. Hyg., 1934, *19,* 343 and 362.
25. Green, Ziegler, Green, and Dewey. Am. Jour. Hyg., 1930, *12,* 109.
26. Kapsenberg. Proc. Soc. Exp. Biol. and Med., 1959, *101,* 611.
27. Leader, Pomerat, and Lefeber. Virol., 1960, *10,* 268.
28. Menegus. N.Y. State Vet. Col. Rpt., 1969–1970, p. 41.
29. Miles, Parry, Larin, and Platt. Nature, 1951, *168,* 699.
30. Morrison and Wright. Res. Vet. Sci., 1976, *21,* 119.
31. Müller and Thordal-Christensen. Nord. Vetmed., 1954, *6,* 767.
32. Poppensiek. Proc. Am. Vet. Med. Assoc., 1952, p. 288.
33. Poppensiek and Baker. Proc. Soc. Exp. Biol. and Med., 1951, *77,* 279.
34. Prier and Kalter. Proc. Soc. Exp. Biol. and Med., 1954, *86,* 177.
35. Riser. North Am. Vet., 1948, *29,* 568.
36. Rubarth. Acta Path. et Microbiol. Scand., Sup. 69, 1947, p. 1.
37. Storm and Riser. North Am. Vet., 1947, *28,* 751.
38. Surdan, Cure, Dumitriu, and Wegener. Acta Virol., 1959, *3,* 115.
39. Swango, Wooding, and Binn. Jour. Am. Vet. Med. Assoc., 1970, *156,* 1687.

Bovine Adenoviruses

Klein (9) first isolated two bovine adenoviruses from USA cattle, and these now represent bovine adenovirus types 1 and 2. They were recovered from cattle during a search for viruses responsible for the production of poliovirus antibodies in cattle. A serotype antigenically distinct from types 1 and 2 was isolated in England from the conjunctiva of a healthy cow (7), and it is now recognized as bovine adenovirus type 3. Other strains have been isolated in Hungary from calves with diarrhea and still others from calves with pneumoenteritis (1). Nine bovine adenovirus serotypes are recognized; it is reasonable to assume others will be recognized as studies progress. A strain of ovine adenovirus isolated from natural disease in sheep is closely related to bovine adenovirus type 2 and produced pneumoenteritis in experimental calves. (2)

Character of the Disease. Bovine adenovirus infection is common in cattle populations in many countries of the world including the United States, Japan, Hungary, England, and Germany. Various serotypes cause a variety of clinical signs such as conjunctivitis, pneumonia, pneumoenteritis, diarrhea, and polyarthritis (weak calf syndrome). Adenovirus types 3, 4, and 5 are the ones usually incriminated in the production of disease in the USA (14, 13, 12). The Hungarian workers who initially had the greatest field experience repeatedly made isolations of bovine adenoviruses from natural cases of pneumoenteritis in calves where the mortality was a significant factor (1). With many of their isolates they fulfilled Koch's postulates by reproducing the disease in colostrum-deprived calves and in susceptible calves 2 to 16 weeks of age.

Bovine adenovirus type 5 causes a mild, self-limiting disease in colostrum-deprived calves characterized by a marked pyrexia, polyarthritis, and occasionally diarrhea. (14, 6). Natural disease is enhanced by cold weather and by other disease agents such as virus diarrhea virus.

In the natural and experimental disease of calves the signs of illness and necropsy findings were similar according to Darbyshire (7). In experimental disease clinical signs referable to the respiratory and digestive tracts were observed 7 days after intranasal or intratracheal injection of virus. At necropsy, varying degrees of consolidation, collapse, and emphysema of the lungs were most prominent 7 days after viral exposure, but these lesions persisted for at least 3 months. Histologic features were proliferative bronchiolitis with necrosis and bronchiolar occlusion resulting in alveolar collapse. Nuclear inclusion bodies are found in the bronchiolar epithelium, septal cells, and bronchial lymph nodes. The viruses are resistant to ether and possess a complement-fixing antigen common to the adenovirus group. Type 1 shows a two-way cross with human and canine adenoviruses (5).

Properties of the Virus. Considerable interest in bovine adenovirus type 3 (BAV 3) as a result of its oncogenic capability has led to detailed studies of its properties. Using purified virus in a cell line derived from calf kidney (CKT1) it was observed that viral DNA synthesis was initiated after 24 hours and its rate was greatest about 40 hours (15). Viral maturation occurred several hours later. Purified virus was separated into four discrete bands in cesium chloride representing complete, incomplete, empty, and degraded virions. The virus is similar in morphology and size to human and avian adenoviruses. There is a 25 percent homology between DNA of BAV 3 and human adenovirus type 5. Complete virions contain at least 10 polypeptides.

Types 1 and 2 agglutinate rat erythrocytes, and type 2 also agglutinates mouse erythrocytes. Neither serotype agglutinates red blood cells of chicks, guinea pigs, cattle, sheep, or human O (9). In morphological studies hexons, groups of hexons, and pentons were found in the soluble fraction, and the presence of free pentons supported the existence of incomplete hemagglutinins in type 1. (10)

Calf-kidney and calf-testes cell monolayers of primary and stable cell cultures show a cytopathic effect after inoculation with bovine adenoviruses. The Hungarian workers made successful isolations only in bovine testicular cultures. The type of cytopathic effect is characteristic of the adenovirus group.

Type 3 virus induced tumors when inoculated into newborn hamsters, but the virus was not recovered (7). Strizhachenko *et al.* (17) believe the antigenicity of spontaneous tumor and its immunologic relationship with the host are probably associated with antigens of cellular origin occurring on the cell membrane as a result of tumor formation rather than with the antigens induced by an etiological agent.

Serotypes 1 and 2 failed to produce infection in suckling and adult hamsters, chicken embryos, guinea pigs, hamsters, or rabbits (9).

Adult hamsters immunized with type 3 virus rejected tumor transplants from suckling hamsters with bovine adenovirus type 3 tumors, whereas transplants were readily made in nonimmune adult hamsters.

Immunity. The mechanism of neutralization of virus by antibody is complex, but the type-specific determinants exposed on the virion must play a critical role (18). Calves inoculated with bovine adenoviruses develop neutralizing antibodies in 10 to 14 days, reaching an approximate level of $10^{2.7}$ to 100 $TCID_{50}$ of homologous virus. Heterotypic responses were not observed. These antibody levels are maintained for at least 10 weeks. Precipitating antibodies appear in 3 weeks with no diminution of titer at 10 weeks (7). At necropsy of 2 young calves with diarrhea and dehydration that failed to respond to therapy, foci of necrosis were found in the abomasum and rumen of each calf, and the intestinal tract contained grayish, turbid fluid. Intranuclear inclusion bodies found in endothelial vessels of the abomasum, rumen, adrenal cortical sinusoids, and renal glomeruli and also in intestinal epithelial cells were identified as adenovirus particles (3).

Complement-fixing antibodies were not always present, but CF antigen was found in various tissues of calves infected with type 3, particularly in the upper respiratory tract (7).

Hemagglutinating antibodies reach a maximum level 7 days after intranasal exposure with type 1 virus which was maintained for at least 6 weeks (7).

The duration of immunity in cattle to BAV 3 after 2 intranasal administrations of attenuated virus 6 weeks apart was at least 21 months. Before challenge with virulent virus at that time local and systemic antibodies were detected in the experimental cattle (20). It is reasonable to anticipate that the duration of immunity after vaccination or natural disease will be quite long lasting and durable. Submucosal application of the virus induces the production of interferon, which undoubtedly also plays some role in adenovirus immunity.

Transmission. From experimentally infected calves virus could be recovered from the conjunctiva, nose, and feces for periods ranging from 10 to 21 days after onset of infection. As carriers are typical of the adenovirus group, more exhaustive studies may show that the virus persists for a longer period of time than 21 days. Present knowledge suggests that the virus is transmitted to susceptible cattle from acutely infected or infected cattle or their contaminated excretions.

Diagnosis. This is one of a number of bovine viruses that produce respiratory signs and, frequently, diarrhea as well. It is difficult to distinguish clinically for this reason. Consequently a positive diagnosis requires assistance from a laboratory that attempts virus isolation in monolayer cell cultures derived from calf testes, preferably, or calf kidney.

The best material for isolation is from exudate of nasal passages and conjunctiva and from feces of acutely ill cattle. Recovery of virus in tissue-culture cells was regularly accomplished from trachea and lungs. The isolate can be identified by the characteristics given in the section on its properties. Particularly, the ability of most serotypes to hemagglutinate rat erythrocytes offers a convenient and quick method for identification. The demonstration of a rising titer with paired serums utilizing the serum neutralization, agar gel precipitation, complement-fixation, passive hemagglutination, fluorscent antibody, or hemagglutination-inhibition tests also is an excellent way to diagnose the disease.

In the serotyping of isolates no cross-reactions are noted in the neutralization test.

Control. There is considerable activity and interest in the production of inactivated and attenuated virus vaccines for the prevention and control of bovine adenovirus infection. Present evidence suggests that these vaccines to either BAV 1 or BAV 3, usually in combination with infectious bovine rhinotracheitis or bovine parainfluenza 3, are safe and provide excellent protection to cattle, for a considerable period of time, against homologous virus (19, 16, 8, 11). Rondhuis (16) believes oil adjuvant vaccines are superior, but considerably more work must be done to prove his arguments. Present evidence suggests that cattle will also have a large number of serotypes with no suggestion of cross protection among them. It seems unlikely that vaccination will ever play a prominent role in the control of the disease unless it is found that a very limited number of serotypes are the significant pathogens, or cross protection does occur with some of the 9 serotypes.

A general characteristic of this adenovirus group is the persistence of the virus which also makes control of these diseases more difficult. Good management, health care, and housing can reduce the severity of the disease, but prevention is difficult, if not impossible, until a practical and economic vaccination program becomes a reality. No vaccines are licensed in the USA at this time.

The Disease in Man. The relationship between bovine adenoviruses and infection in man has not been established. There is no reported evidence of disease in man caused by bovine adenoviruses, but serum-neutralizing antibodies to bovine adenoviruses type 1 and 2 have been found in humans. There is no cross-reaction between these two bovine serotypes with antiserums to human adenoviruses 1 through 18.

REFERENCES

1. Aldasy, Csontos, and Bartha. Acta Vet. Acad. Sci. Hungarscae, 1965, *15,* 167.
2. Belak, Palfi, Szekeres, and Tury. Zentrbl. Vet.-Med., 1977, *24B,* 542.
3. Bulmer, Tsai, and Little. Jour. Am. Vet. Med. Assoc., 1975, *166,* 233.
4. Cabasso and Wilner. Adv. Vet. Sci. and Comp. Med., 1969, *13,* 199.
5. Carmichael. Quoted by Cabasso and Wilner in Adv. Vet. Sci. and Comp. Med., 1969, *13,* 199.
6. Cutlip and McClurkin. Am. Jour. Vet. Res., 1975, *36,* 1095.
7. Darbyshire. Jour. Am. Vet. Med. Assoc., 1968, *152,* 786.
8. Haralambiev. Arch. Exp. Vet. Med., 1975, *29,* 397.
9. Klein. Ann. N.Y. Acad. of Sci., 1962, *101,* 493.
10. Khristov, Ignatov, and Popov. Vet. Med. Nauki., 1977, *14,* 11.
11. Khristov, Karadzhov, Ignatov, and Khristova. Vet. Med. Nauki., 1976, *13,* 36.
12. Lehmkuhl, Smith, and Dierks. Arch. Virol., 1975, *48,* 39.
13. Mattson, Smith, and Schmitz. Am. Jour. Vet. Res., 1977, *38,* 2029.
14. McClurkin and Coria. Jour. Am. Vet. Med. Assoc., 1975, *167,* 139.
15. Niiyama, Igarashi, Tsukamoto, Kurokawa, and Sugino. Jour. Virol., 1975, *16,* 621.
16. Rondhuis. Dev. Biol. Stand., 1975, *28,* 493.
17. Strizhachenko, Graevskaya, Karmysheva, and Syurin. Arch. Geschwulstforsch, 1975, *45,* 324.
18. Willcox and Mautner. Jour. Immunol., 1976, *116,* 25.
19. Zygraich, Lobmann, Peetermans, Vascoboinic, and Huygelen. Dev. Biol. Stand., 1975, *28,* 482.
20. Zygraich, Vascoboinic, and Huygelen. Dev. Biol. Stand., 1976, *33,* 379.

Porcine Adenoviruses

A porcine adenovirus first was isolated from a rectal swab of a 12-day-old piglet with diarrhea (5). Subsequently, porcine adenoviruses were derived from various tissues of normal pigs at slaughter, rectal swabs of healthy pigs, and from the brain of a 10-week-old pig with encephalitis (1, 7–10). During the passage of hog cholera virus in cell cultures from the kidneys of normal pigs taken at a slaughterhouse, an adenovirus as well as particles similar in size to enteroviruses were isolated as latent viruses from the pig kidneys (6). At present, there are 4 recognized serotypes of porcine adenoviruses (2). Reference antisera against human adenoviruses types 1 to 31 failed to neutralize porcine adenovirus serotypes 1, 2, and 3, while neutralizing antibodies to the 3 porcine adenovirus serotypes were present in sera of normal sows (5). The incidence of infection in the pig populations of Hungary and Bulgaria is approximately 20 percent (4). It appears that many strains are of relatively low pathogenicity, and usually serotype 4 is isolated from natural cases of diarrhea or encephalitis. This serotype produced meningoencephalitis in gnotobiotic pigs (3).

The porcine adenoviruses have all the morphological

and biochemical characteristics of the other adenoviruses (4). The strains usually replicate in primary cell cultures of embryonic and piglet kidney, of rabbit kidney, of porcine embryonic lung, and of porcine embryonic testes and also in the stable cell line PK-15. The cytopathology is characteristic of adenoviruses.

REFERENCES

1. Darbyshire, Jennings, Dawson, Lamont, and Omar. Res. Vet. Sci., 1966, *7,* 81.
2. Derbyshire *et al.* Jour. Comp. Path., 1975, *85,* 441.
3. Edington, Kasza, and Christofinis. Res. Vet. Sci., 1972, *13,* 289.
4. Genov and Bodon. Vet. Med. Nauki., 1976, *13,* 31.
5. Haig, Clarke, and Pereira. Jour. Comp. Path. and Therap., 1964, *74,* 81.
6. Horzinek and Uberschän. Arch. f. die gesam. Virusforsch., 1966, *18,* 406.
7. Kasza. Am. Jour. Vet. Res., 1966, *27,* 751.
8. Kohler and Apodaca. Zentrbl. f. Bakt., I. Abt. Orig., 1966, *199,* 338.
9. Mahnel and Bibrach. Zentrbl. f. Bakt., I. Abt. Orig., 1966, *199,* 329.
10. Mayer, Bibrack, and Bachmann. Zentrbl. f. Bakt., I. Abt. Orig., 1967, *203,* 60.

Ovine Adenoviruses

The original isolations of ovine adenoviruses were made from sheep feces by negative contrast electron microscopy for the size and morphology of the virions (3). The feces came from normal and diseased sheep. On the 9 isolates, 3 were serologically distinct. A 4th serotype was isolated and identified by Sharp *et al.* (6). Subsequently a 5th serotype was identified.

In general, it would appear that the ovine adenovirus serotypes produce a mild or inapparent infection associated with respiratory and enteric tracts. Ovine adenovirus 4 infection in specific pathogen-free lambs (7, 5) fails to elicit clinical signs, but pathological changes referable to the respiratory and alimentary tracts were discernible. In all likelihood this infection may predispose the host to more serious infections. Belak *et al.* (1) reported on a natural outbreak of adenovirus disease in suckling and fattening lambs causing pneumoenteritis on 2 large farms with heavy mortality. One isolate typed as ovine serotype from this epizootic produced a similar disease in 3-week-old experimental lambs (4).

On the farm that raised only sheep, a virus was isolated from 6- to 8-week-old Merino sheep with mild respiratory signs of illness that was similar, if not identical, to BAV 2 (2) but different from known ovine serotypes.

REFERENCES

1. Belak, Palfi, and Palya. Zentrble. Vet.-Med., 1976, *23B,* 329.
2. Belak, Palfi, and Tury. Acta Vet. Acad. Sci. Hungaricae, 1975, *25,* 91.
3. McFerran, Nelson, and Knox. Arch. f. die gesam Virusforsch., 1971, *35,* 232.
4. Palya, Belak, and Palfi. Zentrbl. Vet.-Med., 1977, *24B,* 529.
5. Rushton and Sharp. Jour. Pathol., 1977, *121,* 163.
6. Sharp, McFerran, and Rae. Res. Vet. Sci., 1974, *17,* 268.
7. Sharp *et al.* Jour. Comp. Path., 1976, *86,* 627.

Equine Adenoviruses

Adenoviral infection may cause pneumonia in foals, particularly in Arabian horses. In recent years various investigators have isolated an adenovirus from pneumonic cases (9, 8, 3, 5). In one instance 28 Arabian and 3 non-Arabian foals less than 3 months of age developed a disease characterized by pneumonia, lymphopenia, and intermittent fever with 27 Arabian foals dying and 1 Arabian and 2 non-Arabian foals recovering (5).

Studdert *et al.* (7) made antigenic comparisons of 7 strains of equine adenovirus from the United States, Germany, or Australia by the serum neutralization and hemagglutination-inhibition tests. The 7 equine adenoviruses were closely related. Further, these investigators tested 631 equine serums, and 73 percent had antibodies indicating this is a very common infection in horses, suggesting that only in unusual situations or cases do clinical signs accompany the infection. It has been suggested that an autosomal inherited trait is responsible for the susceptibility of Arabian foals to this virus.

In experimental studies with equine adenovirus, neonates developed clinical signs that included fever, nasal and ocular discharge, and dyspnea (6). Older foals were less affected and colostrum-fed foals had a milder illness than colostrum-deprived foals. Neonatal foals that were euthanitized during acute illness had lesions that included hyperplasia, swelling, necrosis, and intranuclear inclusions in epithelial cells of the respiratory tract. Virus was recovered from most experimental foals.

Strains of equine adenovirus have been isolated in fetal or horse kidney cell cultures or in equine fetal dermis cells. The cytopathic alterations in cell culture are characteristic of adenoviruses, and examination by electron microscopy of infective cell cultures confirmed the presence of adenovirus particles and also the presence of equine adeno-satellite viral particles (1). Its other characteristics also were typical of adenoviruses (2, 4).

REFERENCES

1. Dutta. Am. Jour. Vet. Res., 1975, *36,* 247.
2. Harden. Res. Vet. Sci., 1974, *16,* 244.
3. Henry and Gagnon. Can. Vet. Jour., 1976, *17,* 220.
4. Konishi, Harasawa, Mochizuki, Akashi, and Ogata. Jap. Jour. Vet. Sci., 1977, *39,* 117.
5. McChesney, England, and Rich. Am. Jour. Vet. Res., 1973, *162,* 545.
6. McChesney, England, Whiteman, Adcock, Rich, and Chow. Am. Jour. Vet. Res., 1974, *35,* 1015.
7. Studdert, Wilks, and Coggins. Am. Jour. Vet. Res., 1974, *35,* 693.
8. Thompson, Spradborw, and Studdert. Austral. Vet. Jour., 1976, *52,* 435.
9. Whitlock, Dellers, and Shively. Cornell Vet., 1975, *65,* 393.

Other Mammalian Adenoviruses

The murine adenovirus occurs in some mouse colonies. It is eliminated in the urine as it persists in the urinary tract and accounts for the maintenance of virus in a colony. Suckling mice inoculated by various routes suffer fatal infection with disseminated pathological lesions particularly in the brown fat, heart, and adrenals.

The opossum adenovirus was isolated from the kidney-cell culture of this species. As adenoviruses commonly persist as latent viruses in the kidneys of various species, investigators who are using animal kidney-cell cultures must be aware of this situation. The ability of the opossum isolate to produce disease has not been determined.

Presently, there are 31 recognized serotypes of simian adenoviruses. Only a few instances of primate disease attributable to natural adenovirus infection of the respiratory tract or conjunctiva have been reported in the literature. Its physical and chemical properties are typical for the adenovirus group.

From two goats that died from *peste des petits ruminants* in separate outbreaks, an adenovirus was isolated in the large intestine of both goats. The two isolates were considered different serotypes from the sheep and cattle types. The authors (1) suggest the adenoviruses were probably commensals in these cases.

REFERENCE

1. Gibbs, Taylor, and Lawman. Res. Vet. Sci., 1977, *23,* 331.

Turkey Adenoviruses

Adenovirus infection may cause respiratory illness, marble spleen disease, or enteric disease in turkey poults. Various investigators isolated virus from cases with respiratory illness. In some instances the isolate failed to produce signs of illness in experimental poults (7, 8) or only mild illness (2). With another isolate identified as turkey type 1, respiratory signs were severe in day-old poults, and the mortality was 50 percent (1). Itakura and Carlson (6) produced hemmorrhagic enteritis in two turkeys. Clinically, the affected young turkeys showed bloody diarrhea. Birds died acutely. Birds at necropsy had a large number of dark red bloody clots in the intestinal tract, many petechiae in the mucous membrane of small intestine and ceca, and atrophy of the spleen (4). Characteristic histological changes were acute hemorrhagic enteritis, degenerative changes of lymphatic tissue, and proliferation of reticuloendothelial cells with intranuclear inclusion bodies in these cells throughout the host. Viral particles in these cells were characteristic of adenoviruses.

Marble spleen disease (MSD) has been described in young poults, and ring-necked pheasants (5). Morphologically the virus was consistent with that of an avian adenovirus. MSDV antigen showed a cross-reaction with antiserum to turkey adenovirus serotypes TA-1 and TA-2.

Easton and Simmons made an antigenic analysis of several turkey respiratory adenoviruses by reciprocal-neutralization kinetics. These viruses were placed into four serologic groups (3). Certain surveys have been conducted to show that there has been widespread exposure of the turkey population in the USA to these viruses.

REFERENCES

1. Blalock, Simmons, Muse, Gray, and Derieux. Avian Dis., 1975, *19,* 707.
2. Cheville and Sato. Vet. Pathol., 1977, *14,* 567.
3. Easton and Simmons. Avian Dis., 1977, *21,* 605.
4. Fujiwara, Tanaami, Yamaguchi, and Yoshino. Natl. Inst. An. Health Q. (Tokyo), 1975, *15,* 68.
5. Iltis, Daniels, and Wyand. Am. Jour. Vet. Res., 1977, *38,* 95.
6. Itakura and Carlson. Can. Jour. Comp. Med., 1975, *39,* 299.
7. Simmons, Miller, Gray, Blalock, and Colwell. Avian Dis., 1976, *20,* 65.

8. Sutjipto, Miller, Simmons, and Dillman. Avian Dis., 1977, *21*, 549.

Chicken Adenoviruses

Various disease entities are attributed to the 11 avian adenovirus serotypes (8) now known to exist. Ten serotypes have been established in the USA (2), and in all likelihood all 11 serotypes are present. In some instances the adenoviruses are known to cause respiratory disease (10), enteric disease, inclusion body hepatitis (7), egg-drop syndrome (5), atrophy of the bursa of Fabricius (10), and the hemorrhagic-aplastic anemia syndrome (13). Grimes and King described the latter syndrome in an experimental situation as a spontaneous outbreak that could not be attributed to an avian adenovirus (6). There is a suggestion that a duck adenovirus contaminant in a vaccine used for Marek's disease is responsible for some cases associated with the egg-drop syndrome. An adenovirus isolated from a normal turkey caused experimental disease in both chicks and turkey poults (3). In many instances adenoviruses isolated from diseased chickens fail to produce illness in susceptible test birds. This is to be expected because this is characteristic of adenoviruses. Adenoviruses are common infectious agents of poultry and other avian species throughout the world. Limited observations suggest the adeno-associated viruses (parvoviruses) coinfect many chickens that carry adenoviruses (16).

The original type of quail bronchitis virus isolated many years ago produced signs of illness in 4-week-old quail characteristic of quail bronchitis. The experimental disease also transfers readily to susceptible quail with the production of an acute, highly fatal respiratory disease. Quail that recover from experimental disease are resistant to the production of disease, but reinfection does occur despite the presence of neutralizing antibody (11).

The properties of avian adenoviruses have been thoroughly investigated. The avian adenoviruses lack a common complement-fixing antigen shared by all mammalian adenoviruses. The physical and chemical characteristics are typical of the genus (1). Chicken embryos infected with quail bronchitis virus become curled or dwarfed after one or a few serial passages (11). The cytopathic effects of avian adenoviruses in chicken embryo kidney (14) or liver (4) cell cultures are characteristic of the adenovirus group. A microneutralization test, using chicken kidney monolayers as an indicator, now is used to facilitate immunity and serotyping tests with the adenovirus (5). Hemagglutinating activity of an oncogenic strain (Phelps) of avian adenovirus is a function of complete and incomplete particles, and this characteristic facilitates the study of disease in birds (9).

A solid and long-lasting immunity is conferred to monovalent virus. No cross protection is conferred between heterologous serotypes 1, 2, and 3 (15). Maternal antibodies confer temporary protection to young chicks (15, 12). Polyvalent vaccines produced lower virus-neutralizing antibody titers on occasion when compared with chickens given the monovalent vaccines (15). Their vaccines were effective and safe, and vaccine virus was not shed beyond 28 days after vaccination.

Because the duck adenovirus contaminant in Marek's vaccine has caused the egg-drop syndrome in many European flocks along with the problem of high incidence and latent infection characteristic of adenoviruses, an inactivated vaccine is in use in these breeder flocks with probable success.

REFERENCES

1. Cabasso and Wilner. Adv. Vet. Sci. and Comp. Med., 1969, *13*, 159.
2. Calnek and Cowen. Avian Dis., 1975, *19*, 91.
3. Cho. Avian Dis., 1976, *20*, 714.
4. Defendi and Sharpless. Jour. Natl. Cancer Inst., 1958, *21*, 925.
5. Grimes and King. Am. Jour. Vet. Res., 1977, *38*, 317.
6. Grimes and King. Avian Dis., 1977, *21*, 97.
7. Grimes, King, Kleven, and Fletcher. Avian Dis., 1977, *21*, 26.
8. McFerran and Connor. Avian Dis., 1977, *21*, 585.
9. Mishad, McCormick, Stenback, Yates, and Trentin. Avian Dis., 1975, *19*, 761.
10. Mustaffa-Babjee and Spradbrow. Avian Dis., 1975, *19*, 150.
11. Olson. Proc. U.S. Livestock Sanit. Assoc. (Phoenix), 1950, *54*, 171.
12. Otsuki, Tsubokura, Yamamoto, Imamura, and Sakagami. Avian Dis., 1976, *20*, 693.
13. Rosenberger, Klopp, Eckroade, and Krauss. Avian Dis., 1975, *19*, 717.
14. Taylor and Calnek. Avian Dis., 1962, *6*, 51.
15. Winterfield, Fadly, and Hoerr. Poultry Sci., 1977, *56*, 1481.
16. Yates, Rhee, and Fry. Avian Dis., 1977, *21*, 408.

42 The Iridoviridae

African swine fever (ASF) is a member of a new family called Iridoviridae. At present ASF is the only animal virus included in this family that causes disease in a domestic animal. Other members include *Tipula iridescent* (type species), *Sericesthis iridescent, Aedes iridescent, Lymphocystis* (fish), *Amphibian cytoplasmic,* and Gecko viruses. Some members such as ASF have a lipid envelope.

The biophysical and biochemical characteristics for members of this family, which has the single genus *Iridovirus,* can be found in Chapter 36.

African Swine Fever

SYNONYMS: East African swine fever, wart hog disease, Montgomery's disease; abbreviation, ASF

Montgomery (13) first described ASF from Kenya Colony, where it was recognized as an entity in 1910. Later it was studied by Steyn (20, 21) and Walker (22). The disease is an acute, highly fatal disease of domesticated swine of European breeds imported into several areas of east Africa. The signs and lesions are much like those of hog cholera. Montgomery viewed the disease as a hyperacute form of swine fever (hog cholera), but others regarded it as a different malady. It is caused by a virus distinct from hog cholera, and it differs immunologically from European hog cholera. Montgomery was unable to protect against the disease with anti-hog-cholera serum, and he had very little success with East African virus and antiserum. Steyn confirmed these results. When the disease appeared on isolated ranches, almost all pigs died. In several survivors Steyn was able to show that virus was detectable in the blood up to 2 months afterward.

Until 1957, African swine fever was not known to occur in any part of the world other than east Africa. In that year the disease was found in Portugal (18). At first thought to be hog cholera, it was finally recognized to be ASF. Before it was stamped out, 433 herds comprising more than 16,000 pigs had become infected. In 1959 the disease was found in Spain, and in 1960 it recurred in Portugal. The disease was widespread in Cuba in 1971, but was successfully eradicated, although it occurred again in 1979 and was eradicated in May, 1980. In 1978 the disease was introduced into Brazil, the Dominican Republic, and Haiti and is thought to exist still in these countries as well as Iberia, Mozambique, Zambia, South Africa, and Angola (4). Its presence in Latin America, a Caribbean island, and Europe constitutes a threat to the swine industry in Central America, Mexico, Canada, and the United States.

Character of the Disease. ASF is quite similar to hog cholera in some respects. The incubation period is 5 to 9 days, and the onset of illness is characterized by a sudden rise in temperature. Death usually occurs 4 to 7 days later with an exceedingly high mortality as a rule. A day or two before death the temperature falls rapidly. At this time the animal may show some or all of the following signs: labored breathing, depression, weakness, bloody feces, incoordination, reddish discolorations on ears, snout, fetlock, and flanks, coughing, and occasionally a

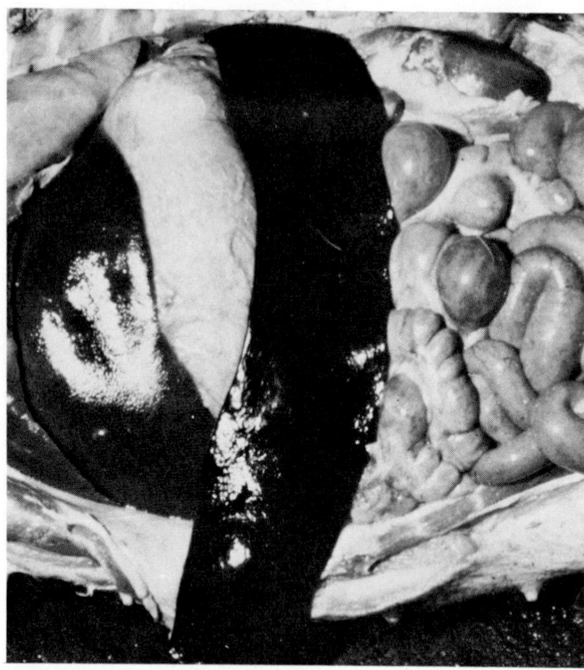

Figure 42.1. African swine fever. The spleen in acute African swine fever is greatly enlarged, friable, and reddish black. (Courtesy D. A. Gregg, Plum Island Animal Disease Center, USDA.)

Figure 42.2. African swine fever. The hepatogastric lymph node in acute African swine fever is enlarged and reddish black. (Courtesy D. A. Gregg, Plum Island Animal Disease Center, USDA.)

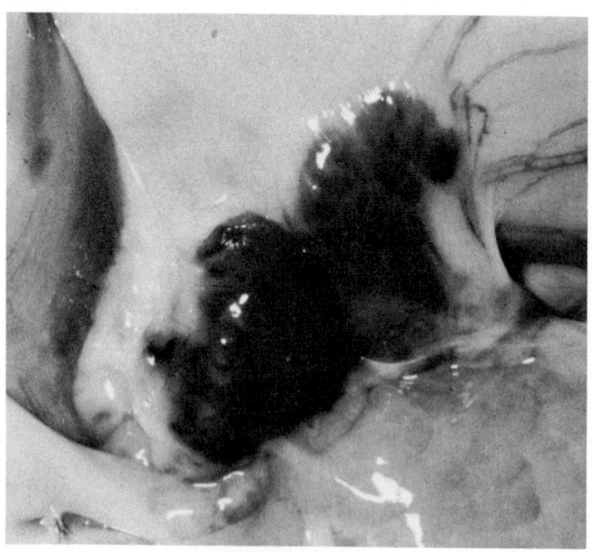

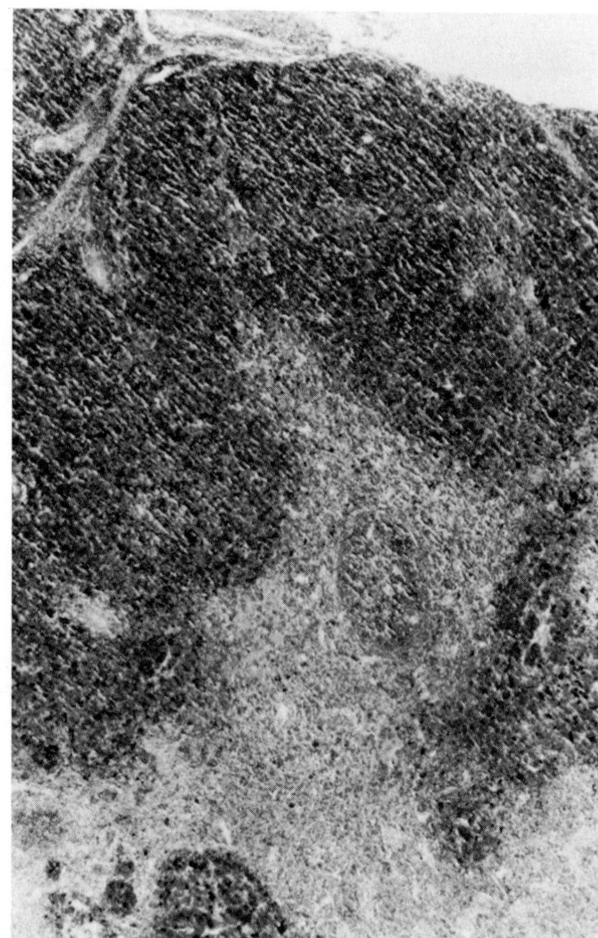

Figure 42.3. Photomicrograph of a section of lymph node from a pig with acute African swine fever. There is extensive hemorrhage in the cortical part of the node. H and E stain. (Courtesy C. A. Mebus, Plum Island Animal Disease Center, USDA.)

sticky ocular discharge. Unlike swine with hog cholera, swine with ASF may continue to eat until death.

DeTray (5) has shown that African swine fever sometimes behaves in European swine in about the same way as it does in native African swine in that surviving animals have a persisting viremia for long periods of time even though they appear well. European pigs that showed no signs of the disease after inoculation nevertheless became virus carriers and had viremia. The animals had antibodies and viremia simultaneously. The antibodies and virus were demonstrated in the serums of these animals for a short period. Virus persisted for a long period afterward, but antibody did not. Immunity to the homologous virus strain seems transient. After infection with virulent virus it is present in all the major blood fractions and was associated with equivalent

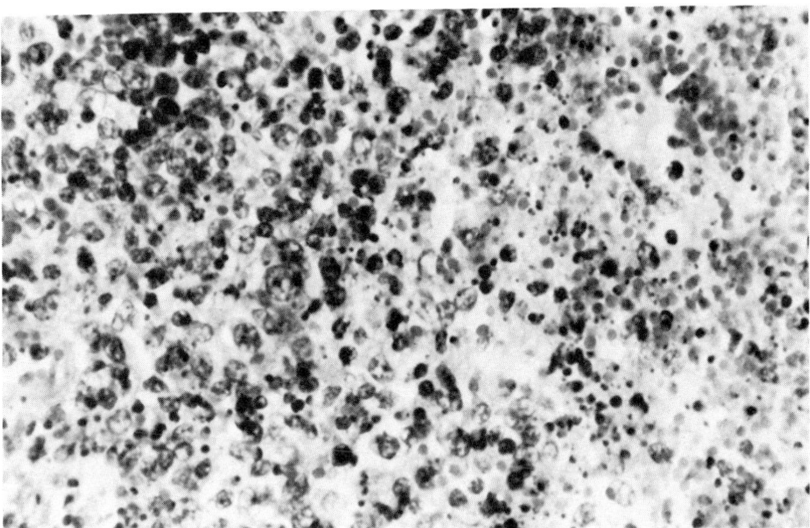

Figure 42.4. Photomicrograph of the cellular stroma in a lymph node from a pig with acute African swine fever. The right side of the photograph has many erythrocytes characteristic of hemorrhage. In the center of the photograph, there are numerous pyknotic nuclei. (Courtesy C. A. Mebus, Plum Island Animal Disease Center, USDA.)

numbers of both red blood cells and white blood cells (23). Ninety percent of the virus is in the RBC. Of the WBC subpopulations virus was definitely associated with lymphocytes and possibly neutrophils.

In comparison with hog cholera, Maurer, Griesemer, and Jones (10) found few differences in the lesions caused by ASF. The primary lesions in cases of fatal ASF are in the spleen, which is greatly enlarged, friable, and reddish black (Figure 42.1), in the lymphatic tissues (Figures 42.2, 42.3, 42.4) with its characteristic hemorrhages, and in the walls of the arterioles and capillaries. A marked difference is the karyorrhexis of the lymphocytes, which occurs in ASF but not in hog cholera.

After ASF is introduced into a susceptible pig population, the acute form of the disease is dominant. With the passage of time coupled in some instances with introduction of attenuated virus vaccine, the chronic form of the disease predominates. Under these circumstances pigs develop a chronic pneumonia (Figure 42.5). The pathogenesis of chronic pneumonia was studied by Moulton *et al.* (14). Interalveolar septums become thickened by accumulation of lymphocytes and monocytes, and focal areas of lymphocytes and macrophages appear in the lungs. Necrosis soon develops in these foci, which then become calcified. The calcified areas are surrounded by mononuclear cells, including plasma cells,

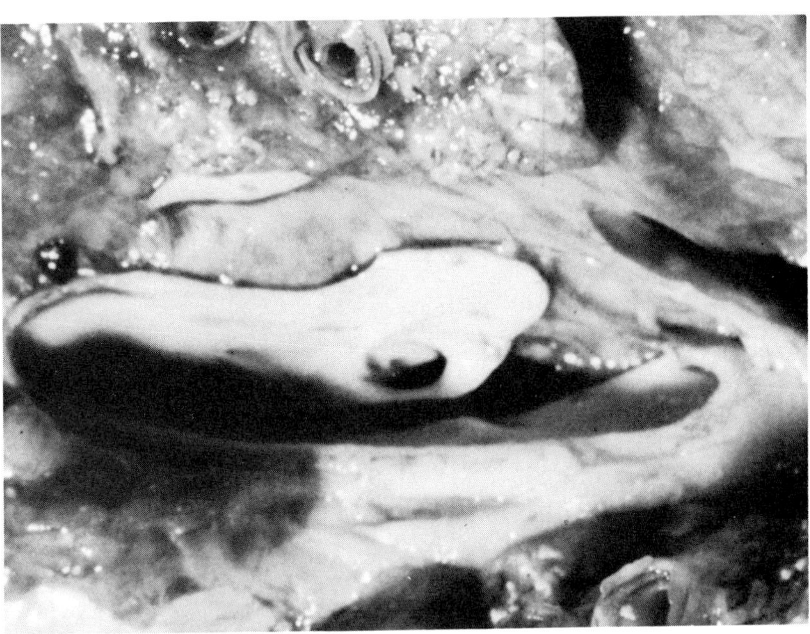

Figure 42.5. Lung lesion in chronic African swine fever. The lesion has a lobular distribution and whitish necrotic appearance. (Courtesy D. A. Gregg, Plum Island Animal Disease Center, USDA.)

and fibrous tissue. Hypergammaglobulinemia accompanied by hypoalbuminemia occurs in chronic ASF. Sufficient protein changes occur in the serum of most chronically infected swine to give a positive iodine agglutination test (17). The viral antigen was seen mainly in the macrophages and cell debris in alveolar walls and lumens (15), suggesting that the virus replicated in the cytoplasm of alveolar macrophages which subsequently degenerated and released the virus. These investigators also showed IgG immunoglobulin is bound to intracytoplasmic inclusion bodies in some degenerating macrophages, indicating that antibody against ASF viral antigen(s) excluded from blood circulation or produced by local immunocytes (or both) reacted with viral antigen at intramacrophage and extramacrophage levels and resulted in the formation of insoluble antigen-antibody (AG-AB) complexes. The participation of complement in the immune complex is evident in the early stage of the pneumonia, but less evident in the subsequent extensive, progressive necrotic processes.

Properties of the Virus. In electron micrographs of thin sections of cells the mature viral particles have a hexagonal outer membrane, 175 to 225 nm in diameter, separated by a clear region from a dense nucleoid, 72 to 89 nm (3). In (Figure 42.6) negatively stained cell-spread preparations, collapsed particles appear to be icosahedral capsids suggesting cubic symmetry (2). Extraction of infectious nucleic acid from ASFV and direct characterization by ultraviolet light and by reaction with RNase and DNase have proved that it is a DNA virus (1). The virus contains a lipid membrane and is ether-sensitive. It is inactivated in 30 minutes at 55 C and in 10 minutes at 60 C; thus it is less heat-resistant than hog cholera virus. The virus survives for years when dried at room temperature or frozen in skin or muscle. It is resistant to most disinfectants, but is inactivated by 1 percent formaldehyde in 6 days, by 2 percent NaOH in 24 hours, and by chloroform and other lipid solvents.

The viral particles appear to be formed in the cell cytoplasm, and they bud out from the cell membrane, many acquiring an added layer (3). Hemagglutination of red blood cells is not reported, but hemadsorption of pig red blood cells is seen in cultures of pig marrow or "buffy coat" (9) (Figure 42.7).

There are several serotypes in Africa, but probably only one in Europe. Specific and group antigens are demonstrated by the complement-fixation, gel-diffusion, and other tests. The CF test is group reactive, but the hemadsorption-inhibition test is specific (8).

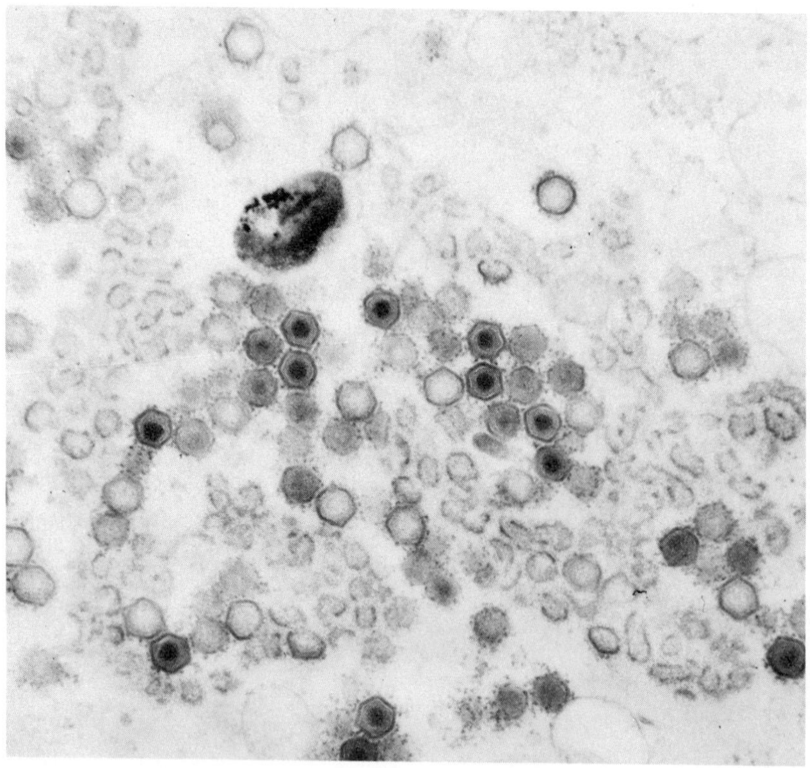

Figure 42.6. African swine viral particles (strain Lisbon 57) in a pig kidney cell culture. × 27,900. (Courtesy S. S. Breese, Plum Island Animal Disease Center, USDA.)

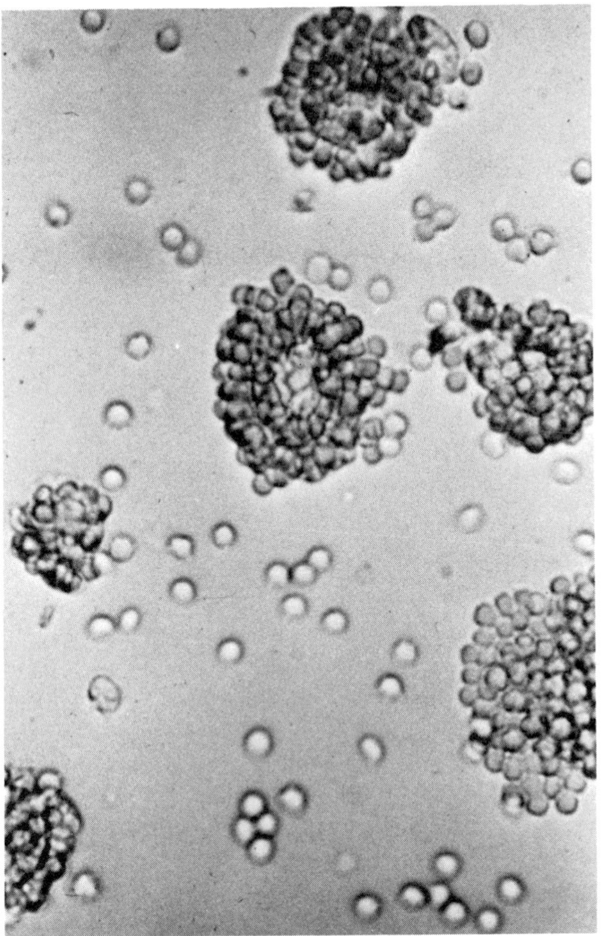

Figure 42.7. Hemadsorption of red blood cells in virus-infected cell cultures used for diagnosis of ASFV. (Courtesy J. J. Callis and staff, Plum Island Animal Disease Center, USDA.)

Cultivation. McIntosh (11) was able to cultivate the ASF virus in chick embryos through 12 transfers by inoculating them into their yolk sacs. The virus is lethal to the embryos, deaths generally occurring on the 6th or 7th day following inoculation. Malmquist and Hay (9) were successful in cultivating the virus in tissue cultures consisting of bone marrow cells or of cells from the buffy coat of swine blood. Cytopathogenic effects and hemadsorption were observed. More recently Malmquist showed that the Hinde Strain produced a cytopathogenic effect in cultures of pig kidney cells.

Wardley and Wilkinson (24) observed a high rate of infection and complete destruction within 2 to 3 days of monocytes in cell cultures derived from pig bone marrow, whereas the macrophages in culture had only a low level of infection and survived to form persistently infected cultures. These observations help to explain the persistence of virus in the pig.

A microplaque assay and conventional plaque assay procedure were reproducible and reliable in titering the virus, but approximately 0.9 log lower in sensitivity in viral detection than the hemadsorption test (16).

Immunity. Immunity to homologous strains seems to be transient. Pigs that recover from the disease often remain carriers of the virus in the blood stream for months. Attenuated strains have been used as vaccines in Spain and Portugal but vaccinated pigs may carry the virus despite the presence of antibody. The cellular immune mechanism is not impaired by ASF infection in pigs as demonstrated by the leukocyte migration inhibition test and the development of delayed hypersensitivity but viremia did persist in the pigs (191).

DeTray and Scott (6) confirmed the work of Montgomery by finding that hyperimmune hog cholera antiserum had virtually no effect on the ASF virus *in vitro* or *in vivo*.

Transmission. Domestic pigs in Africa may contract the infection from carrier wart hogs, and these animals may liberate the virus, particularly during farrowing and other periods of stress. Thereafter, infection is by contact and through fomites. Infected premises remain infective for long periods.

A different cycle of transmission has developed in Europe where the disease became less virulent, and chronically infected pigs perpetuated the infection. This also is true in Brazil and other Latin American countries.

Virus has been recovered from the argasid tick, which may be a factor in the pig disease.

Diagnosis. Differentiating ASF from hog cholera is most important. This must be done by virus isolation or by the demonstration of a rising serum titer utilizing the hemadsorption-inhibition, complement-fixation test, or immunofluorescence test (7).

The enzyme-linked immunosorbent assay (ELISA) is in the process of development. This rapid and automated test procedure would be used in diagnosis and disease eradication where a large number of serums must be tested (4).

Since ASF is so difficult to differentiate from hog cholera in the field many countries in which hog cholera now exists have broadened and improved their vaccination program against hog cholera. This is not as simple as it sounds because attenuated hog cholera vaccines also produce a chronic disease in some pigs under certain conditions in which pigs become stunted and virus carriers.

Control. As yet a satisfactory vaccine has not been developed despite a concerted research effort in several places around the world. Considering the nature of the disease it is unlikely to occur. Some novel approach to immunity of viral, chronic, and degenerative diseases must be developed before success is likely to occur. One cannot be very optomistic at present.

Present control of the disease is based on early reporting and a rapid diagnosis followed by immediate slaughter of all infected and exposed swine coupled with a strict quarantine in the infected area. This is likely to be the approach if the disease is ever introduced into the United States. Success by this approach has been achieved in certain European countries and Cuba in recent years.

The United States imports some processed pork products. Our control officials are concerned about the effects of processing on the presence of ASF fever in these products. It has been shown that virus was recovered from dried salami and pepperoni sausages, but not after the required curing period (12). Partially cooked canned hams did not contain virus.

The Disease in Man. This virus is not known to cause disease in human beings.

REFERENCES

1. Adldinger, Stone, Hess, and Bachrach. Virol., 1966, *30,* 750.
2. Almeida, Waterson, and Plowright. Arch. f. die gesam. Virusforsch., 1967, *20,* 392.
3. Breese and DeBoer. Virol., 1966, *28,* 420.
4. Callis. ASF-Review, Proc. XII Inter-American Meeting, Curaçao, Netherlands Antilles, 1979, Pan Amer. Health Org., Washington D.C.
5. DeTray. Am. Jour. Vet. Res., 1957, *18,* 811.
6. DeTray and Scott. Jour. Am. Vet. Med. Assoc., 1955, *126,* 313.
7. Heuschele and Hess. Trop. An. Health Prod., 1973, *5,* 181.
8. Malmquist. Am. Jour. Vet. Res., 1963, *24,* 450.
9. Malmquist and Hay. Am. Jour. Vet. Res., 1960, *21,* 104.
10. Maurer, Griesemer, and Jones. Am. Jour. Vet. Res., 1958, *19,* 517.
11. McIntosh. Jour. So. Afr. Vet. Med. Assoc., 1952, *23,* 217.
12. McKercher, Hess, and Hamdy. Appl. Environ. Microbiol., 1978, *35,* 142.
13. Montgomery. Jour. Comp. Path. and Therap., 1921, *34,* 159.
14. Moulton, Pan, Hess, DeBoer, and Tessler. Am. Jour. Vet. Res., 1975, *36,* 27.
15. Pan, Moulton, and Hess. Am. Jour. Vet. Res., 1975, *36,* 379.
16. Pan, Shimizu, and Hess. Am. Jour. Vet. Res., 1978, *39,* 491.
17. Pan, Trautman, DeBoer, and Hess. Am. Jour. Vet. Res., 1974, *35,* 629.
18. Ribeiro, Azevedo, Teixeira, Braco, Forte, Ribeiro, Noronha, Pereira, and Vigario. Bull. Off. Int. Epiz., 1958, *50,* 516.
19. Shimizu, Pan, and Hess. Am. Jour. Vet. Res., 1977, *38,* 27.
20. Steyn. 13th and 14th Ann. Rpts., Dir. Vet. Educ. and Res., Union So. Afr., Part I, 1928, p. 415.
21. Steyn. 18th Ann. Rpt., Dir. Vet. Educ. and Res., Union So. Afr., 1932, p. 99.
22. Walker. Proc. 11th Internatl. Vet. Cong. (London), 1930.
23. Wardley and Wilkinson. Arch. Virol., 1977, *55,* 327.
24. Wardley and Wilkinson. Jour. Gen. Virol., 1978, *38,* 183.

43 The Poxviridae

In the family Poxviridae there are two subfamilies: (*a*) Chordopoxvirinae, which includes six genera covering all the animal poxviruses and (*b*) Entomopoxvirinae, which has one genus, *Entopoxvirus*, which includes all the insect poxviruses. This chapter will cover the genera of animal poxviruses: *Suipoxvirus, Orthopoxvirus, Avipoxvirus, Capripoxvirus, Leporipoxvirus,* and *Parapoxvirus*. The diseases in this family are listed in Table 43.1. The taxonomy of this family is based largely on three criteria: (*a*) similar morphology, (*b*) a shared group-specific nucleoprotein antigen, and (*c*) members of each genus having other antigens in common.

The genus *Orthopoxvirus* includes cowpox, vaccinia, variola, alastrim, ectromelia (mousepox), rabbitpox, monkeypox, buffalopox, camelpox, and horsepox. Fowlpox, pigeonpox, turkeypox, canarypox, quailpox, lovebirdpox, sparrowpox, juncopox, and starlingpox comprise the genus *Avipoxvirus*. The genus *Capripoxvirus* contains sheeppox, goatpox, and lumpy skin disease. Myxoma viruses and rabbit, hare, and squirrel fibroma viruses are in the genus *Leporipoxvirus*. The genus *Suipoxvirus* includes swinepox. Contagious pustular dermatitis of sheep (orf), bovine papular stomatitis, sea-lionpox virus, and pseudocowpox (milker's nodules) embrace the genus *Parapoxvirus*. New poxviruses have been isolated from elephants, lions, raccoons, and gerbils, but have not been sufficiently characterized to place into a genus. It is interesting that no poxviruses have been isolated from the dog or domestic cat. It is unclear where *molluscum contagiosum* of humans or Yaba monkey virus fit into the taxonomy of poxviruses.

Formerly, poxviruses were classified on the basis of morphology and the animal species showing disease. The so-called true poxviruses (*Orthopoxvirus* and *Avipoxvirus*) and pseudopoxviruses (*Parapoxvirus*) were readily distinguished by morphology. (See sections on *Orthopoxvirus* and *Parapoxvirus* for figures on size and morphology of particles.) The true poxviruses are slightly larger and less ovoid than the pseudopoxvirus. There is a pronounced difference in the arrangement of the threadlike structures; the true poxviruses display an irregular whorled (mulberrylike) appearance. In contrast, these threadlike structures are wound around the virion creating a highly regular criss-cross pattern characteristic of pseudopoxviruses.

The serological relationships of poxviruses are determined by the use of infected cell extracts (5). In these preparations up to 20 antigens are capable of forming precipitin lines with antiviral serum for orthopoxviruses (1, 6) and for leporipoxviruses (3). One of these antigens is probably responsible for production of neutralizing antibody (2). Viruses of the genus *Orthopoxvirus* differ by no more than one antigenic component according to the gel-diffusion test (7), and the same is true for the genus *Leporipoxvirus* (3). It is generally assumed that these antigens are structural protein components, but this has not been proved. Viruses of the genus *Leporipoxvirus* are not neutralized by vaccinia antiserum, and none of the major antigens is shared by these two groups. The avianpox viruses are not related to other true poxvirus groups. Many poxviruses form a hemagglutinin. Alkaline digestion of all poxviruses yields

Table 43.1. Diseases in domestic animals caused by viruses in the Poxviridae family

Common name of virus	Natural hosts	Type of disease produced
Genus *Avipoxvirus*		
Fowlpox	Chickens, turkeys, pheasants, canaries	Pox lesions appear on comb, wattles, nostrils and eyes; pustules dry into epithelial crusts. Affected animals may become lethargic and die
Pigeonpox	Pigeons	Lesions of mouth region. Occasionally eyes are affected causing blindness
Turkeypox	Turkeys	Disease similar to fowlpox
Genus *Orthopoxvirus*		
Cowpox	Cattle, man	Mild. Affecting teats and udder forming vesicles followed by crusting
Vaccinia	Cattle, man	Mild. Affecting teats and udder forming vesicles followed by crusting
Buffalopox	Cattle, buffalo	No significant information available
Rabbitpox	Rabbit	Acute generalized disease of domesticated rabbits. Wild animals appear immune. High mortality rate in domesticated rabbits
Camelpox	Camel	Acute, highly infectious disease similar to variola in man
Horsepox	Horse, man	Multiple lesions of lips and gums, tongue and cheeks. Pustules form. Fever may develop. There may be mortality among young animals
Genus *Suipoxvirus*		
Swinepox	Swine	Acute infectious disease that affects swine only. Pox lesions found primarily on abdomen and inside thighs and legs
Genus *Capripoxvirus*		
Sheeppox	Sheep	Acute disease—mortality 5% to 50% of infected animals. Lesions occur on mucous membranes in pharynx and trachea. Hemorrhage and inflammation of digestive and respiratory tracts
Goatpox	Goats	Lesions occur on hairless regions. Similar to sheeppox, but not as severe
Virus dermatitis	Goats	Resembles goatpox
Lumpy skin disease	Cattle, buffalo	Nodules in the skin, pathological changes in mucous membranes and viscera
Genus *Leporipoxvirus*		
Myxomavirus	Rabbits, hares	Acute, generalized, highly fatal disease characterized by tumorlike masses having rubbery, gelatinous consistency
Shope fibroma	Rabbits	Fibrous tumor of cottontail rabbit located in subcutaneous tissue
Genus *Parapoxvirus*		
Contagious pustular dermatitis of sheep	Sheep, goats, man	Formation of vesicles on lips and areas of nose and eyes—later forming pustules and scabs. Fatalities occur in sheep and goats from complications
Bovine papular stomatitis	Cattle	Mild. Causes craterlike ulcers of stoma
Pseudocowpox	Cattle, man	Mild. Resembles lesions of cowpox

a fraction called the NP antigen which is shared by all poxviruses. The poxviruses contain 5 to 7.5 percent double-stranded DNA with a molecular weight of 160 × 10^6 daltons. The brick-shaped or ovoid particles are 170 to 250 by 300 to 450 nm. Virions have a complex structure with an external coat surrounding double membrane with filamentous subunits in irregular arrangement and an internal body (core) consisting of a double membrane with cylindrical subunits and containing the DNA. The buoyant density in cesium chloride is 1.1 to 1.33 g per cm^3, and the sedimentation coefficient is 5,000 S. The viruses probably contain enzymes, and some contain RNA polymerase. Some poxviruses are ether-resistant. Members can recombine genetically. All members exhibit nongenetic reactivation. Replication takes place in the cytoplasm of cells, principally in epithelial types. Except for contagious pustular dermatitis of sheep the parasitized cells contain cytoplasmic inclusion bodies which harbor the virus particles sometimes called elementary bodies.

Diseases characterized by the formation of pustules on the skin, with or without general manifestations of illness, occur in all species of domestic animals except dogs and cats. These are the animal poxes. In man, the disease is called *variola*, or *smallpox*. It is believed by some that all of our pox diseases came originally from one or more basic strains, which in the course of time have changed as they became adapted to different hosts. The disease in birds differs from that in mammals in several respects but principally in that the lesions are proliferative and tumorlike rather than pustular. It is seldom possible to establish an infection in a mammal with a bird pox, or vice versa. There are many types of bird poxes, but these are related immunologically, and many of them can readily be adapted to new bird-species hosts. The true pox diseases of mammals show immunological relationships, and in many instances they may be adapted to new mammalian hosts.

Man may be successfully infected with cowpox virus, and cattle can be infected with smallpox. Immunologically these two viruses are very closely related to each other and also to that of horsepox. The pox diseases are quite rare today in mammals, especially in western Europe and North America, but this has not always been the case. The pox diseases of man, sheep, and fowl are severe and destructive.

Pox in fowls, turkeys, pheasants, pigeons, canaries, and many wild birds is seen from time to time in the United States. Immunization of domestic fowls has reduced the incidence and importance of this disease.

Excellent review articles have been written by Joklik (4, 5).

REFERENCES

1. Appleyard, Westwood, and Zwartouw. Virol., 1962, *18*, 159.
2. Appleyard, Zwartous, and Westwood. Brit. Jour. Exp. Path., 1964, *45*, 150.
3. Fenner. Austral. Jour. Exp. Biol. and Med. Sci., 1965, *43*, 143.
4. Joklik. Bact. Proc., 1966, *30*, 33.
5. Joklik. Ann. Rev. Microbiol., 1968, *22*, 1514.
6. Rodriguez-Burgos, Chordi, Diaz, and Tormo. Virol., 1966, *30*, 569.
7. Rondle and Dumbell. Jour. Hyg. (London), 1962, *60*, 41.

THE GENUS *AVIPOXVIRUS*

Fowlpox

SYNONYMS: Chickenpox, sorehead, contagious epithelioma

Fowlpox attacks chickens primarily and occurs in pheasants, other wild birds, and canaries. Occasionally outbreaks in turkeys are observed. The virus differs somewhat in pathogenicity in different species, usually being of greater disease-producing power for the species from which it was recovered than for other kinds of birds. Pigeonpox virus, for example, is only slightly pathogenic for chickens, but it immunizes chickens against fowlpox and constitutes a good vaccine for this purpose. A virus that Brunett (3) isolated from a turkey proved to be identical in every way to that of chickens, but one isolated by Brandly and Dunlay (2) was not typical. Virus recovered from infected pheasants usually is typical of that of fowlpox, but Dobson (4) found a strain in one serious outbreak which resembled that of pigeonpox rather than fowlpox. It seems obvious that all bird poxviruses are closely related but are host-modified. That these modifications become considerable, however, is indicated by the fact that pigeonpox virus does not naturally pass from pigeons to chickens, and that fowlpox virus is transmitted to pigeons by inoculation only with difficulty.

Character of the Disease. Pox in chickens is manifested by characteristic lesions on the head. They appear on the comb and wattles and around the corners of the mouth, the nostrils, and the eyes (Figure 43.1). In some cases the lesions spread into the mouth and even into the trachea, causing whitish lesions that ulcerate forming what are commonly called *cankers*. This form of pox

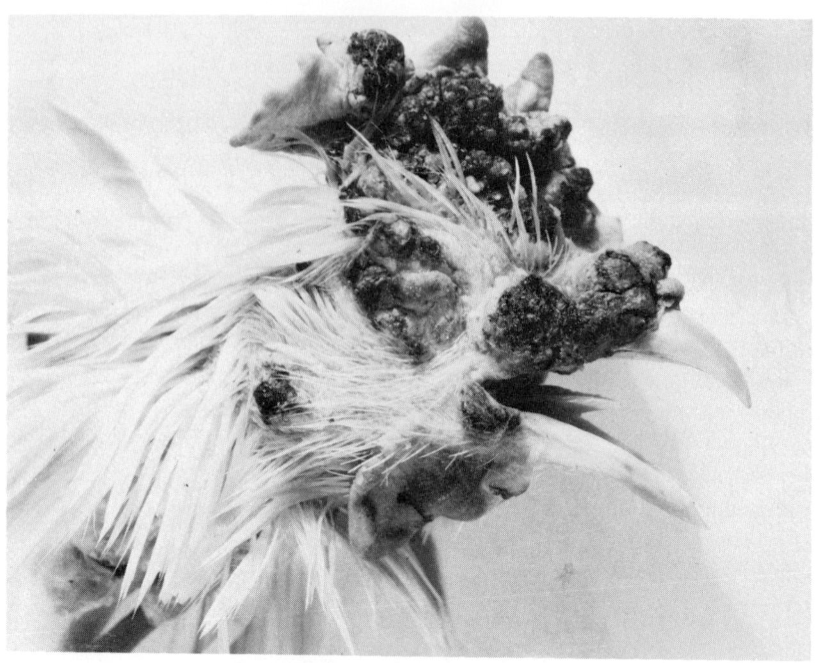

Figure 43.1. Fowlpox, showing characteristic dry scabs on the comb and around the eye, nostrils, and corner of the mouth.

was considered to be a separate disease and was known under the name of *avian diphtheria* for many years. In such infections the infraorbital sinus is frequently involved, becomes greatly distended, and thus distorts the facial features. The content is a yellowish or brownish caseous mass.

The skin lesions consist first of small pustules, which soon dry and become transformed into warty epithelial crusts. These may become quite thick. The affected birds become very ill, refuse to eat, become emaciated, and stop laying; many of them die. The lesions are confined to the featherless part of the head, as a rule, but occasionally pox lesions are found around the vent, and even on the feet. If the infection remains on the skin and does not involve the mucous membranes of the head, the effect on the bird is much less severe and recoveries are more common. In favorable cases the course of the disease is 3 or 4 weeks; in the presence of complications it may be much longer.

Properties of the Virus. In 1902 Marx and Sticker (8) proved that fowlpox was caused by a virus. The Borrel bodies (or elementary bodies) have an estimated diameter of 332 by 284 nm. The elementary bodies have a pepsin-resistant core (11). They are located in the Bollinger body, a cytoplasmic inclusion body which consists of a matrix (Figure 43.2). This matrix is dissolved by sodium lauryl sulfate, but is quite resistant to enzymes. It gives a positive Feulgen reaction after previous extraction of lipoids. The developing elementary bodies initially are poorly defined, but later acquire the characteristic poxvirus appearance of a dumbbell-like structure within an outer membrane. Virions are readily observed by electron microscopy.

Fowlpox virus is resistant to drying. In the dried crusts removed from epithelial lesions, the virulence remains unimpaired for many months providing the drying has been well done. In soil subject to the usual conditions, the viability of the virus is not longer than several weeks as a rule. The disease tends to recur, year after year, on the same premises. It is now known how the virus is preserved in the intervening periods. It is readily destroyed by alkalis and by most disinfectants. It is preserved for long periods by 50 percent glycerol. It is resistant to ether, but is chloroform-sensitive. It is activated by heating for 30 minutes at 50 C, or 8 minutes at 60 C.

Neutralization tests can be performed involving the use of "pock" counting on chorioallantoic membranes. Precipitating antibodies can be revealed by gel diffusion and complement-fixing antibodies by the complement-fixation test. The hemagglutination test can be used to measure virus and detect hemagglutination inhibition (HI) antibody.

Virus neutralization in cell culture is more reliable in differentiating avian poxviruses than the passive hemagglutination (PHA) test as cross-reactions were detected among avian poxviruses.

Cultivation. Goodpasture, Woodruff, and Buddingh (6) cultivated the virus of fowlpox on the chorioallantoic membrane of the developing chick embryo in 1931. Brandly (1) and others have confirmed these findings, and such cultures are now being used for vaccine production.

Fowlpox and pigeonpox viruses produce a cytopathogenic effect (CPE) in chick embryo tissue cultures. More recently, Tripathy *et al.* (12) described the formation of plaques in cell culture.

Immunity. Birds that have recovered from fowlpox are solidly immune thereafter. Both humoral and cellular immunity are involved in protection. There is a possibility of persistence of virus, which might also be a factor in long-term protection. In flocks in which the disease has occurred for some years, the disease is seen only in the young birds. In previously uninfected flocks, birds of all ages develop the disease.

Transmission. Fowlpox is believed to be transmitted principally by direct inoculation from bird to bird through fighting wounds and by the birds' picking at one another. The disease may also be spread by the bites of mosquitoes (7, 9) and possibly by other arthropods. Arthropod transmission is certainly not as important as direct contact in the spread of this disease within flocks, but it may be the usual way by which the infection is spread from one flock to another. Doyle and Minett (5) placed susceptible birds in cages that had just been occupied by infected birds. Transmission did not occur except when the skin or mucous membranes of the susceptible birds had been scarified. Infection seems to depend, therefore, on breaks in the continuity of the skin.

Immunization. Immunization of poultry flocks is encouraged only in regions where fowlpox is prevalent. Two types of vaccine are available for immunizing chickens against fowlpox. Fowlpox virus is propagated in chicken embryonating eggs or in susceptible cell culture.

Oral vaccination with the attenuated HP-1 cell culture strain in the 200th to 400th transfer is both effective and safer (10) in 5-day-old chicks. A second vaccine dose should be given 3 to 4 weeks later. It is essential that the vaccine dose contain 10 $TCID_{50}$ of virus.

Fowlpox vaccines can be combined effectively with Newcastle and/or Marek's virus vaccine, but inoculations usually are given by a parenteral route.

The Disease in Man. Fowlpox does not affect man. The disease in man commonly known as *chickenpox* or *varicella* is not identical with this disease, nor is it contracted from chickens or other fowls.

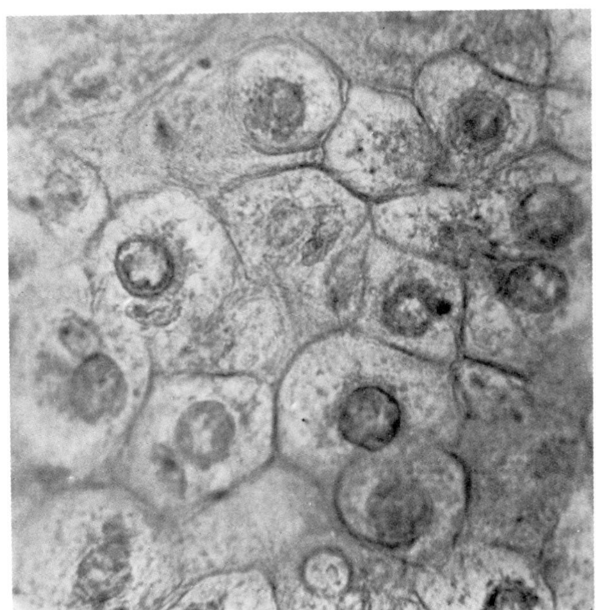

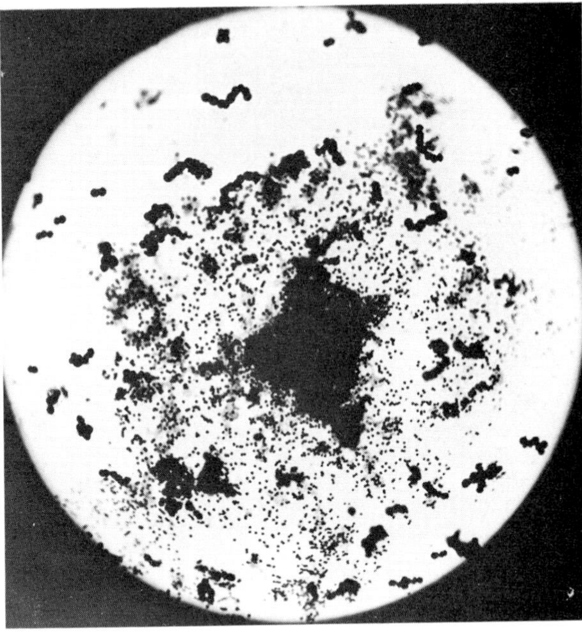

Figure 43.2. (*Upper*) Fowlpox. Swollen epithelial cells in an early lesion show the Bollinger bodies. The inclusion bodies are spherical and prominent in the stained section. In several of the cells the nuclei may be seen crowded against the cell wall. × 465. (*Lower*) The Borrel or "elementary" bodies of fowlpox. These minute spherical bodies were obtained free of tissue debris by tryptic digestion of the Bollinger bodies contained in virus-infected cells. The bodies here are stained after admixture with a *Streptococcus* to indicate comparative size. × 350. (Courtesy E. W. Goodpasture, *Am. Jour. Path.*)

REFERENCES

1. Brandly. Jour. Am. Vet. Med. Assoc., 1936, *88*, 587; 1937, *90*, 479.
2. Brandly and Dunlap. Poultry Sci., 1938, *17*, 511.

3. Brunett. Rpt. N.Y. State Vet. Coll., 1932–33 (1934), p. 69.
4. Dobson. Jour. Comp. Path. and Therap., 1937, *50,* 401.
5. Doyle and Minett. Jour. Comp. Path. and Therap., 1927, *40,* 401.
6. Goodpasture, Woodruff, and Buddingh. Science, 1931, *74,* 371; Am. Jour. Path., 1932, *8,* 271.
7. Kligler, Muckenfuss, and Rivers. Jour. Exp. Med., 1929, *49,* 649.
8. Marx and Sticker. Deut. med. Wchnschr., 1902, *28,* 893.
9. Matheson, Brunett, and Brody. Poultry Sci., 1930, *10,* 211.
10. Mayr and Danner. Dev. Biol. Stand., 1976, *33,* 249.
11. Woodruff and Goodpasture. Dev. Biol. Stand., 1929, *5,* 1; 1930, *6,* 713.
12. Tripathy, Hanson, and Killinger. Avian Dis., 1973, *17,* 325.

Pigeonpox

Pigeonpox frequently causes considerable trouble in squab-raising plants. The squabs may become infected while still in the nest, but more often the disease appears in well-developed birds. Cankers are found in the mouth, and the corners of the mouth are covered with crusts. The eyelids may also become affected and the birds blinded. The legs and toes are sometimes involved. The death rate may be high. Pigeons may be protected against the disease by vaccination with pigeonpox vaccine, used in the same way as for chickens.

THE GENUS *ORTHOPOXVIRUS*

Vaccinia

SYNONYMS: *Vaccinia variolae, Poxvirus officinalis*

In the first half of the 19th century and earlier, evidence indicates that true cowpox prevailed rather frequently in both Europe and America, and that these outbreaks were often related directly to epidemics of smallpox in man (6). This evidence suggests that smallpox infection was not infrequently transmitted from milkers to the cattle that they milked, and that this disease was then known as *cowpox.* There is evidence, too, that horsepox was often transmitted to cattle by the infected hands of milkers, the disease being indistinguishable from that which sometimes came from human beings and sometimes from other cattle. Although smallpox, cowpox, and horsepox are regarded as separate and distinct diseases, it is rather clear that they are related, and differences in the viruses may result from adaptation to different hosts. These relationships were first recognized by Jenner (3), who used the knowledge to immunize man against the deadly smallpox by vaccinating children and susceptible adults with vaccinia or cowpox virus. Some people differentiate between cowpox and vaccinia virus, believing that the latter is really a smallpox virus which has been modified by passage through cattle whereas the former is a true cattle virus (2). The difference does not seem to be very important.

There is no evidence that it now exists in the United States or elsewhere in the world except where smallpox vaccination might be used in rare instances to immunize humans. When it occurred in the past, it was an accidental infection caused by contact between cattle and recently vaccinated humans. A disease commonly called *cowpox* occurs frequently in cattle in the United States and other countries. It is more frequent in dairy cattle. The available evidence indicates that this condition is caused either by cowpox or pseudocowpox virus, separate and distinct agents from vaccinia.

A number of cases were described formerly in the United States in which cattle were infected by recently vaccinated persons (1, 7). The cattle become infected from virus on the hands of the milkers. The disease often spreads to many cows in the milking herd and from these cows to other people. In some cases nearly every unvaccinated person on the farm who had contact with the cows, or who used the raw milk from them, became infected. These individuals developed typical vaccinia lesions on their hands, arms, faces, and other parts of their bodies. It is obvious that recently vaccinated persons should not be permitted to milk or have other close contact with dairy cattle.

Character of the Disease. The lesions of vaccinia occur on the teats and udder (Figure 43.3). They appear as small papules which gradually change to pustules. A reddened areola appears around each lesion. The pustule has a tendency to develop a small pit, or umbilication. The lesions may be numerous, but generally they appear in rather small numbers, most of them being on the teats. The friction of the milking process generally causes the lesions to break, forming raw areas that are very tender. When the lesions are not broken in this way, the pustules dry up and become covered with dry scabs, which fall off in about 10 days leaving an unscarred surface. The healing process is greatly delayed by the friction of milking, and bacterial invasion of the udder often results in mastitis.

The Disease in Experimental Animals. The vaccinia virus can be transmitted experimentally to the skin of

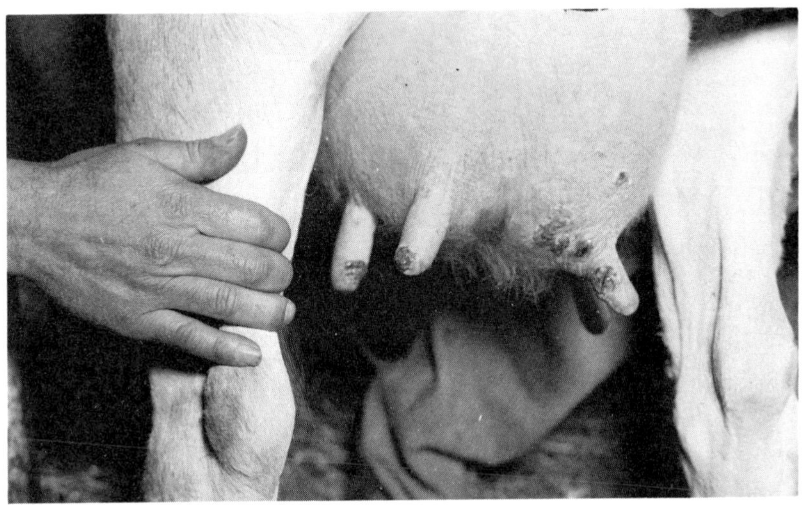

Figure 43.3. Cowpox, showing well-advanced lesion on the teats and udder. (Courtesy Robert Graham.)

many mammals. It can be transmitted readily to the cornea of the rabbit's eye. Paschen (4) believes that the cornea test (Paul's test) is a reliable indicator of the presence of vaccinia or variola virus. This test is performed by placing a suspension of the suspected material on the cornea of a rabbit, introducing it very carefully to avoid mechanical irritation. After 36 to 48 hours the animal is destroyed, and the enucleated eye is placed for a few minutes in a sublimate-alcohol mixture. The presence of poxvirus is indicated by grossly apparent, opaque lesions, circular in outline, which were not apparent before they were acted upon by the fixative solution.

Guinea pigs and mice also react to inoculation with vaccinia. Large doses given intravenously to suckling mice will kill them without the multiplication of virus.

Properties of the Virus. The mature *elementary bodies* known as *Paschen bodies* vary in size from 240 to 380 by 170 to 270 nm (Figure 43.4). The outer membrane is 9 to 12 nm thick, and the virus contains an inner central nucleoid with a smaller body beside it. The nucleoid is probably nucleoprotein. Negative staining subunits exist on the surface of the particle but within the outer membrane. The Paschen bodies probably develop within the cytoplasm causing the formation of large *Guarnieri bodies*. They can be seen readily with light microscopy. The fluorescent antibody test provides another highly effective method for demonstrating the organism in smear preparations.

The virus contains biotin and flavin besides carbon, phosphorous, nitrogen, copper, lipids, carbohydrates, and thymonucleic acid.

This agent is quite stable and resistant. Suspensions of the virus are inactivated in 10 minutes at 60 C, but dried virus withstands 100 C for 10 minutes. It is quite stable between pH 5 and 9. The virus is resistant to ether in the cold, but is inactivated by chloroform. Oxidizing agents such as potassium permanganate or ethyl oxide readily inactivate the particle.

The hemagglutinin is separable from the virus particle, resists boiling, and agglutinates the red cells of some fowls.

The nucleoprotein antigen (NP) is involved in the complement-fixation and precipitation reactions. Neu-

Figure 43.4. Variola-vaccinia-cowpox group negatively stained. × 110,000. (Courtesy Viral Pathology and Viral Exanthems Branches, Center for Disease Control.)

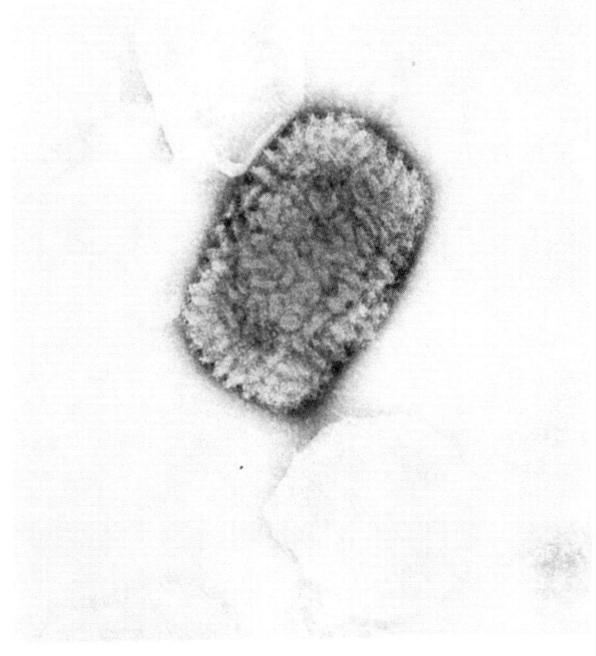

tralizing antibody is demonstrated by the use of tissue culture, embryonated hens' eggs, or rabbit skin reaction. The single radial immunization test has been used for detection of antibodies against vaccinia or variola virus, but the technique requires large quantities of antigen (5).

Interference has been reported between vaccinia and fowlpox, foot-and-mouth disease, and influenza. Interferon has been demonstrated in the latter instance.

Cultivation. Vaccinia grows in primary cultures of chick embryo, rabbit kidney, rabbit testis, bovine embryo skin, and also in continuous cell lines such as HeLa and L. Cell destruction occurs early and includes the formation of giant cells. Plaques are formed in agar overlay systems.

In the embryonated hens' eggs, 7 to 13 days old, the virus grows well on the chorioallantoic membrane producing pocks, the formation of which may be used to titrate the virus. Embryo mortality varies from low to 100 percent depending on the strain and test conditions. Less sensitive routes of inoculation are the allantoic cavity and the yolk sac.

Immunity. After recovery from vaccinia, cattle are immune for a considerable time and perhaps for life. Second attacks have been reported, but these may have been infections of the pseudopox disease. Experimentally, solid resistance is conveyed by one exposure.

Transmission. Vaccinia is clearly transmitted largely in the milking process on the hands of the milker. There is little evidence of any other mode of transmission.

Diagnosis. Except for differential diagnosis between vaccinia and the pseudopox diseases, the diagnosis can readily be made from the appearance of the lesions. Neither of these diseases is particularly serious, and in most instances differentiation is more or less academic. This matter will be discussed further under pseudopox.

Control. Infections of herds with vaccinia virus through exposure to recently vaccinated milkers should be avoided. When the disease appears in a milking herd, affected animals should be segregated from the others as far as practicable. They should be milked last, and the milkers should scrub their hands thoroughly with soap and water after milking them and before handling others.

The use of 5-iodo-2-deoxyuridine for the treatment of vaccinal keratitis is attended with some success.

The Disease in Man. The vaccinia lesion consists of a papule which quickly becomes a pustule. The lesion is reddened about its periphery. Although it itches, it is not particularly painful. The characteristic umbilication appears in most of the pustules. If not rubbed or scratched, the lesion becomes dehydrated after a few days and a scab forms which falls off after 10 to 14 days. The hand lesions usually are not numerous. If the individual suffers from eczema, the disease may spread over large areas of the skin, and there may be fever and illness lasting a few days.

REFERENCES

1. Boerner. Jour. Am. Vet. Med. Assoc., 1923, *64,* 93.
2. Downie. Jour. Path. and Bact., 1939, *48,* 361.
3. Jenner, Edward. An inquiry into the causes and effects of the *variolae vaccinae*. S. Low, London, 1798.
4. Paschen. *In* Kolle, Kraus, and Uhlenhuth. Handbuch der pathogenen Mikroorganismen, 3rd ed. G. Fischer, Jena, 1930, vol. *VIII,* part 11, p. 821.
5. Prakash, Norrby, and Payne. Jour. Gen. Virol., 1977, *34,* 465.
6. Reece. Vet. Jour., 1922, *78,* 81.
7. Sayer and Amos. N.Y. State Jour. Med., 1936, *36,* 1163.

Cowpox

The antigenic properties of this virus are close but distinct from vaccinia as determined by the use of complement-fixation, agar-gel-diffusion, and antibody-absorption tests (1). There is general agreement that the disease is distinct from vaccinia and pseudocowpox.

In general, the features of cowpox virus such as physiochemical properties, hemagglutination red cell spectrum, morphology, and cultivation in tissue culture and eggs are similar to vaccinia.

In cattle the virus affects the skin, particularly the teats and udders of cows. The papules develop into vesicles, followed by crusting which may persist for weeks. Lesions in man resemble those of primary vaccination and may be found on the hands, arms, face, and eyes of the milker (1). The disease may be severe. Man-to-man infection is rare.

The skin or testis are the sites of inoculation for experimental infection of rabbits, mice, guinea pigs, and monkeys (1).

REFERENCE

1. Andrewes, Christopher. Viruses of vertebrates. Williams and Wilkins, Baltimore, 1964.

Horsepox

SYNONYMS: Contagious pustular stomatitis, "grease," "grease-heel"

Horsepox has not been reported from the United States, and it seems to be much less common in Europe that it was a half-century ago.

Character of the Disease. The disease in horses takes two forms. The less important is an infection of the pastern region of horses, apparently spread by the hands of horseshoers and hostlers. This condition is known as *grease* or *grease-heel*. It is manifested by the appearance of a papular eruption on the flexor surface of the joints in the lower part of the leg. The papules change to vesicles, then to pustules, which finally dry up, forming crusts. The legs become somewhat painful, but there is no general reaction as a rule.

The other form is manifested by the appearance of multiple lesions on the inside of the lips and the opposing surfaces of the gums, on the frenum of the tongue, and on the inside of the cheeks. These begin as papules, change to vesicles, and then become pustules. The animal may have some fever, and young animals may become very sick and occasionally die. Food is refused, saliva drools from the corners of the mouth, and the animal likes to dip its mouth in water. Beginning with a few lesions, new crops occur and finally nearly all the mucous membrane of the mouth will be involved. In some cases the lesions are found also in the nasal passages. Virus removed from the horse lesions will infect cattle, and that of cattle will infect horses.

Immunity. Recovery from the disease leaves a substantial immunity. Because lesions on the skin are less severe than those on the mucosa of the mouth, some European authors have suggested vaccination of horses on the skin, claiming good results therefrom. The cow and horse diseases reciprocally immunize against each other, and both will transmit to persons who have not been vaccinated against smallpox and not to those who have been.

REFERENCES

1. De Jong. Jour. Comp. Path. and Therap., 1917, *30,* 242.
2. Zwick. Berl. tierärztl. Wchnschr., 1924, *40,* 757.

Camelpox

This virus causes a highly infectious and generalized disease in camels that transmits readily to susceptible contact animals. It is closely related immunologically to variola (smallpox) virus because protection is provided by this virus upon subsequent inoculation of camels with virulent camelpox virus (1).

REFERENCE

1. Baxby, Hessami, Ghaboosi, and Ramyar. Inf. and Immun., 1975, *11,* 617.

THE GENUS *SUIPOXVIRUS*

Swinepox

This disease has been reported in Europe, Japan, and the United States. It is very common in many of the swine-raising areas of the midwestern states of this country. It has been studied by McNutt, Murray, and Purwin (5), by Schwarte and Biester (8), and by Shope (9) in the United States. For detailed descriptions of this disease the reader is referred to these papers. As it occurs in this country it is not generally considered very important; however, some veterinarians believe that its importance is being underestimated.

Character of the Disease. It affects principally young, growing animals; suckling pigs are especially subject to it. McNutt and associates report that the lesions are usually found on the lower part of the abdomen and inside the thighs and arms (Figure 43.5), but in the outbreak in Iowa described by Schwarte and Biester the lesions were located on the backs and sides. Lesions are not located

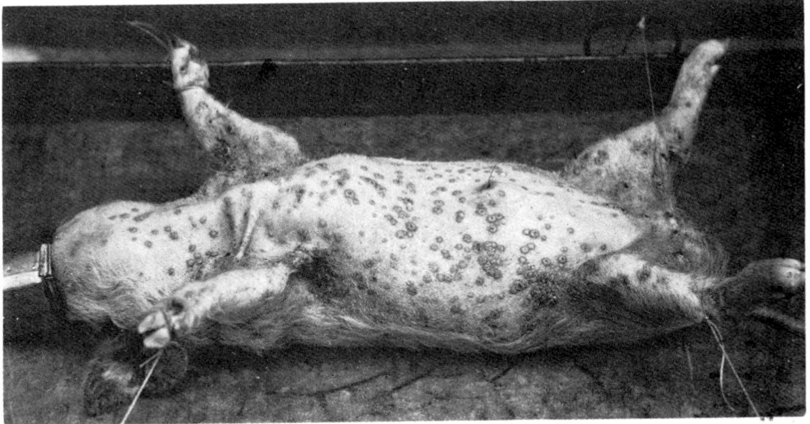

Figure 43.5. Swinepox. (Courtesy R. E. Shope.)

on the head or on the lower parts of the legs, as a rule. They consist of red papules that appear 4 to 5 days after virus is placed on the scarified skin. A slight fever and mild general reaction occur at this time. The lesions rapidly develop into raised, hard elevations, which may be from 1 to 3 cm in diameter. Hard crusts form on these areas, these drop off in a few days, and the whole process is completed in 12 to 14 days. Vesicles and pustules do not ordinarily appear in field cases, but typical lesions that passed through the papule, vesicle, and pustule stages are observed on the abdomen of artificially inoculated pigs.

Two different diseases are known at present under the name of *swinepox*. One of them is caused by vaccinia, the other by an unrelated virus. Manninger, Cosontos, and Salyi (6), who have seen both diseases in Europe, propose to designate as swinepox the one caused by the vaccinialike virus and to call the other a poxlike disease of swine. Schwarte and Biester, who have dealt with the poxlike disease of Manninger, prefer to call the disease swinepox. We concur with Schwarte and Biester. So far as is known, all cases of swinepox occurring in the United States are caused by a virus that is unrelated to the poxviruses of other animals, and this includes vaccinia.

Properties of the Virus. The swinepox virus is 250 nm with surrounding membranes (7). Teppema and DeBoer (10) and Kim *et al.* (4) studied the ultrastructure of swinepox virus. The ultrastructural changes in swinepox-infected cells were as follows: (*a*) intranuclear inclusions consisting of very fine filaments, (*b*) fibrillar structures with cross striations located in the nuclear inclusions, and (*c*) similar striated fibrillar structures in or just adjacent to Cowdry's B type inclusions in the cytoplasm. These observations are in good accordance with descriptions on *in vivo* infection. Vacuoles in nuclei of stratus spinosum cells are observed with swinepox virus infection in pigs, but not in swinepox caused by vaccinia virus, the only other known cause of pox in swine.

The differentiation between vaccinia and swinepox was further elucidated by DeBoer (1) with challenge infections of convalescent pigs and the use of the agar gel diffusion precipitin test and immunoelectrophoresis.

Cultivation. The swinepox virus produces a cytopathogenic effect in porcine kidney, testes, embryonic lung, and embryonic brain cultures (3). Minute plaques are observed in an agar overlay system. Sera from hyperimmunized swine failed to neutralize the virus *in vitro*. Recovered pigs resisted infection to the virus.

Attempts to cultivate the swinepox virus in embryonated hens' eggs, horses, calves, sheep, dogs, cats, fowl, rabbits, rats, mice, and man failed. In contrast vaccinia has a wide experimental host spectrum.

Immunity. Pigs that have recovered from the disease appear to be solidly immune for life. Immunization is not generally practiced, the disease not being important enough for that. The elimination of lice probably would do a great deal to control the disease.

Transmission. Swinepox does not ordinarily pass from one animal to another directly. The transmitting agent usually is the hog louse, *Hematopinus suis*. Because this parasite is found on the lower parts of the animal, on the belly, and in the armpits, and on the inside of the thighs, pox lesions usually are found in these locations. In a large herd studied by Schwarte and Biester, the pigs were free of lice, and the lesions were found largely on the back and sides. This suggested that flies or other insects might be the transmitting agents, and this idea was supported by the fact that the disease disappeared as soon as cold weather eliminated the insects.

Diagnosis. For rapid diagnosis of swinepox virus in the skin lesions of naturally infected pigs, the electron microscope method of negative staining is recommended (2).

REFERENCES

1. DeBoer. Arch Virol., 1975, *49,* 141.
2. Garg and Meyer. Res. Vet. Sci., 1973, *14,* 216.
3. Kazka, Bohl, and Jones. Am. Jour. Vet. Res., 1960, *21,* 269.
4. Kim, Mukhajonpan, Nii, and Kato. Biken Jour., 1977, *20,* 57.
5. McNutt, Murray, and Purwin. Jour. Am. Vet. Med. Assoc., 1929, *74,* 752.
6. Manninger, Cosontos, and Salyi. Arch. f. Tierheilk., 1940, *75,* 12.
7. Reczko. Arch. f. die gesam. Virusforsch., 1959, *9,* 193.
8. Schwarte and Biester. Am. Jour. Vet. Res., 1941, *2,* 136.
9. Shope. Jour. Bact., 1940, *39,* 39.
10. Teppema and DeBoer. Arch Virol., 1975, *49,* 151.

THE GENUS *CAPRIPOXVIRUS*

Sheeppox

SYNONYMS: *Clavelie, Variola ovina*

Of all the animal poxes, sheeppox is the most damaging. Fortunately this disease does not exist in the Western Hemisphere. In past times it has done great damage in Europe, but it has now been controlled or eliminated from the greater part of that area. It continues to exist in

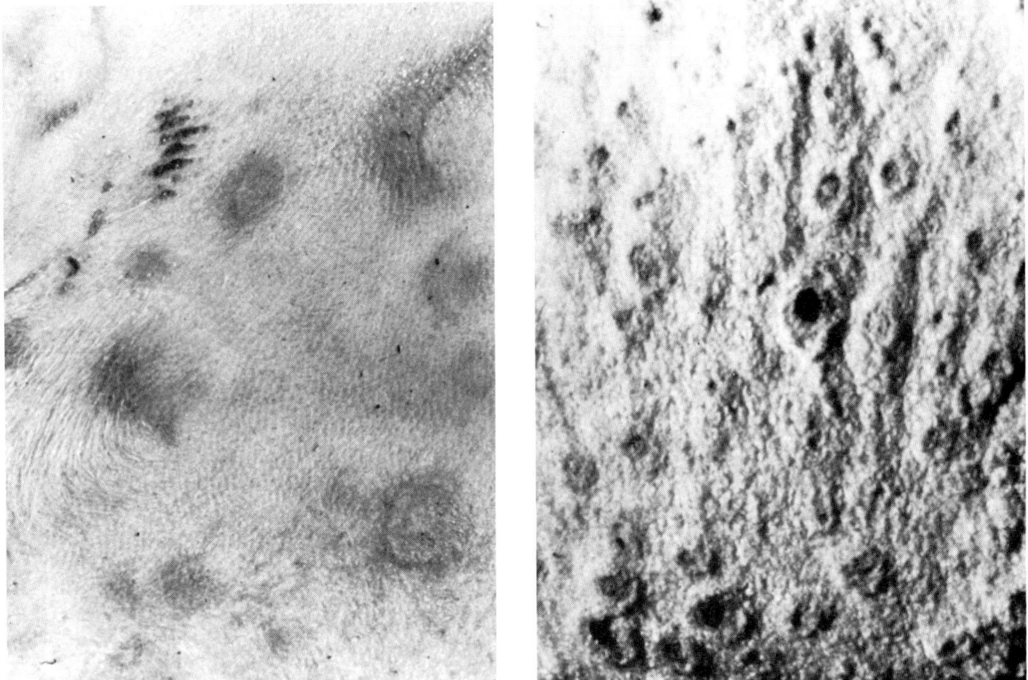

Figure 43.6 (*left*). Sheeppox. Rounded skin lesions in different stages of development. Early lesions are reddened plaques, and older lesions are raised and dark and have an irregular surface. (Courtesy D. A. Gregg, Plum Island Animal Disease Center, USDA.)

Figure 43.7 (*right*). Sheeppox. Old skin lesions characterized by dried necrotic centers with raised edges. (Courtesy D. A. Gregg, Plum Island Animal Disease Center, USDA.)

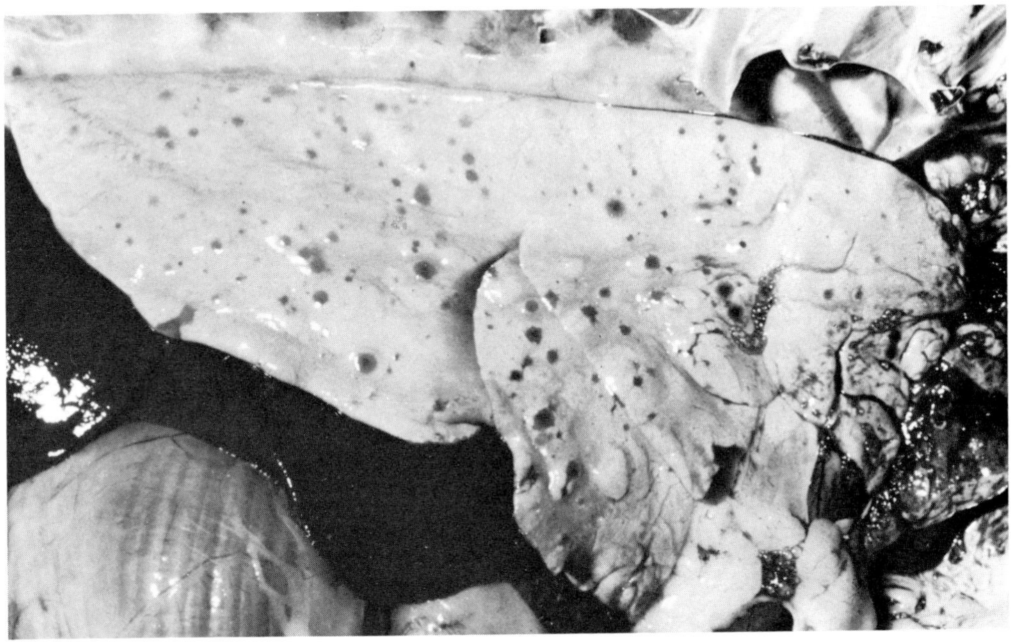

Figure 43.8. Sheeppox lesions in the lungs. Some lesions are firm, whitish nodules, and others are reddened foci with dark red centers. (Courtesy D. A. Gregg, Plum Island Animal Disease Center, USDA.)

southern and eastern Europe, in the Middle East, and in North Africa.

Character of the Disease. A generalized pox eruption occurs on the skin (Figures 43.6 and 43.7), and similar lesions often occur on the mucous membrane of the pharynx and trachea, sometimes even in the abomasum. Hemorrhagic inflammation of the respiratory passages (Figure 43.8) and of the digestive tract occurs. Caseous nodules and areas of catarrhal pneumonia occur in the lungs. The mortality varies from about 5 percent to higher than 50 percent.

Properties of the Virus. The virus is more elongated than other poxviruses and measures 115 by 194 nm (Figure 43.9) (1). It is inactivated in 15 minutes by 2 percent phenol.

All strains are serologically identical, and goatpox virus protects against sheeppox. A complement-fixation test has been reported.

Cultivation. A cytopathogenic effect is produced in the cultures of skin, kidney, and testis of sheep, goats, and calves with no change in virulence for sheep after serial passage (4). An attenuated virus resulted after transfer in sheep embryo cultures (2). The inoculation of strain Perego induced only a local reaction and a temperature rise without generalization after it had undergone serial passage in lamb testes (3).

The virus apparently can be adapted to embryonated hens' eggs with no apparent change in virulence for sheep (6).

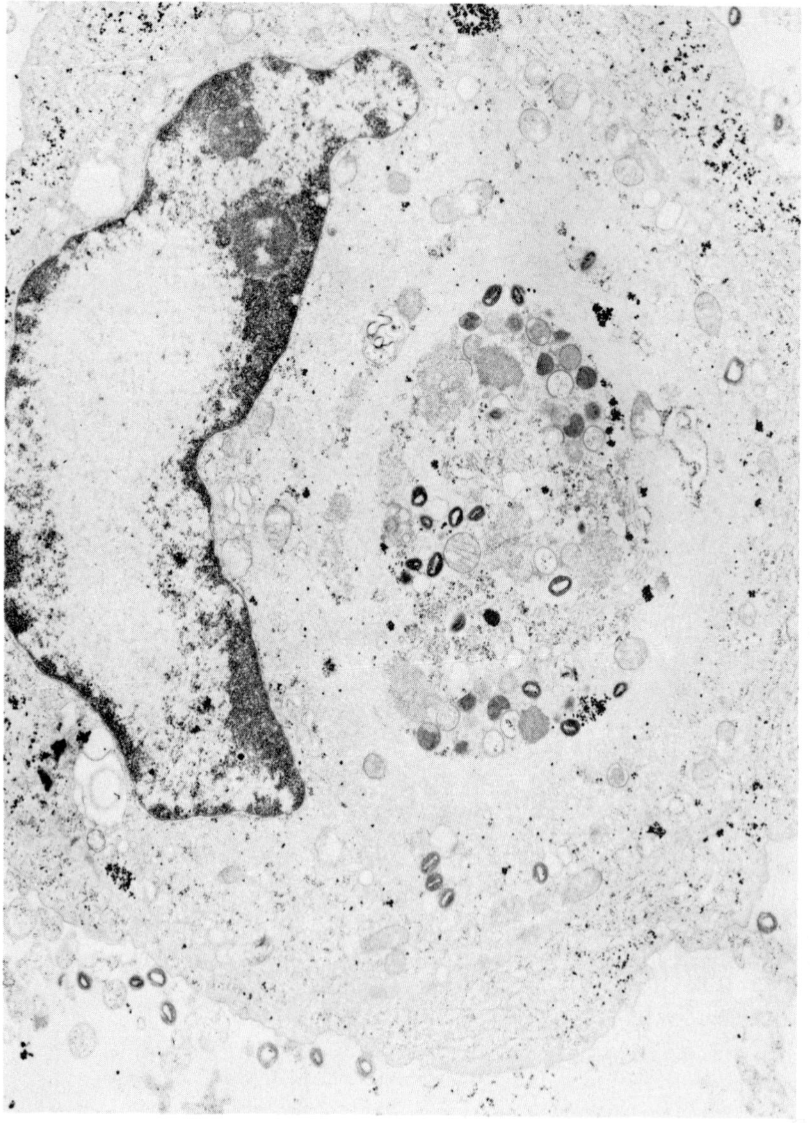

Figure 43.9. Sheeppox in fetal sheep skin. × 8,657. (Courtesy S. S. Breese, Plum Island Animal Disease Center, USDA.)

Control. Vaccination is essential in areas where the disease is enzootic. Various vaccines are used. In Egypt a mild strain from Iran is used to immunize sheep (5). In Turkey a tissue-cultured attenuated vaccine is used with success (2).

REFERENCES

1. Abdusalam and Coslett. Jour. Comp. Path. and Therap., 1957, *67*, 145.
2. Aygün. Arch. Exp. Vet. Med., 1955, *9*, 145.
3. Mateva and Stoichew. Vet. Med. Nauki., 1975, *12*, 18.
4. Plowright and Ferris. Brit. Jour. Exp. Path., 1958, *39*, 424.
5. Sabban. Am. Jour. Vet. Res., 1955, *16*, 209.
6. Sabban. Am. Jour. Vet. Res., 1957, *18*, 618.

Goatpox

The disease is prevalent in North Africa and the Middle East. It also occurs in the Scandinavian countries and Australia. The virus causes generalized pocks on mucous membranes and skin of goats. Typical lesions are shown in Figures 43.10 and 43.11.

The virus produces a cytopathogenic effect and cytoplasmic inclusion bodies in cultures of lamb testis. It causes plaques on the choriollantoic membrane of embryonated hens' eggs (2). Elementary bodies are agglutinated by immune sera.

It is reported that goatpox immunizes against contagious ecthyma of sheep and sheeppox (2); the reverse is not true. It also protects against lumpy skin disease of cattle (1).

REFERENCES

1. Capstick. Quoted by Andrewes, Christopher, in Viruses of vertebrates. Williams and Wilkins, Baltimore, 1964, p. 342.
2. Rafyi and Ramyan. Jour. Comp. Path. and Therap., 1959, *69*, 141.

Virus Dermatitis in Goats

This disease was recently described in India by Haddow and Idnani (1). It is acute and highly fatal. It resembles goatpox, but was considered sufficiently different to warrant another name. A virus is present in the local lesions and in the blood. The incubation period is between 7 and 10 days. Nonpustular, rubbery nodules, 4 to 12 mm in diameter, appear over the body surface and in the mouth. Pneumonia, which was invariably fatal, developed in most cases 1 to 2 days after the appearance of the skin eruption. The few animals that survived developed necrotic tissue in the skin nodules, and these changed into ulcers that healed very slowly. The scabs did not disappear for about 6 weeks.

REFERENCE

1. Haddow and Idnani. Indian Vet. Jour., 1948, *24*, 332.

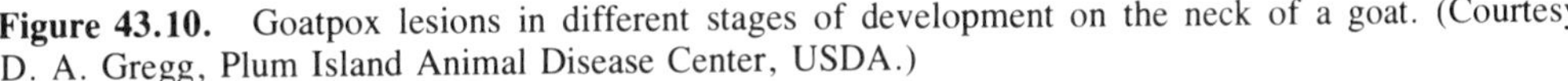

Figure 43.10. Goatpox lesions in different stages of development on the neck of a goat. (Courtesy D. A. Gregg, Plum Island Animal Disease Center, USDA.)

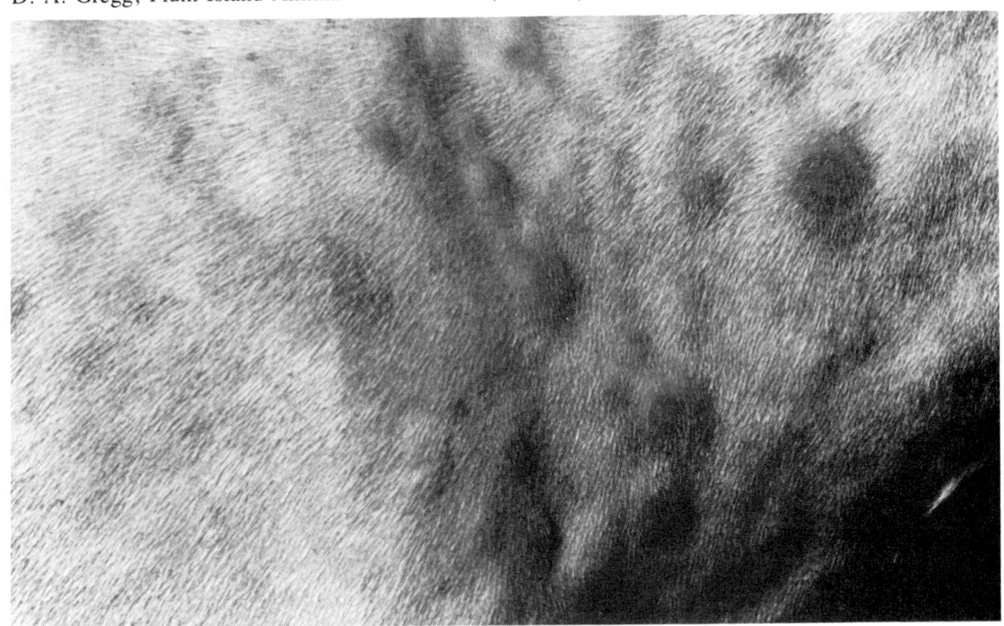

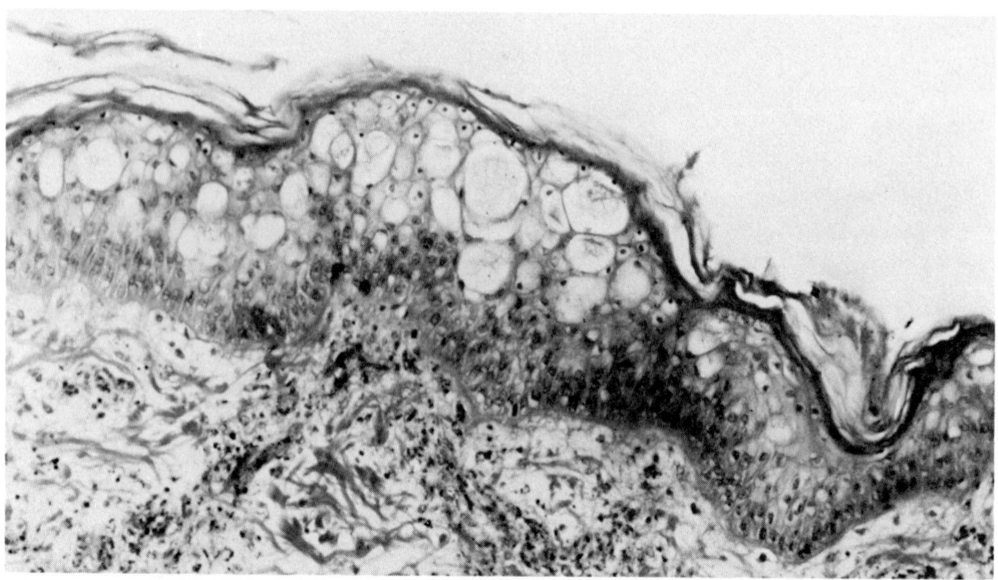

Figure 43.11. Photomicrograph of a section from an early lesion of goatpox in the skin. Cells in the epidermis have undergone hydropic degeneration, and there are microvesicles. In the dermis there is histiocytic hyperplasia and necrosis. H and E stain. × 57. (Courtesy C. A. Mebus, Plum Island Animal Disease Center, USDA.)

Lumpy Skin Disease

SYNONYMS: Lumpy disease, pseudourticaria, *knopvelsiekte*

This condition was first observed in Northern Rhodesia and Madagascar in 1929. It was recognized in Transvaal in 1945 and rapidly spread through southern and eastern Africa. It may occur in buffalo as well as cattle.

Character of the Disease. In cattle a fever develops accompanied by the production of multiple nodules in the skin, pathological changes in the mucous membranes and viscera, and also adenitis. Cytoplasmic inclusions are found in epithelial cells and histiocytes (Figure 43.12).

In past instances the clinical picture in cattle has been complicated by the presence of the Allerton virus, an agent possibly belonging to the herpesvirus group (1).

In rabbits it produces a transient local reaction with some generalized lesions.

Properties of the Virus. Several viruses have been isolated from cases of lumpy skin disease. The Neethling pox strain is closely related to African sheeppox, which is comparable to goatpox (2). It is sensitive to 20 percent ether (3). Figure 43.13 shows its structure and size.

Cultivation. It multiplies in the chick embryo and chorioallantoic membrane producing pocks on the membrane.

After adaptation the virus produces spindle cells within 24 to 48 hours in tissue cultures of embryonic calf and lamb kidney and of calf and lamb testis.

Control. The main control measure is restriction in the movement of cattle from diseased to free areas. The Isiolo or Kedong strains of sheeppox have been used to protect cattle against Neethling virus (2).

Because of the serious economic importance of this disease, cattle from southern Africa should not be exported to other parts of the world until physical examinations and a study of their histories provide assurance that they are not infected.

REFERENCES

1. Andrewes, Christopher. Viruses of vertebrates. Williams and Wilkins, Baltimore, 1964.
2. Capstick. Quoted by Andrewes, Christopher, in Viruses of vertebrates. Williams and Wilkins, Baltimore, 1964.
3. Plowright and Ferris. Virol., 1959, 7, 357.

THE GENUS *LEPORIPOXVIRUS*

Infectious Myxomatosis of Rabbits

This is a highly contagious and almost always fatal disease of domesticated rabbits that was first recognized in South America and later in Mexico and the United

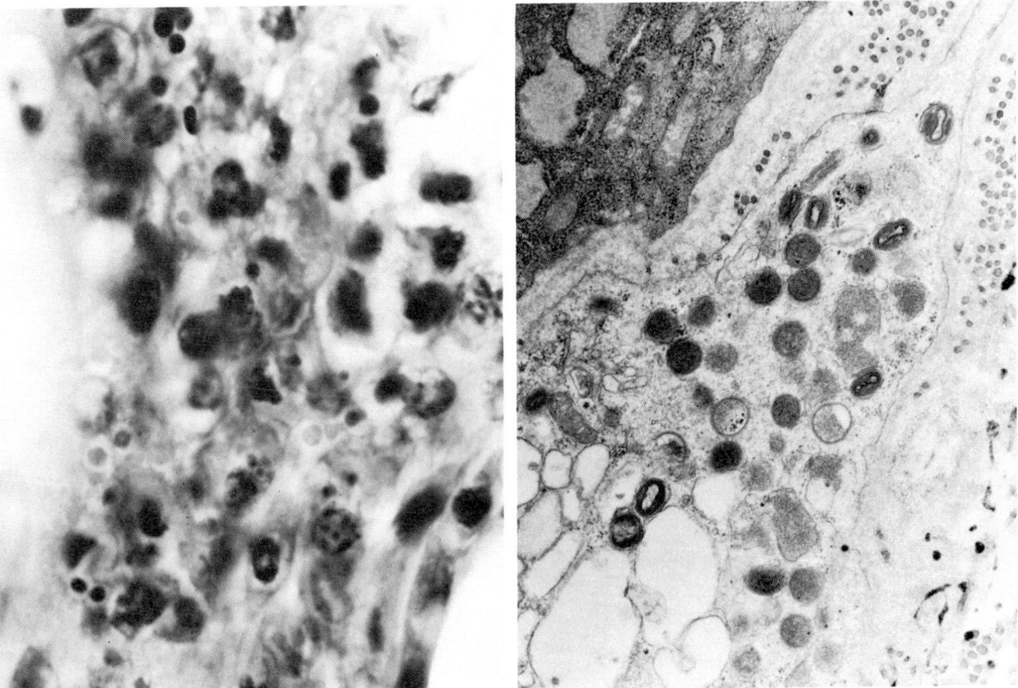

Figure 43.12 (*left*). Photomicrograph of nasal epithelium from a steer with lumpy skin disease. There are several eosinophilic cytoplasmic inclusion bodies in the epidermis. H and E stain. × 300. (Courtesy C. A. Mebus, Plum Island Animal Disease Center, USDA.)

Figure 43.13 (*right*). Lumpy skin disease skin lesions and virus particles. × 16,000. (Courtesy S. S. Breese, Plum Island Animal Disease Center, USDA.)

States (California). The disease often destroys whole rabbitries. In 1976 an epizootic occurred in western Oregon involving 26 rabbitries with mortality ranging from 20 to 50 percent (11).

It was first described in 1898 by Sanarelli (15), who was working in Montevideo, Uruguay. Sanarelli ascribed the disease to a virus since he could not see or cultivate any organisms in the lesions. It is interesting to note that Sanarelli's paper appeared in the same year as that of Loeffler and Frosch, who determined the causative agent of foot-and-mouth disease of cattle to be a virus. The myxoma virus takes its place, historically, as the second animal disease virus to be recognized.

Myxomatosis affects ordinary domestic rabbits, Angora rabbits, Belgian hares, and Flemish giants, but the wild rabbit of Brazil, the common cottontail, and the jackrabbit of the United States are almost wholly resistant. The virus does not affect any animal species other than certain rabbits, and man is also resistant.

Character of the Disease. The disease begins with inflammation of the eyes. The eyelids swell, and a copious discharge from the conjunctival mucous membrane appears. At first the discharge is serous, but shortly it becomes purulent. Within 24 to 48 hours the eyes cannot be opened because of the swelling. A nasal discharge also appears, and swellings are noted involving the skin of the face and ears. The head may become very misshapen; then similar swellings may be noted on other parts of the body. The genital openings become inflamed and discharge a purulent exudate. Finally the tumorous masses may involve nearly the whole body (Figure 43.14); the affected animal appears very ill and almost invariably dies 7 to 15 days after the first signs are noted.

The tumorlike masses consist of tissue having a rubbery, gelatinous consistency. Usually the lungs, liver, and kidneys are normal in appearance, but the spleen is always swollen and the lymph nodes are enlarged and hemorrhagic. Although the external genitalia are inflamed, the testicles, uterus, and ovaries are generally free of lesions. The testicular swelling mentioned by many authors is usually caused by changes in the scrotum rather than in the testicle.

Sections of the myxomata show tissue characteristic of that type of tumor, that is, large stellate cells embedded in a homogeneous, gelatinous substance that is largely if not wholly mucin (Figure 43.15). In addition, however, there is inflammation manifested by engorgement and hemorrhages from the blood vessels and by collections of

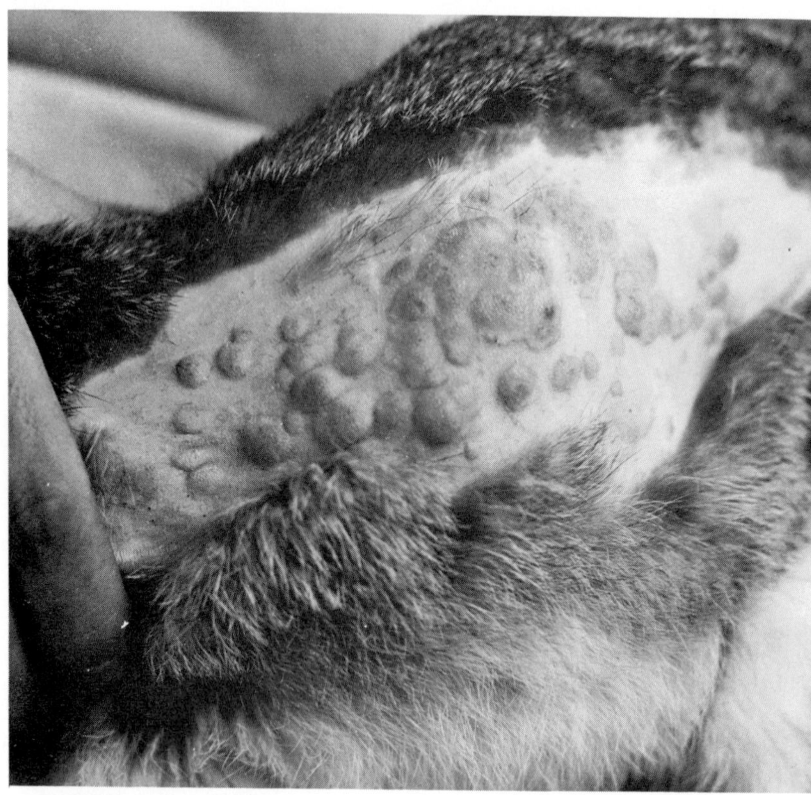

Figure 43.14. Myxomatosis in the rabbit. Multiple primary tumors were induced by virus on the freshly shaved skin. (Courtesy Thomas M. Rivers, *Jour. Exp. Med.*)

neutrophilic leukocytes. Rivers (13) was the first to call attention to another characteristic feature of these virus tumors, that is, a peculiar type of degeneration of the epithelial coverings. The epithelial cells are greatly swollen and vacuolated, and acidophilic bodies rapidly develop in their cytoplasm (Figure 43.16). These bodies contain blue-staining coccoid elements. The whole structure resembles the Bollinger bodies of fowlpox.

Rivers and Ward (14) have found it possible to obtain suspensions of these elementary bodies, which they regard as the virus, in a relatively pure form. Not only are such suspensions highly pathogenic, but the bodies are specifically agglutinated by the serum of recovered or immunized animals.

Properties of the Virus. Because this virus is indistinguishable from vaccinia virus by electron microscopy (4) and it is a DNA virus, it is classified as a poxvirus (1). The cytoplasmic inclusion bodies which presumably contain virus are Feulgen-positive.

It is a reasonably stable virus in glycerol and when frozen or dried. It is inactivated by heat in 25 minutes at 55 C. It survives many months in the skins of affected rabbits that are maintained at ordinary temperatures (8).

The virus is ether-sensitive and in this respect unlike other poxviruses, but similar in that it is resistant to sodium deoxycholate (2). The specific gravity is estimated at 1.3.

The viral antigen produces complement-fixing, precipitating, and neutralizing antibodies. The virus is closely related to the rabbit fibroma.

Cultivation. Hoffstadt and Pilcher (7) have reported successful cultivation of myxoma virus on the chorioallantoic membrane of the developing chick embryo. The virus produces a cytopathogenic effect and grows in cell cultures from cottontail rabbits, squirrels, young rats, hamsters, guinea pigs, and certain human tissues (1). Plaques develop on cell monolayers.

Immunity. Among experimental rabbits the mortality from myxoma infection is so nearly 100 percent that only a few survivors have been available for studies on immunity. These have shown, however, a high grade of resistance to reinfection.

In Australia the initial mortality rates from the induced outbreaks was estimated to be 99.5 percent. It was found, however, in some regions that the mortality rate was not so high in successive seasons; hence a considerable number of survivors were available for study. According to Fenner, Marshall, and Woodroofe (6), these showed serum antibodies that persisted at least 18 months. Inoculation of such rabbits with virulent myx-

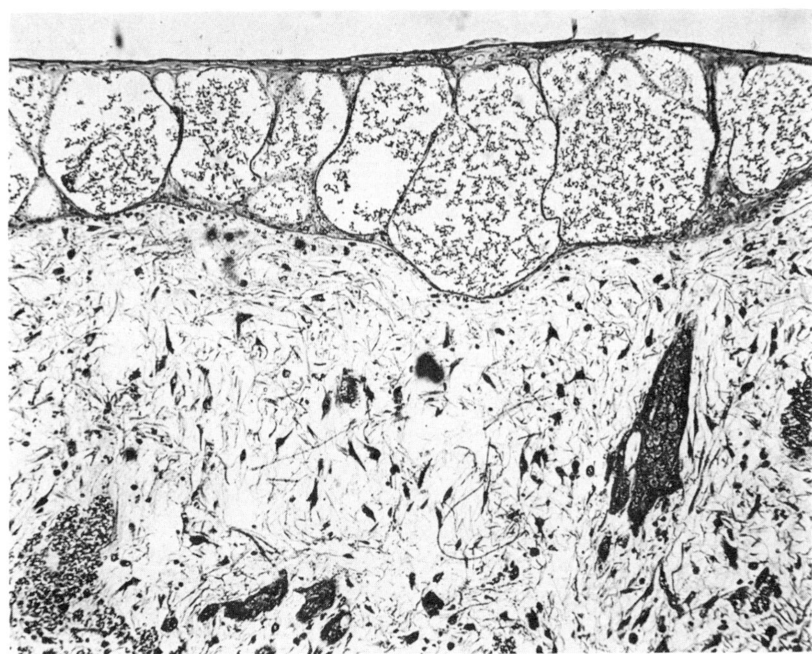

Figure 43.15. Myxomatosis. The virus attacks epidermal cells as well as those of the subcutaneous tissue. In the lower part of the photograph the myxomatous tissue is seen. In the upper part is a series of vesicles—the end result of infection of epithelial cells. × 100. (Courtesy Thomas M. Rivers, *Jour. Exp. Med.*)

oma virus produced a small local lesion in some cases and no lesions at all in others. Fenner and Marshall (5) showed that the young of immune mothers were passively protected, at least in part. In contrast, Sobey and Conolly (18) reported that offspring with maternal antibody to myxoma virus that were exposed to fleas contaminated with myxoma virus and/or had contact with infected rabbits from birth died or became infected before 8 weeks of age. When compared with adult control animals the offspring with maternal antibodies showed no advantage in survival time or recovery rate.

Shope (17) discovered that the virus of the Shope fibroma, which is a benign tumor, immunized rabbits to the virus of myxomatosis. When first reported this interest-

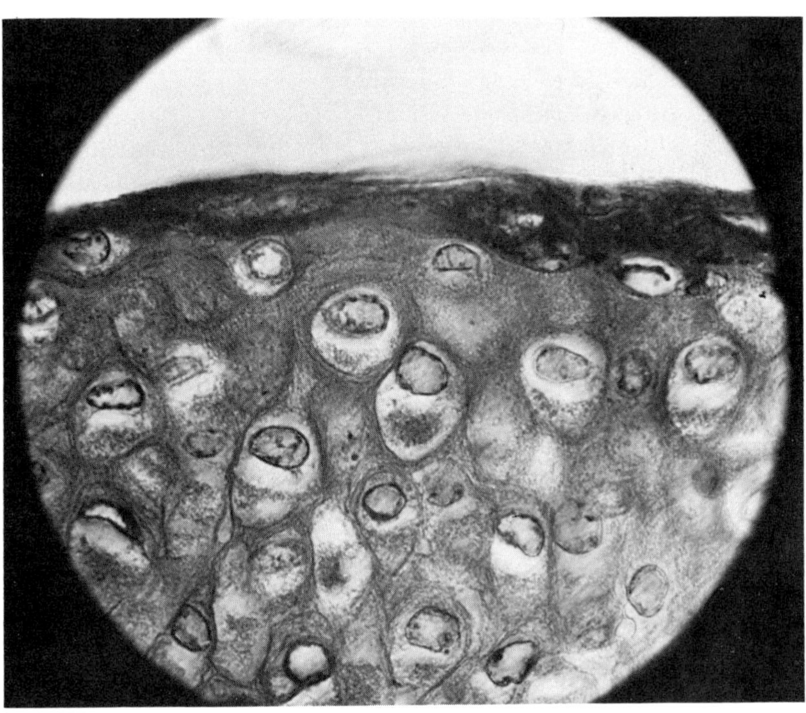

Figure 43.16. Myxomatosis. Epidermis of a tumor shows cytoplasmic inclusion bodies. × 850. (Courtesy Thomas M. Rivers, *Jour. Exp. Med.*)

ing observation was thought to have little practical value. It has since been useful, however, as a means of protecting breeding stocks in Europe since 1953. Ritchie *et al.* (12) report that in England the method gives about 90 percent serviceable immunity, and that few problems have been occasioned by its use. On very young rabbits large tumors may be produced, but on older stock immunity often is obtained without the production of tumors.

Transmission. Myxomatosis spreads readily by contact or close cohabitation of domesticated rabbits. The incubation period is about 5 days.

In attempting to use the virus to destroy wild rabbits that had become a destructive pest in Australia it was learned that rapid spread of the disease occurred only when certain mosquitoes which fed freely on rabbits were present. After several trials had failed, an attempt to set up an epizootic succeeded brilliantly in one of the river valleys where there were many mosquitoes. The rabbit flea (*Spilopsyllus cuniculi*) also is a transmitting agent, but unless rabbit populations are very dense, flea transmission fails to produce epizootics. For papers dealing with the epizootiology of myxomatosis in wild rabbits, see papers by Myers, Marshall, and Fenner (10); Ritchie, Hudson, and Thompson (12); Bull, Ratcliffe, and Edgar (3); Thompson (19); Mead-Briggs and Vaughan (9); and Sheperd and Edmonds (16).

The Use of Myxoma Virus to Destroy Unwanted Rabbit Populations. Reference has been made to the use of this disease to destroy rabbits in Australia. Because this disease is not pathogenic for man or any other animal species, it had often been suggested as a means to control the rabbit population. The wild Australian rabbit is a descendant of European rabbits imported many years ago. Because there are no natural enemies of rabbits in Australia, they thrived remarkably well. It is estimated that the number increased to a total of 1 to 3 billion. They ate a huge amount of vegetation which could more profitably be used for feeding sheep and other animals.

In 1950 myxoma-infected animals were released in seven locations with the hope that the disease would spread from these centers in the form of a great epizootic. In six centers the attempt was a failure. In the seventh, in the Murray River Valley, large numbers of rabbits perished from the disease, and it was here that the importance of mosquito vectors was first appreciated. Hundreds of thousands of acres of land in this valley were cleared of rabbits. The following season, which was hot and dry in the valley, mosquitoes were not numerous, and the disease did not flourish. In other areas, however, where there was more moisture and many mosquitoes, the disease spread rapidly. In later years the kill has been lower, and there is evidence that the host-parasite adjustment is occurring. Virus variants probably will have to be found if the rabbits are to be destroyed, because apparently a resistant population is now developing.

In 1952 a French physician who had retired to his country estate released some infected rabbits, hoping to destroy the rabbits that plagued his gardens. He not only destroyed his own rabbits, but within 18 months the disease had spread through most of France, Belgium, Germany, and Holland; it had even crossed the English Channel into Great Britain. All attempts to stop the disease failed. Only the use of fibroma vaccine saved some of the domesticated species.

REFERENCES

1. Andrewes, Christopher. Viruses of vertebrates. Williams and Wilkins, Baltimore, 1964.
2. Andrewes and Horstmann. Jour. Gen. Microbiol., 1949, *3*, 290.
3. Bull, Ratcliffe, and Edgar. Vet. Rec., 1954, *66*, 61.
4. Farrant and Fenner. Austral. Jour. Exp. Biol. and Med. Sci., 1953, *31*, 121.
5. Fenner and Marshall. Jour. Hyg. (London), 1954, *52*, 321.
6. Fenner, Marshall, and Woodroofe. Jour. Hyg. (London), 1953, *51*, 225.
7. Hoffstadt and Pilcher. Jour. Bact., 1938, *36*, 286.
8. Jacotot, Vallee, and Virat. Ann. Inst. Pasteur, 1955, *89*, 290.
9. Mead-Briggs and Vaughn. Jour. Hyg. (London), 1975, *75*, 237.
10. Myers, Marshall, and Fenner. Jour. Hyg. (London), 1954, *52*, 337.
11. Patton and Holmes. Jour. Am. Vet. Med. Assoc., 1977, *170*, 560.
12. Ritchie, Hudson, and Thompson. Vet. Rec., 1954, *66*, 796.
13. Rivers. Proc. Soc. Exp. Biol. and Med., 1926–27, *24*, 435.
14. Rivers and Ward. Jour. Exp. Med., 1937, *66*, 1.
15. Sanarelli. Zentrbl. f. Bakt., I Abt., 1898, *23*, 865.
16. Sheperd and Edmonds. Jour. Hyg. (London), 1977, *79*, 405.
17. Shope. Jour. Exp. Med., 1932, *56*, 803; Proc. Soc. Exp. Biol. and Med., 1938, *38*, 86.
18. Sobey and Conolly. Jour. Hyg. (London), 1975, *74*, 43.
19. Thompson. Agriculture (Gt. Brit.), 1954, *60*, 503.

The Shope Fibroma of Rabbits

Shope (10) in 1932 described a type of fibrous tumor of the cottontail rabbit which proved to be transmissible

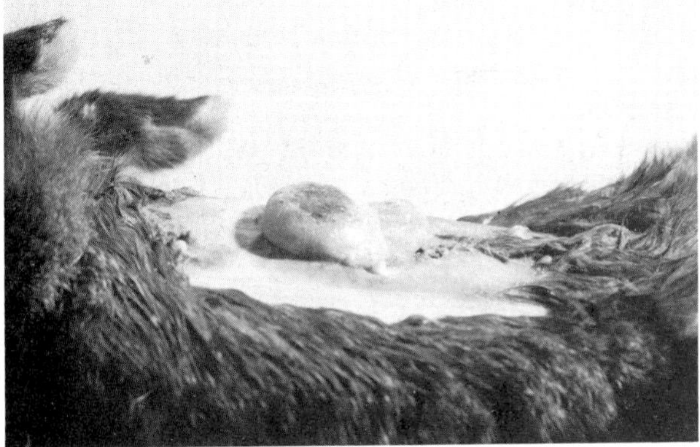

Figure 43.17. The Shope virus fibroma. The tumor on the shaved skin of the abdomen of a rabbit was produced by experimental inoculation 11 days previously. (Courtesy R. E. Shope.)

to other cottontail rabbits and to the domestic species by the injection of cellular suspension and of Berkefeld filtrates. Although of interest on its own account, this virus has attracted much attention because of its relationship to the virus of myxomatosis.

Character of the Disease. The tumor occurs subcutaneously in naturally infected cases. There may be one or several in the same animal. They are firm, spherical masses which can be moved about under the skin because they are only loosely attached (Figure 43.17). Sections show that the masses are made up of spindle-shaped, connective tissue cells, without evidence of inflammatory or necrotic reaction (Figure 43.18).

Filtrates of tumor tissue when injected into the testicles regularly cause the formation of similar tumors. Subcutaneous and intramuscular inoculations frequently, but not always, succeed. Intraperitoneal and intracerebral inoculations fail.

Inoculation transmits the tumors equally well in domestic and cottontail rabbits, but the behavior of the tumors in these species differs. In the cottontail rabbit growth is slow and continues over a long period of months. In the domestic rabbit growth is rapid, but after about 10 days of active proliferation further growth does not occur and retrogression begins.

Properties of the Virus. The virus in rabbit fibromatosis is found only in the tumors. It has not been demonstrated in the blood, visceral organs, or any of the

Figure 43.18. The Shope fibroma virus showing section of a testicular tumor produced by experimental inoculation of a rabbit. × 330. (Courtesy R. E. Shope.)

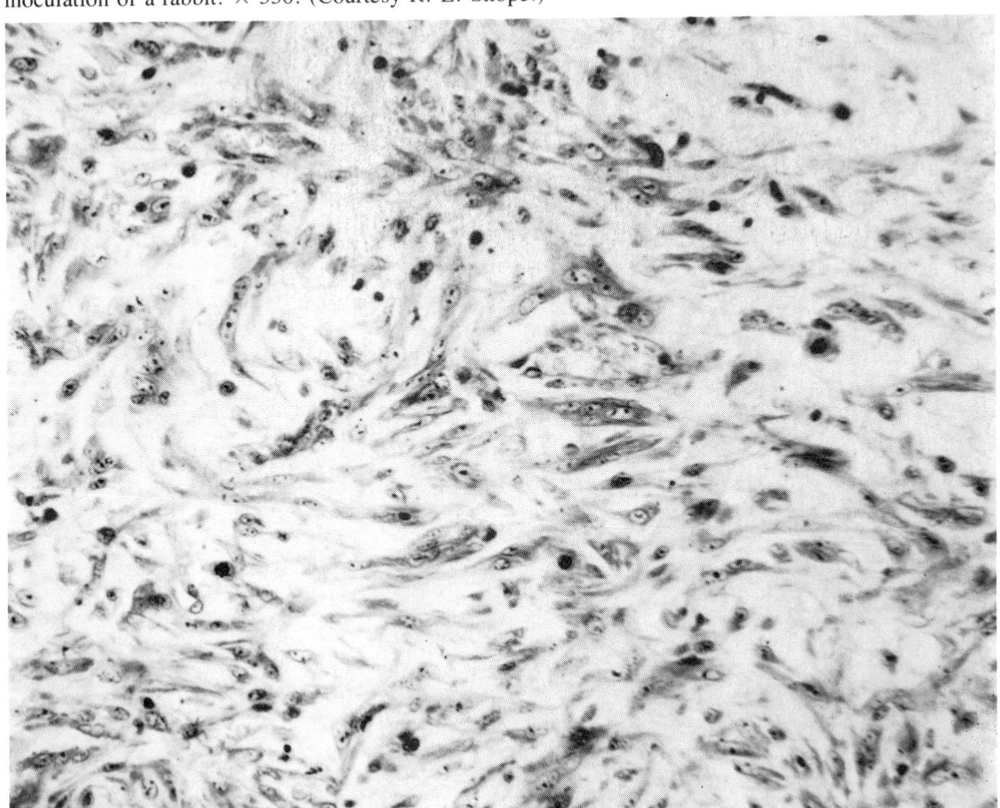

secretions or excretions. In susceptible animals it stimulates a proliferation of the connective tissue at the point where it is deposited. The virus content of the cottontail tumors remains high for a long period (77 days at least), whereas in domestic rabbit tumors it is highest about 7 to 9 days after inoculation and disappears as retrogression occurs (11). Guinea pigs, rats, mice, and chickens proved refractory to inoculation. So far as is known, no animal other than rabbits can be infected with this virus.

This virus resembles vaccinia and myxoma viruses as determined by electron microscope studies. For this reason it is classified as a poxvirus. In thin sections its size is estimated at 200 to 240 nm (2). It is ether-sensitive and quite stable in glycerol and at low temperatures.

Rabbit fibroma virus is closely related immunologically to myxoma virus. Presumably there are minor antigenic differences as determined by the complement-fixation and agar-gel-diffusion tests. Interference is reported by virus III, Semliki forest virus, and Murray Valley encephalitis virus.

Phosphonoacetic acid (PAA) has an inhibitory effect on this virus. A complete suppression of induced tumors was observed when 10 mg of PAA was inoculated into the lesion site for 5 days if treatment was begun 24 hours after virus inoculation (7).

One strain of rabbit fibroma virus, after 18 passages in domestic rabbits, suddenly mutated and thereafter failed to produce tumors but instead caused inflammatory reactions in the injection sites. This change was detected by Andrewes (1) in England, to whom Shope had sent the material. Shope (14) was able to confirm Andrewes's findings. Passage through a series of cottontail rabbits restored part of the tumor-producing power. Other strains have not so changed. The changed strain continued to immunize against the tumor-producing strains.

Cultivation. The OA strain multiplies in the chorioallantoic membrane of embryonated hens' eggs without the production of lesions.

The agent produces a cytopathogenic effect and propagates in cell cultures of tissues from the domestic and cottontail rabbit and also in tissue cultures from the guinea pig, rat, and man (5). Foci appear on rabbit kidney monolayers (9).

Immunity. Shope (11) showed that domestic rabbits in which tumors had formed and retrogressed could not be reinfected with the same virus. To his surprise he found that such rabbits also had a high degree of resistance to the virus of myxomatosis. Whereas myxoma virus is almost always fatal to normal rabbits, it destroyed only 1 of a group of 15 fibroma-recovered animals. These animals then proved to be highly immune to myxoma virus as well as to fibroma virus. One rabbit that recovered from myxoma without having previously been affected with fibroma proved to be resistant to fibroma as well as myxoma (15).

Thinking that fibroma might be the natural reaction of cottontail rabbits to the virus of myxomatosis, Shope (12) attempted to pass the myxoma virus serially through these animals. Only minimal reactions were induced, and these had the character of neither fibroma nor myxoma.

The unexpected finding of the immunological relationship between fibromatosis and myxomatosis suggested that the benign fibroma was caused by an attenuated strain of the malignant myxoma; however, Shope (13) expressed the opinion that such was not the case—that the viruses were qualitatively different.

In 1936 and 1937 Berry and Dedrick (4) and Berry (3) made certain observations on experiments conducted with fibroma virus that have come to be known as the Berry-Dedrick phenomenon. The virus of myxomatosis was heated to 75 C, which appeared to inactivate it completely. When the inactivated myxoma virus was mixed with active fibroma virus, the mixture produced typical myxomatosis in rabbits. It is now known that the nucleic acid of the inactivated myxoma virus is incorporated into the protein overcoat of the fibroma virus. These hybrid particles retain the coding for the myxoma virus and produce myxomatosis when inoculated into susceptible rabbits.

Transmission. The mode of natural transmission is not known. Virus does not transmit from animal to animal by simple contact. Hyde and Gardner (8) found that it was not transmitted from mother to young either through the placenta or through the milk. Experimentally the disease has been produced only by inoculation. In view of what is now known about the transmission of myxoma, it seems to be fairly safe to assume that natural transmission occurs by means of biting insects (6).

REFERENCES

1. Andrewes. Jour. Exp. Med., 1936, *63*, 157.
2. Bernhard, Bauer, Harel, and Oberling. Bull. Cancer, 1954, *41*, 423.
3. Berry. Arch. Path., 1937, *24*, 533.
4. Berry and Dedrick. Jour. Bact., 1936, *31*, 50.
5. Chaproniere and Andrewes. Virol., 1957, *4*, 351.
6. Dalmat. Jour. Hyg. (London), 1959, *57*, 1.
7. Friedman-Kien, Fondak, and Klein. Jour. Invest. Dermatol., 1976, *66*, 99.

8. Hyde and Gardner. Am. Jour. Hyg., 1939 (Sec. B), *30,* 57.
9. Padgett, Moore, and Walker. Virol., 1962, *17,* 462.
10. Shope. Jour. Exp. Med., 1932, *56,* 793.
11. Shope. Jour. Exp. Med., 1932, *56,* 803.
12. Shope. Jour. Exp. Med., 1936, *63,* 33.
13. Shope. Jour. Exp. Med., 1936, *63,* 43.
14. Shope. Jour. Exp. Med., 1936, *63,* 173.
15. Shope. Proc. Soc. Exp. Biol. and Med., 1938, *38,* 86.

THE GENUS *PARAPOXVIRUS*

Pseudocowpox

SYNONYMS: Paravaccinia, milker's nodules

Character of the Disease. This disease clinically resembles cowpox and vaccinia. Pseudocowpox occurs in dairy herds in all parts of this country. The disease, *per se,* has slight effect upon cattle. The lesions resemble those of cowpox except that umbilicated pustules are seldom seen, the lesions progressing from papules to vesicles to raw areas that heal under a dry scab. The disease is very annoying because of the soreness of the teats, which makes the animals difficult to milk. The disease spreads to most of the cows that are milked, apparently on the hands of the milkers or through contamination of the milking machines. Dry cows, nonmilking heifers, and bulls rarely become involved. Mastitis sometimes results, apparently from secondary bacterial infections. Healing occurs after several weeks and the disease then disappears. Antiseptic ointments facilitate healing and make milking less painful.

Properties of the Virus. In 1963 it was shown to be caused by a poxvirus (2). The dimensions are 190 by 296 nm. It has a spiral structure as in contagious ecthyma of sheep and bovine papular stomatitis. It is inactivated in 10 minutes by chloroform.

No cross-immunity has been demonstrated between this virus and cowpox or vaccinia. The virus is probably related to orf and bovine papular stomatitis. It has been suggested that the immunity is transient in cattle.

Cultivation. The virus produces a cytopathogenic effect in bovine kidney cell cultures (2). After cultivation in bovine kidney cell culture, it grew in human embryonic fibroblasts but not in rabbit and rhesus monkey kidney cultures. The infection has not been successfully transmitted to rabbits, mice, guinea pigs, or chick embryos.

The Disease in Man. In man the milker's nodule lesion takes the form of hemispherical cherry-red papules (Figure 43.19) which appear on the hands and sometimes on other parts of the body (1). The lesions begin as papules 5 to 7 days after exposure. They gradually enlarge into firm, elastic, bluish red, smooth, hemispherical masses varying in size up to 2 cm in diameter. They are relatively painless but frequently cause an itching sensation. When fully developed they often show a dimple on the top, but they do not break down with pus formation. They are highly vascular. The tense grayish skin covering them remains intact. The granulation tissue that makes up the mass of the nodule gradually becomes absorbed. The lesions slowly flatten as this occurs, and finally, after 4 to 6 weeks, they disappear. Sometimes there is slight swelling of the axillary nodes, but otherwise there is no evidence of any generalization of the disease.

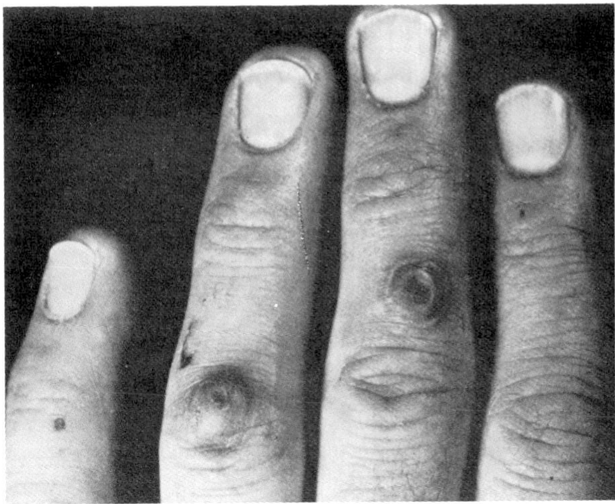

Figure 43.19. Milker's nodules.

REFERENCES

1. Becker. Jour. Am. Vet. Med. Assoc., 1940, *115,* 2140.
2. Friedman-Kiem, Rowe, and Banfield. Science, 1963, *140,* 1335.

Bovine Papular Stomatitis

This disease of cattle is probably the same as erosive stomatitis, stomatitis papulosa, ulcerative stomatitis, or pseudoaphthous stomatitis. There are many discrepancies in the literature, so it is possible that more than one agent is involved in the syndrome. It occurs in North America, Africa, and Europe. Rossi *et al.* (3) in 1977 reported the isolation of a parapoxvirus from a calf with oral lesions and respiratory disease, but they were unable to produce signs of illness or elicit antibody production in experimental calves.

The reported size of the virus varies from 125 by 150 nm in diameter (1) to 207 by 215 nm and the particles are poxlike structures with single or double membranes (2). Two conflicting reports exist on its growth in embryonated hens' eggs. In cultures of calf testis the agent produces foci rapidly after adaptation.

The agent produces an ulcerative stomatitis in cattle. There may be craterlike ulcers 1 cm in diameter. The infection seems to be limited to the stoma. Cytoplasmic inclusions may be found in the infected cells. There is some question whether it can produce an infection in sheep and goats. Transmission to other animals has failed.

REFERENCES

1. Pritchard, Clafin, Gustafson, and Ristic. Jour. Am. Vet. Med. Assoc., 1958, *132,* 273.
2. Reczko. Zentrbl. f. Bakt., I Abt. Orig., 1957, *169,* 425.
3. Rossi, Kiesel, and Jong. Cornell Vet., 1977, *67,* 72.

Contagious Pustular Dermatitis of Sheep

SYNONYMS: Sore mouth, contagious ecthyma of sheep, "scabby mouth," contagious pustular stomatitis, infectious labial dermatitis, orf

This is a poxlike disease of sheep and goats. Occasionally infections of man occur. The disease is frequent on the western ranges during the spring and summer months, and it occurs occasionally in the farm flocks of the eastern part of the United States. It has been reported also in many other sheep-raising countries.

Character of the Disease. In areas where the disease has been well established, it is seen principally in the lambs and kids, the older animals being immune as a result of vaccination or of having suffered from the disease earlier in life.

It is characterized by the formation of papules and vesicles on the skin of the lips and sometimes around the nostrils and eyes (Figure 43.20). These rapidly change to pustules, and finally heavy scabs appear. With their thickened, stiff, sensitive lips, the affected lambs or kids can neither suckle nor graze, and rapid emaciation occurs. Healing usually is complete in about one month, the scabs having fallen off by this time leaving the lips smooth and without scars. It is not uncommon for ewes with suckling infected lambs, to develop lesions on their udders.

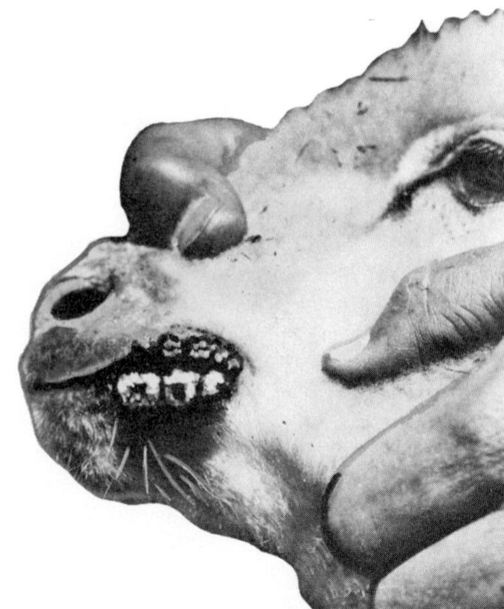

Figure 43.20. Contagious pustular dermatitis (sore mouth) in sheep. (Courtesy Jen-Sal Laboratories, Inc.)

Fatalities are not numerous except in the presence of complications. In the more southerly states these are commonly the result of invasion of the lesions by the larvae of the flesh or screwworm fly (*Cochliomyia hominivorax.*) The losses in young lambs and kids frequently are very great. The disease in older animals is usually less severe, and such animals are better able to resist the damage from the fly larvae. Where the screwworm does not exist, the only serious complication, according to Marsh and Tunnicliff (7), is the invasion of the lesions by the necrosis bacillus (*Fusobacterium necrophorum*).

Properties of the Virus. By electron microscopy its size is 158 by 252 nm, with rounded ends and dense subpolar regions (2) (Figure 43.21). It is an ether- and chloroform-resistant DNA virus.

Boughton and Hardy (4) determined that the virus was destroyed by being heated to 58 to 60 C for one-half hour. It was not destroyed by the same exposure at 55 C.

Of the greatest practical importance is the resistance of this virus to natural conditions. The virus is able to retain viability for very long periods in the dried scabs which fall when the lesions heal. Premises have been known to harbor infection for more than a year after all animals have been removed. Boughton and Hardy showed that such scabs usually lost all virulence when placed on the

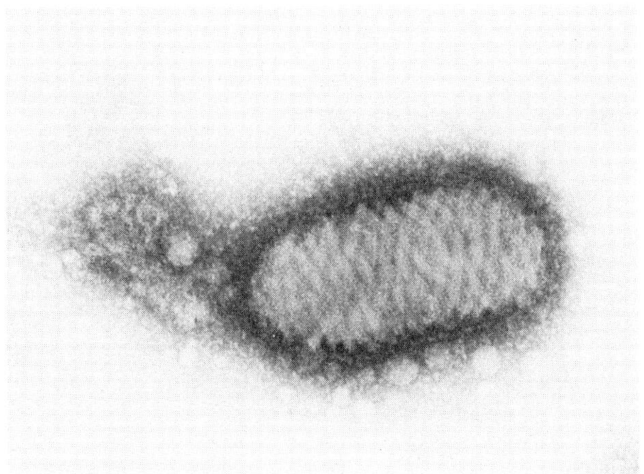

Figure 43.21. Contagious pustular dermatitis of sheep, a parapoxvirus. × 142,500. (Courtesy Viral Pathology and Viral Exanthems Branches, Center for Disease Control.)

surface of the ground during the hot summer period in western Texas for 30 to 60 days, but that if protected they retained their virulence much longer. Scabs placed outside in the fall of the year were found still virulent in the spring. Powdered, dry scab retained virulence for at least 32 months when it was kept in the refrigerator, but it lost it in 54 to 120 days when stored in the dark at an average temperature of 83 F.

Cultivation. Greig (5) has reported success in cultivating the virus of this disease in monolayer cultures of embryonic sheep skin. Three strains were cultivated in this way.

The virus has also been cultivated in embryonic bovine kidney cells with no loss in pathogenicity for sheep (10). Mice, rabbits, guinea pigs, hamsters and chick embryos are refractory to inoculation.

Relationship to Sheeppox. There has been confusion in the past between this disease and pox of sheep and goats. There is no cross-immunization between orf and sheeppox; however, goatpox, which is a much milder disease, appears to give some protection against later exposure to orf.

Immunity. Schmidt and Hardy (9) found that lambs and kids that had recovered from this disease were solidly immune thereafter. Animals that recover from the disease are immune thereafter for periods at least as long as 28 months, and perhaps much longer. As a practical matter, range animals that have had the disease or have been vaccinated are considered immune for life.

Immune sera agglutinate elementary bodies, precipitate soluble antigen, and fix complement (1). The virus shows a small amount of cross-reaction with vaccinia and ectromelia as demonstrated by the complement-fixation and gel-diffusion tests; contagious pustular dermatitis antisera showed some neutralization of ectromelia (11). Goatpox will immunize against contagious pustular dermatitis, but the converse is not true (3); the same situation prevails in the neutralization test. Strains of contagious pustular dermatitis may not be serologically identical (6), but good immunity in sheep between strains from various countries occurs.

Transmission. The evidence indicates that outbreaks are initiated by virus which persists in the soil from one season to the next or by contact with infected animals. Rapid spread, severe disease, and a high morbidity in an Australian herd were attributed to the concentration of sheep around a palatable scrub, *Templetonia retusa,* which caused extensive trauma to mucous membranes during grazing (5).

Diagnosis. The disease is recognized by its characteristic epithelial lesions that show ballooning of cells leading to degeneration, vesicle formation, and possible granulomatous formation. Type B cytoplasmic inclusion bodies are found. Diagnosis is based on the isolation and identification of the virus, or by electron microscopy of negatively stained suspensions from lesions.

There are some similarities to bluetongue in the initial stages of the disease (5) and also to cutaneous anthrax.

Control. In regions where this disease is prevalent, it is wise to vaccinate all lambs or kids each spring before the pasture season begins because the disease tends to recur regularly each year on lands that are once infected.

The Disease in Man. Sheepherders and others who come in intimate contact with sheep infected with sore mouth are apt to develop lesions on their hands or face. Transmission often occurs with apparent ease from infected sheep to humans.

In recent years there have been many reports on the nature of the disease in man. The lesions begin in abrasions, as a rule. They consist of rather large vesicles that may be multiple in structure. The surrounding skin becomes reddened and moderately swollen. The individual may have some fever, there may be swelling of the axillary lymph nodes, and the local lesion is moderately painful. Secondary infection usually occurs and healing is often rather slow (8).

REFERENCES

1. Abdusalam. Jour. Comp. Path. and Therap., 1958, *68,* 23.

2. Abdusalam and Coslett. Jour. Comp. Path. and Therap., 1957, *67,* 145.
3. Bennett, Horgan, and Hasseeb. Jour. Comp. Path. and Therap., 1944, *54,* 131.
4. Boughton and Hardy. Texas Agr. Exp. Sta. Bull. 504, 1935.
5. Gardiner, Craig, and Nairn. Austral. Vet. Jour., 1967, *43,* 163.
6. Greig. Can. Jour. Comp. Path. and Vet. Sci., 1957, *21,* 304.
7. Horgan and Hasseeb. Jour. Comp. Path. and Therap., 1947, *57,* 8.
8. Marsh and Tunnicliff. Jour. Am. Vet. Med. Assoc., 1937, *91,* 600.
9. Newsom and Cross. Jour. Am. Vet. Med., Assoc., 1934, *84,* 799.
10. Schmidt and Hardy. Texas Agr. Exp. Sta. Bull. 457, 1932.
11. Trueblood and Chow. Am. Jour. Vet. Res., 1963, *24,* 47.

44 The Herpesviridae

The family *Herpesviridae* contains many viruses responsible for important human and animal diseases. Provisionally, the family has been divided into 3 subfamilies: Alphaherpesvirinae with human herpes simplex virus as the prototype, Betaherpesvirinae with human cytomegalovirus as the prototype, and Gammaherpesvirinae with Epstein-Barr virus as the prototype. The herpes simplex virus has a higher molecular weight than the human cytomegalovirus, and the Epstein-Barr virus is distinguished from the other two by its T-cell association. Herpesviruses have cuboidal symmetry. The particles are coated with an outer membrane, which makes precise definition of their diameter difficult to ascertain (Figure 44.1). The particle is an icosahedral capsid with a diameter of 100 to 150 nm and is constructed of 162 hollow capsomeres. Each capsomere is about 9 nm across and 12.5 nm deep; the central cavity is about 75 nm in diameter and contains the double-stranded DNA molecule. The molecular weight of the nucleic acid for members of the group varies from 54 to 92 $\times$ 10^6 daltons, which constitutes approximately 7 percent of the particle weight. The buoyant density in cesium chloride is 1.27 to 1.29 per ml. The particles are inactivated by chloroform and usually inactivated by ether.

The development of virus particles begins in the nucleus where it forms an intranuclear eosinophilic inclusion body and the particles become complete by the addition of protein membranes as the virus passes into the cytoplasm. Most viruses in the group had an affinity for epithelial tissue and tend to produce latent infections. In cell culture and on embryonating chicken membranes the members of the group for which information is available produce focal cytopathic effects in the form of plaques or pocks. Some members of the group are strongly cell-associated, requiring special procedures to release the virus into the tissue culture medium in appreciable titers; others readily release virus into the medium. These viruses are rather poor interferon producers.

Few serological relationships have been found among members of the family, but rarely have investigations been done in this regard. Cross-neutralization reactions have been reported between herpes simplex virus and B-virus of monkeys and between herpex simplex virus and canine herpesvirus. Infectious bovine rhinotracheitis and equine rhinopneumonitis viruses share a common antigen demonstrated by complement-fixation and agar-gel diffusion tests, but reciprocal neutralization was not observed. Pseudorabies, herpes simplex virus, and B virus share a common antigen as demonstrated by agar-gel test with no shared antigen from a neutralization standpoint. Pseudorabies virus, when compared with other herpesviruses (such as infectious laryngotracheitis, equine rhinopneumonitis, virus III of rabbits, herpes zoster, and varicella), yielded negative results.

The herpesviruses presently included in this family that cause disease (Table 44.1) are as follows: infectious bovine rhinotracheitis, pseudorabies, feline rhinotracheitis, a feline cytomegalovirus, equine rhinopneumonitis, two other equine herpesvirus groups, canine herpesvirus, malignant catarrhal virus of cattle, bovine ulcerative mammillitis, Marek's disease, infectious laryngotracheitis, atrophic rhinitis virus of pigs, African clawed frog (*Xenopus*) lymphosarcoma, cytomegalo-

Table 44.1. Diseases in domestic animals caused by viruses in the Herpesviridae family

Common name of virus	Natural hosts	Type of disease produced
Subfamily Alphaherpesvirinae		
Infectious bovine rhinotracheitis—infectious pustular vulvovaginitis virus	Cattle	*Respiratory tract form:* Fever, depression, upper and lower catarrhal respiratory signs. Average mortality is 10 percent *Reproductive tract form:* Fever, depression, inflammatory pustular lesions in vulva and vagina of cows and on prepuce and penis of bulls. Negligible mortality *Encephalitis form:* Usually in calves, with high mortality. Morbidity is usually low
Ulcerative mammillitis	Cattle	Ulcerative lesions appear on teats and udder. Slow healing with formation of scabs
Equine rhinopneumonitis (equine herpesvirus type 1)	Horses	Weanlings show fever, respiratory signs, and leukopenia. In mares abortions occur; occasionally develop paralysis
Equine coital exanthema (equine herpesvirus type 3)	Horses	Vesicular or pustular lesions occur in vulva or on penis
Pseudorabies	Cattle, sheep, goats, swine, dogs, cats, and rats	Acute disease in all animals except adult swine. Severe pruritis (except swine), paralysis, cardiac and respiratory distress, convulsions. Mortality high in most species
Canine herpesvirus	Dogs	May cause fatal hemorrhagic disease in infant puppies. Mild signs in older dogs
Feline rhinotracheitis	Cats	Serious disease in kittens. Fever and depression. Signs largely referable to respiratory tract and eye. Pregnant females may abort. Mortality may be appreciable in young cats
Avian infectious laryngotracheitis	Chickens	Acute, highly contagious respiratory disease. Severe respiratory distress results from caseous plugs in trachea that cause death. Mortality can be significant; morbidity is high
Pigeon herpesvirus	Pigeons	Clinical signs of coryza are observed with lesions most prominent in larynx or pharynx

viruses of man and rodents, duck plague, mouse thymic virus, pulmonary adenomatosis of sheep; avian herpesviruses affecting pigeons, owls, parrots, and cormorants; and renal carcinoma of the leopard frog, snake herpesvirus, Epstein-Barr virus associated with infectious mononucleosis and Burkitt's lymphoma of man, varicella, simian herpesviruses including B virus, virus III of rabbits, herpes zoster, and herpes simplex. The character of the diseases caused by this group varies from acute inflammatory conditions to the production of tumors (Table 44.1).

THE SUBFAMILY ALPHAHERPESVIRINAE

Infectious Bovine Rhinotracheitis and Infectious Pustular Vulvovaginitis

SYNONYMS: Infectious bovine necrotic rhinotracheitis, necrotic rhinitis, "red nose" disease, bovine coital exanthema; abbreviations, IBR and IPV

This virus causes disease in cattle, goats, and pigs. The respiratory form usually occurs in the colder months

Table 44.1.—*continued*

Common name of virus	Natural hosts	Type of disease produced
Duck plague	Ducks, geese (rarely)	Acute fatal disease involving the respiratory, enteric, and nervous systems of ducks
Subfamily Betaherpesvirinae		
Atrophic rhinitis	Pigs	The porcine herpesvirus causes lesions in the lamina propria, while *Bordetella bronchiseptica* caused atrophy of turbinate bones in this serious malady of pigs.
Feline urolithiasis (herpesvirus type 2)	Cats	Experimental disease—virus causes urolithiasis often resulting in uremia and death unless appropriate treatment is applied
Subfamily Gammaherpesvirinae		
Malignant head catarrh	Cattle, wildebeest, sheep	Natural disease only in cattle. Wildebeest (in Africa) and sheep have inapparent infection, but serve as carriers. African strains of virus readily produce disease; converse is true with U.S. isolates. It is a sporadic disease with a short febrile period, inflammation of mucous membranes of mouth, nose, and eyes, nervous signs, and a high death rate
Pulmonary adenomatosis	Sheep	In sheep 4 years of age or older chronic progressive disease of lungs that lose their elasticity due to proliferating cells causing consolidation. The tumor is carcinomatous and does metastasize
Marek's disease	Chickens, turkeys, pheasants, quail (principal avian hosts)	Acute fulminating type of oncogenic disease in young chicks that spreads rapidly with a high mortality as a rule. Virus causes various forms of tumors—neurolymphomatosis, ocular lymphomatosis, and visceral lymphomatosis. Arterial sclerosis

of the year. It was first recognized in beef cattle in feedlots of Colorado (29). It was then seen in California and other western states. The virus was recognized in the eastern part of the United States, but manifested itself first as infectious pustular vulvovaginitis (20). On occasions it produces meningoencephalitis in calves (17), keratoconjunctivitis (1), dermal infections, or abortions of pregnant cows (9, 31) as the major herd disease manifestation. The disease causes marked economic loss in some outbreaks.

All forms of the bovine disease now are recognized in the United States, Australia, many European countries, New Zealand, and Japan. It has a worldwide distribution. More than one form of the disease may be observed in a herd outbreak. In the United States the incidence of antibody in the bovine population in various states ranges from 10 to 35 percent. The disease has assumed greater importance in Europe and the USA in recent years.

In goats the virus reputedly causes respiratory disease (32) and has been isolated from two stillborn pig fetuses (16). Infections in various wildlife species have been recorded.

Gibbs and Riveyaniamu (18) have written excellent review articles on the bovine herpesviruses.

Character of the Disease. The respiratory form (IBR) may occur in a very mild, unrecognized infection, or it may be very severe. The acute disease involves the entire respiratory tract with lesser damage to the alimentary

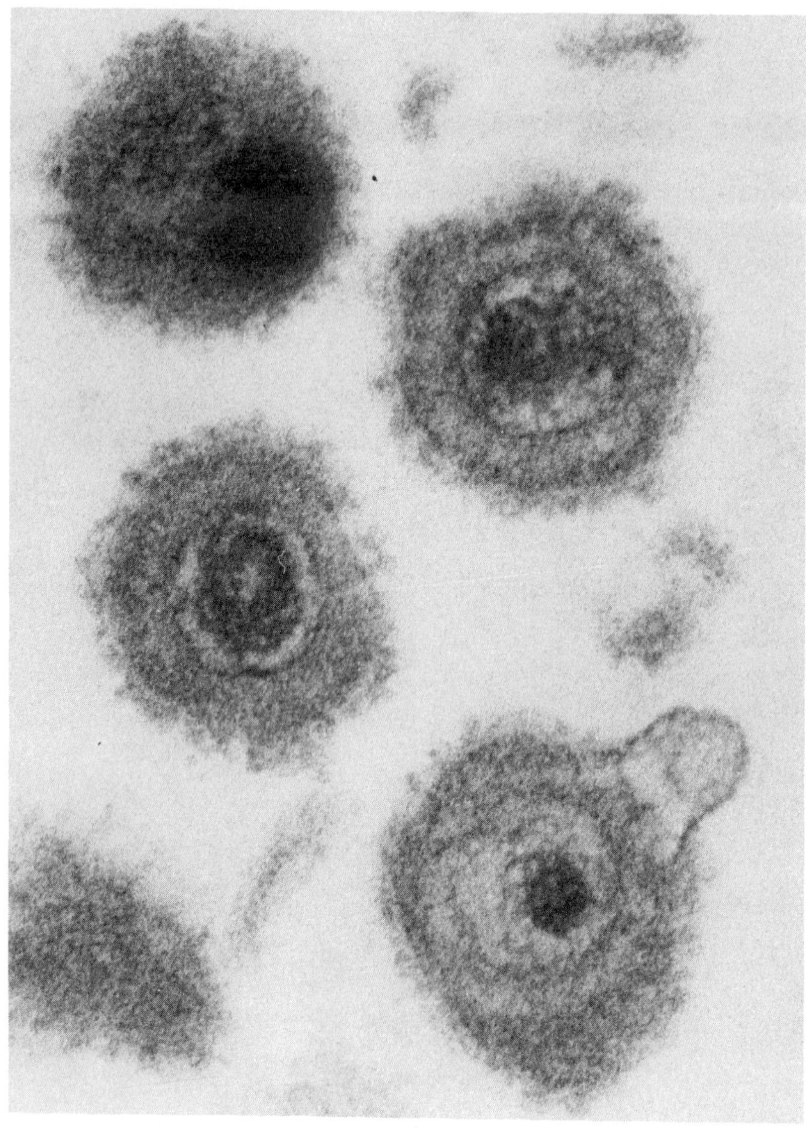

Figure 44.1. Herpes simplex virus particles thin section, lead citrate. × 234,000. (Courtesy B. Roizman and W. Volk. From Wesley Volk, *Essentials of Medical Microbiology,* Lippincott, Philadelphia, 1978.)

canal. It begins with high fever (104.5 to 107.5 F), great depression, inappetence, and the development of an abundant mucopurulent nasal discharge (Figure 44.2). The nasal mucous membranes become very congested, and shallow ulcers appear. Necrosis of the wings of the nostrils and of the muzzle occurs. The highly inflamed tissues gave rise to the name *red nose*. Manifestations of dyspnea and mouth breathing often appear as a result of closure of the nares by inflammatory exudate. Conjunctivitis and lacrimation may be seen, but necrosis of the lacrimal tissues does not occur. The breath usually becomes fetid because of the necrosis of the nasal mucosae. The respiratory rate usually is accelerated, and a deep bronchial cough is frequent. A blood-stained diarrhea is sometimes observed. Abortions may be associated with respiratory disease.

Infectious pustular vulvovaginitis (IPV) occurs in heifers, dairy cows, and bulls (14) (Figure 44.3). The degree of reaction varies greatly in an infected herd. Sometimes the disease spreads rapidly through a herd suggesting transmission by aerosol or by individuals handling the herd. The disease usually begins with a fever, and severely affected cows show considerable anxiety and pain with frequent urination. There is swelling of the vulva, and a sticky exudate may appear on the vulvar hair. The infection usually persists for 10 to 14 days in the herd. Bulls may have lesions on the penis and prepuce similar to those observed in the vulva of cows, and these may persist for 2 weeks or even longer if complications arise. When severe complications result, temporary or perhaps permanent impairment of a bull's ability to mate may result. In general there is disagree-

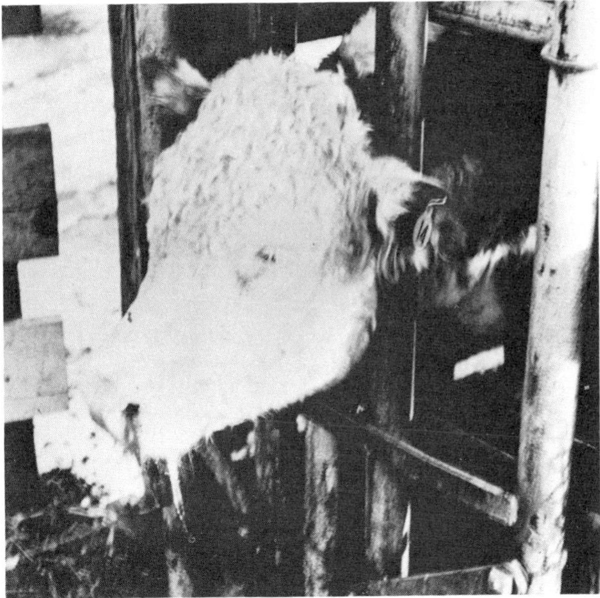

Figure 44.2. Respiratory form of IBR with characteristic hemorrhagic exudate from the nose.

ment on the extent to which infected bulls may be a significant factor in infertility. Certainly every effort should be made to keep a stud free of IBR.

In the naturally transmitted disease the incubation period is from 4 to 6 days. By inoculation intratracheally

Figure 44.3. The vulva of a heifer inoculated 48 hours previously with infectious pustular vulvovaginitis virus. The typical round pustules, some of which are in rows, are present on a reddened mucosa. Near the dorsal commissure the closely spaced pustules have coalesced to form a large, plaquelike lesion. (Courtesy Kendrick, Gillespie, and McEntee, *Cornell Vet.*)

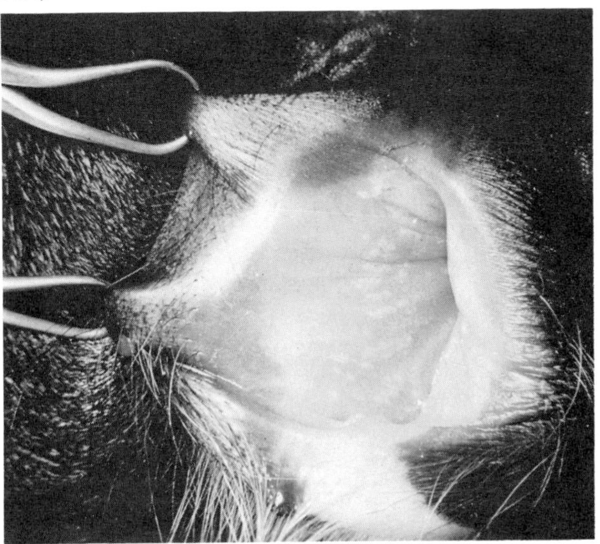

or by nasal or vulvovaginal instillation this period can be shortened to 18 to 72 hours (19). The course of the disease varies widely depending on the severity of the infection. In the milder forms it may hardly be noticed. In the respiratory or brain form some animals may die within a few hours after they are first noticed to be sick; most of them will run a course of a few days.

The mortality varies widely depending on the virulence of the virus, age of cattle, the form of the disease, management conditions, and the condition of the animals. In severe outbreaks in western feedlots 75 percent or more may show respiratory signs with an average mortality of 10 percent. In a susceptible group of calves mortality from the meningoencephalitis form reached 50 percent. Calves that showed nervous signs seldom survived.

The pathogenesis of the various forms of the disease is not fully understood. It is known that a viremia occurs with the dissemination of the virus throughout the body, yet systemic disease is seldom seen except for abortions in pregnant susceptible cows and death in neonates. The encephalitis is believed to gain access to the brain from the oropharynx by way of the cranial nerves. A persistent infection commonly occurs in cattle that can be activated experimentally by synthetic and natural steroids resulting in the release of virus in excretions (14, 38) and occasionally in recrudescence of disease (15).

The characteristic lesions are the highly inflamed mucous membranes of the respiratory tract, with shallow erosions, covered with a glary, fetid, mucopurulent exudate. These lesions may be found also in the pharynx, larynx, trachea, and larger bronchi. There may be a patchy, purulent pneumonia. Ulceration and inflammation of the abomasal mucosa is frequent, and there may be a catarrhal enteritis involving both small and large intestines. Abscesses may form in the lungs and liver of chronic cases.

Cheatham and Crandell (8) and Crandell, Cheatham, and Maurer (11) have described intranuclear inclusion bodies in IBR. They occur in cell cultures of bovine kidney cells and in the epithelial cells of the respiratory tract of infected cattle. It seems that these bodies appear quite early in the course of the disease and disappear before the disease is fully developed clinically.

In the vulva, circumscribed reddened areas become pustules that appear over the lymphatic follicles (27). Many pustules coalesce and a purulentlike exudate appears in the tract. Incomplete healing in some cows results in a condition known as granular vulvovaginitis.

Histologically, there is a predominance of neutrophils and necrosis with a diffuse infiltration of lymphocytes in the connective tissue. Intranuclear bodies appear in the epithelial cells (Figure 44.4).

The brain lesions in cases of meningoencephalitis are quite characteristic of the viral type described by French (17). Intranuclear viral inclusions occur in the astrocytes and neurons. Perivascular edema and cuffing are common in the cerebrum. There are diffuse areas of degeneration of the cerebral cortex with vacuolation around the neurons. The superficial cortical lamina of the cerebrum may show rarefaction necrosis. Aborted fetuses have some focal necrosis in the liver and spleen, and sometimes skin edema, but not consistent or severe enough to be pathognomonic (46). Despite the widespread necrosis that occurs in the tissues of most aborted fetuses, there is little inflammatory reaction. Intranuclear inclusions may be seen in affected cells (18).

In calves this disease may manifest itself as a meningoencephalitis (17). This should not be surprising because it is a herpesvirus and other herpesviruses produce encephalitis in the young.

It also is recognized that this versatile virus has an affinity for mucous membranes and causes keratoconjunctivitis, usually without ulceration of the cornea (1); under certain circumstances field virus or attenuated virus vaccine (31) produce abortions, usually in first-calf heifers in any stage of gestation. Abortions occur sometimes with no signs of illness in the dam.

Baker, McEntee, and Gillespie produced a rather interesting form of the disease in experimental calves only a few days old by feeding, by intravenous injection, and by placing them in contact with infected calves (4) (Figure 44.5). The characteristic pustular lesions, intranuclear inclusion bodies, and necrosis were found in the oral cavity, esophagus, and forestomachs. Necrotic foci were observed in the liver, lungs, and kidneys. Calves that survived the acute infection developed a chronic cough with ensuing pneumonia, but virus could no longer be isolated at this stage. In 1964 Van Kruinigen and Bartholomew (45) isolated IBR virus from a natural case in a calf that was associated with older animals suffering from the respiratory form of the disease. On postmortem examination the calf showed focal necrosis of the liver, necrosis of the suprapharyngeal lymph node, and necrosis of the rumen mucosa.

The Disease in Experimental Animals. Cattle are susceptible to IBR virus. Young goats have been infected experimentally and develop a febrile reaction (30). Rabbits inoculated intradermally or intratesticularly developed local lesions (2), but serial passage of virus was

Figure 44.4. Inclusion bodies in the vulvar epithelium 48 hours after inoculation with infectious pustular vulvovaginitis virus. Two of the inclusion-bearing cells contain double nuclei. Schleifstein's Negri body stain. × 900. (Courtesy Kendrick, Gillespie, and McEntee, *Cornell Vet.*)

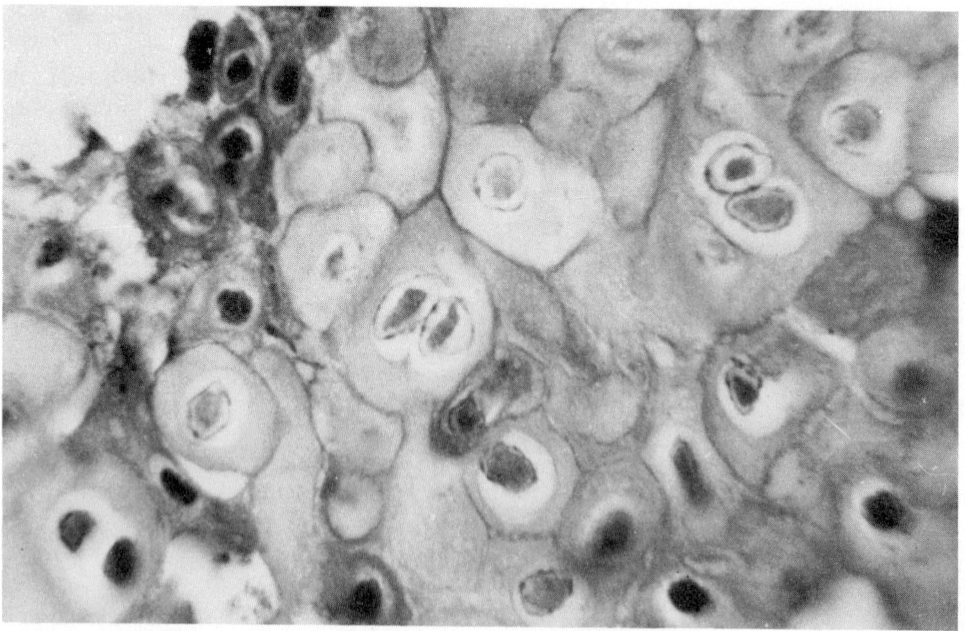

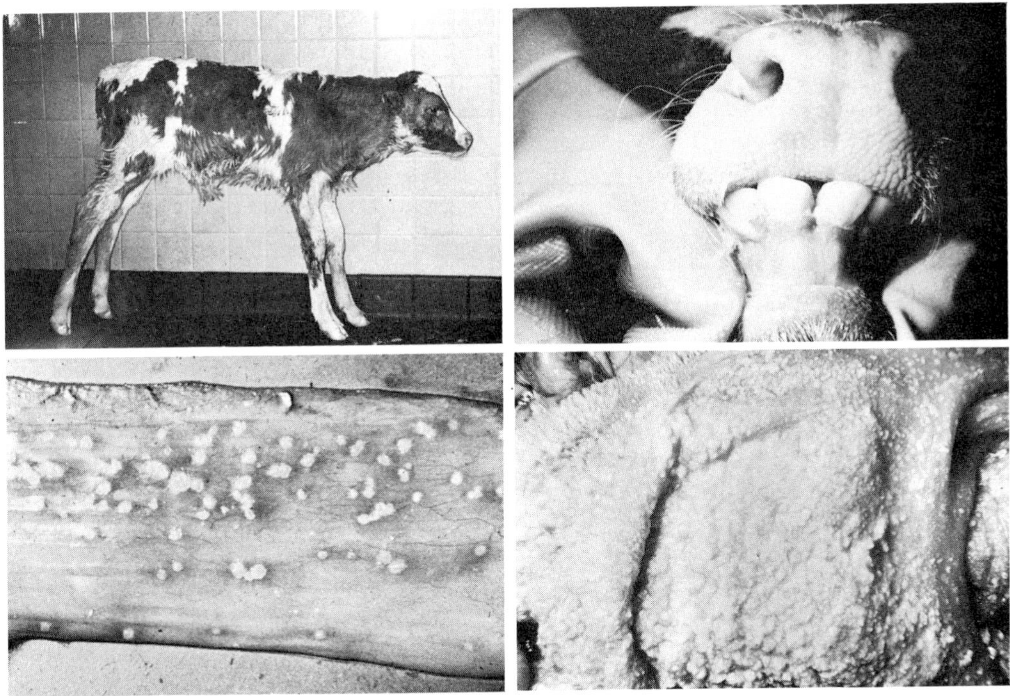

Figure 44.5. IBR-IPV acute disease in infant calves. Calf in typical posture with excessive salivation (*upper left*). Pustular lesions on gum by margin of teeth (*upper right*). Necrotic foci, distal portion of esophagus (*lower left*). Diffuse necrosis in the rumen (*lower right*). (Courtesy J. Baker, K. McEntee, and J. Gillespie, *Cornell Vet.*)

unsuccessful. Newborn rabbits given the LA strain of IBR developed a severe, sometimes fatal, generalized infection with focal and diffuse necrosis of the liver and adrenal glands (26).

Properties of the Virus. Tousimis *et al.* (44), who studied the virus by electron microscopy, determined that the IBR particles produced in bovine kidney cell cultures had a diameter of 145 to 156 nm. In tissue fluids the diameter was determined to be 136± 10 nm. Griffin *et al.* (22) found this virus to be unusually stable when suspended in culture mediums at pH 7.0. The original titer was maintained for 30 days at 4 C. Only one log of infectivity was lost after 5 days at 22 C. Equal parts of virus suspension and either alcohol, acetone, or chloroform caused prompt inactivation. After exposure of some field isolates to 20 percent ethyl ether for 16 hours at 4 C, the majority of isolates were resistant (12). Calcium alginate wool swabs inactivate IBR virus whereas cotton and polyester swabs had little virucidal effect (23). The density of IBRV in the potassium tartrate gradient is 1.22 g per cm^3.

Armstrong *et al.* (2) suggest that this is a DNA virus. Ribonucleotides may be covalently linked to the viral DNA. The mature virion contains 18 structural proteins with molecular weights varying from 29,000 to 250,000 daltons; 8 of them are glycosylated (41). The various strains of IBR virus are antigenically homogeneous, although slight differences between strains have been demonstrated by neutralization tests in tissue culture (47). Carmichael and Barnes showed some relationship to equine rhinopneumonitis by use of the complement-fixation and gel-diffusion tests (7). IBR, Marek's and Burkitt's lymphoma viruses share a common antigen by agar gel diffusion and indirect fluorescent antibody tests. IBR and caprine herpesvirus 1 also possess a common antigen (5).

Cultivation. The IBR virus was first isolated by Madin, York, and McKercher (29) in 1956. In 1957 several groups of workers (21, 42) reported successful cultivation of the virus in bovine embryo tissue culture cells and in bovine kidney cells. The agent of IBR always exhibits strong cytopathogenic effect for practically all cells in which it is cultivated with an apparent cytopathology in 24 to 48 hours. It also grows and produces a cytopathogenic effect in pig, dog, sheep, goat, horse, and WI 38 human diploid kidney cells. Intranuclear inclusion bodies are produced in these cells and can be demonstrated by fixation with Bouin's solution and H and E stains. Plaques may be produced in bovine kidney monolayers and in many other cell cultures (46).

It is possible to establish persistent infection in hamster embryo cell cultures by inoculation of infective viral particles at approximately one-half the number of cells in culture. The persistence of virus is characterized by a minimal degree of cytopathic effect with a low level of released virus (33). Hamster embryo cells showed malignant transformation following IBRV inoculation.

IBR virus grows to high titer, produces intranuclear inclusion bodies, and prevents ciliary activity in nasal and tracheal organ cultures (40).

Cells derived from bovine embryo tissues after freezing provide excellent cultures for the titration of IBR virus.

Immunity. The immune response of cattle to IBRV can be attributed to antibody and cell-mediated components (18). Cattle that recover from natural disease are resistant to challenge by any strain of IBRV regardless of the tissue from which it is isolated. The duration of immunity is long term.

Cattle immunized with attenuated virus are immune to challenge 3 to 4 weeks later with virulent virus by intranasal or intravaginal instillation. It has been observed that a few transient lesions are produced after intravaginal instillation of a massive dose of virulent virus, but no febrile state results (27). The presence of neutralizing antibody has been correlated with protection against clinical signs of illness. An animal with measurable neutralizing antibody against 100 tissue-cultured infective doses ($TCID_{50}$) is immune. Titers occasionally reach 1:256, with the average falling into the range of 1:8 to 1:64. Higher titers can be achieved by adding complement (35). The constant serum-varying virus neutralization test (24) procedure and the passive hemagglutination test (28) reputedly are more sensitive in the detection of antibody. Other procedures used for this purpose are the complement-fixation, gel diffusion and direct and indirect fluorescent antibody tests. Neutralizing antibody can be detected on or about 8 days after infection and without production of apparent disease. The persistence of virus in all likelihood accounts for persisting antibody in most animals, but reexposure to virus resulting in reinfection without disease manifestations cannot be entirely dismissed.

Maternal neutralizing antibodies are readily detected in serum of calves from immune dams. The serum titers are low and sometimes persist until the calf is 4 months old. Maternal antibody interference can interfere with production of an active immunity and must be considered in a herd vaccination program.

In the past the role of antibody in the protection against herpesviruses was questioned because these viruses spread from cell to cell by intracellular bridges (10). It has been shown *in vitro* that it plays an important role in limiting spread by mechanisms of antibody complement lysis and antibody-dependent cellular cytotoxicity. The role of secretory antibody has not been defined in protection of the superficial epithelial tissues involved in some forms of the disease.

To show the role of cell-mediated immunity Rouse and Babiuk (36) developed a viral plaque inhibition assay test which showed that blood lymphocytes from immune animals were able to prevent viral plaque formation in cell monolayers infected with IBRV. The reaction is specific and involves suppression of viral replication rather than the destruction of virus or virus-infected cells. A lymphokine produced by cooperation of macrophages and T-cell lymphocytes from immune animals is involved in the process. This phenomenon has been described as "immune interferon," not to be confused with interferon, which differs in its mode of origin but also in its biochemical and biophysical characteristics.

Interferon production to IBRV has been demonstrated in cattle (34). Interferon produced by an interferon inducer administered 3 hours before infection reduced the severity of the clinical disease in calves when compared with untreated animals (43).

A modified IBR virus has served as a very effective vaccine for this disease (39). It was produced by rapid serial passage in bovine embryo kidney cell tissue culture. In this way the virulence of the virus is almost completely lost for cattle; yet it serves as an effective antigen that will protect against natural exposure and experimental inoculation. The virus probably does not spread from vaccinated to unvaccinated contact cattle. The duration of the immunity is not known; however, vaccine effectively protects cattle for more than the feedlot season, which is all that is required. It should be given, of course, before or at the time the animals are brought in from the range and to nonpregnant animals. Tissue-cultured vaccines produced in other cell cultures are now available. Some vaccines are administered as an aerosal, but there is no evidence the immunity conferred is superior to immunization by the parenteral route. There is rightful concern that vaccine virus may remain latent; a satisfactory inactivated virus vaccine needs to be developed (25).

For complete discussion of the biologics for IBR and their recommended use in a herd health program the reader is referred to the Panel Report, American Veterinary Medical Association Symposium on Immunity to the Bovine Respiratory Disease Complex (21).

Transmission. The disease is readily transmitted by infected cattle. Evidence is now available that certain individuals remain carriers of the virus weeks after acute infection (42). All forms of the disease are transmitted by contact, especially under crowded conditions, and the venereal form can also be transmitted by coitus. The virus has been isolated from semen.

Stress may cause cattle vaccinated with attenuated vaccines to IBR to excrete virus (39), but it has not been established whether the excreted virus regains virulence for cattle. Vaccinated and recovered cattle may contribute to perpetuation of the disease.

Diagnosis. Quite frequently diagnosis can be rendered on the basis of the history and character of the disease. To confirm the field diagnosis, isolation of the virus may be indicated.

For viral isolation the specimens should be collected from body systems displaying the signs and pathological lesions. Virus is most readily isolated in specimens taken during the febrile stage of the infection. In cases of abortion, virus has been isolated from the thoracic cavity fluid of the fetus and from cotyledons but not with high frequency.

IBR virus is readily isolated on bovine kidney cells in tissue culture. It may also be recovered on swine tissue-cultured kidney cells (6, 37) or other cells. The virus may be identified tentatively by its rapid and characteristic cytolytic effects, and also by neutralization and fluorescent antibody tests using tissue culture cells as indicators. Other serological tests used to detect antibody were mentioned earlier under immunity.

Cutaneous reactions to IBRV occur in cattle (13). The accuracy and usefulness of this skin test as a simple diagnostic test under field conditions has not been evaluated.

Control. Vaccination of young cattle before they are put into feedlot in the fall will obviate losses from this disease.

The Disease in Man. The IBR virus is not pathogenic for man.

REFERENCES

1. Abinanti and Plumer. Am. Jour. Vet. Res., 1961, *22,* 13.
2. Armstrong, Pereira, and Andrewes. Virol., 1961, *14,* 264.
3. Babiuk and Rouse. Jour. Gen. Virol., 1976, *31,* 221.
4. Baker, McEntee, and Gillespie. Cornell Vet., 1960, *50,* 156.
5. Berrios and McKercher. Am. Jour. Vet. Res., 1975, *36,* 1755.
6. Cabasso, Brown, and Cox. Proc. Soc. Exp. Biol. and Med., 1957, *95,* 471.
7. Carmichael and Barnes. Proc. U.S. Livestock Sanit. Assoc., 1961, *65,* 384.
8. Cheatham and Crandell. Proc. Soc. Exp. Biol. and Med., 1957, *96,* 536.
9. Chow, Molello, and Owen. Jour. Am. Vet. Med. Assoc., 1964, *144,* 1005.
10. Christian and Ludovici. Proc. Soc. Exp. Biol. and Med., 1971, *138,* 1109.
11. Crandell, Cheatham, and Maurer. Am. Jour. Vet. Res., 1959, *20,* 505.
12. Crandell, Melloh, and Sorlie. Jour. Clin. Microbiol., 1975, *2,* 465.
13. Darcel and Dorwood. Can. Vet. Jour., 1975, *16,* 87.
14. Davies and Carmichael. Inf. and Immun., 1973, *8,* 510.
15. Davies and Duncan. Cornell Vet., 1974, *64,* 340.
16. Derbyshire and Caplan. Can. Jour. Comp. Med., 1976, *40,* 252.
17. French. Austral. Vet. Sci., 1962, *38,* 555.
18. Gibbs and Rweyemamu. Vet. Bull., 1977, *47,* 317.
19. Gillespie, Lee, and Baker. Am. Jour. Vet. Res., 1957, *18,* 530.
20. Gillespie, McEntee, Kendrick, and Wagner. Cornell Vet., 1959, *49,* 288.
21. Gillespie, McKercher, Jensen, Peacock, Bristol, Casselberry, Collier, Fox, Hejl, Mackey, Oberst, Pope, Jones, and Freeman. Jour. Am. Vet. Med. Assoc., 1968, *152,* 713.
22. Griffin, Howells, Crandell, and Maurer. Am. Jour. Vet. Res., 1958, *19,* 990.
23. Hanson and Schipper. Am. Jour. Vet. Res., 1976, *37,* 707.
24. House and Baker. Cornell Vet., 1971, *61,* 320.
25. Kahrs. Jour. Am. Vet. Med. Assoc., 1977, *171,* 1055.
26. Kelly. Brit. Jour. Exp. Path., 1977, *58,* 168.
27. Kendrick, Gillespie, and McEntee. Cornell Vet., 1958, *48,* 458.
28. Kirby, Martin, and Ostler. Vet. Rec., 1974, *94,* 361.
29. Madin, York, and McKercher. Science, 1956, *124,* 721.
30. McKercher. Adv. Vet. Sci., 1959, *5,* 299.
31. McKercher and Wada. Jour. Am. Vet. Med. Assoc., 1964, *144,* 136.
32. Mohanty, Lillie, Corselius, and Beck. Jour. Am. Vet. Med. Assoc., 1972, *160,* 879.
33. Michalski and Hsiung. In Vitro, 1976, *12,* 682.
34. Rosenquist and Loan. Am. Jour. Vet. Res., 1969, *30,* 1305.
35. Rossi and Kiesel. Arch. f. die. gesam. Virusforsch., 1974, *45,* 328.
36. Rouse and Babiuk. Cell. Immun., 1975, *17,* 43.
37. Schwarz, York, Zirbell, and Estela. Proc. Soc. Exp. Biol. and Med., 1957, *96,* 453.
38. Sheffy and Davies. Proc. Soc. Exp. Biol. and Med., 1972, *140,* 974.
39. Sheffy and Rodman. Jour. Am. Vet. Med. Assoc., 1973, *163,* 850.
40. Shroyer and Easterday. Am. Jour. Vet. Res., 1968, *29,* 1355.
41. Sklyanskaya, Itkin, Gofman, and Kaverin. Acta Virol. (Praha), 1977, *21,* 273.

42. Studdert, Wada, Kortum, and Groverman. Jour. Am. Vet. Med. Assoc., 1964, *44,* 615.
43. Theil, Mohanty, and Hetrick. Am. Jour. Vet. Res., 1971, *32,* 1955.
44. Tousimis, Howells, Griffin, Porter, Cheatham, and Maurer. Proc. Soc. Exp. Biol. and Med., 1958, *99,* 614.
45. Van Kruninigen and Bartholomew. Jour. Am. Vet. Med. Assoc., 1964, *44,* 1008.
46. York, Jour. Am. Vet. Med. Assoc., 1968, *152,* 758.
47. York, Schwartz, and Estela. Proc. Soc. Exp. Biol. and Med., 1957, *94,* 740.

Bovine Ulcerative Mammillitis and Allerton Virus

Allerton virus was first isolated in 1957 from lumpy skin disease in the Republic of South Africa by Alexander *et al.* (1). It now is known that the Allerton virus does not cause lumpy skin disease because a poxvirus has been incriminated in the production of that disease.

In 1960 in Ruanda-Urundi Huygelen (7) isolated, from cattle with extensive erosion of the teats, a virus similar to Allerton virus. In 1966 Martin *et al.* (10) reported that bovine ulcerative mammillitis is caused by a herpesvirus which they called bovine mammillitis virus (BMV), also known now as bovine herpesvirus 2. This disease exists in England (14), the United States (16), and Scotland (10), and more recently in eastern and southern Africa, and also in Australia. The Allerton virus and the BMV are indistinguishable antigenically and in physical properties. Neutralizing antibody has been demonstrated in buffalo, giraffes, and other wild animals located in eastern Africa (11). Excellent review articles have been written by Gibbs and Rweyemamu in 1977 (6) and by Cilli and Castrucci (5).

Character of the Disease. *Bovine ulcerative mammillitis.* This condition assumes two forms in a milking herd. In primary herd infections the morbidity rate is high, affecting all ages of milking cows, and there is no mortality. In previously exposed herds the disease is limited principally to first-calf heifers.

The incubation period is 3 to 7 days. Ulcerative lesions appear on the teats and less frequently on the udders of affected milking cows. The infection usually causes gross swelling of the teat wall. Within 48 hours the skin over the affected areas becomes soft and sloughed, revealing an irregularly shaped, painful,deeply ulcerated area that heals slowly with formation of brown scabs within 5 or 6 days after skin lesions are observed (Figure 44.6). The scabs start shedding by day 14. Lymphadenitis occurs. Mastitis follows in approximately 22 percent of the cases.

Histologic changes (9) in the epidermis on the first day of the clinical reaction were severe inflammation accompanied by syncytia and inclusion bodies (Figure 44.7). Inflammatory changes rapidly become more intense in the next few days, with great numbers of polymorphonuclear and other leukocytes appearing in the epidermis and dermis. Syncytial masses containing many

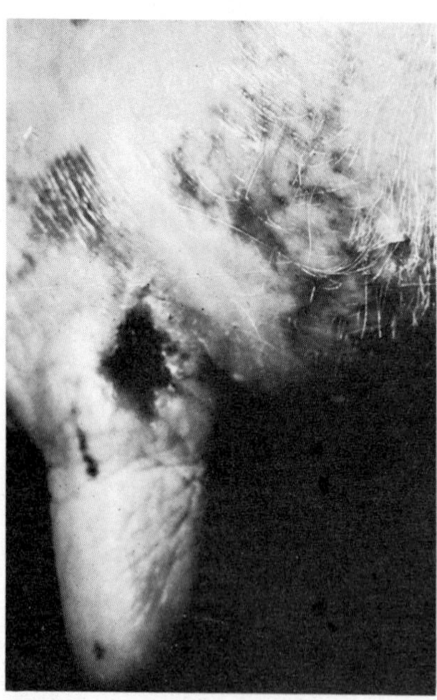
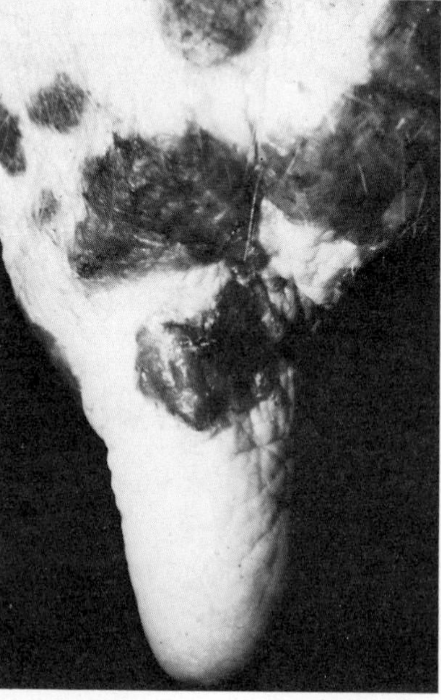

Figure 44.6. Early lesions caused by bovine mammillitis virus (*left*) and later scabby lesions of same teat (*right*). (Courtesy W. B. Martin.)

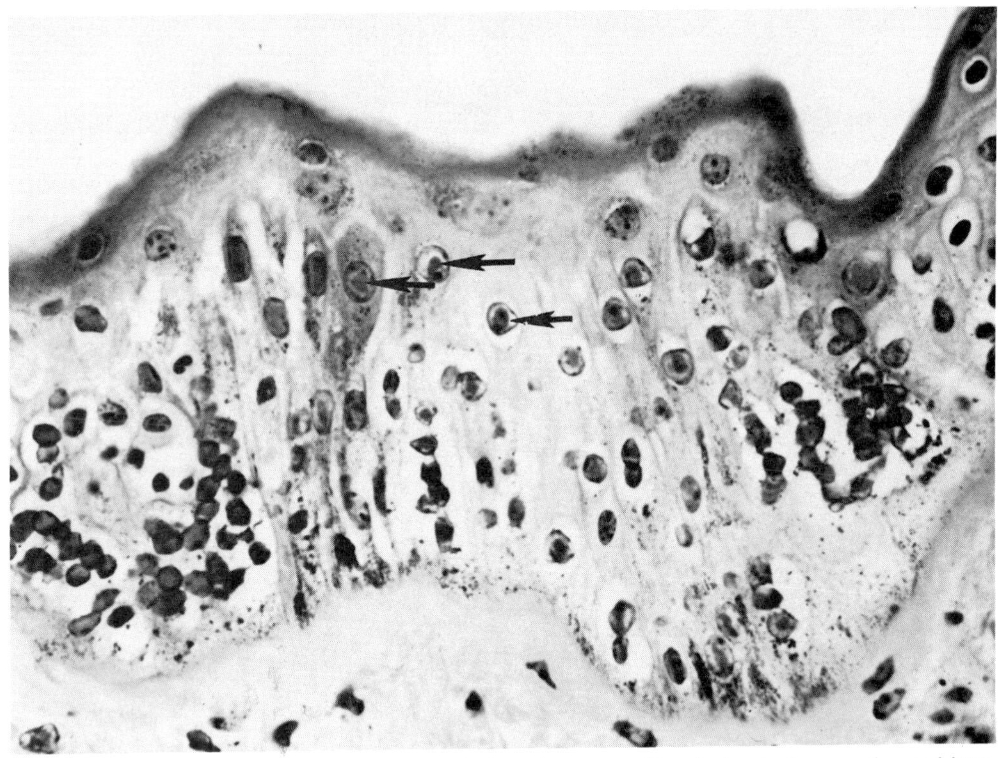

Figure 44.7. Bovine mammillitis. Epidermal lesions from cow. Note hydropic degeneration and intranuclear inclusion bodies (*arrows*). H and E stain. × 660. (Courtesy W. B. Martin.)

nuclei occurred in the lesions during the first few days as well as intranuclear inclusion bodies, which varied somewhat in appearance depending on the age of the lesion.

More mast cells appeared in the dermis during the reaction. Viral particles were found in sections examined with the electron microscope, and particles occurred within the nucleus with single limiting membranes either packed in crystalline array (Figure 44.8) or dispersed irregularly. Particles in the cytoplasm usually had two limiting membranes, with the second one acquired at the nuclear membrane. (Figure 44.9) Teat skin is not particularly susceptible to infection, but skin damage does permit viral entry.

Allerton virus infection. When this virus strain is inoculated into cattle, fever and eruption of skin nodules all over the body ensue. The nodules become necrotic. Lymphadenitis is another feature of the disease.

The Disease in Experimental Animals. One strain of Allerton virus produces skin nodules when inoculated into suckling mice and causes transient lesions when given intradermally to rabbits. It will also infect sheep and probably goats (2).

Day-old rats, mice, and Chinese hamsters are susceptible to BMV infection, characterized by stunting, with or without skin lesions, and high mortality, but older animals are not (14). In rabbits and guinea pigs, which are of lower susceptibility, no difference in age susceptibility was observed.

Properties of the Virus. The Allerton and BM viruses are members of the herpes group. They have all the biochemical and biophysical features of herpesviruses. Iodophors at concentrations used in dairy disinfectants inactivate the virus, but hypochlorite solutions are less effective.

Close antigenic relationships exist between strains of bovine herpesvirus 2 despite some variation in temperature lability (4) in a buffalo strain (3). Early work showed no relationship between this virus and other members of the herpes family including herpes simplex. Recently it was shown by neutralization, complement fixation, immunofluorescence, immunodiffusion, and mouse protection tests that herpes simplex and bovine herpesvirus 2 share at least one common antigen, most likely located in the envelope (15).

Cultivation. The virus replicates in a wide variety of cell cultures, although primary cultures of bovine kidney-tissue develop large sycytia which appear 8 hours after inoculation or as late as 8 days. Soon after formation, cell destruction is complete. Numerous large inclu-

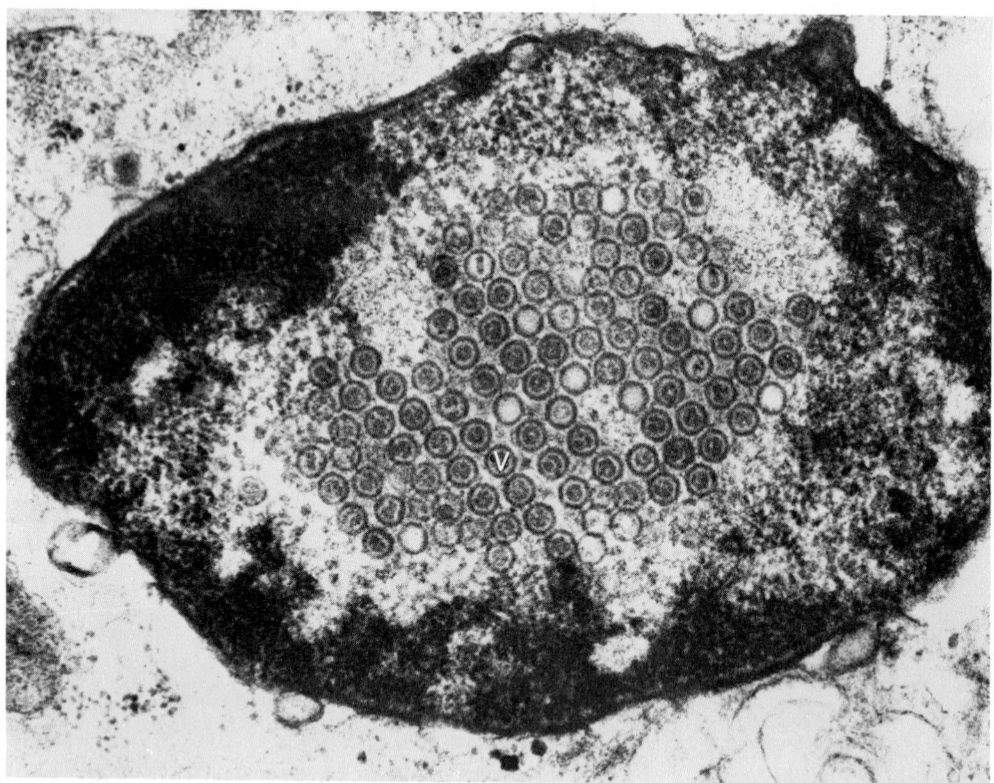

Figure 44.8. Bovine mammillitis. Paracrystalline arrangement of virus particles (*V*) in the nucleus. × 41,800. (Courtesy W. B. Martin.)

sions of Cowdry type A are present in the nuclei. Growth also occurs in baby hamster kidney cells, and Allerton virus is known to multiply also in lamb testes. The BHM-TVA strain produces uniform plaques in bovine cell cultures under carboxymethyl cellulose overlay.

BHV 2 grows to high titer in organ cultures of bovine teat skin; infected explants may excrete virus for up to 165 days (8). Virus also may persist in monolayer cultures.

Immunity. Neutralizing antibodies are found in the sera of recovered cattle. Complete protection results after experience with natural or experimental BMV disease. The duration of protection is unknown, but it persists for at least 8 months (12). This was based on challenge results. Maximal neutralizing antibody titers are achieved 3 weeks after inoculation, but titers did not persist (9). In contrast, following recovery from natural disease, antibody titers persisted for at least 2 years (13). The question of latency has not been resolved, but it seems likely that viral persistence occurs.

Transmission. Transmission of BMV occurs mechanically by means of milkers or by biting flies (10, 14). Insects, such as *Musca fasciata,* may transmit Allerton virus (2).

Diagnosis. In bovine ulcerative mammillitis the lesions are infective from the 1st to the 10th day. High infectivity titers of lesions and of exuding fluid were present during the first 4 days. With this material, virus readily produces a cytopathic effect in cell cultures (discussed in the section on cultivation). By the use of paired sera a rising neutralizing antibody titer can be demonstrated using a cell-culture system.

Paravaccinia, a common cause of teat lesions, can be differentiated from BMV by use of biopsy material before scabbing occurs (14). Paravaccinia causes epithelial hyperplasia, intracellular edema of cells of the stratum spinosum, and cytoplasmic inclusions in the vesicular epithelial cells—this is in marked contrast to lesions described for BMV.

Control. In a study of various experimental vaccine preparations with BMV the most practical virus vaccine was found to be an unaltered virus strain (TV) administered intramuscularly (12). This vaccine was safe in pregnant animals, and there was no evidence of excretion to susceptible contact animals. Protection lasted for at least 8 months. The use of an unattenuated vaccine must be viewed with reservations and only used in infected herds with the recognition that the disease may be

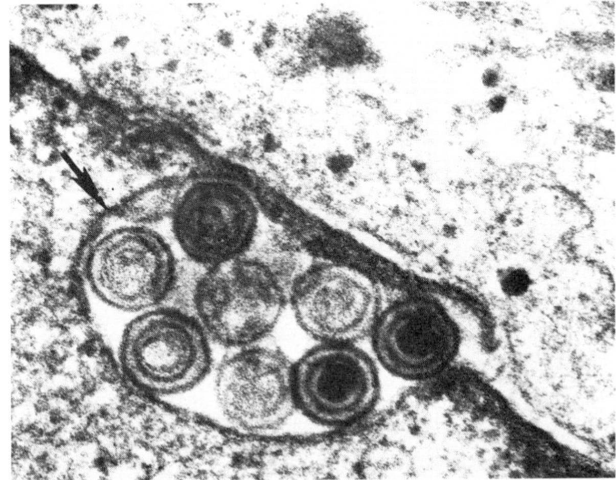

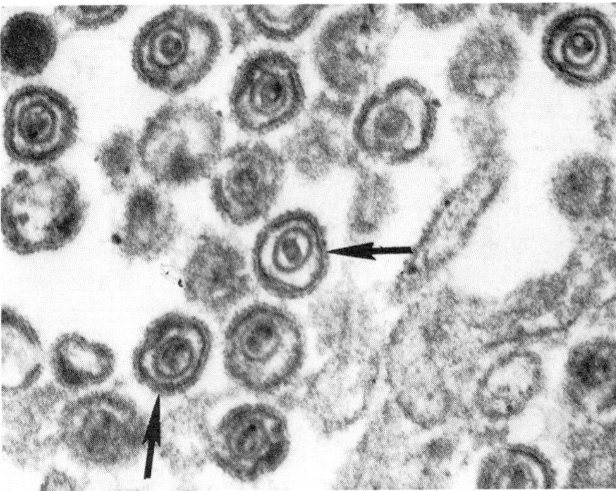

Figure 44.9. Bovine mammillitis. Several enveloped viral particles within a vacuole formed by the nuclear membrane about to leave nucleus (*upper*). Extracellular viral particles (*lower*). × 60,500. (Courtesy W. B. Martin.)

perpetuating on the premises. Certainly a great deal of field study must be done to prove otherwise. Although viral carriers have not been demonstrated with either type of disease, latency is one of the prime characteristics of herpesviruses, so it is reasonable to assume that the carrier status may eventually be demonstrated.

The Disease in Man. There is no evidence that Allerton virus or BMV causes disease in man.

REFERENCES

1. Alexander, Plowright, and Haig. Bull. Epizoot. Dis. Africa, 1957, *5,* 489.
2. Andrewes, Christopher, and H. G. Pereira. Viruses of vertebrates, 2nd ed. Baillière, Tindall, and Cassel, London, 1967.
3. Castrucci, Martin, Pedini, Cilli, and Ranucci. Res. Vet. Sci., 1975, *18,* 208.
4. Castrucci, Pedini, Cilli, and Arancia. Vet. Rec., 1972, *90,* 325.
5. Cilli and Castrucci. Folia Vet. Latina, 1976, *6,* 1.
6. Gibbs and Rweyemamu. Vet. Bull., 1977, *47,* 411.
7. Huygelen. Zentrbl. Vet.-Med., 1960, *7,* 664.
8. James and Povey. Res. Vet. Sci., 1973, *15,* 40.
9. Martin, James. Lauder, Murray, and Pirie. Am. Jour. Vet. Res., 1969, *30,* 2151.
10. Martin, Martin, Hay, and Lauder. Vet. Rec., 1966, *78,* 494.
11. Plowright and Jessett. Jour. Hyg. (London), 1971, *69,* 209.
12. Rweyemamu and Johnson. Res. Vet. Sci., 1969, *10,* 419.
13. Rweyemamu, Johnson, and Laurillard. Brit. Vet. Jour., 1969, *125,* 317.
14. Rweyemamu, Johnson, and McCrea. Brit. Vet. Jour., 1968, *124,* 317.
15. Sterz, Ludwig, and Rott. Intervirol., 1974, *2,* 1.
16. Weaver, Dellers, and Dardiri. Jour. Am. Vet. Med. Assoc., 1972, 160, 1643.

Equine Herpesviruses

At present three separate equine herpesvirus serotypes are recognized. Equine herpesvirus 1 is primarily a respiratory tract pathogen, but it may also cause abortions and nervous manifestations in pregnant mares. Equine herpesvirus 2 often is isolated from the respiratory tract and other sites from normal horses and from others displaying a variety of disease conditions. One group (3) provided some evidence that it may cause pharyngitis in young foals. Because its role in the cause of disease generally is undetermined, it will be given little consideration except where it may be involved with the other equine herpesvirus serotypes. Equine herpesvirus 3 causes coital exanthema in the horse. Diseases caused by equine herpesviruses 1 and 3 are described below.

Equine Rhinopneumonitis

SYNONYMS: Equine virus abortion, equine herpesvirus 1

Dimock and Edwards (13) reported a form of epizootic abortion in mares in Kentucky which was shown to be due to a virus. Their observations were confirmed by Miessner and Harms (36) in Germany, by Hupbauer (29) in Yugoslavia, and by Sedlmeier (41) in Austria. Manninger and Csonotos (34) first called attention to similarities between the viruses of equine influenza and equine virus abortion. Doll and Kintner (19) in the United States made a comparative study of several strains of equine abortion virus with two strains of virus that had been isolated from horses suffering from respiratory infection and that had been regarded as influenza. These strains proved to be identical. Doll, Bryans, McCollum, and Crowe (18) encountered a severe outbreak of abortions in a large group of mares on a brood farm in Ohio, from which a viral agent different from that which had previously been regarded as the influenza virus was isolated. Doll, McCollum, Bryans, and Crowe (20) carried out serological comparisons of it with the viruses of equine, human and swine influenza, among others, and found no relationships. Because equine abortion virus, is essentially a respiratory tract inhabitant and causes abortions secondarily, Doll *et al.* (18) proposed that it be called *equine rhinopneumonitis*. Nervous manifestations occasionally appeared in pregnant mares. The virus also is known as equine herpesvirus 1 (EHV-1).

Natural disease occurs only in horses. It has been described in many areas of the United States and in many European countries and is viewed as an important disease in horses.

Character of the Disease. The disease appears in two different forms—the first in weanlings, the second in pregnant mares.

The weanling disease is manifested by a mild febrile reaction accompanied by a rhinitis or nasal catarrh which appears in the fall months. The disease is so mild as to cause little concern; however, Doll *et al.* (18) showed that it is accompanied by the development of antibodies for the virus of equine rhinopneumonitis. Whereas in September of each year, before the rhinitis appeared, all foals were free of antibodies for this virus, in each successive month while the disease was under way the number of positive animals increased until 80 to 100 percent were positive by December. Doll and associates (18) also showed the etiological connection between this virus and the disease by inoculating sucklings and weanlings with strains of virus obtained from aborting mares. The animals that were inoculated both intravenously and intranasally with virus in fetal tissue responded with a febrile reaction, a mild leukopenia, a mild mucopurulent nasal discharge, and the development of specific antibodies. There was no cough or development of pulmonary or conjunctival involvement. The febrile response appears within 2 to 3 days, generally is diphasic in character, and persists for 8 to 10 days. The mortality in sucklings and weanlings is negligible. The disease originally described in mares consisted of abortions and occasionally nervous signs (15). After the virus was expelled, the genital tract returned to normal rather quickly. Lesions could be found only in the fetus. Abortions occurred in mares with few or no premonitory signs from the 6th month through the remaining period of gestation. Those foals infected very late in pregnancy and born alive generally died within 36 hours. It is believed that abortions in natural outbreaks occur 3 to 4 weeks after a mare is infected. In the abortion disease, mortality in the mares is low, but the loss of foals through abortions may be high. The disease strikes from 10 to 90 percent of the pregnant mares living on the same premises. When the infection appears late in the foaling season after many of the mares have foaled, the incidence of abortion will naturally be much less than when it comes earlier. Some investigators reported numerous cases of meningoencephalitis often were preceded by respiratory signs in pregnant mares residing in Europe and in the United States (12, 16, 31).

In aborting mares without nervous signs, no lesions have been recognized in the dam, but there are characteristic lesions in the fetuses. The most constant of these are multiple focal areas of necrosis in the liver. Many fetuses also exhibit petechial hemorrhages in the heart muscle and in the capsules of the spleen and liver. Edema of the lungs with excessive fluid in the chest cavity is also characteristic. Considered diagnostic of this disease are the inclusion bodies, which in most cases are readily found in the liver and various other organs.

The Disease in Experimental Animals. In mares with nervous manifestations in natural and experimental cases the disease is characterized by horses with ataxia or paresis for up to several weeks. Little and Thorsen (33) mention 12 natural cases with a disseminating necrotizing myeloencephalitis. Necrotic arteriolitis, nonsuppurative necrotizing myeloencephalitis. Necrotic arteriolitis, nonsuppurative necrotizing myeloencephalitis and Gasserian ganglioneuritis were present in a paraparetic horse. In experimental trials with equine herpesvirus 1, a neurologic syndrome was produced in all mares between 3 and 9 months of gestation 6 to 8 days after inoculation (30). Vascular changes and concomitant degeneration were present in the central nervous system of mares with neurological disease.

Doll (17) developed a technique of inoculating the fetuses *in utero* directly through the abdominal wall; this produced abortions in 100 percent of all cases, irrespective of whether the mare was immune to the virus.

The studies of Dimock, Edwards, and Bruner (14), Bruner, Doll, and Hull (4), and Kress (32) indicate that the virus will cause pregnant guinea pigs to abort. When virus material was injected into the fetuses of pregnant guinea pigs on the 35th day of gestation, the fetuses were aborted 7 to 9 days later. The injection of virus-free material into the fetuses of control animals did not cause abortions, and at birth the baby guinea pigs appeared entirely normal (4).

Doll, Richards, and Wallace (21) succeeded in adapting this virus to suckling hamsters, after Anderson and Goodpasture (2) had pointed the way by reporting the finding of intranuclear inclusions resembling those of virus abortion in suckling hamsters. Later Doll and associates succeeded in cultivating, in suckling hamsters, a number of strains of the abortion virus and the so-called influenza virus, which until then was considered to be different. All of these strains produced identical lesions in the hamsters and resulted in their deaths (22). Typical acidophilic intranuclear inclusion bodies were found in the livers of all inoculated individuals, and horse tissues fixed complement with hamster antibodies, and hamster tissues fixed complement with horse antibodies. The virus also has a tropism for the trophoblast cells of the syncytiotrophoblast zone of the placenta (9).

Properties of the Virus. This is a DNA virus that produces intranuclear inclusion bodies (Figure 44.10). Particles have been described in the nuclei of affected hepatic cells of hamsters. The virus bodies are 92 nm in diameter in and outside of the cytoplasm (43). Particles in the nuclei may be in crystalline array. Its morphology is similar to herpes simplex virus, the prototype virus for this subfamily. Homology studies demonstrate that types 1 and 3 exhibit very little genetic homology (1).

Antigenic studies of equine herpesviruses 1, 2, and 3 were undertaken using various serological methods including the neutralization, immunodiffusion, complement-fixation, and direct and indirect fluorescent antibody tests (27). Their studies indicated that each type contains specific antigenic components. EHV-1 and EHV-3 share a common antigen that is not shared with EHV-2. Cross-neutralization was not detected in reciprocal tests among the 3 types. Carmichael and Barnes (11) showed that equine herpesvirus 1 and infectious bovine rhinotracheitis virus share common complement-fixing and precipitating antigens. Complement-fixing antibodies decline more rapidly than other types of antibody, but this is a consistent finding in most viral infections.

Figure 44.10. Characteristic intranuclear inclusions of rhinopneumonitis virus in the epithelium of a bronchus. × 930. (Courtesy Charles C. Randall, *Cornell Vet.*)

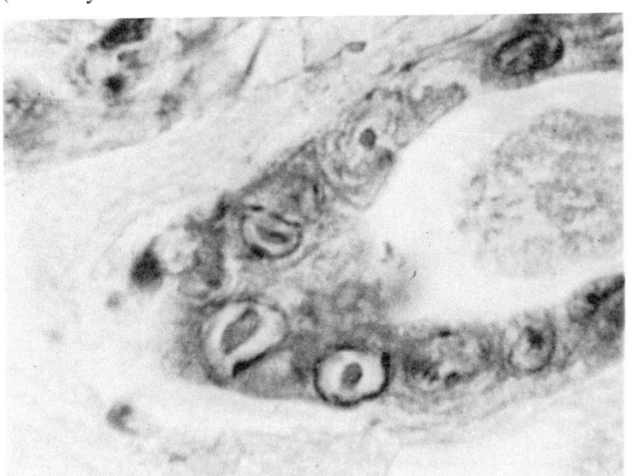

Virus survives for more than 457 days at −18 C. The agent is labile in saline suspensions, and it is inactivated by 0.35 percent formalin. Its density is 1.18 in cesuim chloride.

Horse red blood cells are agglutinated by tissues of affected horses between 4 C and 37 C (35). The hemagglutinin is not neutralized by convalescent horse sera, but inhibition is produced by use of hyperimmune serum from horses given infected hamster tissue.

Cultivation. Strains of equine herpesvirus 1 from the respiratory tract and also from tissues of aborted horse fetuses were adapted to hens' eggs by alternation between the hamster virus and the fertile egg (21).

Equine herpesvirus 1 produces a cytopathic effect in cell cultures of fetal horse kidney, lamb kidney, and rabbit kidney (37), with the production of intranuclear inclusion bodies of varying types depending on the virus isolate (23, 39). With equine herpesvirus 1 the cytopathic effect is rapid and complete. It also produces a cytopathic effect in a number of other cell culture types (19). Plaque-assay methods are available for equine herpesvirus 1, using monolayers of Earle's L cells (40) and horse kidney cells (42).

It is possible to differentiate *in vitro* field strains of virus from a strain adapted to the NL-111 rabbit kidney cells (28). The rabbit-adapted virus produces large, circular plaques, 2 to 3 mm in diameter, in NL-111 rabbit kidney cells whereas field isolates produce small, irregular plaques. This phenomenon provides a mechanism for studying the epidemiology of the disease in areas where horses are vaccinated with rabbit-attenuated virus vaccine.

Immunity. Virus abortions are seldom, if ever, observed in the same mare in two successive seasons, although some have been known to have aborted a fetus several years after the first abortion. This would indicate the presence of an immune mechanism that gives a somewhat transitory resistance, or possibly chance infection with a highly virulent strain.

A serum-neutralizing titer of 10^2 or greater (against 50 to 100 $TCID_{50}$ in a cell culture system) in a mare prevents reinfection by intranasal challenge (7, 8). Horses with lower titers or no measurable neutralizing antibody may develop mild signs of respiratory illness. Occasionally a viremia ensues with certain virus strains localizing in the leukocytes; this may lead to abortion and/or nervous manifestations in pregnant mares. Cell-mediated immunity also plays a significant role in herpesvirus infections such as rhinopneumonitis. The response can be measured by the lymphocyte transformation test (46) or by the *in vitro* cytotoxicity test. It is believed that cytotoxic antibodies or peripheral blood leukocytes could play an important role in restricting virus spread after infection (45). Thus it would appear that neutralizing antibody, cytotoxic antibody, and leukocytes play a combined role in protection against equine herpesvirus 1.

In some sequential infection studies in horses with equine herpesviruses types 1, 2, and 3, it was established that EHV-2 failed to produce a disease in foals. The inoculation of EHV-3 into the genital tract of the same test horses resulted in lesions typical of equine coital exanthema. Intranasal inoculation of EHV-1 produced definite respiratory signs and lesions, but the disease was milder than expected in two of the three foals. Thus the investigators (47) considered the possibility that recent prior infection with EHV-2 and/or EHV-3 may give partial protection against EHV-1.

Transmission. The respiratory disease is undoubtedly transmitted by droplet infection after outbreaks have started. The source of the virus that initiates outbreaks is unknown. Aborted fetuses contain much virus, and aborting mares often bring infections to new premises. There is no evidence, however, to indicate that virus is carried by an aborting mare very long after abortion occurs. It is known, though, that herpesviruses, in general, often persist for long periods after recovery. It is possible that dogs, foxes, and carrion birds may carry infection with fragments of aborted fetuses from one farm to another.

Diagnosis. Clinical diagnosis is usually not difficult. Autopsy of the aborted fetus generally will establish a precise diagnosis. In respiratory cases the lungs are usually edematous, there are hemorrhages on the pericardium, and the liver lesions are most characteristic. The finding of the characteristic inclusion bodies is diagnostic. These are acidophilic, intranuclear, and usually numerous in the liver cells. Often from 50 to 80 percent of the liver cells are necrotic and contain these bodies. They may be found also in the epithelium lining the air passages and the bile ducts and in endothelial cells of the spleen, lymph nodes, and thymus. These were described by Westerfield and Dimock (44). Virus typing may be indicated in certain instances.

Control. Because the disease with equine herpesvirus 1 is highly contagious, isolation of the infected animals is recommended. Indiscriminate movement of infected foals or mares following an outbreak may result in spreading the disease. Following an abortion the stall of the aborting animal should be thoroughly disinfected. This is very important if other pregnant mares are kept in the same stable.

As a prophylactic measure mares have been vaccinated with inactivated virus vaccine (4, 5, 32,), with a hamster-adapted live virus vaccine (Doll and Byrans), with an attenuated vaccine produced in Vero cells (38), and with an attenuated virus vaccine produced in tissue-cultured equine cells (NL-EQ_4) (24). Each product has its advantages and disadvantages, so none is completely satisfactory. Only two products now are in general use. Because the hamster-adapted live virus vaccine may cause a mild disease in many weanlings, it is recommended that the vaccine be given to all horses on a farm late in June and again in October. This procedure has reduced the number of abortions that occur on these farms. The attenuated virus vaccine produced in NL-EQ_4 equine cells does not cause any signs of illness and after 2 injections of vaccine elicits neutralizing antibodies and a cell-mediated immune response. It is generally believed this vaccine affords some protection, yet abortions occur in some vaccinated mares.

Just recently (1979) an inactivated virus vaccine derived from infected hamster cells has been introduced on the market. There has been insufficient time to evaluate its effectiveness as a vaccine.

If equine cytomegaloviruses are found in the United States as a cause of respiratory disease and abortion, the control program for EHV-1 will require considerable modification (6).

The Disease in Man. This disease has not been reported in man. References to an obscure disease of the human fetus in which there are intranuclear inclusion bodies appears in the literature (6).

Equine Coital Exanthema

SYNONYMS: Equine venereal vulvitis or balanitis, equine herpesvirus 3

The disease is characterized by lesions on the vulva of the mare and the penis of the stallion and is spread in a stud by coitus. Gerard, Greig, and Mitchell (25) isolated a herpesvirus from two stud outbreaks which differed immunologically and culturally from equine herpesvirus 1. The signs of illness and lesions are similar to pustular vulvovaginitis in cattle. Early lesions appear vesicular or pustular and occur in the vulva and perineal region in mares and on the penile mucosa of stallions (25). Later, uncomplicated lesions appear circular and pocklike, and as healing progresses, affected areas are depigmented. In the absence of secondary bacterial infection, healing was complete in 10 to 14 days. Infection usually occurs during breeding activities. Lesions may also occur on teats of the mare and the muzzle and lips of the nursing foal. No effects on fertility are apparent, but affected stallions are reluctant to cover mares until healing is complete. The incubation period is 6 to 8 days. There is evidence that virus persists in both the stallion and mare from one breeding season to another (10).

The inoculation of the virus into the amniotic cavity of a pregnant mare (6 to 7 months of gestation) resulted in abortion 11 days later (26). This is an interesting observation, but the virus has not been reported to cause abortions in the field.

EHV-3 will replicate only in cultured cells of equine origin and is known to infect only horses. The virus produces a cytopathic effect in cell culture, but it was slower than EHV-1, and the virus appears to be cell-associated.

Complement-fixing antibodies disappear within 60 days, while neutralizing antibodies persist for at least 1 year. This provides a useful method for establishing recent infections and the temporal incidence of infection in groups of mares.

REFERENCES

1. Allen, O'Callaghan, and Randall. Jour. Virol., 1977, *24,* 761.
2. Anderson and Goodpasture. Am. Jour. Path., 1942, *18,* 555.
3. Blakeslee, Olsen, McAllister, Fassbender, and Dennis. Can. Jour. Microbiol, 1975, *21,* 1940.
4. Bruner, Doll, and Hull. The Blood-Horse, 1949, *58,* 31.
5. Bruner, Edwards, and Hull. The Blood-Horse, 1948, *53,* 666.
6. Bryans. Proc. Am. Vet. Med. Assoc., 1964, p. 112.
7. Bryans. Jour. Am. Vet. Med. Assoc., 1969, *155,* 294.
8. Bryans and Prickett. Proc. 2nd Internatl. Conf. Equine Inf. Dis., ed. John T. Bryans and Heinz Gerber. Karger, Basel, 1969, p. 34.
9. Burek, Roos, and Narayan. Lab. Invest., 1975, *33,* 400.
10. Burrows. Jour. Antimicrobial Rev., 1977, *3,* 9.
11. Carmichael and Barnes. Proc. U.S. Livestock Sanit. Assoc., 1961, *65,* 384.
12. Charlton, Mitchell, Girard, and Corner. Vet. Path., 1976, *13,* 59.
13. Dimock and Edwards. Ky. Agr. Exp. Sta., Bull. 333, 1933.
14. Dimock, Edwards, and Bruner. Ky. Agr. Exp. Sta., Bull. 426, 1942.
15. Dimock, Edwards, and Bruner. Cornell Vet., 1947, *37,* 89.
16. Dinter and Klingeborn. Vet. Rec., 1976, *99,* 1.
17. Doll. Cornell Vet., 1953, *43,* 112.
18. Doll, Bryans, McCollum, and Crowe. Cornell Vet., 1957, *47,* 3.
19. Doll and Kintner. Cornell Vet., 1954, *44,* 355.
20. Doll, McCollum, Bryans, and Crowe. Am. Jour. Vet. Res., 1956, *17,* 262.
21. Doll, Richards, and Wallace. Cornell Vet., 1953, *43,* 551.
22. Doll, Richards, and Wallace. Cornell Vet., 1954, *44,* 133.
23. Erasmus. Proc. 2nd Internatl. Conf. Equine Inf. Dis., ed. John T. Byrans and Heinz Gerber. Karger, Basel, 1969, p. 46.
24. Gerber, Marron, Bass, and Beckenhauer. Can. Jour. Comp. Med., 1977, *41,* 471.
25. Girard, Greig, and Mitchell. Can. Jour. Comp. Med., 1968, *32,* 603.
26. Gleeson, Sullivan, and Studdert. Austral. Vet. Jour., 1976, *52,* 349.
27. Gutekunst, Malmquist, and Becvar. Arch Virol., 1978, *56,* 35.
28. Holmes, Kemen, and Joubert. Am. Jour. Vet. Res., 1979, *40,* 305.
29. Hupbauer. Deut. tierärztl. Wchnschr., 1938, *46,* 745.
30. Jackson, Osburn, Cordy, and Kendrick. Am. Jour. Vet. Res., 1977, *38,* 709.
31. Jeffcoat and Rossdale. Vet. Rec., 1976, *98,* 8.
32. Kress. Wien. tierärztl. Monatschrift., 1946, *33,* 121.
33. Little and Thorsen. Vet. Path., 1976, *13,* 3.
34. Manninger and Csontos. Deut. tierärztl. Wchnschr., 1941, *49,* 105.
35. McCollum, Doll, and Byrans. Am. Jour. Vet. Res., 1956, *17,* 267.
36. Miessner and Harms. Deut. tierärztl. Wchnschr., 1937, *45,* 685.
37. Plummer and Waterson. Quoted by Andrewes, Christopher, in Viruses of vertebrates. Williams and Wilkins, Baltimore, 1964.
38. Purdy, Ford, and Grant. Am. Jour. Vet. Res., 1977, *38,* 1211.
39. Randall. Proc. Soc. Exp. Biol. and Med., 1957, *95,* 508.
40. Randall and Lawson. Proc. Soc. Exp. Biol. and Med., 1962, *110,* 487.
41. Sedlmeier. Munch. tierärztl. Wchnschr., 1938, *89,* 37.
42. Shimizu, Ishizaki, and Matumoto. Jap. Jour. Exp. Med., 1963, *33,* 85.
43. Tajima, Shimizu, and Ishizaki. Am. Jour. Vet. Res., 1961, *22,* 250.
44. Westerfield and Dimock. Jour. Am. Vet. Med. Assoc., 1946, *109,* 101.

45. Wilks. Am. Jour. Vet. Res., 1977, *38,* 117.
46. Wilks and Coggins. Am. Jour. Vet. Res., 1976, *37,* 486.
47. Wilks and Studdert. Austral. Vet. Jour., 1976, *52,* 199.

Pseudorabies

SYNONYMS: Aujeszky's disease, mad itch, infectious bulbar paralysis, *Herpesvirus suis*

This disease occurs naturally in cattle, sheep, goats, dogs, cats, rats, and swine. Cases have been diagnosed clinically in horses, but in the absence of laboratory confirmation there is some doubt about the susceptibility of this species. In all but adult swine it is a highly fatal disease with few or no animals recovering. In adult pigs the signs are very mild and the mortality almost nil. The disease is usually transmitted from infected pigs to other hosts. Swine and dogs may become infected, however, from contact with carcasses of rats and possibly other infected animals. By inoculation the disease can be produced in nearly all warm-blooded animals, including birds. The rabbit is especially susceptible to inoculation and is commonly used in diagnostic work.

The disease was shown to be caused by a virus by Aujeszky (3) in Hungary in 1902. It is known to occur in most European countries and in South America. It has been definitely diagnosed in North America in swine and cattle (21, 23, 24, 26, 27) and in dogs (8). Shope was the first to show that the disease was prevalent in swine in the midwestern states of the United States and that cases in cattle stemmed from the swine reservoir.

Character of the Disease. *In cattle.* The name *mad itch* has been applied to the disease in this species. Intense pruritus of some portion of the skin is the principal manifestation of the disease. This generally appears on one of the flanks, or the hind legs, but it may be on any part of the body. If the part is accessible, the animal begins licking it incessantly until it becomes reddened and abraded. If the victim can reach a wall, post, or fence, it will rub the part until the skin is broken and torn. The itching is so intense as to cause the animal to become frenzied. As the disease progresses, the medulla becomes involved, and this leads to paralysis of the pharynx, salivation, forced respiration, and cardiac irregularities. The animal remains conscious until death approaches. There may be grinding of the teeth, bellowing, mania, and convulsions. Death usually occurs within 48 hours and sometimes much sooner. Occasional cases die within several hours after signs are first observed and without showing the pruritic signs.

In dogs and cats. Cases in these species seem to be common in some European countries; thus Galloway (10) reports that Marek, in Budapest, had seen 118 cats and 29 dogs with the disease in the period between 1902 and 1908. It is not clear why more cases have not been seen in these species in North America. The signs are essentially like those in cattle. The animals are driven into a frenzy because of the intolerable itching and do great damage to themselves by biting and tearing at the affected parts. Bulbar paralysis is generally manifested early; paralysis of the jaws and of the pharynx appears; plaintive cries and howls are emited; and saliva drools from the mouth. The appearance may simulate rabies, but, in contrast to the furious form of rabies, the affected animals show no tendency to attack other animals or man. As in cattle, consciousness is maintained until the end. At no stage is there any fever. In some cases, especially in cats, the disease may progress so rapidly that death ensues before pruritic signs have appeared. Death occurs usually within 24 to 36 hours after signs appear.

In swine. In this species pruritus does not occur. In adult animals the signs may be vague and mild, and recovery is the rule rather than the exception. There may be some fever and mental depression. Some animals vomit. The animals generally recover completely in 4 to 8 days. In some sows respiratory signs signal the onset of the disease (13), and it may be limited to the respiratory tract. At this time the temperature is elevated, and the sows stop eating on the third day after exposure. Constipation and depression may be accompanied by vomition during the next 2 days. If sows are pregnant, about 50 percent will abort and the remainder will farrow. Some pigs will be macerated, others will be normal. A higher percentage of abortions occurs in the first month of pregnancy. Late pregnancies may go as high as 17 days beyond the expected date of delivery. In suckling and recently weaned pigs the death losses may be very severe. According to McNutt (21), Ray (24), and Hirt (14), death losses in pigs less than 15 days old are frequently 100 percent. Such animals usually become prostrate within an hour or so from the time the first signs are observed, and they die in 12 to 24 hours. McNutt says that the losses are directly proportional to the ages of the animals, varying from nil at maturity to 100 percent in the very young.

In goats. The disease is largely referable to the nervous system with extreme signs including restlessness, screaming, profuse sweating, and, in the terminal stage, spasms and paralysis. Death usually occurs in 24 to 48 hours. Pruritus often is conspicuous by its absence. The disease in goats is associated with close proximity to pigs.

The lesions of this disease are not extensive. In those species in which pruritus occurs, the skin and underlying tissues at the point of infection usually are lacerated, torn, and covered with bloody exudate. The subcutaneous tissue of the region usually is very edematous. The lungs often show congestion and edema, and there may be fluid in the pericardial sac and hemorrhages on the epicardium. The other organs usually are normal. In swine, gross lesions generally are absent, but in adults subcutaneous edema and even necrosis may be found.

Infiltrations and necrosis of nerve elements can be seen by microscopic examination of various parts of the nervous system. These begin where the virus was introduced and proceed centripetally along the nerve trunks. Animals often die before the virus has reached the brain, or even the anterior part of the spinal cord. This should be taken into account when tissues are selected for laboratory diagnosis.

The Disease in Experimental Animals. The signs seen in naturally infected cases can be produced experimentally by the inoculation of animals with the virus. A little of the edematous tissue from the lesion in cattle injected subcutaneously in rabbits results in typical mad itch signs. These begin after an incubation period of about 2 days. The animal first licks the point of inoculation, later becomes more frenzied, and bites and tears the skin of this area. This lasts for 4 to 6 hours, by the end of which time the animal is exhausted. It then lies on its side, shows clonic spasms and labored respiration, and dies. Material from cattle will not infect guinea pigs or mice when inoculated subcutaneously, but, curiously, virus that has been passed through a rabbit brain will cause mad itch signs in these animals (29).

According to Hurst (15), who studied the distribution of the virus of pseudorabies in the rabbit, whether the animal is inoculated subcutaneously, intradermally, or intramuscularly, the virus reaches the central nervous system by passage through the peripheral nerves in spite of the fact that virus occurs for a time in the blood. After intracerebral inoculation, virus passes centripetally from the nervous system to the lungs. After intravenous inoculation, the virus rapidly disappears from the blood, forming multiple infective foci in the organs from which it passes through the nerves to the brain. When subcutaneous inoculation is done in an area deprived of its nervous supply, signs are delayed because the virus must then pass from the local area through the blood to establish visceral foci from which the infection of the central nervous system occurs secondarily. Hurst considers this a pantropic virus, that is, one that affects many cells derived from all of the embryonic layers.

When the virus is injected intracerebrally, it is uniformly fatal for rabbits, guinea pigs, rats, and mice. Pruritus of the skin does not occur in such cases. After an incubation period of 24 to 48 hours, signs of excitement are shown, and blindness evidently occurs. The animals run about their cages wildly and injure themselves by running into the walls. Salivation and grinding of teeth frequently occur. Death follows after a short period of coma.

McNutt (21) studied the inoculation disease in swine. When virus was injected into the muscles of one leg, a characteristic behavior pattern was shown which varied according to the size and age of the animal. Those that weighed from 30 to 40 pounds usually became ill after an incubation period of 5 to 7 days and died about 2 days later. Larger pigs usually developed paralysis of the inoculated leg. Some of these died, others remained permanently paralyzed, and others recovered. The paralyzed pigs usually had good appetites, were active, had normal temperatures, and were not noticeably excitable. Virus was not found in the blood of most of these animals, or in the visceral organs. It was found regularly, however, in the nerve trunks of the affected legs, and frequently in the spinal cord and brain. Pigs weighing more than 80 pounds seldom showed any appreciable signs, but virus could be recovered from their nervous systems, and virus was discharged in their nasal secretions.

There is good evidence that natural infection in swine occurs by the nasooropharyngeal route. Gustafson (12) found that intranasal exposure to the virus results in a syndrome seen in natural infections as opposed to those resulting from intramuscular, intratracheal, or intragastric exposures. The primary site of viral multiplication was in the upper respiratory passages and tonsillar tissue. Virus isolations are made as early as 18 hours from olfactory epithelium and tonsils and at 6- to 12-hour intervals thereafter for at least 5 days. Similarly, virus was isolated from the medulla and pons at 24 hours, suggesting transmission from the nasal and oral cavities in the epineural lymph of the 5th and 9th cranial nerves. Virus was not found in the blood during this period.

Ferrets are susceptible to the virus which causes a nonsuppurative meningoencephalitis as well as visceral lesions (1).

Properties of the Virus. Shope (27) reported that virus stored in 50 percent glycerol survives for 154 days with little loss of titer at refrigerator temperature. Virus survives on hay for 30 days in summer and 46 days in winter. It is stable between a pH of 4 and 9. One-half percent sodium hydroxide rapidly inactivates it, but 3 percent phenol is considerably less effective. Lyophilized virus survives 2 years; at low temperatures virus in tissue remains viable many years.

Some strains of virus produce lesions only in the central nervous systems of pigs; others cause rhinitis, pneumonia, and encephalitis (5).

Cultivation. Traub (35) was the first to report success in cultivating the virus of this disease. He succeeded in obtaining multiplication in media containing minced testicular tissue of rabbits and guinea pigs, and also in minced chick embryo medium. Mesrobeanu (22) obtained growth in chick embroyos in 1938, and his work was quickly confirmed by a series of workers. The virus may easily be passed in series in egg embryos after it has once been adapted. Bang (4) called attention to the fact that the lesions which appear as whitish plaques on the chorioallantoic membrane after about 4 days' incubation are quickly followed by invasion of all parts of the central nervous system. Many strains produce hemorrhagic destruction of the nervous system, which leads to protrusion of the cranium of the embryo.

Tokumaru (34) was able to cultivate the virus in monkey kidney cells after it had first been adapted to eggs. Two cytopathogenic varieties were found; one produced typical cytopathogenic effects, the other a cell-rounding type of degeneration which had previously been described in certain other viruses. The virus also grows in cultures of chick, rabbit, guinea pig, and dog tissues. It causes a cytopathogenic effect, and plaques are produced in agar overlays of pig kidney, rabbit kidney, and chick embryo cell cultures. It is suggested that the less virulent strains produce larger plaques (Figure 44.11). Intranuclear inclusion bodies are found in infected cultures and eggs.

Immunity. Shope (32) has shown that swine that have recovered from the disease have neutralizing antibodies in their sera. Using this technique, he was able to show that the European and the American diseases cross-immunized perfectly and the virus strains could be considered identical (28). Shahan, Knudson, Seibold, and Dale (26) showed that, after recovery from the disease, swine are immune to inoculation even by the intracerebral route.

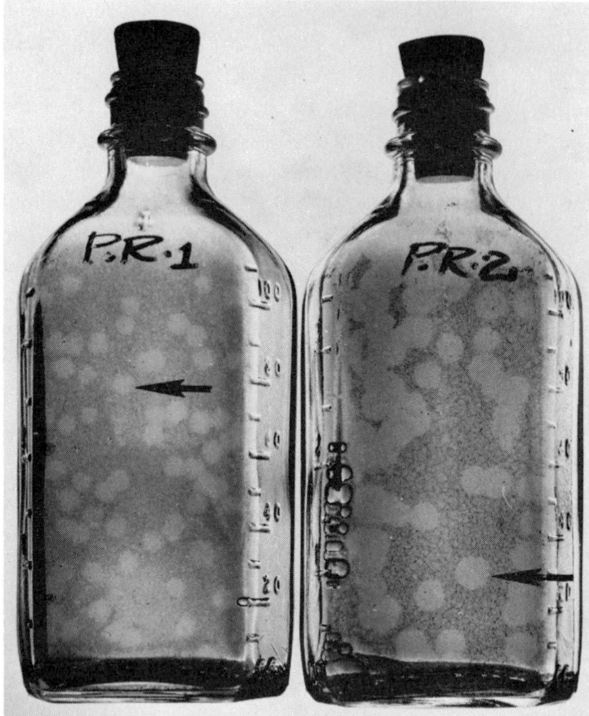

Figure 44.11. Comparison of plaque size (*arrow*) and count of pseudorabies virus on porcine kidney (*PR1*) and rabbit kidney (*PR2*) monolayers 9 days after virus seeding. (Courtesy K. V. Singh, *Cornell Vet.*)

Colostral antibodies have a half-life of 8.5 days and provided protection against virulent virus, but did not prevent the piglets from excreting virus (19).

The first cell-mediated immunity reaction of lymphocytes occurs 4 days after infection, whereas neutralizing antibodies are detected 3 days later reaching optimal titer at day 14 (37). Lymphocytes from the lymph nodes and spleen caused the most marked reaction, blood and thymus lymphocytes reacted less frequently, and those from bone marrow showed no response during the test period of day 7 to 35. Reinfection causes little increase in neutralizing antibody titer, but the sensitivity of the test can be enhanced by the addition of fresh guinea pig complement. Complement-fixing antibodies cannot be detected until 14 days after infection.

A microimmunodiffusion test (MIDT) was developed and evaluated for its sensitivity in detecting antibodies in swine sera (11). The test appears to be as sensitive as the microtiter neutralization test in the detection of antibodies. It also can be used to test sera that are cytotoxic, markedly hemolyzed, or too contaminated with bacteria to use the neutralization test. The MIDT is an accurate, rapid, economical, and sensitive diagnostic test. In contrast, the indirect fluorescent antibody technique is not as sensitive as the microneutralization test for the detection of antibodies (36).

The K vaccine strain grown in Vero cells developed by Bartha was used to vaccinate pigs (20). Following the inoculation of this vaccine virus intramuscularly in pigs, no signs of illness occurred and no virus was excreted. A single inoculation gave good protection against virulent virus challenge. Intranasal vaccine gave similar results except there was some minimal excretion of vaccine virus but also a greater degree of protection against virulent virus challenge. Following vaccination only low levels of neutralizing antibody were detected (geometric mean titer of 1:2) whereas very high levels were found after challenge (GMT > 1,000). Under field conditions the vaccine is very effective in swine even in a contaminated environment (9).The use of the Bartha vaccine in dogs is contraindicated because it caused adverse reactions.

Transmission. The principal natural reservoir of the virus of pseudorabies is in swine. Symptomless animals harbor and transmit the virus. A minor one, but perhaps important so far as its transmission from farm to farm is concerned, is in the brown rat. Other animal species contract the disease from one of these hosts, most often from swine, but the victims do not transmit it to other individuals. The recognition of the reservoir in swine was made by Köves and Hirt (16) and by Shope (31). The European workers assumed that the virus escaped from swine in the saliva and urine. Shope, however, showed that these fluids were not infectious and that the virus escaped only by way of the nasal secretions. Beginning about the 6th day after inoculation, when there is a concomitant temperature rise, and continuing for several days thereafter, virus is demonstrable in the scanty nasal discharge. Rabbits are easily infected by rubbing a slightly scarified skin surface on the snouts of the pigs during this time.

Shope (30, 31) also showed that the ordinary brown rat, which often frequents corn cribs and animal houses, readily develops pseudorabies by ingestion and suggested that such animals may be the means of carrying the disease from farm to farm. Cassells and Lamont (7) and Lamont and Gordon (18) have described cases in dogs (rat terriers) in Ireland in which it was believed that the infection was derived from killing rats on pig farms. Dogs that feed on infected pig carcasses may become diseased.

In the United States mad itch of cattle occurs most often on the feedlots in the midwestern states where range-raised beef cattle are fattened for market. Swine are commonly allowed to run with such cattle to salvage feed wasted by the cattle, and apparently these pigs infect minor wounds on the legs of the cattle.

In coitus, virus may be transmitted from the boar to the sow and vice versa (2). Evidence that this method of transmission takes place was made by the isolation of virus from the prepuce and vagina of infected swine. It is not known whether the virus is secreted with the sperm.

Studies on latency of pseudorabies in swine is under investigation by many scientists. It is possible to establish latent infection in piglets. During acute stages of disease the virus can be isolated readily by swabbing the oropharyngeal region, where replication is initiated, for 10 days. By explantation of tonsils, cervical lymph nodes, nasal mucosa, and Gasserian ganglia, it is possible to isolate virus from these tissues months after the initial infection (25). PRV antigen was seen by immunofluorescence only in explants from Gasserian ganglia where it was localized in the neurons and satellite cells.

Diagnosis. In animals other than swine the clinical signs are quite characteristic and at least suggestive of the diagnosis. The clinician must be aware that pruritis is not observed in all cases in dogs or in goats.

A definite diagnosis can be made in various ways: (*a*) isolation of the virus in rabbits or cell culture, (*b*) demonstration of a rising antibody titer with paired serums, (*c*) fluorescent antibody test (FAT), or (*d*) a skin test in swine.

Edematous fluid of a local lesion, the nerve trunk of the region, parts of the spinal cord, and portions of the brain are appropriate tissues for isolating virus. Virus may be detected in rabbits as easily by subcutaneous as by intracerebral inoculation, and the former method has two advantages: (*a*) intercurrent infections are not so apt to kill the rabbits, and (*b*) the characteristic local pruritus is an aid in recognizing the nature of the virus. For final recognition of the virus, virus-neutralization tests may be conducted using known antiserum against the newly recovered virus.

Acidophilic intranuclear inclusion bodies of the Cowdry A type are usually found in the spinal ganglia, in the posterior horn of the spinal cord, in the glia cells in various parts, and in a variety of cells in the local lesions in rabbits, according to Hurst (15). Such inclusions are found irregularly in cattle and do not occur in swine. The inclusions have little diagnostic importance. There are no cytoplasmic inclusions in any species. Selected cell cultures described under the section on cultivation can be used for virus isolation.

Various serological tests such as microtiter neutralization test, MIDT, and complement-fixation test can be used to demonstrate rising antibody titers.

A skin test provides considerable promise as a diagnostic aid (33). The reaction induced by subcutaneous injection in the lower eyelid is more easily administered and evaluated. A positive response was detected as early as 7 days after exposure, reached near maximal levels by 28 days, and persisted for at least 90 days. Control animals failed to elicit a reaction, so it appears that the test is specific.

Detection of pseudorabies virus in tests can be achieved by using the FAT in tissues, but it is less sensitive than isolation of the virus in cell culture or in rabbits (6). In cell culture systems the plaque method was more sensitive in the detection of virus in meat, organs, and meat products than the cytopathic effect observed in cell monolayers (17).

Control. The available evidence indicates that this disease is transmitted principally by swine, and possibly also by rats. There is little to indicate that other animals are a source of danger. The destruction or control of rats is desirable for many reasons other than their relationship to this disease. Infected lots of swine should be segregated as much as possible from ruminants.

The Disease in Man. The danger to man from this disease is apparently slight, but several human cases have been diagnosed in Europe, from some of which it is claimed that virus was isolated. These usually have involved contamination of skin wounds with tissues of infected animals. No fatalities have been reported, but severe pruritus has been noted in some of these cases. The fact that the disease can be produced experimentally in most warm-blooded animals should serve as a warning that some degree of human susceptibility is probable and that infected animals and their tissues should be handled with caution.

REFERENCES

1. Ahshima, Gorham, and Henson. Am. Jour. Vet. Res., 1976, *37,* 591.
2. Akkermans. Jour. Am. Vet. Med. Assoc., 1963, *143,* 860.
3. Aujeszky. Zentrbl. f. Bakt., I Abt. Orig., 1902, *32,* 353.
4. Bang. Jour. Exp. Med., 1942, *76,* 263.
5. Ben-porat and Kaplan. Virol., 1962, *16,* 261.
6. Biancefiori, Gialletti, Frescura, and Morozzi. Folia Vet. Lat., 1977, *7,* 174.
7. Cassells and Lamont. Vet. Rec., 1942, *54,* 21.
8. Eidson, Kissling, and Tierkel. Jour. Am. Vet. Med. Assoc., 1953, *123,* 34.
9. Elsinghorst, Van der Linden, Van Lieshout, and Schroder. Tijdschr. Diergeneeskd., 1976, *101,* 912.
10. Galloway. Vet. Rec., 1938, *50,* 745.
11. Gutekunst, Pirtle, and Mengeling. Am. Jour.Vet. Res., 1978, *39,* 207.
12. Gustafson. *In* Diseases of Swine 2nd ed., Ed. Howard W. Dunne, Iowa State Univ. Press, Ames, Iowa, 1970.
13. Gustafson, Claflin, and Saunders. Fed. Proc., 1968, *27,* no. 2, 425.
14. Hirt. Arch. f. Tierheilk., 1935, *70,* 86.
15. Hurst. Jour. Exp. Med., 1934, *59,* 729.
16. Köves and Hirt. Arch. f. Tierheilk., 1934, *68,* 1.
17. Kunev. Vet. Med. Nauki, 1977, *14,* 79.
18. Lamont and Gordon. Vet. Rec., 1950, *62,* 596.
19. McFerran. Dev. Biol. Stand., 1975, *28,* 563.
20. McFerran and Dow. Res. Vet. Sci., 1975, *19,* 17.
21. McNutt. North Am. Vet., 1943, *24,* 409.
22. Mesrobeanu. Comp. Rend. Soc. Biol. (Paris), 1938, *127,* 1183.
23. Morrill and Graham. Am. Jour. Vet. Res., 1941, *2,* 35.
24. Ray. Vet. Med., 1943, *38,* 178.
25. Sabo and Rajcani. Acta Virol. (Praha), 1976, *20,* 208.
26. Shahan, Knudson, Seibold, and Dale. North Am. Vet., 1947, *28,* 440.
27. Shope. Jour. Exp. Med., 1931, *54,* 233.
28. Shope. Proc. Soc. Exp. Biol. and Med., 1932, *30,* 308.
29. Shope. Jour. Exp. Med., 1933, *57,* 925.
30. Shope. Science, 1934, *80,* 102.
31. Shope. Jour. Exp. Med., 1935, *62,* 85.
32. Shope. Jour. Exp. Med., 1935, *62,* 101.
33. Smith and Mengling. Can. Jour. Comp. Med., 1977, *41,* 364.
34. Tokumaru. Proc. Soc. Exp. Biol. and Med., 1957, *96,* 55.
35. Traub. Jour. Exp. Med., 1933, *58,* 663.
36. Wirahadiredja and Rondhuis. Tijdschr. Diergeneeskd., 1976, *101,* 1125.
37. Wittman, Bartenbach, and Jakubik. Arch Virol., 1976, *50,* 215.

Canine *Herpesvirus* Infection

A fatal septicemic disease of infant puppies caused by a herpeslike virus was described by Carmichael *et al.* (4). A virus with characteristics of herpesviruses also was recovered by Stewart (10) from young puppies that died of a hemorrhagic disease.

So far as is known, only dogs are susceptible, and fatal infections have been reported only in puppies less than 2 weeks of age. Mild rhinitis and vaginitis are the only signs of illness in bitches inoculated with virus.

The disease has been observed in the United States, Great Britain, and Europe. Serologic studies indicate that the virus is widespread in the eastern and southeastern United States.

Character of the Disease. Severe disease has been recognized only in puppies less than 1 month of age. Fatal illness occurs in those less than 2 weeks of age. The illness in infant puppies starts between the 5th and 14th day after birth with a soft, odorless stool that is yellowish green in color, and with anorexia, labored breathing, abdominal pain, and painful crying as the principal signs.

The incubation period varies between 3 and 8 days in puppies inoculated by intranasal instillation or by intraperitoneal injection. The route of inoculation and virus dose does not appear to be related to the time of onset of signs or the severity of illness.

The course of the disease is short in puppies, most animals die within 24 to 48 hours after the onset of clinical manifestations. Virus has been isolated from the nasopharynx of inoculated dogs for periods up to 21 days.

The disease in older dogs is largely confined to the reproductive system. Usually there are no external clinical signs associated with the genital infection in female dogs, but the vaginal lesions consist of multiple lymphoid nodules in the mucosa interspersed with petechial and submucosal hemorrhages. In the male dogs there is a serous preputial discharge from 3 to 7 days after viral exposure. Occasionally, the infection spreads to the conjunctiva, and like the genital disease it is self-limiting and regresses in 4 to 5 days (6).

Pathologic changes in fatal cases are characteristic. Lesions in inoculated and naturally infected puppies consist of disseminated focal necrosis and hemorrhages. These lesions may be found in virtually all of the organs. Especially noteworthy changes occur in the kidneys, where subcapsular hemorrhages appear as bright red spots on the gray background of necrotic cortical tissue. The lungs are diffusely pneumonic. Focal necrosis and hemorrhages also are common in the liver, intestinal tract, and adrenal glands. Spleens characteristically are enlarged. Meningoencephalitic lesions are frequently found and virus isolated even though clinical signs are lacking (7, 9).

In pathogenesis studies of the dog, Carmichael (3) suggested that virus enters the body by the oral or nasal routes with oral, nasal, and vaginal excretions serving as the source of infection for susceptible dogs. Primary viral replication takes place in the tonsils, nasal turbinate, mucosa, and pharynx. The virus is transported in the blood where it is associated with the leukocytes. Secondary viral replication takes place in blood vessels; reticuloendothelial cells of spleen, liver, and lymph nodes; parenchyma of liver, lungs, kidneys, spleen, and adrenal glands; lamina propria of intestinal tract; meninges; and brain.

Canine herpesvirus-induced retinal dysplasia and associated ocular anomalies were produced in newborn beagle puppies (1). In these studies histologic fluorescent antibody and viral isolation procedures were applied to study the pathogenesis of the eye disease.

Body temperature and its regulation is an important factor in the pathogenesis in infant pups (3, 7). By maintaining puppies that were inoculated with virus at 1 day of age in an environment that increased their body temperature from 38.4 to 39.5 C, survival was prolonged and viral growth was diminished (3). This phenomenon doesn't entirely explain the age resistance associated with canine herpesvirus (CHV) infection in their opinions.

The role of CHV in tracheobronchitis needs to be clarified (9), although it is unlikely that it is involved in the etiology of this disease (5).

Properties of the Virus. Virus particles in thin sections of dog kidney cells have an average diameter of 142 nm. The particles contain a DNA core surrounded by two membranes. The protein coat is composed of 162 subunits, a characteristic shared by other herpesviruses. The virus is inactivated by chloroform and ether, and is destroyed in less than 4 minutes at 56 C. Infectivity is reduced by 50 percent after 5 hours at 37 C. Virus titers are maintained for months at −70 C in virus stocks that contain 10 percent serum. Infectivity is lost below pH 4.5 after 30 minutes. Hemagglutination has not been demonstrated with erythrocytes from a variety of species. The virus is not related serologically to infectious canine hepatitis, distemper, infectious bovine rhinotracheitis, equine rhinopneumonitis, avian laryngotracheitis, or herpes simplex viruses.

Cultivation. This virus grows readily in dog kidney cell cultures. Characteristic cytopathic effects occur in susceptible cell cultures, beginning 12 to 16 hours after inoculation. Cytopathic effects consist of focal areas of rounded and degenerating cells that detach from the glass of the culture tube. Cells occasionally have faintly acidophilic intranuclear inclusion bodies. More typical intranuclear changes, however, consist of dissolution of chromatin and the formation of basophilic nucleoprotein bodies that are often most numerous adjacent to the nuclear membrane.

A plaque reduction test was developed by Binn *et al.* (2) for comparing antigenic relationships of various strains of CHV, and no significant antigenic differences were noted in the comparison of four United States isolates.

Immunity. Puppies from inoculated pregnant females that had antibody titers at the time of inoculation did not develop illness. In contrast, susceptible pregnant females that were inoculated intravaginally with virus gave birth to puppies all of which died within 2 weeks. Virus was recovered from the dead puppies. It has been observed that females whose puppies died naturally of the disease gave birth 1 year later to normal puppies. Neutralizing antibodies develop in older dogs inoculated with the virus; however, the duration of immunity is not known. The need for a vaccine does not presently seem great, and none is available at present (3).

Transmission. The natural route of transmission is by inhalation or ingestion or by vaginal contact. Infections occurred in puppies whose mothers were inoculated intravaginally 2 weeks before whelping. This has also been observed in a naturally infected litter. Transmission by droplet infection has been observed between older inoculated dogs placed in close contact with uninoculated animals.

The problem of latency and carrier animals with this disease has not received much attention as it is not viewed as an important disease of dogs. One report states that virus was isolated from the anterior vagina of a bitch 18 days after whelping a litter of herpesvirus-infected puppies (8).

Diagnosis. The uncomplicated disease in older dogs is so mild that it probably is unnoticed; however, the disease-producing potential of this virus has not been fully explored. Pathological changes in affected puppies are characteristic. Necrotic and hemorrhagic lesions in the liver, lungs, and kidneys of dead puppies suggest this viral infection. Focal renal hemorrhages have not been reported in dogs infected with canine hepatitis or distemper viruses. Microscopic examination will reveal characteristic intranuclear inclusions in cells in areas of necrosis. These must be differentiated from canine hepatitis inclusions. Virus is isolated readily from tissues of dead puppies in dog kidney cell cultures.

The neutralization or complement-fixation tests can be used to demonstrate antibody (7), but CF antibodies are not present in sera of all convalescent dogs, and they often disappear by 1 to 2 months after exposure. Neutralizing antibody titers are produced in low titer, which generally persist longer than CF antibody. Neutralizing titers can be increased two- to eight-fold by the addition of four units of guinea-pig complement (C^1).

The Disease in Man. There is no evidence that the canine herpesvirus is pathogenic for man.

REFERENCES

1. Albert, Lahav, Carmichael, and Percy. Invest. Ophthalmol., 1976, *15,* 267.
2. Binn, Koughan, and Lazar. Jour. Am. Vet. Med. Assoc., 1970, *165,* 1724.
3. Carmichael, Squire, and Krook. Am. Jour. Vet. Res., 1965, *26,* 803.
4. Carmichael. Jour. Am. Vet. Med. Assoc., 1970, *156,* 1714.
5. Gillespie, Carmichael, Gourlay, Dinsmore, Abbott, Binn, Cabasso, Fox, Gorham, Ott, Peacock, Sharpless, Decker, and Freeman. Panel members, Canine Symposium, AVMA. Jour. Am. Vet. Med. Assoc., 1970, *156,* 1669.
6. Hill and Mare. Am. Jour. Vet. Res., 1974, *35,* 669.
7. Huxsoll and Hemelt. Jour. Am. Vet. Med. Assoc., 1970, *156,* 1706.
8. Love and Huxtable. Vet. Rec., 1976, *99,* 25.
9. Percy. Jour. Am. Vet. Med. Assoc., 1970, *156,* 1721.
10. Stewart, David, Ferreira, Lovelace, Landon, and Stock. Science, 1965, *148,* 1341.

Feline Herpesviruses

Feline herpesvirus 1 causes feline virus rhinotracheitis. Another feline herpesvirus associated with feline urolithiasis is described in a later section of this chapter. This latter virus is clearly distinct from feline herpesvirus 1.

Feline Virus Rhinotracheitis

This virus possesses the properties of the genus *Herpesvirus*. The disease occurs in the Eastern and Western Hemispheres, principally, as a respiratory infection.

The virus was first isolated in 1957 by Crandell and Maurer (7) from young kittens with a respiratory disease. The first European isolation was made by Bürki in 1963 (5). It is now recognized that feline viral rhinotracheitis (FVR) is a very important disease of the domestic cat and one of a number of viruses involved in respiratory disease of this species.

An excellent short review of this disease is given by Crandell (6).

Character of the Disease. The respiratory disease varies markedly from an inapparent condition to severe respiratory involvement terminating in death. The disease principally affects the upper respiratory tract and is characterized by sudden onset; transient fever; neutrophilic leukocytosis; paroxsymal sneezing and coughing; nasal, turbinate (Figure 44.12), and conjunctival exudate; difficult breathing; and anorexia and weight loss (4). A similar picture is seen in germ-free cats suggesting that the severity of FVR is not dependent on the secondary activity of respiratory microbes (11). Eosinophilic intranuclear inclusion bodies are associated with extensive nasal epithelial necrosis and focal epithelial necrosis in the conjunctiva, tonsils, epiglottis, larynx, trachea, and rarely bronchi or bronchioles (11). Laryngotracheal lesions usually are mild, and pulmonary lesions are rare with confinement to the bronchi and bronchioles. In natural cases pneumonia may occur as a result of secondary bacterial infection. In separate experimental studies in conventional cats (20) and in germ-free cats (11), lingual ulceration was not observed, but it was observed in feline calicivirus (picornavirus) infection (14) and more recently in a natural case of FVR (18). Intranuclear inclusion bodies were found in the lingual lesions and the multifocal liver lesions of this cat. Naturally occurring dendritic keratitis has been observed in conjunction with FVR in neonatal, juvenile, and adult domestic cats (4).

In addition to resorption of turbinate bone in conventional cats (6) Hoover (11) observed severe osteolytic lesions simulating overt necrosis of bone in the turbinates of some germ-free cats with FVR infection.

In experimental studies pathogen-free queens given FVR virus intravenously in the late stages of gestation (7th or 8th week) had stillborn fetuses (12). Other animal herpesviruses are known to have a similar effect under natural conditions, and it is possible that feline herpesvirus may do likewise. The inoculation of feline herpesvirus intracerebrally causes fatal encephalitis (11),so we may anticipate occasional natural cases, especially in neonatal kittens.

Properties of the Virus. The nuclear particles have an average diameter of 148 nm, consisting of a central dense core surrounded by a clear zone bounded by an outer membrane (6). Cytoplasmic particles vary in size from 128 to 167 nm in diameter while extracellular particles are 164 nm in diameter. The enveloped particle of cubic symmetry has 162 capsomeres. (Figure 44.13) It is a DNA virus (6) that is pH-labile and sensitive to ether and chloroform (1, 6).

The virus is highly species-specific, having been isolated only from the domestic cat. In all likelihood it causes infection in other members of the cat family.

Hemagglutinating and hemadsorbing properties of the virus have been demonstrated by using feline red blood cells (10). A hemagglutination test was developed to detect feline herpes antibodies.

Many strains of feline herpesvirus have been compared by various investigators in the United States and Europe with the conclusion that only 1 serotype of feline respiratory herpesvirus is known to exist. There is no serological relationship between FVR and feline panleukopenia, infectious bovine rhinotracheitis, pseudorabies, certain feline calicivirus strains, and herpes simplex viruses as demonstrated by the neutralization test.

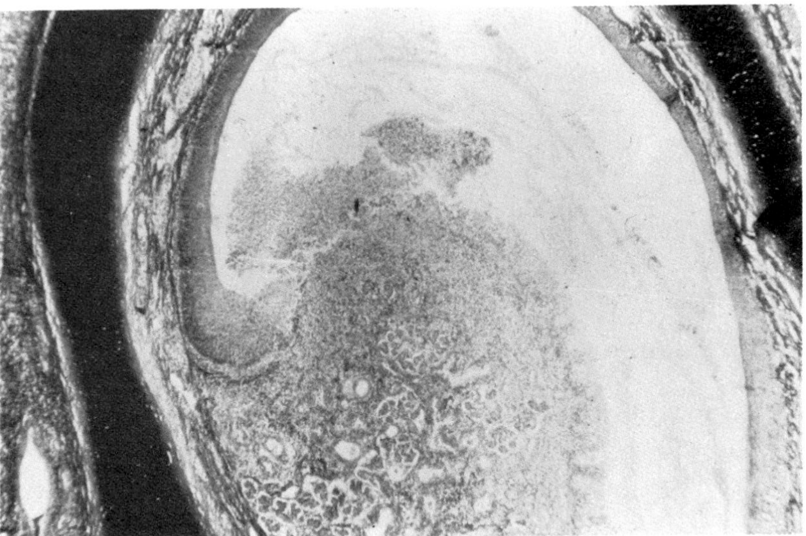

Figure 44.12. Feline herpesvirus infection. Ulcerative area with cellular reaction in the turbinate. H and E stain. × 3.5. (Courtesy T. Walton and J. Gillespie, *Cornell Vet.*)

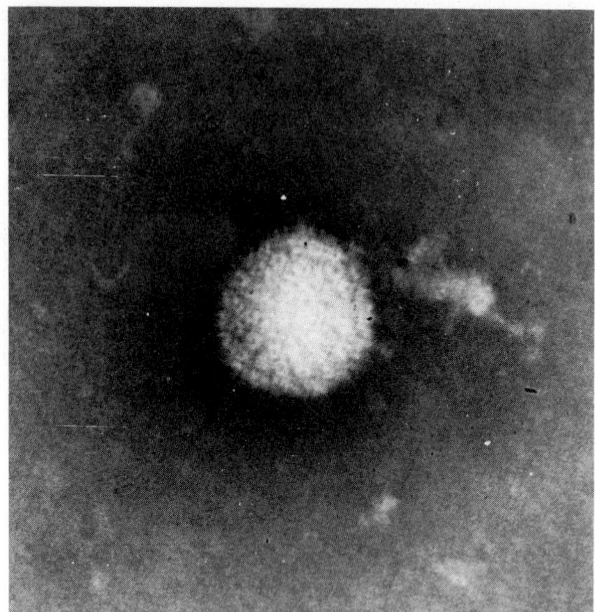

Figure 44.13. Feline herpesvirus particle, stained with phosphotungstic acid, showing capsomeres and other structures characteristic of this genus. × 200,500. (Courtesy J. Strandberg, D. Kahn, P. Bartholomew, and J. Gillespie.)

By complement-fixation test, no antigenic relationship was demonstrated between FVR virus and certain feline calicivirus strains (8) and the human adenovirus group.

Cultivation. The virus replicates and produces a cytopathic effect in cell cultures of feline origin (6) (Figure 44.14). Although tests have not been exhaustive in cell cultures, cytopathology of FVR virus is limited to cultures of feline origin (15).

The characteristic feature of its cytopathic effect is the formation of intranuclear inclusion bodies (Figure 44.15). Multinucleated giant cells or syncytia also are formed in cell cultures. Macroscopic plaques in cultures under agar are readily produced by many strains. The appearance of the cytopathic effect is dose-dependent, but as a rule it is observed within 24 to 72 hours and reaches a maximum titer of 10^4 to 10^6 $TCID_{50}$ per 0.1 ml.

Immunity. Clearly, complete and undisputable knowledge about the immunity to feline herpesvirus in cats is lacking. An evaluation of the present literature suggests that cats in the convalescent stage are completely immune even though some may lack neutralizing antibody at 21 days and a partial but significant immunity still exists after 5 months.

In experimental studies Walton and Gillespie (20) confirmed earlier reports that the initial antibody response after intranasal infection produced little or no neutralizing antibody (1, 6). In addition, the kitten challenged by aerosol route at 21 days did not respond clinically or excrete virus, but serum-neutralizing antibody titers increased significantly (1, 20). When challenged by the aerosol route at 150 days the serum titers of the kittens as a group were significantly lower, and the animals showed only mild signs of illness, with some kittens excreting virus for up to 6 days (20). Johnson and Thomas (13) have associated resistance to infection in older cats with and without detectable antibody levels. A transient antibody response was observed by Povey and

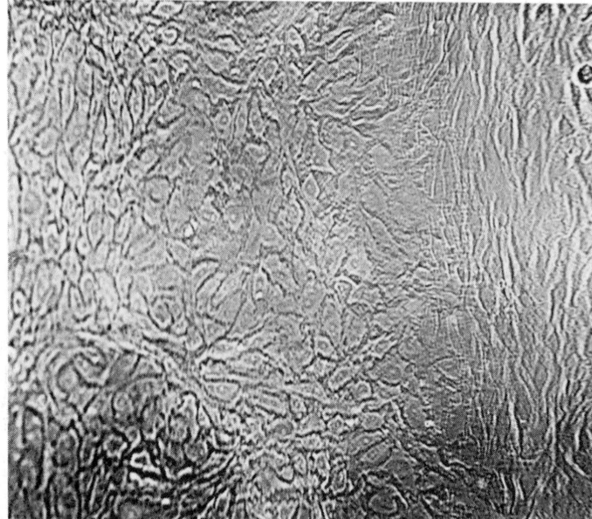

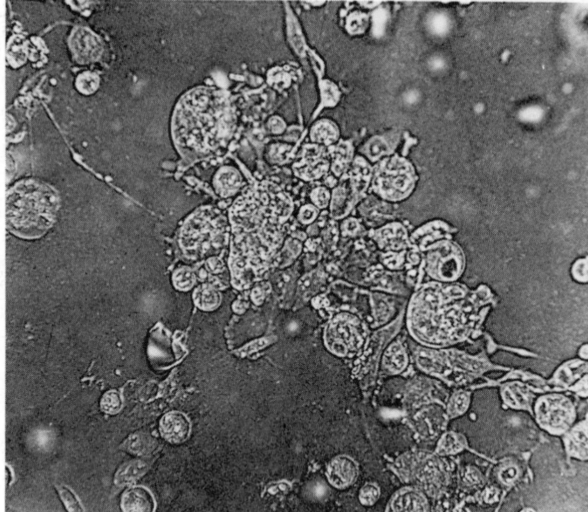

Figure 44.14. Feline herpesvirus in feline kidney cell culture. Uninoculated monolayer (*upper*) and inoculated culture showing characteristic CPE of a herpesvirus (*lower*). × 100. (Courtesy T. Walton and J. Gillespie, *Cornell Vet.*)

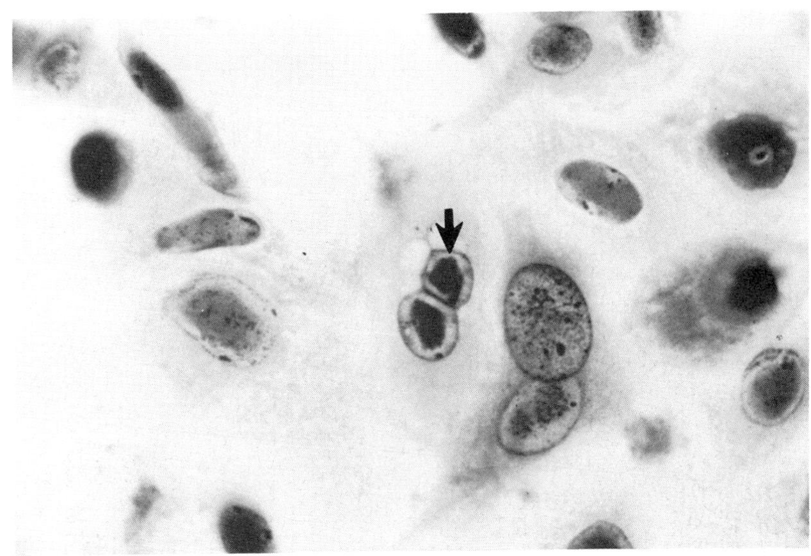

Figure 44.15. Typical Cowdry type A intranuclear inclusion bodies caused by feline herpesvirus. May-Gruenwald-Giemsa stain. × 380. (Courtesy F. Scott.)

Johnson (16) in recovered cats with the development of febrile reaction only upon challenge with virulent virus. They also reported a relatively persistent antibody response in cats that were resistant to challenge. Very little information is available about the serological response following inoculations by routes other than intranasal.

To provide some information on recovery mechanisms from feline viral tracheitis studies were performed in cell cultures (21). It was found that virus-infected cells could be destroyed in three ways: antibody- and complement-mediated lysis, direct lymphocyte cytotoxicity, and antibody-dependent, cell-mediated cytotoxicity. Antibody complement lysis and antibody-dependent, cell-mediated cytotoxicity occurred at 6 hours postinfection when intracellular infections virus spread takes place, while direct cytotoxicity occurred at 8 hours, just prior to extracellular viral spread.

Transmission. All evidence suggests that the infection is transmitted by cats to cats, presumably by the respiratory route. Cats that recover from the disease may become carriers with localization occurring principally in the pharyngeal region (19). The vast majority of cats are viral carriers, and approximately half shed virus spontaneously with or without stress (9). Carriers are probably the most significant source of virus and largely account for the spread of virus.

Diagnosis. To distinguish respiratory disease in the cat caused by FVR virus from other respiratory conditions with other etiologies is difficult, if not impossible in a practice situation.

Successful isolation of the virus is achieved during the acute febrile stage of disease with sterile swabs applied to the pharynx, nasal passages, and conjunctiva in that order. This material is inoculated into cell cultures of feline origin, and with positive material a cytopathic effect is seen. The virus in a tissue-culture system can be quickly identified by a knowledge of its virus properties as described earlier and by the use of the fluorescent antibody test. The latter test can also be applied with good results (2) directly to smear preparations of the conjunctiva, and logically from other infected tissues as well.

Control. Herpesvirus infection in a cattery causes great problems. With the periodic appearance of susceptible kittens in the group that has carriers the disease remains endemic. Because depopulation is often impossible, the disease persists as a major problem.

Attenuated virus vaccines for FVR are now available to immunize cats. The vaccine, singly or in combination with feline calicivirus (FCI), appears to be safe and reasonably efficacious (3, 17). FVR and FCI may also be combined with other agents such as feline panleukopenia and feline pneumonitis (*Chlamydia felis*).

The Disease in Man. There is no evidence that feline herpesvirus causes disease in man.

REFERENCES

1. Bartholomew and Gillespie. Cornell Vet., 1968, *58*, 248.
2. Bistner, Carlson, Shively, and Scott. Jour. Am. Vet. Med. Assoc., 1971, *159*, 1223.
3. Bittle and Rubic. Am. Jour. Vet. Res., 1975, *36*, 89.
4. Bodle. Surv. Ophthalmol., 1976, *21*, 209.
5. Bürki. 17th World Vet. Cong. (Hannover), 5/A/90, 1963, 559.
6. Crandell, Robert. Adv. in vet. sci. and comp. med. Academic Press, 1973, *17*, 201.

7. Crandell and Maurer. Proc. Soc. Exp. Biol. and Med., 1958, *97,* 487.
8. Crandell, Rehkemper, Niemann, Ganaway, and Mauer. Jour. Am. Vet. Med. Assoc., 1961, *138,* 191.
9. Gaskell and Povey. Vet. Rec., 1977, *100,* 128.
10. Gillespie, Judkins, and Scott. Cornell Vet., 1971, *61,* 159.
11. Hoover and Griesemer. Jour. Am. Vet. Med. Assoc., 1971, *158,* 929.
12. Johnson. Jour. Exp. Med., 1964, *120,* 359.
13. Johnson and Thomas. Vet. Rec., 1966, *79,* 188.
14. Kahn and Gillespie. Cornell Vet., 1970, *60,* 669.
15. Lee, Kniazeff, Fabricant, and Gillespie. Cornell Vet., 1969, *59,* 539.
16. Povey and Johnson. Vet. Rec., 1967, *81,* 686.
17. Scott. Am. Jour. Vet. Res., 1977, *38,* 229.
18. Shields and Gaskin, Jour. Am. Vet. Med. Assoc., 1977, *110,* 439.
19. Walton and Gillespie. Cornell Vet., 1970, *60,* 215.
20. Walton and Gillespie. Cornell Vet., 1970, *60,* 232.
21. Wardley, Rouse, and Babiuk. Can. Jour. Comp. Med., 1976, *40,* 257.

Avian Infectious Laryngotracheitis

Until a few years ago a variety of diseases of the respiratory tract of birds were grouped together under the name *roup*. These have been differentiated during recent years into nutritional, bacterial, parasitic, and virus disorders. Infectious laryngotracheitis was shown by Beach (2) in 1930 to be a specific virus disease. First recognized in the United States, it is now known to exist in nearly all parts of the world where poultry are kept. The disease affects chickens, occasionally pheasants, and perhaps Japanese quail.

Character of the Disease. Infectious laryngotracheitis affects chickens of all ages. It is highly contagious, and when it enters a susceptible flock, the disease does not stop until practically every bird has been attacked. Infection occurs through the respiratory tract and the conjunctival sac (14). There is no viremia. The incubation period is short, less than 48 hours as a rule. The course of the disease is acute, some birds dying within 24 hours of the time the infection is first detected, others running a course as long as 5 or 6 days. Birds that do not die during the first 5 days of signs practically always recover. Recovery generally is rapid. Although no single bird will show evidence of disease for as long as a week, the disease may require 3 or 4 weeks to run through a flock. An important fact is that a considerable number of recovered birds continue to harbor the virus, and such birds usually act as centers of new infections when transferred to new flocks, or when new birds are added, perhaps a season or more later (11).

The signs depend on the age of the birds and the season of the year. Young birds during the warm months usually are less severely affected, and the mortality rate is lower than in older birds during cold weather. Affected birds show respiratory distress varying in degree. In severe cases the chickens extend their necks, open their mouths, and inhale in a gasping manner (Figure 44.16). Gurgling and rattling sounds are often heard. Sometimes they are best described as whistling. These sounds are due to partial obstruction of the air passages by exudate. Not all birds show marked respiratory distress since the exudate sometimes is in the nasal passages or nasal sinuses. In mature birds in heavy production the mortality rate may be as high as 70 percent. Death appears to be due largely to suffocation.

The lesions are confined to the larynx, trachea, and bronchi. These are reddened, petechiated, and covered with a slimy exudate containing streaks of bright red blood. Sometimes the exudate is of a caseous nature, and plugs of such material may wholly block the trachea. Histologically, there are surface changes in the trachea including ciliary disruption, luminal debris, and epithelial sloughing (1).

In 1931 Seifried (15) described intranuclear inclusion bodies in the nuclei of the cells of the epithelium of tracheal lesions. Burnet (7) found similar bodies in the ectodermal cell lesions of the membranes of infected eggs.

Figure 44.16. Infectious laryngotracheitis, showing the characteristic gasping type of respiration. (Courtesy E. L. Brunett.)

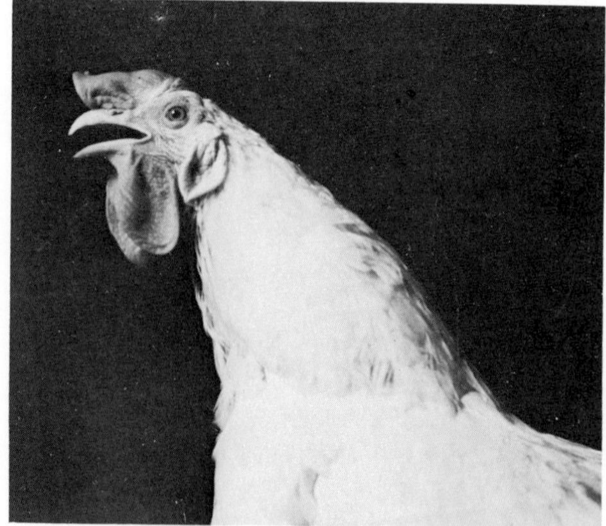

Properties of the Virus. Beach (2), who first identified the virus of this disease, found that it could be filtered readily through Berkefeld V filters but not in every case through Berkefeld N filters. Evidence suggests that the particle is similar in size and structure to other herpesviruses (10). The virus is present only in the air passages and is infective only by introduction in this way, except that, rarely, infections can be established by intravenous inoculation. Injections subcutaneously, intramuscularly, and intraperitoneally are harmless.

The virus is moderately resistant. Premises do not retain effective quantities of virus for long after infected and carrier birds are removed. Beaudette and Hudson (5) reported that egg-propagated virus, when dried and kept in a refrigerator, retained its potency and immunizing properties for 421 days. It is inactivated by a concentration of 3 percent Iosan (iodoform preparation) and 2 percent Bradofen (quaternary ammonium preparation) after 45 minutes of exposure.

Cultivation. The virus of infectious laryngotracheitis was cultivated on the chorioallantoic membrane of developing chick embryos by Burnet (7) in 1934, by Brandly (6) in 1936, and by many others shortly afterward. The virus produces whitish plaques on the membrane. Two kinds of plaques have been described, but immunologically the viruses appear to be identical. Diluted viruses, according to Burnet (8), can be roughly assayed for virulence by counting the number of plaques produced per volume of virus.

Virus replication occurs in avian leukocyte cultures with the production of a cytopathic effect characterized by multinucleated giant cells (9).

Immunity. Birds that recover from this disease are immune for the remainder of their lives. Cell-mediated immunity plays a significant role in this protection. Many of these birds are virus carriers; hence when the disease has once occurred in a flock, annual recurrences of the disease must be expected in the young stock unless they are artificially immunized. In small flocks it is often simpler and less expensive to dispose of all old stock.

The transfer of parental immunity is marginal and is unlikely to inhibit the response to primary vaccination (12).

Beaudette and Hudson (4) developed a method of actively immunizing birds to infectious laryngotracheitis which has proved to be very successful. After trying modified viruses with unsatisfactory results, they hit upon the idea of using fully virulent material on the mucous membrane of the bursa of Fabricius, which is an outpouching of the cloaca. In this location the virus sets up a harmless inflammatory reaction that immunizes solidly. This method has been extensively employed. Its principal objection is that it utilizes a fully virulent disease-producing agent, which, if carelessly used, may do much damage. It should not be used until it is absolutely certain that the flock contains the infection. Full immunity is not developed until about 9 days after treatment (3).

The virus for the cloacal method of vaccination may be obtained directly from the trachea of diseased birds, or it may be virus that has been propagated on egg embryo membranes. Commercially the virus usually is dried and shipped in sealed vacuum tubes with a separate container of glycerol-water mixture in which to suspend it prior to use. The virus mixture is applied with a stiff brush directly on the mucous membrane of the bursa, care being taken not to soil the feathers or to spill any vaccine. Five days later it is well to catch and examine a few birds to make sure that "takes" have occurred. If the vaccine has been potent and the work properly done, most of the birds will show swelling, inflammation, and a small amount of exudate at the point of inoculation. If the vaccine has not produced a high percentage of "takes," the flock should immediately be revaccinated with fresh vaccine, since virus has been introduced into the flock and a serious outbreak of tracheal infections is sure to develop otherwise.

In 1963 Shibley *et al.* (17) described the preparation and standardization of strain 146 for use as a conjunctivally administered vaccine. It causes conjunctivitis without production of permanent tissue damage. Neutralizing antibodies were still present 372 days postvaccination.

Some investigators recommend that broiler flocks be immunized as early as 4 weeks of age with commercial vaccine administered in the drinking water (13, 16).

Transmission. The disease is transmitted naturally through droplet infection.

Diagnosis. Ordinarily after disease is well under way in a flock, a diagnosis can be made easily on the basis of signs and lesions. In individual birds it may not be so simple. If the question is important enough to warrant the trouble, the answer can be obtained by swabbing the larynx of one or two susceptible birds with tracheal exudate from the suspected cases. These birds should develop signs some time between 2 and 5 days later if the disease is laryngotracheitis. If immunized birds are included in the test, they should prove resistant while the others sicken.

Direct electron microscopy of lysed tracheal cells and

the agar-gel diffusion test are methods sometimes used to establish a quick diagnosis (18).

Control. Most producers use commercial vaccine to prevent and control the disease.

The Disease in Man. Infectious laryngotracheitis of poultry does not affect any mammals, including man, so far as is known.

REFERENCES

1. Bayer, Bryan, Chawan, and Rittenberg. Poultry Sci., 1977, *56,* 964.
2. Beach. Science, 1930, *72,* 633.
3. Beaudette. Vet. Med., 1939, *34,* 743.
4. Beaudette and Hudson. Jour. Am. Vet. Med. Assoc., 1933, *82,* 460.
5. Beaudette and Hudson. Jour. Am. Vet. Med. Assoc., 1939, *75,* 333.
6. Brandly. Jour. Am. Vet. Med. Assoc., 1936, *88,* 587.
7. Burnet. Brit. Jour. Exp. Path., 1934, *15,* 52.
8. Burnet. Jour. Exp. Med., 1963, *63,* 685.
9. Chang, Sculco, and Yates. Avian Dis., 1977, *21,* 492.
10. Cruickshank, Berry, and Hay. Virol., 1963, *20,* 376.
11. Gibbs. Jour. Inf. Dis., 1933, *53,* 169.
12. Hayles, Hamilton, and Newby. Can. Jour. Comp. Med., 1976, *40,* 218.
13. Hayles, Newby, Gasperdone, and Gilchrist. Can. Jour. Comp. Med., 1976, *40,* 129.
14. Hitchner, Fabricant, and Bagust. Avian Dis., 1977, *21,* 185.
15. Seifried. Jour. Exp. Med., 1931, *54,* 817.
16. Seimenis and Menasse. Dev. Biol. Stand., 1976, *33,* 328.
17. Shibley, Luginbuhl, and Helmbolt. Avian Dis., 1963, *7,* 184.
18. Van Kammer and Spradbrow. Avian Dis., 1976, *20,* 748.

Herpesvirus Infection in Pigeons

From racing pigeons with a disease resembling ornithosis isolates of a herpesvirus were made by Cornwell and Wright (1). Diphtheric foci were present in the pharynx or larynx of several birds and were associated with intranuclear inclusions in one of them. The herpesvirus produced pocks on the chorioallantoic membrane of the embryonated hen's egg and foci of necrosis in the embryonic liver.

The two strains were pathogenic for young pigeons, but not for chicks (2). Intraperitoneal inoculation of these strains caused pancreatitis, peritonitis, and in some birds hepatic necrosis. Eosinophilic intranuclear inclusions and specific viral antigen were seen in pancreatic acinar and in hepatitic parenchymal cells. Intranuclear inclusion bodies also were observed in the necrotic foci in the laryngeal epithelium after pigeons were given virus by the intralaryngeal route.

In 1975 Vindevogel *et al.* (3) isolated a herpesvirus from pigeons with clinical signs of coryza. Its characteristics are comparable to the virus isolated by Cornwell and Wright. The virus produces cytopathic effect in monolayer cultures in 24 hours. The virus causes disease in experimental pigeons.

REFERENCES

1. Cornwell and Wright. Jour. Comp. Path., 1970, *80,* 221.
2. Cornwell, Wright, and McCuster. Jour. Comp. Path., 1970, *80,* 229.
3. Vindevogel, Pastoret, Burtonbody, Gouffaux, and Duchatel. Ann. Rech. Vet., 1975, *6,* 431.

Duck Plague

SYNONYM: Duck virus enteritis

Duck plague is an acute, highly fatal disease of ducks caused by a herpesvirus, that occurs in the blood and in all organs.

The disease has occurred in the Netherlands, Belgium, India, France, China, the United States, and more recently in Canada. The disease is limited to ducks, and on one occasion it was diagnosed at necropsy in geese.

A recent article describing the disease was written by Jansen (3), who did much of the original work on the disease. Leibovitz and Hwang described the 1967 outbreak on Long Island, New York (6).

Character of the Disease. Naturally and experimentally infected ducks show similar signs of illness characterized by listlessness, ruffled and dull feathers, wet areas around the eyes, which later become mucoid (Figure 44.17); nasal discharge, labored breathing, inappetence, watery diarrhea; and nervous manifestations. Not all of these signs may be present, and ducks frequently show temporary improvement before death occurs in 1 to 3 days. The mortality usually is high, and disease often lasts on a premise about 3 weeks.

At necropsy the most striking lesions are multiple hemorrhages throughout the body, usually most pronounced in heart, serous membranes, and esophageal mucosa. Marked congestion occurs in the ovary that is in production. If the disease becomes subacute, diphtheric membranes may occur on the mucosa of the esophagus and cloaca. These membranes may extend to salpinx and rectum. In many cases there is peritonitis and the liver may be friable. Pathogenesis studies of this disease were undertaken by Proctor using light, electron, and fluorescent microscopy (8, 9) which highlighted the necrosis

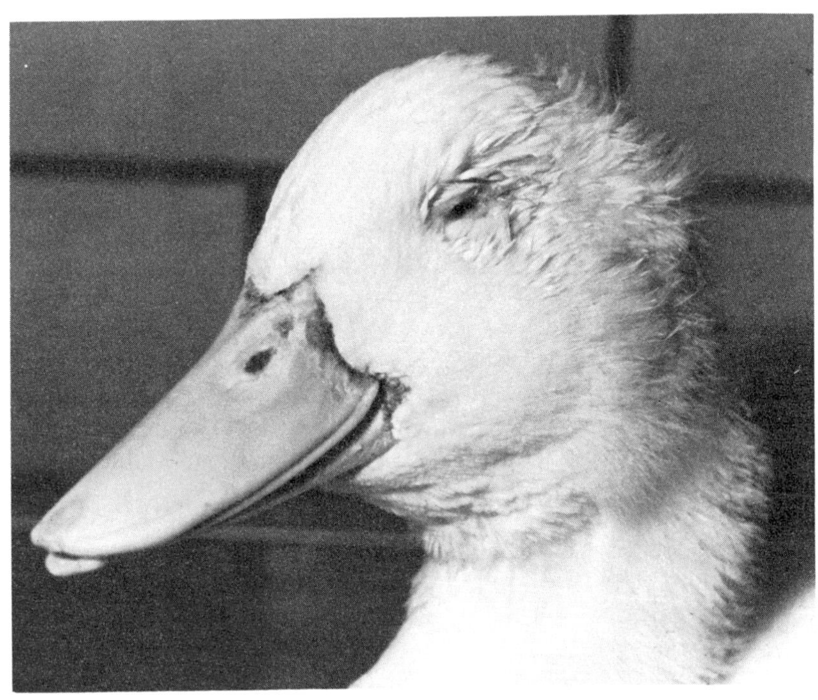

Figure 44.17. Duck with ocular discharge. (Courtesy D. A. Gregg, Plum Island Animal Disease Center, USDA.)

that occurs in many types of cells in the body—lymphocytes, macrophages, fibrocytes, and epithelial cells.

Properties of the Virus. Duck plague virus is a member of the *Herpesvirus* genus (Figure 44.18). There is only one serotype and one immunogenic type as complete cross-immunity has been demonstrated with various isolates by immunity tests in ducks and by neutralization tests in the embryonated duck egg.

Attempts to demonstrate a hemagglutinin have failed (3). The virus is quite stable at −20 C and in the lyophilized state.

Cultivation. The virus can be cultivated readily by inoculation on the choriollantoic membrane of 12-day-old embryonated duck eggs. The embryos die in 4 days, showing extensive hemorrhage (3). Direct cultivation of the virus in the hen's embryonated egg is not possible. Duck-embryo-adapted virus can be established in the hen's embryo. Repeated passage in the latter host produces a virus that is attenuated for ducks (3). Cultivation of the virus in cell culture has been reported by Kunst (5). Kocan (4) compared duck embryo fibroblast cultures from seven species and found that the Muscovy duck and wood duck cells gave the best virus yield and plaque quality.

Immunity. The chick-embryo-adapted strain of duck plaque virus that is avirulent for ducks produces an effective immunity in the duck. It rapidly produces protection as a result of interference. Ducks given this vaccine were immune to challenge 12 to 14 months later, although the majority had no demonstrable neutralizing antibody (3). Dardiri (1) found that a marked anamnestic serologic response resulted from challenge with virulent virus in ducks given chicken embryo attenuated virus vaccine. However, waterfowl that possessed a moderate level of neutralizing antibodies succumbed when secondary or latent microbial invaders were present. This may explain the lack of correlation between these antibody levels and mortality from infection with virulent virus.

There is evidence of parental antibody interference (7).

Transmission. Under natural conditions it is spread by contact because excretions from infected ducks contain virus. Free access to ponds, moats, and pools undoubtedly facilitates spread.

Diagnosis. Duck plague can be confused with fowl chloera, intoxication, or Newcastle disease. Inoculation of rabbits, chicks, and ducks should soon establish the diagnosis as duck plague virus causes disease in ducks only.

Attempts to isolate the virus in embryonating ducks or primary tissue cultures from duck kidney from diseased Muscovy ducks failed (2). Identification of the disease was achieved by serum neutralization with ducklings as the host system.

Control. Because free-flying birds are involved, control is exceedingly difficult other than by a vaccination program.

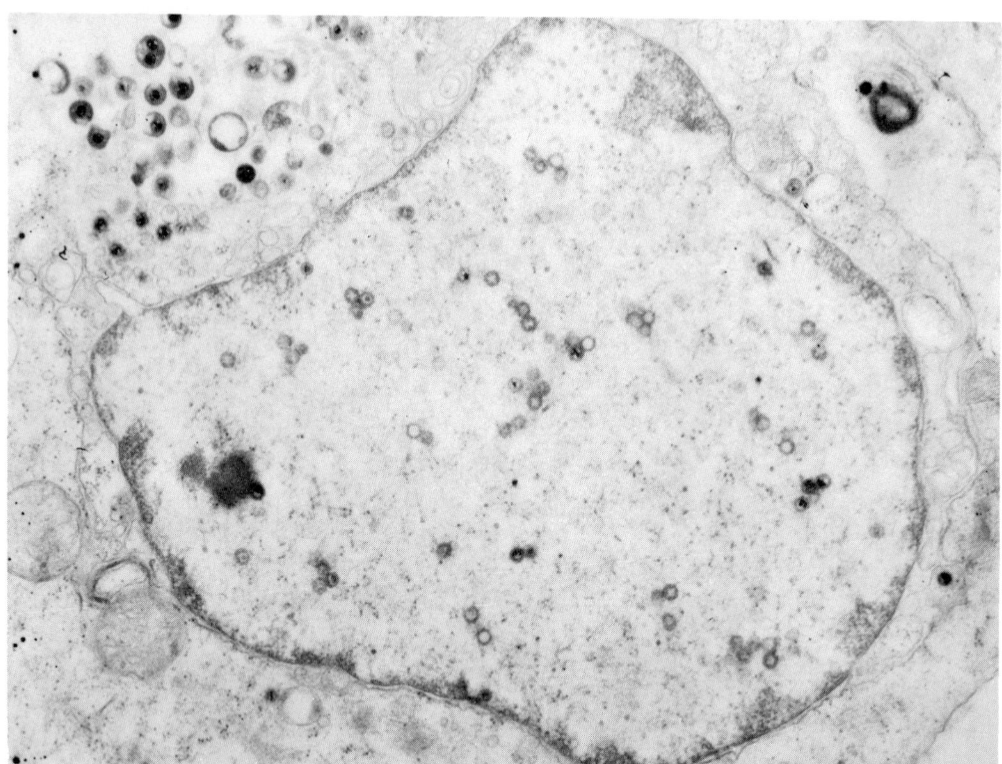

Figure 44.18. Duck plague herpesvirus in duck embryo cells. × 17,100. (Courtesy S. S. Breese, Plum Island Animal Disease Center, USDA.)

The Disease in Man. The disease in man has not been reported.

REFERENCES

1. Dardiri. Am. Jour. Vet. Res., 1975, *36,* 535.
2. Hanson and Willis. Jour. Wildlife Dis., 1976, *12,* 258.
3. Jansen. Jour. Am. Vet. Med. Assoc., 1968, *152,* 1009.
4. Kocan. Avian Dis., 1976, *20.* 574.
5. Kunst. Tijdschr. Diergeneesk, 1967, *92,* 713.
6. Leibovitz and Hwang. Avian Dis., 1968, *12,* 361.
7. Newcomb. Jour. Am. Vet. Med. Assoc., 1968, *152,* 1349.
8. Proctor. Vet. Path., 1975, *12,* 349.
9. Proctor. Am. Jour. Vet. Res., 1976, *37,* 427.

THE SUBFAMILY BETAHERPESVIRINAE

Atrophic Rhinitis

SYNONYMS: Cytomegalic inclusion disease (CID) of pigs, porcine inclusion body rhinitis

This disease is caused by a cytomegalovirus type herpesvirus. It was first described by Done (1). From a clinical standpoint it is principally a disease of the respiratory tract accompanied by anemia in pigs less than 4 weeks of age.

It has been reported in most countries where pigs are raised. The incidence in Great Britain is about 50 percent while in Iowa a 12 percent attack rate has been reported. Infection is probably transmitted by infected sows, with no signs of illness, to piglets by the aerosol route.

The severity of the disease depends on the age of the pig and the amount of acquired immunity by colostrum (4). This observation was confirmed and extended through a longitudinal study in two pig herds with respiratory disease that showed the cytomegalovirus disease was universal in each herd (6). In the acute form of the disease, the signs of illness usually appear between 5 and 10 days after birth. Initial signs include sneezing, presence of nasal exudate, and inappetence probably caused by obstructed nasal passages making suckling very difficult. This is followed by rapid loss of weight, paralysis, and death as early as 5 days later. Survivors are often stunted. Subacute infections generally occur in pigs over 2 weeks of age with clinical signs limited to the respiratory tract. In this age group the morbidity and mortality are low. A severe anemia occurs in clinically affected pigs despite iron therapy.

In some experimental studies on the etiology of atrophic rhinitis it was clear that the porcine cytomegalovirus produced lesions confined to the lamina propria while *Bordetella bronchiseptica* caused atrophy of the turbinate bones and hyperplasia and degeneration of the nasal epithelium. There was exacerbation of the lesions when piglets were given both agents, but the degree of bone atrophy was not increased (2). These studies strongly suggest that *B. bronchiseptica* causes the principal damage to the nasal epithelium and the turbinate bones.

Under experimental conditions susceptible pregnant sows had a mild disease after inoculation with a porcine cytomegalovirus. There was an increased number of mummified and stillborn fetuses in these sows. Virus was isolated from various internal organs of some fetuses indicating that transplacental transmission took place (3). Some survivors excreted virus and transmitted the infection to other noninfected piglets.

At necropsy there is a mucopurulent rhinitis, sinusitis, and sometimes turbinate atrophy in natural cases of atrophic rhinitis. In severe cases piglets may show petechial hemorrhages in kidneys and myocardium. Microscopically, there are intranuclear inclusion bodies in enlarged cells in many organs of piglets including the brain and especially in the tubuloalveolar glands of the nasal mucosa.

The virus is propagated in primary pig-lung cell cultures with the production of a cytopathic effect in 11 to 18 days postinoculation (5). Intranuclear inclusion bodies are formed in cell cultures. The indirect immunofluorescent and serum neturalization tests are used in the study and diagnosis of the virus.

There is no evidence the virus causes disease in man.

REFERENCES

1. Done. Vet. Rec., 1955, *67,* 525.
2. Edington, Smith, Plowright, and Watt. Vet. Rec., 1976, *98,* 42.
3. Edington, Watt, and Plowright. Jour. Hyg. (London), 1977, *78,* 243.
4. Gustafson. Personal communication, 1972.
5. L'Ecuyer and Corner. Can. Jour. Comp. Med. and Vet. Sci., 1966, *30,* 321.
6. Plowright, Edington, and Watt. Jour. Hyg. (London), 1976, *76,* 125.

Herpesvirus-Induced Feline Urolithiasis

During the course of studies on feline urolithiasis, three viruses were isolated from natural cases. The viruses were a feline calicivirus, a feline syncytium-forming virus, and a previously undescribed feline herpesvirus (4). It would appear that this herpesvirus may play a significant role in the urolithiasis syndrome of domestic cats.

An excellent review on urolithiasis in cats was written by Fabricant (2), and this section largely reflects the information available in that review.

Character of the Disease. The disease has a wide geographic distribution including areas in the United States and Europe. Cases occur more frequently in the cold months of the year. Although the disease is assumed to occur in cats fed dry food, cats on a variety of diets contract the disease.

It may occur as an acute disease. The stones or sandy particles that occur most frequently have been identified as triple ammonium magnesium phosphates (struvite). Blockage results in retention of urine and uremia. Death may ensue as a result of a ruptured bladder or azotemia. In cats that recover the condition often recurs.

The etiology of the urolithiasis is complex, and many factors including diet, metabolic disorders, anatomical and physiological reasons, and infection have been suggested as important causes (2). Some or all of these factors may play a role either in primary or secondary ways. Rich (6) eliminated struvite crystals, pH, and bacterial infection as primary causes of the syndrome. After reproducing the disease in conventionally reared male cats with multiple inoculations of filtered urine from obstructed cats, he suspected a possible viral etiology. This led to a series of experiments first in conventionally reared cats and later in specific pathogen-free cats; the conclusion was that the feline herpesvirus alone produces urolithiasis in all of its manifestations (Figure 44.19), but clinical signs of the disease developed earlier with more urinary tract complications when experimental specific pathogen-free cats were inoculated with a feline calicivirus and the feline herpesvirus (1, 2, 7). The significance of the syncytium-forming feline virus as a complicating factor in the disease has not been established yet (2).

Properties of the Virus. The feline herpesvirus associated with this disease has all the physical, chemical, and biological properties of a herpesvirus (4). The average diameter of the viral particles is 115 nm as determined by electron microscopy. The virus is inactivated by ether and chloroform. The nucleic acid was identified as DNA.

This new feline herpesvirus is neutralized by its

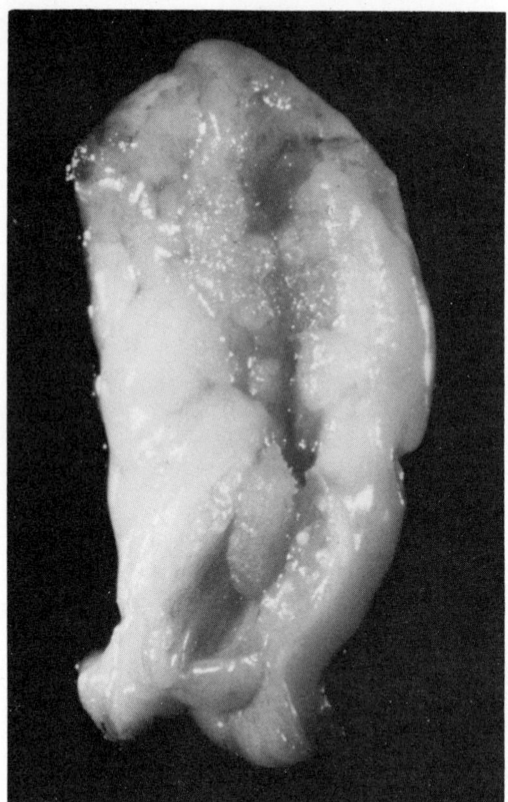

Figure 44.19. Section of urethral plugs from an experimental specific-pathogen-free cat inoculated with feline herpesvirus 2 (cell-associated). (From Catherine G. Fabricant, *Comparative Immunology, Microbiology and Infectious Diseases,* 1979, *1,* 121–34.)

homologous antiserum. At dilutions of 1:2 antisera of various animal herpesviruses including feline rhinotracheitis and herpes simplex failed to neutralize this new feline herpesvirus. As a consequence it should be considered as a candidate in the family herpesviridae as feline herpesvirus 2.

Cultivation. The virus is strongly cell-associated, and viral titers in infected cell cultures prepared by sonically disrupting the supernatant and residual cells varied from $TCID_{50}$ $10^{4.8}$ to $10^{5.8}$ per 0.1 ml.

The cytopathic changes in the Crandell feline kidney cell line and in autogenous heart, bladder, and kidney cell cultures included condensation and reticulation of the nuclear chromatin, often with bizarre nucleolar changes and enlarged and transformed cells. Intranuclear inclusion bodies were seen, but differed from the noted feline herpesvirus 1. Infected cell sheets remained to culture flask surfaces for months without a change of medium, whereas cell sheets or uninoculated cultures detached from the surface in 4 to 8 weeks.

This virus also has induced several types of chemical crystals intracellularly (Figure 44.20) and extracellularly as well as the formation of "tissue culture calculi," a unique finding (5). Cholesterol has been identified as one of the crystals in cell culture (3).

Immunity. There is still a great gap in our knowledge as it relates to the protection this virus may provide to cats against urolithiasis. There is strong evidence to suggest that natural virus persists in cats and under certain conditions the herpesvirus can be triggered by some other mechanism such as another feline virus. Obviously, studies are required to determine the immune mechanism and how it might possibly be manipulated to the advantage of the cat. It is clear that neutralizing antibodies are produced, but in low titer. The role of cell-mediated immunity is entirely lacking, but it is reasonable to expect that its mechanism is similar to other herpesviruses.

Transmission. The virus readily transmits from an infected cat to a susceptible cat. The exact mechanism is unknown, although it is speculated that viral aerosols are produced by cats shedding the virus in the urine (2).

Diagnosis. The diagnosis of the disease in males is simple as the signs of illness are typical. The incidence of the disease may be much higher in females than is generally recognized. The anatomical differences in the two sexes are responsible; castration and the long narrow uretha in males are important factors accounting for urethral blockage by calculi.

Figure 44.20. Intracellular phosphatelike crystals formed in a cell infected with feline herpesvirus 2 (cell-associated). Stained with May-Gruenwald-Giemsa. × 58. (From Catherine G. Fabricant. *Comparative Immunology, Microbiology and Infectious Diseases,* 1979, *1,* 121–34.)

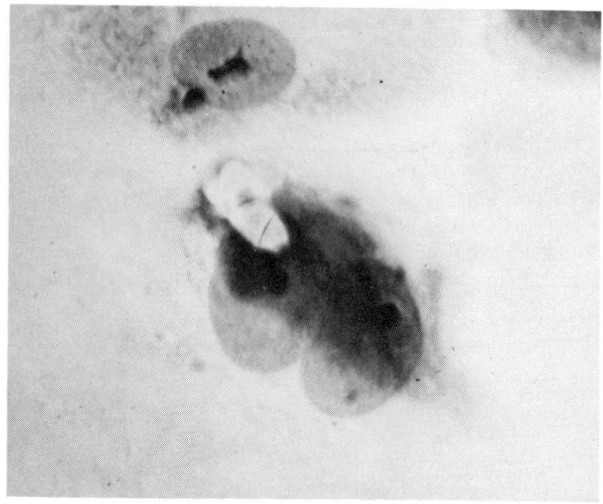

Control. At present herpes-induced feline urolithiasis presents a difficult problem to the veterinary profession. It is a major disease that defies control as long as cats are allowed to have contact with other members of the same species. It is a particular problem in catteries where close contact is constant. This is not the only problem, though; there is evidence that the virus may persist in the ovaries of carrier cats, so vertical transmission also occurs. Horizontal transmission occurs as well, and carrier queens may readily transmit the virus to their nursing progeny. There is good field evidence to support this statement.

Until we learn more about the etiology of the urolithiasis syndrome, we must assume that an infectious agent(s) may be involved and recommend that catteries practice some degree of isolation when a queen is nursing her kittens.

Disease in Man. There is no evidence that this virus causes disease in man.

REFERENCES

1. Fabricant. Am. Jour. Vet. Res., 1977, *38,* 1837.
2. Fabricant. Comp. Immun. Microbiol. Inf. Dis., 1979, *1,* 121.
3. Fabricant, Krook, and Gillespie. Science, 1973, *181,* 566.
4. Fabricant and Gillespie. Inf. and Immun., 1974, *9,* 460.
5. Fabricant, Gillespie, and Krook. Inf. and Immun., 1971, *3,* 416.
6. Rich. Ph.D. thesis, Cornell University, 1969, p. 51.
7. Rich, Fabricant, and Gillespie. Cornell Vet., 1971, *61,* 542.

THE SUBFAMILY GAMMAHERPESVIRINAE

Malignant Catarrhal Fever

SYNONYMS: Malignant head catarrh of cattle, *snotsiekte* (South Africa), bovine epitheliosis; abbreviation, MCF

Malignant catarrhal fever of cattle is, in Europe and America, a sporadic disease, characterized by a short febrile period, inflammation of the mucous membranes of the mouth, nose, and eyes, nervous signs, and a high death rate. The causative agent is a herpesvirus. The disease that exists in Africa is believed to be the same as that occurring elsewhere, but there the disease occurs in epizootics and is more readily transmitted by inoculation. Differential diagnosis of this disease is very difficult, and more than one disease may now be included in this category.

This is a disease of cattle. Sheep and African wildebeests can also be infected, but the signs in these species are vague or absent. Mettam (9) found that wildebeests carried virus without signs of illness and served as the source of outbreaks in cattle. Many Europeans have noted that outbreaks in cattle have frequently followed association with sheep and have thought that the latter carried the virus. Stenius (22), who made an extensive study of the disease in Finland, is one of the latest workers to support the hypothesis that sheep often serve as the reservoir of infection for cattle, but in limited trials Kalunda could not substantiate these findings with the African strain of MCFV (6). It is clear, however, that natural disease occurs in cattle that have had no contact with sheep.

In North America the disease is generally seen in the late autumn and early spring months. Most cases occur in any one herd during a single season. On some farms the disease appears regularly, season after season, occasioning severe losses over a period of years (1). Marshall *et al.* (8) described one outbreak in a large herd that began in the fall and continued until spring. A total of 31 animals died. The disease has been reported in most of the countries of Europe, in South and Central Africa, and in North America.

Neutralizing antibodies to an African strain of MCF were detected in sera from 8 wildebeest from Kenya, 5 of 36 sheep in Australia, and 3 of 6 bovine sera that recovered from MCF-like disease. One of the positive cattle was from New York and 2 from Australia (6). The significance of these results is unclear, but it strongly suggests more sera from U.S. and Australian cattle should be tested for neutralizing antibodies against the African virus.

Character of the Disease. The natural disease begins with a febrile reaction which lasts only 1 or 2 days. During this time the animal refuses feed and water and is greatly depressed. Inflammation of the mucous membranes of the mouth, nasal passages, and eyes appears early (Figure 44.21). Generally there is photophobia, lacrimation, injection of the sclera, cloudiness of the cornea, and even ulceration. There are erosions on the soft palate and tongue with blunting and loss of some conical buccal papillae (Figures 44.22 and 44.23). The nasal mucosa becomes deep red, edematous, and covered with a fibrinopurulent exudate. Because of partial closure of the air passages the animals may have some difficulty in breathing. Ulceration of the nasal mucosa

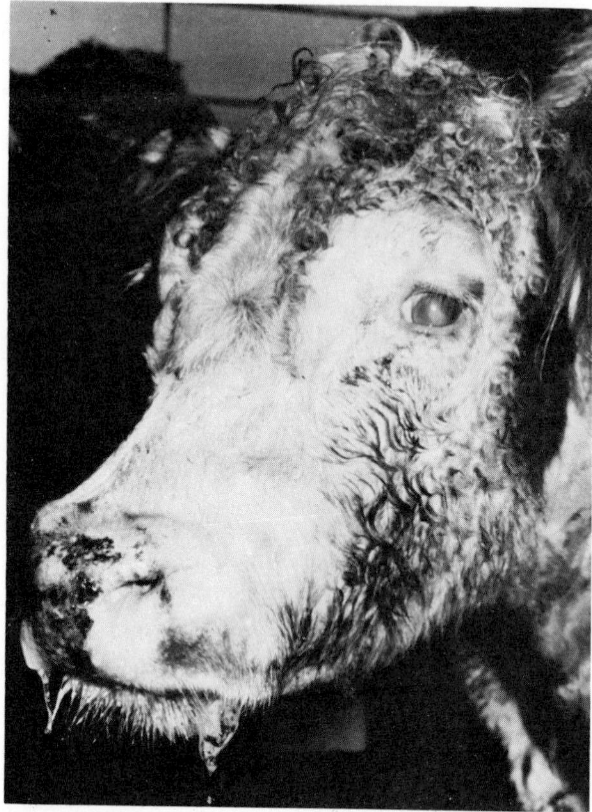

Figure 44.21. Head of a steer infected with an African isolate of malignant catarrhal fever virus. Some characteristic signs are corneal opacity, necrotic skin and exudate on the muzzle, and some slobbering. (Courtesy D. A. Gregg, Plum Island Animal Disease Center, USDA.)

occurs occasionally with hemorrhage, and the breath becomes fetid. A similar process occurs in the mouth and pharynx. Fibrinopurulent pneumonia may occur, if the animal lives long enough.

Nervous signs develop early in most cases. Usually they take the form of great depression or stupor, but sometimes there are signs of excitement. The animal may grind its teeth, bellow, and even charge other animals and human attendants. The victims become dehydrated and lose condition very rapidly.

According to Mettam (9), the incubation period of the African disease, experimentally produced by inoculation, varies from 10 to 34 days. Blood, Rowsell, and Savan (3) in 1961 made four successful transfers in cattle, and the incubation period was 9 to 44 days.

The course of the disease varies greatly. Some of the peracute cases may result in death in 24 hours or less. In the "head and eye" form, the form that is most readily diagnosed and therefore reported most often, the course varies from 5 to 14 days, but a few cases (20) may last much longer. The mortality rate is always high. Goss, Cole, and Kissling (4) reported 16 deaths in 18 sporadic cases. Others report even higher rates.

Except the lesions referable to the general effects of fever, they are largely those of the mucous membranes of the head already described. The dark, swollen, glassy membranes of the turbinates and nasal sinuses are covered with shreds of fibrin and a dirty purulent secretion. Shallow ulcers generally are found on these surfaces. Similar lesions are found in the larynx, trachea, and the larger bronchi, and there may be areas of bronchopneumonia in the anterior lung lobes. The lymph nodes of the head are generally swollen. The mucous membrane of the abomasum often is inflamed, edematous, and sometimes eroded, and there may be similar lesions in the small intestine.

The meninges of the brain often are congested and may show hemorrhages, but the brain itself is usually normal in appearance. Histologically, however, there are lesions of a nonpurulent encephalitis of the virus type, associated in some cases with acidophilic inclusion bodies. Some of the earlier workers reported finding inclusion bodies in the nerve cells of cattle dying from this disease. German workers found intranuclear bodies quite like those found in Borna disease in horses, and the suggestion was even made that this disease might be the same. This idea has not been confirmed elsewhere. Goss, Cole, and Kissling (4) reported the finding of acidophilic, cytoplasmic inclusions bodies in many of the epithelial cells. No confirmation of these findings has appeared. Stenius (22) reported the finding, in all of 50 cases examined, of acidophilic inclusions in degenerated motor neurons, especially in the vagoglossopharyngeal nucleus, and more sparsely in other areas in the medulla oblongata and elsewhere in the brain. These were seen by Schofield (21) and used to diagnose a case of the disease in which the clinical appearances were atypical.

Piercy, (10, 11) and others in Africa apparently have had no particular difficulty in transmitting the disease to cattle, especially when lymph node material has been used for inoculation. According to Kalunda the highest concentration of virus is in the lymph nodes (6). Blood and other organ suspensions also usually transmitted the disease. In one experiment Piercy passed one strain through 19 generations of cattle. In 1961, Blood *et al.* in Canada made four serial transfers in cattle with infective blood (3). Of 41 cows inoculated, all but one contracted the disease. Stenius (22) inoculated a number of sheep

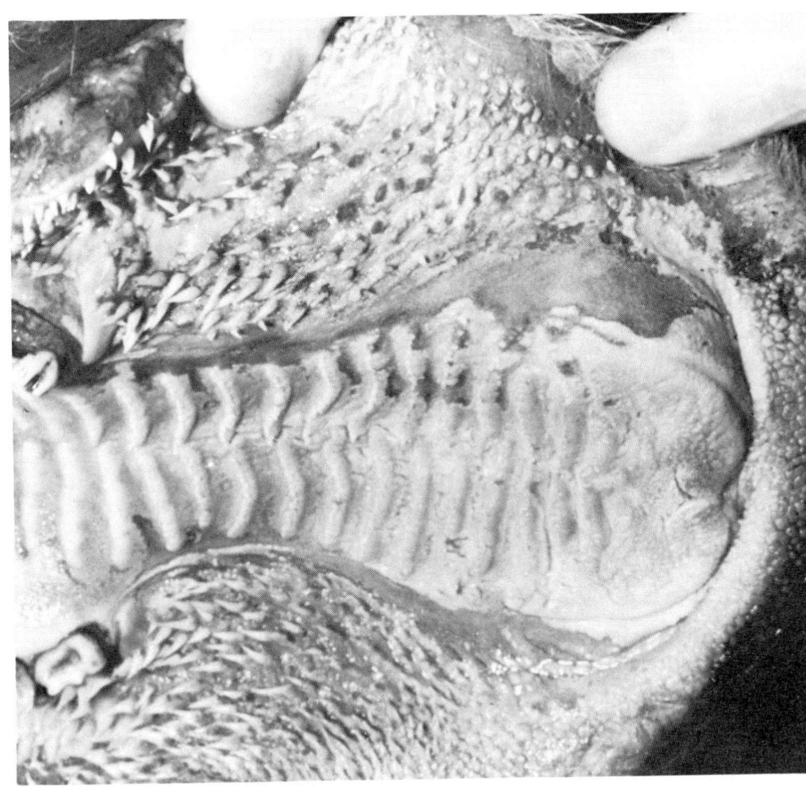

Figure 44.22. Palate and buccal mucosa from a steer infected with an African isolate of malignant catarrhal fever virus. There are erosions on the head and soft palate with blunting and loss of some conical buccal papillae. (Courtesy D. A. Gregg, Plum Island Animal Disease Center, USDA.)

with tissues from diseased cattle and a number of cattle with tissues from the infected sheep. In sheep, he produced an inapparent disease; however, characteristic lesions of a virus encephalitis were present. In cattle, mild lesions of catarrhal fever were produced with materials derived from the infected sheep. Piercy (13), although producing circumstantial evidence that sheep could carry the virus of this disease and serve as the source of bovine outbreaks, was not successful in finding the virus in sheep under natural conditions.

MCF infection was readily reproduced in the United States cattle with the African virus. Forty-seven showed the head and eye form, three had mild signs, and three had inapparent infection. Twenty-eight died (6). Piercy

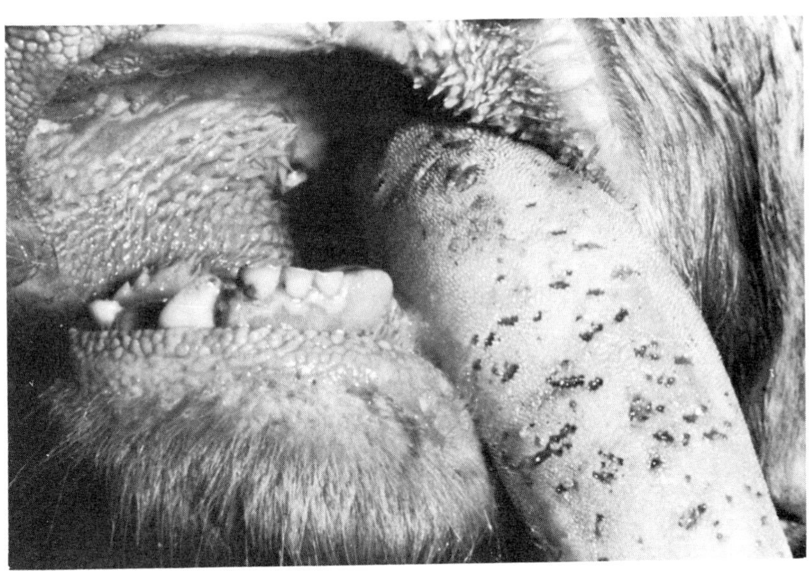

Figure 44.23. Multiple erosions on the tongue of a steer infected with an African isolate of malignant catarrhal fever virus. (Courtesy D. A. Gregg, Plum Island Animal Disease Center, USDA.)

(13) reported that he had been successful on three separate occasions in adapting a bovine strain to rabbits. The response of this species was mild. Plowright (15), employing one of Piercy's strains, reports that in rabbits there was a febrile reaction followed by a mild leukocytosis in nine instances, a mild leukopenia in three, and no blood change in two. In all cases there was an increase in the nongranular cells during the reaction. Using his African strain, Kalunda and coworkers (5) infected guinea pigs, rabbits, and hamsters all of which showed abnormal discharges, paralysis, and death.

The experimental disease in the wildebeest was studied by Plowright (16, 17). A viremic state persisted in one wildebeest calf for 31 weeks and in the other one for 8 weeks. Neither calf showed signs of illness. Bovine calves maintained in contact with the first wildebeest calf during the early weeks of infection (2 to 12) developed typical malignant head catarrh. In conjunction with these studies cultural isolation was made from 7 percent (9) of 282 blood samples from wildebeests in Northern Tanganyika. Some calves were probably infected *in utero* as they were viremic during the first week of life. Transplacental infection occurred as virus was isolated from a fetal spleen.

Properties of the Virus. The virus of this disease is not readily filterable, and some authors, Mettam (9) for example, denied the filterability of the agent and yet believed it is a virus. In blood the virus is closely attached to the cells and cannot be washed off them. Piercy (11) believes the causative agent adheres to the leukocytes. Piercy (12) found it exceedingly difficult to preserve the agent of this disease for more than a few days. Storage at temperatures varying from 5 C to −60 C, lyophilization, and shell-freezing with dry ice and alcohol all failed to preserve viability for more than a very short time. All freezing methods actually seemed destructive to the virus. The best results were achieved with citrated blood stored at 5 C.

Armstrong (2) suggested that this virus was a herpesvirus after electron microscope studies of its structure. Extended studies by E. M. Kalunda (7), clearly showed the presence of viral capsids and enveloped particles in the nuclei of infected bovine thyroid cell cultures. Enveloped particles also were seen in cytoplasmic vacuoles and extracellular space quite characteristic of herpesviruses (Figure 44.24).

Neutralizing, complement-fixing, and precipitating

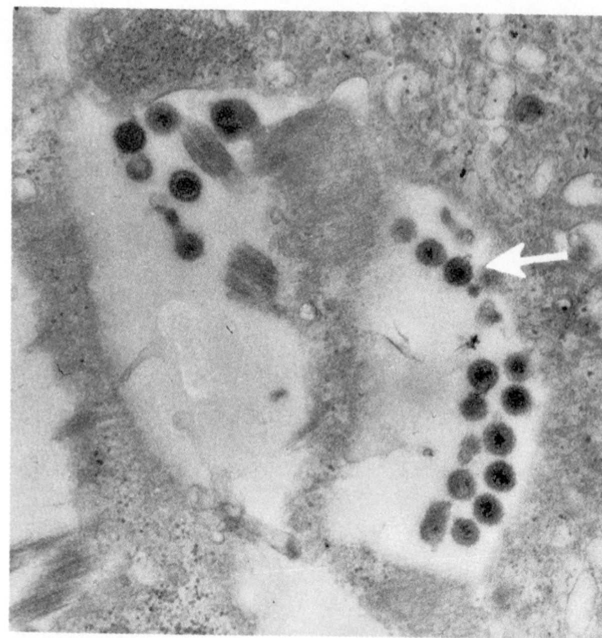

Figure 44.24. An electron microscope photograph showing MCF viral particles (*arrow*) of an African strain inoculated into a bovine thyroid cell culture 8 days previously. × 24,900. (Courtesy S. S. Breese, Plum Island Animal Disease Center, USDA.)

antibodies have been demonstrated in chronic cases and recovered cattle infected with an African isolate (6).

The etiology of MCF in the United States is unclear. Various viruses have been isolated from cattle with MCF, but their role in the production of the disease is uncertain (23).

Cultivation. Plowright, Ferris, and Scott (18) reported that the virus could be grown in thyroid or adrenal gland cultures. Cowdry's type A inclusion bodies and syncytia are produced in these cell cultures. After several cell-culture transfers, the virus could be transferred to calf kidney cultures in which 19 successful passages were made. The adapted virus also grew in cultures of sheep thyroid, calf testis or adrenal gland, and in wildebeest, and rabbit kidney.

Immunity. Because the African strains replicate in cell culture and produce pathologic alterations, it is possible to develop more information about the disease. Herpesvirus isolates associated with MCF-infected cattle in Colorado did not produce disease in experimental cattle and clearly are not related to an African strain of MCF (6). Experimental cattle that recover after inoculation with this African strain have neutralizing, complement-fixing, and precipitating antibodies. Piercy (14) reports that cattle recovering from the natural or artificially produced disease with African virus are resistant to reinfection for periods as long as 4 to 8 months and even longer. He tried a formalinized tissue vaccine and found that his vaccinated animals did not acquire sufficient immunity to resist inoculation of virus, but they appeared to resist field exposure better than others. In contrast, cattle immunized against the herpesvirus of MCF with cell-cultured living or inactivated virus (combined with Freund's adjuvant) produced neutralizing antibody titers, but were susceptible to challenge with virulent virus given parenterally. In a controlled field trial vaccinated cattle showed no evidence of protection against natural challenge by exposure to wildebeest herds (19).

Immunity to the disease as it occurs in North America has been impossible to evaluate because few animals survive the disease, and the precise etiology still has not been ascertained.

Transmission. Transmission occurred when cattle were placed in direct contact with wildebeests in the early stage of infection (17). Attempts to transmit the disease from diseased cattle to contact cattle failed despite the presence of virus in excretions of diseased animals. In this limited trial there was evidence that some contact animals became infected as one calf had a febrile reaction and developed neutralizing antibodies and two others showed resistance to challenge (6). It is known that cattle can be readily infected by the respiratory route. Clearly more studies of this nature must be done to elucidate transmission of this disease.

Some of the African workers believe that arthropods may play a role in transmitting the disease, but the disease in cattle located in North America occurs only during the cold months.

Diagnosis. The specific diagnosis of this disease can be a difficult problem. The clinical signs are similar to those of a composite of diseases that in recent years have been labeled "the mucosal diseases." The sporadic character of malignant catarrhal fever, the presence of eye lesions in most cases, and evidence of encephalitic changes associated with the typical disease tend to differentiate it from the other diseases characterized by mouth, nasal, and intestinal lesions, all much alike.

Control. The sporadic nature of the disease would make control measures difficult even if effective methods were known. In the present state of our knowledge nothing can be done to prevent the development of cases, and therapeutic treatment is hopeless. If multiple cases are occurring on the same premises, and if sheep are also kept, complete separation of the two species should be tried because the cattle may be acquiring the disease from the sheep.

The Disease in Man. No evidence has been found to indicate that man is infected with the agent of this disease.

REFERENCES

1. Anonymous. 31st Ann. Rpt., N. Dak. Livestock Sanit. Bd., 1937, p. 15.
2. Armstrong. Quoted by Andrewes, Christopher, in Viruses of vertebrates. Williams and Wilkins, Baltimore, 1964, p. 233.
3. Blood, Rowsell, and Savan. Can. Vet. Jour., 1961, *2*, 319.
4. Goss, Cole, and Kissling. Am. Jour. Path., 1947, *23*, 837.
5. Kalunda. Ph.D. thesis, Cornell University, 1975.
6. Kalunda, Dardiri, and Lee. Personal communication, 1980.
7. Kalunda, Ferris, and Dardiri. Personal communication, 1980.
8. Marshall, Munce, Barnes, and Boerner. Jour. Am. Vet. Med. Assoc., 1919-20, *56*, 570.
9. Mettam. 9th and 10th Rpts., Dir. Vet. Educ. and Res., Univ. So. Africa, 1923, p. 393.
10. Piercy. Brit. Vet. Jour., 1952, *108*, 35.
11. Piercy, Brit. Vet. Jour., 1952, *108*, 214.
12. Piercy. Brit. Vet. Jour., 1953, *109*, 59.
13. Piercy. Proc. 15th Internatl. Vet. Cong. (Stockholm), 1953, vol. I, p. 528.
14. Piercy. Brit. Vet. Jour., 1954, *110*, 87.
15. Plowright. Jour. Comp. Path. and Therap., 1953, *63*, 318.
16. Plowright. Res. Vet. Sci., 1965, *6*, 56.
17. Plowright. Res. Vet. Sci., 1965, *6*, 69.
18. Plowright, Ferris, and Scott. Nature, 1960, *188*, 1167.
19. Plowright, Herniman, Jessett, Kalunda, and Rampton. Res. Vet. Sci., 1975, *19*, 159.
20. Rines and Barner. Mich. State Coll. Vet., 1955, *15*, 108.
21. Schofield. Rpt. Ontario Vet. Coll., 1950, p. 104.
22. Stenius. Monograph, Bovine malignant catarrh. Inst. Path., Vet. Coll., Helsinki, 1952.
23. Storz, Okuna, McChesney, and Pierson. Am. Jour. Vet. Res., 1976, *37*, 875.

Pulmonary Adenomatosis in Sheep

SYNONYMS: Ovine jaagsiekte (South Africa), progressive pneumonia of sheep, "lungers"

The disease has been recognized in certain parts of continental Europe, in Peru, in Iceland (3), in South Africa (7), in Israel, in India, and in the northern range states of the United States (5). In the United States herders refer to the disease as lungers.

Clinically diseased animals are usually breeding animals, 4 years of age or older. Lesions may be found in younger animals, but in most cases they are not sufficiently advanced to cause signs. When a large portion of the air space of the lungs has been obliterated, the victims become dyspneic. These generally die within a few days to several weeks from anoxia. There are no recoveries from this disease, but many affected animals are marketed before it becomes advanced and general emaciation has occurred.

This is a chronic, progressive disease in which the lungs lose their elasticity due to proliferation of cells in the supporting tissue and gradually the alveoli become filled with proliferating cells causing consolidation of the pulmonary parenchyma; thus it is recognized as a primary lung neoplasm that is transmissible and may be caused by a member of the herpesvirus group. The tumor is carcinomatous in nature and does metastize.

It is a bronchiolar-alveolar cell carcinoma. A-type and C-type viruses were observed in advanced tumors but not in early lesions. Numerous microtubules were found in epithelial tumor cells of early lesions. In advanced tumors cytosome production, surfactant secretion, and glycogen accumulation were observed (4).

The disease has been transmitted with an epithelial cell line derived from lung lesions of a natural case and subcultured *in vitro* for almost 2 years (1). Incubation periods of 10 weeks were recorded when newborn lambs were given intratracheal administration of cells following immunosuppressive therapy. Evidence also was obtained that natural transmission may result from inhalation of viable cells. Cross *et al.* (2) have some evidence that vertical transmission may occur.

In the past some scientists have felt maedi virus may be responsible for pulmonary carcinoma in sheep. Maedi virus clearly is not implicated because no homology sequence was detected when radioactively labeled DNA complementary to the RNA of maedi virus was used to probe for homologous RNA in the polysome fraction of pulmonary carcinomas of Awassi sheep (6).

There is no known way of controlling this disease. Generally, the affected animals are removed from the flocks as soon as they are recognized, for such animals are never profitable to keep and they may spread the disease.

REFERENCES

1. Coetzee, Els, and Verwoerd. Onderstepoort Jour. Vet. Res., 1976, *43,* 133.
2. Cross, Smith, and Moorhead. Am. Jour. Vet. Res., 1975, *36,* 465.
3. Dungal, Gislason, and Taylor. Jour. Comp. Path. and Therap., 1938, *51,* 46.
4. Hod, Herz, and Zimber. Am. Jour. Path., 1977, *86,* 545.
5. Marsh. Jour. Am. Vet. Med. Assoc., 1923, *62,* 458.
6. Perk and Yaniv. Res. Vet. Sci., 1978, *24,* 46.
7. Robertson. Jour. Comp. Path. and Therap., 1904, *17,* 221.

Marek's Disease

SYNONYMS: Polyneuritis, neuritis, neurolymphomatosis, range-paralysis, neural leukosis, skin leukosis, gray eye, fish eye, iritis, and uveitis; abbreviation. MD

There is now rather good proof that two virus groups are involved in the production of the various forms of the avian leukosis complex (1). One group of isolates termed lymphoid leukosis virus, a retrovirus, produces visceral lymphomatosis, erythroblastosis, myeloblastosis, and possibly osteopetrosis (20). In 1962 it was proposed that the nephroblastoma produced by the BAI strain A should be considered an additional tumor in this group (19). The virus strains of the Marek group cause neurolymphomatosis, ocular lymphomatosis, and to a lesser degree a form of visceral lymphomatosis. All the various forms included in the complex have been reproduced by experimental inoculation of filtrates.

The majority of the so-called avian leukosis cases are caused by the avian herpesvirus, a member of the subfamily Gammaherpesvirinae. The chicken is the primary host for the virus, but it also is found in turkeys, pheasants, and possibly quail. Similar lesions are observed in the pigeon, duck, goose, canary, budgerigar, and swan (21). The economic loss in chickens as a result of Marek's disease (MD) is extremely high, and it is a major disease of chicken flocks throughout the world. It is an acute fulminating type of oncogenic disease in young chicks that spreads quite rapidly.

An excellent review article was written recently by Calnek (2). Our knowledge has progressed from the point of complete ignorance regarding the etiology of MD to virtual control of this oncogenic disease by vaccination, saving the poultry industry millions of dollars each year. It is the first oncogenic disease controlled by vaccination. It also serves as an important model for studying viral and host factors which influence the outcome of infection by an oncogenic herpesvirus.

Character of the Disease. Marek's disease consists of inflammatory and neoplastic lesions. It affects primarily the nervous system, but visceral organs and other tissues may also be involved. The disease is seen most often in young birds about the time they are turned out on the range, but it sometimes occurs as early as 3 or 4 weeks and sometimes after a year of age. The disease is manifested by a flaccid or spastic paralysis of a leg, wing, or, less commonly, the neck. Sometimes both legs or wings are affected, but more commonly the disease is unilateral. The affected wing droops and may brush the ground as the bird walks. Affected legs usually are stretched forward or backward, and, when the disease has progressed far, the bird is unable to stand or walk. When the neck is affected, the head is depressed or there may be twisting (torticollis). The location and intensity of the paralysis vary widely in different birds in the same flock.

The gross lesions consist of a grayish white swelling of localized areas of the principal nerve trunks of the region involved. When there is leg involvement, this swelling generally is found in the sciatic nerve on the inside of the thigh. By comparing the size of the nerve trunks on the two sides of the bird, even small tumors can be detected, but generally the growths are sufficiently great to be readily observed. Histological examination of the swollen nerve trunks shows extensive infiltration of small round cells, which generally cannot be distinguished from lymphocytes but sometimes appear like mononuclear cells or histiocytes. The lesion may be edematous, and there may be myelin degeneration of the nerve sheaths, but degeneration of the neuraxons is not conspicuous.

The Marek group of viruses is probably responsible for ocular lymphomatosis. The disease is manifested by a diffuse bluish gray fading of the iris of one or both eyes. Depigmentation sometimes occurs in a spotty fashion and sometimes in the form of annular fading. The pupils frequently become irregular in outline. Histologically infiltrations of lymphocytic or mononuclear cells are found in the iris, and often there are similar infiltrations in the optic nerve. This form of the disease usually occurs in flocks affected with neurolymphomatosis, but the condition generally appears later in life. Many pathologists consider that it represents a latent form of neurolymphomatosis.

The visceral form of lymphoid tumors commonly involves the gonad, liver, lung, and skin. All degrees of severity are seen. In the most acute forms the disease may be observed in birds as early as 6 to 8 weeks of age. Morbidity and mortality may exceed 50 percent of the flock. The disease also may occur in older birds.

The pathogenesis of this disease is reasonably well known (2). Inhalation is the usual means of entry. It is speculated that virus is transmitted by macrophages to lymphoid tissues. Virus replication can be found in the spleen, thymus, and bursa of Fabricius within 3 days. The early infection is characterized by inflammatory, necrotic, and cytolytic (of lymphocytes) pathological changes. When viral activity wanes in the lymphoid organs during the 2nd week of infection, a variety of other tissues, notably those of epithelial origin, become infected. Focal necrosis and intranuclear inclusion bodies may be seen in many organs including the kidney, pancreas, and adrenal gland. In general, infection of the epithelial cells exhibits the productive-restrictive type. The feather follicle epithelium deserves special attention because it is the only tissue in which fully infectious virus particles are released more than 2 weeks after infection, and it represents the mechanism by which the disease is transmitted to susceptible birds (3, 12). The ultimate event is the development of gross tumors in a variety of tissues described above. The neoplastic element of lymphomas is a transformed thymus-derived T lymphoblast.

Recently Fabricant *et al.* (13) reported that grossly occlusive atherosclerosis was observed in a significant number (24 percent) of chickens during a 7-month period after a strain of relatively low oncogenicity was inoculated in newly hatched specific pathogen-free chicks. The lesion type and distribution resembled those seen in human chronic arteriosclerosis. The mechanism of induction is not understood, but the investigators suggested that oncogenic transformation of arterial smooth muscle cells, or a response to direct insult by the virus or to indirect insult by immune complexes, should be considered.

Properties of the Virus. The herpesvirus of Marek's disease belongs to the cytomegalovirus group of cell-associated herpesviruses. All field isolates appear to be antigenically identical as they cross-react in the agar-gel precipitin and fluorescent antibody tests (6, 15); however, some are altered somewhat after cell culture passage (8). A herpesvirus isolated from turkeys is antigenically similar to Marek's disease virus and is nonpathogenic for chickens and turkeys (22). Information

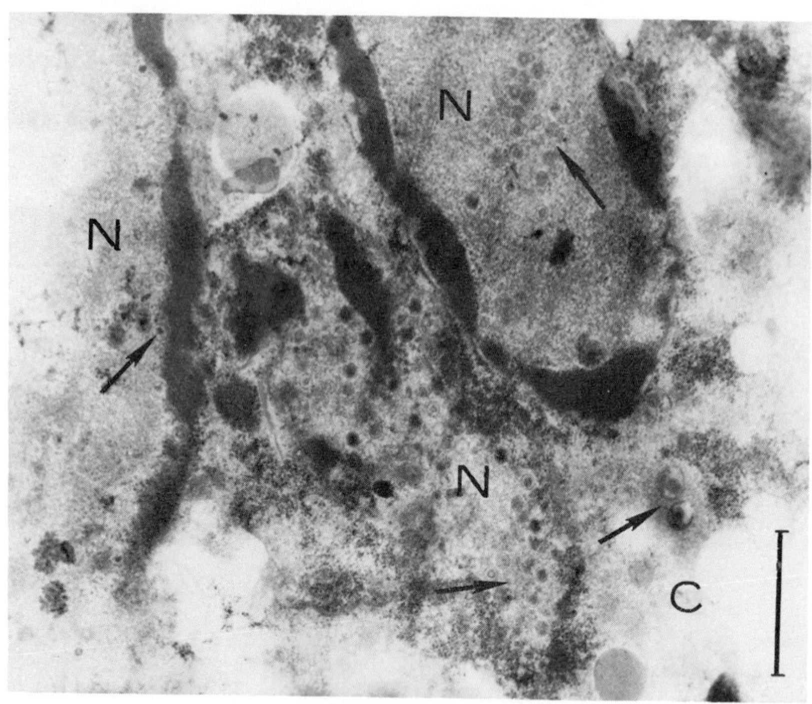

Figure 44.25. Marek's disease. In the nucleus (*N*) naked, incomplete virions are found, but in the cytoplasm (*C*) of the infected feather follicle numerous enveloped particles are observed. Scale—micron. (Courtesy B. Calnek.)

about the biological characteristics of many strains is given by Calnek (2).

The DNA virus particles are 85 to 100 nm in diameter, and the capsid has 162 hollow cylindrical capsomeres. The particles from feather follicles have a similar morphology but a loose irregular envelope up to 400 nm in diameter (Figure 44.25). The extracted DNA has a high guanine-cytosine content.

Marek's disease virus is highly cell-associated, and whole cells must be used as inoculum from all of the infected bird's tissues except from the feather follicles where the virus is excreted (4) (Figure 44.25). Storage of virus-containing cells requires conditions essential for their preservation—the addition of dimethyl-sulfoxide, slow freezing, and holding preferably at 196 C. Viral preparations from feather follicles remain infectious after lyophilization and maintenance at room temperature.

Antibody can be demonstrated in serums of recovered birds by agar-gel precipitin (6), indirect fluorescent antibody (15) or passive hemagglutination tests (12). In the precipitin test up to 6 lines may form; the major line (15) referred to as the precipitin line. This test is most widely used for the detection of antibody to Marek's disease. The indirect fluorescent antibody test is used to distinguish between Marek's disease and the herpesvirus of turkeys.

Cultivation. Marek's disease virus produces cytopathic effect plaques in duck embryo fibroblasts and in chick kidney cell cultures consisting of rounded, highly refractile cells or syncytia or both (Figure 44.26) (7, 18). The plaques appear in 6 to 14 days and consist of rounded and fusiform cells and polykaryocytes containing Cowdry type A intranuclear inclusion bodies. Naked and occasionally enveloped virus particles are seen in the nucleus of the infected cells and occasionally in the cytoplasm.

The virus produces pocks on the chorioallantoic membrane route. The yolk-sac route is preferred.

Immunity. Although there is no effective immunity to infection, resistance of chickens to tumor formation may be affected by the genetic line of the chicken (10, 11), age of infection (17), antibody status of the dam (5), and exposure to avirulent viruses (9, 16, 22). The resistance of chickens to tumor formation may be evaluated by intra-abdominal challenge with virulent virus or by exposure to infected chickens. To be a valid test, known susceptible controls must be challenged in a similar manner at the same time. A satisfactory challenge response is achieved in 6 to 20 weeks depending on the virulence of the challenge virus, age of chicken, and the susceptibility of the chick line (14).

Passive immunity conferred by the dam may persist for 3 weeks after hatching. It will delay the onset and reduce the incidence of disease in birds challenged at 1 day of age by a natural route. It has little effect when birds are challenged intra-abdominally (5).

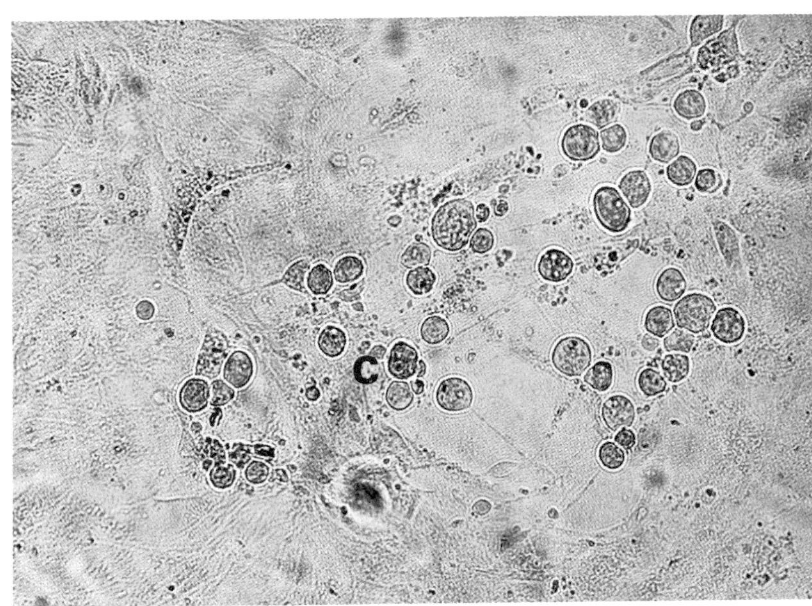

Figure 44.26. Cytopathic effect (*C*) caused by Marek's virus in chicken kidney cell culture, unstained. × 240. (Courtesy B. Calnek and S. Madin, *Am. Jour. Vet. Res.*)

The indirect-hemagglutination antibody titer of chickens infected with Marek's disease virus suggests a direct relationship with the chicken's ability to survive the disease (12).

Transmission. Most birds have antibody to Marek's disease by the time of maturity. Infection persists in birds for long periods of time, possibly for life. Congenital (vertical) infection probably does not occur, so embryos and young chicks are free of virus and susceptible. Consequently, transmission of the disease occurs after the maternal immunity subsides by 3 weeks of age and by exposure to infected chickens or an environment with persisting virus in excreta, litter, and poultry house dust.

Diagnosis. Gross and/or microscopic lesions in nerves or viscera, presence of specific antigen in feather follicles demonstrated by immunofluorescence test, virus isolation in cell culture, or demonstration of antibody are all suitable methods of diagnosis.

Virus isolation can be made in cell culture with infected cells or with virus from feather follicles, but it is 10- to 1,000-fold less sensitive than chicken inoculation (23). Direct cultivation of cells in culture from test chickens is more sensitive than inoculation of cell suspensions on monolayers of susceptible cell cultures.

If the passive hemagglutination test is used, a positive serum has a titer of 1:16 or greater (12). The agar-gel test is most widely used for detection of antibody and also for distinguishing between virulent and attenuated tissue cultured strains.

Control. Present knowledge makes it possible to develop a flock that is free of Marek's disease virus. Such flocks can be kept free of the infection by strict isolation, constant surveillance, and frequent monitoring for virus and antibody.

Three types of commercial vaccines now available are extremely effective. These are (*a*) attenuated oncogenic MD virus, (*b*) naturally apathogenic turkey herpesvirus antigenically related to MDV, and (*c*) naturally apathogenic or nononcogenic MDV. More information about these vaccines is available elsewhere. All vaccines are given subcutaneously. The significant immune responses are probably T-cell mediated since an immunosuppressive drug, Cy, interferes with vaccination response only during the transient period when the drug suppresses T-cell activities. It is clear that the immune responses appear to be aimed at both viral and tumor antigens.

The Disease in Man. It is not known to occur.

REFERENCES

1. Biggs. Brit. Vet. Jour., 1961, *117*, 326.
2. Calnek, Bruce. Marek's disease virus and lymphoma. *In* Oncogenic herpesviruses, ed. Fred Rapp. CRC Press, Inc., West Palm Beach, Florida, 1980.
3. Calnek, Adldinger, and Kahn. Avian Dis., 1970, *14*, 219.
4. Calnek and Hitchner. Jour. Natl. Cancer Inst., 1969, *43*, 935.
5. Chubb and Churchill. Vet. Rec., 1969, *85*, 303.
6. Chubb and Churchill. Vet. Rec., 1968, *83*, 4.
7. Churchill and Biggs. Nature, 1967, *215*, 528.
8. Churchill, Chubb, and Baxendale. Jour. Gen. Virol., 1969, *4*, 557.
9. Churchill, Payne, and Chubb. Nature, 1969, *221*, 744.

10. Cole. Avian Dis., 1968, *12,* 9.
11. Crittenden. World's Poultry Sci. Jour., 1968, *24,* 18.
12. Edison and Schmittle. Avian Dis., 1969, *13,* 774.
13. Fabricant, Fabricant, Litrenta, and Minick. Jour. Exp. Med., 1978, *148,* 335.
14. Nazerian and Witter, Jour. Virol., 1970, *5,* 338.
15. Purchase. Jour. Virol., 1969, *3,* 557.
16. Rispens, VanUloten, and Moss. Brit. Vet. Jour., 1969, *125,* 445.
17. Sevoian and Chamberlain. Avian Dis., 1963, *7,* 97.
18. Solomon, Witter, Nazerian, and Burmester. Proc. Soc. Exp. Biol. and Med., 1968, *127,* 173.
19. Walter, Burmester, and Cunningham, Avian Dis., 1962, *6,* 455.
20. Walter, Burmester, and Fontes. Avian Dis., 1963, *7,* 79.
21. Wight, Vet. Rec., 1963, *75,* 685.
22. Witter, Nazerian, Purchase, and Burgoyne. Am. Jour. Vet. Res., 1970, *31,* 525.
23. Witter, Solomon, and Burgoyne. Avian Dis., 1969, *13,* 101.

SECTION III RNA VIRUS FAMILIES

The nucleic acid core of this group of viruses is ribonucleic acid (RNA). There are 10 families recognized by the International Committee on Taxonomy of Viruses in the RNA group: Picornaviridae, Reoviridae, Togaviridae, Orthomyxoviridae, Paramyxoviridae, Rhabdoviridae, Retroviridae, Bunyaviridae, Arenaviridae, and Coronaviridae. There is one provisional family in the RNA virus group—Caliciviridae.

45 The Picornaviridae

The viruses in the Picornaviridae family are placed in four genera: *Rhinovirus, Enterovirus, Aphthovirus,* and *Cardiovirus*. There are no known diseases of domestic animals in the genus *Cardiovirus*. This is a rather large family with a primary affinity for superficial tissues, and it contains many important animal virus diseases, particularly foot-and-mouth disease (FMD) (Table 45.1).

Most viruses have been well studied in these four genera and share certain biochemical and biophysical characteristics. They contain single-stranded RNA with comparable molecular weight. All are nonenveloped isometric particles of small size that are ether-resistant and are synthesized in the cytoplasm of cells.

THE GENUS *APHTHOVIRUS*

The seven virus types of FMD comprise the only members of this genus. FMD is the most important animal disease in the world because it markedly affects world trade. Countries that are free of the disease limit trade to selected processed foods and to importation of livestock only after rigorous and costly laboratory tests for virus and/or antibody. For this reason, FMD is called a *political* as well as an *economic* disease.

Foot-and-Mouth Disease

SYNONYMS: Aphthous fever, epizootic aphthae, infectious aphthous stomatitis, *Maul-und Klauenseuch* (German), *fièvre aphtheuse* (French), *aftosa* (Italian and Spanish); English abbreviation, FMD

Foot-and-mouth disease occurs in most of the cattle-raising regions of the world. It has never obtained a firm foothold in Australia, New Zealand, Japan, the British Isles, and North America, regions which have long used drastic means of preventing its establishment. The disease is exceedingly contagious. On at least nine occasions it has broken out in the United States, but all of these outbreaks were successfully stamped out without excessive cost. At the time this is written (May, 1980) there have been no outbreaks in this country since 1932. The disease has been of great interest to animal disease control authorities because of the outbreak that occurred in Mexico between 1946 and 1954. In 1951–52 a small outbreak in western Canada, very close to the international border, caused considerable concern in the United States.

Foot-and-mouth disease affects cloven-footed animals, especially cattle and swine. Sheep and goats are also affected, and there have been outbreaks in wild ruminants, particularly deer. Naturally infected hedgehogs have been found in England. An outbreak has been reported in Indian elephants (61). Human cases occasionally occur, but these are rare and rather trivial in nature. Carnivorous animals are resistant, and solipeds are completely resistant.

Character of the Disease. FMD is the most feared disease of cattle in the world. From time to time the disease

Table 45.1. Diseases in domestic animals caused by viruses in the Picornaviridae family

Common name of virus	Natural hosts	Type of disease produced
Genus *Aphthovirus*		
Foot-and-mouth disease, 7 types, innumerable subtypes	Cattle, swine, sheep, goats, deer, hedgehogs, elephants, rarely man	The most important political and economic disease in the world. The disease in cattle is characterized by depression, fever, and the appearance of vesicles first on the mucous membranes of the oral cavity, then in the interdigital skin, and occasionally on the teats and udder. High morbidity with low mortality; death results from cardiac muscle necrosis. The disease is similar in other natural hosts, except that in swine lameness is the most conspicuous sign. It is important to differentiate FMD from vesicular exanthema of swine, vesicular stomatitis, and swine vesicular disease
Genus *Rhinovirus*		
Bovine rhinovirus types 1 and 2	Cattle	Acute disease in cattle with fever, depression, coughing, nasal discharge, and dyspnea. As a rule it is a mild, inapparent disease, and some strains do not produce disease; morbidity is high in affected herds
Equine rhinovirus types 1 and 2; perhaps a third one	Horses	Infected stables have a high morbidity, negligible mortality. Signs referable to upper respiratory tract
Genus *Enterovirus*		
Teschen disease (porcine enterovirus type 1)	Swine	The disease may be acute or chronic, also inapparent. Initial signs are fever, lassitude, and inappetence, followed by nervous signs. No gross lesions except possible myocardial alterations. Microscopic lesions are typical of a diffuse encephalomyelitis

has spread over the entire continent of Europe. These great panzootics usually run a year or two and then seem to disappear. The disease never completely disappears, however, for infected centers always remain somewhere, from which it again spreads when a new, highly susceptible cattle population has been developed. The disease causes its greatest losses in cattle and may be serious in swine, but in sheep and goats it usually is not very important.

The importance of FMD lies not so much in its killing power, for the mortality usually is not great. The importance lies in the moribidity losses—the loss of milk and of flesh, and the long periods in which the affected animals are not productive.

FMD spreads most rapidly during the summer months because of the greater traffic in animals during those months. The disease now would be especially difficult to handle in the United States because of the highly developed transportation system and the practice of shipping animals long distances—from range to feedlots, from feedlots to slaughtering centers, from farms to marketing centers, and back to other farms.

In cattle the disease is characterized by depression, fever, and the appearance of vesicles filled with clear fluid in certain mucous membranes and portions of the skin. The essential pathological change in the tongue is necrosis of epithelial cells in the stratum spinosum, intracellular edema, and granulocytic infiltration (70). Cir-

Table 45.1.—*continued*

Common name of virus	Natural hosts	Type of disease produced
Porcine enterovirus types 2-8	Swine	Some types produce disease; others do not. Most pathogenic strains cause polioencephalomyelitis; others cause abortions, stillbirths, mummification, and infertility (porcine SMEDI groups). One strain causes pneumonitis
Swine vesicular disease (porcine enterovirus type 9)	Swine	This enterovirus causes signs and lesions in pigs similar to FMD. Important vesicular disease in its own right, but must be differentiated from FMD
Bovine enterovirus types 1-7	Cattle	These viruses have been isolated from normal cattle and from cattle with disease. Except for one report, these viruses fail to produce disease in experimental calves
Avian encephalomyelitis	Chicks and pheasants	The disease manifestations occur only in very young birds which show incoordination, ataxia, and rapid tremors of head and neck. The losses may be as high as 50 percent in a given hatch with an average of 10 percent. Characteristic microscopic lesions are found in the central nervous system
Virus hepatitis, 2 types	Ducks	The virus causes disease in young ducklings. Both viral types cause alterations in parenchymatous organs. The major changes are in the liver, which is enlarged with petechial and ecchymotic hemorrhages; there is also focal necrosis of liver cells. High morbidity and mortality
Virus hepatitis	Turkeys	Probable enterovirus. Highly contagious disease with high mortality in poults under 2 weeks of age. Principal lesions are in the liver
Human enterovirus	Dogs	ECHO virus type 6 may cause enteric disease in dogs
Equine enterovirus	Horses	Significance as a pathogen undetermined

cumscribed, slightly elevated, blanched areas termed "initial lesions" develop in the lingual mucosa. Separation of the mucosa from the underlying tissue causes much of this initial lesion to develop into vesicles (Figures 45.2 and 45.3). Some initial lesions fail to separate from the underlying tissue with the result that the desiccating necrotic mucosa becomes discolored without vesicle formation. Failure to vesiculate in the interdigital skin is exceptional, but the initial lesion is similar to the lingual process.

The vesicles appear principally on the mucous membranes of the mouth (tongue, cheeks, dental pad, and gums), on the skin of the muzzle, of the interdigital space, and around the tops of the claws, and on the teats and occasionally the surface of the udder. More rarely they may be seen around the base of the horns and in the pharynx, larnyx, trachea, esophagus, and wall of the rumen, especially around the esophageal groove.

Within 24 to 48 hours after multiplying in the epithelium, which is first invaded, the virus escapes into the blood stream, by which it is carried to all organs and tissues. This often results in the appearance of secondary vesicles in epithelium remote from the point of entry of the virus. The virus does not multiply in the blood, but presumably does in certain organs. It produces degenerative changes in the muscular tissues, particularly those of the heart. Yellow-whitish streaks, foci of parenchymatous degeneration, and sometimes necrosis (Figure 45.4)

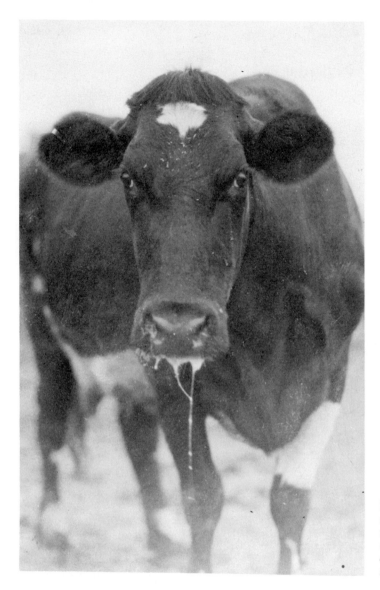

Figure 45.1. Foot-and-mouth disease, showing the characteristic drooling of saliva. Affected animals do not eat because of the soreness of their mouths. They champ their jaws, making a smacking sound. (Courtesy L. M. Hurt.)

are the manifestations of this damage. Severe damage of this type is seen most often in young calves, and this accounts for the greater mortality in young stock than in adult animals. In some outbreaks, the heart damage is greater than usual and the mortality of adult as well as young stock may be much higher than usual. This is said to be the malignant form of FMD. In these outbreaks many of the deaths occur early in the course of the infection and are attributed to the specific action of the virus.

Affected cattle become lame as a result of the foot lesions (Figure 45.5), and they champ their jaws and drool from the mouth because of the mouth soreness. They lie down as much as possible and move with great reluctance. They do not eat, and as a result they lose flesh rapidly and milk secretion diminishes greatly. The vesicles in the mouth rupture within a few hours of the time they are formed, leaving large flaps of whitish, detached epithelium under which are raw, bleeding surfaces. Many times a large part of the tongue is denuded. Secondary bacterial infections of the denuded areas between the claws usually occur, and these result in deep necrosis of tissue and suppurations that frequently undermine the claws, causing them to be loosened from the soft tissues and eventually to be cast off. The mouth lesions usually heal quite promptly so that the soreness disappears within a week, but the foot lesions often require much longer to heal.

Much of the damage in most outbreaks of FMD is caused by bacterial complications. The foot infections have been mentioned. These often require slaughter of

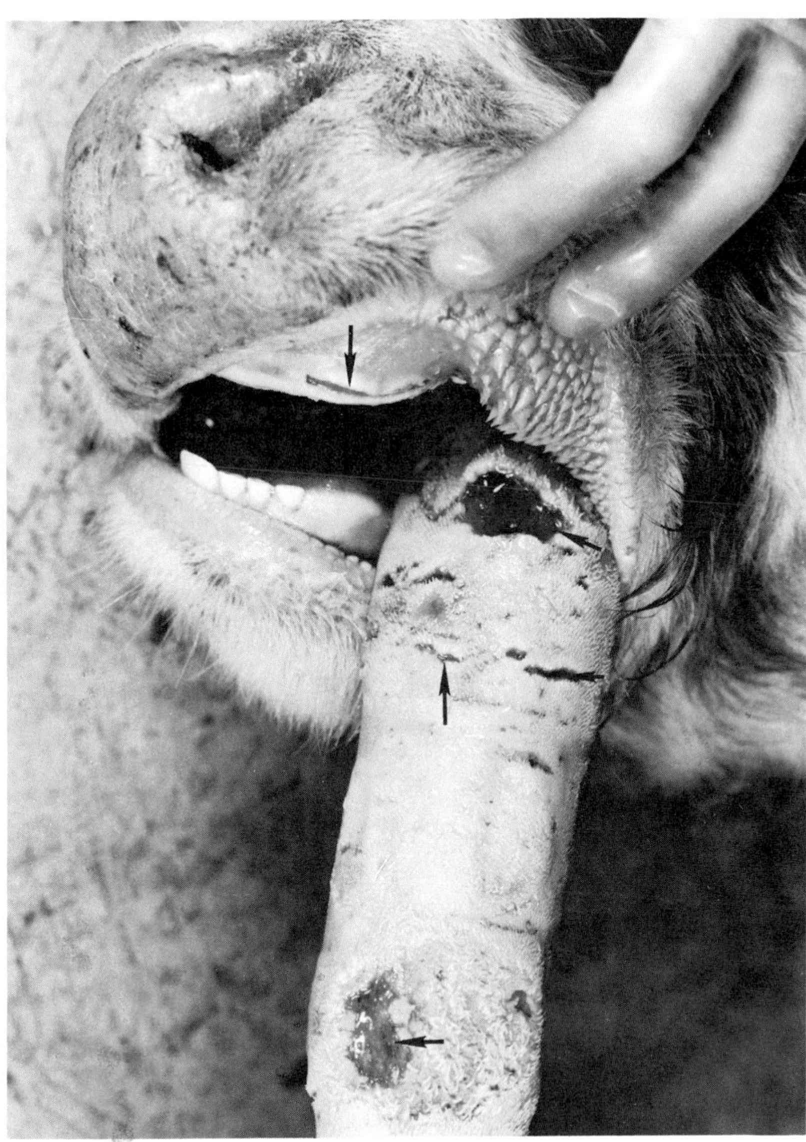

Figure 45.2. Ruptured vesicles (*arrows*) of the tongue epithelium in a steer infected with FMDV. Note ruptured vesicle (*arrow*) on dental pad. (Courtesy J. Callis and staff, USDA.)

the animal. In the few cases in which vesicles develop in the upper respiratory tract, pneumonia may occur. A common and serious complication in dairy cattle is udder infection (Figure 45.6). Early in the course of the disease, acute swelling of the udder is often noticed and the milk becomes thick and viscid, assuming the appearance of colostrum. Whether this is a result of virus action is not clear, but many European workers have so regarded it. In any case streptococcic, staphylococcic, and other bacterial infections often develop, resulting in mastitis.

In swine, lameness is usually the most conspicuous sign and the first noticed. The animals have little appetite, have fever, and move with great reluctance. The lesions in the mouth, between the claws (Figure 45.7), and in the heart muscle are much like those seen in cattle. Large vesicles usually develop in the snouts of pigs (Figure 45.8).

In sheep and goats, lameness is also usually the most conspicuous sign. As a general rule, these animals are not severely affected by FMD. There are exceptions to this rule, however. There have been outbreaks in Europe in which sheep and goats were more severely affected than cattle.

The incubation period in FMD is very short. Inoculated animals develop lesions at the point of inoculation in less than 24 hours, and generalization with fever in less than 48 hours. When cattle and swine are exposed naturally, the incubation period is usually not longer than 4 days and may be shorter than 48 hours.

Cases without complications with pyogenic bacteria

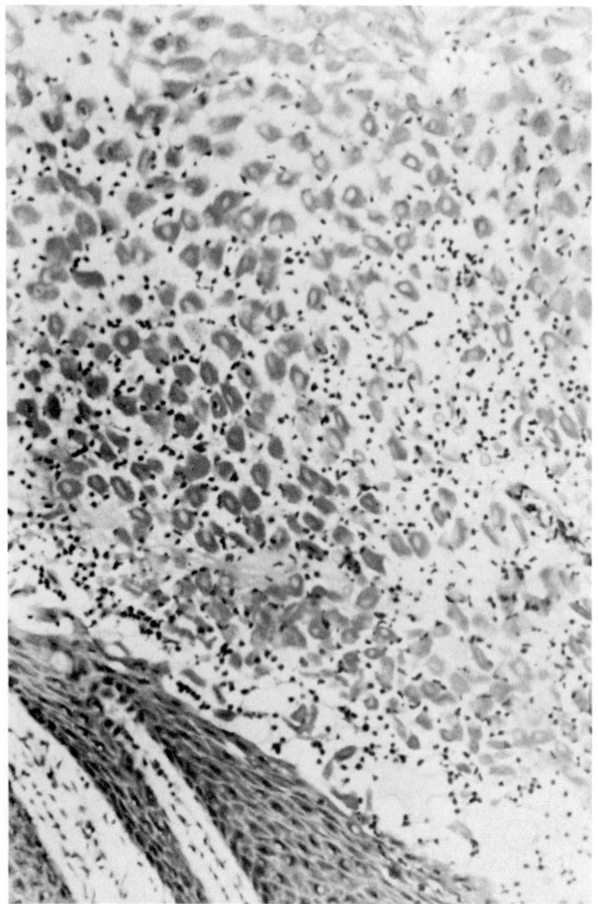

Figure 45.3. Photomicrograph of part of a vesicular lesion of foot-and-mouth disease on the muzzle of a cow. The cells in the stratum spinosum are rounded and separated from each other (spongiosis), and there is a mild leukocytic infiltrate. H and E stain. × 58. (Courtesy C. A. Mebus, Plum Island Animal Disease Center, USDA.)

usually recover completely within 2 to 3 weeks, although milk production may be depressed much longer and recovery of the original body weight may not have occurred at that time. Complications are very common, however, and these may cause trouble for many weeks or months.

In most outbreaks of FMD the mortality is not high. It seldom averages more than 3 percent and often is less than 1 percent. Occasionally it may be much higher, even as great as 50 percent (52). The death rate among young stock is higher than among adults, and somewhat greater in young pigs than in calves. It is usually very low in sheep and goats.

The Disease in Experimental Animals. FMD may be readily produced in naturally susceptible species by inoculation parenterally. Cattle are easily infected by rubbing virus-containing material on the mucous membrane of the mouth. When cattle are used to detect virus in suspected materials, the most sensitive procedure is to inoculate intradermally into the dorsum of the tongue. After inoculation vesicles appear at the point of injection within 10 to 12 hours, and fever and viremia occur within 20 to 24 hours. Secondary vesiculation generally appears in the interdigital space within 2 to 4 days following this method of inoculation. The morphogenesis of vesiculation in cattle infected with FMDV by aerosol was investigated by Yilma (92). Lesions were initiated usually by the infection of single cells in the stratum spinosum adjacent to the papillae. Viremia preceded the development of lesions, and virus appeared to be transported to the epithelium via papillae. Three types of lesions were observed. The first type was a vesicle de-

Figure 45.4. Foot-and-mouth disease. The longitudinal yellow-whitish streaks are areas of myocardial necrosis. (Courtesy D. A. Gregg, Plum Island Animal Disease Center, USDA.)

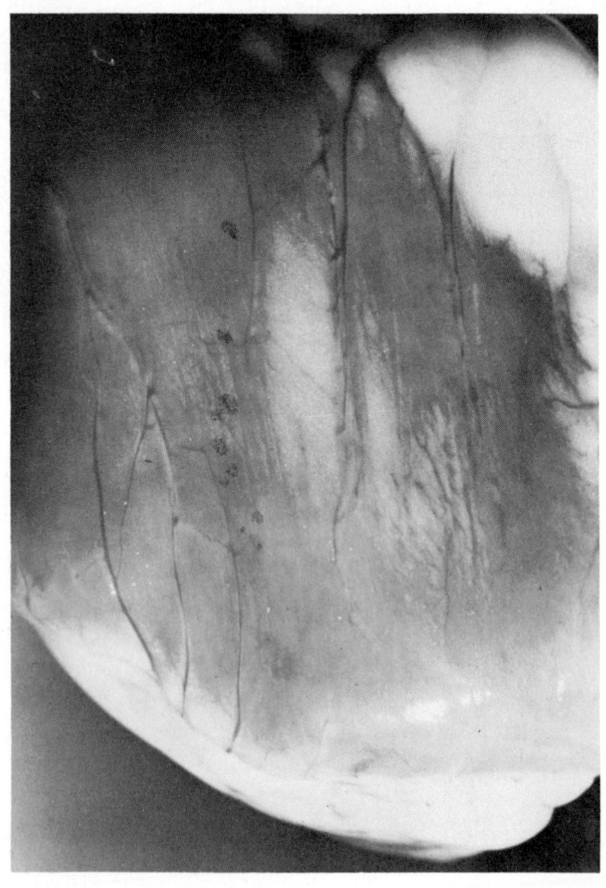

veloped mainly from the lysis of swollen, spherical cells and the release of intracellular fluid. The second type was formed mainly by the accumulation of intercellular edema. The third type was characterized by the absence of a vesicle due to seepage and loss of edema fluid and desiccation of the lesion.

Because infections of small laboratory animals could not be produced, research studies on this disease were greatly hampered for many years, and swine and cattle, which are very expensive, had to be used. Another handicap was the great contagiousness of the disease in these species, which necessitated elaborate equipment and housing facilities to prevent the infection from escaping from the laboratory and from spreading uncontrolled to all susceptible stock brought to the laboratory. The discovery by Waldmann and Pape (90) in 1921 that guinea pigs could be infected with the virus of foot-and-mouth disease by the use of a special technique was an advancement of great importance. These animals can be used to detect virus in animal tissues and in materials that have been in contact with cases. Furthermore, the disease in guinea pigs is not naturally transmissible, and thus the problem of keeping susceptible animals on the premises for experimental work was immediately solved.

Very young and very old guinea pigs are not satisfactory for work with this virus. Half-grown animals weighing about 350 g are best. Inoculation is done by introducing the virus intradermally into the footpads of the hind feet either with a fine hypodermic needle or by scarification. A primary vesicle usually appears at the point of inoculation within 24 hours, occasionally longer. At the time the primary vesicle appears, virus can be demonstrated in the blood. Within 18 to 36 hours, secondary vesicles appear in the mouth, and the virus disappears from the blood. Complete repair of the lesions requires several weeks. Only an occasional animal dies of the disease. There is no evidence that the virus multiplies elsewhere than at the site of the lesions. Recent studies show that intralingual injection is more sensitive than foot-pad inoculation (46). It is not known why the disease in this animal is not naturally transmissible.

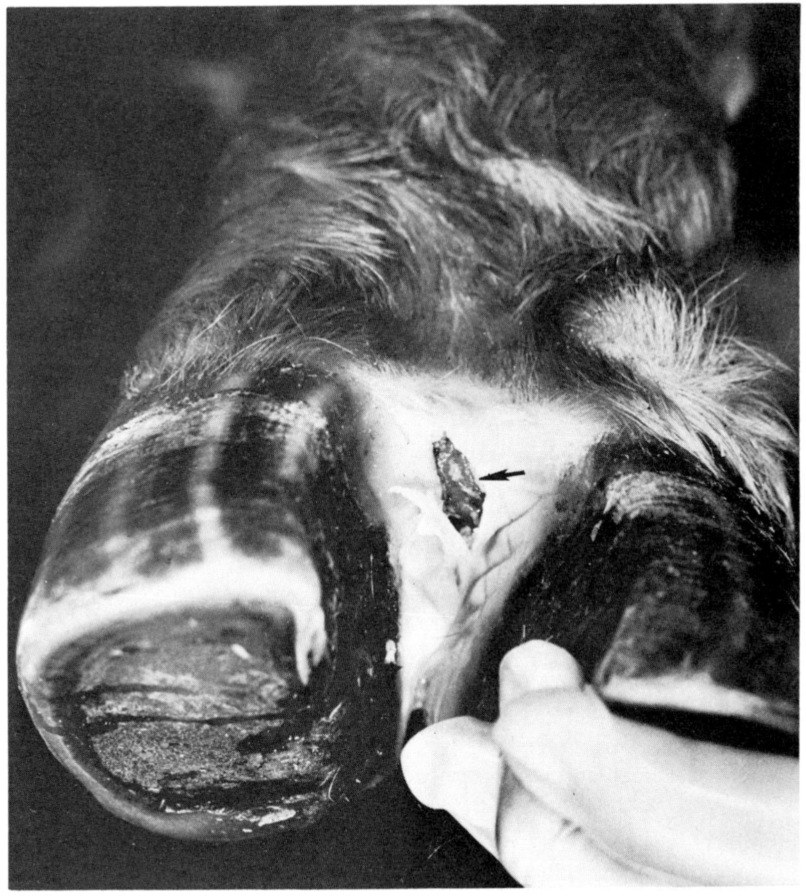

Figure 45.5. Ruptured vesicle (*arrow*) in the interdigital region of a steer infected with FMDV. (Courtesy J. J. Callis and staff, USDA.)

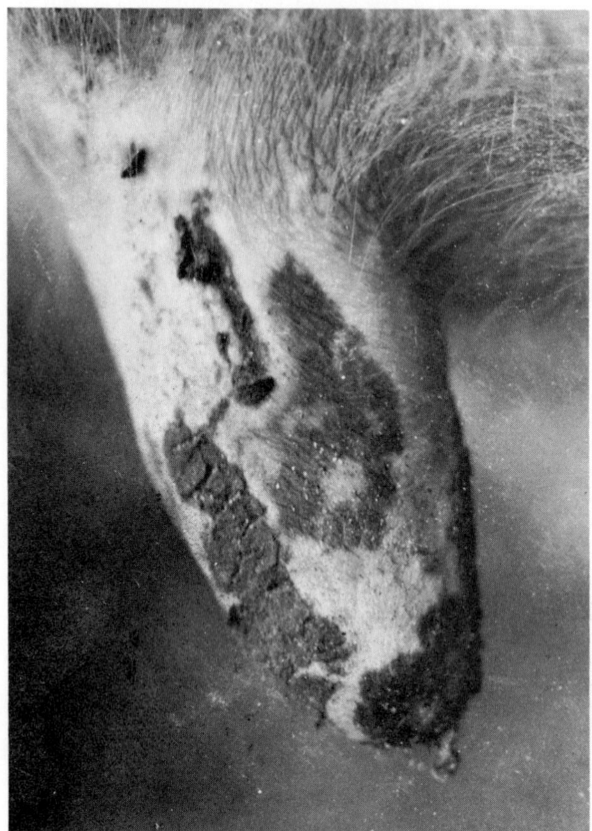

Figure 45.6. Foot-and-mouth disease, showing lesions on the teat of a cow. Beginning as papules which change to vesicles, the latter rupture leaving raw surfaces. These become infected with bacteria, and mastitis often develops as a result of extension of the infection into the teat canal. The surface lesions finally heal under scabs. The lesions here depicted are healing. (Courtesy L. M. Hurt.)

In 1951 Skinner (73) showed that unweaned white mice are very sensitive to foot-and-mouth disease virus and that these animals constitute the best laboratory species for detecting small amounts of virus in suspected materials. The mice are inoculated intraperitoneally. Those from 7 to 10 days old prove most suitable. A spastic paralysis of hind legs generally appears after several days, but some mice die before this sign is exhibited. Those that die or are destroyed after several days show a marked degeneration of the musculature of the hind quarters and often of the lumbar and intercostal regions. Half or more of all animals exhibit myocardial degeneration.

It was shown by Skinner and confirmed by others that unweaned mice were 10 to 100 times more sensitive to foot-and-mouth virus than the guinea pig, (by foot-pad inoculation) and always fully as susceptible, and occasionally more so, than cattle inoculated intralingually. The placenta serves as an active site of infection for FMDV in pregnant mice, but the fetus is relatively resistant to infection (5). Other animals such as armadillos, cats, dogs, hamsters, wildebeests, wild and white rats, deer, and rabbits have been infected artificially.

Various investigators have succeeded in cultivating the virus in birds and chick embryos. In 1954 Gillespie (39) infected day-old chicks with tissue-cultured adapted types A, O, and C FMD viruses and 6-week-old birds with the type A virus. Degenerative gizzard muscle lesions were produced in most chicks and heart lesions in a small percentage. With some cattle strains Skinner (74) infected day-old chicks and observed lingual lesions, injection of FMDV in the tongue or foot pads results in the development of characteristic lesions in bantams, ducks, geese, guinea fowl, and turkeys.

In 1948 Traub and Schneider (83) adapted guinea pig virus to the hen's egg, but this virus was no longer pathogenic or immunogenic for cattle. With chick embryos Skinner (74) succeeded in passing several cattle strains for many generations by intravenous injection. Gillespie (40) did likewise with chick-adapted type C virus by inoculation on the chorioallantoic membrane and noted some attenuation for cattle with the 25th egg transfer. Embryos usually died in 2 to 6 days. Infected embryos showed edema and hemorrhages in the skin, hemorrhages in the liver and kidneys, serous or blood-tinged fluid in the body cavity and pericardial sac and, occasionally, enlarged white areas in the heart muscle. The greatest concentration of virus was in the heart muscle.

Properties of the Virus. The French workers Vallée and Carré (88) in 1922 discovered the existence of two different types of FMD virus. Waldmann and Trautwein (91) in 1926 confirmed the French findings and added a third type. The original French types are now designated A (*Allemand*—French word for "German") and O (for the Oise Valley, from which it came). The German type is known as C. Thus we have three types, O, A, and C, which are known as the European types. Several years ago three new types were found in South Africa. These are designated SAT 1, SAT 2, and SAT 3. The English FMD laboratories reported on a seventh type found in widely separated parts of Asia which they designated the Asiatic type 1.

In addition to the seven basic types, 61 subtypes have been recognized. Some of these have been designated by exponents such as A^5 and O^3. Some of these field subtypes are sufficiently different immunologically from the

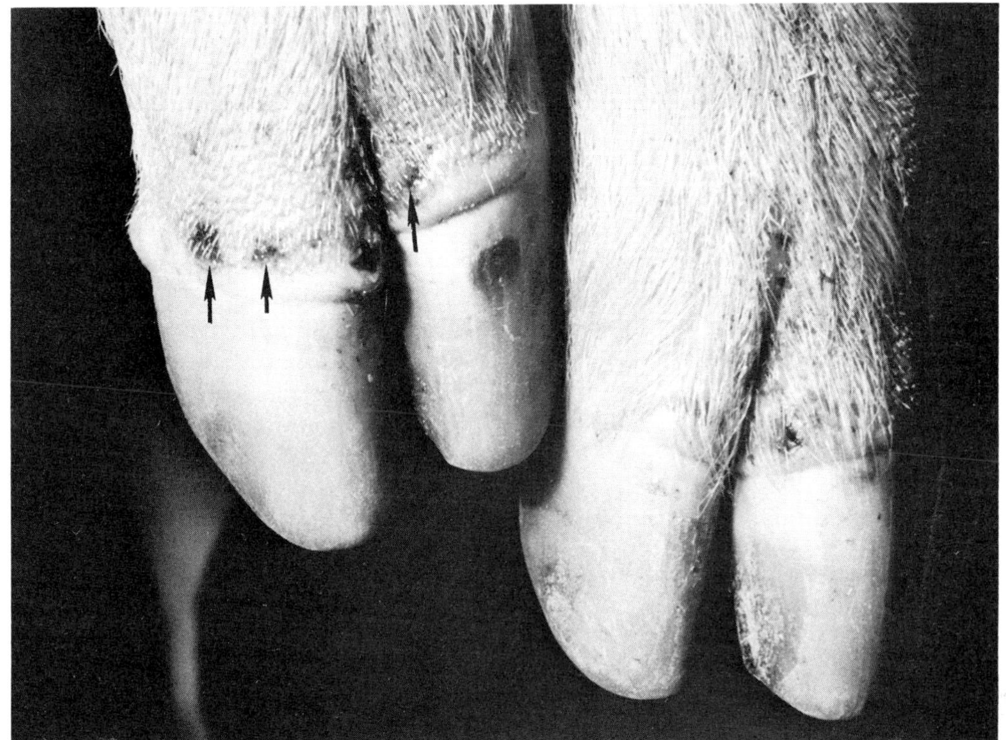

Figure 45.7. Ruptured vesicles (*arrows*) on the coronary band of the feet of a pig infected with FMDV. (Courtesy J. Callis and staff, USDA.)

Figure 45.8. Foot-and-mouth disease. A large unruptured vesicle on a pig's snout. (Courtesy D. A. Gregg, Plum Island Animal Disease Center, USDA.)

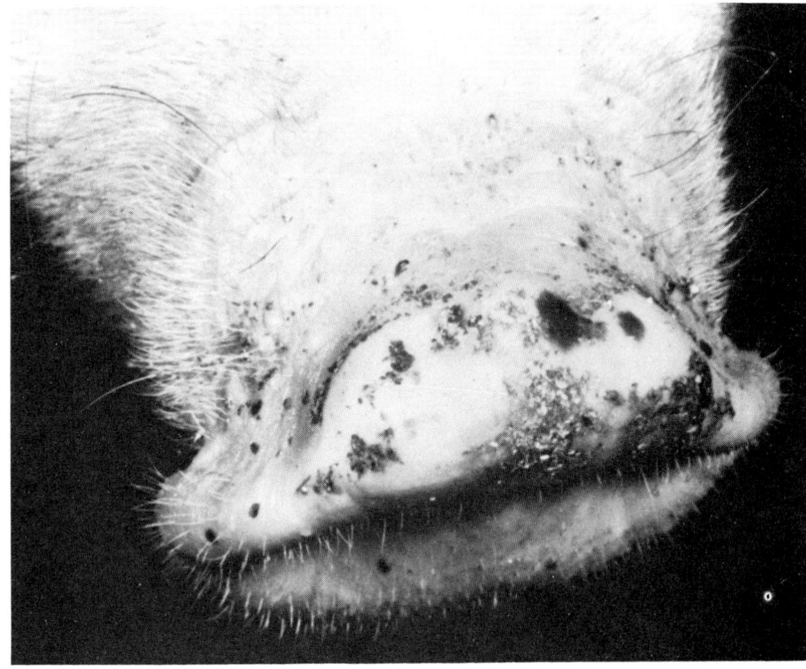

parent strains to make successful immunization dependent upon the use of specific variant vaccines.

The virus of FMD appears to be unusually variable. In later stages of outbreaks in Europe new types or variants appeared which seemed to be derived from the original one rather than introduced from outside. Ramon (62) suggests that such variations may be arising as a result of vaccines which imperfectly immunize animals, thus setting up within them the means for forcing variations in the field strains. In a series of papers a group of investigators (48, 49, 51) studied the evidence for recombination between immunological types of FMDV and developed genetic recombination maps.

Animals that have recovered from FMD caused by one type generally are sufficiently resistant to that type to withstand additional exposure for 6 months to 1 year. Such animals may be immediately infected with one of the other types and exhibit typical signs, however.

The differentiation of types is a laboratory procedure. It may be done with guinea pigs or unweaned mice or by the complement-fixation test. In the animal tests it is necessary to have on hand high-titer immune serum of a known type. The unknown virus is mixed in appropriate dilutions with the known antisera, and the mixtures are injected into the animals. The virus is typed to correspond to the type of antiserum which proves to be able to neutralize it. The complement-fixation test for virus typing has been highly developed and in competent hands has a high order of reliability in differentiating between FMD and other vesicular diseases, with slightly less efficiency in differentiating between the foot-and-mouth virus types. The technique has been extensively studied by Brooksby (22) in England. Confirmation of complement-fixation (CF) typing results are made by cross-neutralizations between virus strains and strain-specific antisera. It has been found that other serological tests such as the indirect complement-fixation (64, 82) and hemagglutination-inhibition (20) tests are comparable to the serum-neutralization test in specificity and sensitivity for detecting virus antibody. The typing of FMDV also may be done by the fluorescent antibody (79) and the radioimmunoassay (33) techniques.

In their excellent review articles on FMD Shahan (54) and Bachrach (6) covered the biochemical and biophysical properties of FMDV. The virus is resistant to alcohol, ether, chloroform, and other fat solvents. Glycerol has a preservative effect, especially if it is mixed with a buffer solution, which prevents the development of acidity. Infected lymph and tissues may be stored for long periods in such a solution without loss of virulence, especially if the solution is kept cold.

In early investigations two complement-fixing antigens were demonstrated in infected guinea pig and cattle vesicular fluids with two different sedimentation coefficients (s rates). The infectious virion (particle) has an s rate of 140 S and a diameter of 23±2 nm (Figure 45.9), and the smaller particle, without infectivity, has an s rate of 12 S with a diameter of 7 to 8 nm. This smaller particle has the properties of a euglobulin and is more

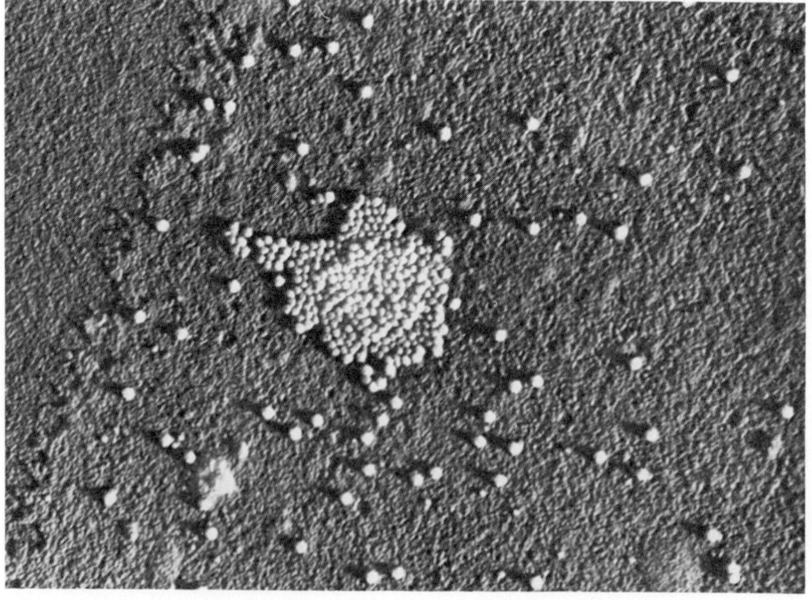

Figure 45.9. Foot-and-mouth disease virus, 23 ±2 nm. (Courtesy H. L. Bachrach and S. S. Breese, *Proc. Soc. Exp. Biol. and Med.*)

stable to heat, acids, and enzymes than the infective particle.

Additional virus-specific antigens have been identified in infected tissues. Graves *et al.* (43) described empty viral capsids with an s rate of 75 S, and Cowan and Graves (32) reported a virus-infection-associated antigen (VIA antigen) with an s rate less than 4.5 S. Empty capsids are precipitated by antibody to virions as well as by antibody to 12 S viral subunit. The VIA antigen is probably enzymatically inactive, FMDV-specific RNA polymerase, because its antibody inhibits polymerase activity. The VIA-RNA polymerase antigen is formed prior to virions and only when virus replicates in cells of animals indicating translation from noncapsid cistrons of the virus genome. Consequently, animals vaccinated with inactivated virus do not produce VIA antigen or its antibody. The test of VIA antibody is a powerful tool in determining whether an animal has ever replicated virus. Thus it is useful in epidemiological studies, in safety evaluation of inactivated virus vaccine preparations, and in detection of infection in an animal population in eradication programs. All VIA antigens are immunologically identical regardless of virus type. VIA antigen as well as 12 S protein subunits interfere with the specificity of complement-fixation tests used for typing FMDV. The adverse effect of these two antigens in this test can be minimized by the use of a short high-temperature test at 37 C for 30 to 90 minutes by the use of high dilutions of antiserum.

All four antigens of the FMD system are active in CF and agar-gel precipitation tests. Only antibodies to 140 S virion are known to be type-specific. The 140 S and 75 S antigens only appear to produce neutralizing antibody and immunity. As little as 0.2 μg of purified 140 S antigen is required to produce measurable neutralizing antibody in guinea pigs. The immunogenic potency of purified 75 S empty capsids has not been determined, but it is anticipated that it would be comparable to infective virus.

The agar-gel-diffusion test coupled with acridine orange staining differentiates the 140 S RNA-containing virions from the other RNA-free 75 S, 12 S, and VIA antigens since the 140 S antigen only fluoresces under ultraviolet light. In contrast the fluorescent antibody (FA) probably is determined by antibody to VIA antigen. Labeling is not type-specific and occurs only with antiserum from animals in which virus replicates. Direct and indirect FA tests detect FMD infection.

Many strains of FMDV have been characterized by their resistance to thermal inactivation (10). There is an initial rapid first-order inactivation of tissue-cultured virus followed by tailing, which suggests the presence of a small, heat-resistant population of virus. The heating of virus yields infectious RNA in absence of RNase. The thermal stability of the FMDV is largely determined by the nature of its protein capsid.

The spherical infectious particle is quite readily inactivated by heat, but its stripped RNA core remains infectious after boiling for 5 minutes. Practical experience over a long period of time has shown that the power to transmit the disease usually is removed from milk by ordinary pasteurization, but not always. Experimentally, however, it has been shown that a minute fraction of active residual virus remains in fluids subjected to much more than pasteurization temperatures for periods as long as 7 hours (7). Virus survived in the milk of acutely infected cows after heating at high-temperature, short-time pasteurization at 7.5 C for 15 to 17 seconds (45) and survived in the pasteurized milk after evaporation at 65 C to 50 percent of the original volume. FMDV survived in the cream after it was heated at 93 C for 25 minutes (18). Other dairy products remain infective depending on the process.

Resistance to drying varies according to the way it is done. If the virus is contained in albuminous material, is dried quickly and completely, and is kept dried, it will persist for very long periods. Virus in epithelial fragments appears to be more resistant than when free in fluids. Schoening (68) found that virus dried on hay and on soil particles remained viable for about a month, and Trautwein (85) found epithelial fragments still infective after being exposed to winter weather for more than 2 months. Gailiunas and Cottral (38) found that virus persisted in bovine skin for varying periods of time after treatment by one of four conventional methods for preservation of hides. The shortest period for viral inactivation was 21 days, and the longest was 352 days. It was indicated that FMDV may survive even longer under field conditions. The virus types isolated from hides stored under experimental conditions were virulent and occasionally highly pathogenic for cattle. The present practice of cattle-hide importation into the United States from countries with FMD obviously poses a potential hazard, although the importation of hides from these countries had continued since 1930 and no outbreak has occurred.

The resistance of the virus of FMD to drying and its persistence in infected tissues are matters of great importance, since they have a distinct bearing on the possibilities of new outbreaks being established in distant regions from accidental transfer of the virus. There is no evidence, for example, that any of the last half-dozen outbreaks of this disease in the United States were the result of importing infected animals. At least two had their origin in imported meat scraps that found their way into garbage and then into native swine (54, 55), and at least one originated in vaccine virus imported from a foreign country (56). The origins of several of these outbreaks were never discovered, but they may well have begun with virus dried on straw packing materials or on other objects contaminated with dried virus.

FMDV is quite sensitive to acid pH. At pH 6.5 there is a 10-fold loss every 14 hours at 4 C, and at pH 6 and pH 5 inactivation rises to 90 percent per minute and second, respectively. It is quite stable at 4 C at pH 7 to 7.5 and only slightly less stable at pH 8 to 9. Purified FMDV-RNA is more stable at pH 4 than crude virus preparations. The RNase present in the latter inactivates the RNA released by acidification of virions.

Phenol and hexylresorcinol release single-stranded infectious RNA from FMDV by stripping the protein coat. The RNA has an s rate of 37 S. RNA extracted from crude virus still contains some RNase to cause slow inactivation, so storage at −196 C or in 70 percent ethanol at −20 C is required to retard inactivation. The FMDV protein is recovered from the phenol phase in pure form by precipitation with methanol and resuspension in phenol, formic acid, or 0.1 percent sodium dodecyl sulfate (11).

Viruses containing RNA, such as FMDV, are inactivated by ultraviolet light through changes in their uracil components. FMDV retains its antigenicity and ability to attach to cells after ultraviolet treatment with the maximum rate of inactivation at 265 nm.

The FMD virion has a molecular weight of 6.9×10^6 daltons and contains 69 percent protein and 31 percent RNA. There are 32 capsomeres which form a symmetrical icosahedral (20 sides) capsid for the RNA core. During replication in tissue culture cytoplasmic crystalline arrays of complete virus (Figure 45.10) and empty capsids may be observed. Its RNA base composition is G.24:A.26:C.28:U.22. Its isodensity in cesium chloride is 1.43 g per cm^3.

FMDV particles contain four major peptides—VP_1, VP_2, VP_3, and VP_4. They also contain two minor polypeptides (65). The N-terminal amino acids for representative strains of FMDV types A, O, and C were glycine in VP_1, aspartic acid in VP_2, and threonine in VP_3. FMDV can be maintained for long periods at low temperatures with little loss of viral infectivity titer (50).

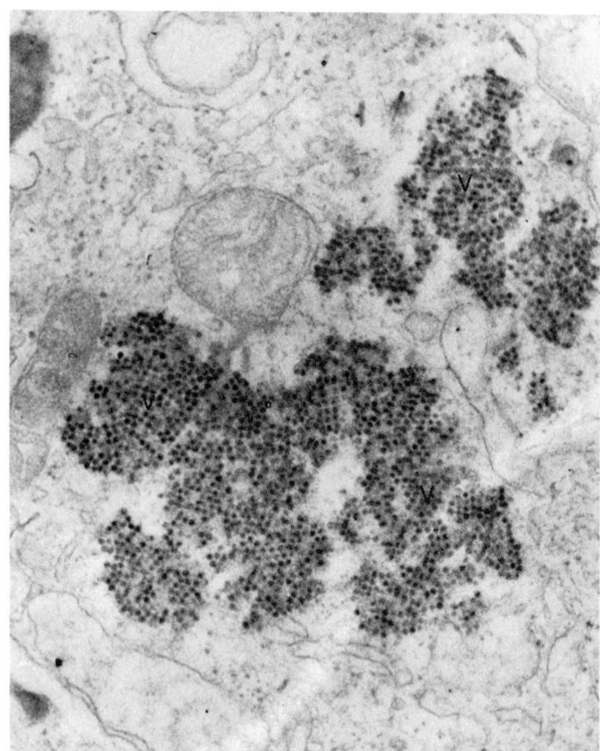

Figure 45.10. Note cytoplasmic crystalline array of FMDV particles (*V*) in a bovine kidney tissue culture cell. × 36,000. (Courtesy S. Breese, USDA.)

FMDV induces the production of interferon in cell culture (34). Medium from infected cultures interferes with heterotypic FMD viruses, as well as parainfluenza, pseudorabies, and bovine enteroviruses. It has been suggested that FMDV with low virulence, or with many defective particles, is a better inducer of interferon than highly virulent strains. Synthetic polyribonucleotide duplexes which produce interferon presumably cause interference with FMDV replication in tissue culture cells. Bögel (19) found a thermostabile inhibitor of FMDV in normal pig serum which is probably a beta-macroglobulin and not interferon. Anderson (2) extended the studies with normal swine sera and concluded that the cross-reactions are the result of immunoglobulin M or a similar macroglobulin. Using the plaque reduction and radioimmunodiffusion tests (1) he examined serums from normal cattle and found high levels of cross-reactions with the various FMD types that were specific but often only with 1 or 2 viruses for a given serum. The incidence of cross-reactions increases after shipping suggesting an infective agent may be responsible (4). A bovine enterovirus (E76T) isolated from a bull in the United States produced serologic cross-reactions to FMD SAT 1 virus but not against representatives of the other antigenic types of FMDV (3).

Cultivation. *In embryonated hens' eggs.* Reference has already been made to the studies in adapting a number of FMDV strains to chick embryos. More recently other investigators have used chick-adapted strains for successful transfer in hens' eggs. Some of these egg-adapted and chick-adapted strains have undergone a marked loss of pathogenicity for cattle.

In tissue cultures. Frenkel and coworkers (36, 37) developed a method by which the virus of FMD may be propagated in tissue culture. The method has been perfected to the degree that it is now used for the commercial production of vaccine. The cultures consist of epithelial tissue from cattle suspended in a solution of peptone, glucose, and salt with small amounts of a number of other substances known as Baker's solution (59). The epithelial tissue is obtained from the tongues of freshly slaughtered cattle. After inoculation with virus, the flasks are incubated at 37 C, and a stream of sterile air bubbled through the medium during incubation. The flasks are harvested after 24 hours' incubation, at which time the virus titer is usually 10^5 to 10^6.

Propagation of FMDV in monolayer cultures of bovine and porcine kidney origin was first reported in 1955 (8, 71). Some other cell cultures that have been used include embryonic bovine skin and muscle, embryonic heart and lung, lamb kidney, fetal rabbit kidney, and murine mammary carcinomatous tissue. The stable line of baby hamster kidney cells (BHK-21) is now commonly used in monolayers and in suspension cultures for research and vaccine virus production, since it is highly susceptible to FMDV. Suspended cell cultures for production of viral vaccine antigen have a number of obvious advantages over monolayer cultures. As a result there is considerable research in progress to improve cell yields, to eliminate serum from the culture media, and to improve viral yields of the various FMDV types (13, 30, 75, 93). Spier and Whiteside (76, 77) have devised a technique to grow BHK-21 C_{13} monolayer cells on the surface of serum-coated DEAE Sephadex A50 beads.

By the use of the plaque overlay method or the production of a cytopathogenic effect, certain cell cultures can be used to assay for virus. The sensitivity and precision of plaque assays for FMDV depends upon the virus-strain cell-substrate system, and on environmental factors (6). The MVPK-1 cell line derived from fetal pig kidneys is equally susceptible to all seven types in a plaque overlay system as bovine kidney cell cultures (81).

Immunity. Cattle that have recovered from FMD generally have enough immunity to protect them from the same type of virus for a year or more, but the resistance is not lifelong. Natural immunity in cattle and swine is negligible, although some individuals have greater resistance than others. Little is known about duration of immunity in swine except it is shorter than in cattle. Even less is known about such other animals as sheep and goats.

Antibodies that develop in immunized or convalescent animals are of two types—early and late (23). The early antibody is present 7 days after inoculation, but persists for 30 days only. It is a 19 S $beta_2$ or $gamma_1$ macroglobulin which adsorbs strongly to DEAE-cellulose and is sensitive to 2 M mercaptoethanol. This antibody neutralizes and precipitates homotypic and heterotypic FMDV but has little or no CF activity. The late-appearing antibody appears in 10 to 14 days and may persist for several months. It is a low molecular weight 7 S $gamma_2$ globulin which adsorbs weakly to DEAE-cellulose and is resistant to 2 M mercaptoethanol. The 7 S antibody possesses neutralizing, precipitating and complement-fixing activities which are type specific. Two or three other late-appearing classes of antibody exist in convalescent cattle sera which have not been fully characterized. Immunity in animals, particularly cattle, can be evaluated by qualitative and quantitative means.

Various qualitative techniques, such as contact exposure, "cloth infection," intranasal or intrapharyngeal instillation, and arbitrary dose of virus on the tongue, are employed. Quantitative methods are more accurate and include (*a*) intralingual titration of virus and (*b*) tongue, intramuscular, or subcutaneous inoculation of a standardized dose of virus. The correlation between pig protection and neutralizing antibody titer is dependent on the strain of virus, so using antibody titer alone for evaluating protection is an unreliable procedure (14).

In 1963 Graves (42) reported that the transfer of neutralizing antibody to calves born of dams vaccinated against foot-and-mouth disease was by colostrum only. Immunoelectrophoretic study showed that calves were born with no gamma globulin in the serum, but it was present 2 hours after the ingestion of colostrum. Transfer of antibody could be blocked by prior feeding of skim milk or immune bovine serum. A passively immune calf did not respond to vaccination until the serum antibody reached low levels, whereas calves of the same age from nonimmune mothers could be vaccinated as evidenced by the production of neutralizing antibody. Piglets derive their maternal immunity through the colostrum.

Immunization. *Passive.* Susceptible animals can be protected against some of the damages of FMD by injection with immune serum just before or simultaneously with the exposure to virus. The protection is short-lived—only 1 or 2 weeks—and often it is not sufficient to prevent infection.

Active. In 1934 Schmidt and Hansen (66, 67) began experiments on the use of adjuvants with inactivated foot-and-mouth disease virus to enhance its immunizing power. Waldmann and Kobe (89) in 1938 reported the successful use of this vaccine in the field. It is now known as the *Waldmann* or *Schmidt-Waldmann vaccine,* and it has been used very successfully in many European countries and in Latin America. A variation known as the *Rosenbusch vaccine* (63) was developed in Argentina. The vaccine used to control the Mexican outbreak was of the Rosenbusch type. Inactivated vaccines of tissue-culture origin are also frequently used now. Three FMD types combined with rabies vaccine or with brucellosis vaccine have comparable efficacy to that of monovalent vaccines (35).

Inactivated vaccines. The production of the Schmidt-Waldmann vaccine differs somewhat from one laboratory to another, but the principles are the same. Virus is obtained by inoculating susceptible cattle with diluted virus. The inoculum is injected in many places over the surface of the tongue, the virus being deposited in the deeper layer of the tongue epithelium. In about 18 hours large confluent vesicles should be present, loosening practically all of the epithelium of the dorsal surface of the tongue. If they have reached a satisfactory stage of development, the animals are slaughtered. If necessary the animals are allowed to live longer, their mouths being examined hourly until the disease has progressed to the desired stage. The tongues are now carefully removed and saved for the harvest of virus. The processed viral suspension is mixed in about 1.5 percent concentration in a colloidal suspension of aluminum hydroxide [$Al(OH)_3$], to the particles of which it is believed that the virus particles are adsorbed. Formalin is added to a concentration of 0.1 percent, and the suspensions are held at 26 C for 24 hours. This constitutes the vaccine. After being appropriately tested both for innocuousness and immunizing ability, it is ready to be bottled for field use. The finished vaccine is an opalescent fluid, the appearance being due to the aluminum hydroxide. The material must be kept cold, but it is spoiled by freezing and by heat. It is injected subcutaneously in a dose of 30 ml.

Immunity develops after 7 to 10 days, but does not reach its peak until 21 days. European workers consider that a serviceable degree of immunity lasts for 1 year in cattle. In Latin America, where management practices are different, cattle must be vaccinated three times per year for maximum protection. In 1963 van Bekkum, Fish, and Dale (16) stated that the serum titers of Dutch dairy cattle given two or more annual vaccinations remained high for at least 2 years.

The Rosenbusch vaccine differs from the Schmidt-Waldmann only in that it contains much more virus material—about 5 percent instead of 1 to 1.5 percent. It is used intradermally, and the dose is 2 ml. The injections are made in the thick skin of the neck just back of the ears. Rosenbusch claims that immunity develops earlier and that it is as solid and lasting as that of the European type.

The method devised by Frenkel (36) of Holland for cultivating the virus of FMD has been described in an earlier section. Frenkel and his coworkers were successful in adapting their methods to mass production of high-titer virus. From this virus, vaccine is made by the same procedures as are used for making the Schmidt-Waldmann vaccine (9, 37). Henderson (44) checked several vaccines made in this way and found them fully as good and perhaps better in some instances than those made from cattle tongues.

Other inactivated virus vaccines have utilized FMDV produced in primary calf-kidney cell cultures in Roux flasks and later in large roller bottles (86). Cell production is limited by the difficulty of processing kidneys and the relatively low cell density reached in the monolayers. The stable baby hamster kidney (BHK) cell line is a vast improvement, as its cell population in roller bottles is eight times greater than primary bovine kidney monolayers, and it can also be grown in 30- to 100-liter submerged cultures with automatic control of temperature and pH (29). Vaccines prepared with BHK cells are as potent as other inactivated vaccines, lack other latent kidney viruses, such as bovine virus diarrhea virus and bovine adenoviruses, and are apparently free of tumorigenicity.

Brown, Hyslop, Crick, and Morrow (24) reported that vaccines prepared by the inactivation of virus with acetylethyleneimine were as potent as the corresponding formalin vaccines. By adding an oil adjuvant, vaccines become more efficient than the standard formalin—Al $(OH)_3$ vaccines because the duration of immunity is lengthened in cattle and pigs. McKercher and Graves wrote a review (53) on the current status of oil adjuvants in FMD vaccines. Binary ethylenimine can be used as the inactivant instead of acetylethyleneimine with comparable results and considerably reduces the potential danger associated with handling pure ethylemine and other aziridines (12).

In summary, tissue-cultured FMDV inactivated by acetylethyleneimine or binary ethylenimine and emulsified with adjuvant provide the most satisfactory virus vaccines for immunization of animals against FMD.

Modified live virus vaccines. The adaptation of FMDV to unweaned mice by Skinner (73) and to chick embryos and day-old chicks by Skinner (74) and by Gillespie (39, 40), to other small animals (72), and to tissue cultures led to the development of modified live virus vaccines. Virulent virus was transferred through one or more of these hosts until the virulence for cattle was markedly reduced. Attenuation for one host does not imply reduction of virulence for another host, or even avirulence for the same host under conditions of stress. There is also a suggestion that in a combined vaccine, two serotypes may interfere with each other to some degree, although this is not true in all instances since it is possible for certain subtypes within serotypes to cross-protect (58). Although modified live virus vaccines undoubtedly confer longer lasting immunity than inactivated vaccines and showed considerable promise under field conditions in certain areas of the world, many problems arose, such as undesirable effects in young cattle, potential activation of other infectious latent agents, and the production of postvaccinal teat lesions leading to mastitis. At the present time (1979) only Venezuela uses modified live virus vaccine in cattle.

Experimental unit vaccines. The VP_3 capsid protein of the FMD virus plays a major role in immunity (9). Purified VP_3 capsid protein of type A_{12} strain 119 emulsified with incomplete Freund's adjuvant inoculated into swine at days 0, 28, and 60 with 100-mg doses provided protection by day 82 against exposure to infected swine. Serums from swine given VP_3 contained viral precipitating and neutralizing antibodies but recognized fewer viral antigenic determinants than antiviral serums. Kaaden *et al.* (47) have studied the immunogenic capacity of cleaved VP_3 from FMDV type O_1 in guinea pigs with similar results. VP_1 and VP_2 are not involved in immune (protective) mechanisms.

Advances with a unit vaccine for the prevention of FMD in cattle and pigs have been made, but the studies with VP_3 and other possible components involved in the immune mechanism require considerably more research. This type of vaccine is highly desirable, though, so these studies must and should continue.

Transmission. Most of the virus in affected animals is concentrated in the epithelial lesions, but during the early febrile period all tissues and organs and all secretions and excretions contain virus. Transmission to susceptible animals near at hand probably occurs through infected saliva. The disease spreads very rapidly to all susceptible animals on infected farms.

Cottral *et al.* (31) demonstrated FMDV in semen before clinical signs appeared and for 10 days after inoculation, and showed that the disease could be transmitted by artificial insemination. This fact should be borne in mind by artificial breeder organizations. No biological insect vector has been identified as important in the spread of FMD. However, there are a few reports that ticks transmitted the disease to cattle. FMD can occur in any season and often seems to be related to the movement of livestock.

Within a comparatively short time after an outbreak on a farm has subsided, or after all infected animals have been removed, the virus disappears. Residual virus may remain in dark damp areas for a long time, however; hence it is very necessary to clean and thoroughly disinfect premises where infection has existed before they are restocked with susceptible stock. It is also wise to allow the premises to remain unstocked for a considerable time after disinfection.

It is the practice of the U.S. Department of Agriculture (87) to permit gradual restocking of premises 30 days after disinfection. A few yearling calves or hogs are first introduced. These are carefully inspected every second day for 10 days, and then semiweekly until the end of the 2nd month. Additional stock may be introduced at this time, but the herd is kept under quarantine and surveillance for a 3rd month. If at the end of 90 days after disinfection there is no evidence of the disease on the premises and no active infection exists on any farms in the immediate neighborhood, the farm is released from quarantine.

It has long been recognized that FMD virus can be shipped to distant parts of the world in infected meat. England has had much experience with this source of infection since it has had to import most of its fresh meat from countries where the disease is enzootic.

The last two outbreaks of FMD in the United States occurred in California in 1924 and 1929. They began in swine fed on ships' garbage that contained scraps of meat from infected areas of the Orient and South America, respectively. The evidence is very strong that the virus was imported in this way. As a result of this experience, ships coming from countries where this disease occurs are no longer allowed to land garbage in any of our ports.

Stockman and Minett (78) studied the survival of FMD virus in carcasses of animals slaughtered while suffering from this disease. They showed that the acidity that develops in muscular tissue after the onset of rigor mortis rapidly destroys any virus it contains. Usually virus cannot be demonstrated after a few days even when the meat is refrigerated normally. Virus in visceral organs, however, and in the marrow of the long bones is not subject to the action of tissue acids, and virus was often demonstrated in such materials for 40 days, and longer when they were kept under refrigeration.

Under a provision of the Hawley-Smoot Tariff Act of 1930, the Secretary of Agriculture of the United States is required to maintain an embargo against the importation of fresh meat, fresh hides, and fresh offal from countries in which FMD is known to exist. This has resulted in the exclusion of meat from these countries, except that which has been canned, dried, or otherwise processed in a way that destroys the virus. The enforcement of this provision is largely responsible for freedom from the disease in the United States since 1929 despite a marked increase of international air and ship traffic. The control officials of the USDA should be congratulated for a job well done despite enormous political pressures to relax their vigilance.

There has been much speculation about the possible role of wild birds in the spread of FMD. Since birds are not naturally susceptible to the virus of this disease, they would have to be mechanical carriers of the virus if they carried it at all. Many species of birds associate closely with farm livestock, and it seems reasonable to believe that they might have some importance in spreading the disease, particularly since no practical quarantine measures have been devised to control their movements. More recently, winds have been incriminated in the spread of FMD by the aerosol route. The initial pattern of outbreaks in England in 1967–68 suggested that spread was airborne. The movement of trucks containing infective milk appears also to have contributed to its spread. Most animals that recover from FMD are not contagious for other animals within a very short time after complete clinical recovery from the disease. The fact that many outbreaks of FMD have occurred in isolated areas, where it has been difficult to explain the origin of the infection, has caused many to believe that recovered animals may continue to harbor virus long after all signs of the disease have vanished, and that such animals often were the cause of new outbreaks. Most attempts to demonstrate virus in recovered animals failed, but van Bekkum (15) demonstrated virus in the saliva of cattle several months after recovery, the virus being capable of infecting unweaned mice and cattle upon inoculation (Figure 45.11). It did not pass naturally to susceptible contact cattle. These studies have been confirmed by many other investigators, Burrows (26) reported on the persistence of FMDV in the tonsils, pharynx, and dorsal surface of the soft palate of sheep for 1 to 5 months. Cattle become carriers after infection with attenuated or virulent virus, and the virus recovered from carriers is more virulent for pigs than cattle (80). In a field study, 1-year-old calves from cows immunized with rabbit-attenuated virus became carriers with the majority lacking demonstrable antibody. Carrier virus in esophageal-pharyngeal fluid may be partially masked by antibodies or other inhibitors, because fluorocarbon treatment increases the infectivity of the test fluid by 10- to 100-fold. It has also been demonstrated that cattle immunized with inactivated virus vaccine may become carriers after exposure to virulent test virus without showing clinical signs of illness. Cattle may be carriers for at least 15 months.

Many unsuccessful attempts to transmit FMDV from carrier to contact cattle under experimental conditions suggest the existence of unknown factors accountable for successful transmission. Carrier cattle undoubtedly contribute to changes in virulence and antigenicity of FMDV, and probably account for the emergence of new viral subtypes where the disease is enzootic and vaccination is practiced. New variants often are available for selection since the mutation rate of some FMDV strains is 1 : 10,000 (60).

Diagnosis. In countries like the United States where FMD does not exist, it is of the utmost importance that cases caused by imported virus be quickly recognized. The stamping-out method is not as costly if the disease has not spread far from the initial site.

Veterinarians and others should always be suspicious of this disease when a number of animals of susceptible species develop stomatitis or lameness about the same time. In these cases the mouths of a number of animals should be examined for evidences of the characteristic vesicles or the denuded areas that follow rupture of the

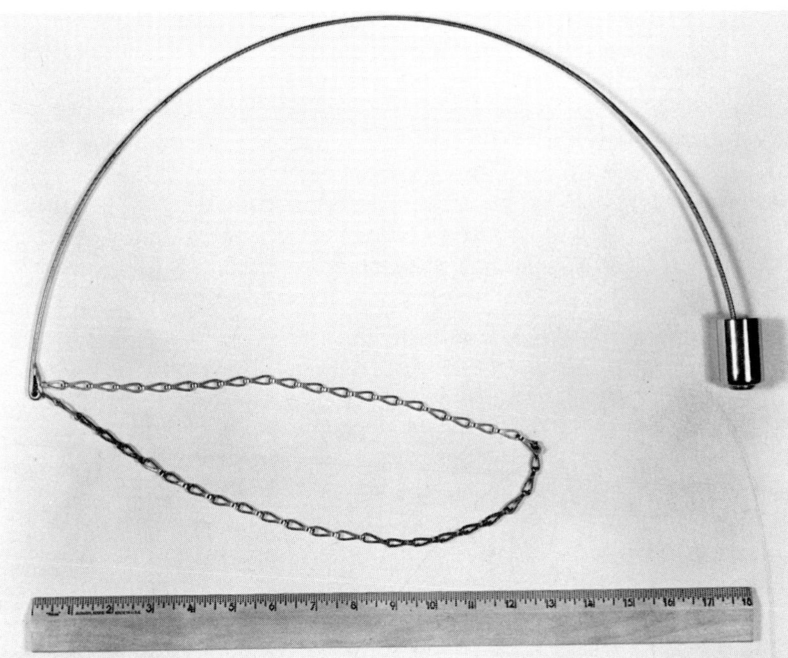

Figure 45.11. Cup probang used for collecting saliva and mucus samples for FMDV isolation from the posterior pharynx and esophagus of the bovine. (Courtesy J. J. Callis and staff, USDA.)

vesicles. The feet should be examined for similar lesions. The epithelial coverings of unruptured vesicles of tongue and feet are the best source of virus (69).

Three other diseases of farm livestock present mouth vesicles and sometimes foot lesions that are not distinguishable from those of foot-and-mouth disease. These are *swine vesicular disease* (SVD), *vesicular stomatitis* (VS) and *vesicular exanthema* (VE). Differentiation of these diseases from FMD is done by laboratory experts. Although the tests are relatively simple, it should be strongly emphasized that the importance of an accurate, early diagnosis is so great that those who have had no experience with them should not ordinarily attempt them. *When a disease that resembles foot-and-mouth disease is seen in any part of the United States, it should be reported promptly to the chief disease-control officer of the state, who will act promptly to have experts assigned to the diagnostic problem.*

Differential diagnosis of these four vesicular viruses by laboratory experts is achieved on the basis of history, clinical signs, and laboratory *in vitro* and *in vivo* tests. When the natural disease occurs in horses, there is no difficulty, for horses are naturally susceptible only to vesicular stomatitis virus. When it occurs in cattle, the question to be decided is whether it is FMD or VS; in swine it may be any of the four viruses.

Both field and laboratory methods are used to reach a decision. If a suitably equipped laboratory is available, not only may these viruses be quickly differentiated from each other by the complement-fixation test, but the virus types may be determined (21, 27, 28). In experienced hands the tests are not only much more rapid than the field or inoculation tests, but they are more accurate and more sensitive.

The field methods of differentiating FMDV, VSV, and VEV depend upon animal inoculation (Table 45.2). The procedures, as recommended by Traum (84), are as follows:

1. Inoculate at least two cattle using fresh vesicular fluid. One should be injected intravenously or intramuscularly; the other should be injected in the mucosa of the tongue, lips, or dental pad, or the fluid may be rubbed into scarified areas.

If the virus is FMD, both animals should develop the disease.

If it is VS, the animal injected intravenously or in-

Table 45.2. Tabular representation of the results of inoculating animals with the viruses of foot-and-mouth disease, vesicular stomatitis, and vesicular exanthema

	FMD	VS	VE
Horse (intradermal-lingual)	−	+	−*
Cow (intradermal-lingual)	+	+	−
Cow (intramuscular)	+	−	−
Guinea pig (intradermal-footpad)	+	+	−

*Small local lesions often produced; no generalization.

tramuscularly will fail to develop the disease; the other should do so.

If it is VE, both animals will fail to develop the disease.

2. Inoculation of swine is useless because the animals usually will develop disease when any of the four viruses is present.

3. Inoculation of horses is very helpful in differentiating between FMD and VS. The horse is susceptible to the virus of VS, but is entirely resistant to that of FMD. The virus of VE is mildly pathogenic for horses. Some animals develop small vesicles near the point of inoculation, others do not. Horses should be injected in the mucous membrane of the dorsum of the tongue, or the virus may be introduced through scarification at this site.

4. Guinea pigs are helpful in differentiating between the virus of VE and the other two viruses, since the former does not cause infections when introduced through the foot pad, whereas FMD and VS quite regularly produce vesicular lesions.

In 1968 Nardelli *et al.* (57) described a vesicular viral disease in Italian pigs which is clinically indistinguishable from FMD, VE, and VS. The Italian virus is classified as an enterovirus, as it has all the characteristics of that genus. By careful study of its properties one can distinguish it from the other vesicular disease viruses of the pig. An approach for differentiation between SVD and FMD is provided by Buckley *et al.* (25). The complement-fixation (CF) test can be used, but its sensitivity is limited, so epithelial diagnostic species should also be inoculated into tube cultures of primary bovine thyroid cells and into 8 oz bottles of $IBRS_2$ line of pig kidney cells. FMDV generally grows causing a cytopathic effect in both types of cell cultures whereas SVD can be detected only in the porcine cells.

Control. The control of FMD is made difficult by four principal factors: (*a*) multiplicity of animal hosts, (*b*) the high contagiousness, (*c*) multiplicity and variability of viral antigenicity, and (*d*) short-lived immunity following infection or vaccination.

In general two methods of control are used for this purpose.

1. *The slaughter method.* This method is the one that has been used in the United States and in other countries sufficiently isolated to make it economically feasible (Figure 45.12). It has been used successfully and often in the British Isles. It has been used less often and with less success on the mainland of Europe.

When this procedure is followed, drastic quarantine measures must be established immediately and enough quarantine officers placed on duty to enforce the regulations. Not only the affected farms but those in a radius of several miles are included in the quarantine. On all the farms of the area the cattle are confined to their stables or corrals, swine are restricted to buildings or small pens,

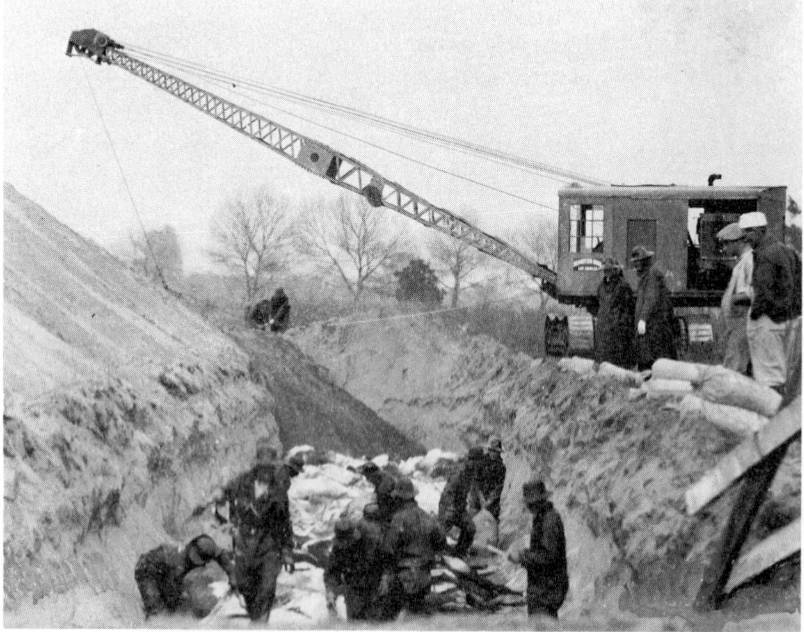

Figure 45.12. Foot-and-mouth disease eradication in the United States. Outbreaks of this disease in this country are stamped out by the drastic method of slaughter and burial on the premises of all infected and all exposed animals. Great trenches are dug, and the cattle are driven into them, slaughtered there, and covered with a deep layer of soil. Before the soil is returned to the trench, the hides of the carcasses are slashed and they are covered with a layer of quicklime. The photograph shows the burial of a herd of infected cattle. (Courtesy L. M. Hurt.)

sheep are restrained, and even dogs and cats are confined to the premises. It is no less important that people be confined and allowed to move from one place to another only by special permission, and then only after thorough disinfection if it is thought that they may have been in contact with infectious materials. The affected animals and all other susceptible stock that may have been in contact with them, whether or not they show any evidence of the disease, are slaughtered as quickly as possible and buried on the premises. The infected premises are then thoroughly cleaned and disinfected with a strong alkali solution. The U.S. Department of Agriculture uses a whitewash made of 5 lb of hydrated or water-slacked (*not air-slacked*) lime, 1 lb of concentrated lye or caustic soda, and 10 gallons of hot water to disinfect floors, stanchions, walls, fences, and any other objects that may have been contaminated with virus. If lime is not available, the lye or soda is used alone at the rate of 2 lb to each 10 gallons of water. This should be applied with a power spray. In any case, all objects should be well soaked with the solution. A 4 percent solution of formaldehyde is considered suitable for harness, blankets, ropes, and finished surfaces that would be damaged by the alkali. Dwellings, milkhouses, and other tight buildings may be fumigated with formaldehyde gas.

Persons whose work requires them to come in contact with infected animals are required to wear rubber clothing—hats, coats, pants, boots, and gloves. These may be disinfected with a 2 percent lye solution or with one of the cresylic acid disinfectants. The lye is caustic and will burn the skin if it is permitted to remain on it. Immediate washing with water is usually sufficient to prevent this; the lye may also be neutralized with vinegar. The alkali solutions may be stored in wooden, earthenware, or metal containers made of any of the common metals except aluminum. Haystacks that may be infected can be made safe by removing the surface layers and spraying the remainder with a 4 percent solution of formalin. Old straw, dried manure, and old wooden structures of small value should be burned. Manure piles may be burned, if sufficiently dry, or the material may be thinly spread on fields to which cattle will not have access and buried by being plowed underground. All procedures must be done very thoroughly.

In the United States the owners of destroyed animals are indemnified from government funds to facilitate the control of FMD. They may also be indemnified for losses of feed, hay, or any other materials destroyed in the course of the cleaning and disinfecting.

All susceptible livestock on farms in the vicinity of infected premises are frequently and thoroughly inspected for evidence of the disease. Milk-receiving stations drawing from the quarantined area are inspected to see that they have suitable equipment, and that it is properly used, to insure that all milk cans returned to farms will be adequately sterilized.

2. *The quarantine and vaccination method.* This method has never been used in the United States. It is unlikely that it ever will be employed in this country unless FMD should become so widespread that the slaughter method would be impracticable. It has been used successfully in some of the countries of continental Europe, and it appears to have contributed to the success of the campaign to stamp out a very extensive outbreak in Mexico. Since the 1967–68 epizootic Britain has maintained stockpiles of vaccine for possible immediate use in conjunction with slaughter in future outbreaks. A similar preparedness policy is under consideration for the United States.

The method consists of rigid quarantine of infected premises with immediate use of inactivated vaccine in all susceptible animals in a zone several miles in width around the center of the infection. This should be done as quickly as the virus type has been determined and vaccine can be procured. When large areas become involved, as in Mexico, all susceptible animals in the entire infected area should be injected.

When vaccines are used, the importance of strict quarantine measures should not be ignored. So far as possible the movement of livestock and of the people who are in contact with livestock should be restricted. The feeding of garbage to swine in such regions should be prohibited unless it is cooked, and unpasteurized milk should not be fed to calves. In 1951–52 an exceptionally virulent and widespread outbreak of foot-and-mouth disease occurred in Europe. Efforts to control this outbreak by vaccination were not very successful as the disease spread faster than animals could be vaccinated. Also, a number of variant types appeared against which the current vaccines were not potent. According to Ramon (62), too little attention was paid to sanitation and quarantine—the old accepted methods—since the opinion existed that these were no longer necessary when the cattle had been vaccinated.

The Disease in Man. Human beings are only slightly susceptible to the virus of FMD. There have been no recognized cases of human infections in any of the more recent outbreaks of the disease in the United States, and none in the last one in Mexico, although countless people have had close contact with active virus. Many of the early reports of foot-and-mouth disease in man must be discounted because of lack of critical evidence that the conditions described were caused by this specific virus.

There are some clear-cut records of the disease in man, however. Gins (41) describes the case of a worker in one of the vaccine laboratories who cut his hand in an accident in which a flask containing vesicular fluid was broken. In this case foot-and-mouth disease virus was identified in the fluid of vesicles that developed along with other symptoms in the individual. There are other authentic cases on record, but the number is less than fifty. The susceptibility of man to the virus of FMD has been reviewed by Betts (17), who concludes that "the number of credible cases in relation to the number of persons exposed is infinitesimal."

The symptoms in man are fever, vomiting, a sense of heat and dryness in the mouth, and the appearance of small vesicles on the lips, tongue, and cheeks. Lesions on the hands have also been described. The course of the disease is short, and there are no records of serious complications or deaths.

FMDV infection in man may be confused with a vesicular exanthema of the hand, foot, and mouth of human beings caused by certain serotypes of Coxsackie virus group A, a subgroup of the genus *Enterovirus*.

REFERENCES

1. Andersen. Am. Jour. Vet. Res., 1975, *36,* 979.
2. Andersen. Am. Jour. Vet. Res., 1977, *38,* 1757.
3. Andersen. Am. Jour. Vet. Res., 1978, *39,* 59.
4. Andersen. Am. Jour. Vet. Res., 1978, *39,* 603.
5. Andersen and Campbell. Am. Jour. Vet. Res., 1976, *37,* 585.
6. Bachrach. Ann. Rev. Microbiol., 1968, *22,* 1508.
7. Bachrach, Breese, Callis, Hess, and Patty. Proc. Soc. Exp. Biol. and Med., 1957, *95,* 147.
8. Bachrach, Hess, and Callis. Science, 1955, *122,* 1269.
9. Bachrach, Moore, McKercher, and Polatnick. Jour. Immunol., 1975, *115,* 1636.
10. Bachrach, Patty, and Pledger. Proc. Soc. Exp. Biol. and Med., 1960, *103,* 540.
11. Bachrach and Vande Woude. Virol., 1968, *34,* 282.
12. Bahnemann. Arch Virol., 1975, *47,* 47.
13. Barteling. Dev. Biol. Stand., 1976, *35,* 55.
14. Bauer, Lorenz, and Wittman. Arch Virol., 1975, *49,* 349.
15. Van Bekkum, Frenkel, Fredericks, and Frenkel. Tijdschr. Diergeneesk., 1959, *84,* 1159.
16. Van Bekkum, Fish, and Dale. Am. Jour. Vet. Res., 1963, *24,* 77.
17. Betts. Vet. Rec., 1952, *64,* 641.
18. Blackwell and Hyde. Jour. Hyg. (London), 1976, *77,* 77.
19. Bögel. Zentrbl. Vet.-Med., 1967, *14B,* 79.
20. Booth, Pay, Hedger, and Barnett. Jour. Hyg. (London), 1975, *74,* 115.
21. Brooksby. Jour. Hyg. (London), 1950, *52,* 394.
22. Brooksby. Agr. Res. Council (Gt. Brit.), Rpt. Series no. 12, 1952, H.M. Stationary Office, London.
23. Brown and Graves. Nature, 1959, *183,* 1688.
24. Brown, Hyslop, Crick, and Morrow. Jour. Hyg. (London), 1963, *61,* 337.
25. Buckley, Osborne, and Pereira. Bull. Off. Int. Epiz., 1975, *83,* 123.
26. Burrows. Jour. Hyg. (London), 1968, *66,* 633.
27. Camargo. Proc. U.S. Livestock Sanit. Assoc., 1954, *58,* 379.
28. Camargo, Eichhorn, Levine, and Giron. Proc. Am. Vet. Med. Assoc., 1950, p. 207.
29. Capstick, Telling, Chapman, and Stewart. Nature, 1962, *195,* 1163.
30. Clarke and Spier. Dev. Biol. Stand., 1976, *35,* 61.
31. Cottral, Gailuinas, and Cox. Arch. f. die gesam. Virusforsch., 1968, *23,* 362.
32. Cowen and Graves. Virol., 1966, *30,* 528.
33. Crowther. Dev. Biol. Stand., 1976, *35,* 185.
34. Dinter and Philipson. Proc. Soc. Exp. Biol. and Med., 1962, *109,* 893.
35. Favre, Valette, Precausta, Roulet, Brun, Terre, Fontaine, and Stellmann. Dev. Biol. Stand., 1976, *35,* 409.
36. Frenkel. Bull. Off. Int. Epiz., 1947, *28,* 155.
37. Frenkel. Am. Jour. Vet. Res., 1951, *12,* 187.
38. Gailuinas and Cottral. Am. Jour. Vet. Res., 1967, *28,* 1047.
39. Gillespie. Cornell Vet., 1954, *44,* 425.
40. Gillespie. Cornell Vet., 1955, *45,* 170.
41. Gins. Klin. Wchnschr., 1924, *3,* 1135.
42. Graves. Jour. Immunol., 1963, *91,* 251.
43. Graves, Cowan, and Trautman. Virol., 1968, *34,* 269.
44. Henderson. Proc. 15th Internatl. Vet. Cong. (Stockholm), 1953, *1,* 191.
45. Hyde, Blackwell, and Callis. Can. Jour. Comp. Med., 1975, *39,* 305.
46. Hyde and Graves. Am. Jour. Vet. Res., 1963, *24,* 642.
47. Kaaden, Adam, and Strohmeier. Jour. Gen. Virol., 1977, *34,* 397.
48. Lake, Priston, and Slade. Jour. Gen. Virol., 1975, *27,* 355.
49. MacKenzie and Slade. Austral. Jour. Exp. Biol. Med. Sci., 1975, *53,* 251.
50. Matheka and Bachrach. Jour. Virol., 1975, *16,* 1248.
51. McCahon, Slade, Priston, and Lake. Jour. Gen. Virol., 1977, *35,* 555.
52. McFadyean. Vet. Rec., 1926, *6,* 358.
53. McKercher and Graves. Dev. Biol. Stand., 1976, *35,* 107.
54. Mohler. USDA Cir. 400, 1926.
55. Mohler. Rpt. Chief, Bur. Anim. Indus., USDA, 1929.
56. Mohler and Rosenau. USDA Cir. 147, 1909.
57. Nardelli, Lodetti, Gualandi, Burrows, Goodridge, Brown, and Cartwright. Nature, 1968, *219,* 1275.
58. Palacios. Rpt. Mtg. Res. Group Standing Tech. Comm., European Comm. Control FMD, Rome, Italy, Paper 8, 1967.

59. Parker, Raymond C. Methods of tissue culture. Paul B. Hoeber, New York, 1938.
60. Pringle. Bull. Off. Int. Epiz., 1964, *61*, 619.
61. Pyakural, Singh, and Singh. Vet. Rec., 1976, *99*, 28.
62. Ramon. Bull. Off. Int. Epiz., 1952, *37*, 625.
63. Rosenbusch. Jour. Am. Vet. Med. Assoc., 1948, *112*, 45.
64. Sakaki, Suphavilai, and Tokuda. Natl. Inst. An. Health Q. (Tokyo), 1977, *17*, 45.
65. Sanger, Rowlands, Cavanagh, and Brown. Jour. Gen. Virol., 1976, *31*, 35.
66. Schmidt. Zeitschr. f. Hyg., 1936, *191*, 1.
67. Schmidt and Hansen. Comp. rend. Soc. Biol. (Paris), 1935, *120*, 1150.
68. Schoening. Jour. Bact., 1927, *13*, 21.
69. Scott, Cottral, and Gailuinas. Am. Jour. Vet. Res., 1966, *27*, 1531.
70. Seibold. Am. Jour. Vet. Res., 1963, *24*, 1123.
71. Sellers. Nature, 1955, *176*, 547.
72. Shahan. N.Y. Acad. of Sci., 1962, *101*, 444.
73. Skinner. Proc. Royal Soc. Med. (Gt. Brit.), 1951, *44*, 1041.
74. Skinner. Nature, 1954, *174*, 1052.
75. Spier. Dev. Biol. Stand., 1976, *35*, 73.
76. Spier and Whiteside. Biotechnol. Bioeng., 1976, *18*, 649.
77. Spier and Whiteside. Biotechnol. Bioeng., 1976, *18*, 659.
78. Stockman and Minett. Second Progress Rpt., Foot and Mouth Dis. Research Comm., H.M. Stationary Office, London, 1927.
79. Sugimura and Eissner. Natl. Inst. An. Health Q., 1976, *16*, 152.
80. Sutmöller, McVicar, and Cottral. Arch. f. die gesam. Virusforsch., 1968, *23*, 227.
81. Swaney. Am. Jour. Vet. Res., 1976, *37*, 1319.
82. Tekerlekov and Mitev. Vet. Med. Nauki., 1976, *13*, 35.
83. Traub and Schneider. Zeitschr. Naturforsch., 1948, *3b*, 178.
84. Traum. Jour. Am. Vet. Med. Assoc., 1936, *88*, 316.
85. Trautwein. Arch. f. Tierheilk., 1926, *54*, 273.
86. Ubertini, Nardelli, Prato, Panina, and Santero. Zentrbl. Vet.-Med., 1963, *10B*, 93.
87. USDA, Bureau of Animal Industry. Instruction for employees engaged in eradicating foot and mouth disease. Washington, 1943.
88. Vallée and Carré. Comp. rend. Acad. Sci., 1922, *174*, 1498.
89. Waldmann and Kobe. Berl. tierärztl. Wchnschr., 1938, *22*, 317 and 349.
90. Waldmann and Pape. Berl. tierärztl. Wchnschr., 1921, 37, 349.
91. Waldmann and Trautwein. Berl. tierärztl. Wchnschr., 1926, *42*, 569.
92. Yilma. Am. Jour. Vet. Res., 1979, In press.
93. Zoletto and Gagliardi. Dev. Biol. Stand., 1976, *35*, 27.

THE GENUS *RHINOVIRUS*

The type-species for the genus *Rhinovirus* is *Rhinovirus* h-1A of man. Other members in the genus are additional human rhinoviruses (more than 100), equine rhinoviruses, and bovine rhinoviruses. The particles contain 30 percent of single-stranded RNA with a molecular weight of 2.4 to 2.8 × 10^6 daltons. Isometric nonenveloped particles are 20 to 30 nm in diameter, probably with icosahedral symmetry. Thirty-two capsomeres seem to form a symmetrical capsid for the RNA core. Ether-resistant particles are labile at pH 3, and some viruses are stabilized by magnesium chloride. They have a sedimentation rate of 140 to 150 S and a buoyant density in cesium chloride of 1.38 to 1.43 g per ml. The viruses multiply in the cytoplasm and normally reside in respiratory and ancillary structures.

Bovine Rhinovirus

Bovine rhinovirus is one of a number of viruses isolated from the respiratory tract of cattle; it was first described by Bögel (1). Its significance as a pathogen of economic importance is still unclear, but fragmentary evidence suggests that it is a widespread infection in the cattle population (2). Limited serological surveys have always found antibodies to rhinovirus in test cattle populations in rather high percentages (2, 5). The virus appears to be highly specific for cattle, with a strict affinity for mucous membranes of the respiratory tract, principally the nasal mucosa.

Character of the Disease. Field experience with respiratory disease caused by bovine rhinovirus is limited, and only a few isolations have been made. It is rarely isolated from bovine respiratory outbreaks, but this failure may be due in part to the difficulties associated with isolating the virus.

In natural and experimental cases the disease is usually characterized by a serous nasal discharge that is seen 2 to 4 days after exposure (2). Other signs of illness may be a rise in temperature, depression, coughing, anorexia, hyperpnea, and dyspnea (6). A pneumonic condition may occur in some experimental calves without other signs of illness (6, 7). In their experiments Mohanty *et al.* (6) observed pneumonia in calves inoculated intratracheally but not in calves exposed to their isolate by the intranasal route. Mayr *et al.* (4) failed to produce disease in calves with their isolate of bovine rhinovirus. Thus, virulence of a strain may play an important role in the production of disease, but a great deal more needs to be learned about host susceptibility and immunity. The principal pathological changes occur in the nasal passages.

Apparently the morbidity in affected herds is high, but the mortality is negligible. The infection has been reported in Western Germany (2), Great Britain (3), and the United States (2, 6).

Properties of the Virus. Bovine rhinovirus is an RNA virus less than 30 nm in diameter. It is resistant to lipid solvents such as chloroform, ether, and sodium dodecyl sulfate. It is inactivated at pH 4 to 5.

The original isolates of bovine rhinovirus were serologically related or identical (2, 3). A second type is now known to exist. In comparative studies with 11 human rhinovirus serotypes no serological relationship was found. More than 100 rhinovirus serotypes have been described in man, so it will not be surprising if additional serotypes are subsequently described in cattle.

Attempts to demonstrate a viral hemagglutinin utilizing red blood cells from various species failed (3).

Cultivation (2). The only known host system available for the cultivation of bovine rhinovirus are bovine kidney-cell cultures. Cytopathogenic effects are observed in monolayer cultures maintained at 33 C 1 to 3 days after inoculation. At 33 C viral replication leads to more marked cytopathic changes and a higher infectivity yield than incubation at 37 C. At 33 C viral titers usually are approximately 10^5 $TCID_{50}$, and disruption of cells produces higher virus yields. Virus plaques are visible in this cell-culture system 4 days after inoculation.

Bovine rhinovirus failed to produce a cytopathic effect in cell cultures of other bovine tissues and kidney cells from other species. Clinical signs were not observed in various aged mice inoculated by various routes. No alterations were observed in guinea pigs or in embryonated hens' eggs injected with bovine rhinovirus.

The virus is quite stable at −60 C for long periods of time. It is readily inactivated by heat.

Immunity. Cattle with low titers of serum-neutralizing antibodies can be infected with challenge virus of the same serotype, and maternal immunity in calves is never complete (2). These experimental observations suggest that cattle may be reinfected with the same serotype if the titer drops to a low level, but this is mere speculation.

In cattle with no serum-neutralizing antibody, active immunity is accompanied by the production of serum-neutralizing titers that range from 1 : 2 to 1 : 100 against 100 $TCID_{50}$ of rhinovirus (2). The mean antibody titer seems to increase with age, possibly as a result of reinfection with some serotype (2).

There is no evidence that recovered cattle are carriers of the virus, although exhaustive studies have not been done. Virus carriers have been detected in other animal species recovered from Picornaviridae infections.

Transmission. Virus can be isolated from the nasal exudate of cattle only for a few days after inoculation. It is obvious that our knowledge of the transmission and maintenance of this virus in the cattle population is extremely limited. Somehow the virus is maintained in nature and commonly transmitted to cattle, as the morbidity in this host is high.

Diagnosis. Clinically, diagnosis of rhinovirus infection from other respiratory pathogens of cattle is difficult if not impossible. The demonstration of a rising serum-neutralizing titer with paired sera is a sound basis for a positive diagnosis. Isolation of the virus in tissue culture is rather difficult, but is the only method available at present. Its identification as a rhinovirus includes resistance to chloroform, sensitivity to acid media (pH 4 to 5), optimum growth at 33 C, and a lack of demonstrable pathogenicity for embryonated hens' eggs or small laboratory animals.

Control. Until we have further information regarding the economic importance of this disease there is no need for a vaccine.

The Disease in Man. There is no evidence that bovine rhinovirus causes disease in man.

REFERENCES

1. Bögel. Zentrbl. f. Bakt., 1962, *187,* 2.
2. Bögel. Jour. Am. Vet. Med. Assoc., 1968, *152,* 780.
3. Ide and Darbyshire. Brit. Vet. Jour., 1969, *125,* Initial Rpt. VII, no. 1.
4. Mayr, Wizigmann, Wizigmann, and Schliesser. Zentrbl. Vet.-Med. 1965, *12B,* 1.
5. Mohanty. Jour. Am. Vet. Med. Assoc. 1968, *152,* 784.
6. Mohanty, Lillie, Albert, and Sass. Am. Jour. Vet. Res., 1969, *30,* 1105.
7. Wizigmann and Schiefer. Zentrbl. Vet.-Med., 1966, *13B,* 37.

Equine Rhinovirus

Equine rhinovirus infection occurs in North America, South America, Europe, and Africa. Holmes, Kemen, and Coggins (5) recently provided information about the incidence of the disease in selected United States horse populations. In most instances the infection in horses is inapparent, but it may cause a mild to severe upper respiratory disease. Plummer first characterized the virus and disease in horses (7, 8). Until recently all subsequent isolates from horses were serologically related to the first isolate of Plummer except one isolated and described in

Canada (3) but no longer available for confirmation of a second type. In 1977, Newman *et al.* (6) isolated and described the properties of a second serotype recovered from sick horses in a Swiss army remount station (4). In 1978, a probable third serotype was reported (10).

Character of the Disease. The incubation period is 3 to 7 days. The signs of illness in natural outbreaks include fever, anorexia, and a copious nasal discharge (3). The discharge is initially serous but later mucopurulent in nature. There may be a mild cough and a marked pharyngitis. Lymphadenitis and abscesses of the submaxillary lymph nodes is sometimes observed as a result of secondary bacterial infection, usually with *Streptococcus equi* or *Streptococcus zooepidemicus,* and this prolongs the disease beyond a few days. Infected stables have a high morbidity but a negligible mortality. Virus is recovered from nasopharyngeal swabs taken from horses with high antibody levels (1, 9).

The Disease in Experimental Animals. Plummer and Kerry (9) described the clinical signs and virological findings of experimental infection in horses. The clinical signs were similar to those observed in natural disease. The majority of susceptible horses developed a viremia which lasted 4 to 5 days, terminating with the appearance of serum-neutralizing antibodies. Virus was recovered from the pharyngeal tissues of slaughtered horses but not from the intestinal tract. It was estimated that virus persisted for at least 1 month in the pharyngeal tissues on the basis of virus recovery from the feces.

Equine rhinovirus differs from human and bovine rhinoviruses in its pathogenicity for other animal species (8). Rabbits, guinea pigs, monkeys, and man are susceptible to intranasal instillation of rhinovirus type 1 (8). Virus was isolated from blood of man and monkeys, and from rabbits, for a few days after virus instillation and from the upper respiratory tract and associated lymph nodes of the laboratory animals for as long as 10 days after infection. Virus also was isolated from the urine and kidneys of some laboratory animals. Neutralizing antibody appeared in the serum of all species about 7 days after exposure.

Unsuccessful attempts to infect mice, hamsters, chickens, and embryonated hens' eggs have been reported (1). A Canadian strain also failed to produce infection in the guinea pig (1).

Properties of the Virus. The physicochemical properties are similar to those of bovine rhinovirus (1). Its particle diameter is 25 to 30 nm with an RNA genome. It is reasonably heat-stable, with little loss of infectivity over several days at 37 C, and with no appreciable loss of titer of two virus strains maintained at 50 C for 1 hour (11). The virus is not stabilized against inactivation at 50 C with 1 M magnesium chloride.

There are two serologically distinct equine rhinoviruses (4)—perhaps three (4). Types 1 and 2 have slightly different sedimentation coefficients and buoyant densities (4). A limited number of base composition analyses also showed differences between the two virus RNAs. The polypeptide profile of each serotype in polyacrylamide gels was similar to those of other picornaviruses, but the two serotypes could be readily differentiated from each other. No hemagglutinin has been demonstrated for these viruses. The serological test presently used is the serum-neutralization test (2).

Cultivation. The equine rhinovirus strains differ from human and bovine rhinoviruses since they will grow in cultures prepared from several animal species (1). A cytopathic effect is produced by equine rhinovirus in primary kidney cultures prepared from the horse, monkey, rabbit, dog, and hamster, in diploid cells of equine origin, and in stable cell lines such as HeLa and HEP-2 from the human, LLC-MK_2 from the monkey, and RK-13 from the rabbit. Field isolations have been made in several of these cell culture types. The cytopathic changes in cell culture are typical of rhinoviruses, and plaques are present under suitable cultural conditions. A temperature of 33 C and the special requirement of low bicarbonate for human and bovine rhinoviruses are not essential for optimum growth with known strains of equine rhinovirus.

Immunity. Our knowledge of immunity to equine rhinovirus is rather limited, and some of our present ideas are based on our general knowledge of immunity as it pertains to other rhinovirus infections of animals and man.

Neutralizing antibody to equine rhinovirus is detected 7 to 14 days after infection, and some horses develop maximum serum titers ($>\log 10^3$) which presumably persist for long periods of time. The persisting titers are based on field observations, so reinfection cannot be excluded as the factor accounting for persisting antibody. The relationship of antibody level and protection against disease is not known for equine rhinovirus infection. There probably is a relationship as established for rhinovirus infections of other species since a low level of antibody ($<\log 10^{0.5}$) does not protect against infection, whereas higher levels do. There is indirect evidence that maternal neutralizing antibody protects, as 22 foals less than 6 months of age had no antibody (3). It is assumed these foals were protected against this common infection without the development of an active immunity and by 5 to 6 months of age lost their maternal antibody. This speculation was confirmed in a study of 5-month-old foals from immune mares that had no antibody (1). In contrast, a high percentage of Thoroughbreds in training had antibody (9). Other small serological surveys have demonstrated that it is a highly contagious and common infection in the horse population.

Transmission. Rhinovirus infections of horses are spread mainly by direct or indirect contact with nasal excretions from infected horses and by aerosol inhalation over limited distances (1). Horses can carry the virus for at least 1 month after infection, so carrier horses as well as horses in the acute stage of infection with or without signs of illness are good sources of virus for perpetuating the disease on a premises. The virus is also quite stable and conceivably could survive on inanimate objects of an infected premises for a long period of time.

Diagnosis. Isolation of the virus from the blood or from the nasal excretions during the acute stage of disease can be readily made in a tissue-culture system. Virus can also be isolated from the pharynx of some horses for as long as 30 days after onset of infection. The virus has the characteristics of a typical rhinovirus; it is a small RNA virus with resistance to lipid solvents, susceptibility to pH 4 to 5, lack of demonstrable pathogenicity for embryonated hens' eggs, and typical Picornaviridae cytopathic effect in cell culture.

The demonstration of a rising serum titer with paired sera is another excellent means of diagnosis. The use of immune electron microscopy offers a rapid means of diagnosis.

Control. Present knowledge suggests that a suitable vaccine could be developed that would protect horses against this disease (1). If a number of serotypes are subsequently found, it may not be feasible. This is the problem in man where at least 100 serotypes are known to exist.

The Disease in Man. Plummer's studies (7, 8) suggest that man can acquire infection without symptoms from contact with diseased horses, but he found no evidence of transmission from man to man or from laboratory animal to laboratory animal.

REFERENCES

1. Burrows, Proc. 2nd Internatl. Conf. Equine Inf. Dis., ed. John T. Bryans and Heinz Gerber. Karger, Basel, 1969.
2. Ditchfield. Jour. Am. Vet. Med. Assoc., 1969, *155*, 384.
3. Ditchfield and MacPherson. Cornell Vet., 1965, *55*, 181.
4. Hofer, Steck, Gerber, Lohrer, Nicolet, and Paccaud. Proc. 3rd Internatl. Conf. Equine Inf. Dis., ed. John T. Bryans and Heinz Gerber. Karger, Basel, 1972, p. 527.
5. Holmes, Keman, and Coggins. Proc. 4th Internatl. Conf. Equine Inf. Dis., ed. John T. Bryans and Heinz Gerber. Veterinary Publications, Inc., Princeton, N.J., 1978, p. 315.
6. Newman, Rowlands, Brown, Goodridge, Burrows, and Steck. Intervirol., 1977, *8*, 145.
7. Plummer. Nature, 1962, *195*, 519.
8. Plummer. Arch. f. die gesam. Virusforsch., 1963, *12*, 694.
9. Plummer and Kerry. Vet. Rec. 1962, *74*, 967.
10. Steck, Hofer, Schaeren, Noclet, and Gerber. Proc. 4th Internatl. Conf. Equine Inf. Dis., ed. John T. Bryans and Heinz Gerber. Veterinary Publications, Inc., Princeton, N.J., 1978, p. 321.
11. Wilson, Bryans, Doll, and Tudor. Cornell Vet., 1965, *55*, 425.

THE GENUS *ENTEROVIRUS*

The type species for the genus *Enterovirus* is *Enterovirus* polio 1. Other members of the genus are at least 63 human enteroviruses including polioviruses, Coxsackie viruses, human hepatitis A virus, and echoviruses; bovine enteroviruses; porcine enteroviruses including Teschen virus and swine vesicular disease; simian enteroviruses; Nodamura virus; murine encephalomyelitis virus; and encephalomyocarditis virus. Other members are duck and turkey hepatitis viruses, avian encephalomyelitis virus, and acute bee-paralysis virus.

The particles contain 20 to 30 percent single-stranded RNA with an appropriate molecular weight of 2.5×10^6 daltons. Nonenveloped isometric particles with icosahedral symmetry are 20 to 30 nm in diameter. The particles have a sedimentation rate of 150 to 160 S and a buoyant density in cesium chloride of 1.34 to 1.35 g per cm^3. Naturally occurring protein shells have a sedimentation rate of 80 S. The particles are naked (no envelope) and inactivated at 50 to 60 C after 30 minutes. The virions are acid-stable at pH 3 and are resistant to ether and other lipid solvents. The virus is synthesized in the cytoplasm and principally resides in the intestinal tract. Replication involves functional protein formation by posttranslational cleavage or an unpunctuated precursor.

Porcine Enteroviruses

Porcine enteroviruses are cytopathogenic agents isolated from the feces, alimentary tract, and the nasopharynges of pigs in cell cultures. The prototype porcine enterovirus is the virus of Teschen disease, porcine enterovirus type 1.

The physiochemical characteristics of porcine enteroviruses are typical of the genus *Enterovirus*. Multiplication of the viruses takes place principally in the alimentary tract, but it can also be recovered from the brains of colostrum-deprived pigs that develop nervous manifestations as a result of experimental infection. All porcine enteroviruses grow well on primary porcine kidney cells. Most isolates replicate well on the PK 15 stable kidney-cell line, but isolation is more difficult to achieve in this line than in primary cultures. The viruses produce two different types of cytopathogenic effect, and most strains will cause plaque formation. The viruses are host-specific, as attempts to adapt them to other hosts have failed except those of Moscovici *et al.* (7), who reported pathogenicity for the hen's embryonated egg, including swine vesicular disease.

There are nine porcine enterovirus serotypes, and some are pathogenic for the natural host. Most pathogenic strains produce polioencephalomyelitis, although others called SMEDI (Stillbirth, Mummification, Embryonic Death, Infertility) viruses are implicated with reproductive disorders. One strain of porcine enterovirus reputedly causes severe pneumonia when instilled into the nostril (6), and other strains produce mild pneumonitis by the same route. (1). Pericarditis and myocarditis have been observed in experimentally infected germ-free pigs that also developed encephalomyelitis (4). Porcine enterovirus type 9 causes swine vesicular disease, and as previously stated porcine enterovirus type 1 causes Teschen disease.

Serological surveys have shown that porcine enteroviruses are worldwide in distribution and the infection rate among pig populations is high. It is extremely difficult to prevent the spread of these agents, and it is rare indeed to find a pig herd without antibodies to one or more of the porcine enteroviruses. The antibody response of the pig to various enteroviruses varies, but in general, higher neutralizing-antibody titers are produced by the pathogens. In some inapparent cases of Teschen disease only low titers of neutralizing antibody are produced and precipitating antibodies are absent (5). Perhaps these infections were limited to the gastrointestinal tract and high titers are associated with those cases in which a viremia is part of the infectious process.

Vaccination against Teschen disease is presently indicated. If virulent strains of Teschen disease virus are not known to exist in a country or territory, there is every justification to guard against introduction of virulent strains. Vaccine trials with inactivated and attenuated virus vaccines have been reported for protection of pigs against porcine enterovirus serotype 2 (T-80 strain) (2, 3).

These viruses are not known to cause disease in humans or in animals other than the pig.

REFERENCES

1. Betts. "Porcine enteroviruses," *in* Diseases of swine, 2nd ed., ed. Howard W. Dunne. Iowa State Univ. Press, Ames, Iowa, 1970.
2. Hazlett and Derbyshire. Can. Jour. Comp. Med., 1977, *41*, 264.
3. Hazlett and Derbyshire. Can. Jour. Comp. Med., 1977, *41*, 257.
4. Long, Koestner, and Kasza. Lab. Invest., 1966, *15*, 1128.
5. Mayr and Wittman. Zeitschr. f. Immunoforsch., 1959, *117*, 45.
6. Meyer, Woods, and Simon. Jour. Comp. Path., 1966, *76*, 397.
7. Moscovici, Ginevri, and Mazzaracchio. Am. Jour. Vet. Res., 1959, *20*, 625.

Teschen Disease

SYNONYMS: Porcine poliomyelitis, Talfan disease, infectious porcine encephalomyelitis

This is a virus-induced encephalomyelitis of swine that has caused serious losses in Czechoslovakia, southeastern Germany, Hungary, Yugoslavia, and Poland. It has also been reported in Switzerland, France, Sweden, Denmark, Great Britain, and Madagascar. In England it became known as *Talfan disease* before its identity became established as a milder form of the disease. This disease has not been recognized in Asia. Mild strains are present in Canada (11), the United States (7), and Australia. A condition described by Thordal-Christensen in Denmark as *benign enzootic paresis of swine* may be a mild form of Teschen disease (12).

The disease was first accurately described in 1929. Teschen is the name of a town in Czechoslovakia where the disease was first recognized. So far as is known, natural infection with this virus occurs only in swine.

Character of the Disease. The incubation period averages about 14 days, though it may be considerably longer or shorter. Sometimes the disease is sporadic, affecting only a few individuals in a herd; at other times it may affect nearly the whole herd. The disease may be acute or chronic, and there is an inapparent form. The prodromal signs are fever, lassitude, and inappetence. This may be followed by a variety of nervous signs—irritability, convulsions, prostration, stiffness, and then paralysis of the legs, particularly of the hind legs. Opisthotonos is frequent. Often the animals lie on their sides and make running motions with their forelegs. Sometimes they squeal when disturbed. The mortality averages about 70 percent, varying from 50 to 90. Animals that recover from the acute stages frequently have residual paralysis. If such animals are carefully nursed, they may live a long time, in which case atrophy of affected muscles may occur. Animals that live more than 1 week often develop pneumonia and succumb.

There are no gross lesions with the possible exception of myocardial lesions. The microscopic lesions are confined to the central nervous system, in which they are typical of a diffuse encephalomyelitis. Cytoplasmic masses occur in nerve cells. With minor exceptions the lesions are confined to the gray matter. Dobberstein (2) was so impressed with the similarity of these lesions to those of poliomyelitis of man that he insisted on calling the disease *porcine poliomyelitis.* Horstmann, Manuelidis, and Sprinz (6), while admitting that the cord lesions have a resemblance to those of poliomyelitis, think that the diffuseness of the lesions and especially their great concentration in the cerebrum make them very different from those of the human disease.

Properties of the Virus. The virus particles are approximately 20 to 25 nm in diameter (5). The viral antigen has been demonstrated in the cytoplasm and to a lesser degree at the periphery of the nucleus (10). Cold phenol has been used to extract the infectious RNA.

It has a wide range of pH stability and shows ether resistance, and it survives well at icebox or low temperatures. A temperature of 60 C for 20 minutes or 0.15 percent formalin inactivates the virus. The International Committee on Taxonomy of Viruses has designated the virus porcine enterovirus type 1. The Teschen and Konratice strains are representative of type 1. The Talfan strain is antigenically identical to the other two strains. The neutralization test in pig kidney cell cultures and the gel-diffusion test demonstrate antibodies.

Cultivation. Fortner was able to obtain growth of the virus in chick embryos. Horstmann obtained survival in tissue cultures for 17 days, but was unable to prove that multiplication had occurred. Mayr and Schwobel (9) were successful in cultivating the virus in swine kidney cell tissue cultures. After some passages the virus grew well, produced cytopathogenic effects, and retained its virulence for swine. It also produces plaques on monolayers.

Immunity. Animals that have recovered from this disease are solidly immune thereafter, at least for a few months. Several attempts have been made to make a brain-virus vaccine. Fortner (3, 4) had only indifferent success with a formalin-treated vaccine. Single injections failed completely. Better but unsatisfactory results were obtained with two injections. Zarnic (13) reported somewhat better results with a formol-treated brain vaccine.

Rapid passage in pig kidney cultures attenuates the virulence of the virus for piglets. This attenuated virus vaccine or formalin-inactivated vaccine using culture virus gave 80 to 86 percent protection (8). Fortner found that the blood serum of recovered pigs had little effect in protecting against virus exposure.

Transmission. The disease apparently is transmitted by direct contact. Experimentally it was shown that it can be transmitted by feeding and by intranasal instillation. Fortner, however, was not able to demonstrate virus in the nasal secretions. The virus is usually a harmless inhabitant of the intestinal tract. Seldom does the disease spread rapidly in a herd. Fortner obtained infection by pen contact in only 3 out of 29 trials.

It was suggested that the disease might be due to the virus of cholera, but Diernhofer (1) found that animals immune to cholera can be infected with the Teschen virus and that animals that have recovered from the latter can be infected with cholera. It seems to be clearly established that the Teschen virus is unique and not related to any other disease-producing agent.

Virus has been inoculated by various workers into mice, rats, guinea pigs, sheep, cattle, and monkeys, generally intracerebrally, with negative results.

REFERENCES

1. Diernhofer. Deut. tierärztl. Wchnschr., 1940, *48,* 213.
2. Dobberstein. Zeitschr. f. Infektionskr. Haustiere, 1942, *49,* 54.
3. Fortner. Deut. tierärztl. Wchnschr., 1941, *49,* 43.
4. Fortner. Zeitschr. f. Infektionskr. Haustiere, 1942, *59,* 81.
5. Horstmann. Jour. Immunol., 1952, *69,* 379.
6. Horstmann, Manuelidis, and Sprinz. Proc. Soc. Exp. Biol. and Med., 1951, *77,* 8.
7. Koestner, Long, and Kasza. Jour. Am. Vet. Med. Assoc., 1962, *140,* 811.
8. Mayr and Correns. Zentrbl. Vet-Med., 1959, *6,* 416.
9. Mayr and Schwobel. Monatsh. f. Tierheilk., 1956, *8,* 49.
10. Mussgay. Zentrbl. f. Bakt., I Abt. Orig., 1958, *171,* 231.
11. Richards and Savan. Cornell Vet., 1960, *50,* 132.
12. Thordal-Christensen. Monograph, Royal Vet. and Agr. College, Copenhagen, 1959.
13. Zarnic. Jugoslav. veterinarski glasnik, 1947, *11-12,* 600

(Abstract in Jour. Am. Vet. Med. Assoc., 1948, *113*, 181.)

Porcine SMEDI Group of Enteroviruses

In 1965 Dunne *et al.* (2) reported on two serologically distinct groups of swine enteroviruses that are associated with stillbirth, mummification, embryonic death, and infertility in swine. These groups were designated as SMEDI A and SMEDI B. During a 6-year period of porcine abortions it was shown that viruses were involved in 22 percent of the cases and enteroviruses (10.9 percent) were most commonly isolated followed by parvoviruses (4.9 percent), reoviruses (4.4 percent), pseudorabies viruses (1 percent), and adenoviruses (0.8 percent) (3).

Character of the Disease. The problem herds from which enteroviruses were isolated had similar disease syndromes and epizootiological pictures (2). The most consistent observation was a decrease or absence of living pigs at birth and the passage of 1 to 12 mummified fetuses of varying sizes. Many pigs alive at birth died a few hours later. The number of live pigs farrowed by infected sows was less than one-half the average number of unaffected sows. Some infected sows that were bred returned to heat but never farrowed. Repeat breedings were more frequent. At no time during the course of infection did sows show signs of illness. No other diseases were observed in these herds, and certain ones such as brucellosis and leptospirosis were eliminated on the basis of serological testing. Both Yorkshire and Berkshire breeds were involved. In one herd two serological types of SMEDI viruses were isolated in kidney cells from fetal or newborn pigs.

At necropsy the gross lesions in experimental and field stillborn pigs were limited to mild edema, particularly of the spiral colon, hydrothorax, and hydropericardium. Preliminary histological studies of a few stillborn pigs included cellular infiltration, edema, and hemorrhage. These lesions were in most but not in all of the stillborn pigs examined. Encephalitic lesions were seen in a number of the animals.

In England, swine herds affected with similar reproductive disorders were studied by Cartwright and Huck (1). Fifteen enteroviruses were isolated and five were placed in the SMEDI A group, three in the SMEDI B group, two in the SMEDI C group, and one in the T80 group of porcine enteroviruses. A parvovirus also was isolated from many of their test materials. Steck and Addy in Switzerland (4) isolated 30 enteroviruses from 47 aborted fetuses. Their isolates fell into two serological groups with some cross-reaction with SMEDI B and SMEDI C groups.

Properties of the Virus. In the tissue culture neutralization test the SMEDI group A and B viruses were compared with many other viruses of swine. The SMEDI group A appears somewhat related to a group of swine enteroviruses not yet fully classified but designated as Group II. The SMEDI group B show some relationship to edema disease virus and the virus of Ontario (Canada) polioencephalitis of swine. There was no relationship of either group with Ontario (Canada) hemagglutinating, Teschen (Talfan), hog cholera, or transmissible gastroenteritis viruses.

Hemagglutination and hemadsorption trials were negative.

Cultivation. The SMEDI viruses were isolated from infected fetuses, still alive or dead for only a short period of time, in kidney cell cultures from healthy fetuses or newborn pigs. The viruses produced a cytopathogenic effect in these cultures.

Immunity. After infection, sows develop a significant neutralizing antibody titer. The importance of these antibodies in terms of protection or its duration have not been ascertained.

Control. No control measures can be suggested because the means of transmission of this disease are not definitely known.

The Disease in Man. There is no evidence that it occurs in man.

REFERENCES

1. Cartwright and Huck. Vet. Rec., 1967, *81*, 196.
2. Dunne, Gobble, Hokanson, Krandel, and Bubash. Am. Jour. Vet. Res., 1965, *26*, 1284.
3. Kirkbride and McAdaragh. Jour. Am. Vet. Med. Assoc., 1978, *172*, 480.
4. Steck and Addy. Personal communication, 1968.

Swine Vesicular Disease

In 1966 swine vesicular disease appeared on two farms in large numbers of pigs; the disease was indistinguishable from other porcine vesicular diseases including foot-and-mouth disease, vesicular stomatitis, and vesicular exanthema (12). The disease was disseminated rapidly to many countries in Europe, including Britain, Japan, and Taiwan. At present there is no evidence of SVD in Britain (7). It has not been observed in pigs from the United States. This virus has been designated porcine enterovirus type 9, and it has a close serological relationship to Coxsackie B_5 virus of humans (2, 5).

Terpstra (13) wrote a comprehensive review on SVD in 1975.

Character of the Disease. The clinical signs include a fever and vesicular lesions on the coronary band and bulbs of the heel and in the interdigital spaces. Vesicles are found also on the snout and on the skin overlying the metacarpals and metatarsals of some animals. Vesicles rupture after 2 to 3 days, and healing is rapid in most animals without secondary bacterial infection. The clinical disease is indistinguishable from the other swine vesicular diseases.

Reports of natural and experimental infections with SVD indicate that some pigs show no clinical signs, but develop significant levels of neutralizing antibody (10, 12). Morbidity rates in natural outbreaks have ranged from 25 to 65 percent. In experimental pigs in contact with clinically affected donors morbidity usually has been 100 percent with pigs showing moderate to severe lesions. Under experimental conditions sows showed slight clinical signs, and lesions were not obvious on casual examination (3).

In a pathogenesis study contact (9) pigs developed vesicular lesions by day 2. Lesions first appeared on the coronary band and then on the dewclaw, tongue, snout, lips, and bulbs of the heels. The onset of viremia coincided with febrile response and the appearance of vesicles. Virus was isolated from the nasal discharge, esophageal-pharyngeal fluid, and feces as early as postinoculation day 1. Greater amounts of virus were isolated from samples collected during the first week of infection, and lesser amounts from samples collected during the second week. The appearance and the distribution of specific fluorescence in various tissues indicated that during the development of swine vesicular disease virus infection, the epithelial tissues were initially involved, followed by a generalized infection of lymph tissues, and, subsequently, a primary viremia. Seroconversion was detectable as early as postinoculation day 4.

A mild, nonsuppurative meningoencephalomyelitis throughout the CNS was observed in both inoculated and contact-exposed pigs. The olfactory bulbs were most severely and most frequently affected, particularly in contact pigs. The most severe brain lesions were found in pigs 3 to 4 days after the onset of viremia; contact pigs showed more severe brain lesions than inoculated pigs. Microscopic changes were also found in the coronary band, snout, tongue, and heart.

The injection of the tongue dermis of a donkey, two cattle, rabbits, and chickens with infective vesicular epithelium failed to induce frank disease. Injection of the footpads of guinea pigs or of the abdominal skin of hamsters failed to elicit an inflammatory reaction. Large doses of tissue-cultured virus given intracerebrally or intraperitoneally in day-old mice produced nervous signs 4 to 5 days after inoculation and death in 5 to 10 days. Virus was distributed in the brain, spinal cord, and muscular tissues. No signs of illness were produced in 7-day-old mice with the same inoculum by the same routes.

Properties of the Virus. This porcine virus has all the characteristics of an enterovirus. It is stable at pH 5, and it is stabilized by 1 M magnesium chloride at 50 C. Its buoyant density in cesium chloride is 1.34 g per cm^3. The virion is resistant to ether. The sedimentation rate is 150 S in sucrose gradients. Viewed with the electron microscope it is roughly spherical, 30 to 32 nm in diameter.

SVDV and Coxsackie B_5 virus were shown to be related but not identical by serological and molecular analysis. Both viruses contain single-stranded RNA and four major polypeptides referred to as VP_1, VP_2, VP_3, and VP_4.

The isolates from the Italian outbreak in 1966 and in Hong Kong in 1971 were different from the isolates of SVDV from England, Italy, and Austria in 1972–73 as determined by polyacrylamide gel electrophoresis. By comparison, there was less antigenic drift between SVD isolates than in the 1952 and 1973 Coxsackie B_5 isolates from humans, and the SVDV isolates were intermediate between the Coxsackie B_5 isolates of 1952 and 1973 (6). Although Coxsackie B_5 virus will not cause vesiculation in experimental pigs, it does produce micropathological lesions in the brain and spinal cord (4, 11).

Various serological tests are used to evaluate the properties of the virus and immunity. The complement-fixation, fluorescent antibody, immunodiffusion, and neutralizing-antibody tests are all used.

Cultivation. The virus produces a cytopathic effect in primary and secondary pig-kidney monolayer cultures and in cultures of pig-kidney cell lines PR 15 and IB-RS-2. No effect was observed in primary calf-kidney or in calf-thyroid monolayer cultures or in first-passaged baby hamster kidney cell-line cultures.

The sequential appearance of SVDV viral antigens and virus (in pig kidney cell line MVPK) was studied by immunofluorescence and electron microscopy (8). The replication cycle was approximately 3 to 4 hours. Viral antigens were demonstrable in the cytoplasm 2 hours after inoculation. After 3 hours, a few viral particles, seen by electron microscopy, were in the cytoplasm. Morphological changes of cells, margination, and condensation of nuclear chromatin occurred at the same time. A compact mass of fluorescence was seen when cells showed cytopathogenic effect at 5.5 hours. Cytoplasmic crystalline arrays of virus were first detected at 7 hours.

Immunity. The duration of immunity to SVDV is unknown. Neutralizing antibodies are formed in the pig after exposure to the virus. Their relationship to protection is not known, but it is reasonable to assume that there is a correlation.

Transmission. The disease appeared on two farms at the same time in the 1966 outbreak in Italy. Both farms received pigs for fattening from the same source. On both farms all introduced pigs were afflicted, and approximately 25 percent of the resident pigs in the same pens showed signs of illness. No new cases were seen after 3 weeks.

Subclinical infection undoubtedly occurs in the field. These pigs also may serve as a means for transmitting the virus, especially if they are stressed.

Diagnosis. The appearance of a vesicular disease in pigs requires immediate contact with a state or federal control official, especially in countries where other diseases such as foot-and-mouth disease, vesicular exanthema, or vesicular stomatitis do not occur. A differential diagnosis can be made only in a laboratory with competent personnel and appropriate reagents available for this purpose. These procedures were discussed in the section on diagnosis of FMDV.

Control. There are no reports in the literature on the development and use of a vaccine against SVD. Britain has controlled the disease by requiring that garbage be cooked and when an outbreak occurred, immediately imposed a strict quarantine and slaughter policy.

The Disease in Man. The close relationship of Coxsackie B_5 virus and SVDV suggests that these viruses could cause disease in both hosts, humans and pigs. Several individuals in a laboratory working with SVDV became ill with symptoms that occur in Coxsackie virus infections, and high levels of antibody to SVD were found in their sera (1). Coxsackie B_5 produces an inapparent infection in pigs.

REFERENCES

1. Brown, Goodridge, and Burrows. Jour. Comp. Path., 1976, *86,* 409.
2. Brown, Talbot, and Burrows. Nature, 1973, *245,* 315.
3. Burrows, Mann, Goodridge, Wrathall, and Done. Zentrbl. Vet.-Med., 1977, *24B,* 177.
4. Garland and Mann. Jour. Hyg. (London), 1974, *73,* 85.
5. Graves, Nature, 1973, *245,* 314.
6. Harris, Doel, and Brown. Jour. Gen. Virol., 1977, *35,* 299.
7. Hendrie, Watson, Hedger, Rowe, and Garland. Vet. Rec., 1977, *100,* 363.
8. Lai, Breese, Moore, and Gillespie. Personal communication, 1979.
9. Lai, McKercher, Moore, Gillespie. Am. Jour. Vet. Res., 1979, *40,* 463.
10. Mann, Burrows, and Goodridge. Bull. Off. Int. Epiz., 1975, *83,* 117.
11. Monlux, McKercher, and Graves. Jour. Vet. Res., 1975, *36,* 1745.
12. Nardelli, Lodetti, Gualandi, Burrows, Goodridge, Brown, and Cartwright. Nature, 1968, *219.* 1275.
13. Terpstra. Tijdschr. Diergeneeskd., 1975, *100,* 555.

Bovine Enteroviruses

Bovine enteroviruses (BE) have been isolated from normal cattle, and from cattle showing various signs of illness. More than 60 isolates in various parts of the world have failed to produce disease in experimental cattle, although Van Der Matten and Packer claim that some of their strains caused diarrhea (7). Anderson and Scott (2) did a serological comparison of the French WD-42 enterovirus isolated with bovine winter dysentery. Their results indicated that the WD-42 isolate failed to produce signs of illness. Serological studies of paired acute and convalescent serum samples from 10 New York State herds naturally infected with winter dysentery essentially showed no relationship to winter dysentery occurring in New York State to WD-42 isolate.

At present, bovine enterovirus types 1 through 7 are recognized by the International Committee on Taxonomy of Viruses. LaPlaca has divided BE into two major groups based on the hemagglutination of rhesus monkey RBC and sensitivity to hydroxybenzylbenzimidole (HBB) (4).

The bovine enteroviruses have the same physicochemical properties as other members of the genus *Enterovirus.* A bovine enterovirus was shown to have 4 major proteins termed VP_1, VP_2, VP_3, and VP_4 (3). BE are present in feces and produce a characteristic enterovirus cytopathic effect in cell cultures of embryonic bovine kidney, calf testicle, embryonic lamb kidney, human kidney, rhesus monkey kidney and testes, rabbit kidney, established bovine kidney, and diploid embryonic bovine trachea (5). Embryonic bovine kidney or calf testicle cell cultures are recommended for initial isolations.

Neutralizing antibody can be produced in various laboratory animals. The rooster and goat are preferred to produce hyperimmune antisera. Rabbits should be avoided because their sera contain a naturally occurring inhibiting substance. Nonspecific inhibitors to bovine enteroviruses have been found in serum, allantoic, and amniotic fluids of bovine fetuses (6). Cross-reactions to FMDV have been observed in normal swine sera using the plaque-reduction neutralization and mouse protection tests (1).

REFERENCES

1. Andersen. Am. Jour. Vet. Res., 1977, *38*, 1757.
2. Andersen and Scott. Cornell Vet., 1976, *66*, 232.
3. Carthew. Jour. Gen. Virol., 1976, *32*, 17.
4. LaPlaca. Arch. f. die gesam. Virusforsch., 1964, *17*, 98.
5. Moll and Davis. Am. Jour. Vet. Res., 1959, *20*, 27.
6. Rossi, Kiesel, and Hubbert. Cornell Vet., 1976, *66*, 381.
7. Van Der Matten and Pecker. Am. Jour. Vet. Res., 1967, *28*, 677.

Avian Encephalomyelitis

SYNONYM: Epidemic tremor of chicks; abbreviation, AE

This avian enterovirus disease was first described by Jones (9) in Massachusetts in 1932. In a more complete description of the disease and the virus that causes it, Jones (10) in 1934 called the disease *epidemic tremor* because of the peculiar vibration of the head and neck that characterizes many cases. Because this sign is not so frequently seen as others referable to damage of the nervous system, Van Roekel, Bullis, and Clarke (21) proposed that it be named *infectious avian encephalomyelitis*. The word *infectious* is now generally dropped from the name.

Character of the Disease. For some years avian encephalomyelitis was believed to be confined to the northeastern part of the United States. In later years, according to Feibel, Helmboldt, Jungherr, and Carson (5), it has been identified in many states across the country, and it has been reported also from Canada, Great Britain, Sweden, South Africa, Korea, and Australia. The disease has a seasonal prevalence in the United States, where it is seen more frequently in the winter and spring months than in the summer.

The disease has been recognized only in very young chickens. It generally makes its appearance when the chicks are 2 to 3 weeks of age, but it may appear earlier or later. Van Roekel and associates have observed signs in chicks as they were removed from the incubator within 24 to 48 hours after they had been hatched. Others have reported cases as late as 42 days after hatching.

The first sign noted is an ataxia or incoordination of the muscles of the legs. The signs become more obvious as the disease progresses, and finally the bird may lose all control of its legs and be unable to stand. Before this stage is reached, the bird is reluctant to move and may walk on its shanks. The characteristic vibration of the muscles of the head and neck usually appears well after the ataxic signs have been noticed. This tremor is periodic, continuing for varying lengths of time. Finally the victim is unable to feed, becomes somnolent, and dies. In many cases the course of the disease is very rapid, somnolence appearing within 24 hours after the first signs are noted.

Chicks infected by intracerebral inoculation rarely show signs in less than 9 or 10 days. There are no data on the incubation period in natural infections; however, it probably is 2 weeks or more.

The course of the disease varies greatly. Many birds become incapacitated so that they cannot reach food and hence die of starvation; others are killed by being trampled by other birds. If separated and given individual care, many severely affected birds will live for a long time, and some even recover.

The losses may be very high, in excess of 50 percent in some cases. The average mortality is about 10 percent.

There are no gross lesions. Microscopically, the islands of lymphatic tissue which, in birds, are scattered throughout the organs, show evidence of marked hyperplasia. The most characteristic lesions, however, are found in the central nervous system. Exceptionally large masses of lymphocytes and monocytes surround all of the blood vessels. Extensive neuronal degeneration occurs especially in the anterior horn of the cord, in the medulla, and in the pons. No specific inclusion bodies have been identified in this disease.

The Disease in Experimental Animals. Avian encephalomyelitis is not known to occur naturally in species other than chickens and pheasants; however, ducklings, turkey poults, and young pigeons may be infected by inoculation. All mammals are refractory. All workers have found that the most certain way of reproducing the disease is by intracerebral injection. Injection of virus peripherally—intravenously, intraperitoneally, or intramuscularly—induces signs in only a small proportion of those inoculated. Chicks from hatching time to 3 weeks of age are most susceptible to inoculation, but Van Roekel (21) and others have succeeded in producing the disease in birds up to 3 months of age, and Feibel (4) has infected birds more than 6 months of age by intraperitoneal injection.

Properties of the Virus. Virus is regularly present in the nervous system of infected birds. Virus suspensions regularly pass V and N Berkefeld filters and Seitz disks. Olitsky and Bauer (18) showed by filtration through Gradocol membranes that the particle size of this virus is about 20 to 30 nm in diameter. The virus is readily preserved for long periods by rapid freeze-drying, and it has retained viability for at least 80 days when suspended in 50 percent neutral glycerol. By the use of polyethylene glycol and fluorocarbon a 50-fold increase of AEV over the original homogenate can be achieved (14). Olitsky (17) found no relationship between the virus of avian encephalomyelitis and that of equine encephalomyelitis. The chick virus proved innocuous for mice, guinea pigs, and monkeys, which are susceptible to the equine virus; furthermore, there were no cross-immunological reactions between the two viruses.

Cultivation. Jungherr, Sumner, and Luginbuhl (11) successfully propagated the virus in embryonated eggs by inoculating them into the orb of the eye. Wills and Moulthrop (23) succeeded by inoculating into the yolk sac and into the allantoic cavity. Kligler and Olitsky (12) failed with chick embryos but succeeded in obtaining growth in a medium consisting of minced chick embryos suspended in a mixture of rabbit serum and Tyrode's solution. Neutralizing antibodies are demonstrable by the use of the cytopathogenic effect produced in monolayers of chick fibroblast cultures (7) and in monkey kidney cell cultures.

Monolayer cell cultures consisting of epithelioid cells from pancreatic tissue of 10- to 13-day-old chicks provided a substrate for the propagation of an embryo-adapted strain of AEV (13).

Immunity. Schaaf and Lamoreux (19) observed that after a flock had suffered from an outbreak of this disease, generally there was very little further trouble from it; apparently the flock had become immunized. Following this observation they injected virus into the birds of the breeding flock when they were 16 to 20 weeks of age. Birds at this age react very mildly to the virus, but they become solidly immune thereafter and apparently do not lay infected eggs when they come into production. Schaaf and Lamoreux claim to have eliminated the disease from a flock by following this procedure. Chicks that have recovered from this disease are resistant to reinoculation, and neutralizing antibodies can be demonstrated in them.

Various test procedures such as the fluorescent antibody (15) immunodiffusion (8), and neutralization tests are available for viral and antibody assay.

In the United States birds approximately 2 to 4 months of age are vaccinated with the embryo-propagated strain 1143 placed in the drinking water. The virus produces no clinical signs of illness in birds of this age and provides protection against infection with natural virus. Other vaccine strains available for use in some other countries include the NSW-1 (22), Philips-Duphar (6), and chicken pancreas cell culture (16).

Transmission. Rather convincing information now exists which shows that horizontal and vertical transmission of the disease takes place. The disease is transmitted from infected chickens of various ages to susceptible birds or by placing susceptible birds in a colony house that previously housed infected chickens (2). Virus has been recovered from the feces of normal chicks. Vertical transmission occurs via infected eggs from carrier birds which produces clinical infection in the progeny (2). Transmission of virus occurs when egg-infected chicks are placed with susceptible contact chicks following exposure within the incubator during hatching (3, 21) or in batteries following hatching with an incubation period of 11 to 16 days following contact (2). Because the disease usually occurs during the winter months, it is unlikely that insect vectors play a role in its transmission.

Diagnosis. Clinical diagnosis of avian encephalomyelitis in young chicks is not difficult. In doubtful cases other chicks may be inoculated intracerebrally with brain tissue. This procedure is not always successful since the viral content of brain tissue of diseased chicks sometimes is below an infectivity level. The presence of blood vessel cuffing, gliosis, and neuronal degeneration points toward a viral encephalitis but does not necessarily indicate this disease. The demonstration of rising antibody titer with paired sera is also useful.

Control. A simple test based on the failure of embryos produced from immune hens to support the growth of virus can be used to select resistant-breeder flocks as a means of avoiding disease in their progeny (20).

It is possible to produce an immune breeder flock by the use of live and inactivated vaccines when used under the appropriate circumstances (1).

The Disease in Man. It is not known to occur in man.

REFERENCES

1. Calnek, Luginbuhl, McKercher, and Van Roekel. Avian Dis., 1961, *5*, 456.
2. Calnek, Taylor, and Sevoian. Avian Dis., 1960, *4*, 325.
3. Doll, Bruner, and Hull. Rpt. of the Director, Ky. Agr. Exp. Sta., 1948, p. 48.
4. Feibel. Thesis, Univ. of Conn., 1951. (*In* Biester, Harry E. and Louis H. Schwarte. Diseases of poultry, 3rd ed. Iowa State Univ. Press, Ames, Iowa, 1952, p. 621.)
5. Feibel, Helmboldt, Jungherr, and Carson. Am. Jour. Vet. Res., 1952, *13*, 260.
6. Folkers, Jaspers, Stumpel, and Wittevrongel. Dev. Biol. Stand., 1976, *33*, 364.
7. Hwang, Luginbuhl, and Jungherr. Proc. Soc. Exp. Biol. and Med., 1959, *102*, 429.
8. Ikeda. Natl. Inst. An. Health Q. (Tokyo), 1977, *17*, 88.
9. Jones. Science, 1932, *76*, 331.
10. Jones. Jour. Exp. Med., 1934, *59*, 781.
11. Jungherr, Sumner, and Luginbuhl. Science, 1956, *124*, 80.
12. Kligler and Olitsky. Proc. Soc. Exp. Biol. and Med., 1940, *43*, 680.
13. Kodama, Sato, and Miura. Avian Dis., 1975, *19*, 556.
14. Matsumoto and Murphy. Avian Dis., 1977, *21*, 300.
15. Miyamae. Am. Jour. Vet. Res., 1977, *38*, 2009.
16. Miyamae. Am. Jour. Vet. Res., 1978, *39*, 503.
17. Olitsky. Jour. Exp. Med., 1939, *70*, 565.
18. Olitsky and Bauer. Proc. Soc. Exp. Biol. and Med., 1939, *42*, 634.
19. Schaaf and Lamoreux. Am. Jour. Vet. Res., 1955, *16*, 627.
20. Taylor and Schelling. Avian Dis., 1960, *4*, 122.
21. Van Roekel, Bullis, and Clarke. Jour. Am. Vet. Med. Assoc., 1938, *93*, 372.
22. Westbury and Sinkovic. Austral. Vet. Jour., 1976, *52*, 374.
23. Wills and Moulthrop. Southwest. Vet., 1956, *10*, 39.

Virus Hepatitis of Ducklings

This disease was first recognized and described by Levine and Fabricant (10) in 1950. The disease had not been seen previously by experienced observers in the duck-raising area on Long Island, where many ducklings have been raised annually for many years. Dougherty (4) has reported finding the disease in Massachusetts and in the western part of New York State. Hanson and Alberts (6) reported an outbreak in Illinois. Asplin and McLauchlin (3) reported the presence of the disease in England. Virus isolated from English birds was neutralized by antiserum obtained from New York. The disease was recognized in Canada in 1957 and the virus isolated (11). It has since been recognized in Michigan and also in various other countries of the world.

This virus affects only young ducklings. There are no signs in adult birds, although such birds often harbor infection. Young chicks and turkey poults have been raised in close association with infected ducks without developing the disease.

Character of the Disease. In the earlier outbreaks, losses occurred only among ducklings between 2 and 3 weeks of age, but later losses were incurred on many farms on birds as young as 3 days. The disease is very acute with a short incubation period of about 2 to 3 days. In most instances signs were not observed longer than 1 hour before death. The affected birds were observed to lag behind the remainder of the hatch; they quickly became somnolent, fell on their sides, and died after a brief struggle. Nearly all deaths in a particular hatch occurred within 4 days, the peak of the death rate usually occurring on the 2nd day. The mortality varies from flock to flock, and from hatch to hatch in the same flock. Sometimes it is as high as 85 to 95 percent of large hatches. In other cases it may be as low as 35 percent.

The principal lesions are found in the liver. Usually it is enlarged and contains petechiae and ecchymotic hemorrhages. Mottling of the parenchyma is commonly seen. Focal necrosis of liver cells occurs. The spleen and kidneys often are swollen. The microscopic changes (5) consist of necrosis of the parenchymal cells and proliferation of bile duct epithelium. These changes are accompanied by varying degrees of inflammatory reaction and hemorrhages. In ducklings that do not die, successful regeneration of liver parenchyma occurs.

In 1969 Toth (14) reported the isolation of an agent from liver suspensions from ducks that died under 2 weeks of age with hepatitis despite a parenteral immunity to duck hepatitis virus (DHV). This agent caused hepatic disease in susceptible ducks and in duck hepatitis virus immune ducks. The clinical signs and lesions were similar but not completely identical to typical virus hepatitis of ducks.

In a recent report (8) it was shown that Toth's agent is a picornavirus that is serologically different from the classical duck hepatitis virus. These investigators recommended that Toth's virus be designated type 3 DHV whereas the classical virus is called type 1 DHV. Type 3 virus had some biological characteristics that differed from type 1.

Properties of the Virus. It is classified as an enterovirus. Electron photomicrographs showed the virus to be spherical and quite small, 20 to 30 nm. It is an RNA virus that is ether-resistant.

Its thermostability at various temperatures was reported by Hwang (9). It resists 0.1 percent formalin held for 8 hours at 37 C.

Attempts to demonstrate hemagglutinins have failed. Two lines of precipitate have been demonstrated in the gel-diffusion test. In 1963 Sueltenfuss and Pollard (13) described a technique for the cytochemical assay of interferon produced by duck hepatitis virus.

Cultivation. The virus can be propagated in developing chick embryos, killing most of the embryos in 4 days without observable lesions. Later deaths showed characteristic lesions consisting of stunting of growth; severe edema; greenish discoloration of the embryo liver, egg fluids, and yolk-sac; and necrotic foci of the liver (10).

In cultures of chick embryo tissues propagation of the virus occurs without production of a cytopathic effect (12).

Immunity. Ducks recovering from the natural disease or from inoculation with egg-propagated virus are resistant to reinoculation, and their sera contain neutralizing antibodies for the virus.

Artificial immunization of ducklings has been attempted. Active immunization with vaccines made from allantoic fluid and embryo livers, inactivated with formalin, and from living virus of egg origin did not give satisfactory results. The failure apparently was due to the fact that the disease usually struck before the animals had had time to produce a protective antibody level. Much better results were obtained with antiserum from ducks that had recovered from the disease. This was secured at the slaughterhouse at the time the birds were dressed for market. This serum, administered intramuscularly in 0.5-ml doses, protected most of the ducklings from the disease when administered at ages varying from 3 to 11 days. In eight trials the treated ducklings showed mortality rates varying from 0 to 19 percent, whereas control ducklings, raised in the same pens, had mortality percentages varying from 26 to 80. This procedure has been used with success on many thousands of ducklings in the concentrated duck-raising area of eastern Long Island, New York.

Asplin (1) has reported success in preventing losses of ducklings by actively immunizing the breeder ducks with virulent virus. He has also reported the successful use as a vaccine of an attenuated strain of virus which had been modified by growth in chick embryos. Ducklings were vaccinated with a needle which was thrust through one of the foot webs after being dipped in virus (2).

Hanson and Tripathy (7) have been successful in immunizing 350,000 ducklings from susceptible and immune breeders by placing an attenuated live duck hepatitis virus in the drinking water. This procedure, if successful, would be ideal as it circumvents handling the birds.

The type 3 DHV (14) is now included in the immunization program for prevention of virus hepatitis in ducks on Long Island. This program now has fewer immunization problems since it has been recognized and included in the vaccine procedures.

Transmission. The means of transmission is not entirely clear. The high incidence of the disease in infected flocks indicates a high rate of transmissibility; yet many instances have occurred in which hatches with a high mortality rate have been kept in the same buildings, and sometimes in the same rooms, with other hatches in which the disease has failed to develop. Transmissibility through eggs has not been proved, and considerable evidence is at hand to indicate that this does not occur. Hatches, and parts of hatches, which have been removed to other premises directly from the incubators have failed to develop the disease, whereas the remainder, kept on the premises, have exhibited a high mortality rate. Present evidence indicates that the disease spreads during the brooding process by contacts other than through droplets.

Diagnosis. The diagnosis is based on clinical signs and is made by inoculation of chick embryos. Inoculations succeed when organ suspensions, blood, or brain material is used for injection.

The Disease in Man. There is no evidence to connect this disease with illness in man. Comparisons of the virus of duck hepatitis with those of virus hepatitis of dogs and man show no serological relationships (5).

REFERENCES

1. Asplin. Vet. Rec., 1956, *68,* 412.
2. Asplin. Vet. Rec., 1958, *70,* 1226.
3. Asplin and McLauchlan. Vet. Rec., 1954, *66,* 456.
4. Dougherty, Ill. Proc. Am. Vet. Med. Assoc., 1953, p. 359.
5. Fabricant, Rickard, and Levine. Avian Dis., 1957, *1,* 257.

6. Hanson and Alberts. Jour. Am. Vet. Med. Assoc., 1956, *128,* 37.
7. Hanson and Tripathy. Dev. Biol. Stand., 1976, *33,* 357.
8. Haider and Calnek. Avian Dis., 1979, *23*, 715.
9. Hwang. Am. Jour. Vet. Res., 1975, *36*, 1683.
10. Levine and Fabricant. Cornell Vet., 1950, *40,* 71.
11. MacPherson and Avery. Can. Jour. Comp. Med., 1957, *21,* 26.
12. Pollard and Starr. Proc. Soc. Exp. Biol. and Med., 1959, *101,* 521.
13. Sueltenfuss and Pollard. Science, 1963, *139,* 595.
14. Toth. Avian Dis., 1969, *13,* 834.

Virus Hepatitis of Turkeys

Two groups of workers in the eastern part of the United States (1, 2) independently and almost simultaneously described a hitherto unknown viral-induced hepatitis of turkey poults. Both were successful in propagating the virus in the yolk sacs of embryonating eggs and in producing the disease in day-old poults by inoculating them into the unabsorbed yolk sacs.

The virus is classified provisionally as an enterovirus. Baby chicks are resistant to inoculation with the virus.

The disease is very contagious and produces a high death rate in poults under 2 weeks of age. Turkeys that recover from infection developed resistance to reinfection, but no serum-neutralizing antibodies were demonstrated in the sera of these birds or in the serum of chickens, turkeys, or rabbits repeatedly inoculated with this virus (3). A common antigen between turkey and duck hepatitis viruses was demonstrated by the agar-gel-diffusion test, but other characteristics of the two viruses are dissimilar (3). Attempts to infect ducklings, quail, and pheasants proved unsuccessful (3).

REFERENCES

1. Mongeau, Truscott, Ferguson, and Connell. Avian Dis., 1959, *3,* 388.
2. Snoeyenbos, Basch, and Sevoian, Avian Dis., 1959, *3,* 377.
3. Tzianabos and Snoeyenbos, Avian Dis., 1965, *9,* 578.

Human Enteroviruses in Dogs

It was reported that the human enteroviruses—ECHO virus type 6, Coxsackie virus B1, B2, and B3—were isolated from nasopharyngeal and rectal specimens of beagle dogs without signs of illness (2, 3). Low neutralizing antibody titers against Coxsackie viruses B1 and B5 were present in some of the sera collected from these dogs. No titers were demonstrated for Coxsackie virus B1 or ECHO virus type 6. There was no correlation between virus isolation and serum titers.

Feeding ECHO virus type 6 to dogs produced signs of enteric disease (4). Although virus was recovered from fecal samples of 5 of the 6 dogs, antibody was not demonstrated.

Neutralizing antibody to poliovirus types 1 and 3, Coxsackie virus A9 and B2, and ECHO virus types 6, 7, 8, 9, and 12 has been found in dog serums (1). Replication of these viruses and the production of disease in the dog by them has not been ascertained.

REFERENCES

1. Gefland. Progr. Med. Virol., 1961, *3,* 193.
2. Lundgren, Clapper, and Sanchez. Proc. Soc. Exp. Biol. and Med., 1968, *128,* 463.
3. Pindak and Clapper. Am. Jour. Vet. Res., 1964, *25,* 52.
4. Pindak and Clapper. Texas Rep. Biol. and Med., 1966, *24,* 466.

Equine *Enterovirus*

An equine enterovirus was isolated from the liver and spleen of an aborted foal (1). The RNA virus is less than 28 nm. It is resistant to ether, chloroform, and trypsin, relatively stable to cations at normal temperatures, and over a wide pH range.

Its significance as a pathogen is yet to be ascertained.

REFERENCE

1. Böhm. Zentrbl. Vet.-Med., 1964, *11B,* 240.

46 The Caliciviridae

This is a new suggested family under consideration by the International Committee on the Taxonomy of Viruses that includes vesicular exanthema of swine virus (VESV), San Miguel sea lion virus (SMSV), and feline calicivirus (FCV). Until recently, it was listed as a possible genus in the family Picornaviridae. Indeed, the caliciviruses do resemble picornaviruses in many respects. They are small, lipid-solvent, ether-resistant viruses that contain a single-stranded, nonsegmented RNA and replicate in the cytoplasm. Yet there are some clear differences; the caliciviruses are larger, with a diameter of 35 to 40 nm. Their capsid is composed of a single major polypeptide (1), and their morphology is distinct and unique with 32 cup-shaped depressions arranged in icosahedral symmetry.

The type species for the family Caliciviridae is vesicular exanthema type A virus. The particles in this family contain single-stranded RNA with a molecular weight of approximately 2×10^6 daltons. The isometric, nonenveloped particles have 32 capsomeres with probable icosahedral symmetry. Their buoyant density in cesium chloride is 1.37 to 1.38 g per cm^3. The particles are unstable at pH 3 and have variable stability at pH 5.

Excellent review articles on the caliciviruses were written by Studdert (14) and by Schaffer (11).

Vesicular Exanthema of Swine

Vesicular exanthema occurs naturally in swine. This disease has been recognized only in the continental United States, Hawaii, and Iceland, where it undoubtedly was carried in American pork. The disease was eradicated in the United States in 1959.

Madin pointed out that VESV is perhaps the only infectious-contagious disease of higher mammals that has run the full cycle from discovery to official extinction in the short space of 27 years. Madin (7) and Smith and Akers (12) postulated that VESV may have arisen from a marine source. This proposition has become more potent because VESV viral antibodies to a number of VESV types also have been demonstrated in marine and feral mammals (13).

Early in 1932 an outbreak of what was regarded as foot-and-mouth disease (FMD) appeared in a number of swine herds in southern California. Seventeen premises eventually became infected, and about 18,000 hogs were slaughtered and buried in an effort to stamp out the disease. It reappeared the following year, but on a much smaller scale, and was again handled in the belief that it was FMD. Investigations conducted during these outbreaks led to the conclusion that the disease was not FMD, but a hitherto unknown, virus-induced malady. The disease was first differentiated from FMD by Traum (15), who proposed the name by which it is now known.

VESV continued to occur in California year after year since little effort was made to control it after it was recognized not to be FMD. In 1952, just 20 years after it had first been recognized, the disease suddenly spread eastward in the United States. Within a few months outbreaks had been reported in 42 states and the District of

Columbia. Vigorous control measures were then initiated, with the result that the disease was eliminated by 1959.

In 1972, the San Miguel Sea Lion Virus (SMSV), a virus isolated from California sea lions, proved to be indistinguishable from VESV (12) when SMSV was injected into swine. Clinical signs of vesicular exanthema developed leading to the conclusion that for all practical purposes, SMSV and VESV were the same. To date, five species of marine mammals and two species of terrestrial mammals, including feral swine, have been shown to possess antibodies to one or more of the four distinct SMSV serotypes. Current evidence suggests that SMSV infections occur among both terrestrial and marine mammals inhabiting the California coastal zones. The practice of shipping frozen meats known to contain SMSV to mink ranches in Utah points to the possibility that domestic swine in the United States are occasionally being exposed to SMSV. Although marine mammals are a source of SMSV, the primary virus reservoir is thought to be one or more submammalian marine species common to the southern California coastline. Such a primary reservoir presumably is the source of a new SMSV serotype infecting marine mammals and may have been the original source of the VESV serotypes that infected swine through the intermediary of raw garbage.

Neutralizing antibodies to some VESV types were found in California sea lions, in certain species of whales, in feral swine, and in one donkey along the coast of southern California (13). These findings clearly show that certain marine and terrestrial mammals are susceptible to either or both viruses—VESV and SMSV.

Character of the Disease. In VESV as in FMD, vesicles of varying size occur on the snout, lips, tongue, footpads, and skin between the claws, around the coronary bands and dew claws, and also on the teats of nursing sows (Figure 46.1). About 12 hours before the lesions appear a febrile period occurs in most animals. Failure of the animals to come for feed when called is frequently the first sign noted. It is then noticed that the animals are lame. This is generally more severe in heavy animals than in those of lighter weight. The foot soreness causes most of the animals to lie down, and they protest by squealing when they are forced to rise to their feet and walk. Sometimes animals will walk knuckled over on their fetlocks to remove weight from their feet. During this time rapid loss in body weight usually occurs. It has been estimated that the weight loss in growing pigs as a result of this disease amounts, on the average, to the equivalent of one month's feeding. All experienced observers agree that the lesions of VESV cannot be distinguished from those of FMD by gross inspection.

According to White (16), the incubation period in this disease usually is about 48 hours, though sometimes it may be as short as 18 hours. In a few instances it has been reported to be very much longer. Apparently it is about the same, as a rule, as that of FMD.

The course of the disease is relatively short. The mouth lesions heal quickly, but the foot lesions may cause lameness of several weeks' duration because of secondary bacterial infections. The disease in an infected herd may last several weeks to several months, because it does not spread as rapidly as FMD. Some animals may escape infection even though they are susceptible.

The death rate among adult animals is very low, but heavy losses often occur among suckling pigs. The baby pigs are believed to die from suffocation because of vesicles that form in their nostrils or from starvation because of failure of lactation in the sows.

The lesions of VESV consist of the vesicles on the skin and mucous membranes already described. As in FMD, these vesicles rupture very easily leaving raw surfaces with ragged margins to which whitish flaps of partially detached epithelium often adhere.

The Disease in Experimental Animals. The disease may readily be produced in swine by inoculation with virus-containing materials or by feeding organs or tissues containing virus. All attempts to infect cattle, calves, sheep, goats, rabbits, rats, mice, hedgehogs, and chick embryos have failed. In horses, intradermal lingual injection gives variable results. Some strains produce vesiculation at the points of injection; others do not. Crawford (5) found that two strains with which he worked regularly produced such lesions and two others did not. Since those that succeeded were of a different serological type than those that failed, it was his belief that the difference was a type characteristic. This has not been confirmed. It may be only a question of relative virulence without reference to serological grouping.

Unlike the viruses of FMD and vesicular stomatitis, the virus of VE does not ordinarily infect guinea pigs. Traum claims that he has seen vesiculation in a few cases at the point of injection. His attemps to adapt some such strains to continued passage in this species have always failed after a few passages.

Bankowski and Wood (3) reported occasional successes in infecting dogs by intradermal lingual injection. The lesions produced at the point of inoculation were mild and characterized by erosion of epithelium and blanching. Often the animals showed some fever. Virus was recovered on one occasion from the spleen of a dog

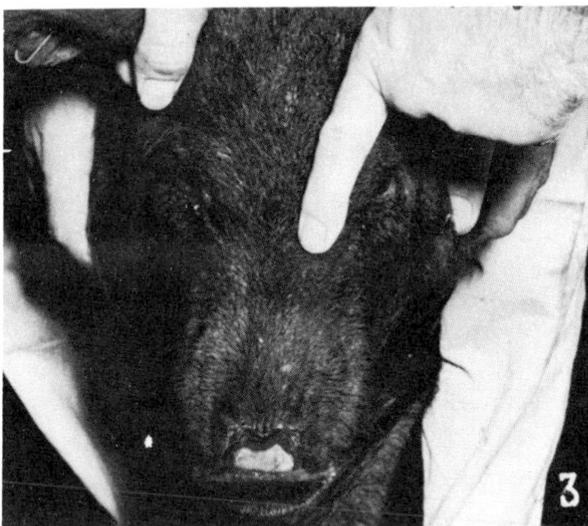

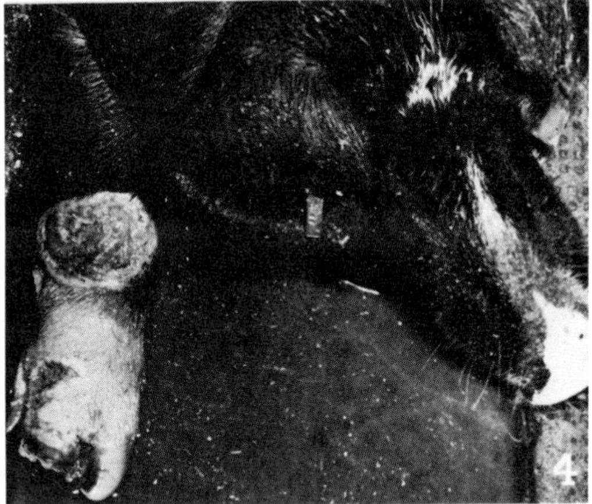

Figure 46.1. Vesicular exanthema, showing ruptured vesicles on the snout (*3*) and on the forelimb (*4*). These lesions cannot be distinguished from those of foot-and-mouth disease. (Courtesy L. M. Hurt.)

16 hours after inoculation. It was not recovered from several others that did not become febrile. Dogs were successfully infected with strains belonging to the three types of virus then known.

Madin and Traum (8) report success in infecting hamsters with VESV virus. With one strain they succeeded in making six serial passages by intradermal inoculation of the skin of the abdomen. The strain then lost its ability to cause further infections. Another strain proved to be regularly pathogenic for hamsters. Secondary lesions were never found. The development of local lesions was definitely associated with a fever curve.

Properties of the Virus. Crawford was the first to show that there was a plurality of viruses in VESV. He identified four serological types, which were designated A, B, C, and D. Unfortunately the strains with which he worked have been lost, so they cannot be identified with relation to present-day strains. Madin and Traum (8) proposed that three types found in southern California be named A, B, and C, and to these Bankowski *et al.* (2) added a fourth, D. More recently at least 9 more types were identified in California, making a total of 13. As in FMD, all of these types are immunologically distinct from each other. No differences in pathogenicity for swine have been recognized among the several types. A protein essential for infectivity is covalently linked to virion RNA (11).

Multiple-virus types have been found only in California. In other areas where the disease has been found since the 1952 spread, only the B type was identified.

Electron micrographs showed that the virus bodies were 35 nm across. Resistance is similar to FMDV. It is inactivated in 60 minutes at 62 C, or in 30 minutes at 64 C. The virus survives 6 weeks at room temperature and 2 years in the refrigerator in 50 percent glycerol. Two percent sodium hydroxide is recommended for its destruction. The virus is not disrupted by mild detergents, but some members are inactivated by trypsin. Thermal inactivation is accelerated in high concentrations of magnesium ions.

Precipitin reactions indicate antigenic relationships among caliciviruses, although the RNAs of the three caliciviruses have similar base compositions. Homology tests show that VESV is closely related to SMSV, but is not related to FCV (4). Tryptic peptide maps of the single major polypeptide compromising the capsid of each virus also show that SMSV and VESV are more closely related to each other than to FCV.

Cultivation. The types grow with considerable ease in kidney, skin, or embryonic tissue cultures of swine, horse, dog, and cat with the production of CPE (7). On monolayers of pig kidney cultures plaques of two sizes occur, the larger ones being more virulent for swine (6).

Immunity. Swine inoculated with any of the types of VESV virus develop, within 3 weeks, a solid immunity to that type which lasts for at least 6 months and perhaps much longer. Animals recovering from infection with one type may, however, almost immediately develop the disease again as a result of infection with one of the other types of virus. Madin and Traum (8) made a formalin-killed vaccine adsorbed to an aluminum gel, by essentially the same technique as that used for the Schmidt-Waldmann vaccine for FMD, and found that it would create a solid immunity. No attempt has been made to make such a vaccine for field use.

Transmission. Nearly all of the past outbreaks of VE have occurred in herds of swine that were fed garbage. White (16) reported that in the 1939–40 outbreak in California, only 8 of the 123 herds involved had not been fed raw garbage, and four of these had had some contact with herds that had been fed garbage. Throughout their entire experience with this disease, it has been recognized that new herd infections are initiated in one of two ways: (*a*) by the introduction of infected animals into the herd, or (*b*) by the feeding of uncooked garbage which originated off the premises.

Garbage-fed swine undoubtedly become infected from pork scraps and trimmings derived from carcasses which contained virus at the time of slaughter. Meat-inspection authorities make efforts to prevent the use of meat from any slaughtered animals that are infected, but it is known that such animals often cannot be detected, and their flesh enters trade channels. It is such meat that, finding its way uncooked into garbage, eventually sets up outbreaks in swine herds.

Since SMSV and VESV infections occur in marine and terrestrial mammals it is clear that hosts other than domestic swine and their byproducts are involved in the ecology of these viruses.

Mott, Patterson, Songer, and Hopkins (9) found that it was difficult to infect susceptible pigs placed in uncleaned pens which had previously contained infected ones. These findings agree with field experience that the disease is not so easily transmitted as FMD.

Diagnosis. As with VESV, the matter of greatest importance is to make sure that the disease outbreak is not, in fact, FMD. In California during the many years when little was done to control VESV, the precaution was taken of requiring those feeding garbage to swine to keep a few young calves in the same pens with the swine. When a vesicular disease struck the herd, authorities felt safe in assuming the disease to be VE rather than FMD if the calves remained free of infection. The differentiation of FMD, VE, and VS is discussed in the section on FMD in Chapter 45.

Control. Since this disease does not have the high level of infectivity that FMD possesses, it has not proved so difficult to control. For 20 years the disease was confined to a single state and very little effort was made to control it after it became known that it was not FMD. When it was thought to be FMD, two attempts were made to stamp it out by the drastic methods employed for that disease. On both occasions all herds in which the disease was recognized were slaughtered and buried, and yet the disease reappeared in other herds the following year. At that time it was assumed that refrigerated pork was responsible for reinfection in the area. Now we recognize that another source may be virus in meat from infected marine or feral mammals.

Experience has shown that VE is more readily controlled than FMD. The methods used since 1952 in the United States are as follows.

1. *Quarantine of infected herds.* Animals from infected herds should not be permitted to go to slaughter until at least 2 weeks (10) after all evidence of active disease in the herd has disappeared. Even this time period may not be safe in all instances. A better procedure is to allow animals from recently infected swine herds or meat from marine and feral mammals to go only to processing plants where all meat is cooked or otherwise processed by methods which will destroy the virus.

2. *The enactment and enforcement of garbage-cooking laws.* This is undoubtedly the most effective and practical single procedure. If such laws were universally enforced, they would quickly eliminate the disease from domestic swine. They would also remove part of the danger of infection with FMD, would greatly reduce the trichinosis hazard in man, and would help in the control of hog cholera. The federal government has assisted by banning the interstate shipment of pork from pigs fed uncooked garbage at any time in their lives unless the meat has been processed in such a way as to destroy any virus it might contain.

The Disease in Man. There is no evidence that VESV is infective for man.

REFERENCES

1. Bachrach and Hess. Biochem. Biophys. Res. Commun., 1973, *55,* 141.
2. Bankowski, Keith, Stuart, and Kummer. Jour. Am. Vet. Med. Assoc., 1954, *125,* 383.
3. Bankowski and Wood. Jour. Am. Vet. Med. Assoc., 1953, *123,* 115.
4. Burroughs, Doel, and Brown. Intervirol., 1978, *10,* 51.
5. Crawford. Proc. U.S. Livestock Sanit. Assoc., 1936, *40,* 380.
6. McClain, Hackett, and Madin. Science, 1958, *127,* 1391.
7. Madin. "Vesicular exanthema," *in* Diseases of swine, 4th ed., ed. Howard W. Dunne. Iowa State Univ. Press, Ames, Iowa, 1975.
8. Madin and Traum. Vet. Med., 1953, *48,* 395.
9. Mott, Patterson, Songer, and Hopkins. Proc. U.S. Livestock Sanit. Assoc., 1953, *57,* 334.
10. Patterson and Songer. Proc. U.S. Livestock Sanit. Assoc., 1954, *58,* 396.
11. Schaffer. "Caliciviruses," *in* Comprehensive virology, vol. 14, ed. H. Fraenkel-Conrat and R. Wagner. Plenum, New York, 1979.
12. Smith and Akers. Jour. Am. Vet. Med. Assoc., 1976, *169,* 700.
13. Smith and Latham. Am. Jour. Vet. Res., 1978, *39,* 291.
14. Studdert. Arch Virol., 1978, *58,* 157.
15. Traum. Jour. Am. Vet. Med. Assoc., 1936, *88,* 316.
16. White. Jour. Am. Vet. Med. Assoc., 1940, *97,* 230.

San Miguel Sea Lion Viruses

This group of caliciviruses perhaps will be best remembered as the first viruses from marine animals that are infectious for terrestrial animals.

Because these viruses have a close relationship to VESV types, the reader should refer to the above section on VESV caliciviruses for the similarities and minor differences. The SMSV are closely related to VESV in every respect—biochemically, biophysically, and biologically.

At present, at least eight serotypes of SMSV are known to exist. These viruses produce the same disease in domestic pigs as VESV. They have been associated with vesicular lesions on the flippers of pinnipeds and with abortions and neonatal deaths in pinniped pups. Marine and terrestial animal transmission is likely with SMSV and VESV.

SMSV has been isolated from California sea lions and northern fur seals. Neutralizing antibody to the virus has been found in Stellar sea lions, northern elephant seals, and California gray whales. SMSV serum neutralizing antibodies have also been in feral swine, sheep, and foxes inhabiting the Channel Islands of California.

Feline Caliciviruses

SYNONYM: Feline picornaviruses;
abbreviation, FCV

Until 1971 the feline caliciviruses were called feline picornaviruses. In most instances the infection is limited to the upper respiratory tract, but it may also produce pneumonia. In 1957 Fastier (13) first isolated and studied a virus representative of this group. Other investigators then made isolations characteristic of the group, and it soon became apparent that many serotypes might exist. A concerted and organized effort by a group of scientists with an interest in feline caliciviruses pooled their efforts as a calicivirus team of the World Health Organization, Food and Agricultural Organization Board on Comparative Virology and showed that there is only one serotype and one variant of that serotype.

A review of this disease was written by Gillespie and Scott (16).

Character of the Disease. The disease is characterized by a diphasic temperature reaction, serous and mucoid rhinitis, conjunctivitis, profound depression, and, in some cats, rales and ulcerative glossitis. Cats that survive 4 to 5 days of illness fully recover in 7 to 10 days. The incubation period is estimated at 2 to 3 days.

This is a common disease in many cats and often is a major disease problem in catteries. In these circumstances the morbidity is high and the mortality usually is low.

The Disease in Experimental Animals. In experimental cats the signs of illness are similar to those observed in cats with natural infection. Kittens show marked and acute signs including dyspnea, depression, and pulmonary rales. Pneumonia was detected by radiography (17).

A pneumotropic strain was used by Kahn and Gillespie to study the pathogenesis of a feline calicivirus (19). At necropsy, pneumonia was the most consistent lesion found at death or when kittens were sacrificed at various times after aerosol exposure to virus. During first days after exposure, the lungs were mottled with reddish-gray areas of congestion and edema. Kittens examined after acute inflammatory response contained slightly elevated, firm areas in the lung, pink gray to pale red in color. The lesions had a patchy distribution. By day 10 the pneumonia was resolving, and by day 34 the lungs were normal. In the oral cavity glossal and palantine ulcers, 2 to 5 mm, were irregular with well-defined margins. The most common site of ulcer formation was the rostrodorsal epithelium of the tongue. Ulcers also were seen on lateral margins of tongue, base of tongue, and beneath the tonsillar folds. The spleens of most kittens had irregular transverse bands, 5 to 10 mm in width. The tissues of experimental kittens were studied further by histopathological examination and by immunofluorescence. Some kittens had a mild fibrinous rhinitis, but lesions in the upper respiratory tract and eye were minimal. Ulceration of tongue epithelium and the hard palate was a necrotic process accompanied by a neutrophilic reaction beneath the lesions. Viral antigen was demonstrated at the base of a tongue ulcer by fluorescent antibody technique (17). The acute inflammatory response in the lungs was maximal by the second day and was followed by hypertrophy of alveolar macrophages which had desquamated into the alveolar spaces. Small accumulations of mononuclear cells were seen in some bronchi. At this stage viral antigen was seen in the cytoplasm of alveolar macrophages. Fluorescence also was observed in bronchial and bronchiolar epithelial cells. Mild hypertrophy and hyperplasia of the epithelium of these air passages also were apparent. By the 5th day, neutrophils were replaced largely by lymphocytes and plasma cells. Specific fluorescence was seen in the cytoplasm of columnar epithelial cells lining bronchiolar passages. The proliferation of mononuclear cells was accompanied by a proliferation of macrophages lining the alveoli resulting in adenomatoid formations. These reactions seemed most prominent between the 7th and 10th days and thereafter slowly resolved. Resolution was still incomplete at 34 days. The spleens had well-developed foci of hematopoiesis and also a reticuloendothelial hyperplasia. Diffuse fluorescence may occur in some kittens. Fluorescence in the tonsillar cells is confined to the epithelium of the tonsillar crypts, and the staining was not intense.

Langloss, Hoover, and Kahn (24) reported that FCV causes direct injury to the alveolar lining, particularly type 1 cells, after aerosol exposure. Necrosis of pneumocytes attended by an acute exudative response in the air exchange tissues was evident from 12 through 96 hours after infection with FCV. The reparative process following alveolar injury was characterized by regenerative hyperplasia of type 11 pneumocytes, proliferation of stromal cells, and infiltration of mononuclear cells. A marked infiltration of neutrophils and immunocytes was observed after FCV injury.

Experimental evidence exists that one feline calicivirus may be involved in the etiology of feline urolithiasis (11, 28). Present studies suggest a complex etiology (11, 12). Certain interesting facts are emerging, and it appears that the calicivirus plays a secondary role to a feline herpesvirus (see Chapter 44).

Attempts to produce disease in such laboratory animals as rabbits, mice, and guinea pigs have failed.

Properties of the Virus. Estimation of the virus particle size has been done by filtration (7, 8) and by electron-microscopic examination (2, 30, 33), and it is generally agreed that its diameter is 37 to 40 nm. The 32 hollow capsomeres are arranged in icosahedral symmetry (2, 33), and Strandberg (30) described the capsomeres as thin and rodlike, 5 nm long and 2.5 nm wide (Figure 46.2). The virions are naked, and this is in accord with their resistance to lipid solvents such as ether, chloroform, and deoxycholate (4, 13). The virus is a single-stranded RNA particle (1, 17). The members of this group exhibit a pH sensitivity that is intermediate between enteroviruses and rhinoviruses. In general the feline caliciviruses are inactivated at pH 3 and stable at pH 4 and pH 5 (7, 8, 18). The virus is resistant to HBB (hydroxybenzylbenzimidazole), guanidine HC1 and 0.2 percent sodium deoxycholate (7). These viruses are inactivated at 50 C in 30 minutes. The presence of $MgSO_4$ or $MgCl_2$ does not stabilize the agents; in fact, $MgCl_2$ enhances thermal inactivation (18).

No hemagglutinin has been associated with feline caliciviruses (9, 14). The WHO/FAO Board on Comparative Virology after years of deliberation on the problem accepted the 20 unit antibody concept of Kapikian *et al.* (23) to classify feline caliciviruses. On the basis of the serological data of many investigators including Povey (26), Kalunda *et al.* (22), and Burki *et al.* (6), it was agreed that there was one serotype with one variant (one-way cross-neutralization test reaction) despite minor antigenic crossings among many strains.

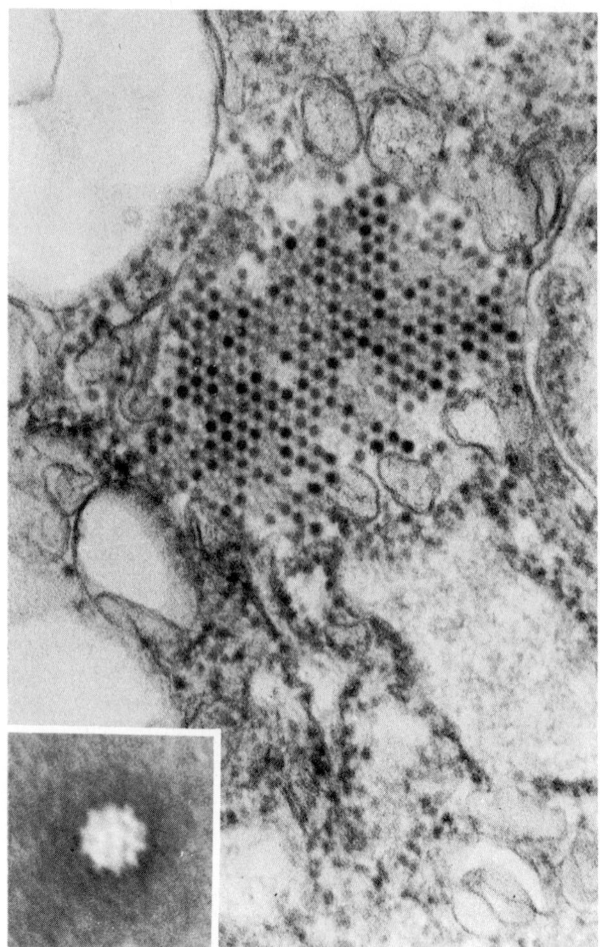

Figure 46.2. Feline calicivirus. Virus crystals. × 69,000. (*Inset*) A single virion of stain KCD showing thin and rodlike capsomeres. Negative stain. × 230,000. (Courtesy J. Strandberg, D. Kahn, P. Bartholomew, and J. Gillespie.)

Cultivation. These viruses originally were isolated in monolayer cultures of feline kidney cells (9, 13). All serotypes tested produce a cytopathic effect, usually within 48 hours, in monolayer cultures of primary and secondary feline kidney cells, of diploid feline tongue and feline thymus cell lines (25), and of established cell lines from feline kidney cells (Crandell) and from embryonic feline lung.

Attempts to cultivate a few strains in monolayer cultures of established cell lines from selected tissues of various hosts other than domestic cat or lion failed (25).

In susceptible cell cultures overlayed with agar or methyl cellulose, feline caliciviruses produce plaques (4, 7, 8) (Figure 46.3). It is sometimes difficult to obtain suitable plaques in successive transfers for plaque purification with certain serotypes (15).

The cytopathology in a tissue-culture system at the ultrastructural level showed that the virus replicated within the cytoplasm of infected cells, forming large crystalline arrays of closely packed particles (31), similar to poliovirus. (Figure 46.4). The infected cells develop large numbers of small, membrane-bound vesicles, myelin figures, and other membranous structures within their cytoplasm. Changes occurring within the nucleus, although secondary to viral infection, included the formation of dense nuclear masses of clumped chromatin.

Immunity. At present it is accepted that FCV viruses represent a single serotype (with a single variant) as established by neutralization test data. It is known that cats are protected against the homologous strain (4), and Povey and Ingersoll (27) and Kahn *et al.* (20) have shown that degrees of heterotypic protection also occur *in vivo*. Homotypic and heterotypic antibody responses correlated well with protection. Kahn *et al.* also mentioned that some cats remain virus carriers for at least 35 days.

Figure 46.3. Agar overlay monolayer cell cultures with clearly defined plaques showing results of a virus titration of a feline calicivirus (strain C14). (*Top left*) An uninoculated control. (*Top right*) A 10^{-7} dilution of virus (0.1 ml of inoculum). (*Lower left*) A 10^{-6} dilution. (*Lower right*) A 10^{-5} dilution.

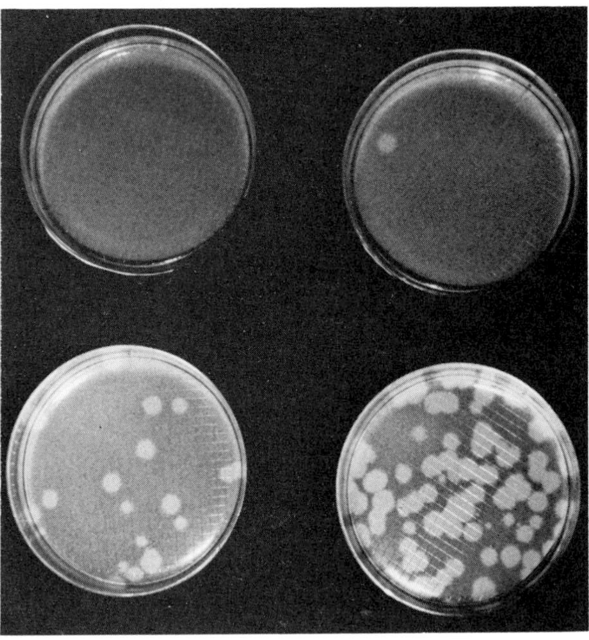

Bittle and Rubic (5) used the F9 strain as an attenuated virus vaccine after modification by passage in cell culture at low temperature (30 to 32 C) and terminal dilution. Following two doses of vaccine given at 27-day intervals cats remained healthy, did not transmit virus to contact cats, developed neutralizing antibody, and resisted challenge to a significant degree. The FCV vaccine has been made available for use alone or in combination with attenuated feline herpes type 1 vaccine and/or inactivated feline panleukopenia. The combined FCV-FVR (feline virus rhinotracheitis) vaccine given intramuscularly appears to be safe without oropharyngeal viral replication and reasonably efficacous (29, 32). Another FCV vaccine is available that provides adequate protection in the cat (10).

Transmission. The feline caliciviruses appear to be limited in nature to the cat family (3). The virus may persist in the pharyngeal region (17, 21), principally the tonsil (2) of recovered cats, so carriers conceivably play the major role in the transmission of the infection.

Diagnosis. The diagnosis of the respiratory disease is difficult for the clinician as a number of other respiratory pathogens produce similar signs of illness in the cat. After the technique is refined, it should be possible to detect the viral antigen in conjunctival scrapings or in tonsillar biopsies by the use of immunofluorescence. A conjugate prepared with antiserum against a single serotype will be sufficient to make a diagnosis for most, if not all, as the feline caliciviruses share a common antigen that is demonstrable by this test (15).

Isolation of the virus can be made in cell cultures of feline origin from nasal excretions, pharyngeal swabs, or conjunctival scrapings during acute stages of respiratory illness. Virus may be found in blood during the acute stage, but it is not a tissue of choice for this purpose. It is not difficult to establish the identity of a tissue-cultured feline calicivirus isolate as a member of that group by using our knowledge of its physicochemical properties and the immunofluorescence test. The complement-fixation and immunodiffusion tests as well as the immunofluorescence test can be used to detect a common antigen(s) of FCV.

Control. Feline calcivirus infections in the cat population are exceedingly difficult to control and treat because of their contagious nature and refractiveness to specific therapy. The husbandry practices used to main-

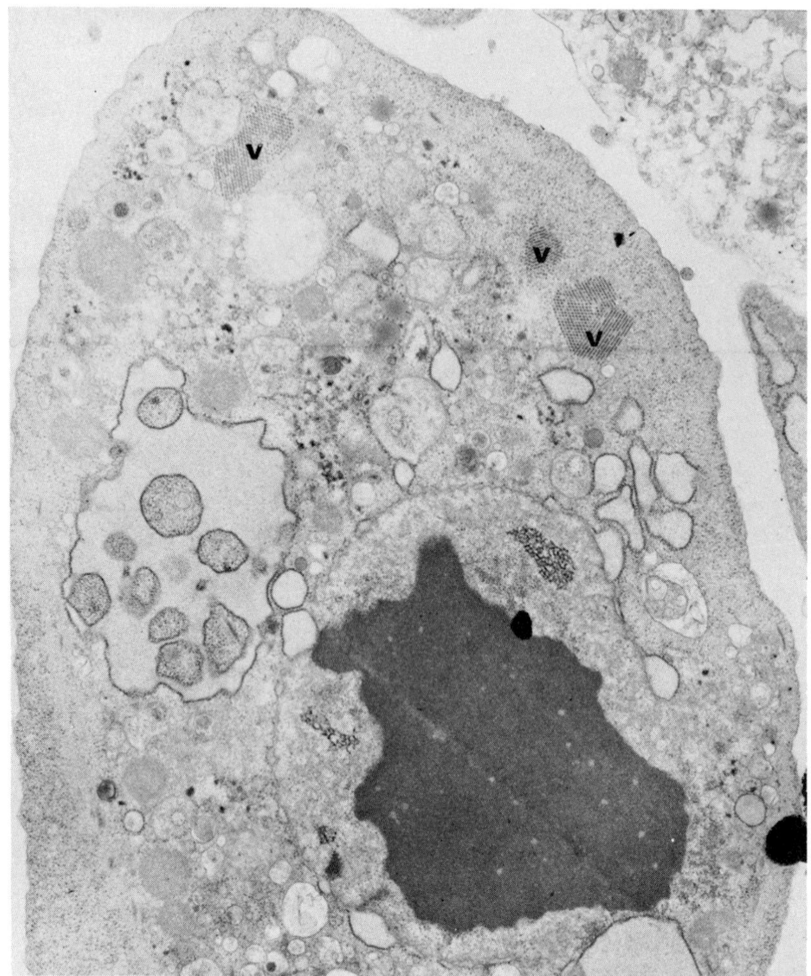

Figure 46.4. Feline calicivirus. Note crystalline array of virus particles (*V*) in the cytoplasm. × 12,560. (Courtesy J. Strandberg, D. Kahn, P. Bartholomew, and J. Gillespie.)

tain cat colonies tend to encourage the dissemination of respiratory illnesses. The existence of carriers and the relative stability of feline caliciviruses further complicate the control. Unless a colony is depopulated and the premises properly disinfected, the infection is likely to persist in cat colonies for an indefinite period of time.

Vaccination with attenuated FCV virus vaccine is recommended as part of a routine feline immunization program (29).

The Disease in Man. There is no evidence that feline calicivirus causes disease in man.

REFERENCES

1. Adldinger, Lee, and Gillespie. Arch. f. die gesam. Virusforsch., 1969, *28,* 245.
2. Almeida, Waterson, Prydie, and Fletcher. Arch. f. die gesam. Virusforsch., 1968, *25,* 105.
3. Archetti and Horsfall. Jour. Exp. Med., 1950, *92,* 441.
4. Bartholomew and Gillespie. Cornell Vet., 1968, *58,* 248.
5. Bittle and Rubic. Am. Jour. Vet. Res., 1976, *37,* 275.
6. Burki, Starstka, and Ruttner. Inf. and Immun., 1976, *14,* 876.
7. Burki. Arch. f. die gesam. Virusforsch., 1965, *15,* 690.
8. Crandell. Proc. Soc. Exp. Biol. and Med., 1967, *126,* 240.
9. Crandell, Nieman, Ganaway, and Maurer. Virol., 1960, *10,* 283.
10. Davis and Beckenhauer. Vet. Med. Sm. An. Clin., 1976, *71,* 1405.
11. Fabricant, Rich, and Gillespie. Cornell Vet., 1969, *59,* 667.
12. Fabricant, Gillespie, and Krook. Inf. and Immun., 1971, *3,* 416.
13. Fastier. Am. Jour. Vet. Res., 1957, *18,* 382.
14. Gillespie, Judkins, and Scott. Cornell Vet., 1971, *60,* 159.
15. Gillespie, Judkins, and Kahn. Cornell Vet., 1971, *60,* 172.
16. Gillespie and Scott. Adv. Vet. Sci., 1973, *17,* 163.
17. Kahn. Cornell Univ. thesis, 1969.
18. Kahn and Gillespie. Cornell Vet., 1970, *60,* 669.

19. Kahn and Gillespie. Am. Jour. Vet. Res., 1971, *32,* 521.
20. Kahn and Hoover. Am. Jour. Vet. Res., 1976, *37,* 279.
21. Kahn, Hoover, and Bittle. Inf. and Immun., 1975, *11,* 1003.
22. Kalunda, Lee, Holmes, and Gillespie. Am. Jour. Vet. Res., 1975, *36,* 353.
23. Kapikian. Nature (London), 1967, *213,* 761.
24. Langloss, Hoover, and Kahn. Am. Jour. Path., 1977, *89,* 637.
25. Lee, Kniazeff, Fabricant, and Gillespie. Cornell Vet., 1969, *59,* 539.
26. Povey. Inf. and Immun., 1974, *10,* 1307.
27. Povey and Ingersoll. Inf. and Immun., 1975, *11,* 877.
28. Rich and Fabricant. Can. Jour. Comp. Med., 1969, *33,* 164.
29. Scott. Am. Jour. Vet. Res., 1977, *38,* 229.
30. Strandberg. Cornell Univ. thesis, 1968.
31. Strandberg, Bartholomew, Kahn, and Gillespie. Unpublished information, 1971.
32. Wardley and Povey. Res. Vet. Sci., 1977, *23,* 15.
33. Zwillenberg and Bürki. Arch. f. die gesam. Virusforsch., 1966, *19,* 373.

47 The Reoviridae

The family Reoviridae consists of three genera now recognized by the International Committee on Taxonomy of Viruses: *Reovirus, Orbivirus,* and *Rotavirus*. In addition, infectious bursal disease (IBD) virus of chickens and infectious pancreatic necrosis virus of salmonids are placed in this family, but they do not fit into the three designated genera because the viruses have no envelope and contain marked differences in RNA segmentation, although IBD virus is provisionally classified as an orbivirus. Reoviridae infections are extremely common in mammals and birds, including many important animal pathogens in domestic animals (Table 47.1). As a consequence, antibodies can be readily detected in all domestic animals.

THE GENUS *REOVIRUS*

Viruses in the genus *Reovirus* are characterized by double-stranded RNA. Their total molecular weight is about 15×10^6 daltons. The particle is an isometric capsid with icosahedral symmetry, usually naked; but a pseudomembrane, probably of host origin, is seen. The capsid diameter is 75 nm. The buoyant density in cesium chloride is 1.36 g per cm^3. The virion resists treatment with lipid solvents. Virus synthesis and maturation occur in the cytoplasm with the formation of inclusions sometimes containing virions in crystalline arrays. Most viruses in this genus have two layered capsids (1).

The type species for this genus is *Reovirus h-1* (human type), one of three mammalian serotypes. Definite members in the genus occur commonly in various species, and they are morphologically and serologically indistinguishable from each other. The natural occurrence of these three serotypes in different species suggests transmission from one animal species to another in nature. Although this has not been demonstrated, it is reasonable to assume that it does occur on occasion. At present the economic importance of these reoviruses as a cause of disease is still largely unknown in our domestic animal species. It is obvious that most infections are mild or inapparent (1).

Some characteristics of reoviruses that help to distinguish them from other mammalian viruses are: (*a*) the rather distinctive cytopathic effects including intracytoplasmic inclusion bodies in cell cultures from a variety of animal species; (*b*) a common complement-fixing antigen; and (*c*) ability to agglutinate human group O and bovine erythrocytes, but not chick or guinea pig erythrocytes.

In his review article Rosen (2) discusses five avian reovirus serotypes that are officially recognized by the International Committee on Taxonomy of Viruses.

REFERENCES

1. Fenner. Intervirol., 1976, *7*, 34.
2. Rosen. *In* Virology monographs, ed. S. Gard, C. Hallauer, and K. F. Meyer. Springer-Verlag, New York, 1968, *1*, 74.

Bovine Reoviruses

Reoviruses 1, 2, and 3 were recovered from the feces of naturally infected cattle (4). Their importance as pathogens in the respiratory syndrome is still undetermined. Bovine reoviruses are widespread in nature, and their incidence in the cattle population is significant.

Character of the Disease. Present evidence strongly suggests that bovine reoviruses cause an inapparent infection in nature (2, 4), although one group (6) reported the production of a mild respiratory disease in calves with a strain (Lang) of reovirus 1 of human origin.

Although no clinical signs of illness were produced in colostrum-deprived calves with reovirus 1 strains of human and bovine origin, macroscopic and microscopic lesions of interstitial pneumonia were seen 4 and 7 days after a combined regimen of intranasal and intratracheal routes of inoculation (1, 2). There also was a nonspecific lymphadenitis of the retropharyngeal, bronchial, mediastinal, and mesenteric lymph nodes and some congestion and degenerative changes in the liver. Virus in low titers was recovered up to day 5 from nasal swabs and for 7 days from rectal swabs. In a viral distribution study, suspensions of respiratory tissues had higher titers than other body tissues (2).

It has been suggested that a strain of *Pasteurella multocida* did not enhance reovirus infection in calves (6). *Pasteurella hemolytica* did enhance reovirus 1 infection in day-old calves deprived of colostrum (2).

Properties of the Virus. Properties of the three reovirus types recovered from cattle are indistinguishable from these same serotypes isolated from other species.

Cultivation. Bovine reoviruses 1, 2, and 3 have been propagated in bovine kidney-cell cultures (4, 5) and also in pig kidney, monkey kidney, and mouse fibroblast (L strain) cell cultures (2). The three bovine serotypes cause a cytopathic effect in these cell cultures, but the bovine kidney-cell cultures seem to be more resistant to pathological change (2).

Immunity. Maternally acquired immunity does not appear to protect calves from infection under natural conditions (5) and perhaps under experimental conditions as well (2).

The degree and duration of protection of cattle after active infection is unknown, but neutralizing antibodies are formed and presumably persist for a period of time.

Transmission. Bovine reoviruses may be detected in the feces of naturally and experimentally infected cattle for as long as 1 month although they usually are present for a shorter period of time (3, 4, 5). Virus also is discharged from the nasal passages and conjunctiva, probably for a comparable period of time. Through contact with these infected sources susceptible cattle may become infected. Although it has not been demonstrated, the possibility exists that cattle may become infected with the three serotypes which are common to many animal species.

Diagnosis. As a potential respiratory pathogen, reoviruses must be distinguished from numerous other microbial respiratory pathogens of cattle. This is a difficult, if not impossible, task unless one resorts to viral isolation or serology.

The only practical means for viral isolation and identification is in a tissue-culture system. The neutralization or hemagglutination-inhibition (HI) test can be used for demonstrating a rising serum titer with paired sera. With the HI test a rise in titer of 4-fold or greater between the acute and convalescent samples is considered positive (2).

The Disease in Man. Although not proved, it is conceivable that the bovine reoviruses may infect man.

REFERENCES

1. Lamont. Proc. Roy. Soc. Med., 1966, *59*, 50.
2. Lamont. Jour. Am. Vet. Med. Assoc., 1968, *152*, 807.
3. Moscovici, LaPlaca, Maisel, and Kempe. Am. Jour. Vet. Res., 1961, *22*, 852.
4. Rosen and Abinanti. Am Jour. Hyg., 1960, *71*, 250.
5. Rosen, Abinanti, and Hovis. Am. Jour. Hyg., 1963, *77*, 38.
6. Trainor, Mohanty, and Hetrick. Am. Jour. Epidemiol., 1966, *83*, 217.

Canine Reoviruses

Reovirus 1 was isolated from dogs with respiratory signs of illness (3). Studies by these investigators with their isolate showed that interstitial pneumonia was produced in naturally and experimentally infected dogs. The inoculation of this same isolate into germ-free and specific pathogen-free dogs failed to produce signs of illness or pathological changes, but it did cause infection as virus was isolated and seroconversion occurred (2). Massie and Shaw (4) recovered reovirus 1 from 4 of 133 dogs. In four experimental puppies one of their isolates produced signs of illness referable to the respiratory and enteric tracts. It is obvious that further studies in conventional and pathogen-free dogs are essential to determine the factors responsible for the pathogenicity of reovirus 1 in dogs.

Reovirus 2 was isolated from the throat and feces of an immature dog with upper respiratory disease (1). Its pathogenicity in experimental dogs was not reported.

Table 47.1. Diseases in domestic animals caused by viruses in the Reoviridae family

Common name of virus	Natural hosts	Type of disease produced
Genus *Reovirus*		
Reovirus types 1–3	Cattle	Usually inapparent disease; possibly mild respiratory disease on occasion
Reovirus types 1 and 2	Dogs	Mild or inapparent upper respiratory infection
Reovirus types 1 and 3	Cats	Mild upper respiratory infection when it occasionally occurs
Reovirus types 1, 2, 3	Horses	Coughing, nasal and ocular discharge
At least 5 avian viral types recognized	Birds	Cloacal pasting; infectious tenosynovitis (4 serotypes recognized)
Genus *Rotavirus**		
Bovine rotavirus infection—single immunogenic type	Cattle	Acute gastroenteritis of neonatal calves
Porcine rotavirus infection—single immunogenic type	Pigs	Acute gastroenteritis of piglets
Equine rotavirus infection—single immunogenic type	Horses	Acute gastroenteritis of neonatal foals and young horses
Ovine rotavirus infection—single immunogenic type	Sheep	Acute gastroenteritis of neonatal lambs
Human rotavirus infection—2 immunogenic types, perhaps 3	Humans	Acute gastroenteritis of infants and occasionally adults
Canine rotavirus	Dogs	Acute gastroenteritis of puppies

REFERENCES

1. Binn, Marchwicki, Kennan, Strano, and Engler. Am. Jour. Vet. Res., 1977, *38*, 927.
2. Holzinger and Griesimer. Am. Jour. Epidemiol., 1966, *84*, 426.
3. Lou and Wenner. Am. Jour. Hyg., 1963, *77*, 293.
4. Massie and Shaw. Am. Jour. Vet. Res., 1966, *27*, 783.

Feline Reoviruses

In 1968 Scott *et al.* (6) isolated reovirus 3 from a cat that was suspected of having died from feline infectious panleukopenia. Cell cultures inoculated with a suspension of intestinal tract from this cat developed intracytoplasmic inclusion bodies. These inclusions were subsequently shown to be produced by reovirus 3. Three subsequent isolations of reovirus 3 from cats were made by Csiza *et al.* (1). Hong (2) also made three isolations of reovirus from feline neoplasm cell cultures, and all were typed as reovirus 1 as determined by the hemagglutination test.

Character of the Disease. The experimental disease produced by feline reovirus 3 is mild (4, 6). The experimental disease is characterized by conjunctivitis, photophobia, gingivitis, serous lacrimation, and depression. A majority of contact cats developed similar signs of illness 4 to 19 days after exposure, and signs persisted from 1 to 29 days. Virus is isolated from the pharynx, eye, and rectum of the experimentally infected cats with 6 to 10 days being the optimal times for isolation. Cytoplasmic reovirus inclusion bodies are found in the bronchiolar epithelium of severely stressed neonatal experimental kittens (2).

Properties of the Virus. Feline reovirus 3 particles in negatively stained preparations have a diameter of 75 nm and exhibit prominent hollow-cored capsomeres (6) (see Figure 47.1). The hexagonal-shaped particle has icosahedral symmetry and is composed of 92 capso-

Table 47.1.—*continued*

Common name of virus	Natural hosts	Type of disease produced
Genus *Orbivirus*		
African horse sickness viruses, types 1–9	Horses; less severe disease in donkeys and mules	Acute form—pulmonary signs. Chronic form—hydropericardium and edema of head, neck, and shoulder regions
Bluetongue, types 1–20	Sheep, cattle, goats, and wild ruminants	Acute form—usually in feeder lambs—characterized by edema erosions in oral cavity, respiratory signs, and stiffness. Abortions in ewes, occasionally other signs. Less serious consequences in cattle as a rule, but disease manifestations are similar
Epizootic hemorrhagic disease (also known as Ibaraki disease in cattle), types 1–3	Deer (*Odocoileus virginianus*), cattle	Acute disease—high morbidity with high mortality in confined deer. Severe shock, edema, and hemorrhages are characteristic
Unspecified genera		
Infectious bursal disease	Young chickens	Highly contagious disease. Enteric disease with bursa of Fabricius as the target organ. Principal lesions in lymphoid structures
Infectious pancreatic necrosis disease	Salmonids	Acute disease—high morbidity, and mortality usually is high in young fish and the disease manifested by catarrhal enteritis and pancreatic necrosis

*In many cases animals in all species have mixed enteric infections and accompanying pneumonia associated with rotavirus disease.

meres. With acridine staining, infected cell cultures have green-staining inclusion masses, and the borders of the cytoplasm fluoresced reddish orange. Viral particles in infected cell cultures examined by electron microscopy were either arranged as closely packed, highly ordered paracrystalline arrays or spread rather diffusely through osmophilic reticular masses (see Figure 47.2). A few cells contain masses of viral particles in membrane-bound cytoplasmic vesicles within their cytoplasm.

The virus is quite thermostabile as there is no loss of virus after heating for 30 minutes at 56 C.

Cultivation. The virus was propagated in primary cultures of feline kidney cells and of bovine fetal kidney cells (6). The feline kidney-cell cultures give a titer of approximately 10^6 $TCID_{50}$ per ml whereas the titer is about 1 log less in the bovine kidney cultures. The virus produces a typical cytopathic effect in unstained cultures. In May-Gruenwald-Giemsa-stained preparations large, irregularly shaped, blue-staining, intracytoplasmic inclusions begin to appear on the 3rd or 4th day after inoculation (Figure 47.3).

Immunity. Little is known about the immunity. Neutralizing antibodies are produced in cats to the homotypic virus. The high incidence of neutralizing antibody in a small population of cats suggests that it is a common disease and the majority of cats are immune. Obviously, considerably more work must be done in this regard.

It is not practical at this time to develop a vaccine against the feline reoviruses until we have more information about the immunity, pathological effects, and pathogenicity of these viruses in cats.

Transmission. The virus is readily transmitted from infected cats to susceptible cats maintained in the same room. At present this is the only known means of transmission.

The incidence of the disease is not known, although it probably is widespread (5). The virus has been isolated from cats in California and New York, and neutralizing

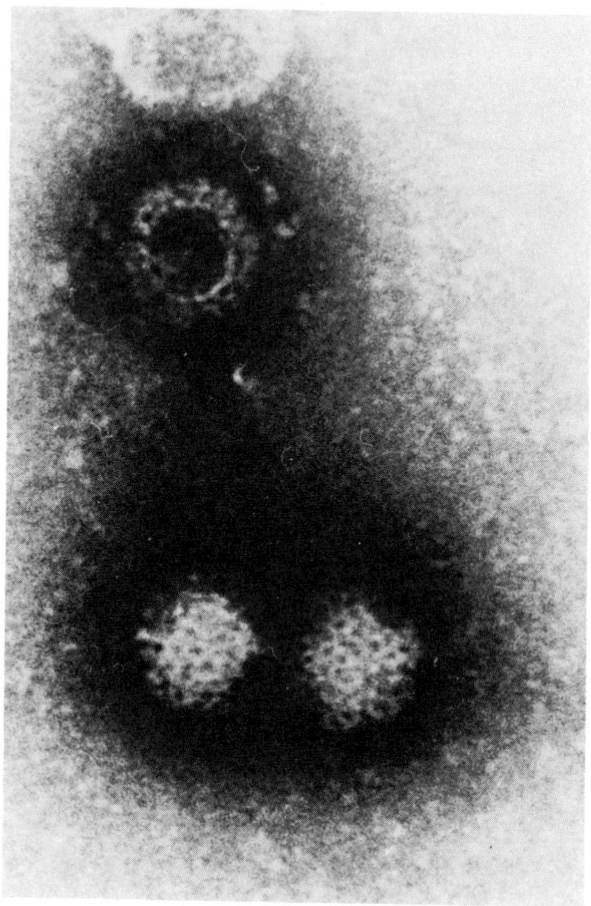

Figure 47.1. Feline reovirus particles. Prominent capsomeres with hollow cores are evident in a negatively stained preparation. (Courtesy F. Scott, D. Kahn, and J. Gillespie, *Am. Jour. Vet. Res.*)

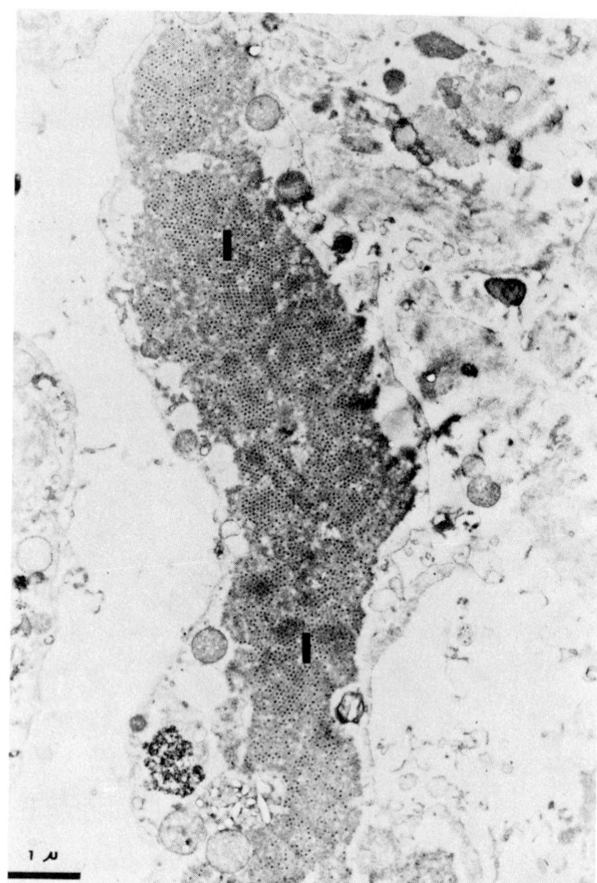

Figure 47.2. Single cytoplasmic inclusion (*I*) of feline reovirus particles in a closely packed paracrystalline array. (Courtesy F. Scott, D. Kahn, and J. Gillespie, *Am. Jour. Vet. Res.*)

antibodies are present in a significant percentage of cats in the Ithaca, New York, area (50 percent for reovirus 3 and 71 percent for reovirus 1).

Diagnosis. Reovirus infection in the cat can be confused with other feline respiratory diseases. Its importance as a feline pathogen is still undetermined. Scott (5) has made the following observations which help to differentiate it from the others. The clinical disease is mild and usually of short duration. The signs of illness are restricted primarily to the eyes; a nasal discharge usually is associated with other respiratory infections. A febrile response, leukopenia or leukocytosis, and anorexia generally are not observed.

Certain ground rules must be observed in attempts to isolate feline reoviruses from feline tissues in cell culture. Because the cytopathic effect in unstained cell cultures may go unnoticed for up to 10 days, cultures must be retained for this period of time. Although not proved, it may be necessary to make blind passages before declaring a test sample negative. At present the cell-culture method would appear to be the method of choice for viral isolation.

Serological methods such as the neutralization and hemagglutination tests can be used to demonstrate a rising titer with paired sera from active cases.

The Disease in Man. The occurrence of reovirus 1 and 3 in cats and humans naturally suggests the possibility of transmission in nature between these species and others that harbor these viruses. Such transmission has not yet been demonstrated, but it is almost inconceivable that it does not occur on occasion (3).

REFERENCE

1. Csiza, Scott, and Gillespie. Quoted by Scott in Jour. Am. Vet. Med. Assoc., 1971, *158*, 944.

2. Hong. Cornell Univ. thesis, 1970.
3. Rosen. *In* Virology monographs, ed. S. Gard, C. Hallauer, and K. F. Meyer. Springer-Verlag, New York, 1968, *1*, 74.
4. Scott. Cornell Univ. thesis, 1968.
5. Scott. Jour. Am. Vet. Med. Assoc., 1971, *158*, 944.
6. Scott, Kahn, and Gillespie. Am. Jour. Vet. Res., 1970, *31*, 11.

Equine Reoviruses

Antibodies to reovirus serotypes 1, 2, and 3 have been found in horses with respiratory disease and also in healthy horses from Germany, Holland, England, and Belgium (1). The incidence in 415 individual sera and 184 paired sera was 23 percent to serotype 1, 7 percent to serotype 2, and 50 percent to serotype 3.

In a respiratory outbreak of horses in an Arab stud both reovirus types 1 and 3 were isolated. The horses showed coughing and also an ocular discharge but no fever. Experimental horses inoculated with reovirus types 1 and 3 showed typical signs of illness and the specificity was confirmed virologically and serologically.

This report clearly demonstrated that reoviruses are one of the causes of upper respiratory disease in horses.

Figure 47.3. Note production of large cytoplasmic inclusion bodies (*arrows*) in a 4-day-old feline kidney cell culture. May-Gruenwald-Giemsa stain. × 650. (Courtesy F. Scott, D. Kahn, and J. Gillespie, *Am. Jour. Vet. Res.*)

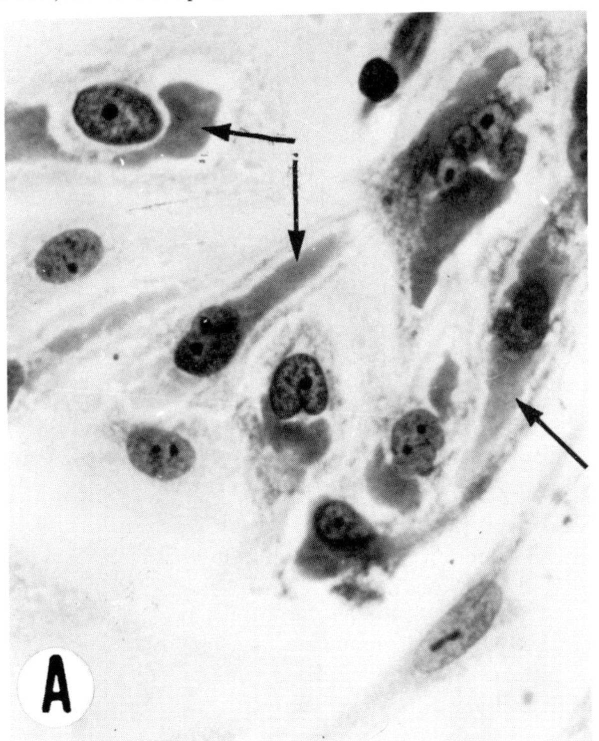

REFERENCE

1. Theil and Mayr. Zentrbl. Vet.-Med., 1974, *21B*, 219.

Avian Reoviruses

Most chicken reoviruses have been recovered from the rectal contents or rectal swabs, but on two occasions reoviruses were isolated from the trachea (6). Reoviruses were isolated from the intestinal tracts of turkeys with bluecomb disease from widely separated geographic areas of the United States and Canada (1). A reovirus (strain WVU-2937) is responsible for viral arthritis in chickens. At present five avian reovirus serotypes are recognized. Many isolates have been made, but a great deal more study is required to establish the precise number of avian reovirus serotypes.

Three reoviruses related to the human reoviruses 1, 2, and 3, as demonstrated by hemagglutination-inhibition, complement-fixation, serum-neutralization, and agar-gel diffusion tests, were isolated from chicks showing severe cloacal pasting (2). No clinical signs were seen in chickens inoculated orally or intravenously with three chicken serotypes isolated by Kawamura (5). Attempts to reproduce cloacal pasting in chicks maintained under isolation with two reovirus isolates from cloacal chick disease were successful but inconsistent (3, 4). The chicks that developed cloacal pasting were depressed and lost weight. In contrast, germ-free chicks failed to develop cloacal pasting. Day-old turkey poults also failed to show signs or lesions after viral inoculation of these cloacal isolates.

The properties of avian reoviruses generally are consistent with reoviruses isolated from other species (6). A major difference is the lack of hemagglutinins that is a characteristic of mammalian reoviruses. Avian reoviruses produce pocks on the chorioallantoic membrane of embryonated chicken egg. The 7-day-old eggs are killed when inoculated by the chorioallantoic membrane, yolk-sac, and allantoic cavity routes. These observations were extended by Deshmukh and Pomeroy, who observed embryo stunting and necrosis of the liver with two of their strains (2). Two reovirus strains associated with chick cloacal disease produced a syncytial type of cytopathic effect in whole chicken embryo primary-cell culture, although the viral titer was not high (3). Plaques also are produced in this type of culture. A similar type of CPE was produced in chicken embryo kidney-cell culture. CPE was not observed in cultures of bovine fetal kidney, liver, endocardial, or corneal cells.

In recent years there have been reports that isolates of avian reovirus may cause viral arthritis (infectious tenosynovitis) in chickens (7, 8, 9, 10). The disease is characterized by tenosynovitis with a generalized infection that largely subsides in 2 weeks, but infection may persist in the tendons, oviduct, and enteric tract up to 30 days. Virus isolation in chick kidney cell culture is more reliable than fluorescent-antibody tests for detection of virus (7). Virus is found in embryos of eggs 8 to 12 days after inoculation of hens (10) but not in chicks hatched from eggs laid 12 to 35 days after inoculation of the breeders (7). Maternal antibodies protect progeny for at least three weeks after oral administration of virus, but subcutaneous injection overrides maternal immunity (11). Virus isolates that can experimentally produce viral arthritis have a common agar gel precipitin line (9). On the basis of the plaque reduction test in primary chicken kidney cells the viruses in the group were placed into four major serotypes (9).

REFERENCES

1. Deshmukh and Pomeroy. Jour. Am. Vet. Med. Assoc., 1968, *152*, 1346.
2. Deshmukh and Pomeroy. Avian Dis., 1969, *13*, 239.
3. Deshmukh and Pomeroy. Avian Dis., 1969, *13*, 427.
4. Deshmukh and Pomeroy. Avian Dis., 1969, *13*, 16.
5. Kawamura. Quoted by Rosen in Virology monographs, ed. S. Gard, C. Hallauer, and K. F. Meyer. Springer-Verlag, New York, 1968, *1*, 74.
6. Kawamura, Shimizu, Maeda, and Tsubahara. Natl. Inst. An. Health Q., 1965, *5*, 115.
7. Menendez, Calnek, and Cowan. Avian Dis., 1975, *19*, 112.
8. Olson and Sahu. Am. Jour. Vet. Res., 1975, *36*, 545.
9. Sahu and Olson. Am. Jour. Vet. Res., 1975, *36*, 847.
10. Van DerHeide and Kalbac. Avian Dis., 1975, *19*, 683.
11. Van DerHeide, Kalbac, and Hall. Avian Dis., 1976, *20*, 641.

THE GENUS *ROTAVIRUS*

A wide range of mammalian species, including calves, piglets, lambs, foals, rabbits, deer, pronghorn antelope, monkeys, and children are infected with rotaviruses (7). Recently, the dog was added to this list. Frequently, other viruses are isolated from feces of animals that show diarrhea and also contain rotavirus.

The resemblance of rotaviruses to reoviruses was recognized early in their history (2, 4). The bovine rotavirus (5) and porcine rotavirus (9) were described as reoviruslike agents. As more information on basic properties was developed, it became clear that rotaviruses were sufficiently different to justify their classification as a separate genus (25). The name was recommended since the virion resembled a small wheel with short spikes and a narrow rim.

The virions are 65 mm with a double capsid shell. The rotaviruses are not related antigenically to the members of the other two genera in the family. Rotaviruses share a common antigen present in the inner capsid, demonstrable by complement fixation, immunofluorescence, immunodiffusion, and immune electron microscopy (7). Rotaviruses from the various animal species are distinguishable on the basis of virus-neutralization test and the blocking test using the enzyme-linked immunosorbent assay technique (ELISA). With the isolates tested there was a lack of cross-neutralization between the bovine and ovine rotaviruses (22), and also between human, porcine, murine, and bovine strains (26). In the latter comparative studies some of the viruses showed a degree of cross-neutralization. This cross-neutralization was restricted to high concentrations of antibody, and homologous titers were 8- to 10-fold higher than heterologous titers. Some degree of specificity can be shown for the outer capsid layer, but this does not correlate entirely with neutralization specificity (19, 32). The serological specificity of neutralization is associated with infectivity and thus with outer capsid polypeptides (19, 26), and it may be correlated with certain RNA virion segments of varying electrophoretic mobility and with the glycosylated polypeptides (18) of the outer capsid for which the RNA may code. Apparently, there are two (perhaps three) immunogenic types of human rotaviruses, but until recently (1979) the rotaviruses isolated from each animal species were a single immunogenic type.

In recent years the importance of rotaviruses in the etiology of diarrheal disease in young animals has been well established. Further, there has been confirmed transmission of human, bovine, porcine, and equine strains to calves, monkeys, and pigs. Not all strains are transferable among mammalian species, and variation in virulence and avirulence is contingent upon the host in which the strain is experimentally cultured (29). Biological differences among strains may be reflected in serological differences, but this must await more extensive study of many strains of rotavirus from the various susceptible hosts.

The natural history of rotavirus diseases in humans,

domestic animals, and others is so similar that, in general, the rotavirus infections of the various species in this genus will be treated as a single entity. Exceptions or differences among the species will be presented. In general, the format used by Woode and Crouch (33) will be followed to cover rotavirus diseases of cattle, sheep, pigs, horses, and dogs. The literature is particularly voluminous on cattle, humans, sheep, and pigs, so most of our knowledge is known about the disease in these four species.

Character of the Disease. Rotaviruses have been isolated from feces of neonatal calves, foals, pigs, and lambs with diarrhea. In this age group the disease is often severe and fatal. Infections occur at all ages, including in adult cattle (30) and young horses. For many years practitioners have been familiar with a disease known as pneumoenteritis in calves and piglets. There is little doubt that rotaviruses, often as mixed infections with other viruses and pathogenic bacteria, are involved in many cases of pneumoenteritis in domestic animals.

As a rule rotavirus infection occurs as a sudden and rapidly spreading epizootic in domestic animals. Viral infection in animals (and humans) is between 90 and 100 percent and usually sporadic and often subclinical in nature. The incubation period of this afebrile disease is 18 to 96 hours followed by depression and then diarrhea. The disease in calves and foals becomes apparent sometime between 3 days and 15 weeks after birth.

In calves on a total milk diet, feces are usually brilliant yellow to white, not always putrid, and similar to classic milk scours. In other calves, feces may be watery, brown, gray, or light green with fresh blood and mucus. The color appears to be dependent on the diet. If the diarrhea is prolonged, dehydration becomes apparent and the calf may die within 4 to 7 days of diarrhea and a significant loss in body weight. Severely ill calves usually recover after administration of glucose and saline mixtures are fed instead of milk. Continued feeding of milk is harmful and probably accounts for the severe epizootics in calves maintained in a cow/calf operation. Inclement weather complicates an outbreak as many calves develop severe pneumonia after the onset of diarrhea and die 2 to 3 weeks later.

There are some points that should be emphasized about the disease in pigs. There is a marked loss in body weight associated with severe cases of diarrhea. Milk should be withdrawn from the diet of suckling or newly weaned pigs and replaced with glucose and saline feedings. A drop of 10 to 20 degrees in ambient temperature increases the mortality. In addition to other signs of illness pigs often vomit prior to the onset of diarrhea.

The virus infects the epithelial cells of the absorptive portion of the villus and not crypt cells. Desquamation of infected cells is followed by the shortening of the villi and proliferation of the crypt cells (Figure 47.4). The epithelial cells in gnotobiotic lambs given human rotavirus contained cytoplasmic vesicles, and rotavirus was observed in these cells and subepithelial phagocytic cells.

Viral replication takes place in the enterocytes of the small intestine throughout its length in fatal cases, but it may extend into the large intestine in lambs. Rotavirus pathogenesis is similar to transmissible gastroenteritis (TGE) in pigs. The diarrhea causes a disordered sodium transport system with a net extracellular fluid-to-lumen flux of sodium ions. Villous tip cells are rich in thymidine kinase rather than sucrase, thus possessing an immature enzyme profile similar to that in crypt cells

Figure 47.4. Scanning electron micrograph of lower ileum from a gnotobiotic calf infected with bovine rotavirus. Shortened villi are covered by irregular-sized epithelial cells. Lips of several villi are denuded. × 100. (Courtesy C. A. Mebus, Plum Island Animal Disease Center, USDA.)

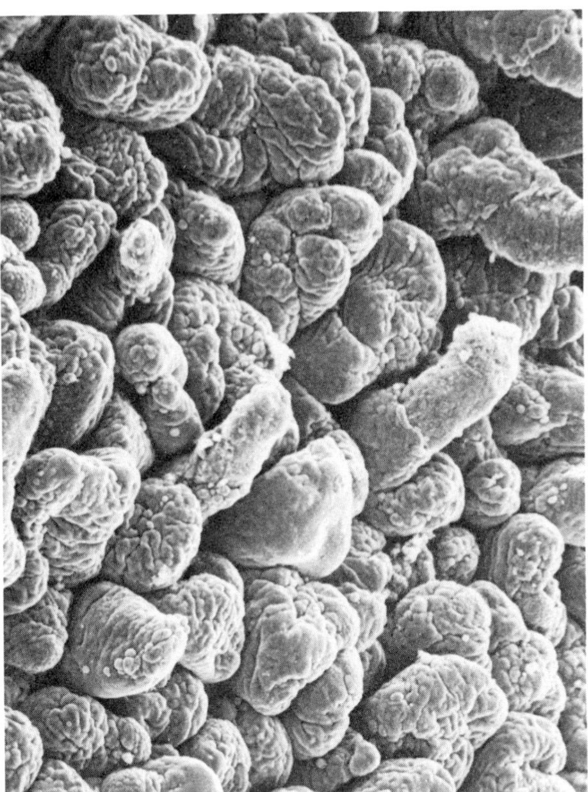

(16). This finding explains the accelerated migration of secretory crypts to the villi normally lined by mature enterocyte cells. The failure of enterocytes to differentiate fully as they migrate up villi appears to be a major factor producing electrolyte transport defect.

The Disease in Experimental Animals. The most satisfactory results are obtained by the use of gnotobiotic animals. Such studies are possible with pigs, cattle, and sheep. To quantitate the effects of diarrhea caused by rotavirus disease in pigs daily weight records were used. The mortality in experimental pigs varied between 0 and 100 percent according to age (31) with some individual variation within litters. Experimentally infected pigs have a shorter period of illness than pigs infected under natural conditions. The same is true for infected calves and lambs. The role of bacteria presumably enhanced the severity of the disease.

Foal, human, or lamb rotaviruses fed to gnotobiotic pigs did not cause disease, but infection occurred and the viruses were excreted in quantities similar to those observed in pigs given virulent porcine rotavirus (32). Another strain of human rotavirus fed to pigs and calves produced diarrhea in the experimental animals (14).

Dual infection in gnotobiotic pigs given porcine rotavirus and transmissible gastroenteritis virus (TGE) produced a more severe disease (33). In another set of animal experiments it was shown that rotavirus infection did not interfere with the virulence of the TGE virus.

Properties of the Virus. In electron microscope studies of the double-stranded RNA of the Nebraska strain of bovine rotavirus, the virus was found to have four size classes of RNA in contrast to the well-described three classes of double-stranded RNA reoviruses. The RNA migration pattern for the Nebraska strain was stable, whereas three different RNA migration patterns in electrophonesis existed among human rotaviruses. These differences do not necessarily imply antigenic difference.

Rotaviruses have a distinctive outer capsid (Figure 47.5) more clearly defined than the reoviruses (Figure 47.1) and differ from the orbiviruses, which have an amorphous outer capsid (Figure 47.14). In other physical and chemical characteristics rotaviruses closely parallel other genera in the family except that they have 5 to 10 structural polypeptides, whereas reoviruses and orbiviruses have 7 polypeptides.

Except for human rotaviruses only one immunogenic type has been described for the rotaviruses of other species.

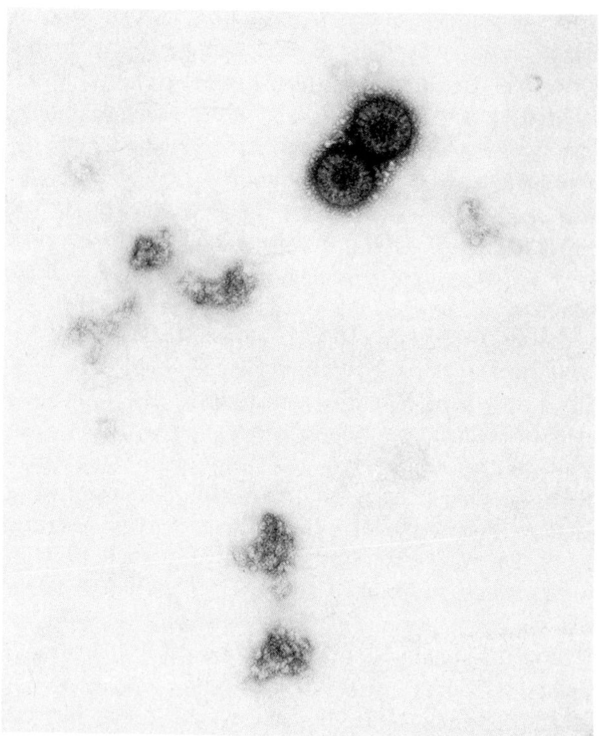

Figure 47.5. Porcine rotavirus. Note sharply defined outer capsid membrane of the virus. × 118,500. (Courtesy R. Sharpee, Norden Laboratories.)

Cultivation. Serious interest in the cultivation of rotaviruses in cell culture did not take place until bovine rotavirus was recognized as a cause of neonatal calf diarrhea (NCD) (11) and adapted to cell culture passage in fetal bovine kidney cells (Lincoln strain). With the production of plaques (12) the cytopathic effect caused by this virus was not readily recognizable, so the fluorescent antibody (FAT) was used to determine the presence or absence of viral antigen in cell systems. Despite this success with NCD virus, the adaptation of rotaviruses of various species met with little or no success. The pancreatic enzymes trypsin and α-chymotrypsin, were found to be important determinants in the replication and adaptation of porcine rotaviruses in porcine kidney cell cultures (24). Specifically, trypsin (15 μg per ml) and α-chymotrypsin (15 μg per ml) were added to sonicated virus laden culture fluid, and this mixture was inoculated on washed monolayers of either primary or cell-line (MDPK-15) pig kidney cells. After 1 hour of incubation, the inoculum was removed and the monolayers were washed once to remove the residual enzymes and then maintained with serum-free medium. At 18 to 24 hours, greater than 90 percent of the cells contained virus as demonstrated by fluorescent-antibody procedure. Using this modified procedure with pancreatic enzymes it was possible to make repeated transfers in cell cultures at 24-hour intervals. It is now recognized that certain influenza viruses (8) and paramyxoviruses (17) require proteolytic cleavage of envelope glycoproteins for the activation of their infectivity; perhaps pancreatic enzymes act similarly on proteins or glycoproteins in the porcine rotavirus capsid. When replication of rotaviruses in cell cultures has met with limited or no success, the use of pancreatic enzymes or lactase, found in microvilli, as a possible receptor for rotaviruses, may facilitate or enhance viral reproduction.

NCD virus formed distinct plaques in monolayers of MA-104 cells, an established macacus rhesus monkey kidney cell line, when diethylamino-ethyl dextran (100 μg per ml) and trypsin (2 μg per ml) were added (10). In this system discrete plaques 2 to 3 mm in diameter were formed with viral plaque titers reaching 1.5×10^7 after 3 to 4 days of incubation at 37 C: the plaques are inhibited by homologous antiserum.

Immunity. Resistance to rotavirus disease appears to be mediated by local immunity at the epithelial surface of the small intestine (23). Unfortunately, the passive protection afforded by the cow's colostrum has limited value. Some dams have low levels of protective antibody in the colostrum, and in the other immune dams the antibody in the milk rapidly declines 10-fold 24 to 48 hours after birth. A similar situation occurs with pigs, yet children maintained on breast feeding in Bangladesh had virtually no rotavirus diarrhea. Using the ELISA blocking test (35), a high level of antibody was found in the colostrum, and the amount fell to lower but detectable levels for 1 year after parturition. There obviously is a difference in hosts. Calves are protected when they are fed colostrum with rotavirus antibody of high content, but it must be fed continuously in the face of constant viral exposure. Similar results occur in lambs infected with lamb or human rotavirus that were fed daily with sheep colostrum or human gamma globulin (20, 23).

There is no direct correlation between rotavirus antibody in serum and protection in domestic animals, yet the antibody classes and subclasses in serum, and particularly in body fluids, have relevance to rotavirus immunity. After rotavirus infection ensues, IgM appears early in the course of the disease and persists in the disease syndrome. IgG usually is correlated with history of exposure. It is likely that secretory IgA antibody plays an important role in protection as it does in the case of transmissible gastroenteritis in pigs (3). Natural or experimental infection by the intestinal route produces higher IgA levels in the colostrum and milk than in the serum and greater protection was afforded than after parenteral injection of virus. IgG also was shown to be protective when antibody was present in high concentrations. Cell-mediated immunity also may have a significant role in protection against intestinal infections, but its mechanism is unclear except that proper T-cell function is essential (28).

Rotaviruses isolated from the various species do not show optimal cross-neutralization activity. Despite this fact there may be some degree of cross-protection between some species. Foal rotaviruses did not induce neutralizing antibodies in calves to a bovine strain, but 30 percent were protected against a virulent bovine rotavirus. Similar results were observed in pigs after inoculation with bovine or foal rotavirus. A bovine strain inoculated into bovine fetuses *in utero* induced resistance to diarrheal disease caused by the human type 2 virus as well as the homologous bovine virus (34).

Active immunization of the newborn is one approach to providing active immunity and protection to the neonate. There is a tissue-culture attenuated vaccine available for calves (13), but its effectiveness has been questioned (1). Passive immunity is another approach, but it is obvious the protection afforded is temporary. Snodgrass *et al.* (21) used various regimens in lambs, such as feeding colostrum with high antibody content on a daily basis throughout the period of greatest risk and thus providing clinical protection while allowing a reduced degree of viral multiplication and permitting the development of an active immunity. Serum or serum products of high antibody titer could replace colostrum if it is not available. Vaccination of the ewes prior to conception may also be a logical approach by increasing the antibody levels in colostrum and milk.

Transmission. The duration of immunity is not known. The period of persistence of virus in the feces of individuals after illness is unknown, but virus persistence certainly occurs. The effectiveness of cell-mediated immunity in individuals apparently has an influence on its persistence. Because immunity may be only partial and not long lasting, adults can become diseased from infected neonates. As the incidence of the disease is extremely high and reinfection in a host may occur, the disease probably is perpetuated through viral persistence within an animal species. There is a possibility that interspecies infection also may be an important factor in disease transmission. It is well documented that rotaviruses of one species can provide another means for transmission and viral existence in nature.

Diagnosis. For the routine diagnosis of rotavirus infection various techniques have been developed such as tissue culture (certain species only), ELISA test, cross-electrophoresis or complement fixation (6). A doubtful positive result obtained by other methods can be confirmed rather quickly by electron microscopy with an excellent photomicrograph as there is a distinct difference in morphology between the diarrheal viruses and reoviruses and orbiviruses, which are all approximately the same size. Specificity of rotaviruses of the various animal species can be determined either by a cross-neutralization test in cell culture (not always possible) or the blocking antibody ELISA test.

In some cases in which new diarrheal epizootics or valuable neonatal animals are involved, fecal specimens should be prepared and examined for viruses (6). In many instances, one or more other potential viral pathogens may be detected, such as coronavirus, adenovirus, and parvovirus in addition to a rotavirus. If mixed viral infections are found in diarrheal disease, this knowledge is useful in applying appropriate control, treatment, and preventive measures.

Control. Neonatal diarrheal disease caused by rotaviruses is most serious, often fatal. Further, it must be reemphasized that the protection against intestinal disease is mediated by a system that operates largely in the enteric tract. As a consequence, colostrum initially is extremely important in the control of this disease. The colostrum must contain reasonably high levels of antibody to the rotavirus involved, and it must be fed every day during the crucial age period of susceptibility to be effective. It has been suggested that a homologous hyperimmune antiserum could be used in lieu of colostrum. In general, this system has its limitations as a practical procedure with most animals.

At present, there is only one licensed vaccine for rotavirus disease in the United States. The bovine attenuated tissue-cultured vaccine is given to day-old calves. Although there is some question about its degree of efficacy, it seems wise to use the product in herds with a serious diarrheal problem. It may save the lives of some calves that would otherwise die.

A combined attenuated vaccine containing bovine rotavirus and coronavirus provides some protection against diarrheal disease (15, 27).

The Disease in Man. Rotavirus infection in infants is a common and serious malady. Two different serotypes (perhaps three) exist in humans that do not provide cross-protection. Because human rotavirus produces disease in newborn monkeys, calves, and pigs, we should not be surprised if the animal viruses eventually are found to cause infection in humans.

REFERENCES

1. Acres and Radostits. Can. Vet. Jour., 1976, *17,* 197.
2. Banfield, Kasnic, and Blackwell. Virol., 1968, *36,* 411.
3. Bohl, Gupta, Olquin, and Saif. Inf. and Immun., 1972, *6,* 289.
4. Derbyshire and Woode. Jour. Am. Vet. Med. Assoc., 1978, *173,* 519.
5. Fernelius, Ritchie, Classick, Norman, and Mebus. Arch. f. die gesam. Virusforsch., 1972, *37,* 114.
6. Flewett. Jour. Am. Vet. Med. Assoc., 1978, *173,* 538.
7. Flewett and Woode. Arch. Virol., 1978, *57,* 1.
8. Lazarowitz and Choppin. Virol., 1975, *68,* 440.
9. Lecce, King, and Mock. Inf. and Immun., 1976, *14,* 816.
10. Matsuno, Inouye, and Kona. Jour. Clin. Microbiol., 1977, *5,* 1.
11. Mebus *et al.*, Univ. Neb. Res. Bull., 1969, *233,* 1.
12. Mebus, Kono, Underdahl, and Twiehaus. Can. Vet. Jour., 1971, *12,* 69.
13. Mebus, White, Bass, and Twiehaus. Jour. Am. Vet. Med. Assoc., 1973, *163,* 880.
14. Mebus, Wyatt, Sharpee, Sereno, Kalica, Kapikian, and Twiehaus. Inf. and Immun., 1976, *14,* 471.
15. Mebus, Torres-Medina, Twiehaus, and Bass. Dev. Biol. Stand., 1976, *33,* 396.
16. Middleton. Jour. Am. Vet. Med. Assoc., 1978, *173,* 544.
17. Nagai and Klenk. Virol., 1977, *77,* 125.
18. Rodger, Schnagl, and Holmes. Jour. Virol., 1977, *24,* 91.
19. Schoub, Lecatsas, and Prozesky. Jour. Med. Microbiol., 1977, *10,* 1.
20. Snodgrass, Madeley, Wells, and Angus. Inf. and Immun., 1977, *16,* 268.
21. Snodgrass and Wells. Jour. Am. Vet. Med. Assoc., 1978, *173,* 565.
22. Snodgrass, Herring, and Gray. Jour. Comp. Path., 1976, *86,* 637.
23. Snodgrass and Wells. Arch. Virol., 1976, *52,* 201.
24. Theil, Bohl, and Saif. Jour. Am. Vet. Med. Assoc., 1978, *173,* 548.
25. Thein and Scheid. Report No. 1 of the WHO Collecting Centre for Collection and Evaluation of Data on Comparative Virology, 1976, p. 34.
26. Thouless, Bryden, Flewett, Woode, Bridger, Snodgrass, and Herring. Arch. Virol., 1977, *53,* 287.
27. Thurber, Bass, and Beckenhauen. Can. Jour. Comp. Med., 1977, *41,* 131.
28. Welliver and Ogra. Jour. Am. Vet. Med. Assoc., 1978, *173,* 560.
29. Woode. Acute Diarrhoea in Childhood (Ciba Foundation Symposium), 1976, *42,* 251.
30. Woode and Bridger. Vet. Rec., 1975, *96,* 85.
31. Woode, Bridger, Hall, Jones, and Jackson. Jour. Med. Microbiol., 1976, *9,* 203.
32. Woode, Bridger, Jones, Flewett, Bryden, Davis, and White. Inf. and Immun., 1976, *14,* 804.
33. Woode and Crouch. Jour. Am. Vet. Med. Assoc., 1978, *173,* 52.

34. Wyatt, Mebus, Yolken, Kalica, James, Kapikian, and Chanock. Science, 1979, *203*, 548.
35. Yolken, Barbour, Wyatt, and Kapikian. Jour. Am. Vet. Med. Assoc., 1978, *173*, 552.

THE GENUS ORBIVIRUS

In this genus there are some important pathogens including African horsesickness, bluetongue in sheep and cattle, epizootic hemorrhagic disease of deer, and Colorado tick fever of man. Morphologically, the particles of infectious bursal disease (IBD) of chickens, infectious pancreatitis necrosis (IPN), and bluetongue viruses are similar, but serologically are not related. It is conceivable that the chicken and trout viruses will be placed in a different taxonomical position after they are more completely studied. Many orbiviruses have been found in wild birds, but do not have any known significance in domestic animals.

The outer capsid of members in the genus is indistinct. The inner capsid has icosahedral symmetry (T=3 plus complex secondary symmetry). The particles, 60 to 80 nm in diameter, are partially resistant to ether, and most are sensitive to acid pH; exceptions are IBD and IPN. They are very resistant to acid pH. Member viruses contain double-stranded RNA, but there may be significant differences in the number of segments in the strands of the viruses now placed in this genus.

African Horsesickness

SYNONYMS: Equine plague, *pestis equorum;* abbreviation, AHS

This is an acute or subacute infectious disease of solipeds which occurs principally in Africa, although it has raged through the Middle East and parts of Asia since 1944. It is unknown in the Western Hemisphere.

Horses are most susceptible and the principal losses occur in them. Mules are considerably more resistant than horses. Donkeys in most parts of Africa are quite resistant, but Alexander (3) found donkeys of the Near East to be fairly susceptible. Outbreaks have been reported in zebras, but generally this species is highly resistant. There have been a few reports of sickness in dogs, the disease generally being attributed to the feeding of infected horse meat. In such districts dogs are not often infected by insects. Angora goats are known to be susceptible. Elephants and zebras are possible reservoirs for virus. (7)

The disease occurs principally in south and central Africa and along the Nile Valley in Egypt. In 1944 cases of horsesickness were diagnosed in Palestine, Syria, Lebanon, and Transjordan. The disease occurs in warm, humid regions, particularly during unusually wet seasons. It is said to be found mostly in relatively flat coastal plains, but it also occurs in level valleys lying at considerable altitudes. It is definitely a seasonal disease, occurring mostly in the late summer and disappearing quickly after frosts come.

The disease remains a threat to Europe and Soviet Russia. With modern transport systems no country is safe from the disease as the vector may survive journey by aircraft.

Character of the Disease. Some cases are very mild, recovery occurring in 3 to 5 days. There is fever (105°F or higher), inappetence, redness of the conjunctivae, and labored breathing. The highly acute form that accounts for most of the deaths is the pulmonary type in which there is severe edema of the lungs and the victims literally drown in their own fluids. There is coughing, severe dyspnea, fever, and copious foamy discharges from the nostrils. A somewhat more chronic form is characterized by the presence of heart lesions and edema of the tissues of the head and neck. Many of these cases recover. A mixture of both forms is most commonly observed in field cases.

In the experimental disease the incubation period generally is about 7 to 9 days, but occasionally it is much shorter or longer. It has been noted that in the natural disease no new cases are seen 9 days after the time of the first severe frost.

In the severe forms of the disease the course is rarely longer than 5 days, since the animal generally dies by that time. In the milder forms the course may be several weeks. The mortality varies considerably. In some outbreaks in which the agent is highly virulent the death rate may be as high as 90 to 95 percent. In others the death rate may be as low as 25 percent.

The lesions depend on the severity of the case. In the acute type the thorax generally contains several liters of fluid, and the lungs are distended with fluid (Figure 47.6). The interlobular tissue generally is separated from the alveolar portions by infiltration of a yellowish fluid. Upon section the lungs do not collapse; the surface is wet, and fluid runs out of the cut surface. The pericardial sac may have some fluid in it, and subendocardial hemorrhages generally are present. Some fluid is usually present in the abdominal cavity, the liver is swollen, and the intestines are reddened.

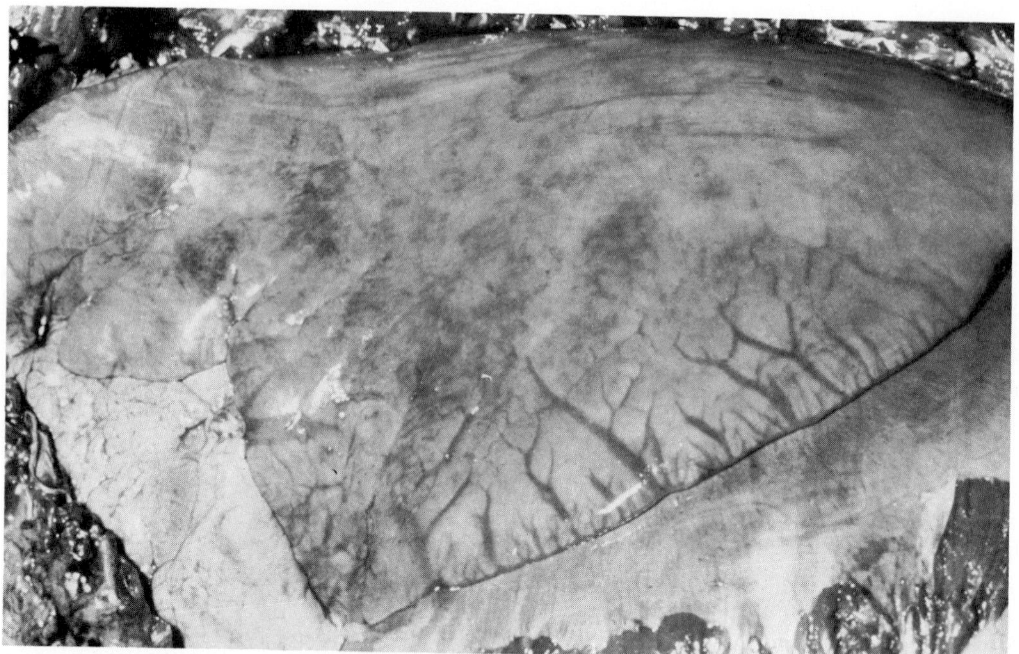

Figure 47.6. African horsesickness. The lung is distended and there is severe pulmonary edema. The edema is manifested by the greatly widened interlobular septa and rounded edge. (Courtesy D. A. Gregg, Plum Island Animal Disease Center, USDA.)

In the more chronic form, characterized by edema of the head, neck, and sometimes the shoulder region, a hydropericardium generally is found and there is hydropic degeneration of the myocardium, but the lungs and pleural cavity show only moderate edema.

The Disease in Experimental Animals. Horses can readily be infected by the injection parenterally of small amounts of blood, tissue emulsions, and bronchial secretions. The urine is infective only occasionally. By feeding, the disease is transmitted irregularly, and only with large amounts of material.

In addition to the animals that are naturally susceptible, the disease can be transmitted by inoculation to goats, ferrets, rats, guinea pigs, and mice.

Properties of the Virus. That the disease was caused by a virus was first shown by McFadyean (11) in 1900. Polson and Madsen (18) suggested that there were two different-sized particles, 50.8 nm and 31.2 nm in diameter.

According to Breese *et al.* (6) the spherical particle has an average diameter of 49 nm in negative-stained preparations and about 71 nm with an inner core diameter of 36 nm in thin sections. The core of AHSV contains RNA (12) and is double-stranded. The particle has 92 capsomeres. Virus particles can be observed in Figure 47.7.

The virus is stable between a pH of 6 and 10, and it survives for years in the cold in an oxalate-phenol-glycerol mixture (1). It is ether-stable and resistant to sodium deoxycholate but readily inactivated by a 1:1,000 dilution of formalin in 48 hours. The virus is relatively resistant to heat. The neurotropic virus is destroyed at 60 C within 15 minutes, but infective virus in tissue-culture medium persists after heating at 50 C for 3 hours or at 37 C for 37 days. At 4 C the cultured virus retains its infectivity for long periods of time. The best method of storage is to freeze-dry the virus with lactone and peptone or to maintain viral suspensions or infected tissues at −70 C. Inactivated virus prepared with 0.4 percent or lower concentrations of betapropiolactone were immunogenic in guinea pigs (15).

There are nine immunological virus types as determined by cross-neutralization tests in mice (10). Each virus strain possesses a common CF antigen which has a diameter of 12 nm (18). The virus in mouse brain tissue also hemagglutinates horse cells at pH 6.4 at 37 C for 2 hours (16).

Cultivation. Various cell lines such as Vero, MS (monkey kidney), baby hamster kidney (BHK), and primary cultures of BHK support replication of AHSV (13). Not all serotype viruses produce a cytopathic effect on first passage of field specimens, but on subsequent passages characteristic CPE may be produced in 48 to 96 hours. The onset of CPE is shortest in MS cell line

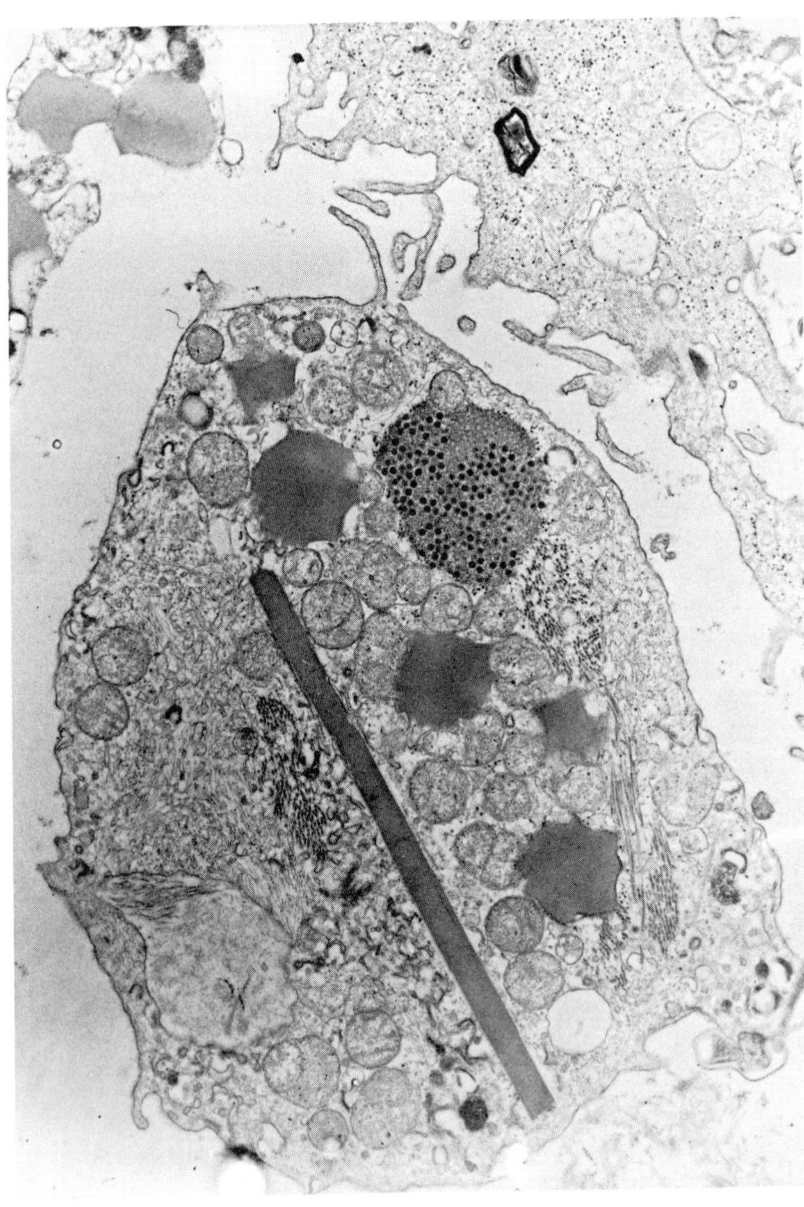

Figure 47.7. African horsesickness type 9 in green monkey kidney cells, 48 hours after inoculation. × 19,100. (Courtesy S. S. Breese, Plum Island Animal Disease Center, USDA.)

and occurs within 24 hours after infection with some strains (12). Plaques are produced in Vero and MS cell cultures (12).

Infected cell cultures have multiple inclusion bodies in the cytoplasm. The inclusions are near the nucleus, and these bodies show immunofluorescence (12). AHS virus propagated in suckling mouse brains may be readily adapted to adult mice and chick embryos.

Immunity. Animals that have recovered from horsesickness are not always permanently immune to the disease. Immune mares convey a passive immunity to their foals, usually protecting them until they are 6 months old. Cases have been reported of animals having the disease a second time. These have been explained by the finding that there are at least nine types of virus, and immunization against one type does not fully protect against all others. Usually second attacks of the disease are mild.

An immune serum serves to provide passive protection from the disease for a limited time. This serum is made by hyperimmunizing recovered horses by transfusing them directly with blood from horses in the febrile stage of horsesickness. To obtain a lasting immunity, horses formerly were given simultaneous injections of large doses of immune serum and small doses of virus. About 85 percent of such horses developed fever, in which case another dose of immune serum was given. A considerable number always developed severe disease, and about a 4 percent mortality was expected. The method has been abandoned in favor of vaccines.

Du Toit, Alexander, and Neitz (9) reported in 1933 on a vaccine for horsesickness made from formalinized spleen pulp emulsion. Four doses were given, the first having been treated by formalin in a concentration of 1:1,000, the second in 1:2,000, the third in 1:3,000 and the fourth 1:4,000. The results were generally satisfactory, but the resulting immunity was not permanent.

Alexander and Du Toit (4), Alexander (2), and Alexander, Neitz, and Du Toit (5) have reported successful immunization of horses with a living vaccine made by modifying the virulence of the horsesickness virus by intracerebral passage through mice. As the virus became adapted as a neurotropic strain for mice, its virulence for mice increased, but that for horses decreased. After it had gone through more than 100 passages in mice, the virulence became fixed for this species and was no longer capable of producing the disease in horses. Because of the several immunological types, it was necessary to make fixed virus from each type. The field vaccine is manufactured from a mixture of nine types, because it was found that a polyvalent vaccine made from nine selected virus strains usually protects against all the types found in South Africa. A single dose of 100 mouse-infecting doses of each type is enough to afford protection.

The mouse brain vaccines have now displaced all others for protecting horses against this disease. The immunity conferred may not be permanent; hence exposed animals should be vaccinated annually before the horsesickness season.

Transmission. Horsesickness is not directly transmissible from animal to animal. Affected animals placed in stables with susceptible horses do not cause outbreaks of the disease. Outbreaks usually occur in warm, damp weather, on swampy, low-lying farms, and only in horses that are pastured at night. These facts indicate that night-flying insects are the probable vectors. Certain species of *Culicoides* (midges), including *C. variipennis,* have been shown to harbor the virus of horsesickness and to be capable of transmitting the infection by bite (8). These insects feed at night and are believed to be the main and perhaps the only vector of the disease. Multiplication and persistence of the virus in *Aedes* mosquitoes has been demonstrated experimentally (14). Mules, asses, elephants, zebras, and dogs, which are not as susceptible to the disease as are horses, have been suggested as possible reservoirs of virus.

There is a suggestion that the virus may be spread to a premise by the wind (17).

Diagnosis. When AHS first appears in a country free of the disease, the condition is frequently diagnosed as equine infectious arteritis, equine infectious anemia, trypanosomiasis, or anthrax as these diseases exhibit similar clinical signs and postmortem findings. Consequently, a field diagnosis should be confirmed by viral isolation and identification or by serological means using paired sera.

Suckling mice are most commonly used for viral isolation from infectious blood or tissues. They are inoculated intracerebrally with 0.03 ml of each preparation. The incubation period may vary from 4 to 20 days, and the mortality may reach 100 percent in the first passage. Serial passages of brain virus shorten the incubation period, and suckling mice die within 2 to 7 days after inoculation. Tissue-cultured cells also may be used for field isolations, but these cells are not as susceptible as suckling mice or horses.

The demonstration of a rising titer utilizing paired serums is ample proof that the disease is AHS. The complement-fixation, agar-gel diffusion, and the immunofluorescence tests are disease-specific as all nine serotypes share a common antigenic component. There are at least two precipitating antigenic components common to the nine serotypes.

Viral typing is usually done by the serum-neutralization test, but the hemagglutination test also may be used. The neutralization tests are performed in mice (1) or in tissue culture. Some cross-neutralization occurs among some of the nine serotypes with the greatest level occurring between types 6 and 9.

Control. Vaccination is the best means of control in infected regions, but nonvaccinated animals can be given protection by stabling them at night in insect-proof stables.

The Disease in Man. This virus has not been reported to cause disease in man.

REFERENCES

1. Alexander. Onderstepoort Jour. Vet. Sci. and Anim. Indus., 1935, *4*, 349.
2. Alexander. Onderstepoort Jour. Vet. Sci. and Anim. Indus., 1936, *7*, 11.
3. Alexander. Onderstepoort Jour. Vet. Sci. and Anim. Indus., 1948, *23*, 77.
4. Alexander and Du Toit. Onderstepoort Jour. Vet. Sci. and Anim. Indus., 1934, *2*, 375.

5. Alexander, Neitz, and Du Toit. Onderstepoort Jour. Vet. Sci. and Anim. Indus., 1936, *7,* 17.
6. Breese, Ozawa, and Dardiri. Jour. Am. Vet. Med. Assoc., 1969, *155,* 391.
7. Davies and Otieno. Vet. Rec., 1977, *100,* 291.
8. Du Toit. Onderstepoort Jour. Vet. Sci. and Anim. Indus., 1944, *19,* 7.
9. Du Toit, Alexander, and Neitz. Onderstepoort Jour. Vet. Sci. and Anim. Indus., 1933, *1,* 25.
10. Howell. Onderstepoort Jour. Vet. Res., 1962, *29,* 139.
11. McFadyean. Jour. Comp. Path. and Therap., 1900 *13,* 1.
12. Ozawa. Arch. f. die gesam. Virusforsch., 1967, *21,* 155.
13. Ozawa and Hazrati. Am Jour. Vet. Res., 1964, *25,* 505.
14. Ozawa, Shad-Del, Nakata, and Navai. Proc. First Internatl. Conf. on Equine Inf. Dis. (Stressa, Italy), 1966, 196.
15. Parker. Arch Virol., 1975, *47,* 357.
16. Pavri. Nature, 1961, *189,* 249.
17. Pedgley and Turner. Jour. Hyg. (London), 1977, *79,* 279.
18. Polson and Madsen. Biochem. Biophys. Acta, 1954, *14,* 366.

Bluetongue

SYNONYMS: Catarrhal fever of sheep, sore muzzle of sheep, range stiffness in lambs

Bluetongue is an infectious viral disease of ruminants transmitted by the insect vector, *Culicoides variipennis.* In sheep the disease is characterized by fever, emaciation, oral lesions, lameness, and a substantial death rate with the heaviest losses in lambs.

The heaviest losses are in sheep, but the disease also occurs in cattle and in goats. It has been suspected that cattle may sometimes be the source of infection for sheep. In certain areas of South Africa, sheep have developed the disease after being brought into areas where no sheep or cattle had existed previously; hence it is highly probable that other natural hosts of this virus such as goats, wild ruminants, and possibly certain wild rodents transmitted the disease. In 1966 Howell (13) reported that at least 18 immunologic serotypes existed worldwide; now there are 20. Using the neutralization test at least six antigenic types were recognized in 1967 in the United States (19). At present (1979), four serotypes are recognized in the USA: 10, 11, 13, 17 (3).

Bluetongue was first reported in South Africa by Theiler (37) in 1905. The disease has constituted a serious disease problem there throughout the years up to the present. In recent years it has been identified in Palestine and on Cyprus. In 1952 a clinical diagnosis of bluetongue in sheep was made in California by McGowan (24), and in the following year the virus was isolated by McKercher, McGowan, Howarth, and Saito (26). These authors sent a strain of their virus to South Africa, where it was compared immunologically with South African strains and the identification confirmed. Soon afterward a disease which had been described by Hardy and Price (10) in the United States in Texas under the name of *sore muzzle* was identified as bluetongue. According to Price (31), by 1954 bluetongue had been identified in sheep by laboratory means, not only in California and Texas, but also in Arizona and Colorado. Since then it has been identified in Kansas, Missouri, Nebraska, New Mexico, Oklahoma, Oregon, Florida, Louisiana, Utah, and other states. Because of its wide distribution it is obvious that the disease was not recently introduced. Apparently it has existed for many years unrecognized on western sheep ranges in the United States.

Character of the Disease. The disease is seen only in midsummer and early fall and is especially prevalent in wet seasons, but seroconversion occurs in some animals during the dry season. It disappears abruptly with the onset of frosts.

In sheep, the principal losses are in feeder lambs, but losses in older animals occur. There is an early temperature reaction which reaches 105 F or higher and lasts only a short time. The victims are greatly depressed, they do not feed, and they lose weight rapidly. Edema of the lips, tongue, throat, and brisket develops in many animals. The buccal mucosa sometimes becomes flushed or even cyanotic. Erosions usually appear on the dental pad, tongue, gums, margins of the lips, and corners of the mouth. The lips bleed easily. Frequently there is a thick, tenacious nasal discharge which dries and crusts on the muzzle. There may be an eye discharge, and edema of the lungs and pneumonia (Figure 47.8) some-

Figure 47.8. Acute, bilateral inhalation pneumonia in a bluetongue-virus-infected sheep that died. (Courtesy T. Walton, Arthropod-Borne Animal Diseases Branch, USDA.)

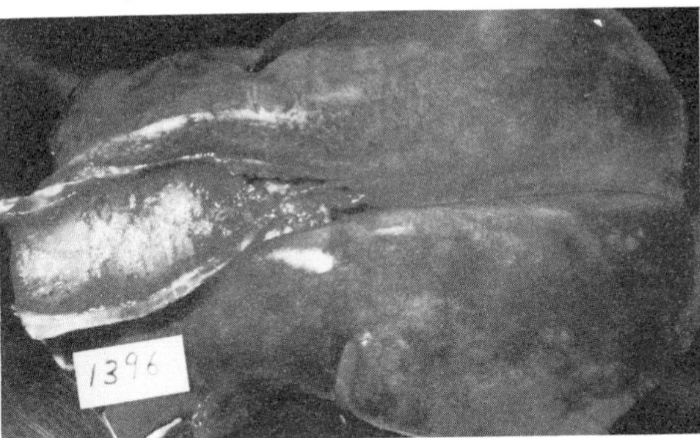

times occur. Occasionally there is a diarrhea, especially in young animals. Abortions may occur in pregnant ewes. Hydranencephaly may occur in infected fetuses.

A characteristic sign is stiffness or lameness due to muscular changes and also, in many cases, to the development of laminitis. Examination of the feet often shows a reddish or purplish line or zone in the skin of the coronet (Figure 47.9), and the hemorrhages frequently extend into the horny tissue. Following recovery, a definite ridge, which persists for many months, may be seen in the horn of the hoof. If animals survive the acute attack, many will need months to reacquire thriftiness.

It should be pointed out that virulence of the causative agent varies widely, and there may be differences in susceptibility in different breeds of sheep. Very young lambs suckling immune ewes are protected by colostral antibodies. Price (31) believes that the syndrome which has long been known in Texas under the name of *range stiffness in lambs* is a mild form of bluetongue contracted by lambs before they have wholly lost their colostral immunity. In most outbreaks many of the older animals have only very mild attacks, manifested principally by a short febrile period.

The mortality varies widely. In Africa, where the virus obviously is much more virulent than in this country, it is said to range from 2 to 30 percent. In California the mortality in 1952 was estimated to be about 5 percent. In Texas the mortality has been considerably less. In a highly susceptible virgin cattle or sheep population the mortality is usually higher.

Experimental studies in sheep indicate that the incubation period in bluetongue is relatively short—from 3 to 10 days. Death seldom occurs before 8 to 10 days following the appearance of the first signs. In many animals the course is much shorter, the mild signs having disappeared after several days. Animals that are severely affected, if they survive, are apt to have a prolonged period of convalescence.

The principal lesions in sheep are cyanosis, edema, and erosions found in the oral mucosa and tongue, edema and hemorrhages in the musculature, hemorrhages on many of the serous membranes, and hyperemia of the mucous membranes of the rumen, abomasum, and intestines. Frequently there are hyperemic areas of the skin, and these may develop into localized areas of dermatitis. The congestion and hemorrhages in the coronary band have already been mentioned. Leukopenia is found in the early stages of the disease. Later there may be leukocytosis and anemia. Congenital deformity and hydranencephaly (Figures 47.10 and 47.11) may occur as a result of *in utero* infection.

The foregoing description of bluetongue has been of the disease as it occurs in sheep. The picture in cattle is quite similar except that cattle generally suffer only mild infections and have a low mortality rate (4, 20). In Africa infections have been confused with foot-and-mouth disease. In many other instances the disease in cattle has been diagnosed only by inoculating sheep. Sometimes there may be frank signs and well-developed lesions.

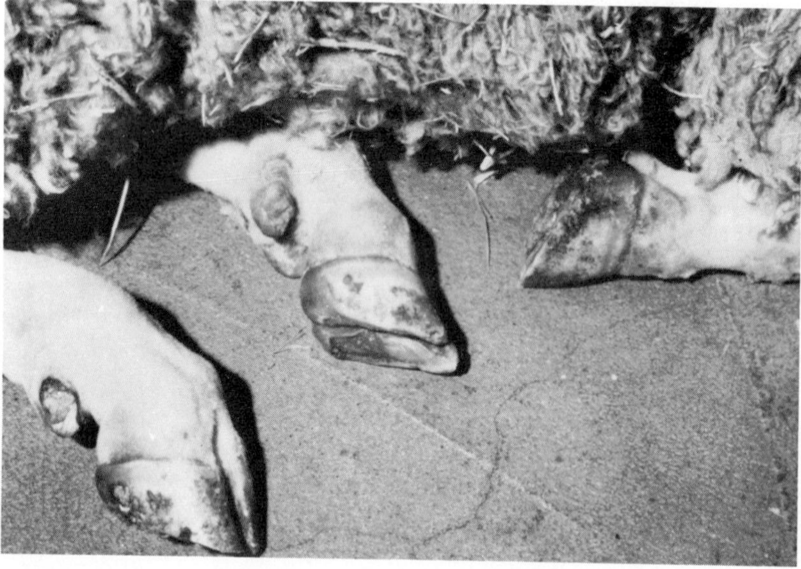

Figure 47.9. Note the coronitis in a bluetongue-infected sheep. (Courtesy T. Walton, Arthropod-Borne Animal Diseases Branch, USDA.)

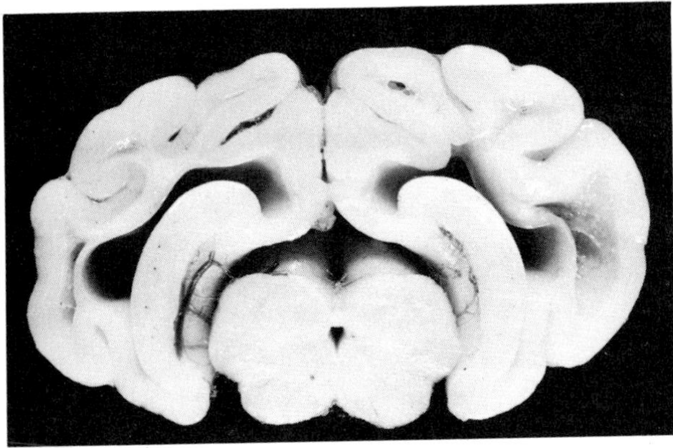

Figure 47.10. Subcortical cavitation (hydranencephaly) in lamb brain following *in utero* bluetongue virus infection. (Courtesy D. Cordy.)

The mouth lesions, the crusts and excoriations on the muzzle, the nasal discharge, the laminitis which is often severe, and an acute dermatitis of a patchy nature involving the flanks, groin, perineum, udder, and teats are characteristic. Necrosis of the skin in the interdigital spaces often occurs. In certain instances a suggested carrier status was established (20). *In utero* transmission occurs in cattle and can result in abortion, hydranencephaly, congenital deformity, and immunologically tolerant calves (Figure 47.12) (11). The virus can produce pathological changes in the reproductive tract of bulls such as focal degeneration of the seminiferous tubules and hemorrhage and hyperemia in the colliculus seminalis.

The Disease in Experimental Animals. The disease may be produced by inoculation of blood or tissues in sheep producing a disease similar to the one observed in nature. The mutton breeds are more susceptible than the wool breeds, and native African sheep are resistant to the disease.

Goats are susceptible to virus, but there is no evidence of clinical signs experimentally or during natural outbreaks. The experimental infection in cattle also is inapparent.

Experimental disease of wild ruminants has been produced in the blesbok and white-tailed deer. Naturally occurring cases have been observed in a bighorn sheep and a captive deer herd. Based on a serological survey for bluetongue in wild ruminants of North America (38) elk, antelope, big horn sheep, Barbary sheep, moose, and three species of deer should be susceptible to the virus. Experimental bluetongue disease in white-tailed deer usually terminates in death (40). The signs of illness and lesions of bluetongue and epizootic hemorrhagic disease are similar. In fatal cases of bluetongue the lesions

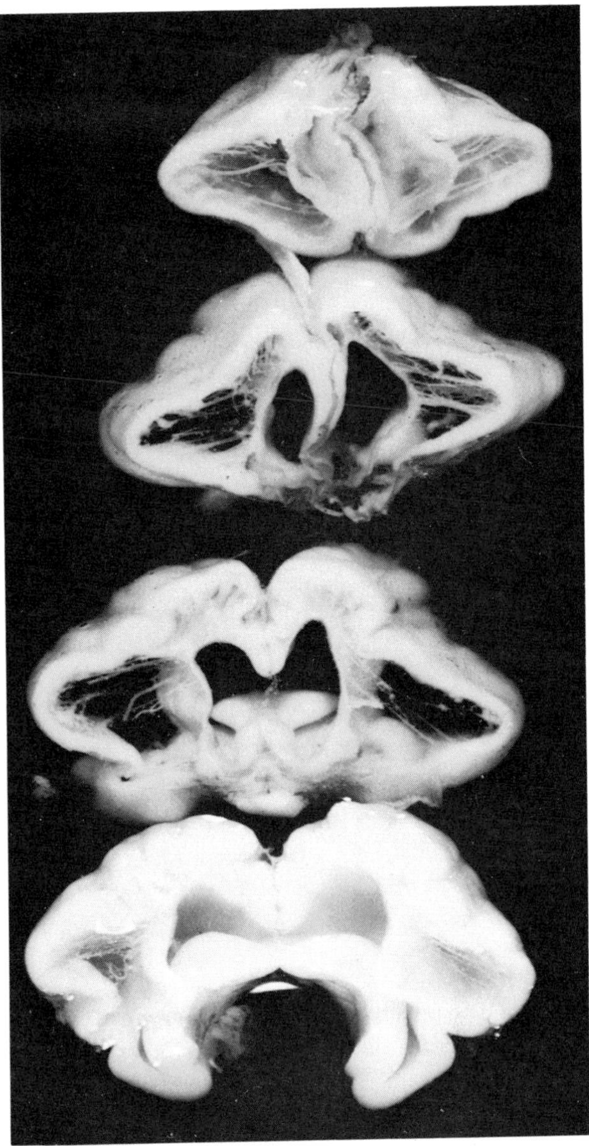

Figure 47.11. Severe hydranencephaly in lamb following *in utero* infection. Secondary hydrocephalus *ex vacus* also is present. (Courtesy D. Cordy, *Jour. Neuropath. and Exp. Neurol.*)

are subendocardial hemorrhages, hemorrhages in the tongue, and enteritis in the small and large intestine. The predominant histological changes are extensive thrombosis with hemorrhages, degenerative changes, and necrosis in affected tissues and organs. Bluetongue virus is readily recovered from the blood and a variety of tissues. Neutralizing antibodies are detected in all convalescent sera.

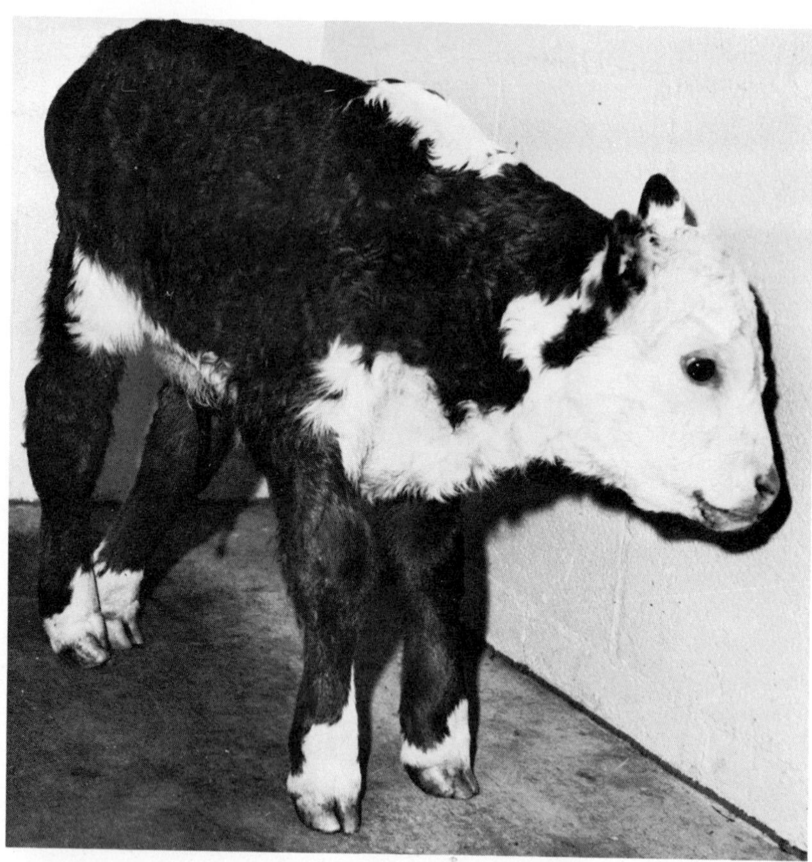

Figure 47.12. Newborn dwarf calf with congenital deformities of the rear legs born to a bluetongue-infected dam. (Courtesy T. Walton, Arthropod-Borne Animal Diseases Branch, USDA.)

Cabasso *et al.* (5) have succeeded in propagating this virus in suckling hamsters, and Van den Ende and coworkers (39) were successful in transmitting it in series in mice by intracerebral inoculation.

Properties of the Virus. Polson and Decks (30) estimated the bluetongue virus to be a sphere 60 to 80 nm (Figures 47.13 and 47.14). Recent information by Els and Verwoerd (8) suggests that bluetongue virus consists of 32 capsomeres rather than the 92 accepted for reoviruses. There is a difference of opinion regarding the presence or absence of a true envelope—it apparently depends on the degree of purification. The virus has a hemagglutinin.

The virus is somewhat resistant to ether, chloroform, and deoxycholate. The virus is sensitive to trypsin and has a narrow zone of pH stability between 6 and 8. It is extraordinarily resistant to influences that destroy most viruses quickly. It will withstand, for example, a considerable amount of putrefaction. The virus has been recovered unchanged by filtering highly decomposed blood. Neitz (27) was able to isolate virulent virus from a lot of infective blood which had been preserved more than 25 years at room temperature in a glycerol-oxalate-phenol mixture. Air-dried virus keeps unusually well, and

Figure 47.13. A cluster of bluetongue virions in pig kidney cell culture, 24 hours after inoculation. × 29,000. (Courtesy S. S. Breese, Plum Island Animal Disease Center, USDA.)

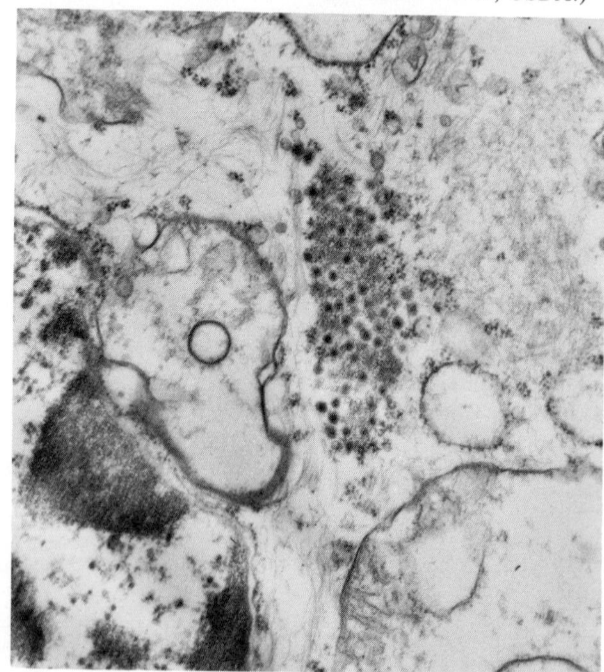

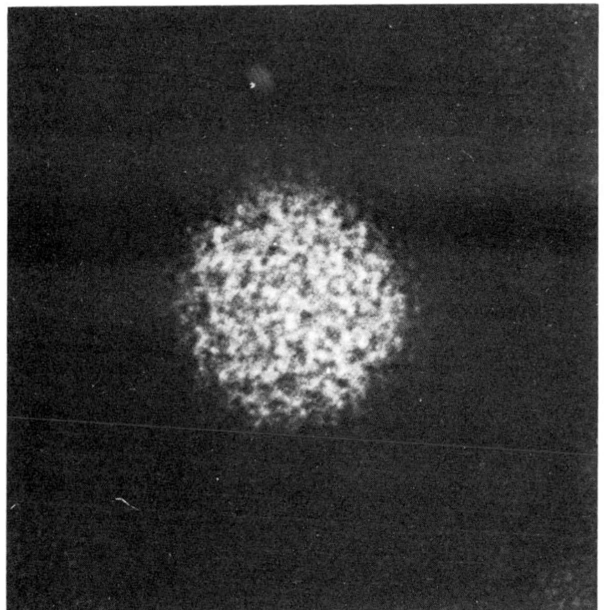

Figure 47.14. A single bluetongue virus particle. × 662,000. (Courtesy T. Walton, Arthropod-Borne Animal Diseases Branch, USDA.)

freeze-dried material remains viable for many months. McCrory, Foster, and Bay (23) found the virus comparatively resistant to several common disinfectants, such as sodium hydroxide, sodium carbonate, and ethyl alcohol. The most effective chemical disinfectant tried was a proprietary preparation known as Wescodyne.

In Africa 19 different antigenic strains of bluetongue virus have been recognized. Price and Hardy (32) compared American virus strains and found that not all were alike; however, they were not sure whether the differences were great enough to warrant considering them as distinct types. At present (1979), serotypes 10, 11, 13, and 17 are known to exist in the USA (3).

Temperature-sensitive mutants of bluetongue virus have been isolated and classified in genetic recombination groups (36). The frequency of recombination varied both within and among groups. The period of incubation required for maximum recombination was 48 hours at 28 C.

The virus has a close affinity for erythrocytes. In attempting isolations of virus from the blood, washed erythrocytes should be used and injected into susceptible lambs rather than cell culture.

Cultivation. Alexander (1) in South Africa showed that bluetongue virus could be propagated readily in chick embryos providing the temperature did not exceed 33.5 C. This is considerably below the optimum temperature for development of the embryo. Serial passage in egg embryos rapidly reduces the virulence of the virus. The yolk sac or intravascular route of inoculation is satisfactory, but the latter method is more sensitive and more time-consuming (20).

Haig *et al.* (9) demonstrated that egg-adapted strains of virus could be cultivated on monolayers of sheep kidney cells and that cytopathogenic activity was exhibited. This activity could be neutralized with homologous antiserum. Cytolytic phenomena were not seen with virulent, unmodified virus on the same cells. Two adapted strains produce a cytopathogenic effect in bovine kidney cells. Since the original studies it has been demonstrated that the virus propagates in various primary and established cell lines including the baby hamster kidney cell line. Using egg-adapted strains of virus it was possible to produce plaques in a mouse fibroblast cell line under agarose (14). Jochim and Jones (16) used a plaque assay system in plastic panels using baby hamster cells grown under an overlay of gum tragacanth. Plaques also are formed by virus in Vero cells (Figure 47.15). Bovine macrophage cultures and organ cultures of tracheal rings were susceptible to bovine bluetongue virus strains (34), and with few exceptions viruses cytopathogenic for bovine embryonic lung cultures also were cytopatho-

Figure 47.15. Plaque formation by bluetongue virus in African green monkey cells (Vero). Stained with neutral red in a Noble agar overlay. (Courtesy T. Walton, Arthropod-Borne Animal Diseases Branch, USDA.)

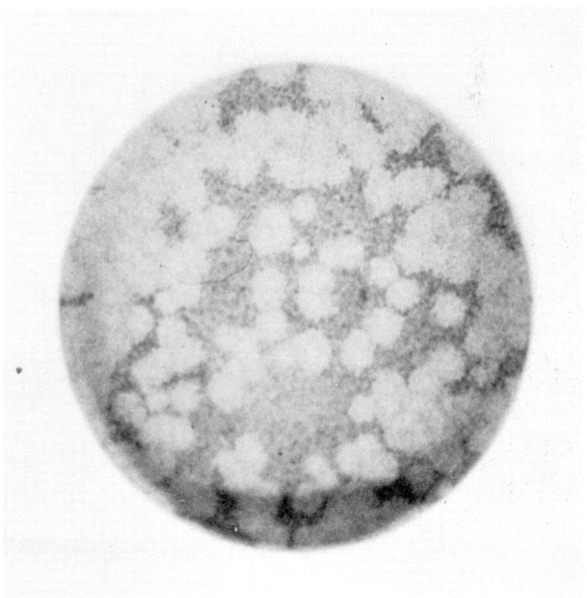

genic for bovine macrophages. Although the viruses were initially cytopathogenic in macrophages, cytopathogenicity was lost upon repeated passages despite replication.

Immunity. Sheep that have recovered from an attack of bluetongue are solidly resistant for a period of months to infection by inoculation with the same virus strain. If more than one type of virus exists in the same locality, second infections may occur within a short time, but this does not happen often since some different types partially immunize against each other. Because there is a plurality of viral serotypes and variability in susceptibility of sheep breeds, no clear pattern of the duration and degree of immunity has been ascertained. Active immunity in sheep produced by virulent virus is associated with the formation of neutralizing and complement-fixation (CF) antibodies (12). Neutralizing antibodies at a high level persist for more than 2 years. In contrast, CF antibodies are detectable for 6 to 8 weeks postinfection but barely detectable at 1 year (12).

Oellermann, Carter, and Marx (28) described a modified hemolytic plaque technique for the detection of bluetongue-antibody-forming cells. It was observed that primary IgM response in mice to sheep red blood cells or virus occurred after 4 days, but declined rapidly to less than 5 percent by day 9. IgG response was detected from day 6 onwards and dominated the response.

Calves that are infected *in utero* may become latently infected, and virus can be isolated from washed erythrocyte samples for over 1 year and in one instance 5 years after challenge with bluetongue virus. The latently infected calves may be immunologically competent or incompetent in producing virus antibodies (21). Cattle that are immunologically tolerant can become competent after repeated exposures by bites of virus-infected *Culicoides variipennis*. These results suggest an overwintering mechanism for viral survival (22).

In South Africa a vaccine was used for many years that had been produced by inoculating virus serially in sheep, without intervention of the natural vector. Attenuation was obtained in this way, and a serviceable vaccine developed. A more uniform, better vaccine was developed by Alexander, Haig and Adelaar (2) in 1947. Their vaccine was a strain of bluetongue virus attenuated by serial passage through chick embryos until it no longer produced signs of illness in sheep. Generally it is necessary to combine several types of strains in a single vaccine in order to give protection against the multiple types found in the field. In 1957 McKercher and coworkers (25) introduced a modified virus vaccine for use in the United States. American strains also were attenuated by serial passage in fertile hens' eggs. A freeze-dried product was tested in the laboratory and field and was found to be very successful. This vaccine produces only nominal reactions when injected into sheep, it does not regain virulence by sheep passage, and it immunizes solidly against massive challenges with virulent virus. When stored under good refrigeration, the vaccine deteriorates very slowly.

In 1968 Leudke and Jochim (19) reported a variation in the clinical and immunologic response of sheep to vaccination. An egg vaccine produced fairly good serum-neutralizing antibody indices, but a tissue-culture vaccine produced little or no antibody response in a 21-day exposure period. A poor correlation also was apparent between the clinical reponse of sheep after challenge and its serum-neutralization index. Obviously, more research must be done in this area. There also was evidence of immunologic nonspecificity for one of the serotypes. Pregnant ewes should not be vaccinated during pregnancy with attenuated virus vaccines.

A bluetongue virus grown in baby hamster kidney cells, inactivated with 0.2 percent betapropiolactone, produced neutralizing antibodies that reached a high level that persisted for at least 1 year (29). After revaccination a secondary response was elicited. Similar results were obtained with a bivalent inactivated virus vaccine.

Transmission. This disease is not transmissible by simple contact. It has long been known that an insect vector must be involved. Mosquitoes were suspected but largely acquitted by experimental work. Du Toit (7) in 1944 showed that gnats (*Culicoides*) were natural transmitters. In this country Price and Hardy (33) found the virus in *Culicoides variipennis,* which happened to be the most common gnat in the infected regions of Texas. *C. pallidipennis* often is involved in transmission. If there are any other natural insect carriers of this disease, they have not yet been identified.

Because of the need for a vector, the disease occurs only in warm weather, generally in midsummer or later when the insect population has built up to maximum heights, and it is generally worst in wet seasons. In California it occurs on irrigated pastures where conditions for insect development are ideal.

The carrier status of cattle after infection and the susceptibility of domestic and wild ruminants, and possibly of rodents, must be considered in the ecology of the disease. The suggestion that the virus may be recovered from the semen of bulls that are immunologically incompetent provides another potential mechanism for the transmission of the virus (22). It is suggested that sheep are not essential for continued survival of bluetongue virus but merely function as accidental hosts.

Diagnosis. In regions where the disease commonly occurs, the diagnosis is usually based upon the clinical signs. Bluetongue resembles, but must be differentiated from, such diseases as foot-and-mouth disease, mycotic stomatitis, infectious bovine rhinotracheitis, bovine virus diarrhea-mucosal disease, rinderpest, Ibaraki, and vesicular stomatitis. Ibaraki disease and bluetongue viruses are similar in morphology, but neutralization tests, complement-fixation tests, and ferritin tagging indicated antigenic differences (6). In newly infected regions, confirmation of bluetongue should be obtained by transmission experiments, serological tests, or serum-protection tests.

Viral isolation from blood or tissues can be done by inoculation of susceptible sheep, of embryonated hens' eggs (18), of susceptible cell cultures (12, 13), and of suckling mice and hamsters (12). The system of choice at present for field isolations is the inoculation of the embryonated hen's egg. If blood is used quantitation of virus is dependent on ultrasonic disruption of blood samples. The use of the glycerol-oxalate-phenol preservative mixture is an excellent stabilizer for the virus and enhances its isolation.

Five separate serological tests can be used in aiding a diagnosis of bluetongue. They are the serum-neutralization (SN) test done in cell culture, microagar-gel diffusion (AGP) test (15), fluorescent-antibody (FA) direct and indirect tests (17), complement-fixation test (20), and the modified complement-fixation test (MCF). The serum-neutralization test has been used most widely in diagnosis and viral typing and is based upon inhibition of cytopathic effects in a cell culture by specific antibody. Because the AGP test is simple, sensitive, and economical it is the *in vitro* test of choice for study of group-specific antigens. The direct FA test can be used for detecting antigen in bovine labile mucosa tissues and chicken embryonic membranes. The plaque neutralization test is the most sensitive serological test for detecting reactors.

Control. Ordinary isolation measures will not stop the spread of bluetongue in regions infested with *Culicoides*. Control must be aimed at reduction of the gnat population, moving the lambs out of the gnat-infested regions, using repellent sprays on the lambs to discourage gnat bites, keeping the lambs indoors from the late afternoon until well into the next day, or immunizing the lambs shortly after they are weaned and before the advent of the gnat season. South African workers claim that gnats, unlike mosquitoes, will seldom enter buildings at night, even though unscreened, unless they are attracted by lights.

Immunization is the most practical scheme, but pregnant ewes must not be vaccinated during early pregnancy (particularly 4 to 8 weeks) as previously mentioned because vaccine virus produced stillborn, spastic "dummy or crazy," putrefied, and deformed lambs (35). Sheep should be vaccinated after shearing as wool fiber breaks occur in severely reacting sheep (12). Maternal immunity protection persists for 3 to 6 months, and this fact must be considered in any immunization program.

The Disease in Man. There is no evidence that the virus causes disease in man.

REFERENCES

1. Alexander. Onderstepoort Jour. Vet. Sci. and Anim. Indus., 1947, *22*, 7.
2. Alexander, Haig, and Adelaar. Onderstepoort Jour. Vet. Sci. and Anim. Indus., 1947, *21*, 231.
3. Barber. Am. Jour. Vet. Res. 1979, *40*, 1654.
4. Bekker, DeKock, and Quinlan. Onderstepoort Jour. Vet. Sci. and Anim. Indus., 1934, *2*, 393.
5. Cabasso, Roberts, Douglas, Zorzi, Stebbins, and Cox. Proc. Soc. Exp. Biol. and Med., 1955, *88*, 678.
6. Campbell, Breese, and McKercher. Can. Jour. Microbiol., 1975, *21*, 2098.
7. Du Toit. Onderstepoort Jour. Vet. Sci. and Anim. Indus., 1944, *19*, 7.
8. Els and Verwoerd. Virol., 1969, *38*, 213.
9. Haig, McKercher, and Alexander. Onderstepoort Jour. Vet. Sci., 1956, *27*, 171.
10. Hardy and Price. Jour. Am. Vet. Med. Assoc., 1952, *120*, 23.
11. Hourrigan and Klingsporn. Austral. Vet. Jour., 1975, *51*, 170.
12. Howell. Bluetongue. Emerging diseases of animals. Food and Agriculture Org., Dept. Vet. Sci., Onderstepoort, 1963, *61*, 111.
13. Howell. Bull. Off. Int. Epiz., 1966, *66*, 341.
14. Howell, Verwoerd, and Oellermann. Onderstepoort Jour. Vet. Res., 1967, *34*, 317.
15. Jochim and Chow. Am. Jour. Vet. Res., 1969, *30*, 33.
16. Jochim and Jones. Am. Jour. Vet. Res., 1976, *37*, 1345.
17. Livingston and Moore. Am. Jour. Vet. Res., 1962, *23*, 701.
18. Leudke. Am. Jour. Vet. Res., 1969, *30*, 499.
19. Luedke and Jochim. Am. Jour. Vet. Res., 1968, *29*, 841.
20. Luedke, Jochim, Bowne, and Jones. Jour. Am. Vet. Med. Assoc., 1970, *156*, 1871.

21. Luedke, Jochim and Jones. Am. Jour. Vet. Res., 1977, *38,* 1697.
22. Luedke, Jones, and Walton. Am. Jour. Trop. Med. Hyg., 1977, *26,* 313.
23. McCrory, Foster, and Bay. Am. Jour. Vet. Res., 1959, *20,* 665.
24. McGowan. Cornell Vet., 1952, *42,* 213.
25. McKercher, McGowan, Cabasso, Roberts, and Saito. Am. Jour. Vet. Res., 1957, *18,* 310.
26. McKercher, McGowan, Howarth, and Saito. Jour. Am. Vet. Med. Assoc., 1953, *122,* 300.
27. Neitz. Onderstepoort Jour. Vet. Sci. and Anim. Indus., 1944, *20,* 93.
28. Oellerman, Carter, and Marx. Inf. and Immun., 1976, *13,* 1321.
29. Parker, Herniman, Gibbs, and Sellers. Vet. Rec., 1975, *96,* 284.
30. Polson and Decks. Quoted by Andrewes, Christopher. Viruses of vertebrates. Williams and Wilkins, Baltimore, 1964.
31. Price. Proc. U.S. Livestock Sanit. Assoc., 1954, *58,* 256.
32. Price and Hardy. Proc. Am. Vet. Med. Assoc., 1954, p. 65.
33. Price and Hardy. Jour. Am. Vet. Med. Assoc., 1954, *124,* 255.
34. Rossi and Kiesel. Am. Jour. Vet. Res., 1977, *38,* 1705.
35. Schultz and Delay. Jour. Am. Vet. Med. Assoc., 1955, *127,* 224.
36. Shipham and DeLaRey. Onderstepoort Jour. Vet. Res., 1976, *43,* 189.
37. Theiler. Ann. Rpt., Dir. Agr., Transvall, 1904–1905, p. 110.
38. Trainer and Jochim. Am. Jour. Vet. Res., 1969, *30,* 2007.
39. Van den Ende, Linder, and Kaschula. Jour. Hyg. (London), 1954, *52,* 155.
40. Vosdingh, Trainer, and Easterday. Can. Jour. Comp. Med. and Vet. Sci., 1968, *32,* 382.

Epizootic Hemorrhagic Disease

SYNONYM: Ibaraki disease of cattle;
abbreviation, EHD

This disease occurs in the Virginia white-tailed deer (*Odocoileus virginianus*) and is caused by a virus classified as an orbivirus.

Shope *et al.* (10) first described the natural disease. It was characterized by an incubation period of 6 to 8 days; severe shock; multiple hemorrhages and associated edema in various tissues and serous sacs; coma; and death. Prothrombin deficiency may cause the hemorrhages (5). Other epizootics have occurred in the United States (4, 9). The clinical signs and lesions were consistent with Shope's original findings. In one instance the infection rate among captive and free-ranging park deer in Mammoth Cave National Park (Kentucky) was high (± 90 percent) with a high mortality (62 percent) in captive deer and with negligible mortality in free-ranging deer. The greatest mortality occurred in fawns and adults, but less in yearlings.

Mule deer and other species are insusceptible to the virus. The biting gnat, *Culicoides variipennis,* is responsible for transmitting the disease. Infection does not occur by direct contact. Intracerebral inoculation of suckling mice causes 100 percent mortality, and after four transfers in this host the virus produced an inapparent infection in deer (6).

The Washington strain of virus replicates in deer fetal cells derived from an entire fetus. The cytopathic effect was characterized by focal development of rounded and clumped cells (4). The staining of infected cells with acridine orange indicated the presence of double-stranded nucleic acid in the cytoplasm. It is known that the New Jersey strain produces a cytopathic effect in Hela cells (6). A similar effect is produced by the South Dakota strain in embryonic deer kidney cells (8).

Using a plaque and neutralization test the existence of two serotypes of EHDV (EHD-Alberta and EHD-New Jersey) was demonstrated (2). Antibodies to both serotypes and bluetongue virus have been found in cattle in the United States. These results emphasize the need to consider both diseases in cattle when either disease agent is suspected as the clinical signs and lesions may be similar.

Ibaraki virus causes a bluetonguelike disease in cattle in Japan. Antibodies to virus are commonly found in cattle in all regions of the United States except the northeastern states (1). There is no antigenic relationship between bluetongue virus and Ibaraki virus, but Ibaraki virus and the two EHDV serotypes are related antigenically as shown by the agar-gel diffusion and immunofluorescent antibody tests for group antigens (3). Yet there is a common complement-fixing antigen shared by the two EHDV serotypes and bluetongue virus serotypes (7). All of these viruses have been placed in a single serological group, but it is clear that considerably more comparative study must be done. Based on plaque neutralization tests it is suggested that Ibaraki virus may be a third serotype of EHD. Its significance as a pathogen in United States cattle is unknown, but judging from its effects in Japanese cattle and its wide distribution in the United States we can anticipate problems similar to those seen with bluetongue in sheep.

REFERENCES

1. Anderson and Campbell, personal communication, 1979.
2. Barber and Yochim. Proc. Am. Assoc. Vet. Lab. Diagnost., 18th annual meeting, 1975, p. 149.

3. Campbell, Barber, and Sochim. Vet. Microbiol., 1978, *3*, 15.
4. Fosberg, Stauber, and Renshaw. Am. Jour. Vet. Res., 1977, *38*, 361.
5. Karstad, Winter, and Trainer. Am. Jour. Vet. Res., 1961, *22*, 227.
6. Mettler, MacNamara, and Shope. Jour. Exp. Med., 1962, *116*, 665.
7. Moore and Lee. Arch. f. die gesam Virusforsch, 1972, *37*, 282.
8. Pietle and Layton. Am. Jour. Vet. Res., 1961, *22*, 104.
9. Roughton. Jour. Wildlife Dis., 1975, *11*, 177.
10. Shope, MacNamara, and Mangold. Jour. Exp. Med., 1960, *111*, 155.

UNSPECIFIED GENERA OF THE REOVIRIDAE FAMILY

Infectious Bursal Disease

SYNONYMS: Gumboro disease, avian nephrosis; abbreviation, IBD

The virus that causes infectious bursal disease appears to possess properties most closely related to the genus *Orbivirus*.

The disease was described as a specific entity by Cosgrove in 1962 (3) and is also termed *avian nephrosis*. As it was first observed in the neighborhood of Gumboro, Delaware, in the United States, *Gumboro disease* became another name for the condition. Winterfield and Hitchner (15) soon confirmed the original observations of Cosgrove and also successfully propagated the virus in chicken embryos. The disease is prevalent in the United States and in other parts of the world in concentrated poultry-producing areas.

Character of the Disease (10). The natural infection occurs in chickens only, and white leghorns show a more severe reaction than the heavy breeds. The disease is principally limited to young chickens with the greatest incidence in chicks 3 to 6 weeks of age. The initial outbreak is usually the most severe. Subsequent outbreaks in succeeding broods are less severe and often are unnoticed.

The incubation period is short, as clinical signs are detected in 2 to 3 days. The birds display ruffled feathers and a droopy appearance. Other signs include soiled vent feathers, whitish or watery diarrhea, anorexia, depression, trembling, severe prostration, and finally death. In affected flocks the morbidity approaches 100 percent and mortality varies from negligible to 30 percent. It has been observed that groups of birds fed the highest protein starter diet (24 percent protein) had a significantly higher mortality and a large number of stunted birds (12).

Birds that die are dehydrated, with discoloration of pectoral muscles that also may show hemorrhages. There is increased mucus in the intestine, and the kidneys are enlarged from the accumulation of urates. The bursa of Fabricius is the target organ for this virus and, initially, it is edematous, hyperemic, and cream-colored with prominent longitudinal striations; by the time of death it is atrophied and gray. The bursa often show necrotic foci and may have hemorrhages on the serosal surface. The spleen may be enlarged with small gray foci on the surface. On occasion, hemorrhages are seen in the mucosa at the junction of the proventriculus and gizzard. The condition is regarded as an infectious lymphocidal disease with the principal histologic lesions appearing in the lymphoid structures such as the bursa of Fabricius, spleen, thymus, and cecal tonsil (6). In neonates the virus produces aplastic anemia, liver necrosis, and hemorrhage.

When mixed infections of IBD occur in young chicks that involve other pathogens such as infectious bronchitis virus, Newcastle disease virus, or *Eimeria tenella* (coccidial agent) the disease is more severe and a higher mortality ensues. When certain attenuated virus vaccines are administered to a flock suffering with IBD, certain problems arise since IBD clearly has a deleterious effect on the immune mechanism.

Properties of the Virus. Information about the physicochemical characteristics is rather limited (2) so its classification as an orbivirus is provisional. It is resistant to ether and chloroform and also to pH 2. It is quite resistant to heat, being viable after treatment for 5 hours at 56 C. The virus is unaffected by exposure for 1 hour at 30 C in 0.5 percent phenol or 0.125 percent merthiolate solutions. There is a marked reduction in virus titer when exposed to 0.15 percent formalin for 6 hours. Chloramine in 0.5 percent concentration destroyed the virus in 10 minutes.

By electron-microscope studies the virus particle is 58 to 65 nm (4, 10). In immune electron microscopy studies negatively stained preparations revealed morphological similarities to both the bluetongue virus group and the infectious pancreatic necrosis virus of salmonids. Small particles found in such preparations are a degradation product of the large particle (5).

Cultivation. Isolation and serial propagation of the virus in 10-day-old embryonated hens' eggs is not difficult if eggs are purchased from a flock free of the disease. Infected chorioallantoic membranes of embryos are used as the source of virus for passage, and the eggs are inoculated on the chorioallantoic membrane (7). Embryo adaptation of the virus by serial passage can result in increased virus titers in amniotic-allantoic fluid (14). Embryo mortality occurs between the 3rd and 7th days after inoculation (7). The dead embryos show edematous distension of the abdominal region, cutaneous congestion and petechial hemorrhages on toe joints and in the cerebral region, occasional necrosis and hemorrhages in the liver, a pale, "parboiled" appearance of the heart, congestion and necrosis of the kidneys, congestion of the lungs, and pale spleen, sometimes with necrotic foci. The chorioallantoic membrane may have hemorrhagic areas, but the bursa of Fabricius does not undergo marked changes.

Landgraf *et al.* (9) reported on the propagation of the virus in monolayer cultures of chick embryo fibroblast. Petek and Mandelli (11) observed cytopathic changes in chick embryo kidney cell cultures.

Immunity. Antibodies are transferred from immune dams to their progeny through the yolk sac of the egg. These chicks with parental antibody are protected for a minimum of 4 to 5 weeks after hatching.

Four-week-old susceptible birds develop an excellent neutralizing antibody response to chicken-embryo-adapted virus with a mean titer of $10^{3.5}$ (14). In contrast 3-day-old chicks had titers between $10^{1.5}$ to $10^{2.0}$. Hitchner (7) observed excellent titers in 12-week-old birds that were about $10^{3.8}$ after 27 weeks. Adult birds usually do not respond as well to virus. The delayed and poor response is probably caused by the absence of an active bursa of Fabricius. Chicks inoculated orally with IBD virus 1 day after hatching showed a 50 percent incidence of immunodeficiency but little mortality. The antibody response to IBD virus and subsequent inoculations with vaccine viruses was suppressed. Serum IgG concentration was decreased while IgM occurred exclusively in its 7S monomeric form. The same IBD virus inoculated into 3-week-old chicks resulted in a 50 percent mortality level but little immunodeficiency (8). Paradoxically the serum IgG concentration was elevated in comparison with normal birds. It appears that bursal but not peripheral B cells are targets of IBDV, and the immunodeficiency results from impaired peripheral seeding of B cells in infected day-old chicks.

Transmission. The disease is highly contagious and spreads readily on an infected farm. The virus is resistant to heat, acids, and many chemicals, so it may remain viable on infected premises for at least 122 days after removal of the infected birds (1).

The existence of carrier birds is unknown, but it is suspected that they exist. The lesser mealworm, *Alphitobius diaperinus,* taken from infected premises 8 weeks after outbreak, was infectious for susceptible chickens. Conceivably, insects may play a role in its transmission.

Diagnosis. In acute outbreaks in susceptible flocks the high morbidity, the rapidity of onset and recovery from clinical signs (5 to 7 days) in 3- to 6-week-old chicks, and the spiked mortality curve should make the diagnostician consider infectious bursal disease. Pathological confirmation can be made by the examination of the bursa of Fabricius and other organs for lesions typical of this disease. Viral particles in smear preparations of infected bursa are readily detected.

Isolation of the virus can be readily accomplished in the embryonated hen's egg for identification by the use of a known positive antiserum against the isolate in the neutralization test. The use of paired sera for demonstration of a rising neutralizing antibody serum could be used as a method of diagnosis but is rarely done because the history, signs of illness, and gross pathological changes, particularly of the bursa, are sufficient to render a correct diagnosis as a rule.

Control. Once infection occurs on premises, control is often accomplished in a natural way because chicks exposed at an early age develop an active immunity without showing signs of illness. The resulting infection without disease may be the result of natural resistance of chicks at an early age or the effect of parental antibody. Vaccination with an attenuated virus vaccine (13) is recommended in flocks in which management practices do not control the disease, especially in the interests of an effective vaccination program involving the use of vaccines for Newcastle disease, infectious bronchitis, infectious laryngotracheitis, Marek's disease, and possibly for other diseases as well.

The Disease in Man. It has not been reported in man.

REFERENCES

1. Benton, Cover, and Rosenberger. Avian Dis., 1967, *11,* 430.
2. Benton, Cover, Rosenberger, and Lake. Avian Dis., 1967, *11,* 438.
3. Cosgrove. Avian Dis., 1962, *6,* 385.
4. Cheville. Am. Jour. Path., 1967, *51,* 527.
5. Harkness, Alexander, Pattison, and Scott. Arch. Virol., 1975, *48,* 63.
6. Helmboldt and Garner. Avian Dis., 1964, *8,* 561.
7. Hitchner. Personal communication, 1971.
8. Ivanyi and Morris. Clin. Exp. Immunol., 1976, *23,* 154.
9. Landgraf, Vielitz, and Kirsch. Deut. tierärztl. Wchnschr., 1967, *74,* 6.

10. Mandelli, Rinaldi, Cerioli, and Cervio. Atti della Soc. Italiana delle Scienze Vet., 1967, *21,* 1.
11. Petek and Mandelli. Atti della Soc. Italiana delle Scienze Vet., 1968, *22,* 875.
12. Proudfoot. Poultry Sci., 1975, *54,* 294.
13. Vielitz and Landgrof. Dev. Biol. Stand., 1976, *33,* 332.
14. Winterfield. Avian Dis., 1969, *13,* 548.
15. Winterfield and Hitchner. Am. Jour. Vet. Res., 1962, *23,* 1273.

Infectious Pancreatic Necrosis Disease

Infectious pancreatic necrosis (IPN) is an acute, highly contagious virus disease of salmonid fishes often causing high mortality and significant economic loss in salmonid hatcheries throughout the world. The disease apparently was first recognized in Canadian hatcheries by M'Gonigle (4), who described it as catarrhal enteritis due to the presence of excess mucus in the stomach and intestines of diseased fish. The disease subsequently was reported in the United States, where it was described as infectious pancreatic necrosis on the basis of histopathological findings (10). Five years later, Wolf, Snieszko, Dunbar, and Pyle (9) were able to demonstrate the viral etiology of IPN using brook trout explants and susceptible brook trout fry, thus making the etiologic agent of IPN the first virus to be isolated from fish. The indiscriminant movement of salmonid fish and eggs on a worldwide basis has resulted in the spread of IPN throughout Europe and Japan.

IPN is a disease that classically causes clinical signs and mortality in very young trout. Outbreaks usually occur shortly after fry have begun feeding and may result in mortality ranging from less than 10 percent to more than 90 percent depending on the virus strain and fish population involved (8). Fish surviving an acute infection with IPN often become persistent carriers and may shed virus in the feces and seminal or ovarian fluids, thus allowing for the horizontal and vertical transmission of IPN. Species reported to be susceptible to infection with IPN virus include brook trout (*Salvelinus fontinalis*), rainbow trout (*Salmo gairdneri*), cutthroat trout (*Salmo clarkii*), and brown trout (*Salmo trutta*) (11). Atlantic salmon (*Salmo salar*) also have been shown to undergo infection following exposure to IPN virus (5).

The virus is easily propagated in many of the piscine cell lines and produces cytopathic effect in 2 to 3 days at 20 C. Classification of the virus has been somewhat controversial, but recent studies indicate that IPN virus is an unenveloped icosahedral virus, approximately 60 nm in diameter and contains two species of double-strained RNA in its genome (1, 3, 6). Underwood *et al.* (6) noted its resemblance to the infectious bursal disease agent based on RNA segmentation and a similar polypeptide composition. Although IPN virus does share certain characteristics with the Reoviridae, differences in capsid structure and nucleic acid may warrant its exclusion from this family in the future.

The diagnosis of IPN is usually made by the isolation of virus from tissues of active cases and its identification using specific antiserum in the serum-neutralization method. High titers of virus are present in tissues from moribund fish, and diagnosis is rarely difficult during acute outbreaks. However, the diagnosis of IPN in apparently healthy carriers remains one of the most perplexing problems associated with this disease. Adult carriers seem to excrete virus only intermittently and are often too valuable to sacrifice in the numbers necessary to sample a population for the presence of IPN. Such nondestructive methods as examining feces, peritoneal washes, and seminal and ovarian fluids all have been employed with varying degrees of success. Serological testing of adult fish has proved inadequate because of the tendency of carriers to be poor antibody producers.

Owing to the absence of vaccines or chemotherapeutic treatments the control of IPN presently is limited to preventive measures and the propagation of virus-free salmonid stocks. Measures employed by hatcheries following IPN outbreaks vary, but total slaughter of infected stock and disinfection of water supply are the only certain means of avoiding recurring epidemics. There is considerable promise in the development of an attenuated vaccine that could be administered at a very early age in the feed. Some progress has been made in the attenuation of certain IPNV strains (2, 7), but the safety and effectiveness of these have not been tested on a field basis. Considering the appearance of multiple serotypes among IPN virus isolates, an additional concern in the development of future vaccines is the degree of protection afforded following exposure to heterologous strains.

REFERENCES

1. Dobos, Hallett, Kells, Sorensen, and Rowe. Jour. Virol., 1977, *22,* 150.
2. Dorson. Bull. Off. Int. Epiz., 1977, *87,* 405.
3. MacDonald and Yamamoto. Jour. Gen. Virol., 1977, *35,* 235.
4. M'Gonigle. Trans. Am. Fish Soc., 1941, *70,* 297.

5. Swanson and Gillespie. Jour. Fish Res. Board Canada., 1979, *36,* 587.
6. Underwood, Smale and Brown. Jour. Gen. Virol., 1977, *36,* 93.
7. Wolf. Adv. Virus Res., 1966, *12,* 35.
8. Wolf, K. *In* Diseases of fish. Zool. Soc. of London 30th Symposium, ed. Lionel E. Mawdesley-Thomas. Academic Press, London and New York, 1972.
9. Wolf, Snieszko, Dunbar, and Pyle. Proc. Soc. Exp. Biol. and Med., 1960, *104,* 105.
10. Wood, Snieszko, and Yasutake. Am. Med. Assoc. Arch. Path., 1955, *60,* 26.
11. Yasutake, W. I. *In* Pathology of fishes, ed. William E. Ribelin and George Migaki. Univ. of Wisconsin Press, 1975, p. 247.

48 The Togaviridae

At present four genera are included in this family. The genus *Alphavirus* includes former members of the arbovirus A group, and the genus *Flavivirus* formerly was called the arbovirus B group. The genus *Pestivirus* consists of hog cholera virus (HCV), also known as swine fever, bovine virus diarrhea-mucosal disease virus (BVD-MDV), lactic dehydrogenase virus, and possibly simian hemorrhagic fever virus and border disease virus. The genus *Rubivirus* includes rubella virus (of man) and possibly equine arteritis virus (EAV).

There are more than 200 recognized arboviruses, and an appreciable number are included in this family. Most arboviruses replicate in arthropod host as well as vertebrates. Because many arboviruses now are better characterized, it is possible to place them in specific genera included in various families. Important diseases of domestic animals caused by members of the Togaviridae family are listed in Table 48.1

THE GENUS *PESTIVIRUS*

Hog cholera virus and bovine virus diarrhea-mucosal disease virus are closely related to each other biophysically, biochemically, and biologically. They share a common soluble antigen. HC, BVD-MD, and border disease of lambs will be the only diseases of this genus covered in this book.

Hog Cholera

SYNONYM: Swine fever (English); abbreviation, HC

Hog cholera is an acute, highly contagious disease of swine characterized by degeneration in the walls of the smaller blood vessels, which results in multiple hemorrhages, necrosis, and infarctions in the internal organs. Affected animals are prone to suffer from the effects of bacterial agents that frequently accompany the virus, but these secondary agents are not necessary for the production of the disease. The cause of the disease is a virus.

The history of HC was reviewed by Kernkamp (37). Hog cholera was first recognized as a separate disease entity by Salmon and Smith (53) in 1885, but it was erroneously believed to be caused by the bacterium that they called *Bacillus cholerae-suis,* now known under the name *Salmonella choleraesuis.* The error was corrected in 1903 when DeSchweinitz and Dorset (18) proved that the disease was caused by a virus and that the "hog cholera bacillus" played a secondary role in the disease.

Hog cholera is a tremendously destructive disease which, despite fairly satisfactory immunization procedures, causes large losses in parts of the world where the disease exists. The disease seems to have been first seen in the state of Ohio in 1833; from there it spread to all parts of the United States through the shipment of stock. Its greatest prevalence in the United States was in the north central states, the so-called corn belt, where the

Table 48.1. Diseases in domestic animals caused by viruses in the Togaviridae family

Common name of virus	Natural hosts	Type of disease produced
Genus *Pestivirus*		
Hog cholera (swine fever)	Swine	Acute, highly contagious disease with variable mortality depending on virus strain and herd susceptibility. Fever, depression, and degeneration of small blood vessels resulting in multiple hemorrhages, necrosis, and infarction characterize the disease.
Bovine virus diarrhea-mucosal disease	Cattle, swine, sheep, deer, and goats	Principally a disease in cattle of all ages. High morbidity, low disease occurrence and mortality as a rule. Fever, leukopenia, depression, excessive salivation caused by erosions in oral cavity, nasal discharge, and abortions in pregnant cows.
Border disease of lambs	Lambs	Border disease in lambs is a mucosal disease caused by a virus antigenically related to BVD-MD virus.
Genus *Rubivirus*		
Equine arteritis	Horses	Acute, contagious disease characterized by fever, stiffness of gait, edema of limbs and around eyes, and abortions precipitated by lesions in the small arteries.
Genus *Alphavirus*		
Western and eastern equine encephalomyelitis	Horses, humans, wild and domesticated birds, invertebrate hosts (mosquitos and chicken mites)	WEE and EEE affect horses of all ages. EEE causes greater mortality than WEE in horses. Epizootics occur during mosquito season. Fever and depression may be followed by signs referable to CNS if the virus invades that system, with death usually resulting 1 to 2 days after nervous signs begin. Can cause encephalitis in humans and pheasants.
Venezuelan equine encephalomyelitis	Horses, humans, many mammals, reptiles, insects	Signs of illness in horses similar to WEE and EEE. May cause encephalitis in humans.

concentration of the swine population is greatest. Cholera was not seen in England until 1862 and on the continent of Europe until 1887. The disease has been eradicated from swine in the United States.

Character of the Disease. Present knowledge suggests that hog cholera virus produces natural disease only in domestic and wild pigs. Outbreaks of the disease in swine have been recorded in nearly all European countries, Africa, Asia, and Australia.

The disease is first manifested by fever (104 F or higher), although often the first sign noticed is loss of appetite. In a fully susceptible herd the disease generally begins in a few animals, then gradually spreads to others until finally practically all are sick. The affected animals appear dull and drowsy; they crowd together in corners or under haystacks or in any other protected place as if chilled. Vomiting is common, a mucopurulent discharge from the eyes frequently is seen, and many suffer from diarrhea. Sometimes the diarrheal attacks alternate with periods of constipation. In white-skinned animals a livid coloring of the skin frequently appears, especially on the abdomen and the inside of the thighs and flanks. Cutaneous hemorrhages may also appear in these areas. If the course of the disease is prolonged beyond 1 week, as it often is, bacterial complications usually occur, principally in the form of pneumonia and ulcerative enteritis.

Table 48.1.—*continued*

Common name of virus	Natural hosts	Type of disease produced
Genus *Flavivirus*		
St. Louis encephalitis	Horses, wild and domesticated birds, humans, insects	Encephalitis in man. Inapparent infections in horses and birds.
Japanese encephalitis	Horses, pigs, cattle, humans, wild birds, insects	Causes encephalitis in man; domesticated animals may occasionally have disease in mild form, with occasional deaths in cattle, swine, and horses. Abortions occur in pregnant sows.
California encephalitis	Foals, suckling pigs, humans, mosquitoes	In humans it causes an influenzalike disease with some individuals developing meningoencephalitis. Antibodies found in foals and suckling pigs, but no disease.
Louping-ill	Primarily sheep, also horses, deer, humans, ticks	Generalized infection in lambs that may involve CNS. Mortality negligible unless CNS signs occur; then death usually ensues. Horse disease similar to disease in sheep. The disease in humans is initially a febrile disease of short duration that may be followed by CNS disease.
Central European tickborne fever	Cows, sheep, goats, humans, ticks	Diphasic disease in man—influenzalike signs followed by CNS involvement. Virus may cause infection in cattle, sheep, and goats and be present in the milk.
Murray Valley encephalitis	Horses, feral pigs, birds, humans, insects	Infection but no disease in horses. Principally a disease of humans; birds and mosquitos play a role in its ecology.
Wesselbron disease	Sheep, cattle, humans, mosquitoes	Causes epizootics in sheep with abortions accompanied by death of newborn lambs and pregnant ewes. Abortions in cattle. In man causes fever and muscular pains.
Turkey meningo-encephalitis	Turkeys	Progressive paralysis associated with a nonpurulent meningoencephalitis.
Powassan disease	Goats, humans	Antibodies to this virus found in a small percentage of goats in New York State. It causes disease in man.

Nervous signs occur quite commonly in hog cholera. These may be manifested by grinding of the teeth, evidence of local paralyses, locomotor disturbances, and occasionally lethargy and convulsions. These are manifestations of an encephalomyelitis that occurs in a large percentage of all cases. Seifried (57) found brain and cord changes in 33 out of 39 cases, although most of the animals had not manifested unusual nervous signs. Macroscopically, hemorrhages are often found in the meninges and in the brain substance. Microscopically, besides the hemorrhages, the usual evidence of encephalomyelitis is found, i.e., perivascular "cuffing" with lymphocytes, mononuclear cells, and a few plasma and eosinophilic cells (Figure 48.1). The glial cells show proliferation both diffusely and in the form of compact nodes. There is degeneration of nerve cells and some neuronophagia. Changes of this type are found in some pigs very early in the disease and before recognizable signs have occurred. They represent a true virus type of reaction.

Inclusion bodies have been recognized in hog cholera. Boynton, Woods, Wood, and Castleberry (7) believed that certain bodies that they saw in the nuclei of epithelial cells of the gall bladder in cholera were of this type. Intranuclear inclusion bodies were observed in reticuloendothelial cells of various organs from more than

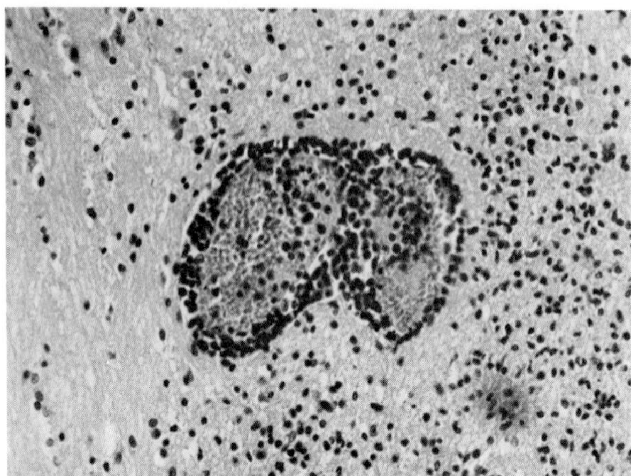

Figure 48.1. Hog cholera, showing lesions of encephalitis, which commonly occur in this disease. Perivascular cuffing and infiltrations of round cells into the nerve tissue are shown. × 210. (Courtesy S. H. McNutt.)

half of the pigs given 3 different strains of virulent virus, but inclusion bodies were not found in pigs injected with various strains of modified HC virus (69).

Congenital infections of the dam cause small litters, fetal deaths, premature births, stillbirths, cerebellar ataxic piglets, and tremors. Congenital disease may occur in immune pregnant sows as well as susceptible dams (8, 70). Some piglets that survive are unthrifty and remain as viral carriers. Those piglets that fail to survive beyond a few weeks have a disease totally different from classical hog cholera (26).

Lewis and Shope (42) called attention to a reaction in hog cholera that apparently had first been noted by Dinwiddie (21) as early as 1914. This is the precipitous fall in the number of circulating leukocytes in the blood—a severe leukopenia. Within 48 hours after the inoculation of the hog cholera virus, the leukocytes, which vary between 14,000 and 24,000 per cu mm in normal pigs, fall to a level below 4,000, and sometimes no leukocytes can be found. So far as is known, no other common disease of pigs exhibits this reaction. Late in hog cholera, when secondary bacterial action plays a prominent part in the disease picture, the leukopenia is replaced by a leukocytosis.

Animals that die within 1 week after first showing signs usually exhibit lesions that are purely of virus origin. The pure virus disease is best seen in inoculated animals held under good hygenic conditions. When these are destroyed at the height of the temperature reaction, which occurs generally on the 5th or 6th day, many will have practically no lesions visible to the naked eye. If lesions are found, they consist only of petechia hemorrhages in the kidney cortex and in the mucosa of the urinary bladder, larynx, and trachea. Sometimes they are found also on some of the serous membranes. Larger hemorrhages often are found in the intestinal mucosa, in the lungs, in the spleen, and especially in the cortex of many of the lymph nodes. These hemorrhages are caused by the rupture of capillaries in which retrogressive changes have occurred as the result of virus action (Figure 48.2). The endothelial linings of the vessels commonly show swelling and proliferation, and many lymphatic channels are plugged with such cells which have desquamated. Many small vessels degenerate into hyaline tubes, which readily rupture allowing blood to leak into the lymph channels. These changes have been minutely described by Seifried and Cain (58).

In the cases that run a longer course, fibrinous pneumonia, often with necrotic foci in the consolidated portions, and fibrinopurulent enteritis with ulceration are commonly found. In these cases the "button" ulcers of the mucosa may appear, especially in the region of the ileocecal valve. Because of the deposition of concentric layers of fibrin over the mucosal perforations, raised, buttonlike deposits are formed—hence the name. These lesions may be associated with the activities of the "hog-cholera bacillus" (*S. choleraesuis*) and the necrosis bacillus (*Fusobacterium necrophorum*). The latter lives saprophytically in the alimentary canal of most swine and causes damage only when the way for it is paved by some other agent such as *S. choleraesuis*.

Following inoculation with virulent virus, pigs remain apparently well for at least 3 days. Field exposures to much smaller quantities of virus by natural routes may cause this incubation period to be prolonged to 6 or 7 days. Most swine die within 7 to 10 days from the time signs first appear. Sometimes individuals will live longer, in which case pneumonia and enteric complications are apt to appear. The mortality in some natural outbreaks is close to 100 percent. Since the introduction of the attenuated virus vaccines, many outbreaks of HC have occurred where the mortality is low. Some individuals suggest that these outbreaks represent strains of attenuated virus that have increased in virulence by transfer in nature.

The Disease in Experimental Animals. Only swine show clinical signs of illness with HC virus. The virus has been adapted to rabbits, and after several passages, the only sign of illness is a slight rise in body temperature (3). Growth of virus has been demonstrated by serial

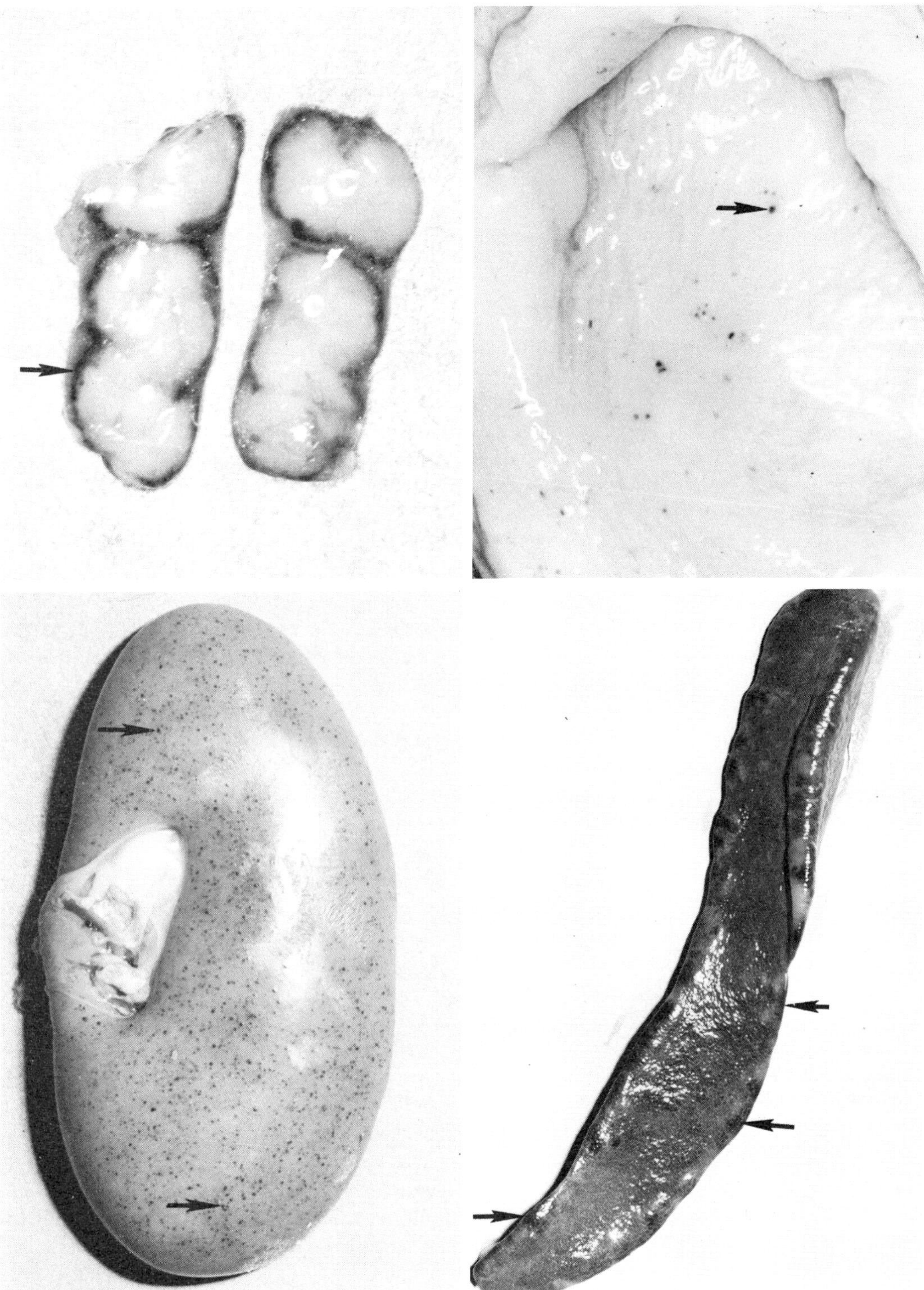

Figure 48.2. Gross lesions in swine associated with hog cholera virus emphasizing the production of hemorrhages. (*Upper left*) Peripheral hemorrhage in cervical lymph node. (*Upper right*) Submucosal hemorrhages in urinary bladder. (*Lower left*) Subcapsular petechiation of kidney. The white areas are photographic artifacts. (*Lower right*) Hemorrhagic areas along margin of the spleen. (Courtesy D. Gustafson.)

transfer in cattle, goats, sheep, and peccaries (37). Significant antibody production was detected in peccaries, calves, goats, sheep, and deer after inoculation with HCV. The inoculated animals failed to transmit the virus by contact to pen-mates of the same species, and calves failed to transmit the infection to susceptible cohabiting pigs (45). Antibody production was not detected in wild mice, cottontail rabbits, sparrows, wild rats, raccoons, or pigeons after HCV inoculation (45).

In experimental studies in pigs, the virus is introduced into the body either by the respiratory system or by the upper digestive tract (27). According to Lin *et al.* (43) the tonsil is a prime target area because the greatest concentration of virus is found there. Infectious virus is present in the blood stream 24 hours after respiratory or tonsillar exposure. Leukocytes of the peripheral blood are infected and capable of viral replication. Regional lymph nodes are the first tissues to show edema and hemorrhage. After intravenous inoculation of HCV, infective virus could not be demonstrated at 0.5, 5, 8, and 13 hours after injection, but blood samples at 16 and 18 hours contained infective virus (27). Apparently many reticuloendothelial cells become infected. Many internal organs contain virus, but not until 48 hours after infection.

Properties of the Virus. The particle size of HCV is generally believed to be approximately 38 to 44 nm (25). Small particles ranging from 3 to 23 nm have been observed in many tissue-cultured HCV virus preparations (25). In some instances they are known to be a parvovirus. A ring of light particle projections observed at the particle surface probably represent the soluble antigen of HCV (51). This RNA virus is spherical with an envelope (20). It is sensitive to ether and chloroform. In a sucrose density gradient the particles are seen as a visible band at a density of 1.13 to 1.14 (11). It is a relatively stable virus. It survives 50 C for 3 days, 37 C for 7 but not 15 days, and −70 C for many years without appreciable loss of infectivity. After an initial drop upon lyophilization it remains viable at 6 C for years. Greatest pH stability of virus in defibrinated blood occurs at pH 5 to 5.5. Dimethyl sulfoxide helps to stabilize the virus (68). Hydrolytic enzymes such as trypsin and phospholipase C reduce viral infectivity, suggesting that it is dependent on the integrity of membrane phospholipids (40). The virus also is inactivated by Roccal, cresol, sodium hypochloride, sodium-o-phenylphenate, and beta-propiolactone.

Strains of HCV were divided into 2 groups, H and B, based on the difference in the neutralization capacity (36). Group H consists of strains reacting poorly in the neutralization test and causing acute illness in experimental pigs. The B group consists of strains reacting well with bovine virus diarrhea antiserum and producing a chronic type of illness in pigs. Pigs immunized with bovine diarrhea virus resisted challenge with a B group virus, but succumbed to challenge with a group H virus. This represents a significant biological difference in HCV strains, yet the attenuated hog cholera virus vaccines clearly protect pigs against challenge with virulent strains (group H). A number of serological methods have been described to study HC antigen and antibody. A conglutination-complement-absorption test for the detection of HC antibody was described by Millian (49). A hemagglutination test was used to measure hog cholera virus and antibody (56). This latter test is based on the linkage of formalinized erythrocytes through diazo bonds with either HC virus or HC antibody. The agar-gel method of Ouchterlony is used to demonstrate a specific antigen-antibody precipitation. The neutralization test in pig kidney cultured cells is possible since the isolation of a cytopathic strain of HC virus by Gillespie *et al.* (30). An indirect neutralization test called the END method was developed by Japanese workers (39), and its cytopathogenicity is based on the exaltation effect of Newcastle virus on HC virus in a tissue culture system. A complement-fixation test is available and was used to demonstrate that HCV and virus diarrhea-mucosal disease virus share a soluble antigen (33). A rapid enzyme-labeled antibody (ELA) microtiter technique for detecting hog cholera antibodies was developed by Saunders (54). It measures the same antibody as the neutralization test, so cross-reactions with antiserums to HCV and BVD-MDV occur.

Cultivation. Virus was found to multiply in embryonated hens' eggs only when freshly minced testicular tissue was placed on the chorioallantoic membrane (67).

HCV was first grown in cell culture by Hecke in Maitland plasma cell type cultures (25). Frenkel *et al.* (25) cultivated the virus in suspended porcine spleen tissue. In general, HC viruses have grown most successfully in primary or stable cell cultures derived from swine tissues. The tissues used include bone marrow, lymph node, lung, leukocytes, kidney, testicle, and spleen. In most instances no cytopathic effect was observed following inoculation with HC virus. A slight cytopathology in spleen cultures was reported by Gustafson and Pomerat (32). A strain (PAV-1) was described in 1960 (30) that produced marked cytopathology in primary swine-kidney cells. This virus also grows in swine testicular cells. Subsequent studies by a Munich group (2) with this cytopathic strain (PAV-1) have shown that it contains no adenovirus, bovine virus diarrhea-mucosal disease virus or *Mycoplasma* agents (6, 35). The Munich group (59) also reported that their viral preparations of PAV-1 had particles of two sizes, 39 to 40 nm and 14 to 16 nm, which both banded in cesium chloride fractions between 1.14 and 1.20 g per ml. The larger ones are believed to be the principal HCV particle since the smaller particles were not found in the Ames or strain A HC pig virus strain preparations (59). The exact nature of the smaller particle or its relationship to the larger HCV particle, if any, has not been ascertained (2). It is unlikely that it is a *Parvovirus* as members of this genus band at 1.4 g per ml in a cesium chloride gradient. Whether the larger particles of the PAV-1 strain have unique cytopathic properties by themselves, or whether the combined efforts of both particles are required for the cytopathic effect in cell culture remains to be determined.

The production of cytopathogenesis by the exalted effect of Newcastle virus on hog cholera was described in 1961 (39). Any strain of virus can be detected in tissue culture by the use of the fluorescent antibody technique (48, 63). The reverse plaque formation (RPF) method was developed as a simple and rapid plaque procedure to assay for HCV in cell culture based on its interference with vesicular stomatitis virus (29, 41).

HCV usually persists in cell cultures without a cytopathic effect. It is known to survive and multiply in leukocyte cultures for more than 2 months (25), and it persisted in subcultural leukocytes for more than 471 days (44).

Immunity. Animals that recover from an attack of HC have a long-lasting and durable immunity. It is generally accepted that a single immunological type of virus exists. In 1949 Dale *et al.* (16) described a variant strain that required larger doses of antisera produced against standard virus for protection against the variant strain than the normal homotypic virus strain. An encephalitic strain described by Dunne *et al.* (28) was only partially neutralized by commercial HC antiserum.

In preliminary tests with the PAV-1 cytopathic strain of HC virus, neutralizing antibody titers were correlated with resistance to hog cholera infection (52). This suggests that resistance is related to the presence of circulating antibody or to its rapid production. The neutralization test is accurate and specific. The presence of antibody appears to be indicative of resistance to HC. It can also be used to test the efficacy of vaccines. Immune serums to all strains of HC virus neutralize the PAV-1 cytopathic strain of virus. It has been used to study maternal and active immunity and also the relation of HC to virus diarrhea virus.

The newborn pig obtains most, if not all, of its antibody from the colostrum of its immune dam. Colostral antibody is lost from the young pig at a constant rate. Its half-life is 13 days, and pigs that have maternal antibody titers of 1:1,000 or above still have some antibody at 4 months. Pigs with maternal antibody titers in this range resist virulent HC virus at 4 months of age (10). Pigs that have sufficient antibody to resist virulent virus become solidly immune following challenge (10).

Colostral or serum antibody may interfere with the development of immunity following vaccination (24). In 1964 Coggins (11) showed that the interference is not an all-or-none phenomenon. Interference is dependent on the amount of antibody in the host and the amount of virus in the vaccine. Tissue culture vaccine containing 10,000 immunizing doses of virus overcame maternal immunity at antibody levels of 1:1,000 or above. It was found that high levels of antibody did depress the antibody response to vaccine and such animals consistently developed lower titers. Thus, the amount of viable virus appears to be the most important single factor in overcoming maternal antibody interference.

Transmission. Hog cholera is transmitted principally by intimate contact with sick animals and directly or indirectly with fresh secretions and excretions. It is not known precisely how the virus is passed from farm to farm in every case. Birds have been suspected of carrying virus on their bodies, and undoubtedly virus may be carried on the shoes and clothing of persons and animals if they travel rather directly from infected to noninfected premises. The disease may be carried to new premises by the careless handling of blood virus, which is used for immunization, or of the bottles that have contained such virus.

Probably one of the most frequent ways by which hog cholera reaches isolated swine herds is through the practice of feeding kitchen scraps or garbage. Birch (5) in 1915 showed that many pigs were slaughtered for food while in the early stages of the disease when their tissues contain a great deal of virus, and that this virus persisted for considerable periods in fresh pork and even in pickled and smoked hams. Trimmings from such materials, finding their way into garbage, can readily start outbreaks. This work was amply confirmed by Doyle (23) in England. Claxton (9) points out that most English outbreaks are initiated in this way. During the period between 1944 and 1949, at the end of World War II, England imported very little pork from abroad, and during this time the incidence of cholera (swine fever) fell far below the usual level. In some recent studies by McKercher, Hess, and Hamdy (47), virus was not recovered from partly cooked hams and from dried pepperoni sausages after the required curing period.

Dunne *et al.* (27) showed that cholera virus, introduced in double gelatin capsules into the stomach, did not infect. Infection was readily accomplished through the tonsils and also through the respiratory tract when precautions were taken to avoid tonsillar infection.

Inasmuch as the virus does not persist on premises after swine have been removed, it has long been a mystery how the annual outbreaks of the disease were initiated. Cholera is largely a seasonal disease. It would be expected to be related to the farrowing seasons because it is the new crops of pigs in which the disease occurs. Most of the sows are bred to farrow in the spring and fall of each year; hence most of the cholera outbreaks occur in those seasons. When new pigs have not been brought to the premises, or other obvious sources of virus have not been introduced, cholera outbreaks generally begin in a single animal, or at least a few animals, the main outbreak appearing some 10 days or more later.

Seeking an answer to the question of how and where virus persists in the relatively long periods that often intervene between frank outbreaks, Shope (62) reported some interesting observations that demonstrate that the virus may be harbored for substantial periods by animals other than swine. He showed that the swine lungworm could serve as a reservoir and intermediate host for the virus of hog cholera. Lungworms in affected pigs may acquire virus which is transmitted through their ova to succeeding generations of worms. The progeny of worms which had acquired virus may infect other swine, susceptible to cholera, without, in most instances, producing the disease. A provoking agent is needed to cause the "masked" virus to emerge as an actively pathogenic agent. One such agent was ascaris larvae. This provocation was effective only during the spring months of the year. Shope was also able to show that suspensions of adult lungworms that were derived from apparently normal, cholera-susceptible swine but which were the progeny of lungworms that had come from cholera-infected animals, could in some instances induce cholera when they were injected intramuscularly into susceptible animals. The mechanism demonstrated by Shope may not operate frequently or effectively in the spread of the natural disease; however, it does mean that hog cholera may not be dependent wholly on a swine reservoir. It is entirely possible that other extraswine reservoirs of virus may be found. Certainly more information is necessary regarding the ecology of this disease.

Mosquitos trapped during an epizootic of hog cholera contained virus (65). Pigs inoculated with positive pools of mosquitos developed chronic hog cholera with a persistent viremia. In experimental studies it was demonstrated that *Aedes aegypti* and *Culex tarsalis* may mechanically transmit the virus to susceptible pigs.

The findings of Baker and Sheffy in 1960 (4) have far-reaching significance in the epidemiology of the disease. They reported that partially attenuated rabbit virus given to some young pigs caused stunting and reverted to virulence while persisting in the blood until the time of death 2 to 3 months later. Consequently, prenatal and neonatal infections that persist in immunologically tolerant piglets may be the principal and perhaps the main means by which HCV is maintained in nature. The success or failure of an HC eradication program probably hinges on this single factor.

Diagnosis. Prompt diagnosis of hog cholera is extremely important because delays often mean the loss of entire herds when many animals might have been saved by prompt use of antiserum. If the diagnosis is in doubt, it is best to treat a disease as hog cholera rather than delay prophylactic treatment for a day or two until the nature of the disease becomes clearer. It is a case of risking the cost of unnecessary serum treatment against that of losing many of the herd.

The fluorescent antibody method is the preferred method with diagnostic laboratories for the detection of HCV. Direct examination of tissues from infected pigs makes a diagnosis possible within a few hours. It appears that field strains of HC virus grow in tissue culture without producing a cytopathogenic effect, but viral activity can be detected by the fluorescent antibody (FA) technique. This method provides a powerful tool for the diagnosis of this disease and its eradication. Solorzano *et al.* (64) tested specimens from 462 cases of suspected hog cholera using the PK-15 cell line for viral propagation and the FA test for identification of viral replication. By this procedure 146 (32 percent) were positive, and 169 (37 percent) were positive when brain lesions were used as diagnostic criteria. The two methods agreed in 82 percent of the cases and disagreed in 18 percent. There were 32 cases (7 percent) positive by the FA that were negative for brain lesions, and 53 cases (11 percent) with brain lesions were not confirmed by FA test. They concluded that the FA method is superior to conventional methods for HC diagnosis. A 2-step technique for the isolation of HCV consisting of an initial culture on buffy coat cultures and subinoculation to PK-15 cell line was a more efficient and sensitive cell culture procedure for isolating virus from field cases, but it is not infallible (38). Pig inoculation with field test specimens is still the most sensitive method for isolating HCV.

The testing of acute and convalescent serum samples for antibody and the detection of a significant rise between the paired sera is another method that can be profitably used for the diagnosis of HC. The serum-neutralization test is usually used for this purpose (30).

The differential diagnosis between hog cholera and acute erysipelas infection often presents serious difficulties even to experienced veterinarians. In erysipelas infections it is not uncommon for several animals to die suddenly with few or no premonitary signs. This does not happen in cholera. In both infections the sick animals have high temperatures, but more animals are apt to develop signs about the same time in erysipelas than in cholera. The sick animals in both cases lie on their bedding, refuse food, and are reluctant to move, but whereas in cholera they are mentally depressed and sleepy, they are mentally alert in erysipelas. The joint swellings that appear in many cases of erysipelas are absent in cholera. Nausea and vomiting occur in both diseases. The characteristic "diamond skin" lesions of erysipelas appear most often in the chronic rather than the acute form of the disease, but they are sometimes seen in acute cases and may be helpful in diagnosis. In some cases of acute erysipelas infection, edema of the lungs develops, and this causes the animals to pant and show evidence of shortness of breath. This is not seen in cholera.

The autopsy findings often are not very helpful in the more acute cases since these diseases may cause only minimal lesions. If facilities for blood counts are available, the leukopenia of cholera contrasts with the leukocytosis of erysipelas. The organism of erysipelas can usually be isolated from the spleen of affected animals, and this constitutes a method of confirmation of the field diagnosis.

The introduction of African swine fever into a country where hog cholera exists poses very serious problems in diagnosis. It is impossible to differentiate these two important diseases in swine except by laboratory tests that are performed by competent laboratory personnel familiar with the test procedures for both diseases.

Immunization. Several methods have been developed for the prophylactic immunization of swine against cholera. Passive immunity is accomplished with a hyperimmune antiserum made from swine. Active immunity may be conferred by simultaneous injection of antiserum and active virus, with vaccines containing only inactivated virus, or with vaccines containing living, attenuated virus. The use of bovine virus diarrhea-mucosal disease virus of cattle as a means of protecting pigs against HC has been proposed by Atkinson *et al.* (1). Another group (36) showed that BVD virus protects pigs against certain biotypes of HCV but not others.

Teehken *et al.* (66) used the FA test to differentiate the effects of virulent, attenuated, and inactivated hog cholera viruses on tonsillar tissue in young swine. Bright cytoplasmic fluorescence was diffusely distributed throughout the epithelial and lymphoid tissues in tonsils of pigs given virulent HCV. After the injection of attenuated HC vaccines bright fluorescence was observed primarily in plaquelike areas in the tonsillar crypt epithelium. In pigs given either of two inactivated virus vaccines fluorescence was granular and limited to the tonsillar germinal centers.

Passive Immunity. The value of the antiviral serum was demonstrated by a group of workers connected with the U.S. Department of Agriculture. The first report was by Dorset, McBryde, and Niles (22) in 1908. The serum is prepared from pigs. As a prophylactic agent it is very effective, the immunity being established immediately. As a curative agent its usefulness is very limited because most animals that show definite signs will die in spite of serum treatment. The principle use of serum alone is at the beginning of outbreaks to protect those animals that have not yet contracted the infection. It is very efficient for this purpose, but the immunity is short-lived.

Dosages of antiserum for hog cholera must be gauged to the body weight of the animal (Table 48.2). It is important that these dosage levels not be under-gauged, particularly when serum is used simultaneously with virus. It is much better to give considerably more serum than needed than too little.

Active Immunity. The simultaneous injection of antiserum and virus was the first method used in the United States to protect pigs against hog cholera. This method sometimes caused a reaction in pigs and occasionally

Table 48.2. The dosage level of hog cholera antiserum required to induce passive immunity in pigs

Pig weight	Minimum dose (ml)
Suckling pigs	20
20 to 40 pounds	30
40 to 90 pounds	35
90 to 120 pounds	45
120 to 150 pounds	55
150 to 180 pounds	65
180 pounds and over	75

caused death, but the survivors are solidly immune. When serum breaks occur, they represent a failure of the antiserum to provide the expected protection against the virus administered. Serum breaks always occur within a few days. Virus breaks are cases in which pigs develop cholera several weeks or months following the simultaneous treatment. These failures occur when the virus lacks proper potency or when pigs fail to react properly to virus. Such animals are only passively immunized and become susceptible 2 to 3 weeks later.

Crystal violet vaccine was a commonly used inactivated virus vaccine. Neutralizing-antibody titers following one injection of crystal violet vaccine are low or undetectable (10). A second injection improved its effectiveness (13). It takes longer to produce an adequate immunity with inactivated virus vaccine, more injections are required, and a dependable immunity does not persist longer than 8 months. Another commonly used inactivated virus vaccine that was used in the United States was the Boynton tissue vaccine. Dhennin *et al.* (19) developed an inactivated virus vaccine produced with virulent virus replicating in PK-15 cells. The virus is concentrated by ultrafiltration and inactivated by glyceraldehyde, then mixed with an oil adjuvant. Protection is reputed to last at least 1 year. Inactivated vaccines are safe, but it is important to establish that residual virus does exist after inactivation. The protection afforded pigs with crystal violet vaccine was variable, and the duration of the immunity is limited. Antiserum will interfere with development of an active immunity from these vaccines and with certain attenuated virus vaccines (13).

The use of BVD-MD virus of cattle for protection against hog cholera has been recommended (1). Vaccination with strain NY 1 of BVD-MD virus protects against some HCV strains that were tested, but not all. This protection is based on the secondary response because immunization with strain NY 1 produces BVD-MD antibody but no hog cholera antibody. Upon challenge with virulent hog cholera virus these pigs usually produce hog cholera antibody quickly, and this antibody may render clinical protection. Its potential use as an immunizing agent has certain advantages: its lack of pathogenicity for pigs; its safety factor, because hog cholera virus is not involved; and with no HC antibodies produced, HC antibody in a pig population can be related to field exposure of HC virus. Recent studies (36) suggest that BVD vaccine might be used with success in areas where the chronic form of hog cholera predominates.

The first attenuated HCV vaccines were modified by rabbit passage (1). Certain attenuated vaccines are given simultaneously with HC antiserum. Serum use was dependent upon their degree of attenuation by rabbit passage or by tissue culture passage (31, 34). The tissue culture vaccines have largely replaced the rabbit-adapted virus vaccines. They cost less to produce and are reputed to contain more virus with higher antigenicity. The use of the cytopathic strain or the fluorescent antibody technique for the detection of noncytopathic vaccine strains makes production control and viral assay much simpler. There is evidence that the rabbit vaccines spread to susceptible pigs. Apparently tissue-cultured vaccines also spread. The immunity derived from these vaccines lasts a long time and is quite durable. Parenteral or intranasal vaccination provide a good systemic and local immune response (15). Maternal immunity may suppress primary antibody response depending on the serum antibody concentration in the piglets. The inhibition of antibody production is either partial or complete, but a primary response of the immune system did occur as evidenced by the clinical signs and the type of immune response following challenge with virulent virus (14). It may be necessary to revaccinate breeder stock. The use of rabbit vaccine virus is contraindicated in pregnant sows during pregnancy because the virus produces a variety of fetal abnormalities with fetal death and partial reabsorption sometimes occurring (55). Low passaged rabbit virus should not be used in young pigs because stunting and death may occur (4). It also would be well to avoid the use of tissue-cultured virus vaccines in pregnant sows.

Serum shock. After pasteurization of anti-hog-cholera serum became a requirement, a type of shock occurring immediately after its injection came to notice. This occurs in only a few animals. The signs vary from animal to animal, but usually consist of rapid respiration and prostration, and sometimes vomiting and convulsions. These signs are seen more often in young animals than in older ones. Deaths are rare; consequently the reactions are not considered to be serious enough to cause hesitancy in the use of serum. The shock-provoking principle can be precipitated from heated serum by ammonium sulfate in concentrations great enough to precipitate the euglobulin. Some evidence indicates that there is a relationship between serum shock and young pig anemia (51). For a discussion of the present status of this problem, see Mathews and Buthala (46).

Control. Hog cholera virus is spread through fresh pork, the trimmings of which often find their way back to swine in garbage. When cholera appears in herds of swine of marketable size, farmers frequently rush their stock to market. In slaughtering establishments under federal meat inspection, efforts are made to prevent the slaughter of swine obviously ill from cholera, but very frequently such animals are not detected in the short time they are held in the yards. This means that many hogs that harbor active virus are slaughtered and enter the trade. Slaughtering establishments that are not under federal control probably distribute more virus through infected pork than those where some, but insufficient, control is exercised.

Laws requiring the cooking of all garbage fed to swine have long been in effect in many European countries, the United States, and Canada. These were enacted in most cases to reduce the hazards of foot-and-mouth disease transmission, but they also serve, of course, to reduce the hazards of other diseases including hog cholera.

Pigs that recover from hog cholera may be carriers of the virus. Some vaccine strains also may persist in immunized pigs. As a consequence, the existence of pigs on any premise that has been exposed to live virus constitutes a potential source of infection for susceptible pigs. At present swine are the only known potential source of virus, but the natural history of this disease has not been completely studied. Other virus reservoirs may exist, although none has been identified with certainty, but we cannot ignore Shope's studies (62).

Hog cholera has been eradicated successfully in various countries of Europe, the United States, and Canada. These procedures are extremely expensive, but control officials believe the benefits outweigh the costs of an eradication program. To effect a successful project requires the unqualified support of the control officials, practitioner, and the swine industry officials. It will require continued vigilance of all parties to remain free of the disease in a given country.

Relationship of HCV to BVD-MD. Using the agar-gel-diffusion test Darbyshire (17) showed that the two viruses were related. The precipitation reaction was specific, and antibody could be absorbed with heterologous antigen as well as with homologous antigen. In neutralization tests their respective antibodies did not cross-neutralize (60). Each virus is capable of stimulating a primary response for the other, and an accelerated antibody to the heterologous virus occurs in 5 to 7 days. In the case of HC in pigs this secondary response confers protection to virulent HC virus but apparently not against all strains (61). In calves, resistance was not clearly demonstrated because calves only have a mild clinical infection when given BVD-MD virus, making challenge evaluation difficult. Nevertheless, an anamnestic type of antibody response was found in these animals. HCV and BVD-MDV each multiply in the rabbit without the production of disease. In these animals heterotypic neutralizing antibody responses were seen irrespective of the virus injected (12).

Knowledge of the physical, chemical, and morphological features of both viruses show that similarities exist. They interfere with each other in tissue culture systems. There is cross-staining when immunofluorescence is employed. Furthermore, heterologous reactions indicate a common soluble antigen (48). This antigen has been used in a complement-fixation test to further characterize their relationship (33). Hyperimmune antiserums contain detectable levels of the heterotypic neutralizing antibody.

The Disease in Man. There is no evidence HC virus causes infection in man.

REFERENCES

1. Atkinson, Baker, Campbell, Coggins, Nelson, Robson, Sheffy, Sippel, and Nelson. Proc. U.S. Livestock Sanit. Assoc., 1962, *66,* 326.
2. Bachmann, Sheffy and Siegl. Arch. f. die gesam. Virusforsch, 1967, *22,* 467.
3. Baker. Jour. Am. Vet. Med. Assoc., 1947, *111,* 503.
4. Baker and Sheffy. Proc. Soc. Exp. Biol. and Med., 1960, *105,* 675.
5. Birch. Rpt. New York State Vet. Coll., 1915–16, p. 60.
6. Bodon. Acta. vet. Acad. Sci. Hung., 1965, *15,* 471.
7. Boynton, Woods, Wood, and Castleberry. Jour. Am. Vet. Med. Assoc., 1942, *101,* 523.
8. Carbrey. Jour. Am. Vet. Med. Assoc., 1965, *146,* 233.
9. Claxton. Agriculture (Gt. Brit.), 1954, *60,* 473.
10. Coggins. Cornell Univ. thesis, 1962.
11. Coggins. Am. Jour. Vet. Res., 1964, *25,* 613.
12. Coggins and Seo. Proc. Soc. Exp. Biol. and Med., 1963, *114,* 778.
13. Cole, Henley, Dale, Mott, Torrey, and Zinober. USDA Inform. Bull. 241, 1963.

14. Corthier. Ann. Rech. Vet., 1976, *7,* 361.
15. Corthier and Aynaud. Ann. Rech. Vet., 1977, *8,* 159.
16. Dale, Schoening, Cole, Henley, and Zinober. Jour. Am. Vet. Med. Assoc., 1951, *118,* 279.
17. Darbyshire. Vet. Res., 1960, *72,* 331.
18. DeSchweinitz and Dorset. U.S. Bur. Anim. Indus. Cir. 41, 1903.
19. Dhennin, Larenaudie, and Remond. C. R. Acad. Sci. D. (Paris), 1976, *283,* 1457.
20. Dinter. Zentrbl. f. Bakt., 1963, *188,* 475.
21. Dinwiddie. Ark. Agr. Exp. Sta. Bull. 120, 1914.
22. Dorset, McBryde, and Niles. U.S. Bur. Anim. Indus. Bull. 102, 1908.
23. Doyle. Jour. Comp. Path. and Therap., 1933, *46,* 25.
24. Dunne, Howard. Sympos. on Hog Cholera, Coll. of Vet. Med., Univ. of Minn., 1961, p. 161.
25. Dunne, Howard. Diseases of swine, 3rd ed. Iowa State Univ. Press, Ames, Iowa, 1970, p. 177.
26. Dunne and Clark. Am. Jour. Vet. Res., 1968, *29,* 787.
27. Dunne, Hokanson, and Luedke. Am. Jour. Vet. Res., 1959, *20,* 615.
28. Dunne, Smith, Runnells, Stafseth, and Thorp. Am. Jour. Vet. Res.. 1952, *13,* 277.
29. Fukusho, Ogawa, Yamamoto, Sawada, and Sazawa. Inf. and Immun., 1976, *14,* 332.
30. Gillespie, Sheffy, and Baker. Proc. Soc. Exp. Biol. and Med., 1960, *105,* 679.
31. Gillespie, Sheffy, Coggins, Madin, and Baker. Proc. U.S. Livestock Sanit. Assoc., 1961, *65,* 57.
32. Gustafson and Pomerat. Am. Jour. Vet. Res., 1957, *18,* 473.
33. Gutekunst and Malmquist. Can. Jour. Comp. Med. and Vet. Sci., 1964, *28,* 19.
34. Hejl. Sympos. on Hog Cholera, Coll. Vet. Med., Univ. of Minn., 1961, p. 169.
35. Horzinek and Uberschär. Arch. f. die gesam. Virusforsch, 1966, *18,* 406.
36. Kamijo, Ohkuma, Shimizu, and Shimizu. Natl. Inst. An. Health Q. (Tokyo), 1977, *17,* 133.
37. Kernkamp. Arch. f. die gesam. Virusforsch, 1966, *18,* 19.
38. Kresse, Stewart, Carbrey, and Snyder. Am. Jour. Vet. Res., 1975, *36,* 141.
39. Kumagai, Shimizu, Ikeda, and Matumato. Jour. Immunol., 1961, *87,* 245.
40. Laude. Ann. Rech. Vet., 1977, *8,* 59.
41. Laude. Arch Virol., 1978, *56,* 273.
42. Lewis and Shope. Jour. Am. Vet. Med. Assoc., 1929, *74,* 145.
43. Lin, Shimizu, Kumagi, and Sasahara. Natl. Inst. An. Health Q., 1969, *9,* 10.
44. Loan and Gustafson. Am. Jour. Vet. Res., 1961, *22,* 741.
45. Loan and Storm. Am. Jour. Vet. Res., 1968, *29,* 807.
46. Mathews and Buthala. Am. Jour. Vet. Res., 1958, *19,* 32.
47. McKercher, Hess, and Hamdy. Appl. Environ. Microbiol., 1978, *35,* 142.
48. Mengling, Pirtle, and Torrey. Can. Jour. Comp. Med. and Vet. Sci., 1963, *27,* 249.
49. Millian and Englehard. Am. Jour. Vet. Res., 1961, *22,* 396.
50. Mohler. Rpt., Chief, Bur. Anim. Indus., USDA, 1931.
51. Ritchie and Fernelius. Vet. Rec., 1967, *69,* 417.
52. Robson, Coggins, Sheffy, and Baker. Proc. U.S. Livestock Sanit. Assoc., 1960, *65,* 338.
53. Salmon and Smith. Rpt., Chief, Bur. Anim. Indus., USDA, 1885.
54. Saunders. Am. Jour. Vet. Res., 1977, *38,* 21.
55. Sautter, Young, Luedke, and Kitchell. Proc. Am. Vet. Med. Assoc., 1953, p. 146.
56. Segre. Am. Jour. Vet. Res., 1962, *95,* 748.
57. Seifried. Jour. Exp. Med., 1931, *53,* 277.
58. Seifried and Cain. Jour. Exp. Med., 1932, *56,* 345.
59. Sheffy, Bachmann, and Siegl. Proc. U.S. Livestock Sanit. Assoc., 1967, *71,* 487.
60. Sheffy, Coggins, and Baker. Proc. U.S. Livestock Sanit. Assoc., 1961, *65,* 437.
61. Sheffy, Coggins, and Baker. Proc. Soc. Exp. Biol. and Med., 1962, *109,* 349.
62. Shope. Jour. Exp. Med., 1958, *107,* 609, and *108,* 159.
63. Solorzano. Penna. State Univ. Thesis, 1962.
64. Solorzano, Thigpen, Bedell, and Schwartz. Jour. Am. Vet. Med. Assoc., 1966, *149,* 31.
65. Stewart, Carbrey, Jenny, Kresse, Snyder, and Wessman. Am. Jour. Vet. Res., 1975, *36,* 611.
66. Teehken, Aiken, and Twiehaus. Jour. Am. Vet. Med. Assoc., 1967, *150,* 53.
67. TenBroeck. Jour. Exp. Med., 1941, *74,* 427.
68. Tessler, Stewart, and Kresse. Can. Jour. Comp. Med., 1975, *39,* 472.
69. Urman, Underdahl, Aiken, Stair, and Young. Jour. Am. Vet. Med. Assoc., 1962, *141,* 571.
70. Young, Kitchell, Luedke, and Sautter. Jour. Am. Vet. Med. Assoc., 1955, *126,* 155.

Bovine Virus Diarrhea-Mucosal Disease

SYNONYMS: Mucosal disease, virus diarrhea of cattle, abbreviation, VD, BVD-MD

In 1946 Olafson, MacCallum, and Fox (38) described a disease of dairy cattle that had a striking resemblance to rinderpest except that it was much milder. They had no difficulty in transmitting the disease with defibrinated blood, spleen tissue, or other organ tissue by parenteral injection, and the disease proved highly contagious under natural conditions (39). In 1956 Pritchard, Taylor, Moses, and Doyle (49) described a similar disease in dairy and beef cattle. It was thought that there were some immunological differences and also some clinical variations between the New York and the Indiana diseases, and for a time they were identified as virus diarrhea–New York and virus diarrhea–Indiana. The original Indiana strains have been lost, but Gillespie and Baker (13) made comparisons of other Indiana and New York strains and found no differences between them. It is now assumed that there is but one type of virus diarrhea in the United States.

All cytopathogenic strains of virus isolated from clinical cases of mucosal disease first described by Ramsey and Chivers (45) are serologically and, when tested, immunologically related to many available cytopathogenic strains of VD virus. As these two entities are now considered clinical variations of the same virus disease, an Ad Hoc Committee on Terminology for the American Veterinary Medical Association Symposium (3) named it bovine virus diarrhea-mucosal disease. An awkward name, perhaps, but it clearly states that the two disease conditions have a common etiology.

Virus diarrhea has been diagnosed in cattle in many countries of the world. The only reported clinical cases of this disease involve cattle. The disease is widespread and is found in the United States, Australia, Canada, Germany, England, Scotland, Sweden, Japan, and Argentina. Strain NY 1 was isolated by Baker, York, Gillespie, and Mitchell (1) from a New York herd, and it was the original type strain until the cytopathogenic strain Oregon (C24V) was isolated by Gillespie, Baker, and McEntee in 1960 (14). The availability of strain Oregon for comparative serological and virological studies has been used by various investigators in the world to evaluate clinical entities that resemble VD (16, 31).

The clinical disease is most frequent in the late winter and spring. Serological surveys have been conducted in various parts of the United States and abroad. In a New York State survey 53 percent of cows selected at random within 500 herds (2 cows per herd) distributed through 53 counties had antibodies (26). Serum samples from cattle in 22 counties of Florida showed that 65 percent of beef cattle and 61 percent of daily cattle were positive for VD antibodies (29). In another survey of states where 100 or more cattle serums were tested, 59 percent in Illinois, 69 percent in Iowa, and 73 percent in Nebraska were positive (36). Incidence studies in Europe yielded similar results.

Neutralizing antibodies have been demonstrated in serums of white-tailed deer from New York State (26). A disease of white-tailed deer and mule deer in North Dakota with lesions similar to VD infection of cattle has been described by Richards *et al.* (46). Antibodies to BVD are found in pronghorns located in Canada (2).

BVD-MD occurs as a natural infection, usually without signs of illness, in domestic swine in the United States (6, 54).

Neutralizing antibodies to BVD virus have been demonstrated in sheep and goats (55). The virus causes an inapparent infection in both species (56). However, there is a condition in lambs resembling border disease characterized by hairiness of the birth coat and poor viability that is caused by a mucosal disease virus that is antigenically related to BVD-MD and HC viruses (41).

Character of the Disease. The disease affects cattle of all ages, but young stock are more likely to show signs of illness. This may be related to the higher susceptibility rate of these animals.

The high incidence of cattle with antibodies suggests that most cattle experience a mild or inapparent infection. When the disease manifests itself in a herd, it may occur as a mild or severe acute infection or occasionally in a chronic form. As a herd disease it varies from one with a high morbidity and a low mortality to one with a low morbidity and a high mortality.

The severely affected cattle have a high temperature and a leukopenia. Other signs of illness include depression, anorexia, scouring, excessive salivation, recumbency, dehydration, reduced milk supply, cessation of rumination, conjunctivitis, congestion and ulcerations in the mucous membrane of the oral cavity, and abortions in pregnant cows. These field observations of abortions were fortified by the isolation of BVD-MD virus from two aborted fetuses representing two New York State dairy herds (15). Lameness, probably caused by laminitis, occurs in some cases. Occasionally there is a mucoid nasal discharge which leads individuals to confuse it with infectious bovine rhinotracheitis, parainfluenza-3 infection, or some other respiratory illness. BVD virus is just one of many bovine viruses involved in neonatal respiratory diseases. Often mixed viral and bacterial infections occur to the detriment of the host.

The gross lesions associated with natural cases were first described in 1946 by Olafson, MacCallum, and Fox (38). The eyes were sunken and the carcasses gaunt and dehydrated. Erosions were found on the dental pad, palate, and lateral tongue surface, around the incisors, and on the inside of the cheeks. Occasionally erosions were seen on the muzzle and at the entrance of the nostrils, and the nasal mucosa was reddened. Ulceration of the pharynx and larynx or diffuse necrosis of the mucous membranes in these regions occurred in some fatal cases.

Secondary pneumonia was observed in some cows in one dealer's herd. Characteristic lesions were irregular, shallow, punched-out erosions of varying sizes and shapes in the mucous membranes of the esophagus, arranged in a linear fashion. Some of the ulcers coalesced, and sometimes the necrotic material remained intact. An occasional calf did not develop oral ulcers. The forestomachs may show small necrotic areas and a few ulcers. The small intestine may have a diffused, reddened mucosa. The cecum often showed petechiae and small ulcers. Hemorrhages were sometimes seen in the subcutaneous tissue, in the epicardium, and in the vaginal mucosa. In subsequent descriptions of the disease other changes were mentioned (7, 43, 45). Hemorrhage, edema, necrosis, and ulceration of the pyloric portion of the abomasum were observed. Similar changes were occasionally noted in the small intestinal tract, with marked lesions in Peyer's patches (Figure 48.3). Other significant lesions were atrophic changes in lymphatic tissues and degenerative alterations in the kidney, skin, and adrenals. Erosions or ulcerations developed in interdigital regions of some cattle, and extensive necrosis may have followed. The lymph nodes often appeared normal, but in some cases they were greatly enlarged and edematous.

Various investigators (7, 45, 57, 62) have reported on the microscopic changes allied with the natural and the experimental disease. The most striking changes occurred in the digestive system. Probably the first change in that portion lined by stratified squamous epithelium was the vacuolation of the cytoplasm in cells, particularly of the stratum germinativum and stratum spinosum. Destruction of the intercellular bridges occurred, and the nuclei became pyknotic. With cellular destruction lesions developed and coalesced with the formation of erosions. In the early lesions there was marked hyperemia with minimal infiltration of mononuclear cells. Some old lesions had deep ulcerations and a marked inflammatory cellular reaction because bacteria invaded the denuded epithelium.

Ulcers, involving the fundus of the abomasum were formed by localized necrosis, erosion of the epithelium, and damage to the lamina propria. Accompanying changes were edema of the lamina propria and submu-

Figure 48.3. Gross lesions in a severe case of BVD-MD of cattle. (*Upper left*) Erosions and hemorrhages of gums. (*Upper right*) Erosions on dorsal surface on the tongue. (*Lower left*) Erosions and necrosis in esophagus. (*Lower right*) Hemorrhage and necrosis of Peyer's patches of intestinal tract. (Courtesy K. McEntee.)

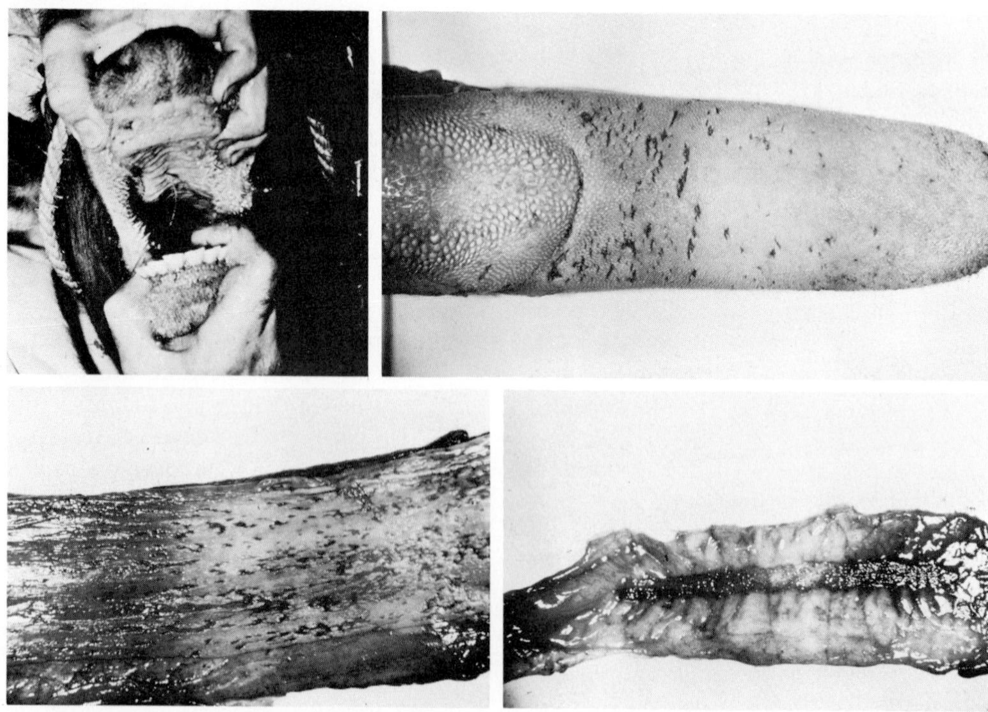

cosa with moderate leukocytic infiltration and hemorrhage. Edema, hemorrhage, erosions, and ulcerations may occur in the pyloric mucosa. Sometimes the lesions were indicative of a necrotic abomasitis.

In severe cases marked changes occurred in the intestinal tract. The crypts of the intestinal glands were filled with mucus, necrotic cells, and varying numbers of leukocytes. Edema was evident in some cases. Destruction of the glandular epithelium occurred, especially in acute cases. In the submucosa lymphatic tissue, necrosis sometimes initiated changes which led to erosion formation. Depletion of lymphocytes in Peyer's patches may be prominent. Ulcers were especially evident over Peyer's patches. Similar changes could be found in the colonic mucosa. Severe cecitis, colitis, and proctitis, varying from a catarrhal inflammation to a necrotic inflammation, were often found.

The thymus was smaller than normal and may contain grayish-white foci. There was a loss of differentiation between the medulla and cortex and a widespread depletion of thymocytes. Lymphocytes were replaced by large mononuclear cells in the tonsils.

There was a hyperplasia of the myeloid elements of the bone marrow with a decrease in the normal amount of fatty marrow.

Subepicardial and subendocardial hemorrhages were observed. Vessel changes occurred only in the media of the arterioles in the submucosa of the digestive tract where severe changes occurred, especially in the germinal centers. The subcapsular sinus may be extended and filled with leukocytes. Neutrophiles occasionally infiltrate the cortex and the medulla. Similar histological changes occurred in the spleen and hemal nodes.

The Disease in Experimental Animals. Susceptible cattle are infected by mouth and parenteral injection. The incubation period is 2 to 3 days after parenteral injection. The first temperature response usually lasts for 1 to 2 days; the second response starts 2 to 3 days later and persists 2 to 3 days with temperatures ranging from 104 to 107 F. A leukopenia occurs which may be followed by a leukocytosis. Diarrhea seldom is noted, and reddening and ulceration of the gums sometimes occurs (1).

Using a noncytopathic strain (Studdert) of BVD-MD virus isolated from an aborted fetus (15), Ward *et al.* (61) inoculated 11 pregnant dairy cows intravenously at varying stages of gestation (150 to 217 days). The fetus that was 150 days old at time of viral injection showed ataxia, blindness, and buccal lesions at birth. Two other neonatal calves had buccal lesions at birth, and the 8 other calves were normal. All 11 calves had BVD-MD antibodies at birth including 4 from whom blood samples were collected before suckling. The antibody levels persisted for 6 months without decline, and 6 of these calves failed to develop signs of illness when given virulent virus at that time. This evidence gives substantial proof that the bovine fetus produces active antibody against BVD-MD virus as early as 5 months of embryo development. Subsequent experimental studies by Scott *et al.* (51, 52) extended these studies. These investigators gave the same Studdert strain intravenously to susceptible cows 3 to 5 months pregnant. Infection in the cows was followed by fetal death, fetal mummification, abortion, or birth at term of calves with cerebellar or ocular defects. Kahrs *et al.* (28) made similar observations in natural disease of a dairy herd: BVD-MD virus was isolated from one aborted fetus, and rising serum-neutralizing antibody titers were demonstrated in some cows. These results suggest that BVD-MD virus causes abortions and congenital defects in the cattle populations. In pathogenic studies of the bovine fetus acute ocular lesions occurred in fetuses taken 17 to 21 days from susceptible pregnant cows given BVD virus at approximately 150 days of gestation (5). The acute lesions were characterized by a mild to moderate retinitis. After 28 days the acute lesions were beginning to resolve, and in newborn animals focal to total retinal atrophy was seen. Sheep and goats are susceptible to experimental inoculation with BVD-MD virus. An English strain produces a rise in temperature that occurs between the 5th and 8th day (24). Lack of appetite and diarrhea also were noted in the sheep. Ward inoculated pregnant sheep and reported the occurrence of congenital anomalies and antibody response in the fetus (60).

Strain NY 1 has been maintained in rabbits for more than 100 transfers and strain Indiana for more than 20 transfers without producing signs of illness in this species.

In experimental pigs BVD-MD virus replicates, and specific antibodies are formed. No signs of illness occur.

The virus fails to elicit a response in white mice.

Properties of the Virus. BVD-MD virus is an RNA-helical-enveloped virus. Both 5-iodo-deoxyuridine and 5-bromo-deoxyuridine fail to inhibit the Oregon strain of BVD-MD (23). Inactivation occurs after treatment with chloroform and ether (18, 23). The sedimentation coefficient of the virus particle is 80 to 90 S. In a sucrose-density gradient its buoyant density is 1.13 to 1.14 g per cm^3 (11). Gratzek (20) reported a 10-fold loss of virus in 24 hours at 26 C or 37 C. Coggins (unpublished data,

1964) found no loss of strain Oregon virus in 24 hours at 25 C. The virus is readily maintained in lyophilized or frozen state (−60 to −70 C) for many years.

Electron photomicrographs of strain Oregon shadowed with chromium reveal somewhat spherical particles that are 35 to 55 nm in size (29). Ultrathin sections of viral pellets also reveal spherical particles approximately 40 nm in diameter (23). In studies by Ritchie and Fernelius (47), three major size classes of particulate entities were observed by EM of negatively stained (phosphotungstic acid) crude and partially purified preparations of one noncytopathic and two cytopathic (including strain Oregon) BVD-MD strains cultured in embryonic bovine kidney cells: (*a*) 15-to-20-nm virus-specific precursor particles considered to represent a ribosomelike soluble antigen—although quite similar in size to the 15 to 16 nm unknown particlelike entities associated with the PAV-1 strain of hog cholera virus, these BVD-MD particles were different in appearance; (*b*) 30 to 35 nm particles, a heterogenous population of three types of particulate entities; and (*c*) 80 to 100 nm pleomorphic membrane-bounded particles. The two larger components had infectious particles, and the surface of the largest unit generally was smooth with rare prominent projections. In other studies (34) with concentrated and purified strain Oregon involving the use of ultracentrifugation, density-gradient centrifugation in potassium tartrate, and rate-zonal centrifugation in sucrose, the virion of strain Oregon stained with uranyl acetate consisted of an envelope without projections and a nucleocapsid probably displaying a cubical symmetry. The particle was 57 ± 7 nm with the core accounting for 24 nm ± 4 nm. In general, the measurements from electron micrographs are in fair agreement among the various investigators, and the differences may be the result of different procedures of viral preparation for electron microscope study.

Ultrafiltration experiments with Millipore filters indicate that some infectious particles are less than 50 nm in size (23).

Strains of BVD-MD virus are closely related serologically, and cross-protection tests in cattle further confirm this close relationship (8). The virus produces neutralizing, precipitating, and complement-fixing antibodies. No hemagglutination has been associated with the BVD-MD virus particle.

Cultivation. Isolates of BVD-MD virus are either cytopathic or noncytopathic in various tissue culture systems. Strain NY 1 multiplies in bovine embryonic skin-muscle cells or embryonic bovine kidney cells without cytopathic changes (33). Similar results in embryonic bovine kidney cells were obtained with strain

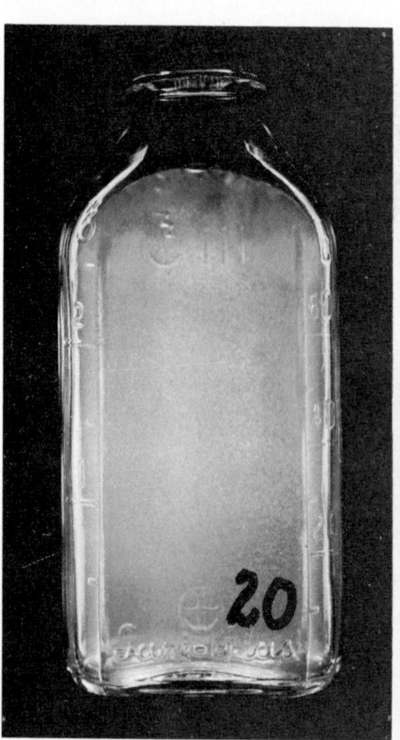

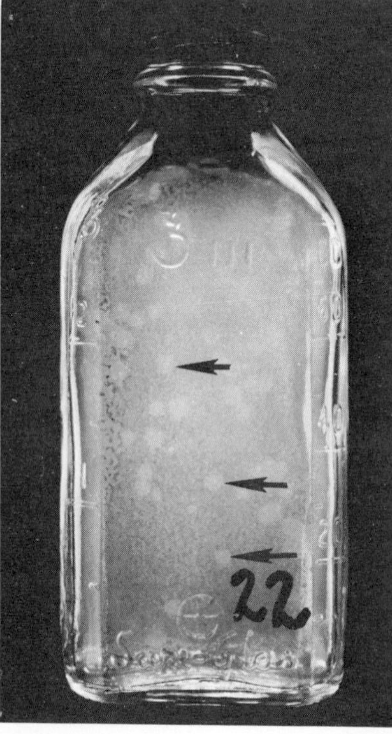

Figure 48.4. Interference test for BVD-MD virus. (*Left*) Culture first inoculated with noncytopathic virus followed by 50 PFU of cytopathic virus 3 days later. No plaques are visible as interference with viral replication occurred. (*Right*) Plaques (*arrows*) are clearly visible as this control culture was only inoculated with 50 PFU of cytopathic virus.

Indiana 46 and the Saunders strain (10). Noncytopathic virus is most conveniently demonstrated in tissue culture by the interference phenomenon (17, Figure 48.4), by the exaltation effect produced by the addition of Newcastle disease virus (25), or by the immunofluorescence test (21).

Noice and Schipper (37) and Underdahl, Grace, and Hoerlein (58) isolated cytopathogenic strains of virus from cases described as mucosal disease. Gillespie, Baker, and McEntee (14) isolated a cytopathogenic strain from the spleen of a calf supplied by investigators at Oregon State University which was designated strain Oregon of BVD-MD virus (Figure 48.5). This strain produced experimental infection in calves and neutralized the homologous antiserum as well as antisera produced in calves that were inoculated with the NY 1 strain, Indiana strain, and others. These same investigators and additional ones soon isolated many cytopathogenic strains from field cases.

Some of the viruses produce a cytopathogenic effect quicker than others and completely destroy the cell sheet. Nuclei of bovine kidney cells become pyknotic and also marginated, and vacuolization occurs. Various strains produce plaques, and this method can be used for more accurate viral titration (17, 30). Throughout the growth cycle the fluid phase of the culture has a greater concentration than the cells, and this suggests that the completely infective particle is formed in the cytoplasm (18). Other monolayer cell cultures of bovine origin that support viral replication include bovine fetal lung (19), fetal endometrium (53), and blood macrophages (50). The virus also replicates in bovine tracheal-ring organ cultures and readily destroys ciliary activity (50).

Figure 48.5. (*Upper*) Uninoculated 8-day-old tissue culture of embryonic bovine kidney cell. H and E. (*Lower*) Eight-day-old virus diarrhea virus culture on embryonic bovine kidney cells. Note cytopathogenic effect. H and E stain. (Courtesy Gillespie, Baker, and McEntee, *Cornell Vet.*)

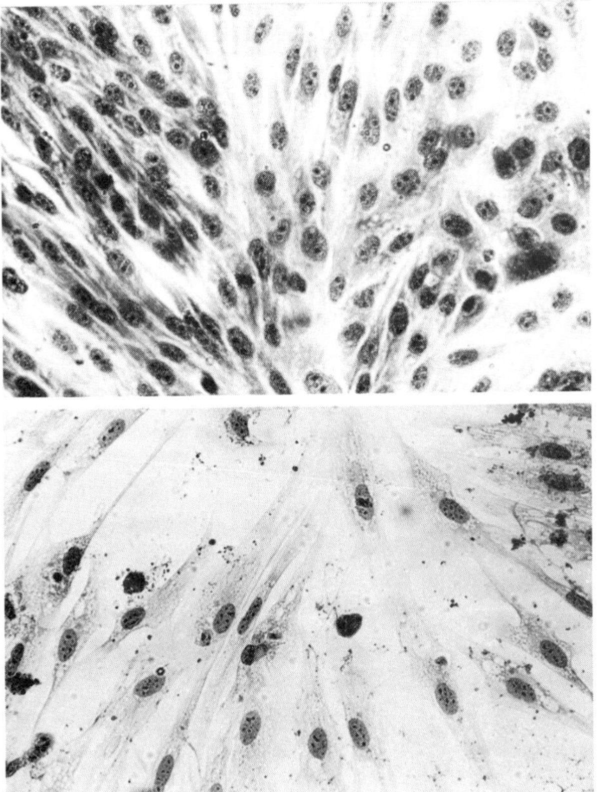

All investigations except one (6) have failed to propagate BVD-MD virus in the hens' embryonated eggs.

Endogenous bovine virus contaminants occur in commercially supplied fetal bovine serum (32), and this includes BVD-MD virus. Noncytopathic virus constitutes the gravest problem since it could go undetected but it would interfere with viral assay of cytopathic strains. Fetal serum also may contain BVD-MD antibody and also interfere with viral or antibody assay procedures for this infection.

Immunity. The high incidence of our bovine population with neutralizing antibodies and the viremic nature of the disease together suggest that animals develop a long and solid immunity after exposure to BVD-MD virus. The MD England LS strain provided protection for two cattle that were challenged with virulent virus at 13 and 22 months following inoculation (24). Cattle immunized with strain Indiana 46, strain New York 1, or strain Oregon were resistant to virulent virus for at least 12 to 16 months (42). Calves that were infected with virus *in utero* had an active immunity at 6 months of age and were resistant to challenge (61).

After inoculation with BVD-MD virus no serum-neutralizing antibodies are detectable at 1 week postinoculation, but the titers at 2 weeks ranged from 80 to 280 and at 4 weeks between 210 and 2,500 (49). High concentrations of IgG are present in the serum and follicular fluid (63). IgG, IgM, and IgA concentrations are low in uterine and vaginal secretions. Interferon can be produced by BVD-MD virus in heifers or fetuses in mid-second trimester (48).

Serum-neutralizing antibody resulting from an active immunity is a good indication of protection in cattle. The relationship between this test and immunity to challenge with virulent virus in a sequential experiment showed that the neutralization test is at least 95 percent accurate, and thus is usable as a substitute for direct challenge (49). To assure reasonable accuracy the test was standardized by the use of 100 $TCID_{50}$ of cytopathic virus against serial 3-fold dilutions of test serum (14). The serum titer varies according to the amount of virus in the test with an increase of 1 log of virus causing a decrease of 0.44 log of serum titer (9). The neutralization test is quite accurate, varying as little as 0.26 log within tests and 0.41 log between tests.

Calves given BVD-MD virus formed complement-fixing antibodies before serum-neutralizing antibodies, and the CF antibodies remained at high levels for at least 15 weeks (21).

Its immunological relationship to hog cholera virus was described earlier (p. 675). Although rinderpest virus produces similar pathological changes, no immunological relationship between VD and rinderpest viruses could be established (12, 59).

Maternal immunity studies were performed by Kahrs *et al.* (27), Brar *et al.* (4), and Malmquist (35). Antibody titers persist for 6 to 9 months in calves whose dams are immune. The half-life of maternal antibody to BVD-MD virus is 21 days. Calves respond to virus before they entirely lose their maternal antibody with the production of an active immunity. Production of an active immunity may not result if the antibody titer derived from its dam is sufficiently high.

Transmission. Because this is a viremic disease, it is assumed that the excretions contain infective virus during the acute stage of infection. Fecal material, blood, and splenic tissue contain virus during this state. Despite the presence of serum-neutralizing antibodies BVD-MD virus was isolated from buffy coat of cattle given virus 3 weeks earlier (21). Infection can be produced with infective virus by the oral route or by parenteral injection. There is excellent field evidence that the infection can be carried readily from one herd to another by mechanical means.

Natural BVD-MD infection probably occurs in sheep and goats, and they may play a role in transmission of the virus to cattle. It occurs as a natural infection in swine so transmission with other susceptible animals is possible. Neutralizing antibodies have been found in a small percentage (7) of New York white-tailed deer (26). A disease resembling BVD-MD has been described in white-tailed and mule deer in North Dakota (46). One or more of these wildlife hosts may play a significant role in the ecology of this disease.

It is known that the virus may persist in recovered or chronically ill cattle and serve as a potential source of infection to other susceptible livestock.

Diagnosis. The diagnosis generally is based on clinical signs and more specifically on lesions. This disease can be readily confused clinically with malignant catarrhal fever or rinderpest in some instances, and on occasions with bovine respiratory infections.

As far as we know, all noncytopathic and cytopathic field isolates replicate in tissue-culture systems including embryonic bovine cultures of kidney, spleen, testicle, and trachea. Virus has been isolated from the blood, urine, nasal, or ocular discharges of acute cases. At necropsy spleen, bone marrow, or mesenteric lymph nodes are good sources for virus. If cytopathic changes are not observed after three passages in cell culture, noncytopathic strains can be identified by the immunofluorescence test, by the END method, or by the cellular resistance test.

The demonstration of a rising titer with paired serums in the serum-neutralization or complement-fixation test constitutes a good method for diagnosis, but, in practice, the serum-neutralization test is preferred. Because serological variants do occur, one strain may not detect antibody to a heterologous virus if the antibody titer is low. This problem can be circumvented to a large degree by adding complement to the neutralization test system (22).

Fluorescent antibody conjugate for HCV also detects BVD-MD antigen. In some instances it is important to distinguish the virus. As a consequence, it is sometimes necessary to run test serums from pigs against HCV and BVD-MD antigens in neutralization tests (6).

Immunization. No alteration in virulence in calves was noted with strain New York after 100 transfers in embryonic bovine kidney cells (Gillespie, 1965). In contrast, strain Oregon showed attenuation for calves by the 32nd passage in this same cell system and did not spread to a limited number of contact calves (10). Laboratory and field tests of this strain by other workers confirmed these observations and recommended its use in the field (64). This vaccine strain is produced by commercial firms and probably produces a long-lasting immunity. Another attenuated virus vaccine that was modified by passage in a continuous porcine cell line has been described for vaccination of cattle (40). It is reputed to be safe and efficacious in cattle without spread to contact animals.

The immunization of calves with an ethanol saponin vaccine against BVD-MD causes the formation of neutralizing antibodies in high titers (65). The vaccinated calves were resistant to challenge with virulent virus of BVD-MD. The duration of immunity is unknown.

At an AVMA Symposium on Bovine Diseases in 1967 a panel included BVD-MD vaccine in their recommendations in their herd health programs. In beef cattle a herd health program includes the following. In a preconditioning program for calves on the ranch BVD-MD modified living virus of tissue culture origin singly or in combination with *Leptospira pomona* bacterin should be given to 5-month-old calves. Calves that arrive at feedlots without preconditioning should not be given BVD-MD vaccine unless a given feedlot has had previous problems with BVD-MD, and then only 48 hours or more after arrival, depending upon recovery from the stress of shipping.

In the self-contained dairy herd inoculate calves with BVD-MD vaccine at 6 to 8 months of age only if the disease is prevalent in the area. Additions to the open herd should be kept in isolation for 30 days and immunized with BVD-MD vaccine if the disease is common in the herd.

The panel (3) recognized that BVD-MD modified living vaccines are quite effective and relatively safe for most cattle under field conditions. Reports following field use indicate that in some cattle this vaccine may be a predisposing factor or possibly the primary cause of severe reactions. Such adverse reactions, which usually involve low morbidity and high mortality, may be the combination of stress and/or other infectious agents and of the vaccine. It is known that the BVD-MD virus has an immunosuppressive effect, and the combined factors may tip the balance with frank disease ensuing after vaccination. In consideration of these reactions, BVD-MD vaccine is recommended only where previous or anticipated disease problems are of sufficient magnitude to warrant the risk involved. It should be recognized that BVD-MD antibody of maternal origin may persist in a small percentage of calves at detectable levels up to 9 months of age.

It is now known that BVD-MD virus causes abortions and congenital anomalies, so the use of vaccine in pregnant cows is ill advised.

Control. The economic importance of this disease has been reasonably well established, particularly in feedlot operations. Because it causes abortions and congenital anomalies, there is little doubt of its economic significance in dairy cattle as well. Regular vaccination with the present vaccine is not advised despite the high incidence of infection in cattle populations unless it manifests itself as a serious disease malady in a given area or herd. There is a clear need for an improved vaccine that is safe and efficacious.

Great care should be exercised by individuals who go from one herd to another to avoid carrying the virus.

The Disease in Man. There is no evidence to suggest that man is infected with this virus.

REFERENCES

1. Baker, York, Gillespie, and Mitchell. Am. Jour. Vet. Res., 1954, *15*, 525.
2. Barrett and Chalmers. Jour. Wildlife Dis., 1975, *11*, 157.
3. Bovine Respiratory Disease Symposium. Panel Report., Jour. Am. Vet. Med. Assoc., 1971, *152*, 940.
4. Brar, Johnson, Muscoplat, Shope, and Meiske. Am. Jour. Vet. Res., 1978, *39*, 241.
5. Brown, Bistner, DeLahunta, Scott, and McEntee. Vet. Pathol., 1975, *12*, 394.
6. Carbrey, Stewart, Kresse, and Snyder. Jour. Am. Vet. Med. Assoc., 1976, *169*, 1217.
7. Carlson, Pritchard, and Doyle. Am. Jour. Vet. Res., 1957, *18*, 560.
8. Castrucci, Avellini, Cilli, Pedini, McKercher, and Valente. Cornell Vet., 1975, *65*, 65.
9. Coggins. Cornell Univ. thesis, 1962.
10. Coggins, Gillespie, Robson, Thompson, Wagner, and Baker. Cornell Vet., 1961, *51*, 540.
11. Coggins. Unpublished data.
12. DeLay and Knaizeff. Am. Jour. Vet. Res., 1966, *127*, 512.
13. Gillespie and Baker. Cornell Vet., 1959, *49*, 439.
14. Gillespie, Baker, and McEntee. Cornell Vet., 1960, *40*, 73.
15. Gillespie, Bartholomew, Thomson, and McEntee. Cornell Vet., 1967, *57*, 564.
16. Gillespie, Coggins, Thompson, and Baker. Cornell Vet., 1961, *51*, 155.
17. Gillespie, Madin, and Darby. Proc. Soc. Exp. Biol. and Med., 1962, *110*, 248.
18. Gillespie, Madin, and Darby. Cornell Vet., 1963, *53*, 276.
19. Goldsmit and Barzilai. Am. Jour. Vet. Res., 1975, *36*, 407.
20. Gratzek. Univ. of Wis. thesis, 1961.
21. Gutekunst and Malmquist. Can. Jour. Comp. Med., 1963, *28*, 19.
22. Haralambiev. Arch. Exp. Veterinaermed., 1975, *29*, 777.
23. Hermodsson and Dinter. Nature, 1962, *194*, 893.
24. Huck. Vet. Rec., 1957, *69*, 1207 and 1213.
25. Inaba, Omori, and Kumagai. Arch. f. die gesam. Virusforsch., 1963, *13*, 245.

26. Kahrs, Atkinson, Baker, Carmichael, Coggins, Gillespie, Langer, Marshall, Robson, and Sheffy. Cornell Vet., 1964, *54,* 360.
27. Kahrs, Robson, and Baker. Proc. 70th Ann. Meet. U.S. Livestock Sanit. Assoc., 1967, 145.
28. Kahrs, Scott, and de Lahunta. Jour. Am. Vet. Med. Assoc., 1970, *156,* 1443.
29. Knaizeff. Quoted by Pritchard in Advances in veterinary science, ed. C. A. Brandly and E. L. Jungherr. Academic Press, New York, 1963, p. 8.
30. Knaizeff and Walker. Quoted by Pritchard in Advances in veterinary science, ed. C. A. Brandly and E. L. Jungherr. Academic Press, New York, 1963, p. 8.
31. Knaizeff, Huck, Jarret, Pritchard, Ramsey, Schipper, Stoeber, and Liess. Vet. Rec., 1961, *73,* 768.
32. Knaizeff, Wopschall, Hopps, and Morris. In Vitro, 1975, *11,* 400.
33. Lee and Gillespie. Am. Jour. Vet. Res., 1957, *18,* 952.
34. Maess and Reczko. Arch. f. die gesam. Virusforsch., 1970, *30,* 39.
35. Malmquist. Jour. Am. Vet. Med. Assoc., 1968, *152,* 763.
36. Newberne, Robinson, and Alter. Vet. Med., 1961, *56,* 395.
37. Noice and Schipper. Proc. Soc. Exp. Biol. and Med., 1959, *100,* 84.
38. Olafson, MacCallum, and Fox. Cornell Vet., 1946, *36,* 205.
39. Olafson and Rickard. Cornell Vet., 1947, *37,* 104.
40. Phillips, Heuschele, and Todd. Am. Jour. Vet. Res., 1975, *36,* 135.
41. Plant, Littlejohn, Gardiner, Vantsis, and Huck. Vet. Rec., 1973, *92,* 455.
42. Pritchard. Adv. Vet. Sci., 1963, *8,* 2.
43. Pritchard, Taylor, Moses, and Doyle. Ann. Rpt. Dept. Vet. Sci., Indiana Agr. Exp. Sta., 1954, p. 724.
44. Pritchard, Taylor, Moses, and Doyle. Jour. Am. Vet. Med. Assoc., 1956, *128,* 1.
45. Ramsey and Chivers. North Am. Vet., 1953, *34,* 629.
46. Richards, Schipper, Eveleth, and Shumard. Vet. Med., 1956, *51,* 538.
47. Richie and Fernelius. Arch. f. die gesam. Virusforsch., 1969, *28,* 369.
48. Rinaldo, Isackson, Overall, Glasgow, Brown, Bistner, Gillespie, and Scott. Inf. and Immun., 1976, *14,* 660.
49. Robson, Gillespie, and Baker. Cornell Vet., 1960, *50,* 503.
50. Rossi and Kiesel. Am. Jour. Vet. Res., 1977, *38,* 1705.
51. Scott, Kahrs, de Lahunta, Brown, McEntee, and Gillespie. Cornell Vet., 1973, *63,* 536.
52. Scott, Kahrs, and Parsonson. Jour. Am. Vet. Med. Assoc., 1970, *156,* 867.
53. Soto-Belloso, Archbald, and Zemjanis. Am. Jour. Vet. Res., 1976, *37,* 1103.
54. Stewart, Carbrey, Jenny, Brown, and Kresse. Program, 108th Ann. Mtg., Am. Vet. Med. Assoc., 1971, 163.
55. Taylor, Okeke, and Shidali. Trop. An. Health Prod., 1977, *9,* 171.
56. Taylor, Okeke, and Shidali. Trop. An. Health Prod., 1977, *9,* 249.
57. Trapp. Iowa State Univ. thesis, 1960.
58. Underdahl, Grace, and Hoerlein. Proc. Soc. Exp. Biol. and Med., 1957, *94,* 795.
59. Walker and Olafson. Cornell Vet., 1947, *37,* 107.
60. Ward. Cornell Vet., 1971, *61,* 179.
61. Ward, Roberts, McEntee, and Gillespie. Cornell Vet., 1969, *59,* 525.
62. Whiteman. Iowa State Univ. thesis, 1960.
63. Whitmore and Archbald. Am. Jour. Vet. Res., 1977, *38,* 455.
64. York, Rosner, and McLean. Proc. U.S. Livestock Sanit. Assoc., 1960, *64,* 339.
65. Zwetkow. Arch. Exp. Vet., 1975, *29,* 761.

Border Disease of Lambs

Border disease, also known as "hairy shaker" disease, is a neonatal condition of lambs characterized by excessive hairiness of the birth coat, poor growth, and nervous abnormalities. The disease occurs in Australia, the United States, New Zealand, the British Isles, and a number of other countries. The incidence is low.

The disease in lambs often occurs in flocks with abortions that may take place during any stage of gestation. An acute focal necrotizing placentitis develops about 10 days after maternal infection (2).

The disease can be transmitted experimentally with crude suspensions of brain, spinal cord, and spleen from affected lambs by the intraperitoneal or subcutaneous inoculation of pregnant ewes sometime between the 7th and 85th day of gestation (3). Susceptible sheep in contact with hairy lambs become infected with a mucosal disease virus. Experimentally infected ewes develop antibodies and are immune to subsequent challenges during pregnancy.

All present evidence would suggest that border disease is caused by a mucosal disease virus (1) that shares many of the characteristics of BVD-MD and HC viruses. Sheep that recover from natural or experimental border disease contain precipitating and neutralizing antibodies to the other two viruses. Pregnant cattle inoculated early in gestation with tissues from affected lambs with border disease frequently abort and develop antibodies to BVD-MD virus. The border disease virus replicates in cell culture and is regarded as similar, if not identical, to BVD-MD virus (4). All of these facts point to a close antigenic relationship between border disease virus, BVD-MD, and HCV.

REFERENCES

1. Acland, Gard, and Plant. Austral. Vet. Jour., 1972, *48,* 70.
2. Barlow and Gardiner. Jour. Comp. Path., 1969, *79,* 397.

3. Gard, Acland, and Plant. Austral. Vet. Jour., 1976, *52*, 64.
4. Harkness, King, Terlecki, and Sands. Vet. Rec., 1977, *100*, 71.

THE GENUS *RUBIVIRUS*

Equine Arteritis

SYNONYMS: Epizootic cellulitis-pinkeye syndrome, *rotlaufseuche;* abbreviation, EA

It may be the same disease that was described by German scientists as *rotlaufseuche* and by English writers as epizootic cellulitis-pinkeye syndrome or typhoid fever. In 1953 the virus was isolated from outbreaks in Ohio (USA) that were characterized by illness in horses and abortions in the mares (4). Since then virus has been isolated from three other epizootics in the United States by these same investigators. The first isolation of EA virus in Europe was made in Switzerland (3) and later in Vienna, Austria (3). There is serological evidence for the disease in India (3).

In the past this disease has been confused with equine influenza and equine rhinopneumonitis. The horse is the only susceptible animal, and the principal natural infections have been observed only on breeding farms (2).

Character of the Disease. The horses develop a fever, stiffness of gait, edema of the limbs, and swelling around the eyes. The disease spreads rapidly to susceptible horses on the premises. Pregnant mares abort, and this was the essential feature of the disease in the four natural outbreaks. Stallions may also contract the disease. It usually occurs on breeding farms, and no fatalities are observed, nor does it cause residual damage.

The Disease in Experimental Horses. Inoculation of the virus into pregnant mares or young horses causes death in almost 50 percent of the animals (4). Abortions were produced in the mares. These experimental effects suggest that this virus conceivably could cause mortality under unfavorable circumstances.

The incubation period is 3 to 5 days (4). Fever is a constant sign, and the other signs were dependent on the site and amount of damage to the arteries. Other signs in fatal cases included pronounced conjunctivitis, palpebral edema and edema of the nictitating membrane, and excessive lacrimation. The nasal membrane became congested, and a serous nasal discharge was noted. Pulmonary dyspnea was frequent, and there was marked depression and muscular weakness. Mild or severe colic may be accompanied by watery diarrhea. There was edema of the limbs. On occasions keratitis, hypopyon, icterus, edema of the abdomen, and marked loss of weight were observed. Panleukopenia characterized by lymphopenia occurs in affected horses.

The basic lesions involve small arteries about 0.5 mm in diameter, and these arteries are the smallest vessels that possess well-developed muscular coats (6). The arterioles (less than 0.3 mm in diameter) and the large muscular and elastic arteries are free of specific lesions. Veins and lymphatics are often distended with blood or lymph, respectively, but were neither inflamed nor necrotic. The specific lesions in small arteries are distributed at random in segments of the arterial system throughout the body. Arterial lesions were found in every organ, but more conspicuously in the cecum, colon, spleen, lymph nodes, and adrenal capsule.

The specific microscopic lesion starts with necrosis of muscle cells in the arterial media (6). Edema and a few leukocytes then appear in the adventitia. The arterial media becomes edematous and infiltrated by lymphocytes, some with karyorrhectic or pyknotic nuclei. Initially, these changes may be limited to one microscopic segment of the artery viewed in cross section. As the lesion progresses, most of the arterial media is involved and replaced by edema and leukocytes. At this stage the artery is tortuous, and the intact endothelium becomes surrounded by leukocytes and edema which replaces the media and adventitia. The lumen usually is empty and contains a few erythrocytes. In the large intestine and spleen, frank thrombosis and infarction occur. Consequently, the effect of these arterial changes is most often edema and hemorrhage. The mechanism of death is not definitely known, but the probable changes in electrolytes in cells and tissue fluids might be important (6).

The gross lesions are explained entirely on the basis of distribution of the lesions in small arteries (6). Edema and petechiae are conspicuous in adult animals and fetuses. Fetuses are particularly edematous, but no distinct microscopic lesion is found in the arteries. Edema is found in the subcutis of the legs and abdomen, adjacent to the injection site, and in the adjacent fascia. Edema and petechiae are also found in the omental, mesenteric, and perirenal fat, subpleural and interlobular septums of the lungs, in the intraabdominal lymph nodes, the broad ligament, and the adrenal cortex. Similar hemorrhages and edema are evident along the course of the ileocecocolic and anterior mesenteric arteries. The intestines, especially the cecum and colon, are severely involved with sharply demarcated segments, 1 to 2 meters long. The entire wall is edematous and the mucosa markedly hemorrhagic. These lesions are related to typical changes in submucosal arteries with thrombosis in most vessels. Sharply demarcated, often elevated hemorrhagic infarcts are seen in the spleen, particularly in younger horses.

Properties of the Virus. The incorporation of 5-iodo-2-deoxyuridine in tissue cultures does not inhibit the replication of virus, presenting indirect evidence that EAV is an RNA virus (3). The virus is readily inactivated by lipid solvents and by sodium deoxycholate. It survives 20, but not 30, minutes at 56 C (10). The virus is quite stable at low temperatures. It is resistant to trypsin. In sucrose gradients its density is 1.18 to 1.20 g per cm^3(7).

By Millipore filtration the particle size is estimated from 50 to 100 nm (3). Virus was concentrated and purified by ultracentrifugation and again by zonal centrifugation in sucrose gradients (7). This preparation was treated with uranyl acetate and phosphotungstic acid. The negatively stained particles observed in the electron microscope were spherical and had an average diameter of 60 $\pm$ 13 nm. The inner core of the virion had an average diameter of 35 $\pm$ 9 nm. In the cytoplasm of infected tissue-cultured cells virus particles located in the cytoplasmic vacuoles are 43 $\pm$ 2 nm, with a core diameter of 35 $\pm$ 2 nm (1). These particles are observed at 18 hours postinoculation but not at 12 hours. The viral particles are found in increasing concentration and in increasing numbers of cells at 24, 30, 34, and 43 hours postinfection.

The virion apparently lacks a hemagglutinin, but does contain a complement-fixing antigen component. Only one immunogenic type of virus is known to exist, and it produces neutralizing antibodies. The prototype virus is the Bucyrus strain (4).

Cultivation. Attempts to propagate EAV in the hen's embryonated egg and in laboratory animals have failed (4). It produces a cytopathogenic effect in cultures of horse kidney cells and becomes attenuated so it can be used for immunization (10). It also grows in hamster kidney cells (12) and in rabbit kidney cells (9). This virus produces plaques in overlay cultures. Thus far, only cells of equine origin show a cytopathic effect (CPE) upon inoculation with material from infected horses. Adapted strains replicate in tissue cultures from other species. In cell culture the Bucyrus strain usually yields 10^6 $TCID_{50}$ per ml. Enhancement of equine arteritis viral replication in RK-13 cells was achieved by pretreatment of cells with 6-azauridine (11). Sonified tissue-cultured preparations are used as a good source of CF antigen (3).

Immunity. Horses that recover from infection or immunization with a modified live virus have a solid immunity. Vaccinated horses are immune for at least 1 year to virulent virus challenge and presumably for many years (8). Antibodies against EAV can be demonstrated by the CF and neutralization tests.

The Bucyrus strain was modified by transferring it 131 times in primary cell cultures of horse kidney followed by 111 transfers in primary cell cultures in rabbit kidney. As little as 200 $TCID_{50}$ of virus by the intramuscular route protected horses against challenge with virulent virus. Vaccine administered by the intranasal route failed to immunize horses effectively. The virus protected pregnant mares without causing any ill effects on their fetuses. Newborn foals from two vaccinated mares were not protected by colostrum when they were challenged at 5 and 9 days of age. These studies should be expanded to include greater numbers and also serology correlated with challenge before any definite conclusion on maternal immunity can be ascertained.

Serial passage of the vaccine virus did not restore its virulence. The vaccine virus did not spread to susceptible horses maintained in direct contact with the vaccinated horses.

Transmission. The virus is spread by aerosol and contracted by inhalation (2). The virus is in the nasal secretions for 8 to 10 days. The tissues and fluids of infected aborted fetuses contain virus.

Diagnosis. Arteritis occurs sporadically, and in the typical outbreak mortality does not occur, but abortions occur in 50 to 60 percent of pregnant mares. The aborted fetuses often are autolyzed in contrast to the fresh aborted fetuses usually associated with rhinopneumonitis virus infection.

For diagnosis by virus isolation samples may be taken from the nostrils, blood, or conjunctival sac. The nasal or conjunctival exudate is placed in Hanks' balanced salt solution with antibiotics and 1 percent bovine albumin. These specimens can be stored at −20 C for weeks. At necropsy, many different organ tissues can be used for virus isolation. Virus isolation attempts are made in primary cell cultures of horse origin or by horse inoculation. The demonstration of a rising antibody titer by the use of the complement-fixation test or neutralization test is another suitable means for making a diagnosis.

Control. According to the Panel of the American Veterinary Medical Association Symposium on Immunity to Selected Equine Diseases (5) the disease may be prevented and controlled by good management practices and vaccination. It was their recommendation that the attenuated HK-131 RK-111 Bucyrus virus vaccine be licensed when justified by supplementary data received by the Veterinary Biologics Division, U.S. Department of Agriculture, from potential commercial producers (5). The panel also recommended continued research of an inactivated virus vaccine.

The Disease in Man. It is not known to occur.

REFERENCES

1. Breese and McCollum. Proc. 2nd Internatl. Conf. Equine Inf. Dis., ed. J. T. Bryans and H. Gerber. S. Karger, Basel, 1969, p. 133.
2. Bryans. Proc. Am. Vet. Med. Assoc., 1964, p. 112.
3. Bürki. Proc. 2nd Internatl. Conf. Equine Inf. Dis., ed. J. T. Bryans and H. Gerber., S. Karger, Basel, 1969, p. 125.
4. Doll, Bryans, McCollum, and Crowe. Cornell Vet., 1957, *47,* 3.
5. Equine Disease Symposium. Panel Report. Jour. Am. Vet. Med. Assoc., 1969, *155,* 237.
6. Jones, Doll, and Bryans. Cornell Vet., 1957, *47,* 3.
7. Maess, Reczko, and Böhm. Proc. 2nd Internatl. Conf. Equine Inf. Dis., ed. J. T. Bryans and H. Gerber. S. Karger, Basel, 1969, p. 130.
8. McCollum. Jour. Am. Vet. Med. Assoc., 1969, *155,* 318.
9. McCollum, Doll, Wilson, and Cheatham. Cornell Vet., 1962, *52,* 454.
10. McCollum, Doll, Wilson, and Johnson. Am. Jour. Vet. Res., 1961, *22,* 731.
11. Tozzini. Boll. Inst. Sieroter Milan, 1976, *55,* 279.
12. Wilson, Doll, McCollum, and Cheatham. Cornell Vet., 1962, *52,* 200.

THE GENUS *ALPHAVIRUS*

The type species for the genus is *Alphavirus sindbis.* Some members in the group are as follows: Aura virus, Chikungunya virus, eastern equine encephalomyelitis virus, Getah virus, Mayaro virus, Middleburgh virus, Mucambo virus, Ndumu virus, O'Nyong-nyong virus, Pixuna virus, Ross River virus, Semliki forest virus, Una virus, Venezuelan equine encephalomyelitis virus, western equine encephalomyelitis virus, Whataroa virus.

These viruses contain 4 to 6 percent of single-stranded RNA with a molecular weight of approximately 3 x 10^6 daltons. They are spherical enveloped particles, with a diameter between 25 to 70 nm. They contain lipid and are sensitive to ether. The buoyant density in cesium chloride is 1.25 g per cm^3. Trypsin does not destroy the infectivity of the particle. Hemagglutination is not inhibited by phospholipids. The hemagglutination reaction occurs over a rather narrower range of temperature and pH than with flaviviruses. Alphaviruses are less inhibited by bile salts than flaviviruses. The virion replicates in the cytoplasm, and maturation occurs by budding. All members of the genus *Alphavirus* show cross-reactions in the hemagglutination-inhibition test but not with members of the genus *Flavivirus.* All members replicate in arthropod vectors including the mosquito.

Three viruses in this genus are pertinent to a discussion of infectious diseases of domestic animals—eastern equine encephalomyelitis (EEE), western equine encephalomyelitis (WEE), and Venezuelan equine encephalomyelitis (VEE).

Western and Eastern Equine Encephalomyelitis

It appears certain that an enzootic encephalomyelitis of horses of virus origin has occurred in the United States for many years. In the late summer and early fall of 1912 large numbers of horses were lost in Kansas, Nebraska, Colorado, Oklahoma, and Missouri from what was most certainly virus encephalitis, although it was not recognized as such at the time. The outbreak and the characteristic lesions were described by Udall (54). It is estimated that 35,000 horses died of the disease from midsummer until heavy frosts in October put an end to the outbreak. In later years small outbreaks of the malady have appeared in many of the western states.

In July 1930 the disease appeared among horses in the San Joaquin Valley in California. The outbreak continued through August, reached its peak in September, and disappeared with the advent of cool weather in November. It was studied by Meyer, Haring, and Howitt (43), who estimated that 3,000 horses and mules perished from this disease, this number being about one-half the total of recognized cases. These workers isolated and studied the virus of the disease. The following year the disease recurred in the same area and appeared for the first time in several of the neighboring states. The disease reappeared each successive summer, spreading over a larger and larger area. In 1937 the disease was recognized in every state west of the Mississippi River and in several east of it. The peak in the disease incidence occurred in 1938, when 184,000 horses were estimated by the United States Bureau of Animal Industry to have died from it. By this time every state west of the Appalachian Mountains had cases.

In 1933 an isolated focus of the disease appeared along the coastal plains of Delaware, Maryland, Virginia, and southern New Jersey, and at least 1,000 horses died of the disease in that year. The signs of illness of affected animals were much like those exhibited by horses in the western parts of the country, but the mortality rate was much higher, approximating 90 percent. It was generally believed at first that the disease was identical to that which prevailed in the country west of the Appalachian Mountains, but Ten Broeck and Merrill (53) pointed out that the virus was immunologically different, because animals immunized to the virus of the eastern disease were not protected against the virus of the western disease, and vice versa. These results were quickly confirmed by others, and it was generally accepted that there were two types of the disease in the country differentiated by the names *western type* and *eastern type*. Both types produce encephalomyelitis in horses; the signs of illness and pathological changes are practically identical. The principal differences are that the eastern type is much more virulent for horses, most experimental animals, and man, and that there is little or no cross immunity between the two types.

In 1941 Randall and Eichhorn (47) recognized a small outbreak in the vicinity of Brownville, Texas, as caused by eastern-type virus. More recently the eastern-type virus has been found in Michigan, Wisconsin, Missouri, and other midwestern states. Large and severe outbreaks have occurred in Louisiana.

The virus of equine encephalomyelitis, western type, has caused outbreaks in horses and man in all states of the United States west of the Appalachian Mountains, and outbreaks have also been recognized in western Canada. The western-type virus was not recognized on the eastern seaboard until 1954, when it was isolated from sparrows in New Jersey by Holden (20) and later in Florida chukars. Late in 1955 the North Carolina State Board of Health reported finding virus of this type in a number of mosquitoes trapped in that state. WEE is a rare disease in horses or man along the eastern seaboard.

The U.S. Department of Agriculture has collected statistics on the yearly occurrence of equine encephalomyelitis. It is recognized that these figures are not complete; nevertheless they give an indication of the importance of this disease in the United States. The latest figures are given in Table 48.3 and a map provides information about its distribution in 1976 (Figure 48.6).

Table 48.3. Reported annual cases for equine encephalomyelitis in U.S. horses for the period 1971–1979

Year	WEE	EEE	VEE
1971	4	76	139
1972	446	31	–
1973	119	196	–
1974	312	27	–
1975	703	59	–
1976	38	7	–
1977	617	4	–
1978	17	4	–
1979	71	8	–

Courtesy R. P. Jones, Animal and Plant Health Inspection Service, USDA.

An encephalomyelitis of horses occurs in Brazil. According to Carneiro and Cunha (6), the virus is closely related, if not identical, to the eastern type of North America. Livesay (35) and Mace, Ott, and Cortez, (37) have reported the eastern-type virus in native Philippine monkeys (*Macacus philippensis*) suffering from a disease which resembled poliomyelitis. This disease has not been recognized in Philippine horses, but Mace and coworkers found neutralizing antibodies for eastern-type virus in 26 of a series of 86 horses.

Equine encephalomyelitis occurs in Argentina. According to Meyer, Wood, Haring, and Howitt (44), the Argentina virus is very closely related, or perhaps identical, to the western-type virus of North America.

Character of the Disease. In the United States and Canada this disease is distinctly seasonal. In all but the most southerly parts of the United States it occurs from June to November; in the warmer states sporadic cases may be seen during the winter months. As a rule, the disease is sporadic during the early summer, assumes epizootic proportions during August and September, and diminishes in intensity afterward. In most of the country all outbreaks cease by the middle of November, because the mosquito population has been killed by frosts.

Horses of all ages may succumb to the disease, but younger animals appear somewhat more susceptible than older ones. It is unusual for more than 20 percent of the horses on any one place to become affected, and considerable periods often elapse between cases on the same farm.

The incubation period is from 1 to 3 weeks. In this respect the American forms of encephalomyelitis differ markedly from the German Borna disease, in which it is from 4 to 7 weeks or more.

It is known from observations on experimental animals that a febrile reaction is the first manifestation of

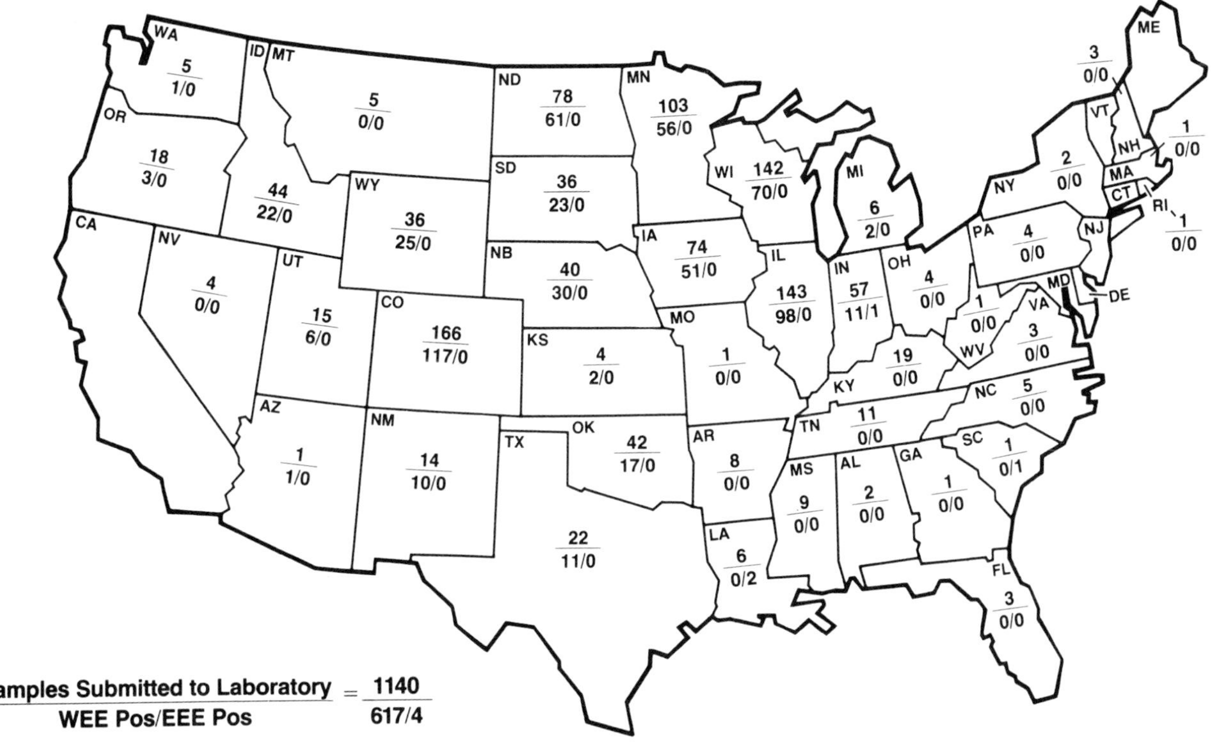

Figure 48.6. Equine encephalitis serology (calendar year 1977). (Courtesy R. P. Jones, Animal and Plant Health Inspection Service, USDA.)

the infection. The depression that occurs at this time may be so mild as to be unnoticed. At this stage there is a viremia—an opportunity for bloodsucking insects to obtain virus. Invasion of the nervous system does not occur in all animals. If it does not occur, the animal is not observed to be ill, but will possess neutralizing antibodies in its blood serum for some time thereafter. When involvement of the nervous system occurs, the signs are, in general, those of deranged consciousness. The fever has disappeared by this time, and the blood is no longer infective. In the early stages of neural involvement, the victim may show signs of restlessness and mild excitement. The animal may walk in circles or crash through fences or walk aimlessly into obstacles of any kind. It may shy at low doorsills and jump high in clearing them. It refuses food and water. Later a sleepy attitude develops, and it stands with head depressed, resting it on the manger or on a fence (Figure 48.7). It can be aroused, but it quickly relapses into the sleepy posture when not prodded into activity. It may sit on its hind quarters, or stand with its front legs crossed, or assume other unusual and unnatural postures. Finally, evidence of paralysis of portions of the body may become evident: its lower lip often becomes pendulous, its tongue may be protruded, or it has difficulty in walking because of lack and full control of its hind legs. Finally, the paralysis may become general: it lies on the ground and is unable to rise. Death usually occurs within a day or two after the nervous signs begin. The horses that recover frequently show permanent cerebral damage, manifested by loss of ability to react to normal stimuli. Such animals are often called *dummies* by horsemen.

The course of the disease varies widely. In some cases animals die within a few hours from the time that the first signs are noted. At the height of outbreaks most deaths occur within 2 to 4 days. Animals that survive the effects of the virus may develop terminal pneumonia and die from this after a week or more. Others may recover completely, or show various paralytic effects for many weeks, or permanently.

The eastern-type virus is considerably more virulent for horses than the western type. In the former the death rate generally exceeds 90 percent; in the latter it may be as high as 50 percent, but averages from 20 to 30 percent.

There are no characteristic gross lesions in animals dying of this disease. Hurst (24), who studied the histology of the lesions in the central nervous system, says that the gray matter is affected to a greater extent than the white and that the lesions are most marked in the cerebral

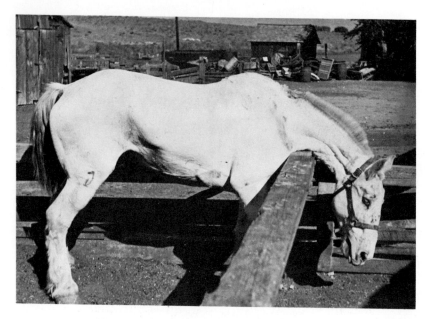

Figure 48.7. Equine encephalomyelitis. (Courtesy Edward Records.)

cortex, thalamus, and hypothalamic regions, with the brain stem and spinal cord as a rule being less involved. The lesions consist of degeneration of the nerve cells, perivascular cuffing with mononuclear and polymorphonuclear cells in varying proportion, polymorphonuclear leukocyte infiltrations into the gray matter, and proliferation of glial cells (Figure 48.8). The lesions produced by the western-type virus are, as a rule, less intense than those caused by the eastern type.

The Disease in Experimental Animals. Meyer, Haring, and Howitt (43) found that guinea pigs were highly susceptible to intracerebral inoculation with virus of equine

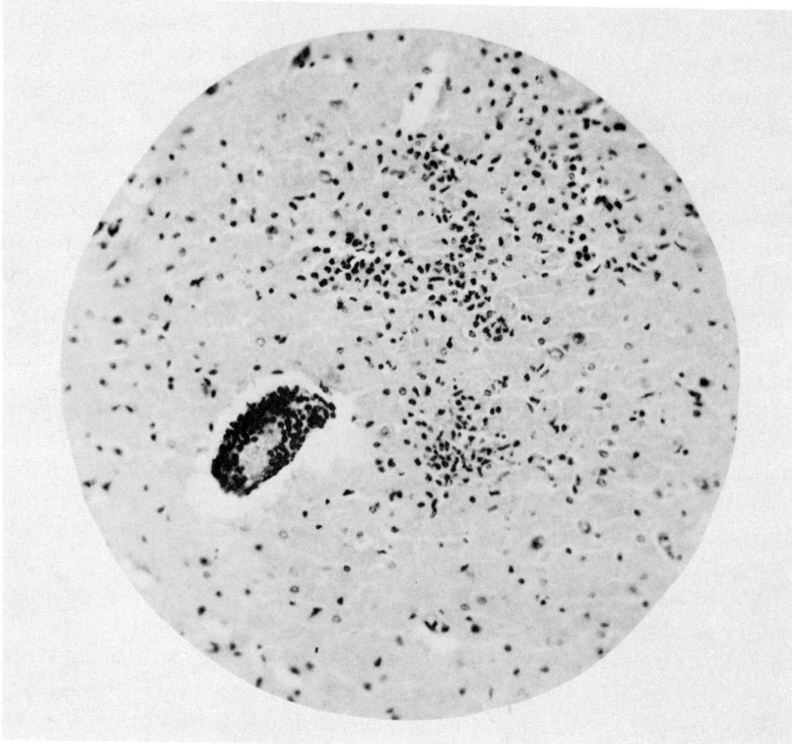

Figure 48.8. Equine encephalomyelitis, showing brain of a guinea pig inoculated with the western-type virus. There are cellular infiltrations of both gray and white matter and perivascular cuffing. × 180. (Courtesy S. H. McNutt.)

origin, and these animals were the most suitable for diagnostic work. Death occurs in 4 to 6 days, as a rule, and is preceded by an early febrile reaction followed by muscular tremors, flabbiness of the abdominal muscles, salivation, and trotting movements after the animal becomes prostrate. Rabbits are much less susceptible. A febrile reaction occurs and virus exists in the blood, but signs are very mild or absent, and recovery generally occurs. White mice are very susceptible. They may be infected by intracerebral inoculation and also through the undamaged nasal mucosa. According to Mediaris and Kebrick (39), suckling mice are even more susceptible to this virus than hens' eggs and constitute the most sensitive means of detecting virus. Calves can be infected by intracerebral inoculation. These animals display marked nervous signs beginning about the 5th day. By the 14th day recovery usually is complete, according to Giltner and Shahan (13). These authors found that sheep, dogs, and cats were refractory to inoculation. The common ground squirrel of the western states (*Citellus richardsoni*) may readily be infected by intracranial inoculation.

Karstad and Hanson (27) showed that swine were highly susceptible to infection with the virus of eastern encephalomyelitis, either naturally or by inoculation. No signs were exhibited by the infected animals, but high antibody titers were quickly developed. Inasmuch as they were unable to demonstrate a viremia in swine, it was concluded that this species probably has little or nothing to do with the natural propagation of this virus.

The eastern-type virus generally produces fatal infections when inoculated into pheasants, quail, pigeons, blackbirds, cardinals, cedar waxwings, sparrows, juncos, thrushes, young chicks, ducklings, chukar partridges, and young turkey poults. Adult domesticated fowl, turkeys, and some wild birds are resistant to inoculation. Ordinarily these birds do not show recognizable signs, but high-titer viremias generally develop for a day or two, and these are followed by high antibody titers.

The subcutaneous inoculation of Texas tortoises (*Gopherus berlandieri*) with WEE virus results in a prolonged viremia of up to 105 days duration (4). The nature of the viremia is markedly affected by environmental temperature.

Properties of the Virus. Member viruses are isometric and enveloped ranging from 50 to 70 nm (Figures 48.9 and 48.10). The capsids have icosahedral symmetry. Alphaviruses replicate in vertebrate and arthropod hosts. Its RNA central core is infectious. Its specific gravity is 1.13, and the particle is inactivated in 10 minutes at 60 C. The virus withstands freezing and thawing and is readily maintained at low temperatures. Ether and desoxycholate inactivate the agent. The virus disappears rapidly in tissues after death probably because of the acidity. The virus is readily destroyed by formalin but not phenol. A hemagglutinin has been demonstrated, and a hemolysin also exists. By the use of CF tests and with neutralization tests in mice by intracerebral inoculation and with plaque inhibition in tissue culture the virus is distinct from other arboviruses. In hemagglutination-inhibition tests some common antigenic components are

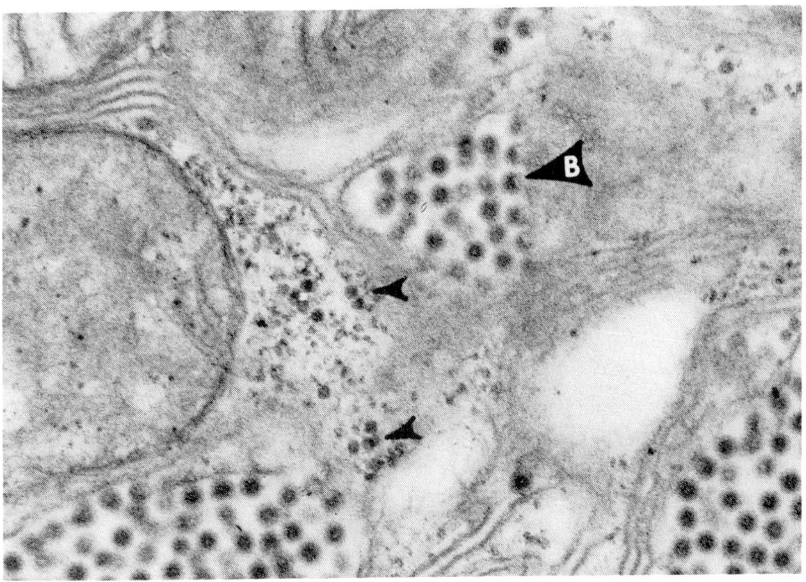

Figure 48.9. Eastern equine encephalitis virus in a mosquito salivary gland. Nucleocapsids (*B*) differentiated from ribosomes (*arrows*) in the cytoplasmic matrix. Distension of reticulum appeared to be consequence of accumulation of enveloped virus. Budding. × 74,300. (Courtesy S. G. Whitfield, F. A. Murphy, and W. D. Sudia, Center for Disease Control.)

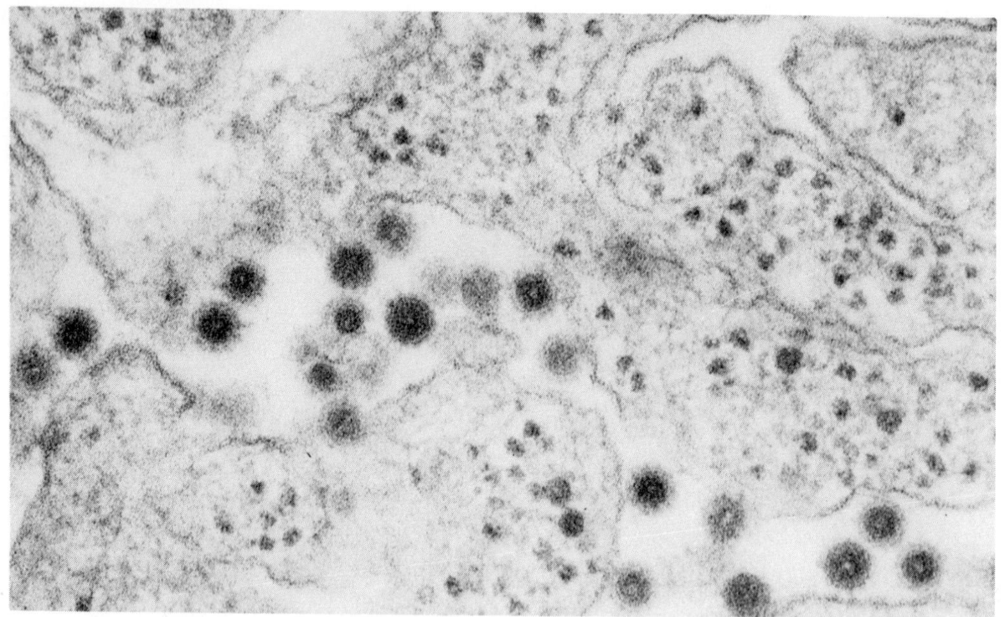

Figure 48.10. Higher magnification of eastern equine encephalitis virus–infected mouse brain cell. Nucleocapsids, clearly distinguishable from ribosomes. Typical extracellular enveloped EEE virus particles with dense center and enveloped surface with projections. × 90,000. (Courtesy F. A. Murphy and S. G. Whitfield, Center for Disease Control.)

demonstrated with other alphaviruses. Some slight antigenic variations are demonstrated between strains of EEE virus coming from different areas. Interference, probably through the production of interferon, occurs between this virus and certain other arboviruses, myxoviruses, and picornaviruses.

Western equine encephalomyelitis (WEE) virus is essentially the same size as EEE and shares most of its physical-chemical characteristics. It has been estimated that 100 infectious particles are released from an infected cell, but only a few at a time. It is more closely related to Sindbis virus than other alphaviruses as determined with the plaque inhibition test. In addition, this has been established by the use of the hemagglutination-inhibition test, which also shows some crossing with other alphaviruses. This virus also produces interferon in appreciable amounts so that it is commonly used to study this nonspecific protein substance produced in tissue culture by many viruses.

Cultivation. In 1935 Higbie and Howitt (19) reported successful cultivation of both eastern and western types of equine encephalomyelitis virus in chick embryos. Minute amounts of brain virus placed on the chorioallantoic membrane resulted in deaths of the embryos in from 15 to 24 hours, the embryonic tissues being saturated with virus of a very high titer. The sensitivity of chick embryos to the virus of this disease is very great; less than 0.1 MLD for the guinea pig is frequently sufficient to infect. Both viruses produce a cytopathogenic effect in hamster kidney cell cultures (29). They also grow in cell cultures from many species. Plaques are produced on monolayers of chick embryo cells. A color test in tissue culture depending on a change of pH has been used as means of titration of WEE virus.

A method for the germ-free cultivation of the mosquitos *Aedes aegypti* and *Aedes trisbriatus* was developed so primary tissue cell cultures could be prepared from minced larvae of both insect species (26). The Louisiana strain of EEE grew in larval tissue cultures of both mosquitoes. There was some evidence of a virus-inactivating substance in the cultures of both mosquito species.

Immunity. The immunity to WEE and EEE persists for years after natural infection and after vaccination with attenuated virus vaccines. Foals of dams that have had an exposure to WEE are temporarily protected by colostral antibody. There is a suggestion that an active immunity is produced by inactivated virus despite the presence of colostral antibodies in the foal.

Inactivated virus vaccine currently is licensed in the USA for use in horses against WEE and EEE using infected tissue-cultured cell culture fluids (15). Formerly, other vaccines using inactivated virus or attenuated virus were recommended for use in horses. The inactivated chick embryo vaccine virus was quite effective, but complications sometimes arose when it was given via subcutaneous rather than intradermal route. The malady characterized by icterus, constipation, nervous signs, and often death usually occurred 30 days after vaccination (30).

The immunity induced by inactivated virus vaccine is excellent and persists during an epizootic season. Annual vaccination usually is practiced in those areas where the disease is expected. Foals vaccinated during the first 8 months of life should be vaccinated again at 1 year of age.

Vaccines prepared from the envelope component of WEE and EEE viruses stimulated the production of humoral antibodies in mice with varying degrees of homologous protection upon challenge (46).

At one time an encephalomyelitis antiserum was available, but apparently its manufacture has been discontinued by American biological supply companies. Large doses of such sera will protect horses for a short time against homologous viruses. After nervous signs have appeared, antisera have little or no value.

Transmission. Vawter and Records (55) showed in 1933 that horses could be readily infected by intranasal instillation of virus, and transmission in this way probably occurs at times. The epizootiology of the disease indicates, however, that this is not the usual way. Transmission by bloodsucking insects, particularly by mosquitoes, had previously been suspected, but Kelser (28) was the first to show, in 1933, that mosquitoes could be infected and could convey the disease from animal to animal. In his work he used yellow-fever mosquitoes (*Aedes aegypti*), which, 6 to 8 days after they had been allowed to feed on infected guinea pigs, were capable of infecting other guinea pigs and a horse. Merrill, Lacaillade, and Ten Broeck (40) in the following year showed that the ordinary salt marsh mosquito (*Aedes sollicitans*) was capable of transmitting both the eastern and western types of virus. Another salt marsh mosquito (*Aedes cantator*) proved capable of transmitting the eastern-type virus but not the western. *Anopheles quadrimaculatus* and *Culex pipiens* were incapable of transmitting either type. Madsen and Knowlton (38) in 1935 showed that local species of *Aedes* mosquitoes in Utah, *Aedes dorsalis* and *A. nigromaculis*, were capable of transmitting the western-type virus. Others have shown that *Aedes albopictus*, *A. taenioryнchus*, and *A. vexans* were able to transmit the western-type virus. Merrill and TenBroeck (41) proved that the virus multiplies in the affected *A. aegypti*.

It was in the summer of 1941 that naturally infected

wild mosquitoes were detected. In that year Hammon, Reeves, Brookman, Izumi, and Gjullin (18) demonstrated the western-type virus in one lot of mosquitoes (*Culex tarsalis*) caught in the Yakima Valley in Washington during the course of an outbreak of the disease in horses. This species is widely distributed in the states west of the Mississippi River. It is known to feed upon man, horses, mules, cattle, and various birds. A number of other species of mosquitoes have been found naturally infected with the western-type virus. Hammon, Reeves, Benner, and Brookman (17) found *Culiseta inornata* and *Culex pipiens*, besides *Culex tarsalis*, infected in the Yakima Valley, but *C. pipiens* proved incapable of transmitting the virus. The first isolation of eastern-type virus from naturally infected mosquitoes was reported by Howitt, Dodge, Bishop, and Gorrie (23) in 1949. The species was *Mansonia perturbans*, and the mosquitoes were captured in Georgia. During the previous year the same workers (22) reported the finding of naturally infected chicken mites (*Dermanyssus gallinae*) and chicken lice (*Menapon pallidum* and *Eomenacanthus stramineus*) taken in Tennesee. The virus was the eastern type. Neutralizing antibodies for this virus were found in one cow and a few chickens in the locality where the strain originated.

Although equine encephalomyelitis can be transmitted by a considerable number of species of mosquitoes, it has become obvious that the western type is transmitted to both birds and mammals principally by *Culex tarsalis*, and the principal vector of the eastern type to birds but not to mammals is the fresh-water swamp mosquito, *Culiseta melanura*. It is not yet clear whether there is a principal transmitter of the eastern-type virus from the bird reservoir to horses and man, but it cannot be *C. melanura*, since this species attacks only swamp-inhabiting birds (7).

In 1940 Kitselman and Grundmann (31) demonstrated the western-type virus in a large bloodsucking insect known as the *assassin bug (Triatoma sanguisuga)* captured in a pasture in Kansas. Since this insect is common in many parts of the west and is known to feed upon horses, it is possible that it sometimes plays a part in the transmission of the virus.

In 1944 Smith, Blattner, and Heys (49) and in the following year Sulkin (51) reported the recovery of western-type virus from the chicken mite (*Dermanyssus gallinae*). Since chicken mites will feed upon horses stabled near chicken houses, they may be of some importance in conveying the disease. Furthermore, it is possible that this virus may be harbored from one season to the next in this mite, as has been found to be true of the virus of St. Louis encephalitis.

Syverton and Berry (52) showed in 1937 that the spotted fever tick, *Dermacentor andersoni,* could serve as a vector for the western type of equine encephalomyelitis virus. Adult and nymphal stages of this tick were allowed to feed on recently infected guinea pigs. At intervals varying from 32 to 80 days thereafter, successive stages in the developmental cycle of these ticks were allowed to feed on normal guinea pigs and ground squirrels. The disease was conveyed to these animals. Continuity of the virus through all stages, including the eggs, was demonstrated. At the time of the report virus had remained in these ticks for 130 days, a period sufficiently long to suggest that this might be one way by which the virus was preserved from one season to the next. The essential details of this work were confirmed by Gwatkin and Moore (16).

Through the work of many investigators it is clear that this disease is transmitted primarily by mosquitoes of various kinds. Transmission by direct contact and by other arthropods undoubtedly occurs, but this is of slight importance in the total picture. There is experimental proof that the disease may be transmitted from infected horses to others by mosquitoes, but many workers believe that the virus reservoir in horses is much less important than that in various wild and domesticated birds. The known presence of virus in hibernating *Culex tarsalis* in all months except December and the experimental overwintering of virus in garter snakes appears to be important in setting the stage for epidemics in horses and man. Moreover, the transmission of WEE to snakes by infected *Culex tarsalis* takes place quite readily (12).

Diagnosis. Although the clinical signs are characteristic, they are not always diagnostic, especially in isolated cases. Several cases thought to be equine encephalomyelitis have turned out to be dumb rabies.

For a specific diagnosis, the virus must be isolated. This is best done by intracerebral injection of animals, preferably guinea pigs, or of embryonated eggs. Fresh brain material should be used for this purpose. The virus is not always isolated, even when other indications make it clear that virus encephalitis is present, for virus often disappears from the tissues very quickly after death. For laboratory confirmation it is best to destroy the animal when it is obvious that it is not going to survive, rather than to let it die naturally. The brain should be removed promptly, cooled quickly, and delivered to the laboratory as soon as possible.

If the virus is isolated, it often becomes desirable to determine whether it is of the eastern or western type. This is most readily accomplished by inoculating several guinea pigs that have been previously immunized with eastern-type vaccine and several more that have received vaccine of the western type. Since there is relatively little cross immunization between these virus types, the homologous animals should survive and the heterologous die. Another approach is to incubate the unknown virus in antisera specific for each viral type and inject the mixtures into a susceptible laboratory animal or a susceptible tissue culture system to establish which of the two specific antisera causes virus neutralization.

The microscopic lesions in the brain are characteristic of virus encephalitis. In diagnostic work it is well to fix material for sectioning, in case virus isolation fails. The histological changes never prove the precise type of virus involved, but the findings can be strongly indicative of this disease.

Meyer, Haring, and Howitt (43) were unable to find inclusion bodies in this disease and made a point of this fact in differentiating it from the Borna disease of Germany. During the Kansas horse plague of 1912 a number of workers, including Joest, sought unsuccessfully to demonstrate inclusion bodies similar to the Joest bodies of Borna disease. Hurst (24), on the other hand, has described acidophilic intranuclear bodies in some of the degenerated neurons.

A new diagnostic procedure for the identification of WEE, EEE, and VEE may replace the use of laboratory animals and also provide a quicker answer (34). The method uses virus precipitation with fluorescein-conjugated gamma-globulin followed by cellulose acetate electrophoresis. Clinical specimens are inoculated into primary duck embryo cell culture, and there is sufficient virus for detection by microprecipitation within 24 hours.

Control. So far as horses are concerned, annual vaccination with inactivated virus vaccine is highly satisfactory. Because the transmitting agents are a number of species of mosquitoes, antimosquito measures undoubtedly help to reduce the incidence of the disease.

The Disease in Man. In 1932 Meyer (42) reported three cases of encephalitis in persons who had associated with horses suffering from the western type of encephalomyelitis. One proved fatal. Virus was not isolated from any of these cases. The first human cases proved to be caused by the equine encephalomyelitis virus were described by Fothergill, Dingle, Farber, and Connerley (11) in the late summer of 1938. Shortly afterward others were reported by Wesselhoeft, Smith, and Branch (57). These cases occurred in eastern Massachusetts during the height of the outbreak in horses. At least 40 human cases occurred, and virus was isolated in nine cases. Webster and Wright (56) proved by neutralization tests on laboratory animals that the virus was of the eastern type, and Schoening, Giltner, and Shahan (48) showed that the human virus would kill unprotected horses as well as one immunized to the western-type virus but was innocuous to horses immunized against the eastern-type virus. The persons affected were mostly children. There were no multiple cases in families, and none had had any contact with horses. The season had been very wet, however, and mosquitoes were common.

The onset of EEE in humans was sudden and was characterized by high fever, convulsions, vomiting, and drowsiness, which rapidly progressed to a comatose condition. Nearly all patients died. The high death rate distinguishes this illness from other forms of virus encephalitis in man which ordinarily have a much lower mortality rate.

In 1938 Howitt (21) reported the first proved case of equine encephalomyelitis virus infection in man caused by WEE virus. This was in a 20-month-old-infant who died after an illness of 5 days. In 1941 the most extensive outbreak of human encephalitis ever recorded was reported by Leake (33) in the north central part of the United States. Nearly 3,000 human cases were recognized. In general, the cases were mild; however 195 deaths occurred. During the same period Jackson (25) reported numerous human cases in the province of Manitoba, Canada, which lies just north of the epidemic area in the United States. Most of these were in infants under 1 year of age and in old persons. Cox, Jellison, and Hughes (9) isolated the western type of equine encephalomyelitis virus from eight fatal cases, and virus neutralizations with sera of recovered cases leave no doubt that the equine virus was the cause of the outbreak. The disease in horses at the time of the human outbreak was not nearly so prevalent as it had been in several preceding years when human cases were not recognized. It was a rather damp summer, however, and mosquitoes were unusually numerous. An interesting feature of this outbreak was that cases were more than twice as numerous among males as in females, which means, presumably, that men working in the harvest fields were more exposed to mosquitoes than were women.

Following the demonstration that an effective vaccine could be made for protecting horses from the virus propagated in developing chick embryos, a number of laboratories began manufacturing the vaccine in 1939. Very soon several fatal human infections occurred in these laboratories. The manufactures then began to immunize their workers with a somewhat refined vaccine of the type used on horses (1). This has proved effective and has not caused unusual discomfort or resulted in undesirable sequelae. The vaccine is recommended for persons unusually exposed to danger of infection. Laboratory workers who are exposed to both western and eastern types of virus should use a mixture of both types of vaccine.

In the epidemic area in Manitoba in the summer of 1941, Jackson (25) reported the vaccination of more than 3,000 adult humans with the chick embryo vaccine. There were no untoward results, although more than one-half suffered from mild vaccine reactions.

Venezuelan Equine Encephalomyelitis

This virus is a member of the genus *Alphavirus* and often called VEE or VE. It was first isolated from an outbreak of virus encephalomyelitis of horses in Venezuela. Beck and Wyckoff (2) compared the virus with WEE and EEE. The viruses shared many physical, biochemical, and biological characteristics, but VEE was immunologically distinct from WEE and EEE.

In 1943 an explosive outbreak of equine encephalomyelitis appeared on the island of Trinidad, which lies off the coast of Venezuela. Gilyard (14) isolated the virus, which proved to be of the Venezuelan type, and vaccine made from this type of virus brought the outbreak under control. The virus was obtained from a local mosquito, *Mansonia titillans,* but other types were not excluded as vectors. A seaman of the United States Navy stationed on the island died of encephalitis about 6 weeks before the animal outbreak. The Venezuelan type of virus was isolated from his brain. This is the first reported case of human infection with virus of this type. Later experiences showed that this type of virus is very highly infectious for man.

In 1962–64 there was severe epidemic by VEE subtype 1 B in Venezuela and Colombia causing innumerable cases in horses and 30,000 cases in humans with 300 deaths. In 1960–64 VEE antibodies were found in Seminole Indians of Florida, and virus later was isolated from rodents, mosquitoes, and three human cases. This strain causes a mild disease in horses, but it produces an immunity.

In 1968 the VEE subtype 1 B appeared in Central America where it spread rapidly and caused severe disease in horses and man. This subtype then appeared in Mexico in 1970 and by midsummer of 1971 was diagnosed in Texas horses and in human patients residing in that state. The disease moved northward into the United States despite an effort to control the disease in Central America and Mexico by the use of a modified VEE vaccine (developed for man) in horses and the use of a spraying program. In certain localities these efforts were begun too late or with logistical problems that decreased the effectiveness of the planned control procedures. The disease moved very fast, and it was essential to move well ahead of the disease front and vaccinate most, if not all of the horses, and also spray with effective insecticides to control the mosquito population. Obviously the introduction of this disease into the United States caused considerable havoc in the horse population, and marked concern on the part of public health authorities. With its multiple-host distribution among mammals, reptiles, and insects, the elimination of this disease from a given area is extremely difficult. Consequently, the disease usually must be controlled by vaccination and by mosquito control.

Character of the Disease. The signs of illness in horses are similar to WEE and EEE. The fever is accompanied by a viremia for approximately 5 days. Marked diarrhea and neurological manifestations usually occur on the 5th or 6th day, and fatal cases usually die 1 to 2 days later. Not all fatal cases show nervous manifestations. Survivors have detectable antibodies within the first 2 weeks after the onset of illness.

The gross and microscopic lesions (Figures 48.11 and 48.12) are typical of a viral encephalitis with no distinguishing features that separate it from WEE, EEE, and most other encephalitides.

Properties and Cultivation of the Virus. In general, properties of the VEE virus are similar to WEE and EEE viruses (Figure 48.13). There is evidence that VEE virus

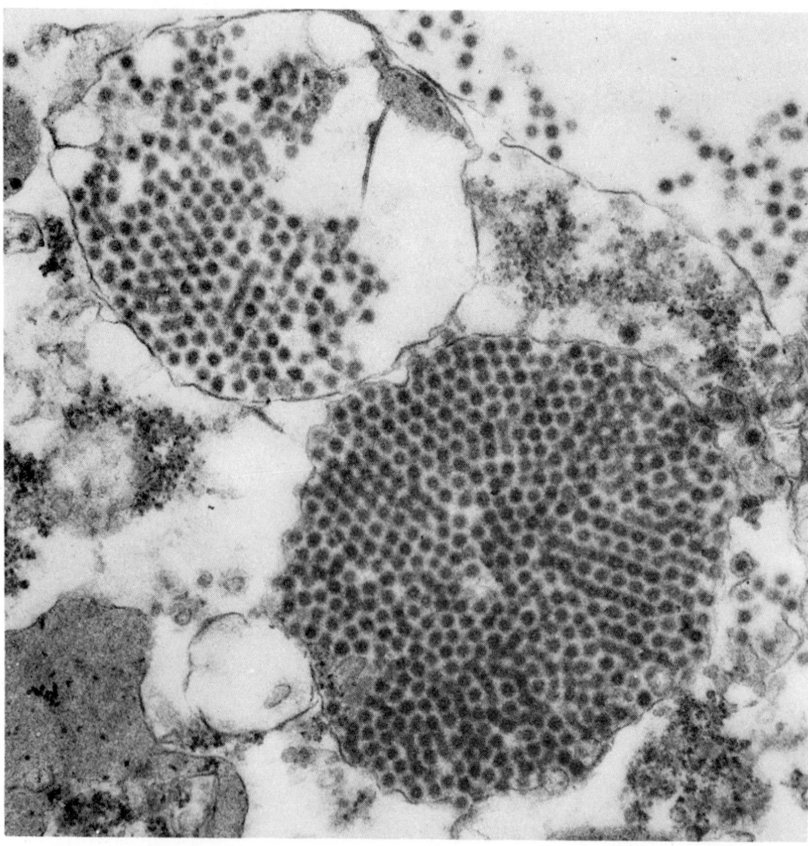

Figure 48.11. VEE. Accumulation of enveloped particles in an area where brain cells were completely disrupted. Apparently, virus particles budding into vacuoles are then trapped there upon disruption of the host cell. × 44,500. (Courtesy F. A. Murphy and A. K. Harrison, Center for Disease Control.)

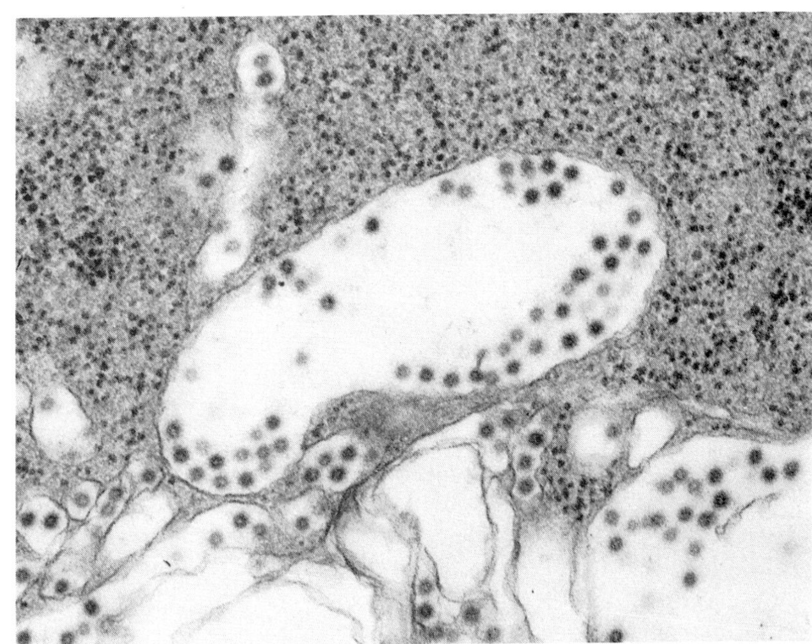

Figure 48.12. VEE. Mononuclear inflammatory cell (monocyte-macrophage) containing numerous mature virus particles within vacuoles. × 38,000. (Courtesy F. A. Murphy and A. K. Harrison, Center for Disease Control.)

is not inactivated by the same treatment with formalin as EEE and WEE viruses (32, 58). In each situation safety tests indicated there was no residual VEE virus, but the use of the inactivated vaccine resulted in clinical disease. This problem led to the development of an attenuated virus vaccine for man.

VEE virus has essentially the same mammalian host range and tissue-cultured cell range as WEE and EEE viruses, so comparable methods are used for its cultivation and assay.

Immunity. VEE virus produces a solid and long-lasting immunity.

An attenuated viral vaccine produced by U.S. Army scientists (3, 36) for use in man was used to control the 1969 Central America epizootic in horses (50). Vaccination of the horse population at the periphery of the epizootic was performed to create an artificial barrier to limit the spread of VEE. Vaccination of horses was also practiced within the epizootic area. Within 7 to 10 days after vaccination, even on ranches where the disease was

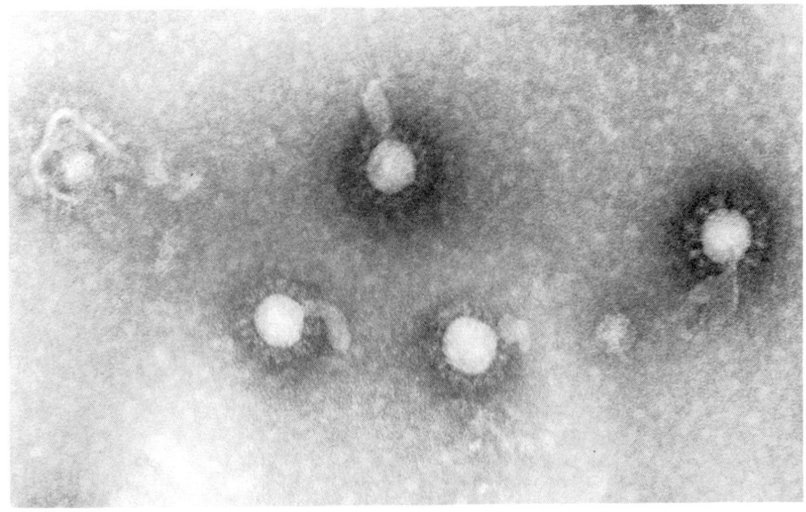

Figure 48.13. Negative stain of VEE virus revealing spherical particles with surface projections ranging from precise, post-like structures to a halo of massed filamentous material. × 158,500. (Courtesy F. A. Murphy and A. K. Harrison, Center for Disease Control.)

rampant, all equine cases subsided. Complete protection occurred in areas where horses were vaccinated and also prevented the spread of VEE into Guatemala by an immune barrier of vaccinated horses, 50 kilometers wide, established on the Pacific Coastal Plain. In 1970 this virulent strain somehow breached the immune barrier and became established in Costa Rica, then Mexico, reaching the USA in 1971; yet no epizootic occurred in 1970 or 1971 in either Guatemala or Nicaragua, evidence which strongly supports the view that the attenuated virus vaccine gives a lasting protection against the disease. Vaccination of pregnant mares may have undesirable effects on the developing fetus.

Primary chicken embryo cell cultures were evaluated as an alternate cell culture system for the production of attenuated VEE (TC-83 strain) vaccine (8). It remained biologically stable through 10 serial passages.

There is no evidence that vaccination against EEE or WEE provides protection against VEE. Previous claims that the combination of EEE and WEE vaccines or multiple doses will provide protection probably are not correct, so it is advisable to use a VEE vaccine to protect horses and man against this specific virus. There is a suggestion that the presence of WEE or EEE antibody in a horse may suppress the development of detectable vaccine-induced VEE antibody (5, 45). As a consequence revaccination of horses in high-risk areas is recommended (45).

Transmission. The culicine mosquitoes *Aedes taeniorhynchus* and *Masonia titillans*, and Tabanid flies, are known field vectors of VEE, and there may be others. Experimental horse transmission of VEE with *Aedes triseriatus* has been accomplished. *Masonia indubitans, Masonia perturbans,* and *Psorophora ferox* are susceptible to laboratory infection with VEE virus. The genus *Aedes* is very abundant in the United States; *M. perturbans* and *P. ferox* are common in southeastern United States; and *M. indubitans* and *M. titillans* occur in Florida. Tabanid flies are found throughout the United States.

Many birds are susceptible to VEE, including migratory birds. Birds generally have lower virus levels than certain mammals (such as rodents) which suggests that the natural cycle more likely occurs in mammals and insects than birds.

Direct-contact transmission occurs between horses, presumably by the respiratory route. VEE virus is found in mouth, nasal, and eye excretions and in milk and urine of infected horses.

The disease coincides with mosquito activity so it is a seasonal disease in colder climates.

Diagnosis. The disease is identifiable as one of the viral encephalitides by the typical neurologic signs in horses; however, fatal cases can occur without neurological signs.

A specific diagnosis can be made only by laboratory procedure, either by the isolation of the virus from central nervous tissue, blood, or nasopharyngeal washings or by the demonstration of a rising serum-neutralization or complement-fixing antibody titer. Serological confirmation is difficult or impossible to achieve since animals often die before a convalescent serum can be obtained. Because the virus is hazardous to humans, few laboratories are willing to attempt viral isolation unless special facilities and vaccinated personnel are available. Erickson and Mare have recommended a combined tissue-culture and fluorescent-antibody system to isolate and identify VEE virus (10). A similar system was described in the section on WEE and EEE that also works for VEE (34).

Certain other diseases can be confused with VEE. Toxic encephalitis causes similar nervous manifestations, but occurs commonly in the fall and winter as the result of eating moldy corn or fodder. Purpura head swellings are similar in appearance, but VEE fails to cause respiratory distress or hemorrhages common to purpura. Rabies may be confused with VEE, but the history often aids in differentiating the two diseases. African horse sickness (AFS) virus produces head swellings, but it is very difficult to differentiate from the encephalitides, including VEE, because AFS has many immunologic types. Mineral poisoning and botulism can be differentiated from VEE chiefly by their nonseasonal nature and history.

Control. Vector control should be given first consideration, but to be effective it must be complete. If vaccination of horses is permitted, then it should be a part of the control program.

Suspected cases should be reported immediately to the proper control agencies so early typing of the virus as well as immediate quarantine can be instigated. Isolate acutely ill animals in separate stalls that are mosquito-proof, if possible.

The Disease in Man. Naturally occuring epidemics of VEE in man have been reported in Columbia, Panama, Venezuela, Mexico, and the state of Texas in the United States. Serological evidence indicates that the infection has occurred in Brazil and in the state of Florida.

Numerous infections in laboratory workers attest to the marked susceptibility of man to this agent. Further evidence is the production of disease in man with inactivated virus vaccines that pass the safety tests in animals. The isolation of VEE virus from the upper respiratory tract of an infected laboratory worker has important epidemiological implications. There is strong field evidence that the disease can be transmitted from man to man.

REFERENCES

1. Beard, Beard, and Finkelstein. Science, 1938, *88*, 530.
2. Beck and Wyckoff. Science, 1938, *88*, 530.
3. Berge, Banks, and Tigertt. Am. Jour. Hyg., 1961, *73*, 209.
4. Bowen. Am. Jour. Trop. Med. Hyg., 1977, *26*, 171.
5. Calisher, Sasso, and Sather. Appl. Microbiol., 1973, *26*, 485.
6. Carneiro and Cunha. Arch. Inst. Biol., Sao Paulo, 1943, *14*, 157.
7. Chamberlain. Ann. New York Acad. Sci., 1958, *70*, 312.
8. Cole, Pedersen, Robinson, and Eddy. Jour. Clin. Microbiol., 1976, *3*, 460.
9. Cox, Jellison, and Hughes. Pub. Health Rpts. (U.S.), 1941, *56*, 1905.
10. Erickson and Mare. Am. Jour. Vet. Res., 1975, *36*, 167.
11. Fothergill, Dingle, Farber, and Connerley. New Eng. Jour. Med., 1938, *219*, 411.
12. Gebhardt, Stanton and St. Jeor. Proc. Soc. Exp. Biol. and Med., 1966, *123*, 233.
13. Giltner and Shahan. Science, 1933, *78*, 63.
14. Gilyard. Bull. U.S. Army Med. Dept., 1944, *75*, 96.
15. Gutekunst, Martin and Langer. Vet. Med., 1966, *61*, 348.
16. Gwatkin and Moore. Can. Jour. Comp. Med. and Vet. Sci., 1940, *4*, 78.
17. Hammon, Reeves, Benner, and Brookman. Jour. Am. Med. Assoc., 1945, *128*, 1133.
18. Hammon, Reeves, Brookman, Izumi, and Gjullin. Science, 1941, *84*, 328.
19. Higbie and Howitt. Jour. Bact., 1935, *29*, 399.
20. Holden. Proc. Soc. Exp. Biol. and Med., 1955, *88*, 490.
21. Howitt. Science, 1938, *88*, 455.
22. Howitt, Dodge, Bishop, and Gorrie. Proc. Soc. Exp. Biol. and Med., 1948, *68*, 622.
23. Howitt, Dodge, Bishop, and Gorrie. Science, 1949, *110*, 141.
24. Hurst. Jour. Exp. Med., 1934, *59*, 529.
25. Jackson. Am. Jour. Pub. Health, 1943, *33*, 833.
26. Johnson. Am. Jour. Trop. Med. and Hyg., 1969, *18*, 103.
27. Karstad and Hanson. Jour. Inf. Dis., 1959, *105*, 293.
28. Kelser. Jour. Am. Vet. Med. Assoc., 1933, *82*, 767.
29. Kissling. Proc. Soc. Exp. Biol. and Med., 1957, *96*, 290.
30. Kissling, Chamberlain, Sikes, and Eidson. Am. Jour. Hyg., 1954, *60*, 251.
31. Kitselman and Grundman. Kan. Agr. Exp. Sta. Tech. Bull. 50, 1940.
32. Kubes. Science, 1944, *99*, 41.
33. Leake. Pub. Health Rpts. (U.S.), 1941, *56*, 1902.
34. Levitt, Miller, Pedersen, and Eddy. Am. Jour. Trop. Med. Hyg., 1975, *24*, 127.
35. Livesay. Jour. Inf. Dis., 1949, *84*, 306.
36. McKinney, Berge, Sawyer, Tigertt, and Crozier. Am. Jour. Trop. Med. and Hyg., 1963, *12*, 597.
37. Mace, Ott, and Cortez. Bull. U.S. Army Dept., 1949, *9*, 504.
38. Madsen and Knowlton. Jour. Am. Vet. Med. Assoc., 1935, *86*, 662.
39. Mediaris and Kebrick. Proc. Soc. Exp. Biol. and Med., 1958, *97*, 152.
40. Merrill, Lacaillade, and Ten Broeck. Science, 1934, *80*, 251.
41. Merrill and TenBroeck. Jour. Exp. Med., 1935, *62*, 687.
42. Meyer. Ann. Int. Med., 1932, *6*, 645.
43. Meyer, Haring, and Howitt. Science, 1931, *74*, 227.
44. Meyer, Wood, Haring, and Howitt. Proc. Soc. Exp. Biol. and Med., 1934, *32*, 56.
45. Moore, Moulthrop, Sather, Holmes, and Parker. Pub. Health Rpts. (U.S.), 1977, *92*, 357.
46. Pedersen. Jour. Clin. Microbiol., 1976, *3*, 113.
47. Randall and Eichhorn. Science, 1941, *93*, 595.
48. Schoening, Giltner, and Shahan. Science, 1938, *88*, 409.
49. Smith, Blattner, and Heys. Science, 1944, *100*, 362.
50. Spertzel. U.S. An. Health Assoc., Proc. 74th Ann. Mtg., 1970, p. 18.
51. Sulkin. Science, 1945, *101*, 381.
52. Syverton and Berry. Jour. Bact., 1937, *33*, 60.
53. TenBroeck and Merrill. Proc. Soc. Exp. Biol. and Med., 1933, *31*, 217.
54. Udall. Cornell Vet., 1913-14, *3*, 17.
55. Vawter and Records. Science, 1933, *78*, 41.
56. Webster and Wright. Science, 1938, *88*, 305.
57. Wesselhoeft, Smith, and Branch. Jour. Am. Med. Assoc., 1938, *111*, 1735.
58. Young and Johnson. Am. Jour. Epidemiol., 1969, *89*, 286.

THE GENUS *FLAVIVIRUS*

In this genus there are a number of arthropod-borne viral encephalitides of man in which domestic animals are involved. The viral encephalitides described in this section include St. Louis encephalitis, Japanese encephalitis, California encephalitis, louping-ill of sheep, Central European tick-borne fever, Murray Valley encephalitis, Wesselsbron disease, Israel turkey meningoencephalitis, and Powassan.

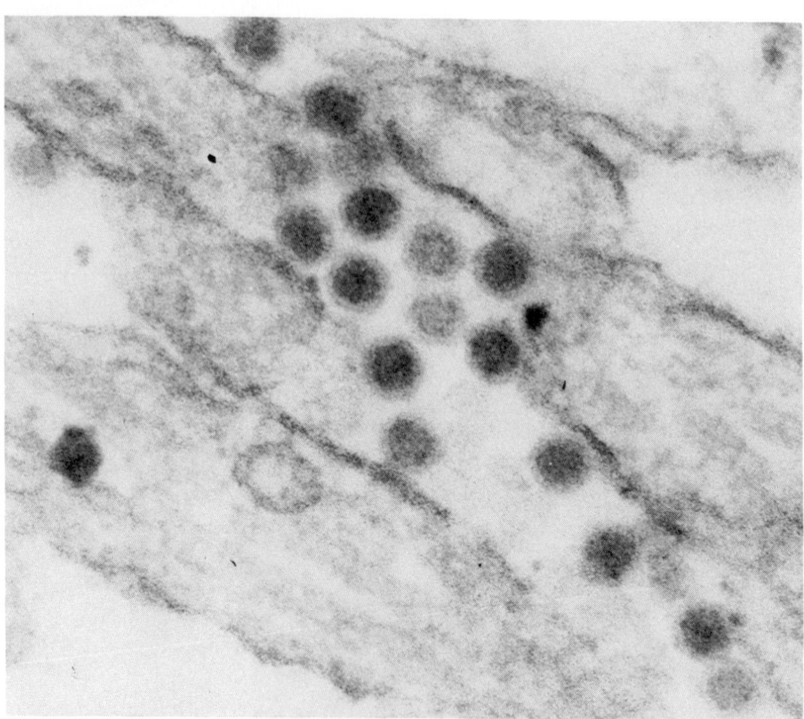

Figure 48.14. St. Louis encephalitis virus, a flavivirus, free in extraspace. Virions consisting of an electron dense core or a closely bound lucid halo or envelope, 38 nm in diameter. × 226,000. (Courtesy F. A. Murphy, A. K. Harrison, G. W. Gary, Jr., S. G. Whitfield, and F. T. Forrester, Center for Disease Control.)

The type species for the genus is *Flavivirus febricis,* otherwise known as yellow fever virus. A typical member of the group contains approximately 7 to 8 percent of single-stranded RNA. Its molecular weight is 3×10^6 daltons. Spherical enveloped particles, ±40 nm (Figure 48.14), have a buoyant density in cesium chloride of 1.25 g per cm^3. The particles contain lipid and are sensitive to ether and trypsin. The particles contain a hemagglutinin. The virions multiply in the cytoplasm and mature by budding. Not all viruses in this genus are proved to replicate in arthropods, but all are serologically related.

St. Louis Encephalitis

This is a warm-weather virus disease which occurs sporadically in the central and western parts of the United States. It was first identified as the cause of a rather large outbreak in and around St. Louis, Missouri, in the summer of 1933, hence its name. It occurs in the late summer and early fall. A number of species of mosquitoes, including many of those that transmit western equine encephalomyelitis, are known to be transmitting agents, and it is believed that they ordinarily convey the disease to man. Hammon and Reeves (10) isolated this virus from eight pools of *Culex tarsalis* captured in the Yakima Valley in 1941, 1942, and 1944, and from other species elsewhere. They found that chickens were easily infected with this virus, a viremia of 2 to 3 days duration being induced. The infected birds showed no clinical signs. Neutralizing antibodies were found in large numbers of chickens in areas where the disease was occurring in man. Smith, Blattner, Heys, and Miller (22) showed that certain mosquitoes could easily be infected by being fed on virus-containing materials and that such insects could transmit the infection to chickens and hamsters for periods of several weeks thereafter, a viremia but no encephalitis being produced. They also demonstrated that the chicken mite (*Dermanyssus gallinae*) could be infected with the virus and that this could be transmitted through the eggs from generation to generation. Infection in these mites could continue indefinitely. It was suggested that this may be the way the virus is maintained from one season to the next. It also is known that the virus can be present in *Culex pipiens* in temperate zones during the winter months, constituting another means for the dissemination and persistence of virus in nature (1).

In an epidemiological study of the 1962 epidemic of St. Louis encephalitis in Florida involving four counties, 222 laboratory-confirmed cases occurred in humans, with 43 deaths (4). The virus was recovered from four humans and from 42 mosquito pools of which 40 were *Culex nigripalpus*. All fatal cases occurred in persons over 45 years of age, and death rate was unusually high in persons 65 years of age and over. Widespread viral activity in nature was demonstrated by mosquito collections and serologic findings in wild or domestic birds in these four counties.

Whenever this disease appears in man, neutralizing antibodies, hemagglutination antibodies, and inhibition antibodies may be found in horses and some other vertebrates. Urban surveillance through wild birds such as immature house sparrows is used (17). The appearance of antibodies in birds often precedes the disease in man, so monitoring may provide a clue about an impending epidemic in man. This may be averted by intensifying mosquito control activities in an area.

Hammon, Carle, and Izumi (9) inoculated horses with virus freshly isolated from mosquitoes. No signs were produced, but viremias occurred in some of the animals and high antibody titers in all. There is no evidence that horses ever suffer from a clinically recognizable disease as a result of infection with this agent or that they play any significant role in the propagation of the human outbreaks. The virus was isolated from the brain of a California gray fox, *Urocyon cimereoargenteus* (5). It was also isolated from the Mexican free-tailed bat, *Tadarida b. mexicana*, during an outbreak in Texas in 1964 (24).

Trent *et al.* (26) described a micro solid-phase radioimmunoassay test (SPRIAT) for antibodies reactive with nonstructural viral protein that is as specific and sensitive as the plaque reduction neutralization test. The test, using wells precoated with purified SLE viral antigen, can be completed in 1 day and can be adapted to use in testing a large number of sera.

Japanese Encephalitis

This is a virus-induced encephalitis that occurs in man in Japan, Korea, Manchuria, Malaya, China, Indo-China, and Sumatra; it has been classified as a member of the B group of arboviruses. It is probable that a disease called Australian X-disease is identical with it. Large outbreaks with high mortality rates have occurred from time to time. A milder form evidently exists since large numbers of people in the Orient carry neutralizing antibodies for this virus. It is reported, for example, that more than 90 percent of all Koreans exhibit antibodies. The attention of western workers was called to this infection when American military personnel went into the infected regions during World War II. The disease was found in Guam in 1948.

The disease is mosquito-borne. Hammon, Tigertt, Sather, and Schenker (14) confirmed earlier Japanese findings that *Culex tritaeniorhynchus* and a local variety of *Culex pipiens* were capable of transmitting the virus, and they captured virus-carrying mosquitoes of the first species in the wild in areas where the disease was endemic. In Japan and neighboring regions the disease occurs only during the summer months. In Guam and other tropical regions the disease may occur the year round.

Hodes, Thomas, and Peck (15), Sabin (19), and Hammon (8), working at different times on the island of Okinawa, showed that most of the horses, pigs, and cattle carried neutralizing antibodies. They all agreed that chickens rarely had such antibodies; apparently these birds do not play the same role that they have in the dissemination of the western equine encephalomyelitis and the St. Louis viruses. Hammon, Reeves, and Sather (11) found that certain wild birds (finches and red-winged blackbirds) circulated more virus following inoculation than did chickens and thus concluded that some wild birds have at least a potential importance in the propagation of this disease. In Sarawak, it appears that the pig acts as a maintenance host of Japanese encephalitis in a cycle involving *Culex gelidus* mosquitos and towards the end of the year in a cycle involving *Culex tritaeniorhynchus* (21). More than 50 percent of fresh-water turtles (*Trionyx sinesis* Wiegman) from China have either or both HI and VN antibodies, and there are no obvious differences in percentage positives between spring/summer and autumn/winter seasons (20).

The various surveys in the endemic areas showing the high incidence of horses, cattle, and swine with high antibody titers indicate that the infection must occur frequently in a mild form. Infections in pregnant sows may cause stillbirths and constitute a significant loss in herds in the Orient. There also is evidence that this virus may produce fatal disease in all of these species. Patterson *et al.* (18) described deaths of a number of race horses in Malaya, and Japanese authors have described fatal cases in cattle and swine. By intracerebral inoculation all of these species show fatal susceptibility.

Two attenuated virus vaccines for protection against Japanese encephalitis have been developed in cell culture systems (6, 7). Both are reputed to be safe and efficacious in test animal systems. Fujisaki *et al.* (6) performed extensive experimental testing in piglets and pregnant sows with excellent results, so it is presumed the S-strain is safe for use in swine practice. Vaccination of gilts prior to mating with the M-strain of vaccine virus developed by Halle and Zebovitz (7) has resulted in marked reduction of stillbirths at a large breeding farm on Taiwan (16).

California Encephalitis

In 1952 Hammon, Reeves, and Sather (12) isolated a new virus from mosquitoes (*Aedes dorsalis* and *Culex tarsalis*) in Kern County, California. Encephalitis, sometimes fatal, developed in mice, cotton rats, and hamsters following inoculation, especially when the inoculum was introduced intracerebrally. The signs and lesions in the experimental animals were indistinguishable from those induced by the equine encephalomyelitis and St. Louis viruses. Guinea pigs, rabbits, ground squirrels, a calf, and a monkey gave serological responses to the injection of the virus, but these animals exhibited no signs. Squirrel and rabbit reactions were of particular interest since both developed viremias which could infect mosquito vectors. Chickens proved to be wholly refractory.

Both species of mosquitoes that had been found to harbor this virus in nature could readily be infected by feeding, and they maintained the virus for at least 7 to 8 days. In one instance it was established that the artificially infected *Aedes dorsalis* could transmit the infection to a rabbit. More recently a virus of this group was isolated from the mosquito *Culex inornata*.

California encephalitis is caused by the La Crosse virus in the north-central part of the United States, and transovarian transmission of the virus in *Aedes triseriatus* is the mechanism for its survival during the winter season (27). Venereal transmission of La Crosse virus from male to female *A. triseriatus* has been shown by experimental studies (25). Human cases of encephalitis have been associated with the isolation of virus from various stages of *A. triseriatus* that were present in tree holes close to their residences (2, 27).

The Tahyna virus is a member of the California group of flaviviruses and occurs in practically all European countries (3). Antibodies to the virus have been found in foals, suckling pigs, and hares. In humans it causes an influenzalike disease; some cases showing meningoencephalitis and atypical pneumonia.

A case of nonfatal encephalitis in man was suspected to have been caused by this virus, since neutralizing antibodies were demonstrated after recovery. The authors believed that the evidence at hand indicated that this virus has a natural reservoir in wild and perhaps also in domestic mammals; the infection is propagated by mosquitoes. Cross-neutralization tests indicated a close relationship with a virus that caused an outbreak of human encephalitis in Barnes County, North Dakota, in the summer of 1949. This outbreak was described by Wenner, Kamitsuka, Cockburn, Krammer, and Price (28).

Other viral isolates have been made that are closely related to the original California isolate. In addition to the five previously recognized viruses in the group, two of which were from the United States, there now appear to be at least eight antigenic types in the United States (13). A member of this group has been isolated from a pool of 23 *Aedes cenerus* mosquitoes in New York State that was antigenically different from the prototype BFS-283 strain for the group (29). The complement-fixation test for the 8 reference viruses in the California group viruses of North America is relatively specific, although only 2-fold differences were observed reciprocally with the closely related La Crosse and snowshoe hare viruses (23).

REFERENCES

1. Bailey, Eldridge, Hayes, Watts, Tammariello, and Dalrymple. Science, 1978, *199,* 1346.
2. Balfour, Edelman, Cook, Barton, Buzicky, Siem, and Bauer. Jour. Inf. Dis., 1975, *131,* 712.
3. Bardos. Munch. Med. Wchnschr., 1976, *118,* 1617.
4. Bond, Quick, Witte, and Oard. Am. Jour. Epidemiol., 1965, *81,* 392.
5. Emmons and Lennette. Proc. Soc. Exp. Biol. and Med., 1967, *125,* 443.
6. Fujisaki, Sugimori, Morimoto, and Miura. Natl. Inst. An. Health Q. (Tokyo), 1975, *15,* 15.
7. Halle and Zebovitz. Arch Virol., 1977, *54,* 165.
8. Hammon. Proc. 4th Internat. Cong. Trop. Dis. and Malaria, 1948, p. 568.
9. Hammon, Carle, and Izumi. Proc. Soc. Exp. Biol. and Med., 1942, *49,* 335.
10. Hammon and Reeves. Am. Jour. Pub. Health, 1945, *35,* 994.
11. Hammon, Reeves, and Sather. Am. Jour. Hyg., 1951, *53,* 249.
12. Hammon, Reeves, and Sather. Jour. Immunol., 1952, *49,* 493 and 511.
13. Hammon and Sather. Am. Jour. Trop. Med. and Hyg., 1966, *15,* 199.
14. Hammon, Tigertt, Sather, and Schenker. Am. Jour. Hyg., 1949, *50,* 51.
15. Hodes, Thomas, and Peck. Science, 1946, *103,* 357.
16. Hsu, Chang, Lin, Chuang, Ma, Inoue, and Okuno. Bull. World Health Org., 1972, *46,* 465.
17. Lord, Calisher, Chappel, Metzger, and Fischer. Am. Jour. Epidemiol., 1974, *99,* 360.
18. Patterson, Ley, Wisseman, Pond, Smadel, Diercks, Hetherington, Sneath Witherington, and Lancaster. Am. Jour. Hyg., 1952, *56,* 320.
19. Sabin. Jour. Am. Med. Assoc., 1947, *133,* 281.
20. Shortridge, Oya, Kobayashi, Yip, Southeast Asian Jour. Trop. Med. Pub. Health, 1975, *6,* 161.

21. Simpson, Smith, Marshall, Platt, Way, Bowen, Bright, Day, McMahon, Hill, Bendell, and Heathcote. Trans. R. Soc. Trop. Med. Hyg., 1976, *70,* 66.
22. Smith, Blattner, Heys, and Miller. Jour. Exp. Med., 1948, *87,* 119.
23. Sprance and Shope. Am. Jour. Trop. Med. and Hyg., 1977, *26,* 544.
24. Sulkin, Sims, and Allen. Science, 1966, *152,* 223.
25. Thompson and Beaty. Am. Jour. Trop. Med. and Hyg., 1978, *27,* 1.
26. Trent, Harvey, Qureshi, and Lestourgeon. Inf. and Immun., 1976, *13,* 1325.
27. Watts, Thompson, Yuill, DeFoliart, and Hanson. Am. Jour. Trop. Med. and Hyg., 1974, *23,* 694.
28. Wenner, Kamitsuka, Cockburn, Krammer, and Price. Pub. Health Rpts. (U.S.), 1951, *66,* 1075.
29. Whitney, Jamnback, Means, Roz, and Rayner. Am. Jour. Trop. Med. and Hyg., 1969, *18,* 123.

Louping-ill

SYNONYM: Infectious encephalomyelitis of sheep

Louping-ill has occurred in the highland sheep of Scotland and the northern part of England for more than a century. It also exists in Ireland. Only recently has it been tentatively identified with a disease of man occurring in Czechoslovakia and Russia known as spring-summer encephalitis. It is not known to occur in the Western Hemisphere. The disease receives its name from the peculiar leaping gait of the ataxic animals. It was shown to be inoculable by intracerebral injection by Pool, Brownlee, and Wilson (10) in 1930. Greig, Brownlee, Wilson, and Gordon (7) proved, the following year, that the causative agent was a filterable virus.

The disease is primarily one of sheep, but it occasionally affects cattle pastured on the same lands with affected sheep. Timoney *et al.* (14) described an outbreak in a group of free-range horses in Ireland. Because wild red deer in Scotland have antibodies to the virus, they may serve as a tangential host (1). Human infection also occurs.

Character of the Disease. Under conditions of natural exposure, the incubation time in sheep is from 6 to 18 days. The earliest signs are dullness and a high temperature, which may be 107 F or more. At this stage virus is present in the blood. The temperature generally falls after a day or so, and the animal appears better, but improvement is only temporary for a second temperature rise usually occurs about the 5th day. At this time involvement of the nervous system may occur. If it does not, the animal recovers rapidly and thereafter is immune. Those that develop nervous signs begin with muscular incoordination, tremors, cerebellar ataxia, and finally paralysis. A high percentage of those that show nervous signs eventually die; those that do not die usually are permanently damaged. In very acute cases death may occur within a day or two of the time the first signs are observed. In chronic cases paralytic changes may exist for months. The disease resembles poliomyelitis of man in that it is always a generalized infection in the beginning which may or may not be followed by an invasion of the central nervous system.

If only generalized or viremic changes occur, without nervous system involvement, the death rate is practically nil. In the highly infected areas of the British Isles it has long been recognized that sheep more than 1 year old seldom develop the disease; they are immune as a result of unrecognized infections. This disease is seen mostly in young lambs.

The disease in horses was characteristic of a louping-ill disease in sheep (14). Three horses displayed signs of central nervous system disturbance, and two died after 2 and 12 days of illness respectively. Virus was isolated from the brain and cervical cord. Serum samples from the infected horses contained hemagglutination-inhibition, complement-fixing, precipitating, and neutralizing antibodies to louping-ill virus.

The lesions of terminal cases are typical of a virus-type encephalomyelitis and meningitis. Degeneration of neurons, and particularly of the Purkinje cells of the cerebellum, is characteristic. There are no typical gross lesions.

The Disease in Experimental Animals. By intracerebral inoculation of brain virus the disease can be produced in sheep, cattle, swine, mice, hamsters, and monkeys. Rabbits and guinea pigs do not appear to be susceptible. According to Galloway and Perdrau (5), monkeys and mice can be readily infected by instilling virus in their nostrils. The incubation period in these cases varied from 13 to 22 days, averaging 17 days. Hurst (8) found characteristic cytoplasmic inclusion bodies in the brain of mice, but he could not find them in monkeys, and others have not been able to find them in other species. Edward (3) was able to produce encephalitis in only 44 percent of susceptible lambs by inoculating virus subcutaneously. The injection of sterile starch solution intracerebrally 3 days after inoculation of the virus subcutaneously increased the number of cases of encephalitis to nearly 100 percent.

Properties of the Virus. The virus has properties characteristic of flaviviruses. The particles are spherical.

Infectious RNA has been extracted from the particle. The virus hemagglutinates rooster red blood cells. Crossing occurs with the other flaviviruses in the hemagglutination inhibition tests, but not to the same degree as with other members of the genus. The agent is well preserved by freezing and glycerol, but deteriorates rapidly in saline or broth, especially in dilute and somewhat acid suspensions.

A complement-fixation test is available, but CF antibodies are transient, so the test has limited value in diagnosis and research (15).

Cultivation. Rivers and Ward (13) were successful in obtaining artificial cultures of the virus on minced chick embryo medium. The virus also grows in cultures of pig kidney. Edward (4) grew it in embryonated eggs by inoculating either the yolk sac or the embryo.

Immunity. Recovery from natural or artificial infections always results in a solid and enduring immunity. Young suckling lambs whose dams are immune are protected by colostral antibody (11). A vaccine developed by Gordon (6), consisting of formalinized nerve tissue, provides effective protection to young lambs. Vaccinated lambs will succumb if inoculated with virus intracerebrally because the protection is due to circulating antibodies, which prevent the initial build-up of virus in the blood stream.

Transmission. Experimentally it has been shown that monkeys and man can contract infection by inhaling infective droplets. This may sometimes happen in sheep, but most transmissions occur through the agency of bloodsucking arthropods. McLeod and Gordon (9) in 1932 showed that in the louping-ill districts of the British Isles the principal transmitter was the castor bean tick, *Ixodes ricinus*. The larval ticks, feeding on infected sheep, convey the infection to new hosts when they next feed as nymphs; or if the tick becomes infected as a nymph, it conveys the disease to a new host as an adult. The disease is prevalent in the early summer, subsides during midsummer, and reappears in early fall. These periods correspond to the seasons of tick activity in the area.

Diagnosis. Diagnosis from the clinical signs may be difficult unless the animals are in a louping-ill district. Virus may be most readily demonstrated by inoculating mice intracerebrally with nerve tissue. Serological tests may be necessary to make a definitive diagnosis in many cases.

Control. Louping-ill may be controlled in two ways: (*a*) by immunizing all newborn lambs with nerve-tissue vaccine shortly after weaning, and (*b*) by dipping the flocks to remove all castor bean ticks.

The Disease in Man. Although louping-ill has occurred for many years, human infections were not recognized until recently. The first cases, described by Rivers and Schwentker (12), were three laboratory workers engaged in research work on the disease in the Rockefeller Institute in New York City in 1933. The illness was of an influenzal nature. Virus was not recovered from these patients, but neutralizing antibodies appeared in their sera shortly after recovery.

Several cases have been recognized in the British Isles. One described by Brewis, Neubauer, and Hurst (2) is typical. A young shepherd whose flock was affected by the disease was the victim. His disease was biphasic. An initial febrile illness of short duration was followed by apparent recovery. About 1 week later, he became delirious and comatose for a period of 36 hours. Virus was recovered by the inoculation of mice with cerebrospinal fluid, intracerebrally and intramuscularly, and neutralizing antibodies later appeared in his blood. He recovered almost completely except for some mild symptoms of ataxia.

REFERENCES

1. Adam, Beasley, and Blewett. Res. Vet. Sci., 1977, *23,* 133.
2. Brewis, Neubauer, and Hurst. Lancet, 1949, *1,* 689.
3. Edward. Brit. Jour. Exp. Path., 1947, *28,* 368.
4. Edward. Brit. Jour. Exp. Path., 1947, *28,* 237.
5. Galloway and Perdrau. Jour. Hyg. (London), 1935, *35,* 339.
6. Gordon. Vet. Jour., 1936, *92,* 84.
7. Greig, Brownlee, Wilson, and Gordon. Vet. Rec., 1931, *11,* 325.
8. Hurst. Jour. Comp. Path. and Therap., 1931, *44,* 231.
9. McLeod and Gordon. Jour. Comp. Path. and Therap., 1932, *45,* 240.
10. Pool, Brownlee, and Wilson. Jour. Comp. Path. and Therap., 1930, *43,* 253.
11. Reid and Boyce. Jour. Hyg. (London), 1976, *77,* 349.
12. Rivers and Schwentker. Jour. Exp. Med., 1934, *59,* 669.
13. Rivers and Ward. Proc. Soc. Exp. Biol. and Med., 1933, *30,* 1300.
14. Timoney, Donnelly, Clements, and Fenlon. Equine Vet. Jour., 1976, *8,* 113.
15. Williams. Am. Jour. Vet. Res., 1968, *29,* 1619.

Central European Tick-Borne Fever

SYNONYMS: Diphasic milk fever, Russian spring-summer encephalitis (western form)

This member of the tick-borne encephalitis complex produces a diphasic disease in man. The initial phase is influenzalike, and the second stage, after a 4- to 10-day afebrile period, is characterized by meningitis or meningoencephalitis. Virus may be present in the milk of infected goats and thus infect man (2). Experimentally, virus may localize in the mammary glands of infected goats, cows, and sheep and be present in the urine. The vector is *Ixodes ricinus*, and it probably is the most important reservoir of infection for man. An attenuated virus vaccine is being tested for immunization of cattle, sheep, and goats (1).

REFERENCES

1. Blaskovic. Symposium on biology of viruses of the tick-borne encephalitis complex. Academic Press, New York, 1962.
2. Van Tongeren. Arch. f. die gesam. Virusforsch., 1955, *6*, 158.

Murray Valley Encephalitis

SYNONYM: Australian X disease;
abbreviation, MVE

This virus is a flavivirus with the usual characteristics attributed to this genus. The encephalitis in man resembles Japanese encephalitis and occurs in certain areas of Australia and Papua. Horses may be infected, but do not develop encephalitis (1, 4), and horses do contain antibodies to MVE virus. Based on the hemagglutination-inhibition (HI) test antibody was found in 58 percent of feral pigs in New South Wales (3). Liehne *et al.* (6) found antibodies to MVE virus in humans, birds, and cattle in the Ord River area in Australia. The important vector is *Culex annulirostris* (7).

The virus has the properties of flaviviruses. It replicates in various cell culture systems such as Vero cells and also the embryonated hens' egg. For isolation of field virus, the hen's egg seems more sensitive (5). For information about the proteins of MVE virus read the paper by Westway (8). Clinical cases of MVE in humans can be diagnosed by the detection of MVE immunoglobulin M (9).

A survey of antibody in domestic fowls may suggest widespread activity of virus in a given area and serve as a warning to health authorities to take immediate action to reduce the mosquito population before the first encephalitis case occurs in a human (2).

REFERENCES

1. Anderson. Jour. Hyg. (London), 1954, *52*, 447.
2. Doherty, Carley, Kay, Filippich, and Marks. Austral. Jour. Exp. Biol. and Med. Sci., 1976, *54*, 237.
3. Gard, Giles, Dwyer-Grey, and Woodroofe. Austral. Jour. Exp. Biol. and Med. Sci., 1976, *54*, 297.
4. Gard, Marshall, Walker, Acland, and Saren. Austral. Vet. Jour., 1977, *53*, 61.
5. Lehmann, Gust, and Doherty. Med. Jour. Austral., 1976, *2*, 450.
6. Liehne, Stanley, Alpers, Paul, Liehne, and Chan. Austral. Jour. Exp. Biol. and Med. Sci., 1976, *54*, 505.
7. McLean. Austral. Jour. Exp. Biol. and Med. Sci., 1953, *31*, 481.
8. Westway. Jour. Gen. Virol., 1975, *27*, 293.
9. Wiemers and Stallman. Pathology, 1975, *7*, 187.

Wesselsbron Disease

This virus is a member of the genus *Flavivirus*, and the disease occurs in South Africa, Rhodesia, and Mozambique. The virus may infect man producing fever and muscular pains. It is known to cause epizootics in sheep, with abortions and death of newborn lambs and pregnant ewes a characteristic feature. Jaundice and hemorrhages may occur and meningoencephalitis in fetuses. It probably causes abortion in cattle as well. The virus has a diameter of 30 nm (2), grows in the chick embryo after yolk-sac inoculation, and propagates in cultures of lamb kidney. The mosquitoes *Aedes caballus* and *A. circumluteolus* (1) are primarily responsible for virus transmission.

REFERENCES

1. Kokernot, Smithburn, Patterson, and Hodgson. So. African Jour. Med. Sci., 1960, *34*, 871.
2. Weiss, Haig, and Alexander. Onderstepoort Jour. Vet. Res., 1956, *27*, 183.

Israel Turkey Meningoencephalitis

In 1960 Komarov and Kalmar (1) described a disease of turkeys in the Shomron area of Israel. It was characterized by a progressive paralysis associated with a nonpurulent meningoencephalitis. The agent is a filterable virus, cultivable in embryonated hens' eggs, and produced plaques on chick embryo cell culture monolayers. Turkeys and mice were susceptible to the virus, whereas chickens, ducks, pigeons, hamsters, and guinea pigs were resistant. Turkeys which recovered were resistant to reinfection.

Following serial passages of the virus in chicken eggs, modification of its virulence for turkeys and mice resulted without loss of antigenicity.

Preliminary studies suggest that a species of mosquito may be involved in its transmission. Mice immune to the turkey virus were susceptible to representative members of groups A and B arboviruses. In 1961 Porterfield (2) showed that this virus falls in the genus *Flavivirus*.

REFERENCES

1. Komarov and Kalmar. Vet. Rec., 1960, *72*, 257.
2. Porterfield. Vet. Rec., 1961, *73*, 392.

Powassan Disease

The virus is a member of the genus *Flavivirus*. It causes disease in man. In a serum survey of 499 goats in New York State, nine animals had neutralizing antibodies to the virus (1). The positive goats came from widely scattered areas in the state, including counties where human cases were confirmed. A lactating goat with a 74-day-old kid inoculated with mouse virulent virus developed infection without disease. Its nursing progeny became infected, but also failed to show clinical signs of illness.

REFERENCE

1. Woodall and Roz. Am. Jour. Trop. Med. Hyg., 1977, *26*, 190.

Spontaneous Virus Diseases of the Nervous System of Experimental Animals

No attempt will be made here to describe in any detail the spontaneous encephalitides that occur in animals commonly used for the isolation and study of viruses of man and animals. It is desired merely to mention that such viruses exist and may affect an investigator's experimental results.

Viruses causing spontaneous encephalitis have been found in rabbits, guinea pigs, and mice and occur occasionally in all species. These viruses often are latent or masked and become evident only when inoculations containing foreign material act as a local irritant to the nerve tissue. Having been activated in this way, such viruses may then be passed readily from animal to animal in series. Römer (4) has described a virus of guinea pig paralysis, and Traub (5) demonstrated that the virus of lymphocytic choriomeningitis may sometimes occur spontaneously in colonies of white mice. The herpes simplex virus of man has been found occurring spontaneously in rabbit colonies.

In the study of neurotropic viruses it sometimes happens that two or more viruses exist in the same material, or a virus may become contaminated with another that existed spontaneously in some animal through which the original material was passed. While studying the etiology of St. Louis encephalitis in man, Armstrong and Lillie (1) first encountered the virus that is now known as that of lymphocytic choriomeningitis. In another instance Dalldorf, Douglass, and Robinson (3) produced a nervous disease in monkeys by injecting them with canine distemper virus. This surprising discovery was explained later when Dalldorf (2) found that the distemper virus had been contaminated with the virus of lymphocytic choriomeningitis, and that the signs of illness were caused by the LCM virus.

REFERENCES

1. Armstrong and Lillie. Pub. Health Rpts. (U.S.), 1934, *49*, 1019.
2. Dalldorf. Jour. Exp. Med., 1939, *70*, 19.
3. Dalldorf, Douglass, and Robinson. Jour. Exp. Med., 1938, *67*, 323.
4. Römer. Zentrbl. f. Bakt., 1911, *50*, Beihefte, p. 30.
5. Traub. Jour. Exp. Med., 1936, *63*, 533.

49 The Orthomyxoviridae

Members of the family Orthomyxoviridae contain 1 percent of single-stranded RNA. The molecular weight is approximately 4×10^6 daltons. Its helical capsid is 6 to 9 nm, probably in eight separate pieces. The enveloped particle, 80 to 120 nm, is spherical or elongated with numerous hollow and cylindrical spheres about 9 nm long and 1.5 to 2 nm wide (Figure 49.1). The virion contains lipid, carbohydrate, and neuraminidase. Virus particles are ether-sensitive, heat-sensitive, and acid-labile. Hemagglutination occurs at neuraminidase-sensitive receptors. Replication is inhibited by dactinomycin. Nucleocapsids form in the nucleus, and maturation takes place by budding at the cell surface. Genetic recombination is common since the RNA genome contains eight segments and antigenic variation frequently occurs (Figure 49.2). There are three discrete antigenic types distinguished by the specificity of the ribonucleoprotein (or soluble) antigen. Antigenic crossing does occur among subtypes of the three types. The hemagglutinin subunits are likely composed of two different hemagglutinins in the viral envelope of influenza A viruses and constitute the main component of the spikes. They carry the specific receptors for the mucins and also the subtype- and strain-specific antigens commonly called "V" antigens. Antibodies are formed to these antigens and are demonstrated by serum-neutralization, hemagglutination, and complement-fixation tests against homologous antigen.

The neuraminidase subunits are most likely located between the spikes of the envelope, a double-membrane that is 6 to 7 nm thick. On the basis of neuraminidase (NASE) thermostability, sensitivity to pH treatment, and specific enzymatic activity (NASE activity per 1 hemagglutinin unit) influenza viruses are placed in two groups by a revised World Health Organization (WHO) nomenclature. Neuraminidases represent the enzymatic activity of the virus and contain antigens that differ from

Figure 49.1. Influenza virus, A2/Hong Kong/1/68; negatively stained particles from chick embryo chorioallantoic fluid illustrating typical pleomorphism. All influenza virus strains are 80 to 120 nm in diameter and have prominent surface projections or spikes covering a membranous envelope. × 142,000. (Courtesy F. Murphy.)

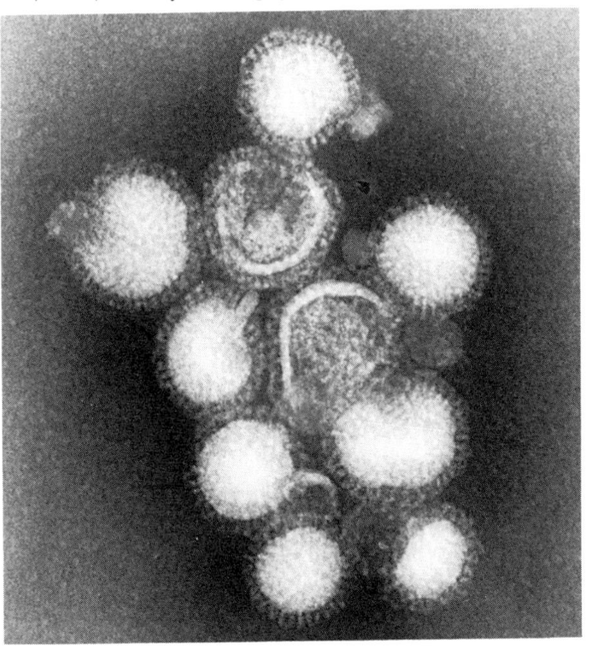

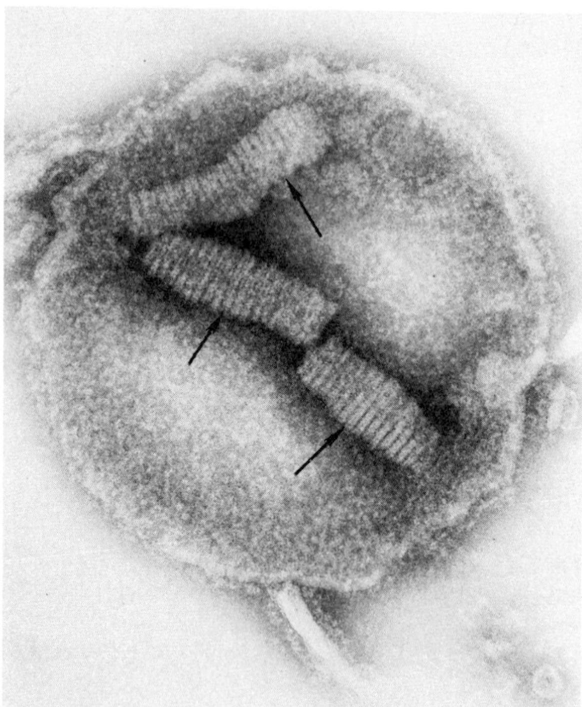

Figure 49.2. Influenza virus, A2/Aichi/2/68; an unusually large particle with three ribonucleoprotein (RNP) capsid coils (*arrows*). The RNP helix consists of a varying number of turns of a 9-nm diameter strand, which replicates as eight separate pieces of RNA and thus makes genetic recombination (and antigenic variation) common. × 138,750. (Courtesy F. Murphy.)

the hemagglutinins. Antibodies to the enzyme inhibit neuraminidase activity but not viral infectivity, although they do delay or even prevent liberation of infectious particles from cells.

The type species for the genus *Orthomyxovirus* is Orthomyxovirus h-A (human influenza A). Other members are as follows:

Type A: Human influenza viruses = A/PR8/34, Al/Cam/46, and A2/Singapore/1/57. Equine influenza viruses = A/Equi-1/Praha/56 and A/Equi-2/Miami/63. Porcine influenza viruses = A/SW/Iowa/31, A/SW/Wis/61, and A/SW/Wis/68. Avian influenza viruses = Fowl plague/27, A/Duck/Czech/56, A/Duck/Eng/56, A/Chick/Scot/59, A/Turkey/Can/63, and A/Quail/Italy/1117/65.

Type B Human = B/Lee/40, B/Johannesburg/59, and B/Taiwan/62.

Type C Human = C/Taylor/1233/47.

The RNA genome is coated with basic proteins. They carry the type-specific antigen referred to earlier. This antigen can be detected by the complement-fixation or flocculation test. As a rule, antibodies against this antigen are developed only after infection. Consequently they are not produced in animals given inactivated or disrupted viruses unless a special procedure is used (5).

The principal diseases in domestic animals caused by members of the genus include equine influenza, swine influenza, and avian influenza (fowl plague) occurring in chickens, turkeys, and ducks. In mammals the disease syndrome is largely confined to the respiratory tract, from which virus can be isolated in high titer and in low titer from bronchial lymph nodes.

Excellent review articles of orthomyxoviruses are available to the reader (1–4).

REFERENCES

1. Andrewes, Christopher and H. G. Pereira. Viruses of vertebrates, 2nd ed. Baillière, Tindall, and Cassell, London, 1967.
2. Chanock and Coates. *In* Newcastle disease virus: An evolving pathogen, ed. Robert P. Hanson. Univ. of Wisconsin Press, Madison, Wis., 1964.
3. Wildy. Monographs in Virol., 1971, *5*, 1.
4. Kaplan and Webster. Scientific Am., 1977, *237*, 86.
5. Zavadova, Kutinova, and Bonka. Arch. f. die gesam. Virusforsch., 1967, *20*, 421.

Equine Influenza

SYNONYMS: Shipping fever, stable pneumonia, pinkeye, epizootic cellulitis of horses

The disease known as equine influenza resembles influenzas in swine and man. It is also included in the influenza A viruses and is a member of the orthomyxovirus genus. Two immunological types are known to exist; they have been designated as A/Equi-1/Praha/56 and A/Equi-2/Miami/63 equine influenza viruses (5).

The disease spreads rapidly among susceptible horses. It affects animals of all ages, but occurs mostly in young animals that have been moved into new surroundings, particularly when they come in contact with older animals. In the past it has given much trouble in sales stables, in dealers' herds, and in army remount stations (8). In centers where fresh "green" horses are arriving from time to time, the newly arrived, highly susceptible stock serves to keep the disease alive and in very virulent form. Under such conditions the death rate may be very high. Like influenza of man, this disease in the past has a history of great panzootics on various continents in which nearly every horse in these areas was a victim of the disease. The last one of this kind in the United States occurred in the winter of 1872–73. At that time traffic in many of our large cities was nearly stopped because of the lack of horses well enough to do their normal work of drawing horsecars, drays, and delivery wagons. Like human influenza, the horse disease formerly occurred every year in a milder, less contagious form, and few horses escaped the disease.

As the horse population decreased in the cities and on the farms, equine influenza was less important as a disease in the horse. With increasing numbers of horses in recent years, its importance and incidence has increased, particularly as it affects the Thoroughbred and Standardbred horse populations.

At present only members of the equine family are known to be susceptible to the two equine serotypes.

Character of the Disease. The disease is highly contagious; practically every young horse and many of the older ones are attacked when the disease appears on the premises. Usually the mortality rate is moderate, and the chief loss is from inability of the victim to work for periods varying from 1 to 3 weeks, occasionally even longer (9).

The disease affects only horses, asses, and mules. The onset is sudden and is manifested by a high temperature—103 to 106 F—which lasts about 3 days. Equine 2 virus causes higher temperatures than equine 1 virus (11). At the same time there is inappetence and great mental depression. The animal stands with head down and with ears depressed, taking little interest in its surroundings. Coughing is the most common sign of illness.

Photophobia and lacrimation are usually exhibited, and often the congested conjunctivae protrude from between the closed eyelids because of the infiltration of the tissues. A mucopurulent discharge from the eyes appears, the corneas often become clouded, and occasionally the function of one or both eyes is lost. Nasal catarrh is usually present, and the lymph nodes of the head may become swollen. Pneumonia occasionally occurs, in which case the victim usually dies, as a rule from secondary bacterial infection.

In some cases edematous swellings appear on the ventral parts of the trunk and especially in the legs, where the tendon sheaths often are inflamed. This form of the disease has been called *epizootic cellulitis*. Mild icterus is not infrequent. Catarrhal and even hemorrhagic enteritis occur in some cases, and kidney damage is not uncommon. Leukopenia appears in the early stages of the modern disease and presumably was present also in the classical disease.

In the accounts of the old classical equine influenza, abortions in mares are mentioned, but one does not gain the impression that this was a frequent happening.

The period of incubation varies from 1 to 3 days with extremes of 0.5 days and 7 days. Its course varies greatly depending on whether or not complications occur. Uncomplicated cases may be essentially well again within 1 week.

The general mortality of naturally occurring cases probably does not often exceed 5 percent. In some outbreaks the virulence becomes exalted and the losses may be very much higher.

The principal lesions in fatal cases are in the lungs, in which there may be extensive edema or a bronchopneumonia with pleurisy. The thorax is usually filled with fluid. Gelatinous infiltrations around the larynx and in the legs are common. Usually there is swelling of the lymph nodes.

The Disease in Experimental Animals. In experimental horses influenza virus is recoverable for 5 days after intranasal instillation (5). Edema of the throat and the intermandibular lymph nodes occurs in some animals. A thick purulent nasal discharge usually follows the acute stage, and it is associated with secondary bacterial infection.

Horses given equine influenza 2 virus by the intranasal route develop an elevated temperature 2 to 3 days later followed by coughing and other signs of illness referable to the lower respiratory tract 2 or 3 days after the onset of fever (3). A contact horse also developed the disease. Virus was readily recovered from the nasal mucosa during the first 5 days postinoculation and also from the contact horse. Other horses given the same virus intramuscularly did not develop signs of illness.

The virus has been adapted to produce pneumonia in mice after intranasal instillation, and encephalitis results after intracerebral inoculation of suckling mice. It causes inapparent infection of ferrets.

Properties of the Virus. All equine cases belong to type A and presumably have the main characteristics described for the type species of the genus, human influenza A (15).

Based upon hemagglutination-inhibition (HAI) tests equine influenza viruses are placed into the two subtypes. Variants showing slight antigenic differences are distinguished in A/Equi-2. No antigenic relationship has been demonstrated between the hemagglutinin and neuraminidase antigens of these two subtypes using antisera produced in laboratory animals. However, horses recovering from A/Equi-2 infections may have antibody rises to A/Equi-1 strains, to certain human A-2 strains, and to the infecting virus suggesting existence of shared minor antigens.

Certain antigenic relationships have been observed among the equine viruses, influenza A avian strains, and strains of human origin. A/Equi-1 is antigenically related to fowl plague/27 and Turkey/Can/63 viruses, including both hemagglutinin and neuraminidase antigens. Influenza equine 1 (A/Equi/Praha/56) has a hemagglutinin that is antigenically related to the hemagglutinin of fowl plague virus strain Rostock and a neuraminidase that cross-reacts with the enzyme of virus N (A/chick/Germany/49) (17). A/Equi-2 virus shows some crossing with avian virus N and Quail/Italy/1117/65. A/Equi-2 shows some cross-reaction with the human A2/Hong Kong/1/68 hemagglutinin antigens.

Like other influenza viruses (19), both equine subtypes hemagglutinate erythrocytes of a wide range of species; the highest titers are attained with pigeon cell suspensions (15).

In an assessment of some equine influenza viruses, the properties of their neuramidases, such as pH sensitivity, thermostability, and specific activities, are attributed directly to the properties of the subunits, such as glycoprotein entities rather than dependent on some association with hemagglutinin (12).

Cultivation. Andrewes and Worthington (1) cultivated the A/Equi-1 virus in fertile eggs and in tissue cultures of bovine kidney, chick embryo kidney and fibroblasts, and rhesus monkey and human embryo kidney. Equine viruses are usually isolated and propagated in the hen's embryonated egg. A/Equi-2 is usually isolated in the egg without difficulty. In contrast, A/Equi-1 is rather difficult to isolate.

In general, isolation of virus in cell cultures is more difficult than isolation in the embryonated egg. A/Equi-2 viruses are isolated in primary cultures of monkey kidney cells, but other primary kidney-cell cultures of bovine, equine, and human origin are not satisfactory for this purpose (15). The equine influenza viruses have been cultivated in the Madin-Darby canine kidney cell line (14). Certain strains can be adapted to replicate in chick and bovine cell cultures.

Immunity. Infected animals generally produce antibodies to the three major components of the viral particle. The horse given inactivated or disrupted virus produces antibodies against the main envelope antigens, hemagglutinins and neuraminidase. CF antibodies against type-specific S antigen may be detected as early as 4 to 6 days after illness has begun, reach their peak at 12 to 20 days, and usually are not detectable after 8 to 12 weeks. CF antibodies against strain-specific V antigen, serum-neutralizing antibodies, and HI antibodies develop later than S-specific CF antibodies but reach their peak at 15 to 20 days and decline until the 3rd month. The HI and serum neutralization (SN) antibodies level off at this time and remain constant for years. The V-specific CF antibody is no longer detectable as a rule at the 6th month.

It is generally agreed that antibody on the respiratory mucosa surface confers protection against this pneumotropic infection. The mucous titer is a good index for determining the level of protection. Although the mucous titer does not always parallel the serum titer, the serum titer gives an approximate idea of the measure of resistance in man, and the same is likely to be true of equine influenza (2). This applies to vaccinated and unvaccinated individuals. Older horses that have had the disease earlier in life usually escape infection later. In times of past epizootics this immunity was frequently not adequate to protect horses completely. Information on the duration of immunity is based on field observations; it is reported that natural infection produces a rather solid immunity that persists for 1 year (11).

Transmission. It is presumed that the respiratory form of the disease occurs as a result of droplet infection. Numerous reports have appeared of the transmission of this disease by stallions used for breeding purposes months after having recovered from influenza. Several reports of the demonstration of virus in the semen of such animals for periods varying from 1 to 6 years are in the literature (10). Schofield (18) in Canada observed two outbreaks apparently initiated by breeding stallions that had had the disease some months previously. The examination of the semen of one of these animals 6 months later failed to show the presence of the virus. A-Equi 2 virus has been isolated from a dead foal.

The pattern and incidence of infectious disease among horses are influenced by the immune status of the population, its concentration of antibody, and the antigenic characteristics of the virus. Although natural resistance to influenza does not seem to be an important factor, it may account for a certain number of horses that show no signs of illness during epizootics (11).

When the disease occurs in a susceptible population, it is explosive and the rapid aerosol spread is principally due to the strong and frequent cough. The short incubation period and the high concentration of virus in the respiratory tract also account for its rapid transmission from horse to horse.

Diagnosis. Equine influenza is generally diagnosed on clinical evidence. When the disease occurs in epizootic form, the signs of illness and high degree of contagiousness are generally sufficient to make a diagnosis. When brood mares abort as a result of this infection, they are sick at the time the abortions occur.

Positive diagnosis can be assured only by isolation of the virus or by the demonstration of a rising hemagglutination or by neutralizing antibodies with paired sera. In an initial outbreak there is a need to isolate the virus for typing. This information is essential to a vaccination program in an area, and also to a correct diagnosis. If a new type is involved, serology alone will not give a satisfactory answer.

Prevention and Control. Inactivated and attenuated virus vaccines have been used for immunization of horses against influenza.

At least two types of inactivated virus vaccine are available (6, 16). According to Bürki *et al.* (7) inactivated vaccines must contain both equine types 1 and 2 and an adjuvant. Two doses are required for basic immunization. In young horses the doses should be spaced 3 months apart, but 2 weeks apart in older horses with unknown immunity status. Until horses are 2 years old, they should be revaccinated twice yearly, preferably in January and July. An annual booster in older horses should be given every January. This schedule would not interfere with vaccination for rhinopneumonitis infections, which are prevalent in the fall.

Attenuation of equine virus is achieved by serial passage on allantois in the presence of normal horse serum (4). Colts immunized by the intranasal route were completely protected while one-third of those immunized orally shed small quantities of virus after challenge.

In outbreaks, isolation and quarantine measures are advised in addition to vaccination.

The Disease in Man. There is a minor antigenic relationship between A/Equi-2 and A-2/Hong Kong (human) strains, but there is no evidence that the A/Equi-2 produces infection in man; nor does the reverse occur (13).

REFERENCES

1. Andrewes and Worthington. Bull. World Health Org., 1959, *20,* 435.
2. Beveridge. Proc. 2nd Internatl. Conf. Equine Inf. Dis., ed. J. T. Bryans and H. Gerber. S. Karger, Basel, 1970, p. 119.
3. Blaskovic. Proc. 2nd Internatl. Conf. Equine Inf. Dis., ed. J. T. Bryans and H. Gerber, S. Karger, Basel, 1970, p. 111.
4. Boudreault, Boulay, Marois, and Pavilanis. Dev. Biol. Stand., 1976, *33,* 171.
5. Bryans. Proc. Am. Vet. Med. Assoc., 1964, 119.
6. Bryans, Doll, Wilson, and McCollum. Jour. Am. Vet. Med. Assoc., 1966, *148,* 413.
7. Bürki, Sibalin, and Jaksch. Zentrbl. Vet.-Med., 1975, *22B,* 15.
8. Dale and Dollahite. Jour. Am. Vet. Med. Assoc., 1939, *95,* 534.
9. Doll, Bryans, McCollum, and Crowe. Cornell Vet., 1957, *47,* 3.
10. Gaffky. Zeitschr. f. Vetkde., 1912, *24,* 209.
11. Gerber, Proc. 2nd Internatl. Conf. Equine Inf. Dis., ed. J. T. Bryans and H. Gerber. S. Karger, Basel, 1970, p. 63.
12. Lipkind, Tsvetkova, and Muraviyov. Dev. Biol. Stand., 1977, *39,* 447.
13. McQueen, Kaye, Coleman, and Dowdle. Equine Dis. Supp., Jour. Am. Vet. Med. Assoc., 1969, *155,* 265.
14. Nath and Minocha. Am. Jour. Vet. Res., 1977, *38,* 1059.
15. Paccaud. Proc. 2nd Internatl. Conf. Equine Inf. Dis., ed. J. T. Bryans and H. Gerber. S. Karger, Basel, 1970, p. 81.
16. Peterman, Fayet, Fontaine, and Fontaine. Proc. 2nd Internatl. Conf. Equine Inf. Dis., ed. J. T. Bryans and H. Gerber, S. Karger, Basel, 1970, p. 63.
17. Rott, Becht, and Orlich. Med. Microbiol. Immunol. (Berlin), 1975, *161,* 253.
18. Schofield. Rpt. Ontario Vet. Col., 1937, p. 15.
19. Tumova and Fiserova-Sovinova. Bull. World Health Org. 1959, *20,* 445.

Swine Influenza

SYNONYM: Hog "flu"

Swine influenza is an acute disease of the respiratory organs which occurs in the colder months of the year. The onset of the disease is sudden, and practically all animals in an affected herd show signs almost simultaneously. They are quite similar to those of epidemic influenza of man, and the virus of swine influenza is closely related to that of human influenza.

The disease was first recognized as an entity in the midwestern part of the United States in the fall of 1918, when a pandemic of human influenza was under way. The similarity of the diseases in man and pigs was recognized. Koen is credited by Dorset, Niles, and McBryde (4) as being the one who suggested the name *flu* or *influenza* for the disease, since he was convinced that it had been contracted from human cases. Much later, when the etiological agents of the two diseases were better understood, the concept that swine may have become infected from man, thus giving rise to a new disease in the species, became much more plausible than before. The swine virus is more closely related to type A human virus than the three human virus types are to each other. Many adult human beings carry antibodies that neutralize, in part at least, the virus of swine influenza. This has been regarded by some as evidence that these persons have been infected at some time in the past with the same type of virus that exists in pigs. This idea was supported by the isolation of a strain of swine influenza virus from a soldier who died of influenza at Fort Dix, New Jersey, in the United States, in 1976. This same strain, Hsw 1/Nsw 1, was isolated from five other soldiers, but at the same time A/Victoria/3/75 also was infecting service personnel. Serological investigations showed that approximately 500 personnel at Fort Dix developed antibodies to the swine strain. Fortunately, this swine strain did not spread further. There have been other recent incidents on farms in which the swine strain has infected humans, but they were self-limiting. Naturally, public health officials are concerned about swine strains because the possibility always exists that a given strain may have an unusual capacity for dissemination and for virulence in humans and create a pandemic comparable to the 1918 episode. Another cause for concern is the isolation of A-2 Hong Kong/1/68 (H3N2) influenza virus from pigs in Hong Kong in 1977, which had not been isolated from humans for several years and the simultaneous occurrence of A/Victoria/3/75 during 1977 (24).

Character of the Disease. Swine and, to a lesser degree, humans appear to be naturally susceptible to the virus of swine influenza. In the United States the disease occurs primarily in the midwestern and north central states, but there is serological evidence for its existence in every state. The virus has also been isolated in England, Russia, Poland, Kenya, Italy, Germany, and Czechoslovakia. It usually occurs in the fall and early winter months, rarely occurring as a disease during the warm months, and only sporadically in European countries (8).

The disease usually appears suddenly in swine herds, and whole groups commonly develop signs of illness almost simultaneously. The development of the disease in many animals at almost the same time has commonly been attributed to an extreme degree of contagiousness, but Shope has put forward another concept—that the disease-producing agent spreads widely without producing obvious disease and that a precipitating agent is responsible for the simultaneous development of many cases. It was suggested that the precipitating agent in this case might be the advent of cold, wet weather with consequent chilling of the animals.

The disease begins with fever, anorexia, extreme weakness, and prostration. The animals crowd together, lying down, and are moved only with difficulty. When moved or handled they exhibit evidence of muscular stiffness and pain. Other cases develop edema of the lungs and bronchopneumonia and usually die. At the height of the disease the animals exhibit a jerky type of respiration, caused by spasms of the diaphragm, which is commonly known as *thumps*. Bronchitis is indicated by coughing. When the animals are in good condition in the first place and are kept during the course of the disease in a dry fairly warm place, well bedded with straw, the principal losses from this disease usually are in retardation of growth and decrease in weight.

The period of incubation is very short—from a few hours to several days. In uncomplicated cases the disease runs a course varying from 2 to 6 days; recovery occurs almost as suddenly as the disease begins. When pneumonia develops, the course will be longer. As a rule the mortality rate does not exceed 4 percent if the animals are given good care. In some instances it has been as high as 10 percent.

Animals killed at the height of the disease exhibit no significant lesions outside the chest cavity. The lung lesions are characteristic. They are limited, as a rule, to the cephalic, cardiac, and azygos lobes. Sometimes all five of these lobes are involved; sometimes only part of them. Usually the involvement is bilateral, but in some cases it is unilateral, the lobes of the right side being involved more frequently. These portions are collapsed, deep purplish red in color, and do not crepitate. They are not pneumonic. The condition is an atelectasis caused by a thick, mucilaginous exudate in the bronchioles and bronchi of the parts (20). The remainder of the lungs is usually pale because of the interstitial emphysema. The cervical, bronchial, and mediastinal lymph nodes are swollen and filled with fluid. In the cases in which pneumonia occurs, the consolidated portions are the same as the atelectatic in the milder ones. The nonpneumonic lung portions in these cases are congested and edematous. The spleen often is moderately enlarged. There is hyperemia of the mucosa of the stomach in most cases. The other abdominal organs generally are normal.

Virus pneumonia of pigs presents lesions that can easily be confused with those of influenzal pneumonia.

The Disease in Experimental Animals. Andrewes, Laidlaw, and Smith (1) demonstrated that the virus of swine influenza was pathogenic for mice when introduced by a special technique into the nasal passages. The virus also causes pneumonia in ferrets and lambs and a respiratory disease in squirrel monkeys.

Mouse-passage virus retains its virulence for swine indefinitely (22). The virulence of *Hemophilus (influenza) suis* may decline, however, in which case new cultures are needed to supply the necessary bacterial factors for producing a more severe form of the swine disease. The virus alone administered to normal pigs in an area where swine influenza does not exist produces a very mild, almost inapparent disease, which surely would be overlooked on the farm (10). *H. suis,* on the other hand, is virtually nonpathogenic for swine. When both agents are given simultaneously, however, typical influenza results. The experimental disease is a result of the concurrent action of two agents, a virus and a bacterium. In natural outbreaks *H. suis* is not always isolated. Scott (19) reported the isolation of *Pasteurella multocida* and influenza virus and others (13, 27) reported the isolation of influenza virus only.

Properties of the Virus. Shope (21) isolated the virus in 1931 and at the same time determined that *H. suis* was regularly present (11). The virus is type A.

It shares a common ribonucleoprotein (S) antigen with the human, equine, and avian members of the type A influenza viruses (6). Among the swine influenza viruses, insufficient antigenic differences have been observed to justify designation of subtypes. Three antigenic groupings have been made on the basis of HI and strain-specific CF reactions (6, 10). The representative strains of the three groups are A/SW/Iowa/31 (the original Shope isolate), A/SW/Wis/61, and A/SW/Wis/68. Accumulated evidence suggests that swine influenza virus represents or is closely related to the 1918 pandemic virus of human influenza. More recently, an antigenic relationship between swine influenza virus and the A/Chick/Scot/59 virus of chickens has been described (26). Using polyacrylamide gel electrophoresis Palese and Ritchey (15) succeeded in establishing a complete genetic map for influenza A viruses. On a farm two isolates from pigs and one isolate from a human possessed identical RNA patterns which differed from other recent swine isolates. This suggested the swine virus was transmitted to man and that swine viruses may occasionally infect humans without causing pandemic. It also is interesting that the Hong Kong strain has caused disease in dogs and in cattle in the USSR.

By use of the hemagglutination test 11 influenza A swine strains could be divided into three antigenic subgroups (3). Neuraminidases are placed into 2 subtypes—N1 and N2—yet there is considerable heterogeneity within subtype N1. When an antigenic change is gradual, it is called a *drift,* while a sudden complete or major change in either or both antigens is called a *shift.* A drift is usually attributed to the selection of preexisting mutants by pressure from increasing immunity in a population. An antigenic shift is less clear, but it may occur from mammalian or avian reservoirs or by genetic strains (5).

These viruses are stable at −70 C and in the lyophilized state for years. Most are inactivated at 56 C for 30 minutes, but some require a longer period. Phenol, ether, and formalin inactivate the virus.

Cultivation. In affected pigs the virus is found in the nasal secretions, in the tracheal and bronchial exudate, in the lungs, and in the lymph glands draining the lungs. It is not ordinarily found in the blood, spleen, liver, kidneys, mesenteric lymph glands, and brain (14).

Köbe and Fertig (9) and Scott (18) reported the successful cultivation of the virus of swine influenza on the chorioallantoic membrane of the developing chick. Scott reports that his cultures as far as the 50th generation were virulent for mice and swine, but that the 85th and later generations had lost their virulence. Intra-allantoic or intra-amniotic routes of inoculation into 10- to 12-day-old embryonated hens' eggs are the most commonly employed methods for cultivation of the virus. The virus is not lethal for the embryo, but it is readily detected by its hemagglutinating property. Strain A/SW/Wisc/1/68 had higher hemagglutination and egg infectivity titers when the embryonated eggs were incubated at 33 C (16).

Various tissue-culture monolayer systems involving primary or stable cell cultures have been used for propagation and assay (6). Depending on the culture system, the virus is recognized by plaque production or by hemadsorption of red cells in positive cultures. The virus also propagates in organ cultures of fetal pig tracheal, lung, or nasal epithelial tissue (13).

The immunofluorescence test has been used extensively in the study of influenza viruses, including swine influenza virus (13).

Immunity. Various serological methods, including the complement-fixation, hemagglutination-inhibition, serum-neutralization, and hemadsorption-inhibition tests have been used in swine-influenza immunity studies.

Based on present evidence it is believed that swine recovered from influenza are refractory to subsequent infection. Shope has reported that swine fully recovered from swine influenza are immune. Subsequent respiratory outbreaks in a herd in a given season mean that one of the outbreaks is caused by another pathogen. There is no unanimity of opinion on this point. According to Scott, experimental pigs with neutralizing antibody are not necessarily immune to challenge by the intranasal route with virus and *H. suis* combined. Pigs exposed to aerosols of virus 83 days after earlier intranasal and aerosol exposure all had HI titers of 80 or above at the time of challenge and resisted that challenge. Increasing evidence suggests that local antibody is very important in influenzal immunity, as local and systematic cell-mediated responses were detected by *in vitro* transformation tests during the second week after intranasal inoculation (2). In addition local and serum-neutralizing antibodies also appeared.

Maternal immunity plays a role in the epidemiology of the disease. Piglets from immune sows are protected from disease as long as 13 to 18 weeks depending on the serum titer level of the dam. In addition to providing protection, colostral antibody often inhibits propagation of the virus in the host and development of an active immunity. Infection of piglets with low titers led to immunologic priming (17). A second exposure to virus produced a secondary response which resulted in a mild clinical disease of shorter duration than in piglets in which antibody completely blocked viral replication.

Transmission. Swine influenza appears each autumn in the midwestern United States. The epizootics coincide with the onset of autumn rains and marked fluctuating temperatures. The disease appears simultaneously on many farms, suggesting that the virus is widely seeded before the outbreak and then provoked by climatic conditions and management procedures. It appears that all pigs become ill at the same time on individual farms, but more astute owners often report that one or a few pigs are ill 2 to 5 days before the diffuse herd disease.

The ecology and epidemiology of swine influenza is complex and not completely understood. The question of how the disease is maintained through the nonepizootic portions of the year when the disease is not seen has possibly been answered by Shope (23), who has demonstrated that the lungworm and the earthworm can harbor the virus for long periods of time. Lungworms, living in the bronchi of affected pigs, ingest virus, and the virus is carried through the eggs and into the larvae of the parasite. These, hatching out in the air passages of the pig, are coughed up and swallowed, eventually reaching the ground in the feces. Here they are ingested by earthworms in which the larvae lodge, most of them being found in the heart and calciferous glands. They may remain in the worms from one season to the next. If the earthworms are fed to swine, as was done by Shope, the pigs show no ill effects. However, if the pigs are then given several intramuscular injections of *H. suis,* about one-half of them will suddenly develop typical swine influenza, and both virus and bacterium will be found in the lungs. Shope regards the injection of the bacterium merely as a precipitating or provoking agent, since he was able to provoke a similar effect in a few cases by injecting calcium chloride into the pleural cavity. He has repeated these experiments successfully many times in the late fall, winter, and spring months but never in the summer. He speaks of the virus in the earthworms as existing in a ''masked'' form.

Subsequent observations have shown that Shope's complex biological cycle is not necessary as an interim reservoir (23). It has been shown that pigs free of parasites can be infected and transmit infection to contact pigs kept with them for at least 3 months thereafter. Nakamura and Easterday (13) extended these findings in a study of the natural history of the disease.

Diagnosis. Swine influenza is suspected in a herd with respiratory disease in the fall or early winter. A clinical diagnosis is presumptive because influenza doesn't always follow the typical pattern and other respiratory diseases are similar (7).

A definitive diagnosis requires virus isolation or the demonstration of a rising titer with paired serum samples. In the past, intranasal inoculation of mice or ferrets was used, but the generally accepted method is allantoic or amniotic inoculation of the 10- to 12-day-old embryonated hen's egg. Nasal exudate from a febrile egg or lung tissue usually contain virus. Proper treatment to eliminate bacteria and molds from test material is desirable to enhance viral isolation. After 72 to 96 hours of incubation the allantoic and amniotic fluids are tested for HA activity. If positive, the isolate is tested against influenza antisera for specificity.

The HI test is used most frequently in diagnosis when serology is applied. Paired sera are used. The first serum sample is taken during the acute phase of illness, and the second one is obtained 2 to 3 weeks later. A rising titer constitutes a positive test. The serologist must be aware of the possible presence of nonspecific inhibitors of hemagglutination and the methods by which the sera can be treated to remove them (12).

Prevention. Experimental vaccines have been produced with swine influenza virus, including a subunit vaccine, but none has been effective enough to become an article of commerce. Although the economic aspects of the disease are not known, it would appear there is a need for a safe and efficacious vaccine which probably would be more effective if administered by the respiratory route. Furthermore, techniques now are available for producing strains in the laboratory by recombinations that are safe and immunogenic (7), so it should be only a matter of time before a satisfactory vaccine is available to immunize pigs.

Careful nursing is important through the provision of comfortable and draft-free quarters with clean, dry, and dust-free bedding. Fresh, clean water and a good source of feed are essential. The animals should not be disturbed or moved during this period. Antibiotics and sulfonamides are useful on a herd basis to control secondary bacterial infections.

There is a considerable amount of research on potential antiviral substances that would effectively control influenza A viruses. All strains of influenza A continue to be sensitive to amantadine-HC1, but until now this drug has not been used in outbreaks of swine influenza. Antiviral activity was observed for 5-iododeoxyuridine in swine with influenza, but toxicity also was observed (25).

The Disease in Man. In recent years swine influenza virus has infected man. Antibodies in the serum of aged persons suggests that they had an infection with a swine influenza virus many years ago or with a human influenza virus that shared a common antigen(s) with the early swine strain. More recently influenza A viruses isolated from swine have transmitted the infection to man. Fortunately, no pandemics have been associated with these episodes (8).

REFERENCES

1. Andrewes, Laidlaw, and Smith. Lancet, 1934, *2*, 859.
2. Charley. Ann. Microbiol. (Paris), 1977, *128B*, 95.
3. DeJong and DeRonde-Verloop. Dev. Biol. Stand., 1977, *39*, 453.
4. Dorset, Niles, and McBryde. Jour. Am. Vet. Med. Assoc., 1922, *62*, 162.
5. Dowdle and Schild. Bull. Pan Am. Health Org., 1976, *10*, 193.
6. Easterday. In Diseases of swine, 3rd ed., ed. Howard W. Dunne. Iowa State Univ. Press., Ames, Iowa, 1970, p. 127.
7. Easterday. Swine Disease Supp., Jour. Am. Vet. Med. Assoc., 1972, *160*, 645.
8. Kaplan and Webster. Scientific Am., 1977, *237*, 86.
9. Köbe and Fertig. Zentrbl. f. Bakt., I Abt. Orig., 1938, *141*, 1.
10. Leif. Center for Disease Control, Zoonoses Surveil., Rpt. 5, 1965.
11. Lewis and Shope. Jour. Exp. Med., 1931, *54*, 361.
12. Nakamura and Easterday. Bull. World Health Org., 1967, *37*, 559.
13. Nakamura and Easterday. Cornell Vet., 1970, *60*, 27.
14. Orcutt and Shope. Jour. Exp. Med., 1935, *62*, 823.
15. Palese and Ritchey. Dev. Biol. Stand., 1977, *39*, 411.
16. Pirtle and Ritchie. Am. Jour. Vet. Res., 1975, *36*, 1783.
17. Renshaw. Am. Jour. Vet. Res., 1975, *36*, 5.
18. Scott. Jour. Bact., 1940, *40*, 327.
19. Scott. Vet. Extension Quart., June 1941, 1.
20. Shope. Jour. Exp. Med., 1931, *54*, 349.
21. Shope. Jour. Exp. Med., 1931, *54*, 373.
22. Shope. Jour. Exp. Med., 1935, *62*, 561.
23. Shope. Science, 1939, *89*, 441; Jour. Exp. Med., 1941, *74*, 49.
24. Shortridge, Webster, Butterfield, and Campbell. Science, 1977, *196*, 1454.
25. Steffenhagen, Easterday, and Galasso. Jour. Inf. Dis., 1976, *133*, 603.
26. Tumova and Pereira. Bull. World Health Org., 1968, *38*, 415.
27. Urman, Underdahl, and Young. Am. Jour. Vet. Res., 1958, *19*, 913.

Fowl Plague

SYNONYMS: Fowl pest, avian influenza virus(es)

Fowl plague usually is an acute, highly fatal disease of chickens, turkeys, pheasants, and certain wild birds. Ducks, geese, and other waterfowl are less susceptible but develop the disease at times. Natural infection among pigeons is uncommon. Artificial infection of ducks, geese, and pigeons by the injection of large amounts of virus from naturally infected chickens often fails. The signs of illness and lesions of fowl plague are similar to those of fowl cholera. It is caused by a virus that occurs in the blood and all organs and is readily filterable.

Fowl plague has been known since about 1880, when it was recognized in Italy as a separate disease. Early in the present century it spread throughout the greater part of Europe. The virus was brought into the United States illegally in 1923 by a laboratory worker. In the fall of 1924 the virus escaped from the laboratory into the New York poultry market, where it has been estimated to have killed more than 500,000 birds (16). From this market it spread to a considerable number of eastern poultry farms, probably on the contaminated crates of dealers, causing large losses. The disease was stamped out within 1 year by rigid quarantine methods. In 1965 in Canada (11) and later in the United States (18, 21) it was reported as an acute respiratory disease in turkeys with a high morbidity and a low mortality (21). Apparently it still exists in these countries and in most countries, if not all of the world. The disease in chickens occurred in laying flocks in 1976 with a substantial mortality and severe drop in egg production (9).

In recent years molecular virologists have used the fowl plague virus to study the genetics, biochemistry, and replication of influenzal viruses because convenient and accurate *in vitro* and *in vivo* systems exist to elucidate these areas of interest. As a consequence the literature on fowl plague virus has been quite voluminous, but it is outside the realm of this book to cover in depth these areas of molecular virology.

Character of the Disease. *In chickens.* The period of incubation is rather short—3 to 5 days as a rule. Inoculated birds may show signs with 24 to 36 hours. A high temperature rapidly develops (110 to 112 F), the appetite is lost, and the birds rapidly become lethargic. The comb and wattle commonly have whitish, necrotic areas of skin (Figure 49.3). A mucoid nasal discharge appears, and often edema of the head and neck develops. The hock may be swollen and discolored because of subcutaneous hemorrhage and edema (Figure 49.4). The course of the disease often is very rapid, death usually occurring within a few hours after the appearance of the first signs. The temperature commonly falls to subnormal shortly before death. The mortality rate sometimes is close to 100 percent.

The lesions generally are not numerous in acute cases. They consist of petechial hemorrhages on the heart, on the fatty tissue around the gizzard, on the serosa of the body cavity, and on the mucous membranes of the proventriculus. In some cases a serofibrinous exudate appears in the pericardial sac. The principal organs may show petechiae and cloudy swelling. The nervous system appears normal, but microscopic examination shows a diffuse encephalitis with cuffing of the blood vessels, degeneration of nerve cells, and necrotic foci around

Figure 49.3. Fowl plague in a chicken. The comb and wattles have whitish, necrotic areas of skin. (Courtesy D. A. Gregg, Plum Island Animal Disease Center, USDA.)

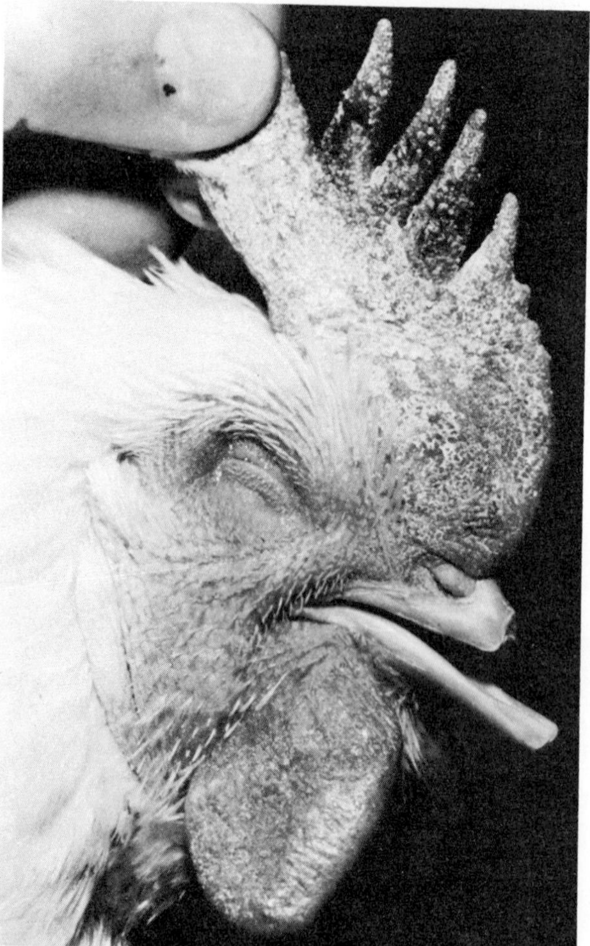

Figure 49.4. Fowl plague in a chicken. The hock is discolored, swollen, and hemorrhagic. (Courtesy D. A. Gregg, Plum Island Animal Disease Center, USDA.)

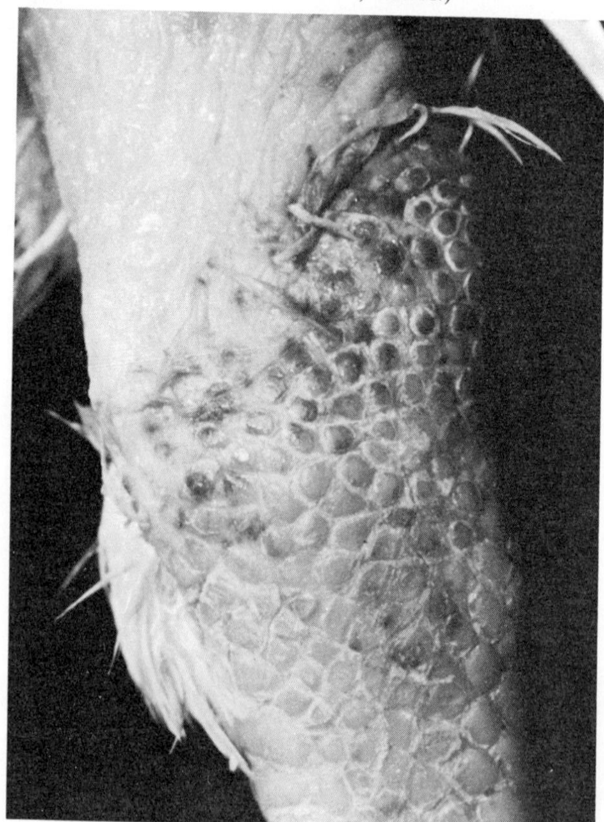

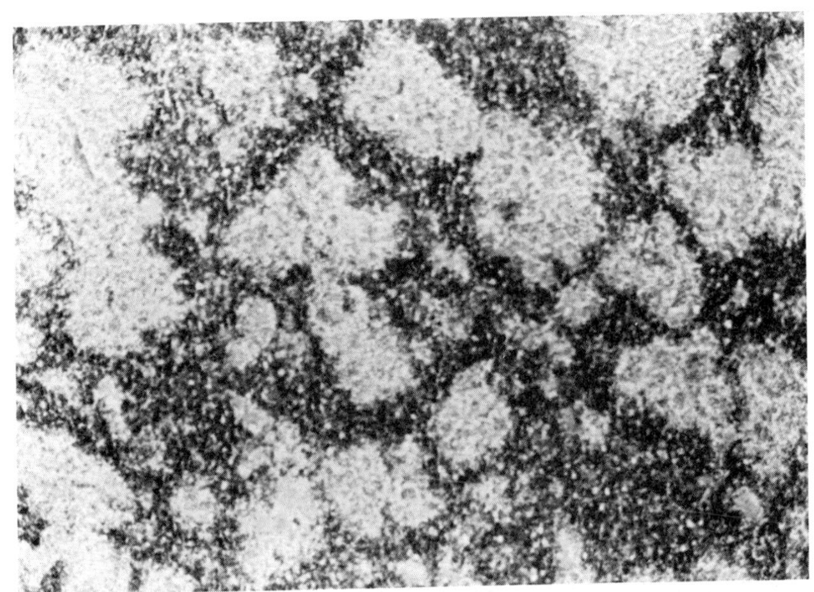

Figure 49.5. Photomicrograph of a spleen from a chicken infected with fowl plague virus. The light areas are necrotic lymphoid nodules. H and E stain. (Courtesy C. A. Mebus, Plum Island Animal Disease Center, USDA.)

which there is proliferation of glia cells. The spleen shows necrotic lymphoid nodules (Figure 49.5).

In turkeys. The first outbreaks in Canada occurred as an acute respiratory disease and a severe production problem in turkeys (11). The viral isolate designated A/Turkey/Can/63 (Wilmot) was related to the influenza A group of viruses. In transmission experiments the virus regularly produced sinusitis in turkey poults under 4 weeks of age but was apathogenic for older turkeys and chickens of any age. In contrast, a later isolate designated A/Turkey/Ontario/7732/66 was highly pathogenic for turkeys and chickens (12).

A Massachusetts isolate produced an air-sac disease in semimature turkeys characterized by depression and sudden but slight mortality (18). Its antigenic relationship to the Canadian Wilmot virus was demonstrated by the HI test.

The Wisconsin isolate is a type A influenza virus that produced an acute respiratory disease in turkeys (21). The disease, with a high morbidity and low mortality, was seen in nine breeding flocks in northwestern Wisconsin, and serologic evidence was demonstrated in 11 turkey flocks.

Properties of the Virus. Various test procedures are common for the study of avian influenza viruses, such as the complement-fixation, enzyme-linked immunosorbent assay, counterimmunoelectrophoresis, electron microscopy, indirect hemagglutination, hemagglutination, and serum-neutralization tests. The avian influenza viruses are members of the *Orthomyxovirus* Type A group. There is a wide range of antigenic variation, but no distinct subtypes have been designated. Six avian influenza virus strains have been listed as representative of the group: fowl plague, A/Duck/Czech/56, A/Duck/Eng/56, A/Chick/Scot/59, A/Turkey/Can/63 (Wilmot), and A/Quail/Italy/1117/65. Nine different hemagglutinins variant types have been recognized. Variant types 1 and 5 are pathogenic, but they must be present in the cleaved form indicating that the hemagglutinin alone is not responsible for pathogenicity—it is a sum of the total genome. Rott *et al.* (19) have provided conclusive evidence that the neuraminidase of influenza viruses plays a significant role in protection.

The virus particles are spherical, 80 to 100 nm in diameter (Figure 49.6). Associated filaments average 80 nm in diameter and are up to 8 μm in length (5). By electron microscopy Waterson *et al.* (22) showed that the avian virus resembled influenza A virus.

The ribonucleoprotein is a continuous strand, 6 nm in diameter, that is formed in the nucleus of infected cells (1), and the hemagglutinin is developed in the cytoplasm (3). Hemagglutination of red blood cells from fowl, rhesus monkeys, horses, and cattle has been demonstrated.

The avian viruses have a complement-fixing antigen common to the influenza A virus group. They also share hemagglutinins and neuraminidases with other species.

Cultivation. The virus multiplies readily in embryonated hens' eggs. A cytopathogenic effect is produced in cell cultures of various fowl and mammalian tissues. Attenuation of virus for fowls is reported after transfers in chick, pigeon, and human cell cultures (8).

Noninfectious virus particles produced by fowl plague virus in infected Ehrlich ascitic carcinoma cells have the

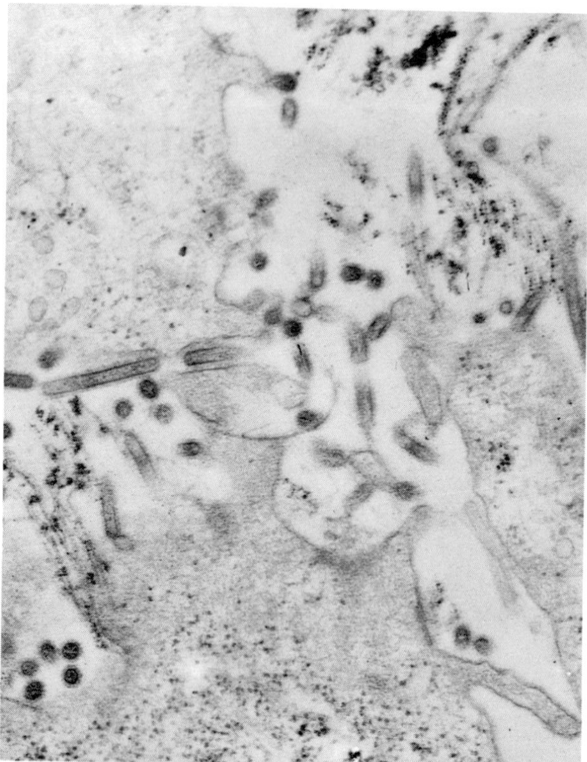

Figure 49.6. An electron microscope micrograph of fowl plague virus particles in infected cells of a chick embryo cell culture. × 38,400. (Courtesy S. S. Breese, Plum Island Animal Disease Center, USDA.)

same morphology, size, and sedimentation rate as standard virions. Apparently the particles are very fragile. In isopycnic fractionation the particles are detected in two forms. Particles with a density of 1.23 g per cm^3 retain their hemagglutinating but not neuraminidase activity. The other form has a density of 1.27 g per cm^3 but lacks both hemagglutinating and neuraminidase activity (7).

The virus has been known to grow in mouse peritoneal macrophages *in vitro,* and Lindenmann *et al.* (14) did some experiments to show that macrophages and resistance of mice are two facets of the same phenomenon.

Immunity. Recovered birds are solidly immune for several months at least. The serum of recovered birds will give a considerable degree of immunity to susceptible fowls, but, because the immunity probably is short-lived and the amount of such serum that can be obtained from immune birds is small, the method has no practical value.

There is a rather large European literature on vaccines for fowl plague. Attempts have been made to produce vaccines from blood and from tissues. Treatment with heat, phenol, glycerol, ether, and formaldehyde will weaken and finally destroy the virus. Moses, Brandly, Jones, and Jungherr (17) obtained a high degree of immunity, which persisted for 18 to 21 weeks, following vaccination with whole-egg adjuvant vaccines (inactivated virus) and with living variant virus. Daubney, Mansi, and Zaharan (4), in experiments designed to improve the quality of the inactivated fowl plague vaccines, noted that serial passage of one strain of plague virus through pigeon embryos resulted in a mutant which is completely nonpathogenic for domestic fowls, turkeys, and young pigeons, but which induces solid immunity against virulent fowl plague virus. A cold variant which is an attenuated virus derived by genetic recombination at 25 C in embryonating eggs provides protection against infection with virulent virus (15). There may be some reservation about its use as a vaccine because virus could be recovered from lung and turbinate (20). Through recombination of fowl plague virus with other influenza A viruses nonpathogenic for fowl, it is possible to produce a number of antigenic hybrids that are nonpathogenic for chickens. From these results it was concluded that the surface components do not by themselves determine the pathogenicity of influenza A viruses.

Transmission. Migratory birds are probably responsible for the spread of avian influenza viruses throughout the world (10). These birds can harbor the virus without showing signs of illness. Further, it has been shown that the virus can replicate in the intestinal tract of feral ducks and shed virus in high concentrations into water where it remains viable for days or weeks depending on water temperature (24). As a consequence, there is a real possibility that influenza viruses are transmitted between wild birds and domestic birds and eventually to mammals, including man, which helps to explain the epidemiology of the influenza viruses. Various investigators, including Fukumi *et al.* (6), have reported that some species of migrating ducks, such as pintail, mallard, widgeon, and falcated teal, possess in their sera antibodies against hemagglutinin antigens of human or avian influenza viruses. Kaplan and Webster conclude that, from an evolutionary point of view, the family of influenza viruses originated in the bird kingdom, an animal group some 100 million years old, and these birds now live in harmony with most of the influenza viruses without the production of disease.

Diagnosis. The enzyme-linked immunosorbent assay for antibodies is an excellent test whose sensitivity is 100 times greater than the complement-fixation or hemagglutination-inhibition tests (13). The isolation of virus also provides a positive approach in the diagnosis of the disease. The embryonating hen's egg is the most sensitive substrate for this purpose, although tissue culture can be employed as well.

Control. After the 1924–25 outbreak, fowl plague was diagnosed in the United States by Beaudette, Hudson, and Saxe (2) in 1929. The second outbreak was a small one, involving only a few flocks in New Jersey. It was brought under control, as was the earlier, larger outbreak, by rigid quarantine measures. These involved controls for shipping birds and also cleaning and disinfecting poultry crates, egg crates, and other objects that might carry virus from infected flocks to others. Vaccination methods were not used.

During the 1920s the disease was readily recognized by its characteristic signs and lesions and its high mortality in chickens. The infections in turkeys in the 1960s were clinically ill defined and moderate in severity and in two instances occurred as inapparent flock infections. To eliminate the disease in its present form from Canada and the United States would be formidable in costs and effort. Naturally, our government control officials are concerned with the potential danger that these avian influenza viruses pose to our commercial poultry flocks.

Vaccines could be used in outbreaks, but the constant drift and shift of influenza viruses pose a special problem, and the stockpiling of appropriate antigens for this purpose is not scientifically feasible at present (1979).

The Disease in Man. Epidemiological studies suggest that avian influenza viruses could conceivably infect man because avian and human strains may share common hemagglutinins. Recently a human case of keratoconjunctivitis that was caused by a fowl plague virus (HAV/1/NEQ/1) occurred as the result of a laboratory accident. The ease by which antigen hybrids of influenza viruses can be produced *in vivo* adds support to the concept that new influenza viruses can arise in nature that cause disease in humans (23).

REFERENCES

1. Almeida and Brand. Jour. Gen. Virol., 1975, *27,* 313.
2. Beaudette, Hudson, and Saxe. Jour. Agr. Res., 1934, *49,* 83.
3. Breitenfeld and Schäfer. Virol., 1957, *4,* 328.
4. Daubney, Mansi, and Zaharan. Jour. Comp. Path. and Therap., 1949, *29,* 1.
5. Dawson and Elford. Jour. Gen. Microbiol., 1949, *3,* 298.
6. Fukumi, Nerome, Nakayama, and Ishida. Dev. Biol. Stand., 1977, *39,* 475.
7. Gitel'man, Martynenko, Molibog, and Vorkunova. Vopr. Virusol., 1976, *6,* 713.
8. Hallauer and Kronauer. Arch. f. die gesam. Virusforsch., 1959, *9,* 232.
9. Johnson and Maxfield. Avian Dis., 1976, *20,* 422.
10. Kaplan and Webster. Scientific Am., 1977, *237,* 86.
11. Lang, Ferguson, Connell, and Wills. Avian Dis., 1965, *9,* 495.
12. Lang, Narayan, Rouse, Ferguson, and Connell. Can. Vet. Jour., 1968, *9,* 151.
13. Leinikki and Passila. Jour. Inf. Dis., 1977, *136,* 294.
14. Lindenmann, Deuel, Fanconi, and Haller. Jour. Exp. Med., 1978, *147,* 531.
15. Merritt and Maassab. Health Lab. Sci., 1977, *14,* 122.
16. Mohler. Jour. Am. Vet. Med. Assoc., 1925, *67,* 764.
17. Moses, Brandly, Jones, and Jungherr. Am. Jour. Vet. Res., 1948, *9,* 399.
18. Olesuik, Snoeyenbos, and Roberts. Avian Dis., 1967, *11,* 203.
19. Rott, Hecht, and Orlich. Jour. Gen. Virol., 1974, *22,* 35.
20. Rott, Orlich, and Scholtissek. Jour. Virol., 1976, *19,* 54.
21. Smithies, Radloff, Friedell, Albright, Misner, and Easterday. Avian Dis., 1969, *13,* 603.
22. Waterson, Rott, and Schäfer. Zeitschr. f. Naturforsch., 1961, *16,* 154.
23. Webster and Campbell. Virol., 1972, *48,* 528.
24. Webster, Hinshaw, Bean, Turner, and Shortridge. Dev. Biol. Stand., 1977, *39,* 461.

50 The Paramyxoviridae

In the family Paramyxoviridae there are three genera: *Paramyxovirus, Morbillivirus,* and *Pneumovirus*. The genus *Paramyxovirus* includes a number of pathogens including Newcastle disease virus, parainfluenza viruses 1-4, turkey paramyxovirus, Yucaipa virus, and mumps virus. A triad of important virus diseases—canine distemper, rinderpest, and measles—in addition to *peste de petite* ruminant virus comprises the genus *Morbillivirus*. Bachmann *et al.* (1) have isolated a paramyxoviruslike virus from the brain of a 15-month-old heifer with signs of encephalomyelitis. Tentatively it is placed in the genus until more information can be developed about its characteristics and relationship to other viruses and to disease. The syncytial-forming viruses of cats and cattle are included in the genus *Pneumovirus*. Important pathogens with salient features are listed in Table 50.1.

Viruses in this family contain 1 percent single-stranded RNA of a molecular weight 4 to 8 $\times$ 10^6 daltons. The spherical, enveloped particles range from 100 to 300 nm in diameter, with characteristic projections. The helical capsid is approximately 18 nm in diameter and 1 μm long. Some particles contain more than one nucleocapsid. The particles are ether-sensitive, but they are antigenically stable. There are two main serological subgroups. Some viruses possess neuraminidase. All accepted members cause hemagglutination except that some such as canine distemper and rinderpest viruses do not contain hemagglutinins. Mostly, the nucleocapsids develop in the cytoplasm and are resistant to dactinomycin. Genetic recombination does not occur.

REFERENCE

1. Bachmann, Ter Meulen, Jentsch, Appel, Iwasaki, Meyermann, Koprowski, and Mayr. Arch Virol., 1975, *48*, 107.

THE GENUS *MORBILLIVIRUS*

Canine Distemper

SYNONYM: Carré's disease; abbreviation, CD

Distemper is a worldwide disease of young dogs. It is highly contagious and manifested by a diphasic fever curve, acute coryza, and later bronchitis and catarrhal pneumonia, severe gastroenteritis, and nervous signs. The initiating agent is a filterable virus, first described by Carré (13), but many of the pathological changes in naturally occurring cases are due to bacterial complications. Carré's studies were not generally accepted until the classical reports of Laidlaw and Dunkin (18, 19, 39, 40, 41). Investigators in England in 1948 (43) described a disease in dogs which they termed *hard pad disease*. This is simply one of the many manifestations that CD produces.

There are many review articles about canine distemper (2, 4, 21, 27). The authors used these, and the AVMA canine distemper symposium proceedings, to good advantage in preparing this section (11).

Character of the Disease. CD causes the death or permanent disability of more young dogs than any other disease. The disease also occurs in wolves, foxes, jackals, badgers, stoats, weasels, grisons, lesser pandas, kinkajous, coatis, coyotes, dingoes, raccoons, and mink Ermine and martens are said to be susceptible by inoculation. Ferrets are exceedingly susceptible to distemper virus and almost always die of the disease. For this reason they are used frequently as experimental animals. There is an infectious disease of cats which is sometimes called *distemper,* but this disease has a different etiology. None of the other domesticated animals or man is susceptible to the virus of canine distemper, although inapparent experimental infection has been produced in the domestic cat (2).

CD occurs in all parts of the world where dogs are raised. It is a disease of young dogs that is especially common in cities, dog colonies, or other places where there are many contacts with other dogs. Puppies born of immune mothers acquire a passive immunity through the colostral milk which protects them until that immunity is lost. Unless the young dog is raised in relative isolation from other dogs, it is likely to develop the disease at this time. Farm dogs, which often live in relative isolation, may escape distemper entirely, or perhaps have it when they are old. Old dogs are not immune to distemper because of age, but only because they have had previous contacts with the virus.

The onset of the disease is usually manifested by a watery discharge from the eyes and nose, lassitude, inappetence, and fever, which may reach 105 F or higher. The lachrymal discharge may become purulent within 24 hours. The initial temperature rise lasts about 2 days and is followed by a period of 2 or 3 days in which the temperature may be nearly or quite normal. During this time the animal may feel better and may eat its food. This is followed by a secondary temperature rise which may last for several weeks. Again the dog feels badly, there is no appetite, vomiting usually occurs, pneumonia frequently develops, and in many cases a severe, fetid diarrhea appears. The feces are watery, mixed with mucus, offensive, and often bloody. Under these conditions the dog loses weight rapidly and usually becomes a sad spectacle. The death rate is high; hence the prognosis should be guarded.

In a few young dogs affected with distemper, a skin eruption appears with the initial temperature. This consists of pustules, which occur on the abdomen, the inside of the thighs, and elsewhere. As the animal recovers, these dry up and disappear. Because these lesions are not seen in the pure virus infections, they must be looked upon as secondary bacterial infections.

Nervous manifestations may occur. There seem to be enzootics, cyclic in nature, during which numerous puppies show nervous signs. On occasions catarrhal signs are not severe and the nervous signs predominate. Dogs with nervous manifestations have a syndrome characterized by several or all of the following signs: depression, myalgia, myoclonus, incoordination, circling, epileptiform convulsions, and coma. In general when dogs show convulsions, death results. In some cases chorea and paralysis may remain after other signs subside. Old dog encephalitis also may be another form of canine distemper.

In the early febrile stage of the disease leukopenia occurs, but later if bacterial infection is not controlled by treatment, a marked leukocytosis appears.

Dunkin and Laidlaw (19), who worked with a pure virus and with dogs raised in strict isolation, were able to show that the uncomplicated virus infections produced severe signs in many cases but with a relatively low death rate. The high mortality usually seen in this disease was undoubtedly due, in most cases, to complications of bacterial infections to which the animal is predisposed by the action of the virus before the introduction of the sulfonamides and antibiotics. Now, mortality is usually the result of viral action on the central nervous system.

It has become obvious in recent years that another virus disease, *infectious canine hepatitis,* is often confused with distemper and that both diseases may occur in a dog simultaneously. There is no interference between the viruses of these two diseases, according to Gillespie, Robinson, and Baker (26). In experiments, dogs infected with both viruses develop a more severe type of illness than is seen in others receiving only one virus. Both viruses are recovered from the blood of such dogs, and the typical inclusion bodies of both viruses are found in their tissues.

Dunkin and Laidlaw found the incubation period to be remarkably constant. In most dogs the febrile reaction began on the 4th day following exposure. Rarely it occurred on the 3rd day, occasionally on the 5th, and rarely on the 6th.

The course of the disease varies greatly, depending on the character and severity of the secondary complications. In uncomplicated cases the dogs may show very mild signs, which may not be recognized, or the animal may suffer a febrile illness, which may last 2 weeks or longer. When complicated with catarrhal pneumonia and enteritis, the course may be much longer. Nervous signs may be evident for many weeks after recovery from all other signs.

Table 50.1. Diseases in domestic animals caused by viruses in the Paramyxoviridae family

Common name of virus	Natural hosts	Type of disease produced
Genus *Morbillivirus*		
Canine distemper	Dogs, other canines, ferrets, and mink	Highly contagious disease of young dogs manifested by diphasic temperature curve, acute coryza, followed by bronchitis and catarrhal pneumonia, severe gastroenteritis and, occasionally, nervous signs. Morbidity high; mortality varies, largely dependent on development of nervous manifestations
Rinderpest	Cattle, water buffaloes, sheep, and perhaps goats	A very important disease in cattle and water buffaloes that occurs in Asia and and Africa. It is an acute febrile disease with lesions largely confined to the digestive tract with ulceration and hemorrhages in the pharynx and larynx and throughout the rest of the tract including Peyer's patches. The respiratory tract shows reddening and often petchiation and a patchy pneumonia. In a susceptible population it is explosive with a high morbidity and mortality
Genus *Paramyxovirus*		
Newcastle disease	Chickens, turkeys, guinea fowl, ducks, geese, pheasants, and many wild avian species	The intensity of the disease varies markedly depending on the virulence of the viral strain involved. The disease usually begins with respiratory signs followed by diarrhea and then nervous signs, particularly by involving younger chickens. The disease spreads rapidly with a high morbidity and a variable mortality
Parainfluenza 3	Cattle	One agent involved in shipping fever syndrome of cattle. Acute respiratory signs and distress accompanied by fever, inappetence, and depression. Morbidity and mortality likely to be high. Stress and concurrent infections contribute to the severity of the disease

The death rate varies widely depending on the breed, age, kind of nursing care, and treatment given. It probably averages about 20 percent.

Distemper virus has an affinity for lymphatic and epithelial cells. The viral antigen first appears in the bronchial lymph nodes and tonsils 24 hours after exposure to virus as determined by immunofluorescence. It appears in the mononuclear cells of the blood by the second or third day followed by widespread dissemination by the ninth day. This accounts for the widespread appearance of lesions in the dog. In the skin a vesicular and pustular dermatitis occur. These changes are confined to the Malpighian layer of the epidermis, but congestion of the dermis usually occurs and lymphocytic infiltration may occur. Proliferation of the keratin layer of the footpad epidermis results in a hardened pad which British investigators have termed *hard pad disease*. The urinary epithelium may show vascular congestion with cytoplasmic and intranuclear inclusion bodies. These occur particularly in the bladder and renal pelvis. Few

Table 50.1.—*continued*

Common name of virus	Natural hosts	Type of disease produced
SV-5 parainfluenza	Dogs	In outbreaks the disease is severe and probably involves other pathogens as well. There is a sudden onset, copious nasal discharge, fever, and coughing resembling a disease called *kennel cough*
Parainfluenza 3	Sheep	Respiratory disease comparable to parainfluenza 3 infections in cattle. Virus strains in sheep comparable but not identical to bovine and human PI-3 viruses
Parainfluenza 3	Horses	Rather obscure disease. Respiratory signs observed in diseased foals or yearlings. The infection may be common in horses
Sendai virus (parainfluenza virus 1)	Swine, humans	In swine, reputedly causes bronchopneumonia in young pigs and abortions in sows in Japan
Yucaipa	Chickens	Causes respiratory illness
Mumps	Cats, dogs, humans	Present evidence suggests that cats and dogs are susceptible to mumps and it occasionally can produce clinical disease
Genus *Pneumovirus*		
Feline syncytium-forming viruses	Cats	Although the virus has been associated with various disease entities, its role as a pathogen has never been established, but it may act in concert with other proven viral pathogens
Bovine syncytium-forming viruses	Cattle	Certain viral isolates produce respiratory disease characterized by pyrexia and rhinitis and histological evidence of pneumonia. The human respiratory syncytial virus causes disease in experimental calves; it is not known if BSV causes disease in man

lesions are observed in the stomach and intestine; however, cytoplasmic acidophilic inclusion bodies may be found in the epithelial lining. Intranuclear acidophilic inclusions also may be seen occasionally in these cells. Excessive mucus is often seen in the large intestine. A catarrhal or purulent bronchopneumonia where bronchi and alveoli are filled with exudate was found more commonly before the introduction of the sulfa drugs and antibiotics. In other cases mononuclear cells lining alveolar walls or partially filling the alveoli are the only evidence of involvment. Epithelioid cells with fused cytoplasm (giant cells) line the bronchioles and alveoli adjacent to the pleura, and it appears microscopically as a giant-cell pneumonia. Inclusion bodies are found in giant cells, other mononuclear cells, and bronchiolar and bronchial epithelium. The spleen may be grossly enlarged, and congested necrosis of lymphoid cells in the splenic follicles may be observed microscopically. In uncomplicated cases the most significant change is a size reduction of the thymus gland, which may be gelatinous. Degenerative changes may occur in the adrenal, usually in the cortex.

Intraocular lesions associated with CD were described by Jubb *et al.* (32). Leukocytes infiltrate the ciliary body. Exudative or degenerative changes are seen in retinal ganglion cells and proliferation in pigment epithelium. Edema causes focal retinal detachments. Ulcerative keratitis sometimes complicates a purulent conjunctivitis.

The urinary and reproductive organs may show lesions. The transitional epithelium of the urinary tract appears swollen and hydropic. Urinary bladder and kidney pelvis epithelium have many inclusion bodies. Mild interstitial epididymitis and orchitis are common.

Dogs with nervous manifestations may show perivascular cuffing, nonsuppurative, leptomeningitis, and vacuoles in the white matter. Many Purkinje cells show degenerative changes. Numerous cells show pyknosis whereas other cells appear swollen and their Nissl granules are small and indistinct. Some Purkinje cells fade so that they are almost unrecognizable. Gliosis is seen in the cerebellum and is most marked in those dogs that develop nervous manifestations a considerable time after onset of infection. Degenerated myelin is not demonstrable in the cerebellum of experimental dogs that are destroyed after displaying nervous signs 7 to 16 days after intracerebral inoculation with Snyder Hill strain (25). Demyelinization accompanied by usual gitter cells and by intranuclear inclusion bodies in glial cells are found in the cerebellums of dogs with nervous manifestations observed at the longer intervals. These data lend support to the concept that demyelinization may be the response of a self-imposed antigen-antibody reaction. However, a direct effect by the virus on oligodendroglia cells that produce myelin has to be considered. By electron microscopy, crystal-like structures similar to CD nucleocapsid are seen in the cytoplasm of endothelial and adventitial cells of meningeal veins and arteries, in the endothelium of cortical and plexus capillaries, in mononuclear cells within the lumen of blood vessels, in histiocytes and macrophages within the arachnoid space, in reactive microglia cells, and in ependymal cells (5).

The Disease in Experimental Animals. *In ferrets.* Ferrets are exceedingly susceptible to the virus of CD (18). Natural outbreaks of the disease often occur, and the mortality is very nearly 100 percent. The disease is readily transmitted through the air. Dunkin and Laidlaw (18) found that they could not keep normal ferrets in the same building with those infected with virus, no matter how much care was used to prevent the spread of the virus. They concluded that the virus was airborne.

The incubation period is about 10 days as a rule, but may occasionally be 1 or 2 days shorter. A watery discharge from the eyes and the nose indicates the onset of the disease. This quickly becomes purulent, and the eyelids become swollen and pasted together. The chin becomes reddened and small vesicles form around the mouth where the hair meets the naked skin of the lips. The feet swell, the footpads become red, and sometimes the skin of the abdomen reddens. On the 3rd day the vesicles on the chin become pustules and the animal remains curled up in the cage, refusing all food. It becomes weaker and generally dies on the 5th or 6th day. Occasionally one lives longer and develops pneumonia or nervous signs, but ultimately it almost always dies.

Heath (31) has described a neurotropic strain of CD virus. After a few passages in ferrets in which typical signs were produced, the signs changed suddenly and nervous manifestations predominated in ferrets inoculated thereafter. The incubation period became longer (about 16 days). Some animals died suddenly without manifesting any signs. Others exhibited intermittent convulsions and died 2 to 4 days after the first spasms were seen.

In dogs. Susceptible dogs will exhibit the typical picture of acute distemper when inoculated with virus. Some virus strains develop neurotropic properties for dogs and will cause a high percentage of cases in which nervous signs are prominent (25, 44). In susceptible puppies 1 to 2 weeks of age, the only signs of illness are hemorrhagic diarrhea, dehydration, and inappetence, terminating usually in death 2 weeks after the onset of illness (23). In studies with the R252 strain, 85 percent of gnotobiotic dogs less than 1 week of age died of acute encephalitis 2 to 5 weeks after infection. The percentage of mortality was considerably lower in older dogs. Physiological immaturity may account for the difference (37).

The distribution of CDV in the CNS was examined in 11 dogs with demyelinating encephalitis by the direct fluorescent antibody test (55). In the gray matter there was a good correlation between the presence and severity of lesions and presence and amount of viral antigen. Large amounts of virus were found in the neurons and their processes. In most demyelinating lesions small amounts of viral antigen were found and mostly located in the astrocytes which presumably play an important part in this process.

In hamsters. Cabasso, Douglas, Stebbins, and Cox (9) reported success in adapting a chick-embryo-adapted strain of CD virus to suckling hamsters. At the time of their report they had passed it through 16 generations. The infected animals died 4 to 7 days following inoculation. Proof of the identity of strain was provided by serum-neutralization tests and by the successful immunization of ferrets.

In suckling mice. CD virus was first adapted to suckling mice by Morse, Chow, and Brandly (45). Intracerebral inoculation of chick-embryo-adapted strains into suckling mice produced nervous manifestations and death.

In nonhuman primates. Encephalomyelitis was induced by a neurovirulent strain of CDV (59). Intracerebral inoculation produced histologic lesions in monkeys comparable to those described in the dog.

Properties of the Virus. Ultrafiltration experiments by Palm and Black (48) gave a particle size between 115 and 160 nm in diameter. Subsequent electron-microscope photomicrographs of Cruickshank *et al.* (16) showed that most particles ranged between 150 and 300 nm. Electron-microscope photomicrographs show that the central core contains helices 15 to 17 nm in diameter (16) (Figure 50.1). Filamentous forms of virus are described. It is an ether-sensitive RNA virus.

The virus remains viable for years at −70 C. Lyophilization provides a convenient method to preserve CDV in the laboratory and for commercial use. Either lyophilized virulent or attenuated virus, provided the moisture content is low, can be maintained at approximately 6 C for years with little or no loss of titer.

Various chemical compounds have virucidal activity for CD virus, including 0.75 percent formalin (14). Hydroxylamine inactivates the virus under certain conditions. Beta-propriolactone in a final concentration of 0.1 percent inactivates CDV within 2 hours at 37 C (7).

A complement-fixing antigen can be demonstrated in infective spleen and in the chorioallantoic membrane of infected hens' eggs. Phillips and Bussell (49) separated three stable CF antigens by cesium chloride gradient centrifugation of the Onderstepoort egg-adapted strain of CDV. One antigen probably is a protein with a buoyant density of 1.289, and the other two probably are lipoproteins with densities of 1.234 and 1.140.

The plate and microscope slide procedures of the agar-gel diffusion test of Ouchterlony have been used to study CDV. Soluble antigens distinct from the infective particle precipitate specific antibody. Antigen can be derived from tissue fragments of mesenteric lymph node or spleen of infected animals or from supernatant fluid of infective tissue-culture fluids. An electroprecipitin test also has been reported for viral detection by Zydeck (60).

The immunofluorescence test has been used effectively in pathogenesis studies of the dog because viral antigen is readily demonstrated in tissue cells (2). It has been located in inclusion bodies of infected dog tissues (46) and also in the raccoon (Figure 50.2). Yamanouchi *et al.* (58) claimed V and S antigen formed in cytoplasm because intranuclear fluorescence in tissue-cultured cells appeared only after 48 to 72 hours and a single growth cycle is approximately 18 hours. Complete virus on cell surfaces fluoresced indicating activity against V antigen. Activity against S antigen was not observed.

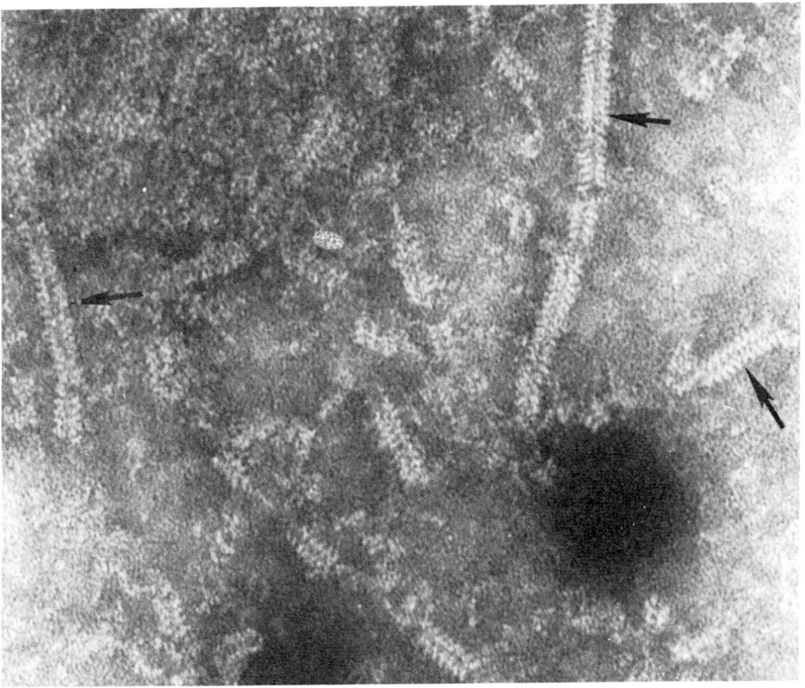

Figure 50.1. Helical cores (*arrows*) of CDV. × 225,000. (Courtesy J. Almeida.)

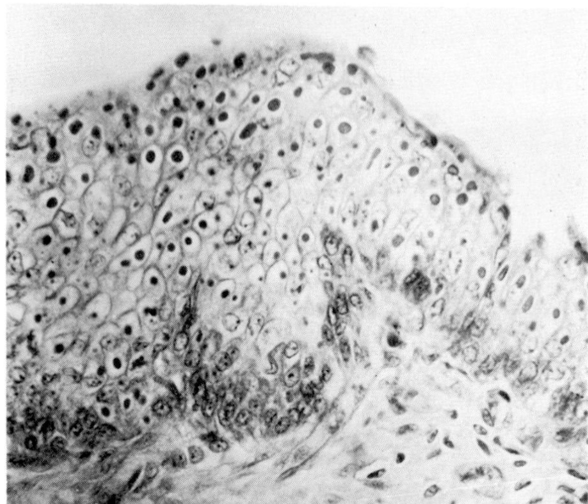

Figure 50.2. Canine distemper inclusion bodies in the urinary bladder of a raccoon. The bodies are located in the epithelial cells. They are not always as numerous as in this case. × 600.

Vladimirov (56) has reported that CDV causes hemagglutination of human and frog erythrocytes at dilutions of 1:40 and 1:320. These results have not been confirmed. The blood cells from many other animal species including the dog are not hemagglutinated by CDV.

The virus of CD, like measles virus, is sensitive to light in fluid suspension and during viral replication. Calf serum or glutathione reduced the inactivation rate of CDV. Certain components of tissue-culture media enhanced light sensitivity, but their presence was not essential for light inactivation. It has been suggested that a substance derived from the host cell that is incorporated into the viral overcoat serves to make CDV light-sensitive (2).

Neutralizing antibodies are formed and can be demonstrated in various systems such as the embryonated hens' eggs, suckling hamsters, suckling mice, ferrets, dogs, and various tissue culture systems. The chick embryo system has been used mostly for immunity studies in the dog. The agar-gel diffusion test has been used to study the viral antigenicity.

With various serological tests and protection tests in animals it has been possible to determine that the viruses of measles, canine distemper, and rinderpest of cattle share some common antigenic material. There is some similarity in the lesions which they produce in their respective susceptible hosts and in certain tissue-culture systems.

Cultivation. Haig (30) in 1948 reported success in cultivating a ferret-adapted strain of CD virus on the chorioallantoic membrane of embryonated chicks. The lesions appear as grayish white thickenings. He had carried the strain through 30 generations at the time of his report. During the following year Cabasso and Cox (8) reported success with a dog-passage strain. This strain retained virulence for ferrets until the 24th to 28th serial passage, when it lost virulence but retained immunizing properties. This strain is the basis of a commercial vaccine.

In 1951 Dedie (17) reported successful cultivation of CD virus in tissue culture. Rockborn (54) propagated the virus in dog kidney monolayer cultures, and it produced syncytia, intranuclear and cytoplasmic inclusion bodies, and stellate cells. In chick embryo cell cultures, egg-adapted virus produced cellular granulation and fragmentation without the formation of syncytia (33). Isolation of virulent CDV in tissue culture is difficult, although it has been done in various cell systems. Dog lung macrophages give good results (Figure 50.3). Once adapted to embryonating eggs or tissue culture the virus can be propagated in a large number of primary and stable cell cultures derived from canine, mustelid, avian, bovine, simian, and human tissues (2). Karzon and Bussell (33) used the plaque overlay method to quantitate virus or antibody.

Immunity. Dogs that recover from an infection with canine distemper virus usually are immune for life. CDV produces an antibody-mediated and a cell-mediated response, while measles virus causes only a cell-mediated response in dogs (20). Antibody titers vary inversely with the disease severity. Recovered dogs have the highest titers, whereas fatally infected dogs have little or no antibody activity. Dogs with chronic persistent infection form a third group with intermediate antibody levels. The inability to produce antibodies to envelope antigens may be a crucial factor in the establishment of a persistent infection (38). Although immunodepressive effects can be demonstrated *in vitro,* complete suppression of immune functions in the course of CDV infection in the dog does not occur (34). A rapid method for the *in vivo* assessment of cell-mediated immunity in the dog are the intradermal mitogen tests (35).

The virus is so widespread that most dogs, except a few that lead sheltered lives, have had the infection before they are 1 year old and are immune. The duration of immunity persisted in dogs retained in isolation for at least 7 years (2). Occasionally older dogs with a history

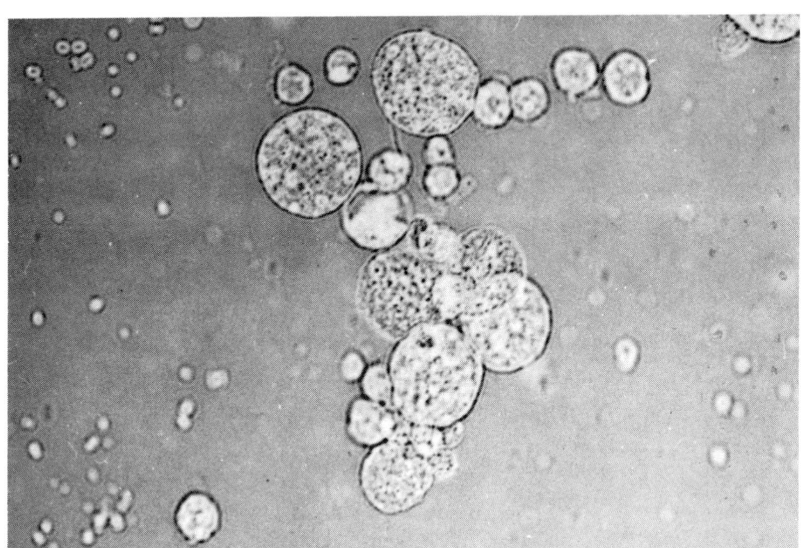

Figure 50.3. The effects of Snyder Hill strain of CDV in dog macrophage culture. × 360. (Courtesy M. Appel.)

of previous vaccination that reside in an urban community develop clinical distemper. Immunity challenge in dogs is difficult to evaluate because contact-exposure to diseased dogs is unreliable and parenteral inoculation does not result in frank disease in some susceptible dogs. A more reliable method is the intracerebral challenge with brain-adapted strains of CDV. Ferrets are often used as test animals as the mortality ranges between 90 and 100 percent. Ferrets given egg-attenuated virus vaccine are immune for at least 5 years.

Neutralizing antibody has been used as a means of evaluating the duration of immunity. Concurrent with protection in dogs, neutralizing antibody appears which at present serves as the only *in vitro* method for measuring immunity. A maternal antibody titer of 1:100 or greater can be correlated with absolute protection against intracerebral or aerosol challenge with the Snyder Hill strain of CDV. Dogs with maternal titers of less than 1:20 are susceptible. On the other hand, dogs given inactivated CD virus or measles virus had little or no measurable neutralizing CD antibody. When these dogs are challenged, no frank disease is produced and they react with an anamnestic antibody response. Consequently, the amount of neutralizing antibody is only a relative index of protection in the dog.

At an American Veterinary Medical Association symposium on canine distemper, the Committee on Standardized Methods and Test Procedures made recommendations for the standardization of the neutralization test (11). These recommendations were based on the statistical evaluation tests of Robson *et al.* (53). Neutralization tests are performed in various tissue-culture systems: embryonated hens' eggs, mice, ferrets, dogs, and suckling hamsters with the properly adapted viral test strain used in each system. Neutralizing antibodies first appear in the circulation 8 to 9 days after aerosol exposure to virulent virus with maximal titers reached at 4 weeks with serum levels ranging from 1:300 to 1:3,000 when tested against approximately 10^2 EID_{50} (egg infective $dose_{50}$) of virus. Titers to vaccine virus are slightly lower. The main fraction of CD-neutralizing antibody is found in gamma globulin fraction of the serum. CD-neutralizing antibody is found in the cerebral spinal fluid of most dogs with demyelinating CD encephalitis. The majority of these dogs have a marked elevation of IgG and also an increase in IgM in the CSF.

Complement-fixing antibodies develop 3 to 4 weeks after initial infection but persist for only a few weeks thereafter. Consequently, this test offers a means by which a recent initial infection can be diagnosed. Dogs given inactivated virus develop CF antibodies that rapidly disappear. Upon challenge with virulent virus a few months later CF titers appear in 4 to 8 days which persist for at least 7 months at significant levels (24).

CD distemper antibody produced with the Rockborn strain of CDV inhibits the hemagglutination of monkey erythrocytes by Tween 80 ether-treated measles virus. In contrast, CD distemper antibody produced by the Snyder Hill strain of CDV failed, yet the serum-neutralization tests of both antiserums were similar.

Puppies, born of immune mothers, obtain an effective immunity from the mother, but this is passive antibody and disappears within a few weeks. This passive neutralizing antibody is transferred *in utero* (3 percent) (Figure 50.4) and by combined placental and colostral antibody transfer equivalent to 77 percent of the mother's

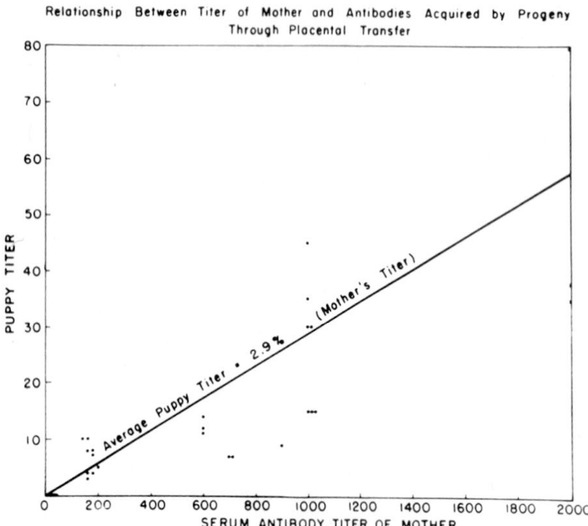

Figure 50.4. Canine distemper. Relationship between titer of mother and antibodies acquired by progeny through placental transfer. (Courtesy J. Gillespie, J. Baker, J. Burgher, D. Robson, and B. Gilman, *Cornell Vet.*)

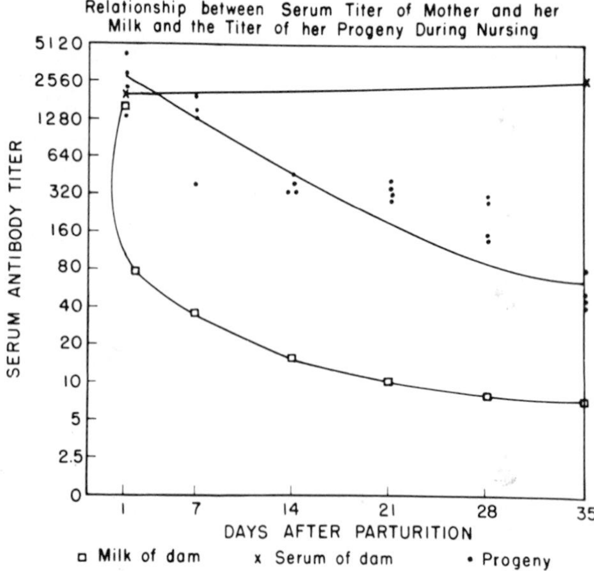

Figure 50.5. Canine distemper. Relationship between serum titer of mother and her milk and the serum titer of her progeny during nursing. (Courtesy J. Gillespie, J. Baker, J. Burgher, D. Robson, and B. Gilman, *Cornell Vet.*)

serum titer. The half-life of maternally transferred distemper antibody is 8.4 days (23) (Figure 50.5).

Until recently it was believed that very young puppies were not capable of producing distemper antibodies. These failures now can be attributed to maternal immunity interference or improper immunization. No effect of age on distemper antibody was discernible when the nomograph was used to determine this age (Figure 50.6). Titers produced in puppies of any age group to egg-virus vaccine are identical (23). Puppies that do not suckle their immune mothers and receive no colostrum can be vaccinated at 2 weeks of age because the amount of antibody transferred *in utero* is relatively small.

Transmission. This disease is transmitted principally by droplet infection, virus being present in abundance in the serous excretions which run from the eyes and nose during the early febrile stage of the disease. Dunkin and Laidlaw found that it was impossible to keep susceptible dogs in the same room with infected dogs without the former becoming infected, no matter what precautions were taken. In their experimental work they set up individual kennels 100 to 150 feet apart, depending upon air dilution to prevent the passage of virus from one to another. This generally succeeded, but there were some instances when they believed that infected droplets had bridged these gaps.

The urine and fecal material contain virus and are capable of transmitting the disease. Kennels, runs, and other places haunted by dogs generally harbor virus. Arthropod carriers of this virus have not been found.

There is a suggestion that transplacental transmission of CDV in dogs may occur (36).

Diagnosis. A positive diagnosis is assured by the isolation of CD virus. The finding of typical cytoplasmic or intranuclear inclusion bodies in affected tissues is presumptive evidence for a definite diagnosis. The possible persistence of inclusion bodies could conceivably lead to a false-positive diagnosis unless supported by serological or virological evidence.

Distemper is a pantropic infection, so virus can be readily isolated from the blood, lymph nodes, spleen, lung, liver, and other visceral organs during the acute stage of infection by ferret or dog inoculation. It has also been isolated from the brain of dogs with epileptiform convulsions long after it was possible to isolate virus from the blood (25). No virus was isolated from the blood, urine, and brains of fully recovered dogs injected with virulent virus 30 days earlier.

The fluorescent antibody technique is used to demonstrate the presence of antigen in inclusion bodies observed in mononuclear cells in the blood (15). This method is used to diagnose distemper.

Generally, susceptible dogs or ferrets are used for the primary isolation of CD virus. The response in dogs can

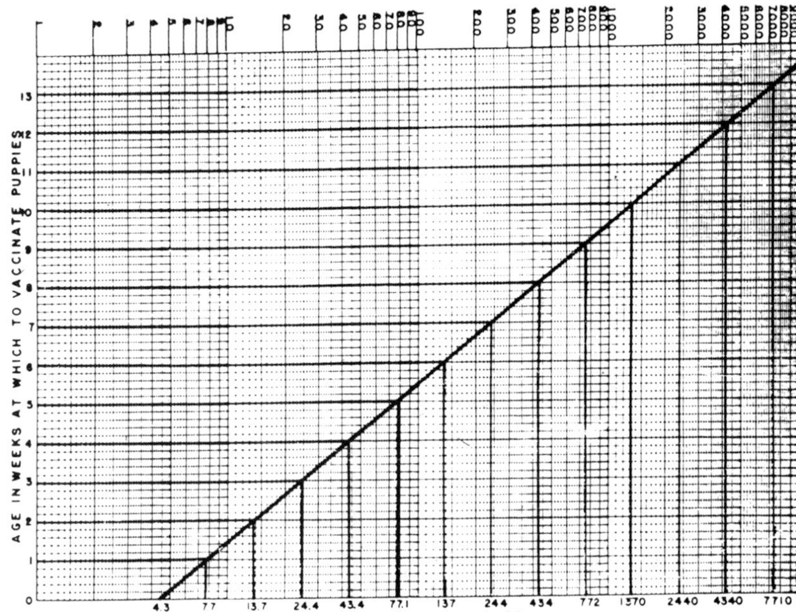

Figure 50.6. A nomograph for CD showing relationship between serum titer of mother and the age in weeks at which to vaccinate her progeny. (Courtesy J. Baker, D. Robson, J. Gillespie, J. Burgher, and P. Doty, *Cornell Vet.*)

be slight, so the use of paired sera samples to demonstrate a rising antibody titer is essential in these instances. Less reliable results are obtained by isolation attempts in dog tissue culture systems unless dog macrophages are used. The use of hens' eggs, suckling mice, and suckling hamsters for primary isolation is inadvisable because these hosts respond only to adapted strains.

The clinical diagnosis of canine distemper has, in the past, been considered a relatively simple matter. It is now quite certain that under this single designation several different diseases of dogs have been included in the past. Probably the most important of these is infectious hepatitis, although the enteric viruses have assumed great importance. A specific diagnosis of distemper, obviously, is not simple. It has already been pointed out that neither signs of illness nor lesions are pathognomonic of the disease.

The Relationship of the Virus of CD to Certain Other Viruses. In 1957 Adams and Imagawa (1) found that a strain of the virus of human measles was neutralized by the serum of ferrets which had been actively immunized against CD virus. The serum of normal ferrets had no such effect. These neutralization studies were conducted in a tissue-culture system. In animal studies, ferrets that had been immunized with measles virus showed partial protection when challenged with CD virus. Also, a mouse-adapted strain of CD virus was completely neutralized by measles antiserum prepared in ferrets.

Pursuing the matter further, Cabasso, Kiser, and Stebbins (10) found that puppies vaccinated against CD developed high levels of homologous antibodies but failed to develop either neutralizing or complement-fixing antibodies for measles virus. Similarly chickens, hyperimmunized against CD virus, did not develop antibodies for measles, although their homologous titers were high.

Most dogs immunized with measles virus developed low distemper neutralizing titers and excellent homotypic antibody titers (24). On challenge with a brain-adapted strain of CD virus all dogs were protected, but the controls sickened and some died. The mechanism of protection depended on a rapid secondary response of distemper antibody following the distemper challenge (24).

The relationship of measles virus (MV) and CDV in animal species is variable (2). Monkeys infected with MV react like humans and produce antibodies to both viruses. Infection of ferrets, rabbits, and guinea pigs with MV produce measles antibody titers but only low distemper neutralizing antibody titers in some of the animals, even after two infections with MV. Ferrets immunized with MV are partially protected against DV challenge. When CDV is inoculated into various species, production of MV antibody is found less frequently and protection against MV less effective.

Polding and Simpson (51) in East Africa, noting that a group of dogs that were constantly in intimate contact with cattle suffering from rinderpest remained free from CD, wondered if the apparent protection stemmed from exposure to rinderpest virus. They tested the hypothesis by injecting rinderpest virus into a group of CD-susceptible dogs and, after 25 days, inoculated these and a similar group of nontreated dogs with CD virus. Those injected with rinderpest virus remained healthy; those that were not so treated developed distemper. Later, Polding *et al.* (52) inoculated cattle with CD virus. No clinically recognized response was elicited, and all later proved susceptible to rinderpest when challenged with virus. Again, a group of dogs given a single dose of rinderpest virus later proved refractory to CD virus, but it was observed that other dogs, given large doses of antirinderpest immune serum, received only slight protection against a subsequent inoculation with CD virus.

For more information about CDV, MV, and rinderpest the reader is referred to the monograph by Appel and Gillespie (2).

Immunization. At the American Veterinary Medical Association symposia (1965 and 1969) the panels made recommendations for the immunization of dogs against canine distemper, and these recommendations are still valid. The recommendations have led to a more standardized approach by the veterinary profession to the prevention and control of this most important disease. The panels' recommendations are incorporated into this section on immunization.

Passive immunization of dogs. The first individuals to produce an antiserum for CD were Lockhart, Ray, and Barbee (42) in 1925. These workers hyperimmunized immune dogs by injections of virus-blood removed from susceptible dogs that had been injected with virus and were suffering a febrile reaction.

Laidlaw and Dunkin (39) prepared an immune serum by hyperimmunizing dogs that had recovered from an injection of virus about 1 month previously. The hyperimmunization was accomplished by making two subcutaneous injections, on successive days, of 20 ml of a 10 percent emulsion of spleen and lymph node tissue that were removed from distemper-affected dogs early in the course of the disease when the virus content of these organs is highest.

CD antiserum may protect susceptible dogs from the disease for a limited time. It is used in some animal hospitals for protecting young canine patients, which may not have had distemper, from infection which they are likely, otherwise, to contract there. If the animal comes in contact with the virus while protected by the serum, it may develop an active enduring immunity. Usually one 10-ml dose of serum is given for a few days' stay in the hospital or at a dog show. If the sojourn is prolonged, another dose is given about the 10th day. Immune serum sometimes is used to protect valuable puppies while they are susceptible. Puppies that are raised in relatively good isolation usually are untreated until they are old enough for the active immunization.

Some manufacturers immunize their serum-producing dogs with the bacteria commonly found as secondary invaders in distemper as well as with the virus of Carré, in the belief that antibodies against these organisms may assist in combating the secondary infections. So far as we know there is no proof that these sera are better than those prepared against the virus alone, but there may be some merit in the idea, and certainly there are no objections.

One manufacturer in the United States (6) produced a canine globulin concentrate of distemper immune serum. It is claimed that the gamma globulin does not contain all of the immune bodies, that there are significant amounts in the beta fraction as well. Hence the product is a mixture of these two fractions. It is claimed that much extraneous material is eliminated and a more concentrated product obtained. It is freeze-dried for the trade and reconstituted just before use.

According to the AVMA panels (11, 12) there is evidence that the routine prophylactic use of agents that passively immunize pups against CD has less merit than multiple doses of attenuated live virus vaccines. Because it may block active immunization, the use of antiserum or concentrated antiserum for short-term protection is to be discouraged. Antiserum or concentrated antiserum is of questionable value in the treatment of dogs with clinical signs of distemper.

Active immunization of dogs. Vaccination of animals represents the most effective means for the prevention of distemper. Seven vaccine methods have been used in the dog: (*a*) formalin-treated virus vaccines, (*b*) ferret-passaged modified vaccine, (*c*) modified hen's egg virus vaccine, (*d*) combined use of distemper antiserum and virulent distemper virus (DV), (*e*) modified cell culture virus vaccines, (*f*) dual virus vaccine utilizing various combinations for distemper and infectious canine hepatitis (ICH), and (*g*) measles vaccine.

Immunization of dogs is a controversial subject, but most individuals including the AMVA panels feel that under normal conditions the modified virus vaccines of chick embryo or tissue culture origin are more desirable. Alone or in combination with modified infectious canine hepatitis virus and leptospirosis, the distemper component does not cause illness, is efficacious, does not spread to susceptible dogs, and gives a relatively long immunity. Immunity after vaccination can be assessed by determining humoral antibody levels and also by the use of the skin-test or lymphocyte transformation test to evaluate the cell-mediated immune (CMI) response.

The formalin-inactivated virus vaccines are usually made with infective dog spleen. Usually three injections at 2-week intervals are recommended for the dog. Neutralizing-antibody titers reach their maximum 30 days after the last injection. The titers seldom rise much above 100 and are no longer measurable 16 weeks after the first injection. Dogs are still sensitized to the distemper antigen 3 to 6 months later, and a secondary antibody response occurs which confers clinical protection when challenged with virulent virus (22). Some veterinarians may still use inactivated virus vaccine, especially in the larger cities where repeated exposures to virus are likely to occur assuring immunity—hopefully without the production of frank disease.

Ferret-passaged modified vaccine produces an immunity which is believed to be solid and enduring, although serological studies have not been reported. Dogs should be in excellent condition at the time of vaccination. In some instances the dog has a reaction, but usually it is mild. Some veterinarians use this product to treat early cases of distemper, although there are questions as to its validity. The procedure is based on the virus interference studies of Green and Stulberg (29).

The combined use of distemper antiserum and virulent distemper virus is no longer employed in the United States.

As distemper virus causes the greatest mortality in young dogs, protection is desirable at an early age. Interference with active immunity by maternal antibody complicates a vaccination program because the immune status of a pup is variable. To overcome the problem, vaccination with MV seemed to be an ideal solution. Despite considerable research and field study the results are equivocal. The confusion formerly apparent in this situation may be circumvented by more complete studies of the CMI response. It has been shown that maternal measles antibody will interfere with an active immunity to that virus. Consequently the presence of maternally derived measles antibody must also be considered as well as distemper antibody in a distemper immunization program.

There has been much controversy in the past about the best age at which to immunize young animals. There are still differences of opinion, and it is not always possible to decide this for an individual animal with precision.

It has been pointed out that, when the mother is immune to CD, antibodies are stored in the colostral milk and these convey a passive immunity to the puppies. The concentration of antibodies in the colostrum varies in different immune bitches, however, and this affects the length of time the sucklings will have sufficient antibodies to protect them against natural exposure. If active immunization is attempted while the young animals retain substantial antibody levels derived from their mothers, enduring immunity will not result since the antigenic properties of the vaccines are wholly neutralized by the passively acquired antibody. On the other hand, if the mother is not immune to CD, there will be no antibody in her colostrum and her puppies will at once be highly susceptible to the disease.

Young dogs, therefore, may contract CD at any age, depending on what level of colostral antibodies they possess. Because immunization will fail if done too early, and will fail also if it is deferred too long allowing natural infection to intervene, the selection of the best time for proceeding with artificial immunization is a difficult individual problem. Gillespie *et al.* (23) and Baker *et al.* (3) have attempted to solve this problem by developing a nomograph which relates the serum antibody titer of the dam to the time after birth when, in most instances, the antibody titers of its offspring will have decreased to the point that artificial active immunization is effective. The system predicts when the antibody loss of the young brings them into the period of susceptibility. The system is based on sound scientific facts and generally is quite effective, but it is more expensive than many dog owners will accept since it involves taking a blood sample from the dam before the birth of its offspring and having its virus-neutralizing titer determined by laboratory tests in infected eggs.

Then, too, individuals often purchase a puppy without the opportunity of determining the serum titer of its mother. Under these circumstances vaccination of puppies at 9 weeks of age with egg or tissue culture virus vaccine immunized approximately 82 percent of the puppies at this age (23). Revaccination at 15 weeks of age took care of the other 18 percent that failed to respond earlier because of maternal antibody interference. One-third of these puppies have titers of less than 1:100 at 1 year of age (53). At 2 years of age another third have titers below this figure. A serum titer of 1:100 is used as the standard level for indicating immunity to CD, although it is recognized that some dogs with lower titers may be immune. It was recommended that dogs be vaccinated yearly with modified virus vaccine until a more sensitive test can be devised that will measure cellular immunity as well as neutralizing antibody. In lieu of this procedure yearly blood tests can be performed. If the serum titer falls below 1:100, revaccination is indicated. More than 90 percent of vaccinated dogs will show a significant rise in titer above the 1:100 level: the absolute criterion that a dog will withstand challenge with virulent CDV.

Vaccination procedures recommended by the AVMA panels. (11, 12) Based on the knowledge available to the two panels concerned with canine distemper immunization, the following recommendations were made as guidelines for the employment of professional judgment in canine distemper immunization. These recommendations have had general acceptance by the veterinary profession in the United States and are as follows.

> The Panel recommends the use of modified live-virus vaccine of chicken embryo or tissue culture origin. There is no evidence that the vaccine will cause untoward reactions in parasitized, malnourished, or otherwise debilitated dogs, or interfere with the natural course of distemper in previously exposed animals.
>
> The Panel recommends annual vaccination of all dogs. Although present evidence of untoward effects on the fetus is inconclusive, vaccination of pregnant bitches should be avoided.
>
> When feasible, a nomograph should be used that predicts the age at which pups should be vaccinated against distemper.
>
> Ideally, vaccinated dogs should be serologically tested 30 days after initial vaccination and revaccinated if so indicated by serologic test. Pups of unknown immune status and more than 3 months old should be given one dose of vaccine. If younger than 3 months, two or more doses should be administered; the first dose should be given after the pup is weaned and the last dose at 12 to 16 weeks of age. Administration of a dose of vaccine at 2-week intervals more nearly approaches the ideal.
>
> Orphan pups that do not get colostrum can be vaccinated as early as 2 weeks of age with modified live-virus vaccine.
>
> No dog should be admitted into an area of possible exposure to distemper without immediate vaccination with modified live-virus vaccine of chicken-embryo or tissue-culture origin, unless the dog has been given such a vaccination within the past 12 months.
>
> Immunization of pups in the presence of homologous antibodies, either with modified canine distemper virus vaccine or attenuated measles virus vaccine, has not always been successful. Evidence indicates that measles vaccine was less effective in pups under 8 weeks old than in those over 8 weeks old. Consequently, the use of modified distemper vaccines may be preferred in pups under 8 weeks old.

Immunization of foxes, mink, and ferrets. Canine distemper virus causes natural epizootics among foxes, mink, and ferrets raised in captivity, the losses often being very great. The virus is the same as that which occurs in dogs, and the disease can be transmitted easily from any of these species to any other. In foxes the heavy losses occur in the fall when the animals are turned loose on the fur ranges.

For fox immunization, the process is best done shortly before the animals are turned on the range. The Laidlaw-Dunkin vaccine has been used successfully. Ott (47) reported success by using antiserum alone, but vaccines appear to be better and less expensive. Green and Carlson (28) were able to show that these losses could be greatly reduced by treating all animals with distemperoid, ferret-passage virus, and West and Brandly (57) had excellent success with formalin-inactivated vaccines made from virulent fox tissues (lungs, liver, spleen, kidneys, urinary bladder, and lymph nodes). A 20 percent suspension of these tissues was used, and the dose was 5 ml given subcutaneously or intramuscularly. Some of the vaccines that contained adjuvants (alumina gel and fatty agents) were somewhat more effective than those that did not contain them.

Distemper infection in foxes must be differentiated from that of fox encephalitis caused by infectious canine hepatitis virus and with which it may exist concurrently. Green states that this may be done by inoculating ferrets, which are susceptible to distemper but resistant to the other virus. He also points out that a search for inclusion bodies is helpful. Typical intracytoplasmic inclusion bodies, resembling those seen in dogs, may be found in the epithelial cells of the air passages and urinary bladder in cases of distemper, whereas they are not found in these cells in encephalitis infection.

Laidlaw and Dunkin (39) found it possible to immunize ferrets much more easily than dogs. A vaccine was prepared from the spleens of ferrets, removed on the 4th or 5th day of illness, by grinding them finely and making them into a 20 percent suspension. Formalin was added to these suspensions in a concentration of 0.1 percent, and the material was allowed to stand for at least 4 days, at which time viable virus had disappeared. When 2 ml of this suspension were injected subcutaneously into susceptible ferrets, they became solidly immune after a few days. After 2 weeks the immunity was made permanent by giving them a small dose of active virus, which they withstood without evidence of a physical reaction in most instances.

Pinkerton (50) reported satisfactory results in immunizing mink by the use of tissue vaccine made from lung tissue of infected milk. At the beginning of an outbreak on a ranch, some of the first animals were used as a source of vaccine virus. The finely ground tissue was made into a 10 percent emulsion, which was treated with 0.3 percent formalin. Several injections were given of 2 to 4 ml at weekly intervals. One commercial company produces a 5 percent ferret spleen vaccine that has been inactivated with ultraviolet light.

The manufacturers of the egg-adapted vaccine claim that it has been used with complete satisfaction for immunizing ferrets and minks. They also say that gratifying results were obtained in stopping outbreaks of mink distemper with it.

The Disease in Man. So far as is known, the virus of CD is nonpathogenic for man.

REFERENCES

1. Adams and Imagawa. Proc. Soc. Exp. Biol. and Med., 1957, *96,* 240.
2. Appel and Gillespie. Handbook of virus research, ed. S. Gard and C. Hallauer. Springer-Verlag, Vienna and New York, 1972.
3. Baker, Robson, Gillespie, Burgher, and Doughty. Cornell Vet., 1959, *49,* 158.
4. Bindrich. Kleintierpraxis, 1962, *7,* 161 and 181.
5. Blinzinger and Deutschländer. Verh. Deut. Ges. f. Path., 1969, *53,* 283.
6. Brueckner, Taylor, Schroeder, and Koehler. Proc. Soc. Exp. Biol. and Med., 1959, *102,* 20.
7. Bussell. Personal communication. Quoted by Appel and Gillespie in Handbook of virus research, ed. S. Gard and C. Hallauer. Springer-Verlag, Vienna and New York, 1972.
8. Cabasso and Cox. Proc. Soc. Exp. Biol. and Med., 1949, *71,* 246.
9. Cabasso, Douglas, Stebbins, and Cox. Proc. Soc. Exp. Biol. and Med., 1955, *88,* 199.
10. Cabasso, Kiser, and Stebbins. Proc. Soc. Exp. Biol. and Med., 1959, *101,* 227.
11. Canine Distemper Symposium. Jour. Am. Vet. Med. Assoc., 1966, *149,* part 2.
12. Canine Infectious Diseases Symposium. Jour. Am. Vet. Med. Assoc., 1970, *156,* part 1.
13. Carré. Comp. rend. Acad. Sci., 1905, *140,* 689 and 1489.
14. Celiker and Gillespie. Cornell Vet., 1954, *44,* 276.
15. Cello, Moulton, and McFarland. Cornell Vet., 1959, *49,* 127.
16. Cruickshank, Waterson, Kanarek, and Berry. Res. Vet. Sci., 1962, *3,* 485.
17. Dedie and Klopotke. Arch. Exp. Vet. Med., 1951, *4,* 137.
18. Dunkin and Laidlaw. Jour. Comp. Path. and Therap., 1926, *39,* 201.
19. Dunkin and Laidlaw. Jour. Comp. Path. and Therap., 1926, *39,* 213.
20. Gerber and Marron. Am. Jour. Vet. Res., 1976, *37,* 133.
21. Gillespie. Ann. N.Y. Acad. Sci., 1962, *101,* 540.
22. Gillespie. Cornell Vet., 1965, *55,* 3.
23. Gillespie, Baker, Burgher, Robson, and Gilman. Cornell Vet., 1958, *48,* 103.
24. Gillespie and Karzon. Proc. Soc. Exp. Biol. and Med., 1960, *105,* 547.
25. Gillespie and Rickard. Am. Jour. Vet. Res., 1956, *17,* 103.
26. Gillespie, Robinson, and Baker. Proc. Soc. Exp. Biol. and Med., 1952, *81,* 461.
27. Gorham. *In* Advances in Veterinary Science, vol. 6, ed. C. A. Brandly and E. L. Jungherr. Academic Press, New York, 1960, p. 287.
28. Green and Carlson. Jour. Am. Vet. Med. Assoc., 1945, *107,* 131.
29. Green and Stulberg. Science, 1946, *103,* 497.
30. Haig. Onderstepoort Jour. Vet. Sci. and Anim. Indus., 1948, *23,* 149.
31. Heath. Can. Jour. Comp. Med., 1940, *4,* 352.
32. Jubb, Saunders, and Coates, Jour. Comp. Path. and Therap., 1957, *67,* 21.
33. Karzon and Bussell. Science, 1959, *130,* 1708.
34. Krakowka, Cockerell, and Koestner. Inf. and Immun., 1975, *11,* 1069.
35. Krakowka, Cockerell, and Koestner. Am. Jour. Vet. Res., 1977, *38,* 1539.
36. Krakowka, Hoover, Koestner, and Ketring. Am. Jour. Vet. Res., 1977, *38,* 919.
37. Krakowka and Koestner. Jour. Inf. Dis., 1976, *134,* 629.
38. Krakowka, Olsen, Confer, Koestner, and McCullough. Jour. Inf. Dis., 1975, *132,* 384.
39. Laidlaw and Dunkin. Jour. Comp. Path. and Therap., 1926, *39,* 222.
40. Laidlaw and Dunkin. Jour. Comp. Path. and Therap., 1928, *41,* 1.
41. Laidlaw and Dunkin. Jour. Comp. Path. and Therap., 1928, *41,* 209.
42. Lockhart, Ray, and Barbee. Jour. Am. Vet. Med. Assoc., 1925, *67,* 668.
43. MacIntyre, Trevan, and Montgomerie. Vet. Rec., 1948, *60,* 635.
44. Mansi. Brit. Vet. Jour., 1951, *107,* 214.
45. Morse, Chow, and Brandly. Proc. Soc. Exp. Biol. and Med., 1953, *84,* 10.
46. Moulton and Brown. Proc. Soc. Exp. Biol. and Med., 1954, *86,* 99.
47. Ott. Jour. Am. Vet. Med. Assoc., 1939, *94,* 522.
48. Palm and Black. Proc. Soc. Exp. Biol. and Med., 1961, *107,* 588.
49. Phillips and Bussell. Personal communication, 1971.
50. Pinkerton. Jour. Am. Vet. Med. Assoc., 1940, *96,* 347.
51. Polding and Simpson. Vet. Rec., 1957, *69,* 582.
52. Polding, Simpson, and Scott. Vet. Rec., 1959, *71,* 643.
53. Robson, Kenneson, Gillespie, and Benson. Proc. Gaines Vet. Sympos., 1959, *9,* 10.

54. Rockborn. Arch. f. die gesam. Virusforsch., 1958, *8,* 485.
55. Vandevelde and Kristensen. Acta Neuropath. (Berlin), 1977, 40, 233.
56. Vladimirov. Veterinariya (Moscow), *26* (7), 59. (Original not seen, cited in Vet. Bull. 1951, *21,* 77.)
57. West and Brandly. Cornell Vet., 1949, *39,* 292.
58. Yamanouchi, Kobune, Fuduka, Hayami, and Shishido. Arch. f. die gesam. Virusforsch., 1970, *29,* 90.
59. Yamanouchi, Yoshikawa, Sato, Katow, Kobune, Kobune, Uchida, and Shishido. Jap. Jour. Med. Sci. Biol., 1977, *30,* 241.
60. Zydeck. Experientia, 1970, *26,* 88.

Rinderpest

SYNONYMS: Cattle plague, oriental cattle plague

Rinderpest is an acute, febrile disease of ruminants characterized by a rapid course and a high mortality rate (25). Excellent review articles have been prepared by Plowright (29) and Scott (32).

Character of the Disease. The disease affects principally cattle, hence its name. In the orient, water buffaloes are frequent victims. Sheep, yaks, and goats are fairly resistant to natural infection and seldom are seriously affected, although a few large outbreaks have been reported. Some wild ungulates, swine, camels, and even warthogs are said to be mildly susceptible.

The disease is enzootic in parts of Asia and Africa. It has spread from Asia on many occasions in the past, especially in times of war, to Europe, where it has affected cattle principally. The results of these epizootics have often been devastating. On some occasions a large portion of the entire cattle population has perished. Only once has the disease appeared in the Western Hemisphere. In 1921 it appeared in Brazil, where it apparently had been imported in zebu cattle. This outbreak was quickly recognized and stamped out after fewer than 1,000 cattle had developed the disease, and about 2,000 additional animals that had been exposed were slaughtered. Rinderpest could do great damage to the cattle population of North and South America should it ever gain a secure foothold. Veterinarians should constantly be on guard to detect it early if it should occur. Modern air travel has greatly increased the hazard of its bridging the oceans which have been our protectors in the past.

The virulence of rinderpest virus (RV) varies greatly from time to time and from place to place. The susceptibility of animals differs widely also. European and American cattle, which have had no contacts with the disease for many years, are generally highly susceptible. In Asia, where the disease is enzootic, the native cattle are much more resistant. Probably this is because the more susceptible strains of such cattle have gradually been weeded out through many years of exposure. Some breeds of cattle appear to be more susceptible than others. In India the so-called hill cattle are usually much more susceptible than the plains cattle. In the same outbreak the mortality of the former may be high and that of the latter light or negligible. The carabao, or water buffalo, the common beast of burden in much of southern Asia, is susceptible to rinderpest, sometimes more so than the native cattle (20, 27).

When the resistance of the host is high and the virus comparatively mild, the signs may be so slight as to be overlooked. It is thought that such animals often are the means of importing the disease into new localities or countries. They acquire permanent resistance as a result of the experience. Young calves from immune mothers often suffer only slightly from rinderpest but acquire an immunity because ot it.

Acute rinderpest is the most common form, and the only one that is likely ever to be seen in European cattle or in those of the Western Hemisphere, where this disease does not exist and where susceptibility is high.

Rinderpest is usually quite explosive; large numbers of animals are likely to exhibit signs almost simultaneously. High fever (104 to 108 F) is an early sign. This is seen about the 3rd day of the disease; later the temperature falls and usually becomes subnormal before death. Rumination is suspended; there is dullness, and the coat becomes rough. The buccal mucosa becomes very congested. Early in the disease often there is constipation. The victim strains in defecating, and the bowel discharges are dry, often coated with mucus and sometimes with blood. Later there is severe diarrhea, the feces becoming quite fluid and very fetid. Frequently there is a profuse nasal discharge and lacrimation. The breath becomes very offensive because of the development of many shallow erosions on the lips, dental pads, and gums. The abdomen becomes very tender, the animal moans, becomes very dull, goes down, and is unable to rise; death usually occurs between the 2nd and 6th day after the first signs are exhibited.

The incubation period in naturally acquired rinderpest is from 3 to 8 days. Only occasionally is it a little longer.

Affected animals usually die in 1 week or less after signs are first observed. Some of the more resistant breeds may linger for 2 or 3 weeks. In some outbreaks

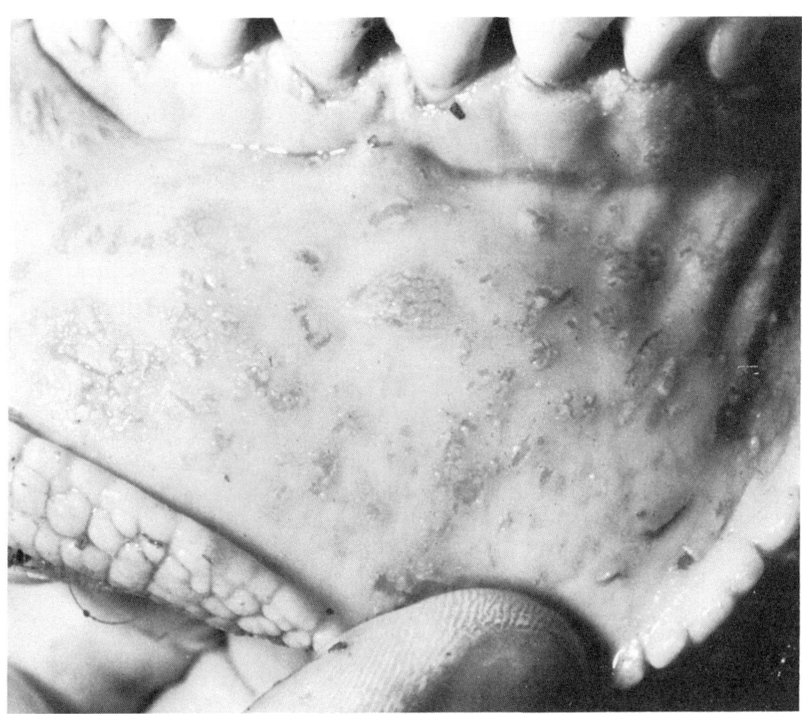

Figure 50.7. Rinderpest in a steer. Multiple focal areas of necrosis on the mucosa of the lower lip. (Courtesy D. A. Gregg, Plum Island Animal Disease Center, USDA.)

the virulence of the virus is low, and many animals may show a longer course than usual. The mortality varies, although it is almost always high. In European and American cattle a mortality rate of 90 to 100 percent must always be expected. It is lower than this in regions where the disease is enzootic.

The gross and microscopic lesions of rinderpest are well described by Maurer, Jones, Easterday, and DeTray (18). The principal lesions are found in the digestive tract. Shallow ulcers are usually found in the mucosa of the mouth—in all parts except the dorsum of the tongue (Figures 50.7 and 50.8). Such ulcers may also be found in the pharynx and esophagus. These are shallow, have a "punched out" appearance, and are filled with whitish caseous material. The mucosa of the abomasum is usually deeply congested. The livid membrane has areas of blood extravasation and dark purplish stripes. Ulceration of the pyloric orifice and the folds is frequent. Sometimes the inflammatory exudate forms a false membrane which may easily be peeled off. The small intestines may exhibit similar lesions. The fluid content usually is very fetid. Lesions in the large intestines include hemorrhages (Figure 50.9), and the rectum often shows linear, bright red stripes—the so-called *zebra striping*. The Peyer's patches are usually ulcerated, and ulcers may be found on other parts of the mucosa.

The respiratory tract shows deep reddening of the upper passages and often petechiation. A patchy pneumonia sometimes develops, a purely secondary lesion. If the animal has lived more than a few days after becoming infected, there will be marked dehydration of all tissues and extreme emaciation.

Plowright (28) reported that degenerative changes in lymphoid tissues also occur. Formation of syncytia with cytoplasmic inclusion bodies has been demonstrated in the stratum spinosum of stratified squamous epithelia of the buccal mucosa and upper alimentary tract and in lymphoid tissues (Figures 50.10 and 50.11) (28, 38). Intranuclear inclusion bodies *in vivo* have been described by Thiery (38).

The Disease in Experimental Animals. For many years it was thought that rinderpest could be transmitted only to cattle, water buffaloes, and a few other species of ruminants. A few authentic outbreaks of rinderpest in sheep were recognized, but these animals and goats were known to be sufficiently resistant to the virus to enable them to escape the disease when it occurred in cattle kept in close association with them. Edwards (11) in 1930 adapted rinderpest virus to goats by serial passage and found that the goat virus could be used as a vaccine for cattle. White-tailed deer given a virulent strain succumbed to experimental infection after showing typical signs of rinderpest (14).

In 1938 Nakamura, Wagatsuma, and Fukusko (24) succeeded in adapting several strains to rabbits so the virus could be propagated in that species. In the early

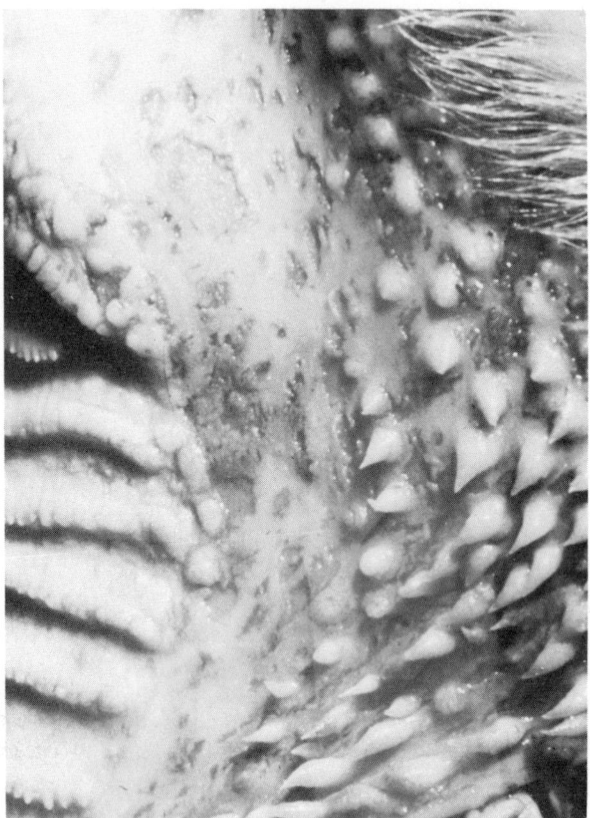

Figure 50.8. Rinderpest in a steer. Multiple erosions on the labial and buccal mucosa. (Courtesy D. A. Gregg, Plum Island Annual Disease Center, USDA.)

passages there were no signs except a slight temperature rise which could easily be overlooked. After the virus has passed through several generations of rabbits, however, the animals show a sharp temperature rise during which they exhibit lassitude, inappetence, increased respiratory rate, and sometimes diarrhea. The febrile state lasts only about 36 to 48 hours, after which the signs subside and the animals again appear to be normal. Animals destroyed at the height of the temperature reaction often exhibit small necrotic areas in the intestinal mucosa, especially in the Peyer's patches. During this time there is a marked leukopenia. Further passage of the Nakamura III strain of lapinized rinderpest virus causes a very high mortality—greater than 95 percent. It is a very useful system to study rinderpest immunity.

In 1946 Baker also adapted a strain of rinderpest virus to rabbits (1) and guinea pigs (2). It also proliferates in mice, hamsters, dogs, ferrets, giant rats, and susliks (28).

Properties of the Virus. The morphological characteristics have been well described by Plowright (28) and Breese and de Boer (5) (Figure 50.12). The particles are pleomorphic with an average diameter of 120 to 300 nm. Like other paramyxoviruses it has an internal helical component and it is 17.5 nm in diameter with a periodicity of 5 to 6 nm. There is an enclosing membrane, and it has filaments that are similar to those observed for influenza A virus and Newcastle disease virus (Blacksburg strain, 28).

It is an ether-sensitive RNA virus. It does not hemagglutinate red blood cells. The virus attaches itself to the leukocytes in blood (8).

The virus is quite stable after lyophilization and at very low temperatures (−70 C or less). High passaged tissue-cultured virus is relatively stable between pH 4 and 10 with the greatest stability between pH 7.2 to 7.9. Virulent strains are less stable under comparable conditions. The virus is stable in glycerol. Strong alkalis are the best disinfectants for its destruction. Certain chemicals, such as phenol, chinosol, formalin, and betapropiolactone, inactivate rinderpest-infected tissues without loss of antigenicity. Trypsin and 1 M hydroxylamine also inactivate the virus. A small fraction of tissue-cultured virus survives heating at 56 C for 50 to 60 minutes and at 60 C for 30 minutes.

Virus is inactivated rather quickly (in 1 or 2 days) in dried secretions, but in the presence of moisture it retains its activity somewhat longer. Boynton (3) found that virus could never be detected by placing susceptible animals in corrals from which infected animals had been removed longer than 36 hours previously, even when water was present and parts of the area were shaded from the sun. He concluded that rinderpest virus does not survive long in pastures after affected animals are removed from them.

The virus contains antigens that produce neutralizing, complement-fixing and precipitating antibodies. Double diffusion in agar reveals a heat-stable and a heat-labile antigen. There is evidence that the viruses of measles, canine distemper, and rinderpest share a common antigen (4). Rinderpest virus protects dogs against a challenge with virulent canine distemper virus. Interference with Rift Valley fever virus occurs, and attenuated rinderpest strains interfere with virulent ones. No hemagglutinin has been unequivocally demonstrated for rinderpest virus, but it has been suggested by Provost and Borredon (31) that RV hemagglutinates erythrocytes of the monkey *Erythrocebus patas*. Infected cell cultures do not cause hemadsorption of erythrocytes.

The *peste des petite* virus causes a rinderpestlike dis-

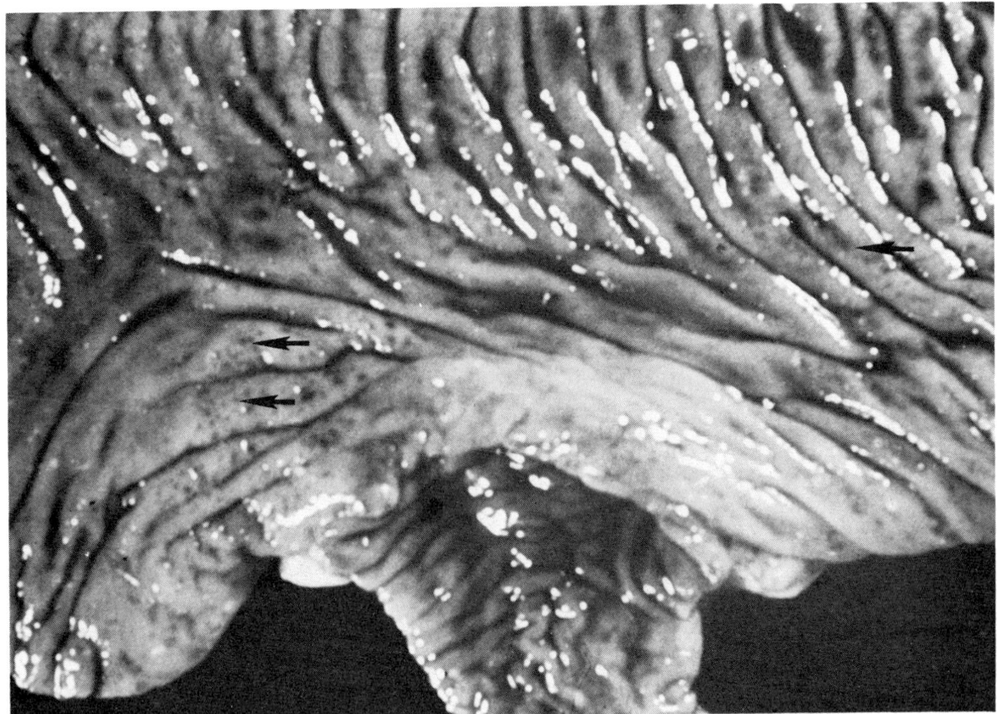

Figure 50.9. Rinderpest. Petechial and ecchymotic hemorrhage areas in mucosal wall of gastrointestinal tract. (Courtesy J. J. Callis and staff, Plum Island Animal Disease Center, USDA.)

Figure 50.10. Rinderpest. The epithelial cells in the stratum spinosum of the buccal cavity of a steer are enlarged, and some have formed syncytia. Notice heavy infiltration of leukocytes in the epithelium on the left side. H and E stain. × 160. (Courtesy C. A. Mebus, Plum Island Animal Disease Center, USDA.)

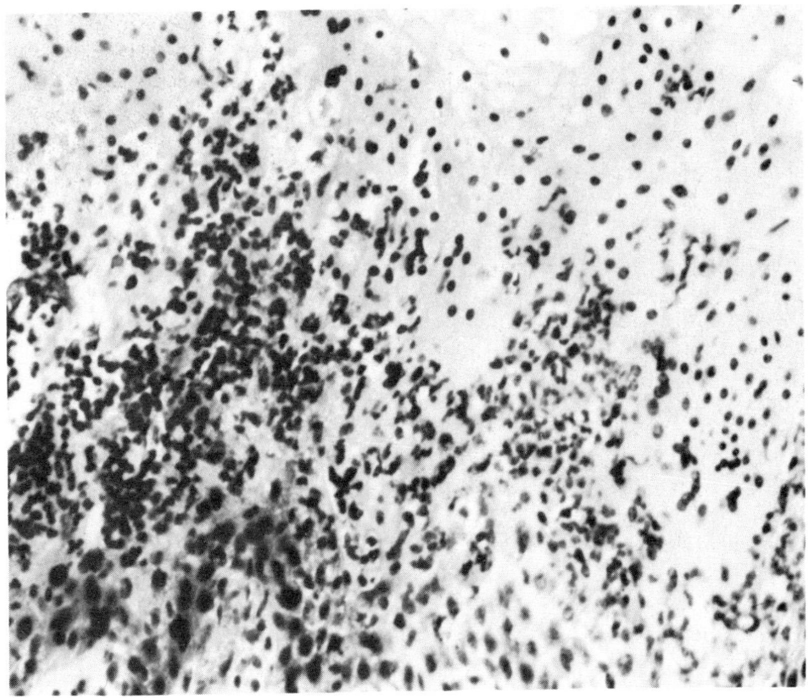

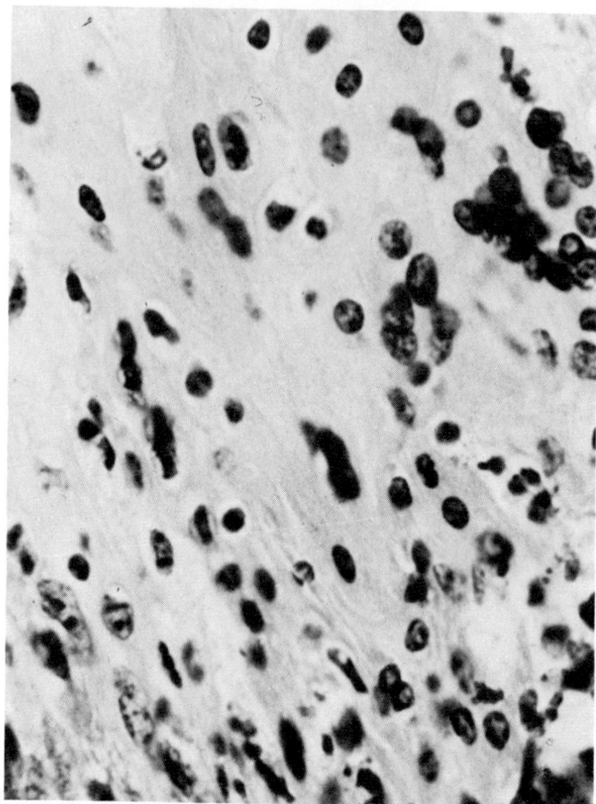

Figure 50.11. Higher magnification (× 400) showing the same changes as Figure 50.10. (Courtesy C. A. Mebus, Plum Island Animal Disease Center, USDA.)

ease in goats and sheep in Western Africa. It has all the characteristics of rinderpest virus (15). It now is classified as a strain of rinderpest that readily causes disease in goats and sheep, but has lost its ability to infect cattle under natural conditions.

Cultivation. Shope *et al.* (34, 35) succeeded in cultivating an African strain (the Kabete strain) on the chorioallantoic membranes of embryonated hens' eggs. They were not successful in adapting several other strains. Later Nakamura, Agric, and Miyamoto (21) reported success in the egg cultivation of a strain of lapinized virus. When the membranes were inoculated, the virus failed to infect the embryos, according to Shope. After several transfers on the membranes, the virus multiplied when inoculated into the yolk sac, and then could be maintained indefinitely in series by yolk-sac inoculation. In embryonated eggs inoculated into the yolk sac, the virus multiplied in the embryo, the fluids, and the egg membranes. Rinderpest virus of direct bovine origin injected into 7-day-old embryos by way of the yolk sac infected the embryos, but it was not possible to transmit this virus in series. Even the egg-adapted strain did not seriously damage the embryos since they regularly hatched. Chicks from such eggs never contained virus. Subsequently Furutani *et al.* (12), following the technique of Nakamura and Miyamoto, observed that the Nakamura III strain of lapinized virus produced embryo deaths and reddening and swelling of embryonic spleens.

Kabete "O" strain of rinderpest virus multiplies and produces a cytopathic effect in primary monolayer cultures of calf and lamb testes; bovine embryonic kidney cells; bovine skin-muscle tissue; pig, goat, sheep, and hamster kidneys; calf thyroid; and dog kidney (28). Virulent field strains selected from tissues of infected cattle regularly produce a cytopathic effect in primary calf kidney cultures (28). Attenuated virus strains do not proliferate (28). The cytopathogenic strains in calf kidney monolayers produce syncytia or multinucleated giant cells together with eosinophilic cytoplasmic and type B intranuclear inclusions. Recently isolated strains of low cattle virulence have a tendency to produce stellate-type cells, which are large and sometimes multinucleated. There is more free virus in culture than cell-associated virus until the 9th day when the titers are comparable and rapidly dropping (28).

Initially, immunofluorescence antigen was not found in the nuclei except for a few granules in the later stages of infection. Using air-dried instead of acetone-fixed preparations, Liess (17) showed fluorescent particles in the nucleus of infected cell cultures as early as 8 hours, often acompanied by perinuclear fluorescence. Cytoplasmic fluorescence was first noticed at 19 hours. It was concluded that the first synthesis of virus-specific materials probably occurred in the nucleus.

The Pendik strain of RV in primary monolayers of bovine kidney cells produced plaques that become visible by 7 to 8 days and attain a diameter of 3mm by day 12 and 5 mm by day 19 (19). The optimum concentration of Noble agar is 1 to 1.5 percent, and a 1:5,000 dilution of neutral red or the lack of immune serum in the overlay had no effect on the results. Virus assay by plaque formation gives lower titers (approximately 2 $\log_{10}$ units) than 50 percent end points in monolayers. Plaque inhibition by specific immune serum is a usable system for virus identification.

Interferon produced in calf kidney cells by Sindbis virus suppresses the growth of a small amount of virulent RV in the same cell type (29). It suppressed the yield of

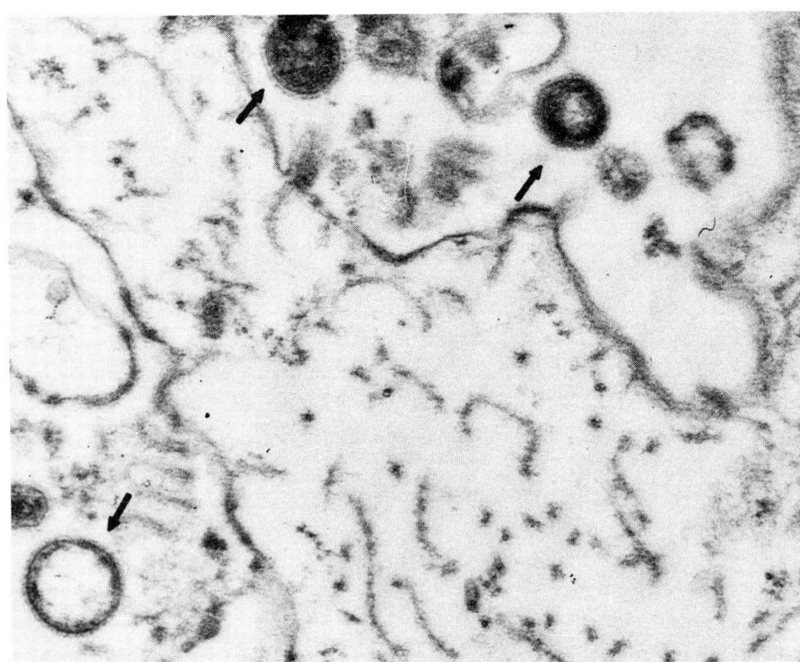

Figure 50.12. Rinderpest virus particles. Two mature particles at top with *arrows* (dark center) and one immature particle at bottom with *arrow* (ghost particle) in cell vacuoles. × 48,000. (Courtesy S. Breese, Plum Island Animal Disease Center, USDA.)

released virus more than the cell associated virus replication for which there is no explanation.

Immunity. Animals surviving an attack of rinderpest to a living virus preparation are generally permanently immune thereafter. Nakamura *et al.* (22), however, claim that the immunity is not always permanent and that it is possible to break it down in some animals by inoculation with highly virulent materials. Immunity to rinderpest is proved by the parenteral inoculation (usually subcutaneous) of 10^4 $TCID_{50}$ or more of a strain which produces severe clinical reactions and high mortality in cattle. Production of significant levels of neutralizing antibody is indicative of resistance to test virus, although a small percentage of resistant animals may have no detectable circulating antibody.

The hemagglutination-inhibition test, using measles virus hemagglutination, is applicable for detection of hemagglutination inhibition antibodies, but its sensitivity is inferior to the neutralization test. Complement-fixing antibodies appear irregularly in the sera of recovered or vaccinated cattle, and they persist for only a short period of time; thus the test is suitable as a diagnostic test on a herd basis but not for epidemiological surveys.

Immunization. Methods for artificially immunizing animals both actively and passively are available. The earliest method was by injecting nasal and ocular secretions under the skin of the dewlap. This method often served to propagate the disease, and the reactions usually were very severe. It is no longer used. Robert Koch in 1897 introduced a great improvement when he showed that cattle could be successfully immunized with bile obtained from animals killed on the 5th or 6th day of the disease. Normal bile is of no value. More than 2 million cattle in South Africa were successfully immunized by this method in a 2-year period. It has now been abandoned in favor of better vaccination procedures.

The methods used for artificially immunizing cattle against rinderpest today differ markedly in different parts of the world. Procedures that seem to be very satisfactory in one area often prove too drastic or ineffective in others. Obviously the virus strains in different regions differ greatly in virulence, and breeds of cattle differ greatly in susceptibility. For these reasons it appears that methods have to be adapted to the particular areas and breeds involved.

Passive immunization. Serum from animals that have recovered from the disease possesses antibodies that are protective for susceptible animals. The value of such sera is greatly increased by hyperimmunization. Hyperimmune serum will give immediate protection, but the resistance can be expected to last for only 10 days to 2 weeks. Immune serum has no value in treating the disease. Its principal use is to protect cattle against transient exposure, such as when they are driven or shipped through infected regions, and to stop the progress of the disease in recently infected herds.

Calves born of immune mothers obtain transient immunity through the colostral milk of their dams. Such animals will resist infection. Active immunization of calves from immune mothers is unsuccessful because maternal antibody interferes with active immunity.

Active immunization: Inactivated virus vaccines. A number of these have been used with success. All are prepared by chemical treatment of tissue suspensions. They have the advantage of safety but the disadvantage that the immunity produced is not lasting. Generally they protect against ordinary exposure for periods up to 1 year. Because they did not give permanent immunity, these vaccines have been largely supplanted by attenuated virus vaccines.

Active immunization: Host-adapted vaccines. These vaccines contain living virus which has been altered in virulence by being serially passed through alien hosts. They cause mild, active infections which generally immunize cattle and carabao permanently, or at least for several years.

1. Caprinized (goat-adapted) vaccines. A serious disadvantage of using bovine blood and tissues for the immunization of cattle against rinderpest in most areas where the disease is enzootic is the fact that such materials often contain other disease-producing agents such as those of babesiosis and anaplasmosis. In an effort to propagate the virus in a host which would eliminate these extraneous infections, Edwards (11) in India discovered that goat-propagated virus gradually lost virulence for cattle and suggested that such virus be used as a vaccine for cattle. Stirling (36) used the material successfully in India in 1932. Pfaff (26), who worked in Burma, developed a goat-adapted vaccine, which was used extensively in that area. The earlier workers used citrated or defibrinated blood as the vaccine, but this material had poor keeping qualities. Later workers found that dried tissue vaccines, generally prepared from spleen pulp, were more stable.

The goat-tissue vaccine has been used with success on many millions of cattle and carabao and appears to be most popular in southern Asiatic countries. In some highly susceptible breeds the vaccine may cause too much mortality. This could be offset in some cases by administering a small dose of antiserum with the vaccine. Daubney (9), who tested the Indian strain of goat-adapted virus, found that it was too virulent in eastern Africa, especially for cattle with some European blood, in which the mortality rate was sometimes as high as 25 percent.

2. Lapinized (rabbit-adapted) vaccines. In 1938 Nakamura *et al.* (24) attenuated the rinderpest virus by 100 passages in rabbits. The vaccine was made from the mesenteric lymph nodes of the infected rabbits. No preservatives were added. This virus keeps its viability for a short time only; hence it must be used promptly. It was employed extensively in China and Korea. Korean cattle are more susceptible to rinderpest than those of Manchuria, where the disease is enzootic. The vaccine alone served satisfactorily on the latter, but for the Korean cattle it was necessary to give a small dose of antiserum simultaneously. This vaccine is claimed to be less virulent than goat vaccine. Nakamura and Kuroda (23) were unable to transmit the infection by contact of normal calves with others that were sick and dying of lapinized virus infection. Infected cows did not transmit the infection to their suckling calves.

Cheng and Fischman (7) vaccinated many cattle and carabao in China with a lapinized virus produced in the field. They reported excellent results. When vaccine was needed, the vaccine strain was inoculated into rabbits. On the 3rd or 4th day, when the temperature reaction was at its height, the rabbits were bled to death from the heart. The spleen and lymph nodes were pooled, finely ground, and diluted with the defibrinated blood in the proportion of 1:4. Next the mixture was diluted 1:100 with saline solutions. It was then ready for use which was always within 8 hours of the time of its preparation. The vaccine was also made by lyophilization of tissues. This would keep satisfactorily for several months in the refrigerator.

3. Avianized (chick-embryo-adapted) vaccines. Jenkins and Shope (16) attenuated the Kabete strain of rinderpest virus by adapting it to develop in egg embryos. After 19 to 24 passages by yolk-sac inoculation the strain had lost enough virulence for cattle while retaining antigenicity to make it useful as an immunizing agent for cattle. After 50 to 60 passages the strain lost its immunizing properties. At the appropriate passage level, the strain solidly immunized calves against inoculation with fully virulent spleen virus. Vaccinated calves do not transmit the virus to susceptible animals, and thus this vaccine can be safely used in noninfected areas. The vaccine deteriorates very rapidly; thus lyophilization must be resorted to, and even then it must be stored and handled carefully. Hale and Walker (13) have described in detail large-scale production of the vaccine. Field tests in eastern Africa were satisfactory.

It has already been pointed out that not every strain of rinderpest virus will grow in eggs. Nakamura *et al.* (21) have succeeded in avianizing a strain which had already been lapinized, and with this strain they were successful in immunizing cattle in Asia. Brotherston (5) has propagated the Nakamura lapinized strain of rinderpest virus in eastern Africa and has used it very successfully on many thousands of cattle of many different breeds. Most cattle show very little reaction to the vaccine but are solidly immunized by it. Vaccinated cattle were tested by subcutaneous inoculation with virulent virus 8 to 15 months afterward and were found to be solidly immune. Natural exposure of 13 months likewise failed to break the immunity.

4. Tissue-cultured vaccines. After 70 or more passages in calf kidney monolayers the virulent Kabete "O" strain produced no detectable clinical reaction in eastern African cattle and was stable on serial cattle passage. The duration of immunity was probably at least 4 years, and the infective titer for cattle with this modified strain was comparable to the tissue culture infectivity titer.

Cattle with East Coast fever have a diminished response to rinderpest vaccination caused by massive lymphoid cell involvement. (39).

Transmission. Rinderpest can be transmitted to susceptible animals by feeding them with blood, urine, feces, nasal discharges, and perspiration. Natural transmission apparently occurs through direct contact with these infected secretions and excretions. The urine is believed to be especially important in the transmission of this disease. Some animals of the more resistant types may suffer from the disease and eliminate virulent infectious material while showing only mild signs themselves. When these animals are driven to market, or shipped to distant points, they may introduce the disease into new localities. Because the virus is not very hardy, infected premises usually become free of infection within a relatively short time after diseased animals have been removed from them. There is little evidence that droplet infection plays any part in transmission, but infected meat may, since European pigs can acquire the disease by ingestion of infected meat and the infected pigs spread the virus by contact to other pigs or to cattle or vice versa (10, 33). It has been suggested that virus produces an exceedingly mild infection in pigs that may be overlooked and presumably the virus may persist in this host for as long as 36 days.

In cattle the disease is usually found in yearlings with no maternal immunity. It is of a mild type, especially in the resistant native breeds. Control is also made more difficult in Africa where large populations of susceptible wildlife have the infection without any detectable mortality or morbidity.

Field experiments in Nigeria showed that recent isolates can spread, although irregularly, by close contact from cattle to sheep and goats and then among small ruminants, but spreading from sheep to cattle was not demonstrable and there was infrequent transfer from goats to cattle (29). It is concluded that immunization of sheep and goats is not necessary once the disease is eliminated from cattle. Obviously, there is a slight element of risk, but the economics involved warrant the risk in some countries.

Diagnosis. In areas where rinderpest is indigenous, the diagnosis usually presents few problems. It is based on signs and the lesions found at autopsy, and also on the fact that the disease is evidently highly contagious. In regions where the disease is not known, the diagnosis should be based on one or more of the following techniques (29): (*a*) the isolation of the virus from sick or dead animals; (*b*) the detection of virus-specific antigens in the tissues; (*c*) the demonstration of antibody production; and (*d*) histological examination of tissues for virus-specific changes.

A tentative diagnosis is possible on the basis of gross examination and specific cytological changes including the formation of syncytia and the presence of eosinophilic intracytoplasmic and perhaps intranuclear inclusion bodies as well (29). The best tissues for histological examination are lymphoid-epithelial such as the tonsil, Peyer's patches, and lymph nodes and also lesions of the tongue, palate, and cheek papillae.

Studies in East Africa (30) show that naturally occurring strains can be readily recovered from the blood of infected cattle or wild animals in primary calf kidney cultures making this a simple, rapid, and excellent aid in the diagnosis of rinderpest. The neutralization of the isolate with rinderpest antiserum confirms the characteristic cytopathic effects if they are not considered to be adequate proof. The fluorescent antibody test also may be applied for the detection of rinderpest virus after its probable development.

It is possible to biopsy nodes of infected cattle and test for antigen by the gel-diffusion agar technique (6). A rapid complement-fixation test for the diagnosis of rinderpest by the use of tissue extracts of biopsied lymph nodes from infected cattle gave excellent results (37).

The testing of paired serum samples by the neutralization tests in cell cultures and in embryonated hens' eggs are also useful in its diagnosis.

A disease that closely resembles rinderpest, except that the mortality rate is much lower, was first described in 1946. It is commonly called *virus diarrhea-mucosal disease of cattle*. Virus diarrhea and malignant head catarrh may have lesions that resemble rinderpest.

Control. In western Asia, India, and parts of Africa where rinderpest is indigenous, the disease is controlled principally by prophylactic vaccination. For this purpose the modified viruses seem to be the safest and most effective. In other parts of the world, including the Western Hemisphere, a complete embargo on the shipment of susceptible animals from infected areas is enforced and has generally succeeded in excluding this disease. Because the virus is a rather delicate one which does not remain viable very long outside the body of infected animals, there appears to be relatively little danger of infection being imported into areas remote from enzootic regions by means of meat, hides, or other contaminated objects. The principal danger appears to be in the importation of live animals of the more resistant types which sometimes suffer from rather chronic, almost inapparent infections.

If the disease should manage to reach the United States, or any other country that is remote from the enzootic regions, it would undoubtedly be dealt with as foot-and-mouth disease has been handled in this country—by quarantine and slaughter. In countries free of the disease for long periods, or which have never been infected, rinderpest can be rapidly and completely eliminated by quarantine and vaccination as in the Philippines in 1955, by movement restrictions and slaughter as in Brazil and Australia, or by quarantine, slaughter, and antiserum as in Belgium (29).

The Disease in Man. There is no evidence that rinderpest virus causes disease in man.

REFERENCES

1. Baker. Am. Jour. Vet. Res., 1946, *7,* 179.
2. Baker, Terrence, and Greig. Am. Jour. Vet. Res., 1946, *7,* 189.
3. Boynton. Philipp. Jour. Sci., 1928, *36,* 1.
4. Breese and de Boer. Virol., 1963, *19,* 340.
5. Brotherston. Jour. Comp. Path. and Therap., 1951, *61,* 289.
6. Brown and Scott. Vet. Rec., 1960, *47,* 1055.
7. Cheng and Fischman. Proc. FAO Conference on Rinderpest, Nairobi, Kenya, 1948.
8. Daubney. Jour. Comp. Path. and Therap., 1928, *41,* 228.
9. Daubney. Ann. Rpt. Vet. Dept., Kenya, for 1938, p. 70.
10. Delay and Barber. Proc. U.S. Livestock Sanit. Assoc., 1962, *66,* 132.
11. Edwards. Imp. Inst. Agr. Res., Pusa (India), Bull. 199, 1930.
12. Furutani, Ishii, Kurata, and Nakamura. Bull. Nat. Inst. Anim. Health, Tokyo, 1957, *32,* 137.
13. Hale and Walker. Am. Jour. Vet. Res., 1946, *7,* 199.
14. Hamdy, Dardiri, Ferris, and Breese. Jour. Wildlife Dis., 1975, *11,* 508.
15. Hamdy, Dardiri, Nduaka, Breese, and Ihemelandu. Can. Jour. Comp. Med., 1976, *40,* 276.
16. Jenkins and Shope. Am. Jour. Vet. Res., 1946, *7,* 174.
17. Liess. Arch. Exp. Vet. Med., 1964, *20,* 157.
18. Maurer, Jones, Easterday, and DeTray. Proc. Am. Vet. Med. Assoc., 1955, p. 201.
19. McKercher. Can. Jour. Comp. Med., 1963, *27,* 71.
20. Naik. Indian Vet. Jour., 1946, *23,* 203.
21. Nakamura, Agric, and Miyamoto. Am. Jour. Vet. Res., 1953, *14,* 307.
22. Nakamura, Fukusko, and Kuroda. Jap. Jour. Vet. Sci., 1943, *5,* 455.
23. Nakamura and Kuroda. Jap. Jour. Vet. Sci., 1942, *4,* 75.
24. Nakamura, Wagatsuma, and Fukusko. Jour. Jap. Soc. Vet. Sci., 1938, *17,* 185.
25. Nicolle and Adil-Bey. Ann. Inst. Past., 1902, *29,* 429.
26. Pfaff. Onderstepoort Jour. Vet. Sci. and Anim. Indus., 1938, *11,* 263.
27. Pfaff. Onderstepoort Jour. Vet. Sci. and Anim. Indus., 1940, *15,* 175.
28. Plowright. Comp. virology. N.Y. Acad. Sci., 1962, *101,* 548.
29. Plowright. Virology monographs, ed. S. Gard, C. Hallauer, and K. F. Meyer. Springer-Verlag, New York, 1968, *3,* 27.
30. Plowright and Ferris. Res. Vet. Sci., 1962, *3,* 172.
31. Provost and Borredom. Rev. d'Elevage., 1968, *21,* 33.
32. Scott. Adv. Vet. Sci., 1964, *9,* 113.
33. Scott, DeTray, and White. Bull. Off. Intl. Epiz., 1959, *51,* 694.
34. Shope, Griffiths, and Jenkins. Am. Jour. Vet. Res., 1946, *7,* 135.
35. Shope, Maurer, Jenkins, Griffiths, and Baker. Am. Jour. Vet. Res., 1946, *7,* 152.
36. Stirling. Vet. Jour., 1932, *88,* 192; 1933, *89,* 290.
37. Stone and Moulton. Am. Jour. Vet. Res., 1961, *22,* 18.
38. Thiery. Rev. d'Elevage., 1956, *9,* 117.
39. Wagner, Jessett, Brown, and Radley. Res. Vet. Sci., 1975, *19,* 209.

THE GENUS *PARAMYXOVIRUS*

Newcastle Disease

SYNONYMS: Pseudoplague of fowls, pseudo fowl pest, pneumoencephalitis, Ranikhet disease; abbreviation, ND.

The disease was first encountered by Kraneveld (21) in Java and reported in 1926. In 1927 Doyle (9) described the disease in a flock of chickens in Newcastle-on-Tyne, England, and announced the cause to be a virus. By 1940 Newcastle disease had been recognized in the Philippines, Asia, Australia, and Africa. Later it appeared in continental Europe. Its identification in California in 1944 marked the first recognition of the malady in the Western Hemisphere (2). It is widely scattered in the United States. Although the virus frequently produces grave epizootics and high mortality rates among fowls in the Eastern Hemisphere, the percentages of losses in the Western world vary considerably depending on many factors.

Chickens, turkeys, guinea fowl, ducks, geese, pigeons, pheasants, partridges, crows, sparrows, mayas, and martins, as well as unidentified species of free-flying birds, have been reported as affected during natural outbreaks (6). The virus sometimes causes conjunctivitis in man.

Character of the Disease. Outbreaks of Newcastle disease vary greatly in intensity. In some instances, particularly in adult birds, the signs may be hardly recognizable; this is termed the *lentogenic form*. In other cases, the disease may be very severe, resulting in deaths of the majority of those affected, and is called the *velogenic form*. The *mesogenic form* causes a disease that usually does not have more than 25 percent mortality. All ages are susceptible, but young birds are usually more severely affected than older ones. The disease usually begins with respiratory signs often followed by diarrhea.

The incubation period varies from 4 to 14 days, with an average of about 5 days. The disease has been observed in 2-day-old chicks. Upon experimental inoculation chicks usually develop signs within 4 days.

The severity of the disease in a flock depends on the age and immunity status, strain virulence, route of infection, and concurrent infections. In chicks, from a few days to a few weeks of age, the disease begins with respiratory signs often followed by profuse diarrhea. The infection spreads rapidly, and respiratory distress is evidenced by gasping, which may be accompanied by moist râles and crackling sounds. In many outbreaks nervous signs appear a few days after the onset of the respiratory syndrome. Very young chicks may show a profound stupor. They often rest on their hocks with toes slightly flexed, head depressed, and eyes closed, or they appear to be unable to use one or both legs and remain in lateral recumbency. Others may show signs of ataxia, such as staggering, torticollis (Figure 50.13), opisthotonos, and posterior propulsion. Handling them often intensifies the nervous manifestations. The death rate usually is high, and those that survive often are useless. In the velogenic form in adult birds the signs are quite comparable with a mortality of 90 to 100 percent. The mesogenic form causes a less severe disease, and in laying flocks there is a sudden drop in egg production with grossly abnormal eggs. The eggs that are laid after the nonlaying period frequently are misshapen and usually have soft and imperfectly formed shells. Often the only change observed

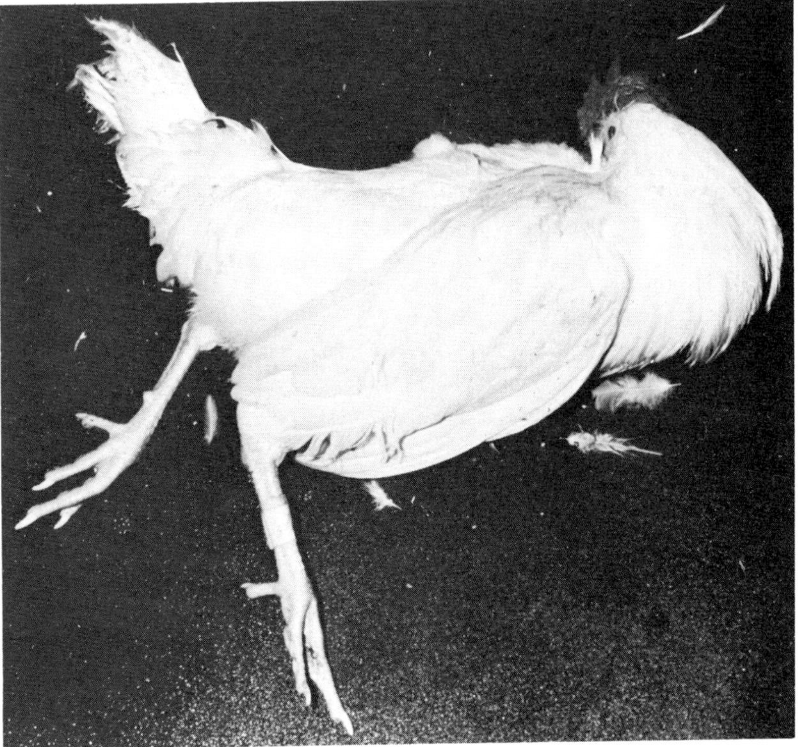

Figure 50.13. Torticollis in a chicken after inoculation with Texas GB strain of Newcastle disease virus. (Courtesy D. A. Gregg, Plum Island Animal Disease Center, USDA.)

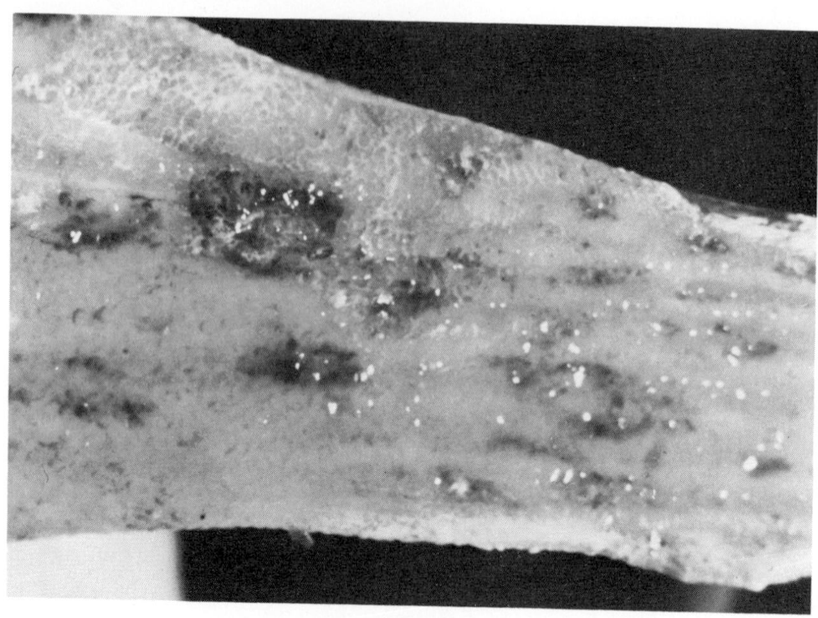

Figure 50.14. Cloaca of a chicken showing hemorrhagic areas and shallow erosions on mucosal surface after inoculation with a velogenic strain of Newcastle disease virus. (Courtesy D. A. Gregg, Plum Island Animal Disease Center, USDA.)

in a laying flock with the lentogenic form is a slight reduction in egg production. Flocks may not return to their former level of egg production for 4 to 8 weeks after recovery.

The nature and extent of the lesions are governed by the pathogenicity of the disease. In mild cases the only changes may be cloudy air sac membranes, an enlarged spleen, and fluid or mucus in the trachea. In the velogenic form petechial hemorrhages may be present in the mucosa of proventriculus, cloaca (Figure 50.14), gizzard, and intestinal tract and sometimes erosions. The spleen may be enlarged and other organs congested. In the laying hen there often is an accumulation of fresh, watery yolk in the ovum and accompanying congestion of the ovarian blood vessels. When nervous signs are observed, microscopic lesions of mild encephalitis usually are found. No inclusion bodies have been seen.

In turkey poults the disease may be severe and result in a 50 percent mortality.

The Disease in Experimental Animals. The disease can be produced by inoculation in a wide series of wild and domesticated birds. Reagan, Lillie, Poelma, and Brueckner (26) successfully carried the virus through 12 Syrian hamsters by serial intracerebral inoculations. Brandly (5) cites Upton as having successfully achieved serial transfer of this virus in suckling mice.

Properties of the Virus. On the basis of filtration trials with graded collodion membranes, Burnet and Ferry (8) estimated the size of Newcastle virus to be 80 to 120 nm. The virus will pass Seitz pads, Berkefeld N and W candles, and Chamberland L_3 and L_5 filters. It is destroyed by pasteurization and exposure to ultraviolet light. Pulp of infected organs dried *in vacuo* over P_2O_5 and stored in the refrigerator remains virulent for years. Allantoic-amniotic fluid from infected embryonated eggs retains its virulence for several years if stored in the moist or lyophilized state at −70 C. Boyd and Hanson (4) studied the survival ability of the virus in soils at varying temperatures and humidities. In the presence of some moisture the virus proved to be surprisingly resistant. Ether treatment disrupts the virus into the V-antigen (hemagglutinating rosettes and the internal symmetrical helical components resembling the S-antigen of influenza virus).

Newcastle virus is the type species of the *Paramyxovirus* genus. It has the same structural features as other members of this genus. It is an RNA virus that is inactivated by formalin and by heating to 60 C for 30 minutes. It is immunologically distinct from other members of the genus except for a possible hemagglutination-inhibition test relationship with mumps virus of man. Immunological strain differences of Newcastle virus have been suggested.

Burnet (7) was the first to show that Newcastle disease virus has the property of agglutinating chicken erythrocytes and that antiserum will neutralize this property. The property of hemagglutination inhibition has proved valuable in diagnosis.

Cultivation. Newcastle disease virus is readily cultivated in embryonated chicken eggs. Bacteriologically sterile suspensions of virus-containing material are inoculated through the chorioallantoic membrane. The virus kills the embryo in about 2 to 6 days. In eggs dead on the 3rd day or later and occasionally in eggs dead on the 2nd day, a small opaque area is found on the chorioallantois at the point of inoculation. Sometimes the membrane is edematous. The yolk sac vessels are congested, and the embryo is reddened, especially in the feet and legs. The skin around the head often shows hemorrhages, and the liver is usually congested.

Newcastle virus produces a cytopathogenic effect in cell cultures of certain chick tissues. In some cell lines the cytopathogenic effect is only visible microscopically. Cultivation is also reported in cell cultures of monkey kidney cell, HeLa cells, calf kidney cells, and many other types of cells. Cytoplasmic inclusion bodies and multinucleated cells also occur in cultures. Occasionally, well-defined intranuclear inclusion bodies are observed. Cell-cultured tissues may become chronically infected with or without viral release and frequently show no cytopathic effect. In cases in which interferon mediates persistent infections, the cells usually are resistant to other closely related viruses.

Immunity. Fowls recovered from Newcastle disease are immune for years. The hemagglutination-inhibiting and serum-neutralizing antibodies are criteria of immunity, and they both persist for years. Birds without antibody may withstand exposure to virulent virus, however, indicating that humoral and cell-mediated mechanisms are involved in protection of birds against NDV.

In mammals the antibody activity in secretions is associated with secretory IgA. This is also true in chickens, except the chicken IgA lacks the secretory component (17). After injection with Newcastle disease virus, there is an increase in total serum protein parallel to an increase in serum-neutralizing (SN) hemagglutination inhibition (HI) and precipitating (P) antibodies. The SN, HI, and P antibodies were detected in both IgM and IgG immunoglobulins. Serum IgM appeared during the first week after injection of virus, then diminished and rose again after secondary vaccination (18).

Mechanism of host resistance to inactivated and mesogenic strains of Newcastle disease virus were studied in normal and immunodeficient birds (24). Most normal birds resisted mesogenic NDV, but T-cell-deficient birds were more susceptible and agammaglobulinemic birds were extremely susceptible. There was no difference in the kinetics and levels of HI activity of plasma in control, irradiated, and T-cell-deficient birds or between dying and surviving birds. Agammaglobulinemic chickens can be partially protected against a lethal challenge following immunization with lentogenic NDV or beta-propiolactone inactivated NDV mixed with complete Freund's adjuvant. Chickens immunized with a lentogenic strain of NDV 2 to 9 weeks before challenge with virulent virus remain normal, but virus can be found in the circulating leukocytes for as long as 10 days (27).

Various vaccines have been used with varying degrees of success in the last 20 years. Formalin-inactivated vaccines were generally regarded as not conferring sufficient immunity, and modified virus vaccines have been most popular in recent years. Hofstad (14) showed that two doses of an inactivated virus vaccine would confer a solid immunity, but he did not determine its duration.

In 1940 Iyer and Dobson (16) reported that certain English Newcastle strains had become avirulent by serial passage through embryonating eggs. They used these strains for immunization purposes and noted that only occasional fatalities occurred. Later it was shown by Komarov (19) that these vaccines could be used successfully to vaccinate day-old chicks from immune parents but produced high mortality when applied to chicks from susceptible parents. Further studies also showed that parental immunity usually interfered with immunity response and that chicks that gave no reaction to the vaccine soon became susceptible to infection.

Komarov and Goldsmit (20) modified Newcastle virus by serial passage in duck eggs. A vaccine prepared from infected eggs was used with apparent success in vaccinating young and adult chickens.

Beaudette, Bivins, and Miller (3) screened 105 strains of Newcastle disease virus to find one sufficiently nonpathogenic to be used for immunization purposes. The vaccine consisted of undiluted allantoic-amniotic fluid and was used to vaccinate chicks at 30 to 36 days of age by the "stick" and intramuscular methods. Losses from vaccination were very low, and the chicks developed solid immunity. Vaccination of three successive lots of chicks, even after the disease had appeared in them, resulted in a marked reduction in the mortality compared with previous nonvaccinated lots. A few adult birds vaccinated at the beginning of the period of egg production showed a decrease in production on the 5th or 6th day, but these returned to normal within 2 weeks after vaccination.

Hitchner (13) and Bankowski (1) have developed modified virus vaccines that have been used with success. Hitchner's vaccine was made from 20 percent suspensions of infected chick embryos. Given to chicks less than 1 week of age, it produced no signs, and the birds were solidly immunized for as long as 1 year. Bankowski's vaccine was made by growing an attenuated strain in minced chick embryo tissue cultures.

A nonavian tissue-culture-modified Newcastle disease vaccine developed by Gale *et al.* (12) had no detrimental effect on fertility and only a slight effect on hatchability and egg production. The vaccine virus did not spread to unvaccinated pen-contact control chickens. Upon challenge with the GB (intramuscular) and DK (intranasal) virulent test strains vaccinated hens showed only a slight decline in egg production; thus the vaccinated hens were well protected.

Transmission. The disease spreads readily by direct contact. Chicks may carry the virus from an infected hatchery, or from contact with diseased fowl while en route, to the poultry farm. Susceptible birds will contract the disease from infected excretions or organs of diseased fowl, from water contaminated by such fowl, and from infected feed bags, feed containers, and the like. Eggs laid by hens during acute infection may contain virus; after a flock has returned to full production, no virus is found in the eggs.

Diagnosis. Newcastle disease should be suspected when a respiratory disease in chicks is associated with or followed by nervous or paralytic signs and when there are tracheal exudates and clouded air sacs on autopsy. Since the disease is primarily a respiratory infection in this country, in the absence of nervous signs it is most likely to be confused with infectious bronchitis. Laryngotracheitis also exhibits respiratory signs, but gasping is more pronounced and respiration more rhythmical. Nervous signs appear in vitamin-deficiency diseases of chicks and in encephalomyelitis (epidemic tremor), but in these diseases no initial respiratory signs are seen. The fowl plague syndrome also simulates that of Newcastle disease and must be considered in the differential diagnosis in countries where it exists.

Virus isolation and identification or serum-neutralization tests establish the identity of the Newcastle disease. Early in the course of the disease good sources of the virus are tracheal exudate, spleen, and brain. Within a few days after the onset surviving birds will show positive serum-neutralization reactions.

Fabricant (10) compared the results of hemagglutination-inhibition (HI) and serum-neutralization (SN) tests in infected chickens and found that the HI test reached a positive level sooner than the SN test. His studies indicated that the HI titer became positive from 2 days before to 5 days after (average 2 days after) the first appearance of respiratory signs. This test has proved quite satisfactory for rapid diagnosis of Newcastle disease.

Control. Newcastle disease is higly contagious and spreads readily through direct contact. It appears to be scattered throughout the poultry-raising areas of the United States. In an outbreak of the disease, removal of the infected unit may eliminate the infection, but frequently it has spread so quickly that all units on the premises are exposed by the time it is diagnosed. Levine, Fabricant, Gillespie, Angstrom, and Mitchell (22) concluded that birds recovered from Newcastle disease do not harbor sufficient virus to infect susceptible birds 1 month after the flock recovers from respiratory signs.

It appears that the most effective vaccines contain live virus, and vaccination introduces this virus into the flock. Beaudette *et al.* (3) believed, however, that their nonpathogenic vaccine did not produce carriers but that the vaccinated flock was a source of infection for about 3 weeks only.

Annual replacement of the laying flock at the end of the first laying year, with segregation of the replacement stock and the application of all sanitary precautions, has proved effective in controlling the disease on certain poulty farms.

Subtilin, a peptide antibiotic, inactivates Newcastle disease virus in allantoic fluid under well-defined conditions of subtilin concentration, pH, and the amount of allantoic fluid in the reaction mixtures (23). At present it has no application in the control of the disease.

Raggi and Lee state that viable infectious bronchitis (IB) virus interferes with Newcastle disease (ND) virus replication (25). The practice of combining IB and ND vaccine should be discouraged.

The Disease in Man. Although there are reports in the literature that Newcastle disease virus has caused generalized disease in man, it appears that this is not true. The virus causes conjunctivitis in man, and several reports of its isolation from this condition have been published (11, 15) Patients show acute, unilateral or bilateral conjunctivitis. No systemic symptoms appear, and no ill effects are noted other than a mild irritation of about 3 to 7 days' duration.

REFERENCES

1. Bankowski. Proc. Soc. Exp. Biol. and Med., 1957, *96,* 114.
2. Beach. Science, 1944, *100,* 361.
3. Beaudette, Bivins, and Miller. Cornell Vet., 1949, *39,* 302.
4. Boyd and Hanson. Avian Dis., 1958, *2,* 82.
5. Brandly. *In* Diseases of poultry, 3rd ed., ed. Harry E.

Biester and Louis H. Schwarte. Iowa State College Press, Ames, Iowa, 1952, p. 541.
6. Brandly, Moses, Jones, and Jungherr. Am. Jour. Vet. Res., 1946, *7*, 243.
7. Burnet. Austral. Jour. Exp. Biol. and Med. Sci., 1942, *20*, 81.
8. Burnet and Ferry. Brit. Jour. Exp. Path., 1934, *15*, 56.
9. Doyle. Jour. Comp. Path. and Therap., 1927, *40*, 144.
10. Fabricant. Cornell Vet., 1949, *39*, 202.
11. Freymann and Bang. Johns Hopkins Hosp. Bull., 1949, *84*, 409.
12. Gale, Gard, Ose, and Berkman. Avian Dis., 1965, *9*, 348.
13. Hitchner. Cornell Vet., 1950, *40*, 60.
14. Hofstad. Am. Jour. Vet. Res., 1956, *17*, 738.
15. Ingalls and Mahoney. Am. Jour. Pub. Health, 1949, *39*, 737.
16. Iyer and Dobson. Vet. Rec., 1940, *52*, 889.
17. Katz and Kohn. Dev. Biol. Stand, 1976, *33*, 290.
18. Khare, Kumar, and Grun. Poultry Sci., 1976, *55*, 152.
19. Komarov. Refuah Vet. 1947, *4*, 96.
20. Komarov and Goldsmit. Cornell Vet., 1947, *37*, 368.
21. Kraneveld. Hemera Zoa (N.I. Bl. v. Diergeneesk.), 1926, *38*, 448.
22. Levine, Fabricant, Gillespie, Angstrom, and Mitchell. Cornell Vet., 1950, *40*, 206.
23. Lorenz and Jann. Am. Jour. Vet. Res., 1964, *25*, 1285.
24. Perey and Dent. Proc. Soc. Exp. Biol. and Med., 1975, *148*, 365.
25. Raggi and Lee. Avian Dis., 1964, *8*, 471.
26. Reagan, Lillie, Poelma, and Brueckner. Am. Jour. Vet. Res., 1947, *8*, 136.
27. Turner, Spalatin, and Hanson. Avian Dis., 1976, *20*, 375.

Parainfluenza Infection in Cattle

Present evidence suggests that parainfluenza 3 (PI-3) virus of cattle plays an important role in acute bovine respiratory diseases commonly termed shipping fever, shipping pneumonia, stockyard fever, or the pneumonic or pectoral form of hemorrhagic septicemia. *Mycoplasma* and particularly *Pasteurella* species also are involved in the etiology with parainfluenza 3 virus. In some respiratory cases concurrent infection of PI-3 with bovine virus diarrhea-mucosal disease, infectious bovine rhinotracheitis, enteroviruses, hemolytic cocci, *Alkaligenes* species, and *Actinobacillus actinoides* has been found.

The disease has been recognized for many years and has been the cause of heavy losses, especially in cattle shipped during the cold months. It formerly was believed to be caused by organisms of the *Pasteurella* group, particularly *P. multocida*. Inasmuch as it was not possible to reproduce the disease with these organisms, it has long been suspected that other etiological agents are involved in the disease. Some think that this organism has nothing to do with the disease, and some cases have been reported in which it seemed to be absent; however, it is present in many cases and generally is found in great numbers in the fibrinous exudate in the alveoli of the lungs and in the pleural cavity. It is difficult to believe that *Pasteurella* species do not have an important role in the terminal lesions of the disease, if not in the initiation of the infection.

Collier, Chow, Benjamin, and Deem (3) suspected that some cases of shipping fever might be the result of a combined infection with the virus of infectious bovine rhinotracheitis (IBR) and *Pasteurella* organisms, particularly *P. hemolytica*. Their experiments supported this belief to the extent that cattle were more severely affected when both agents were given simultaneously than when either was given alone. The disease produced was nonfatal, and while the authors say that the signs were typical of shipping fever, they are careful not to claim that they reproduced that disease.

Reisinger, Heddleston, and Manthei (15) also isolated the virus of IBR from cattle that were showing signs considered to be typical of shipping fever. They also isolated a hemagglutinating virus, a myxovirus belonging to the parainfluenza 3 group, which they identified as SF-4 and with this they were able to produce mild but typical cases of shipping fever. There was no cross-neutralization with IBR virus. These workers isolated *Pasteurella* organisms from 65 percent of the animals in herds where shipping fever occurred and in 50 percent of those that had not been affected. Studies by these same investigators indicate that perhaps *Pasteurella* species alone may cause respiratory infection in cattle under various stressing conditions.

Character of the Disease. Shipping fever seldom occurs naturally in calves. In adult cattle it takes the form of a fibrinous pneumonia. The animals cough, show very high temperatures (107 F and higher), and soon exhibit signs of great respiratory embarrassment. Often they stand with the forelegs held wide apart and the neck extended far forward. The breathing may become stertorous, and often through the mouth. Foamy saliva frequently is blown on the floor and walls before the animal. Such animals usually die within a few hours after the severe respiratory embarrassment is seen, and within 3 or 4 days from the time the first signs of illness are observed.

In typical cases of shipping fever the lesions are located in the respiratory tract, all others being secondary. The lungs often fill the thorax and are covered with a white fibrinous mass that may be peeled off the surface like coagulated egg albumen, the underlying surfaces being rough and congested. The lungs, especially the main lobes, may be very solid and heavy. Cut sections show deep-red lobules and grayish ones separated by interlobular tissue which has been greatly thickened by infiltration of coagulated exudate like that on the serous surface. Histologic examination reveals broncheolitis, alveolitis, serocellular exudate in the lung, intracytoplasmic acidophilic inclusion bodies in nasal and bronchial epithelium, and alveolar macrophages, together with marked fluorescence with specific antibody (23).

The Disease in Experimental Cattle (23). The first signs of illness occur in calves 24 to 30 hours after exposure. The signs may include increased temperature, lacrimation, serous nasal discharge, depression, and dyspnea followed by coughing. The signs may be mild and easily missed in some animals. A calf can have a marked pneumonia with meager clinical signs. A more severe disease results when *Pasteurella multocida* is given intranasally 24 to 48 hours following exposure to PI-3 virus. One strain produces diarrhea.

Colostrum-deprived calves have a mild illness after intransal inoculation of PI-3 virus (26). *In utero* injection of virus into pregnant cows produces pathological changes in the fetus (18), but there is no evidence that the virus has an effect on natural breeding efficiency (2).

In pathogenicity studies with PI-3 certain facts have emerged. The virus inhibits the clearance of *Pasteurella hemolytica* from the lungs of infected calves, but within the limitations of the experiment there did not seem to be a correlation between pulmonary retention of the bacteria and the development of pathological changes. (16). The cytotoxic cells in lung washings of calves are alveolar macrophages, and they cause destruction of viral-infected calf kidney cells in culture and reduce the yields of virus. In infected bovine tracheal organ cultures there is an initial reduction in virus yield, but the macrophages become infected in 2 to 3 days and there is a reduction in toxicity in the cultures (14). Epithelial cells of the respiratory tract are the primary target cells for PI-3 virus with more productive infection in the bronchoalveolar regions and the trachea. The replication of virus in the alveolar type 2 cells suggests that changes in surfactant production may occur during the peak of infection. Virus budding through the basement membrane of small bronchioles and the presence of particles in the interstitial regions imply the basement membrane may be impaired (20).

The PI-3 virus has been isolated from man, cattle, water buffaloes, horses, and monkeys. Guinea pigs, hamsters, sheep, and swine are susceptible to experimental infection.

Properties of the Virus. The intact virus particles vary from 140 to 250 nm. It is an RNA virus that is labile at pH 3 and in the presence of ether or chloroform. The virion causes hemagglutination of red blood cells from birds, cattle, swine, guinea pigs, and human beings. Guinea pig cells are most sensitive. Infected cell cultures show the phenomenon of hemadsorption. The virus produces interferon in fetal bovine kidney cell cultures (17). The human, bovine, and sheep PI-3 viruses are closely related but not identical. The human and bovine strains were differentiated by neutralization, hemagglutination-inhibition, and complement fixation (CF) tests with guinea pig antiserum (10). Strains differ in the neuraminidase activity. The whole virion and the peplomers are active as antigens in the leukocyte migration inhibition, lymphocyte stimulation, and skin hypersensitivity tests (9).

Cultivation. The virus replicates in many types of cultured cells including bovine, swine, equine, and rabbit kidneys, and also in cells from the chicken embryo. Multiplication in cell cultures usually produces syncytia and intracytoplasmic and intranuclear inclusion bodies. Plaques are produced in 3 to 5 days in agar overlay preparations. The virus also replicated in calf alveolar macrophages from the lung but to a higher titer at 32 C than at 37 C (19). The virus also replicates and produces alterations in bovine fetal tracheal mucosa and bovine fetal lung organ cultures (11) (Figures 50.15 and 50.16).

Immunity. The antibody level for bovine PI-3 in the cow increases prior to parturition and decreases to former levels during lactation. Antibodies are transferred in the colostrum resulting in blood levels equal to or greater than that of the mother. This passive antibody decreases with age and is no longer detectable by weaning at 6 to 8 months of age. This antibody does not interfere with exposure to virus by the aerosol route, but the infection was less severe than in calves deprived of colostrum. The immunological response in calves with colostrally acquired maternal immunity was less as the levels of serum and nasal secretion neutralizing antibody were lower than in colostrum-deprived calves (12).

Active antibody develops in calves when the animal comes in contact with PI-3 virus. After intranasal infection IgA was found in the nasal secretions and IgM and

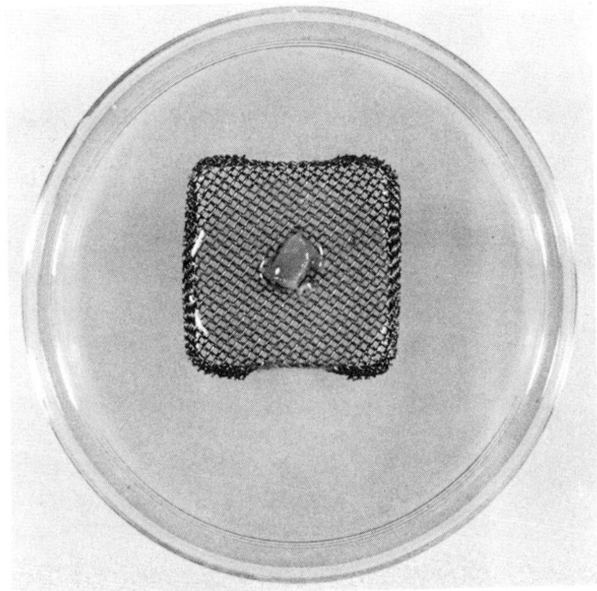

Figure 50.15. Bovine parainfluenza virus 131. An organ culture of bovine fetal lung mounted on a wire grid and partially submerged in tissue culture media. (Courtesy J. Kita, R. Kenney, and J. Gillespie, *Cornell Vet.*)

IgG immunoglobulins were demonstrable in the serum (13). Most investigators agree that the IgA antibodies presumably synthesized locally contribute heavily to the total antibody activity present in the secretions of the respiratory tract and to the protection provided to the animal (21, 24, 27). In parainfluenza 3 infections, reinfections are common and seem to depend more or less on circulating antibody levels (5).

The antibody levels may determine whether an anamnestic response occurs, and, on occasion, mild clinical signs may also occur (7, 8). It seems reasonable to assume that reinfections occur as the majority of adult beef and dairy cattle have demonstrable HI antibody.

Transmission. Natural transmission in susceptible calves exposed to clinically ill calves excreting virus occurs in 5 to 10 days. Virus can be isolated from the nasal excretions for 7 to 8 days after infection and from the lungs for 17 days and perhaps longer despite the presence of serum antibodies. Infected cattle probably are the

Figure 50.16. (*Left*) Bovine parainfluenza 131. Bovine fetal lung organ culture, 14 days. Uninoculated. Note apparent cell viability with occasional large basophilic nucleoli and infrequency of pyknoses. Fixed in alcohol. H and E stain. × 1,100. (*Right*) Replicate culture, 13 days after inoculation with C3F-11 strain of bovine parainfluenza virus. Note many intranuclear inclusion bodies (*arrows*), pyknosis, and karyorrhexis. Fixed in alcohol. H and E stain. × 1,100. (Courtesy J. Kita, R. Kenney, and J. Gillespie, *Cornell Vet.*)

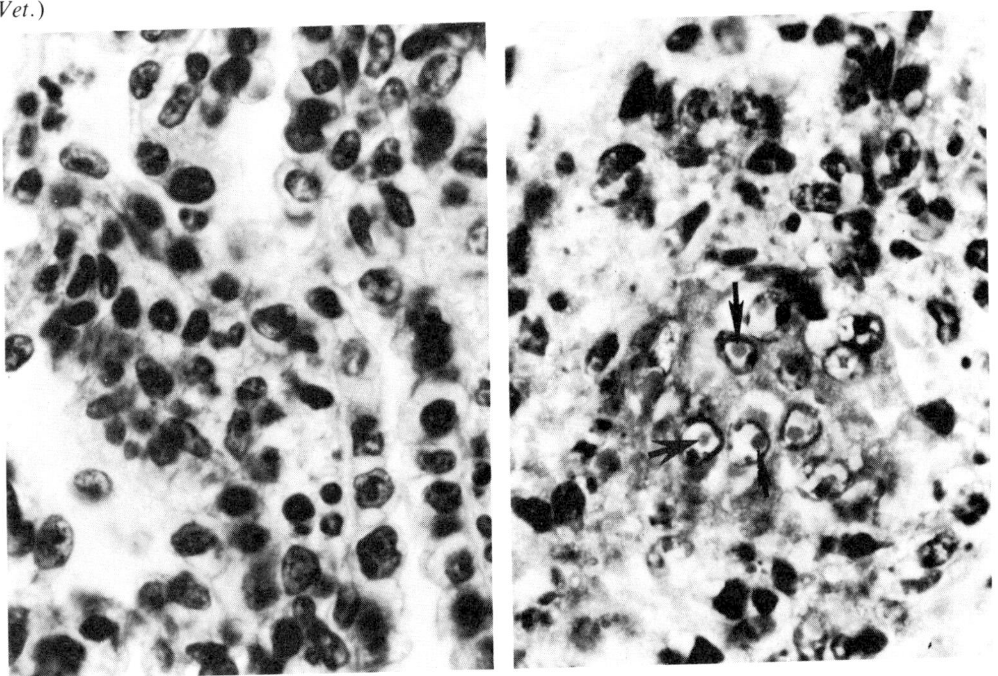

prime source for the continuity of the bovine PI-3 virus in nature.

PI-3 antibodies are found in man, horses (4), guinea pigs, swine, deer, and bighorn sheep. Their role in the transmission of the disease is unknown, but they may be involved in the ecology of the cattle disease which has a world-wide distribution.

Diagnosis. The virus can be readily isolated from respiratory tract exudates in tissue culture. In tissue culture the virus can be identified by a combination of features: (*a*) the production of syncytia and cytoplasmic and intranuclear inclusion bodies, (*b*) a hemadsorbing virus, (*c*) fluorescence by a specific conjugate, and (*d*) neutralization of the isolate by specific antiserum.

The demonstration of a rising titer with paired sera is another method, although it doesn't eliminate the presence of a concurrent infection.

Certain clinical features may vary from those of other specific respiratory diseases of cattle, yet there is considerable overlap in the signs, making a positive diagnosis by this means often impossible (1).

Prevention and Control. The recommended procedures based on our present limited state of knowledge for the prevention and control of bovine PI-3 in beef and dairy cattle was outlined by the Panel, Bovine Respiratory Disease Symposium, American Veterinary Medical Association, in 1968 (1). The reader is strongly urged to consult that reference for details, especially since the approach is different in dealing with dairy and beef herds.

In brief, the panel recommended that beef calves be given PI-3 vaccine and *Pasteurella* bacterin at 4 months of age. One month later another injection of virus vaccine and *Pasteurella* bacterin should be administered. In open and closed dairy herds it is well to vaccinate the calves at 6 to 8 months of age with PI-3 and *Pasteurella* bacterin.

Studies by Woods *et al.* (25) and Gale *et al.* (6) show that two injections of inactivated virus vaccine are required to produce high HI titers. The vaccine produced by Gale *et al.* also contains *Pasteurella* bacteria as well as PI-3 inactivated virus. Some investigators have indicated that the vaccine does not always inhibit the disease in beef cattle but the disease in the vaccinates is less severe and weight loss, if any, is minimal. The unvaccinated cattle have a considerable loss in weight.

Attenuated PI-3 virus vaccines used singly and in combination with attenuated infectious bovine rhinotracheitis and bovine adenovirus 3, have been used to immunize calves by the intranasal route. These vaccines are safe and efficacous (22, 24, 27). The duration of protection against virulent virus has not been ascertained. There is no doubt that these vaccines are useful in dairy and beef practices when properly and appropriately used.

The shipping of cattle, inclement weather, and the associated stress have a marked influence on the severity of disease. Every effort should be made to make the cattle as comfortable as possible.

Clinical evidence indicates that animals sometimes may be successfully treated for shipping fever if treatment is begun early in the course of the disease. The tetracycline compounds appear to be useful, also several of the sulfonamides. Since these agents do not have any appreciable effect on most viruses, their virtue probably lies in their effect on the bacterial agents, especially the *Pasteurella*, which are known to be especially susceptible to these compounds.

The Disease in Man. There is no evidence that the bovine strains of parainfluenza 3 virus produce illness in man, nor has the reverse been proved.

REFERENCES

1. Bovine Respiratory Disease Symposium. Jour. Am. Vet. Med. Assoc., 1968, *152*, part 2.
2. Call, Smart, Blake, Butcher, and Shupe. Am. Jour. Vet. Res., 1978, *39*, 527.
3. Collier, Chow, Benjamin, and Deem. Am. Jour. Vet. Res., 1960, *21*, 195.
4. Ditchfield, Zbitnew, and MacPherson. Can. Vet. Jour., 1963, *4*, 175.
5. Fukumi. Dev. Biol. Stand., 1975, *28*, 159.
6. Gale, Hamdy, and Trapp. Jour. Am. Vet. Med. Assoc., 1963, *142*, 884.
7. Gillespie. Unpublished data, 1957.
8. Hamparian, Washko, Ketler, and Hilleman. Jour. Immunol., 1961, *87*, 139.
9. Hoglund, Moreno-Lopez, and Morein. Arch. Virol., 1977, *53*, 323.
10. Ketler, Hamparian, and Hilleman. Jour. Immunol., 1961, *87*, 126.
11. Kita, Kenny, and Gillespie. Cornell Vet., 1969, *54*, 355.
12. Marshall and Frank. Am. Jour. Vet. Res., 1975, *36*, 1085.
13. Mukkur, Komar, and Sabina. Arch. Virol., 1975, *48*, 195.
14. Probert, Stott, and Thomas. Inf. and Immun., 1977, *15*, 576.
15. Reisinger, Heddleston, and Manthei. Jour. Am. Vet. Med. Assoc., 1959, *135*, 147.
16. Ropez, Thomson, and Savan. Can. Jour. Comp. Med., 1976, *40*, 385.
17. Rosenquist and Loan. Am. Jour. Vet. Res., 1967, *28*, 619.

18. Sattar, Bohl, Trapp, and Hamdy. Am. Jour. Vet. Res., 1967, *28*, 45.
19. Tsai. Inf. and Immun., 1977, *18*, 780.
20. Tsai and Thomson. Inf. and Immun., 1975, *11*, 783.
21. Todd. Dev. Biol. Stand., 1975, *28*, 473.
22. Todd. Dev. Biol. Stand., 1976, *33*, 391.
23. Woods. Jour. Am. Vet. Med. Assoc., 1968, *152*, 771.
24. Woods, Crandell, and Mansfield. Res. Commun. Chem. Path. Pharmacol., 1975, *11*, 117.
25. Woods, Mansfield, Segre, Holper, Brandly, and Barthel. Am. Jour. Vet. Res., 1962, *23*, 832.
26. Woods, Sibinovic, and Starkey. Am. Jour. Vet. Res., 1965, *26*, 262.
27. Zygraich, Vascoboinic, and Huygelen. Dev. Biol. Stand., 1976, *33*, 379.

SV-5 Respiratory Disease of Dogs

In 1967 a parainfluenza virus closely related to SV-5 parainfluenza virus of monkeys, a member of parainfluenza type II virus group, was implicated in an epizootic of respiratory disease in laboratory dogs (6). Two separate outbreaks occurred 1 year later in military dogs in the United States and these isolates were identical (7, 10).

Character of the Disease. The disease syndrome in field outbreaks is severe and probably involves other pathogens as well as SV-5 virus (1). The disease is characterized by sudden onset, copious nasal discharge, fever, and coughing in some dogs. Canine SV-5 virus can produce a disease that looks like "kennel cough" if *Mycoplasma* and certain bacterial organisms are also involved in the disease (2).

The Disease in Experimental Animals. With his original isolate, Crandell (10) produced mild respiratory signs in dogs exposed intranasally. The young dogs had tonsilitis and a slight nasal discharge but no fever. Others (8) observed similar signs in dogs exposed to Crandell's isolate by intranasal or intratracheal routes.

In a pathogenesis study Appel and Percy (1) inoculated dogs by various routes. Intramuscular and subcutaneous inoculation did not cause infection. In contrast, aerosol or contact exposure produced disease restricted to the respiratory tract. Virus inoculated into the urinary bladder directly resulted in local viral replication only and cystitis. By aerosol exposure to 10^4 $TCID_{50}$ of virus a slight rise in temperature was noted in the majority of their experimental dogs (1) that occurred 2 to 3 days after exposure and persisted for 1 to 2 days. There was a slight nasal discharge in a few dogs, and slightly less than 50 percent developed a slight nonproductive cough which could be forced by laryngeal palpation. The cough never persisted more than 1 week. At necropsy there were no lesions except for a few petechial hemorrhages in a few dogs sacrificed 4 days after exposure. Microscopic catarrhal changes are evident in the upper and lower respiratory tract and in regional lymph nodes. Virus is isolated from the oronasal specimens between the 1st and 8th day after exposure, but not from the blood. The highest titers are found from respiratory specimens occurring between the 3rd and 6th days. Viral antigen as demonstrated by the immunofluorescence test is observed in the epithelial cells of nasal mucosa, trachea, bronchi, bronchioli, and peribronchial lymph nodes from 1 to 6 days after exposure, with considerable reduction in fluorescence by the 6th day.

When *Mycoplasma* and *Bordetella bronchiseptica* were given intransally after aerosol exposure to canine SV-5 the respiratory illness was more severe in all dogs with a dry cough, persisting in some dogs for several weeks (2). All dogs exposed to canine SV-5 virus developed serum-neutralizing antibody, but levels declined thereafter with little or no antibody 3 to 4 months later.

Properties of the Virus. The canine strains are closely related to parainfluenza virus (2). The canine strains share a common complement-fixing antigen with SV-5 virus isolated from monkeys, but use of the hemagglutination-inhibition and serum-neutralization tests gave negative results (7, 10).

Other limited studies of properties place the virus in the *Paramyxovirus* genus. Its hemagglutinin and hemadsorbing properties are used in the study and diagnosis of the virus and disease.

Cultivation. The canine SV-5 virus replicates in cultures of primary dog kidney, of African green monkey kidney, of rhesus monkey kidney, and of human embryonic kidney cells. The virus produces multinucleated giant cells and eosinophilic inclusion bodies in the cytoplasm of the renal cells.

Propagation of the virus in the amniotic cavity of the hen's embryonated egg was demonstrated by hemagglutination (10). No embryonic deaths were observed. Both amniotic and allantoic fluids contained virus with an HA titer of 1:128. The virus failed to replicate when inoculated into the allantoic cavity.

Immunity. Dogs infected by the respiratory route are fully immune to challenge by this same route 3 weeks later. There are no signs of illness, and virus is not isolated from the respiratory tract. In contrast, dogs given virus parenterally develop good antibody titers, but are not completely protected by an aerosol challenge (1).

Neutralizing antibody may persist for 3 to 4 months (2) and perhaps for 6 months (4). Its relationship to immunity has not been ascertained as yet. The serum-neutralization test is slightly more sensitive than the standard hemagglutination inhibition test (8).

The level and frequency of neutralizing antibody in the dog population is such that maternal immunity does not play a significant role in protection or in immunization (2).

Transmission. The infection is readily transmitted from dogs in the acute stage to susceptible dogs. It is an important disease where there is an assembly of dogs into a new environment such as laboratories or military service (5).

Virus cannot be recovered from the respiratory tract beyond 9 days after exposure. Natural infections in the dog seem to be limited to the respiratory tract. Serological evidence indicates that the incidence of the infection in the general canine population is quite low—less than 5 percent. Despite these two apparent facts, the virus persists in nature and under certain environmental conditions causes a severe disease in the dog.

The host range for SV-5 is unclear, but probably includes monkeys, man, and dogs. The present information suggests that monkeys are principally infected by man (3), or perhaps by dogs, as monkeys residing in the jungle lack antibody.

Diagnosis. To differentiate this viral disease from others in the dog at the clinical level is extremely difficult. There are many other canine viruses which produce comparable respiratory signs of illness.

Field strains from dogs grow quite readily and produce a cytopathic effect in cell cultures. A further distinguishing feature is its hemadsorbing effect. Consequently tissue culture is an excellent method for virus isolation and identification. The use of paired sera in the HI and SN test and the demonstration of a rising antibody titer serves as another means of diagnosis.

Control. At an American Veterinary Medical Association symposium on canine infectious diseases, a panel recommended that a vaccine be developed to assist in the prevention and control of this disease (9). Emery *et al.* (11) have since developed an attenuated virus vaccine that may be given subcutaneously or intramuscularly. The vaccine is safe and provides a sufficient immunity to protect dogs against an aerosol challenge with virulent virus. An anamnestic response occurs in vaccinated dogs after challenge exposure. The duration of immunity has not been ascertained.

Because secondary microorganisms often appear to be involved in the disease process, the use of antibiotics and sulfa compounds may aid in reducing the severity of the disease.

Concentrations of Ribavirin as low as 1 microgram per ml showed some *in vitro* activity against canine parainfluenza virus, but its effectiveness in a clinical situation has not been evaluated (12).

The Disease in Man. In studies of the epizootiology in military dogs, handlers were not infected (10). The exact role of dogs in the epizootiology of SV-5 in other species, including man, is unknown.

REFERENCES

1. Appel and Percy. Jour. Am. Vet. Med. Assoc., 1970, *156,* 1778.
2. Appel, Pickerill, Menegus, Percy, Parsonson, and Sheffy. Gaines Vet. Symposium, 1970, *20,* 15.
3. Atoynatan and Hsiung. Am. Jour. Epidemiol., 1969, *89,* 472.
4. Binn and Lazar. Quoted by Bittle and Emery in Jour. Am. Vet. Med. Assoc., 1970, *156,* 1771.
5. Binn and Lazar. Quoted by Bittle and Emery in Jour. Am. Vet. Med. Assoc., 1970, *156,* 1774.
6. Binn, Eddy, Lazar, Helms, and Murnane. Proc. Soc. Exp. Biol. and Med., 1967, *126,* 140.
7. Binn, Lazar, Rogul, Shepler, Swango, Claypoole, Hubbard, Asbill, and Alexander. Am. Jour. Vet. Res., 1968, *29,* 1809.
8. Bittle and Emery. Jour. Am. Vet. Med. Assoc., 1970, *156,* 1771.
9. Canine Infectious Diseases Symposium, Jour. Am. Vet. Med. Assoc., 1970, *156,* 1661.
10. Crandell, Brimlow, and Davison. Am. Jour. Vet. Res., 1968, *29,* 2141.
11. Emery, House, Bittle, and Spotts. Am. Jour. Vet. Res., 1976, *37,* 1323.
12. Povey. Am. Jour. Vet. Res., 1978, *39,* 175.

Paramyxovirus Infection in Other Domestic Animals

Sheep. Parainfluenza 3 virus was isolated from the pneumonic lungs of five sheep in three flocks in Australia (13). A mild pneumonia was produced in sheep when they were exposed to one of the isolates (CSL 6) under experimental conditions. It would appear that a PI-3 of sheep origin produces disease in sheep, probably playing a comparable role in the acute respiratory diseases of sheep that bovine parainfluenza viruses play in cattle respiratory diseases.

In the United States serological surveys utilizing the hemagglutination-inhibition and serum-neutralization tests show that PI-3 is a common infection in sheep and widespread in the United States. The CSL 6 strain is closely related antigenically to two bovine and one human PI-3 viruses, but not identical. An epidemiological investigation in one sheep herd demonstrated that new lambs become infected in the fall.

Smith and his colleagues have published a series of papers on the immune response of sheep to virulent, inactivated, and attenuated PI-3 virus (9–12, 15). The nature of immunity is similar to that observed for PI-3 infection in cattle. The concentration of antibody in the respiratory tract and anamnestic response governed by cell mediation both play a significant role in protection against the subsequent respiratory disease. These investigators reported that immunity to challenge as assessed by viral shedding from the nose was conferred by attenuated virus administered by intranasal or intramuscular route, by two doses of inactivated virus in Freund's complete adjuvant (FCA) given intramuscularly, and by intramuscular injection of inactivated virus in FCA followed by intranasal instillation of inactivated virus.

Horses. Information about parainfluenza 3 virus in the horse is rather sparse. The virus was first isolated in 1961 from yearling Thoroughbred horses with acute upper respiratory disease (3). A serologic survey of the premises showed that a large number of horses 2 years or older had hemagglutinating inhibition antibodies to a virus isolate. In a reciprocal HI test with HA-1 (human type) and SF_4 (bovine type) PI-3 strains the equine PI-3 strain (RE 55) gave virtually identical results with the HA-1 strain and similar, but not identical, results with the SF_4 strain.

A PI-3 virus was isolated from four colts in Illinois (8) that had a disease diagnosed as strangles. All the animals in the herd of 10 horses had a mucopurulent discharge and/or a history of a recent respiratory disease. Significant serum HI titers were demonstrated in six of the colts.

Complement-fixing antibody apparently disappears about 4 months after infection. In contrast the HI and neutralizing antibody persisted for at least 1 year (2). Sibinovic *et al.* (8) tested 130 horse sera from 14 counties in Illinois and approximately one-half had high HI titers to equine PI-3 virus. Lief and Cohen (5) found CF antibodies in 20 percent of 129 Philadelphia, Pennsylvania, area horses. Although Todd (14) had negative test results for PI-3 neutralizing antibodies in his serological survey, it is likely that PI-3 infection is common in horses. However, its significance as a pathogen is yet to be ascertained as it relates to horses, human beings, and other animals.

Pigs. The hemagglutinating virus of Japan (HVP), or Sendai virus, is a parainfluenza 1 virus that infects mice and perhaps swine and man. In swine, Sendai virus reputedly causes bronchopneumonia in young pigs, although there is no serological evidence in the swine population in Japan to support this contention. In pregnant sows inoculation of the virus early in pregnancy produces mummified fetuses and stillborn pigs (6, 7).

Greig *et al.* isolated a parainfluenza 3 virus from the brain of a pig (4). It crosses antigenically with parainfluenza 2 virus. Its pathogenicity for swine has not been ascertained.

Chickens. A hemagglutinating agent designated Yucaipa (MVY) virus was isolated from chickens with a mixed respiratory infection (1). It is immunologically and serologically distinct from other known avian viruses and the paramxyoviruses of mammals. This paramyxovirus causes a mild respiratory disease in chickens by the intratracheal route.

The virus can be propagated in chicken embryos and in tissue cultures (1). Infected fluids from embryos hemagglutinate chicken erythrocytes. Chickens produce a specific hemagglutination-inhibiting antibody distinct from Newcastle disease virus and other agents of the paramyxovirus group.

REFERENCES

1. Bankowski and Corstvet. Avian Dis., 1961, *5*, 251.
2. Ditchfield. Jour. Am. Vet. Med. Assoc., 1968, *155*, 384.
3. Ditchfield, MacPherson and Zbitnew. Can. Vet. Jour., 1963, *4*, 175.
4. Greig, Johnson, and Bouillant. Res. Vet. Sci., 1971, *12*, 305.
5. Leif and Cohen. WHO Informal Meeting on Coordinated Study of Animal Influenza, 1964 (July), Geneva.
6. Sasahara, Hayashi, Kumagai, Yamamoto, Hirasawa, Munakata, and Okaniwa. Virus, 1954, *4*, 131.
7. Shimuzu, Kawakami, Fukuhara, and Matomoto. Jap. Jour. Exp. Med., 1954, *24*, 363.
8. Sibinovic, Woods, Hardenbrook, and Harquis. Vet. Med., 1965, *60*, 600.
9. Smith. Res. Vet. Sci., 1975, *19*, 56.
10. Smith, Dawson, Wells, and Burrells. Res. Vet. Sci., 1976, *21*, 341.
11. Smith, Wells, Burrells, and Dawson. Arch. Virol., 1975, *49*, 329.

12. Smith, Wells, Burrells, and Dawson. Clin. Exp. Immunol., 1976, *23,* 544.
13. St. George. Austral. Vet. Jour., 1969, *45,* 321.
14. Todd. Jour. Am. Vet. Med. Assoc., 1968, *155,* 387.
15. Wells, Sharp, Burrells, Rushton, and Smith. Jour. Hyg. (London), 1976, *77,* 255.

Mumps Virus Infection in the Domestic Cat and Dog

Clinical observations by veterinary practitioners (4) suggest that both cats and dogs are susceptible to human mumps virus. A number of cases of parotitis have been seen in pet cats or dogs at the same time that members of the household were infected with mumps virus (4).

Mumps virus was isolated from the saliva of two dogs with swollen parotid glands (6). Both cases occurred during outbreaks of mumps in two households. These isolates produced cytopathic effect in HeLa cells, and the hemagglutinating properties of the virus were inhibited by human mumps antiserum. Stone (8) reported that mumps virus may produce meningoencephalitis in the dog without involvement of the parotid gland. Morris *et al.* (5) reported that 38 of 209 dog sera collected at random from a population fixed complement in the presence of mumps virus. In another study Cuadrado (2) found that the sera of 20 dogs had HI titers greater than 1:20 against mumps virus. Mumps virus given to dogs by the intraparotid route failed to produce signs of illness and virus was not recoverable from the saliva, but dogs did develop mumps antibody. Binn (1) suggests that observations on mumps virus should be viewed with caution especially because SV-5 virus antigens are commonly noted in monkey kidney cell cultures and SV-5 antibodies are often seen in guinea pig serum used as a source of complement in the CF test (3).

Wollstein published two reports (9, 10) which reported on the infectiousness of human mumps virus for the domestic cat. When bacterial sterile saliva from infected humans was inoculated into the parotid salivary gland and the testes of kittens, orchitis and parotitis resulted. The experimental cats had a febrile response, leukocytosis, tenderness, and swelling of the injected glands and histological lesions similar to human mumps.

Scott, Schultz, and Gillespie (7) showed that mumps virus replicated in feline kidney and feline lung cells *in vitro*. They also demonstrated that direct inoculation of virulent mumps virus into the parotid salivary gland and testes of an adult male cat resulted in parotitis and orchitis. Infection spread to the opposite gland, and virus was recovered from the parotid salivary gland 59 days after inoculation. Oral and intravenous inoculation of pregnant cats with mumps virus resulted in viral replication within the fetuses, indicating that virus had crossed the placenta.

Present evidence would suggest that mumps virus infection does occur as a natural infection in dogs and cats. Its true significance as a pathogen and its incidence in these hosts are yet to be ascertained as well as its importance in the transmission of this virus to man.

REFERENCES

1. Binn. Jour. Am. Vet. Med. Assoc., 1970, *156,* 1672.
2. Cuadrado. Bull. WHO, 1965, *33,* 803.
3. Hsuing, Isacson, and McCollum. Jour. Immunol., 1962, *88,* 284.
4. Kirk. Personal communication, 1970.
5. Morris, Blount, and McCown. Cornell Vet., 1956, *46,* 525.
6. Noice, Bolin, and Eveleth. Jour. Dis. Child., 1959, *98,* 350.
7. Scott, Schultz, and Gillespie. Unpublished findings, 1972.
8. Stone. Jour. Small Anim. Pract., 1969, *10,* 555.
9. Wollstein. Jour. Exp. Med., 1916, *23,* 353.
10. Wollstein. Jour. Exp. Med., 1918, *28,* 377.

THE GENUS *PNEUMOVIRUS*

The syncytium-forming viruses detected by their characteristic cytopathic effect in tissue-cultured systems have been isolated from tissues of many different species, including cattle and domestic cats. The isolates, in many instances, came from cats or cattle with disease, but not all strains from cattle are recognized as respiratory pathogens.

Based on our limited knowledge of their properties the syncytium-forming viruses are placed in the family Paramyxoviridae as a member of a new genus, *Pneumovirus*.

Feline Syncytium-Forming Viruses

At least 30 isolations have been made by research workers in California, Ohio, and New York (8). Isolates have come from cats with respiratory infections (3), urolithiasis (2, 9), feline infectious peritonitis (3), neoplasms (5, 6, 7), ataxia (1), and no illness (1). Most isolates are made by direct cultures from feline tissue, but some have been made from nasal or pharyngeal swabs or urine.

Character of the Infection. The syncytium-forming viruses are associated with various diseases of the cat, but experimental inoculation in cats has not produced clinical signs of illness (1, 5, 6). Virus was recovered from all of the numerous tissues examined by direct cell culture from cats sacrificed at 14, 29, and 56 days post-inoculation (1) and also readily from the blood of carrier cats by cocultivation of infected leukocytes with feline fibroblastic cells (3).

The role of a syncytium-forming virus in urolithiasis is unknown, but their presence in natural and experimental cases is very interesting. Further studies in disease-free cats under isolation are required to assess their real importance in this most important disease of cats.

Limited studies suggest it is ubiquitous in nature and can persist in the tissues of cats for long periods of time. Using the agar-gel technique (Figure 50.17), Gaskin (3) has shown that there is a close relationship between the persistence of precipitating antibody and infectious virus in the cat. Consequently, a single test is now available to test for antibody and virus in cat populations.

Properties of the Virus. The feline syncytium-forming viral isolates are sensitive to ether, chloroform, heat, and acid (5, 6). The viral particle contains RNA, and the infectious virion appears to be cell-associated (6). Naked viral particles in the cytoplasm are approximately 45 nm in diameter with an electron-lucent center (1, 7, 8). As the particles bud through the cell membrane into vacuoles, they acquire an outer protein coat with projections in the process. The complete particles are 110 nm in diameter. The feline syncytium-forming isolates may be confused with feline leukemia-sarcoma viruses. They are about the same diameter, but the syncytium-forming virus particles show initial formation as a core in the cytoplasm, lack C-type particles, and display studs or spikes that are absent on the outer membrane of feline leukemia-sarcoma particles. In mixed infections of cell cultures containing both viruses, one finds particles with characteristics of both—in addition, fragments and abnormally constructed particles are common (4). Thus, one must proceed with care when relying entirely on electron microscopy for identification and differentiation (4).

Figure 50.17. Immunodiffusion test depicting the development of precipitating antibody in a cat inoculated with the feline syncytium-forming virus. Serial weekly serum samples starting with the 3rd week postinoculation (*1*) are reacted with antigen (*center well*) prepared from infected tissue-cultured cells. Precipitating antibody develops during the 4th week postinoculation (*2*) and forms a line of identity with one of three lines characteristically formed by the serum of a chronically ill cat (*6*). (Courtesy J. Gaskin.)

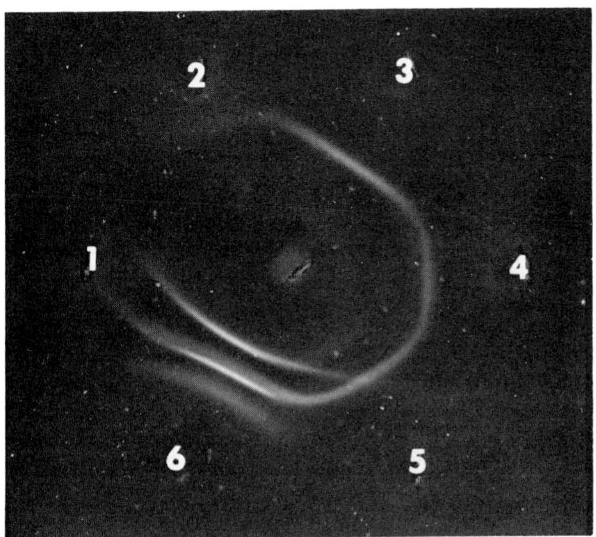

All isolates except one fail to hemagglutinate or hemadsorb cat, chicken, guinea pig, or human O erythrocytes (6, 7). The exception occurred when one of the isolates caused some hemagglutination after sonication (2).

Riggs *et al.* (7) have tested about 10 isolates with the serum-neutralization test. Seven isolates were similar, one was clearly different, and two others may be different (4).

Feline syncytium-forming isolates appear to contain an RNA polymerase common to RNA type C oncogenic viruses and visna virus. There is great interest in this finding as the syncytium-forming viruses could conceivably act in concert with these viruses that have oncogenic capabilities.

Cultivation. Feline syncytium-forming viruses replicate in cell cultures derived from cat, dog, chicken, horse, pig, monkey, and man (7, 8). Most of the isolates produce characteristic syncytium formation in these cultures (Figure 50.18). Multinucleated cells may contain 80 or more nuclei (1). Many cultures do not contain syncytia until 7 and 10 days, with maximum titers attained at 10 to 14 days (7). Occasionally 3 to 4 weeks are required before syncytia become evident. The use of direct cell cultures enhances success of viral isolation.

Immunity. Antibody persists after exposure to the virus, but the virus apparently also persists in most, if not all, cats. At present this causes no concern, as the viruses are not known pathogens.

Transmission. The mode of transmission of this agent is not definitely known (3). Although virus can be iso-

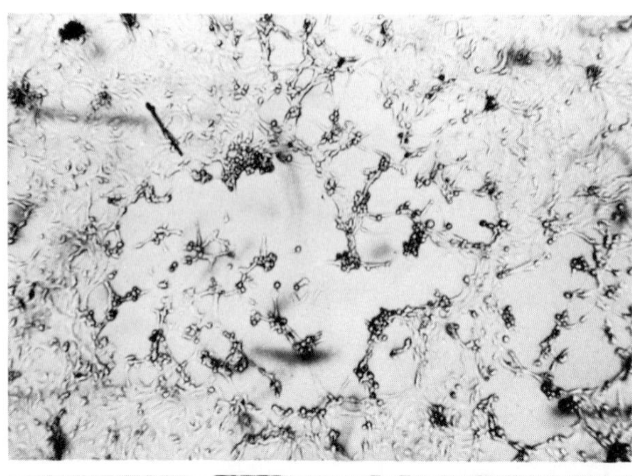

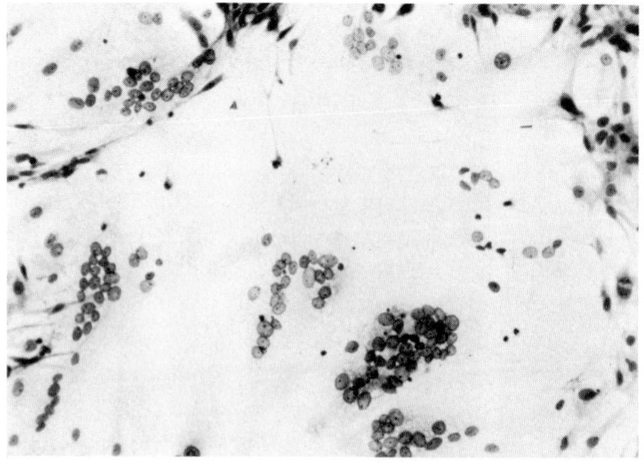

Figure 50.18. The production of syncytia in feline cell cultures by a feline syncytium-forming virus. (*Upper*) Unstained. × 77. (*Lower*) Stained with May-Gruenwald-Giemsa. × 218. (Courtesy C. Fabricant.)

lated from pharyngeal swabs from carrier cats, the infection does not seem to spread readily to uninfected cats housed in the same quarters. Feline syncytium-forming virus is associated with leukocytic cells, and it seems likely that infection may occur early in life by movement of such cells from dam to offspring either in the uterus or via the milk.

The Disease in Man. At present there is no evidence that the feline syncytium-forming viruses cause disease in humans.

REFERENCES

1. Csiza. Cornell Univ. thesis, 1970.
2. Fabricant, Rich, and Gillespie. Cornell Vet., 1969, *59*, 667.
3. Gaskin and Gillespie. Am. Jour. Vet. Res., 1973, *34*, 245.
4. Hackett and Manning. Jour. Am. Vet. Med. Assoc., 1971, *158*, 948.
5. Kasza, Hayward, and Betts. Res. Vet. Sci., 1969, *10*, 216.
6. McKissick and Lamont. Jour. Virol., 1970, *5*, 247.
7. Riggs, Oshiro, Taylor, and Lennette. Nature, 1969, *222*, 1190.
8. Scott. Jour. Am. Vet. Med. Assoc., 1971, *158*, 946.
9. Shroyer and Shalaby. Am. Jour. Vet. Res., 1978, *39*, 555.

Bovine Syncytium-Forming Viruses

In the course of studies with bovine leukemia Malmquist *et al.* (3) isolated a syncytium-forming virus from a case of bovine lymphosarcoma. Paccaud and Jacquier (6) isolated a respiratory syncytium-forming virus from cattle in two herds with respiratory disease. Scott *et al.* (8) isolated syncytium-forming viruses from the lung and kidney of a cow with winter dysentery, from the uterus of a cow, and from the buffy coat of a cow with respiratory signs of illness. Gaskin has also isolated the virus from the buffy coat of cattle (personal communication, 1971).

Within the last few years it has been recognized that some isolates of bovine respiratory syncytial virus cause clinical illness. This is the conclusion of research workers in Europe, the United States, and Japan. It has been reported that the incidence of infection can be reasonably high in cattle populations (1, 4, 9, 10).

Character of the Disease. The natural and experimental disease in cattle is characterized by pyrexia and rhinitis. Histological changes indicative of pneumonia, along with multinucleated cells, were observed in alveolar lumen (4). There also is a focal degenerative rhinitis and a catarrhal bronchiolitis (2).

Pathogenesis studies in bovine fetal tracheal organ cultures suggest that the tracheal epithelium may not be an important target as more viral antigen was seen in the peritracheal connective tissue than in the ciliated epithelium as determined by the fluorescent antibody technique (11).

Properties of the Virus. Various serological procedures now exist to study the antigenic relationship of the many bovine isolates and syncytium-forming viruses of other vertebrate species. They include the fluorescent-antibody, complement-fixation, agar-gel diffusion and serum-neutralization tests. Unfortunately, viruses of bovine origin have not been compared from an antigenic standpoint. Takahasi *et al.* (10) have shown by the microtiter complement-fixation test that a bovine isolate and the Long strain of human respiratory syncytial virus share a common antigen.

There is little information available about the physical

and biochemical properties of bovine isolates. Their size and morphology are comparable to the feline syncytium-forming virus.

Cultivation. The nature of the cytopathic effect in bovine kidney, bovine embryonic lung cells, and Vero cell cultures is similar to the feline virus (10). The use of diethylaminoethyl-dextran (DEAE-D) in the inoculum and the passage of infected cells instead of viral suspension was the quickest and most effective method for producing cell-cultured virus of the highest titer—1 × $TCID_{50}$ $10^{5.5}$ per ml (7). The virus is rather cell-associated, so sonication of infected cultures increases viral titers.

The bovine syncytial virus grown in organ cultures of bovine fetal trachea cultures at 37 C reached maximum titers up to 1 × 10^5 PFU per ml between 11 and 21 days after inoculation (11). The yield could be increased threefold by incubation at 33 C. Histological changes involved slight flattening of the epithelium and the appearance of inclusion bodies.

Immunity. The disease can occur in the presence or absence of circulating antibodies, but there is no evidence of exacerbation of the disease caused by preexisting serum antibody (5). Nasal secretory antibody appears to protect against the disease as calves previously exposed to virus are immune to challenge.

Serum antibody responses to virus or formalin-inactivated viral antigen have not been consistent, but it is believed that moderate serum antibody levels are indicative of protection (1).

Diagnosis. There is difficulty in differentiating this respiratory disease from other bovine respiratory diseases such as infectious rhinotracheitis, bovine adenovirus disease, and bovine rhinovirus disease. A positive diagnosis can be made by isolating the virus in cell culture and identifying it by serological procedure. Virus can be recovered at a high frequency when specimens of nasal secretion are inoculated into susceptible cell cultures within one hour after collection (5). The demonstration of a rising serum antibody titer using acute and convalescent sera provides another positive way to provide a diagnosis.

Control. Until more is learned about the duration of immunity, effectiveness of the inactivated virus vaccine, carrier status of recovered calves, and the pathogenesis and nature of the disease, meaningful recommendations for its control are impossible to provide to the veterinarian.

The Disease in Man. The human respiratory syncytial virus causes a mild respiratory disease in gnotobiotic, colostrum-deprived, and conventional calves (2). Whether the cattle virus causes respiratory disease (or infection) in man is not known.

REFERENCES

1. Jacobs. Dev. Biol. Stand., 1975, *28*, 609.
2. Jacobs and Edington. Res. Vet. Sci., 1975, *18*, 299.
3. Malmquist, Van Der Matten, and Boothe. Cancer Res., 1969, *29*, 188.
4. Mohanty, Ingling, and Lillie. Am. Jour. Vet. Res., 1975, *36*, 417.
5. Mohanty, Lillie, and Ingling. Jour. Inf. Dis., 1976, *134*, 409.
6. Paccaud and Jacquier. Arch. f. die gesam. Virusforsch., 1970, *30*, 327.
7. Rossi and Kiesel. Arch Virol., 1978, *56*, 227.
8. Scott, Shively, Gaskin, and Gillespie. Arch. f. die gesam. Virusforsch., 1973, *43*, 43.
9. Smith, Frey, and Dierks. Arch. Virol., 1975, *47*, 237.
10. Takahasi, Inaba, Kurogi, Sato, and Goto. Natl. Inst. An. Health Q. (Tokyo), 1975, *15*, 179.
11. Thomas, Stott, Jebbett, and Hamilton. Arch. Virol., 1976, *52*, 251.

51 The Rhabdoviridae

The most important animal pathogen in this family, which consists of the single genus *Rhabdovirus,* is rabies virus, although the type species is *Rhabdovirus* b-1, commonly known as vesicular stomatitis virus. Some other members include cocal virus, Hart Park virus, Kern Canyon virus, Flanders virus, infectious hematopoietic necrosis virus, hemorrhagic septicemia virus of trout (Ectved), Sigma virus, *Drosophilia* virus, Lagos bat virus, Mount Elgon bat virus, shrew virus (Iban 27377), bovine ephemeral fever virus, spring viremia of carp, pike fry rhabdovirus, rhabdovirus of eels (American and European), Duvenhage, Mokola, Obudhiang, and kotonkan viruses and perhaps the Marburg virus. There also are plant viruses as well as a large number of animal viruses in this family. Important viral diseases of domestic animals in the Rhabdoviridae family are given in Table 51.1. A typical member of this family contains 2 percent single-stranded RNA with a molecular weight of 3 to 4 $\times$ 10^6 daltons. There is a helical nucleocapsid surrounded by a shell with an envelope containing 10 nm spikes. The whole particle is bullet-shaped, measuring 60 by 180 nm. In cesium chloride it has a buoyant density of 1.20 g per cm^3. Infectivity is destroyed by lipid solvents and a low pH. Some members of the genus contain a hemagglutinin. Maturation of virus particles occurs at the cytoplasmic membrane. Most members multiply in arthropods as well as vertebrates. Antigenic relationships occur among some members.

Each virus particle contains five different proteins besides the single-stranded RNA in unsegmented, linear form. The proteins have been named L (large), G (a single glycoprotein that consists of 500 copies), N (nucleoprotein), M_1 and M_2 (matrix proteins). In addition, the particle contains lipid in the membrane structure and carbohydrate in the fringelike surface projection.

Rabies

SYNONYMS: Hydrophobia, *Tollwut* or *Wut* (German), *le Rage* (French)

Rabies has been known since ancient time in Europe and Asia. Apparently its principal reservoir for many centuries was in wild animals, although dog infections were well known. For the last two centuries in Western Europe the principal reservoir was in dogs until World War II. Since that time sylvatic wildlife rabies has been the principal virus reservoir in Western Europe, Canada, and the United States, principally in the fox and, to a lesser degree, in badgers.

Character of the Disease. The virus of rabies will usually produce fatal disease, by inoculation, in all warm-blooded animals. In the more densely populated parts of the world the disease occurs principally in dogs and cats. It is widespread over the world in wildlife. Foxes, badgers, wolves, skunks, mongooses, bats, and other wild carnivora are the principal host reservoirs in various parts of the world. Cases in man are never very numerous in terms of the whole population, but the fear of the disease, instilled by general knowledge of the dreadful signs and its uniform fatality, makes it of far greater importance to mankind than the incidence suggests.

Rabies occurs on all the continents of the world, ex-

Table 51.1. Diseases in domestic animals caused by viruses in the Rhabdoviridae family, genus *Rhabdovirus*

Common name of virus	Natural hosts	Type of disease produced
Rabies	Humans and all warm-blooded animals, principally dogs, sylvatic wildlife, and bats	The disease occurs on all continents except Australia. The incubation period varies markedly, and two major types of nervous manifestations result: (*a*) furious form and (*b*) paralytic or dumb form. Animals or humans that show nervous manifestations rarely recover. Lagos bat and shrew viruses show some degree of cross-reactivity, so the 3 viruses form a distinct subgrouping
Vesicular stomatitis	Horses, cattle, swine, feral swine, and deer	The principal lesions are in the oral cavity, and secondary vesiculation routinely occurs on the feet of swine and rarely on the feet of cattle or horses. The lesions are indistinguishable from those of foot-and-mouth disease
Ephemeral fever	Cattle	Widespread disease in Africa and similar diseases have been observed in tropical and semitropical regions of the Eastern Hemisphere. Fever, increased respiratory rate, dyspnea, and some degree of lameness are typical signs. At necropsy, generalized lesions are found involving many organ systems
Viral hemorrhagic septicemia	Salmonids, particularly brown and rainbow trout	Enzootics in Europe occur in 1- to 2-year-old trout. The disease occurs in three stages: acute, chronic, and nervous, in that order
Infectious hematopoietic necrosis	Salmonids, primarily in juvenile trout and salmon	It is enzootic in western Canadian and United States coastal areas. High morbidity and mortality as a rule
Spring viremia of carp	Carp	Causes abdominal dropsy

cept Australia, from which it has been successfully excluded by rigid quarantine requirements. Many islands such as New Zealand, Hawaii, and Great Britain are now free of the disease, and also the Scandinavian countries of Europe. It is a very common disease in Mexico. It occurs in varying degrees in most parts of the United States and Canada. In general, the incidence is highest in late winter or early spring. A possible reason for this may be the more promiscuous mixing of animals during breeding season. The disease occurs, it will be noted, in all climates from tropic to frigid.

Rabies in humans in the United States has decreased from approximately 22 cases per year from 1946 to 1950 to one to three cases since 1960. Similarly, rabies in dogs has decreased dramatically from more than 8,000 cases in 1946 to 129 in 1975. As a consequence, exposure of humans to rabies by domestic animals has markedly decreased, but bites by dogs and cats continue to be the principal reason for antirabies treatment. In 1975 only Idaho, Vermont, Hawaii, and the District of Columbia reported no wildlife rabies.

The signs of illness of rabies are similar in all species, but those in individuals vary widely. Two forms are generally recognized: (*a*) the furious form, and (*b*) the paralytic or dumb form. Actually, most cases exhibit some manifestations of both forms. When the stage of excitation is very marked, the first term is applied; when it is not, the second is used. The paralytic is always the terminal stage. Some animals die in convulsive seizures during the furious stage and do not exhibit the final stage. Many exhibit few or no signs of excitement, the clinical signs consisting wholly of paralytic signs. Rarely, affected animals die suddenly, exhibiting few or no signs.

In the stage of excitation many animals become aggressive and dangerous. While in this stage, carnivorous animals may snap at imaginary objects and bite other animals and man. In this way the disease is transmitted. Within a few hours these signs give way to those of the final stage, which usually lasts only a day or two and terminates in death.

An earlier stage is recognized in the disease in man, and this may also be recognized in pet animals that are well known and closely observed. This is called the prodromal stage, since it precedes the other signs described. In this stage vague changes in temperament occur. In man, the individual feels restless, uneasy, and apprehensive. Dogs that are normally affectionate may hide away and shun company; others may become unusually attentive and affectionate, a manifestation probably of a feeling of insecurity. This stage, if it occurs in other species, is not recognized.

In dogs furious rabies is manifested by restlessness, nervousness, and a developing viciousness. At first this is more apt to be manifested toward strangers, but later the animal apparently does not recognize its human friends and is as apt to injure them as others. If the animal is free, it may often leave home and travel great distances, biting and snapping at anything that attracts its attention. If restrained, it will chew viciously on metal chains or the bars of the cage that confines it. The dog may inflict severe bite wounds on itself; it often breaks its teeth, lacerates its lips and tongue, and froths at the mouth, the frothy saliva usually being tinged with blood. The dog seems quite oblivious to pain. It frequently utters strange cries and hoarse howls because of partial paralysis of its vocal cords. Usually it shows no interest in food at this stage, and frequently it is unable to swallow because of paralysis of the muscles of deglutition. The lower jaw often hangs for the same reason. The eyes are usually staring because of dilatation of the pupils. Sometimes the dog is unable to close its eyes, and the cornea becomes dry and dull. It often swallows pieces of wood, stones, its own fecal material, and other foreign bodies. There does not seem to be any real hydrophobia (fear of water) as there is in man. Convulsive seizures often precede the appearance of muscular incoordination, which is the first sign of the final stage of the disease.

The dumb form of rabies in dogs is much less spectacular and often is not diagnosed. Paralysis usually appears first in the muscles of the head and neck. The victim cannot chew its food; it cannot swallow water or does so with much difficulty. Its lower jaw hangs; it cannot close its mouth. A ropy saliva drools from its mouth. The owner often thinks that a bone or other object has become lodged in the dog's throat. In trying to examine the animal's mouth for an object that is not there, the animal's human friends often expose themselves to the disease by scratching their hands on its teeth, or by merely bathing hands that are abraded in the copious saliva. The signs of local paralysis are quickly succeeded by more general signs of like nature, and the animal usually dies within 48 hours of the time the original signs were observed.

In cats the disease generally takes the furious form and the signs are similar to those in dogs. Rabid cats are dangerous animals for human attendants because of their viciousness and quickness of action.

In horses the first manifestation frequently is evidence of itching at the site where the bite wound occurred. The animal rubs and bites the part and often tears the flesh. Frequently it is unusually alert and tense, holding its ears erect and moving them quickly back and forth as if to listen to sounds from many directions. Genital excitement often is evident. The horse may try to break or bite through its halter rope and may attack the manger with such force that it breaks its teeth or even its lower jaw. It refuses food but may swallow bits of wood, manure, or other foreign bodies. The first signs of paralysis usually appear in the throat. The horse may try but cannot swallow food and water. Generally it drools saliva. Locomotor difficulties then appear, and finally it becomes recumbent. Death follows in a few hours.

In cattle the signs often are particularly vague and confusing until late in the course of the disease. If the furious form occurs, the animals bawl, paw the earth and, if not restrained, may attack attendants or other animals. More often they show no evidence of excitement. Salivation is seen in many but not all cases, depending on whether or not pharyngeal paralysis develops. Perhaps the most common sign is tenesmus. Many cattle will strain more or less constantly for many hours as if to defecate. Usually air is aspirated into the rectum when there is relaxation between the straining periods. Beginning paralytic signs are often associated with locomotor difficulties. A frequent sign is knuckling over of the hind fetlocks. The tail often becomes paralyzed. In bulls, the penis may be protruded in a flaccid state. Cases diagnosed as indigestion, milk fever, and acetonemia when first seen often turn out to be rabies. The form of rabies that is transmitted by the vampire bat in Central and South America is almost invariably the paralytic type in all species (47).

In sheep rabies is not often encountered. One outbreak was described by Darbyshire (19) in Rhodesia. A large number of Merino sheep were bitten by a rabid ratel (honey badger). Clinical signs were exhibited by 44 animals. The first case appeared on the 19th day, 19 on the 25th, 7 on the 27th, and the others later. The course was usually 5 or 6 days. The signs were twitching of the lips, restlessness, and excitement. Many showed sexual excitement. Some developed wild and staring eyes. Only one animal exhibited marked salivation, and only one became aggressive.

The incubation period in rabies varies widely in all species. Experimentally it has been shown that the period of incubation varies inversely with the size of the inoculum, and this, no doubt, is also a factor in the natural disease. In man, it has long been recognized that bites in the region of the head and neck, particularly those which result in severe lacerations, are likely to have a higher rate of infectivity and a shorter period of incubation than those which occur on other parts of the body. *In man* the incubation period may vary from 10 days to 6 months or more. Nearly half of all cases develop signs during the 2nd month after exposure. *In the dog* the incubation period averages somewhat shorter than in man, although the extremes are about the same. The majority of exposed dogs develop signs within 3 to 6 weeks and very few after 6 months. Data on farm animals are rather meager. *In cattle* considerable experience with a fox-borne outbreak in central New York indicates that the incubation period may be as short as 13 days and as long as several months, but the average is about 3 weeks. *In horses and swine* it is believed that the period is about the same as for cattle.

In contrast to the usual long incubation periods are the short periods of signs of illness. In dogs and other carnivorous animals, the course of the disease is rarely longer than 5 days, though a few may linger a day or two longer but rarely more than 11 days. The course of the disease in cattle is about the same as in dogs.

A peculiar situation exists as to rabies in vampire bats, which may have the disease in latent form for many months. Pawan (53) has shown that inoculated and naturally infected vampires alike may harbor rabies virus and be active transmitters of the disease for many months while apparently living a normal existence. He showed conclusively that many of these bats were capable of transmitting rabies several months before they died. They generally died suddenly without showing any signs of rabies. Negri bodies and virus could usually be demonstrated in their brains. On the other hand, many of these creatures have been observed showing signs of furious rabies, and these generally died within a few days. Those affected in this way flew about in bright sunlight, attacked animals and man in the daytime, and, when captured, were unusually vicious and aggressive.

There is still a great deal to be learned about the pathogenesis of rabies before we can develop a sound program for the postexposure treatment in humans, but some facts about the pattern of infection are known. When rabies virus is inoculated into one of the body extremities, it may be demonstrated several to many days later in the nerve trunks of that extremity even though no virus then exists in the spinal cord or the brain. Sometimes it may be demonstrated in the posterior part of the cord when it is absent in the anterior portion and in the brain. Apparently virus travels from the bite wound, not through the blood and lymph, but through the nerve trunks to the central nervous sytem, but there is a suggestion virus may remain outside the nervous system for some period of time and then is accessible to IgG antibody. The virus is very seldom demonstrable in the blood or the principal body organs except the salivary gland late in the disease (Figure 51.1). It is a true neurotropic virus. The relatively long and variable period of incubation may be due, in part at least, to the peculiar and relatively slow way in which the infective agent travels from its introductory point to vital centers.

It is generally considered that rabies is invariably fatal in all species. It is true that there has been only one proved case of a human recovery, but there is evidence that animals may sometimes recover. (21, 61). These cases are so rare as to be negligible. For practical purposes we may consider rabies in man and the domesticated animals as invariably fatal.

There are no pathognomonic gross lesions in rabies. The finding of foreign materials such as stones, wood, and fecal material in the stomach of dogs is suggestive. There may be some congestion of the meninges of the brain, and the brain tissue itself may be unusually pink because of congestion. Microscopic evidence of en-

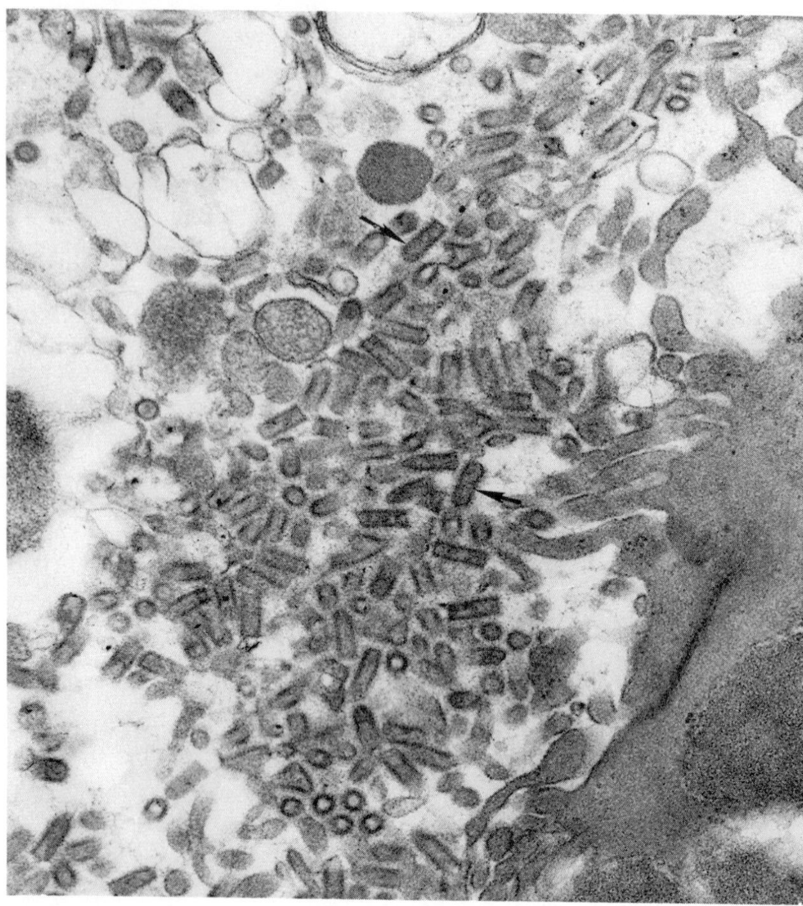

Figure 51.1. Rabies virus in fox salivary gland. Magnification (× 41,300) shows detail of the numerous bullet-shaped virions. (Courtesy F. Murphy, Center for Disease Control.)

cephalitis is present (Figure 51.2), but the lesions cannot be distinguished from some other virus infections.

Properties of the Virus. By the use of the electron microscope the virus particle size is estimated to be 75 × 180 nm in a mouse neuron (Figure 51.3). The virus particle clearly is bullet-shaped, and its size is typical for this family. The antigen can be located in Negri bodies and other particulate matter in the cytoplasm of nerve cells by the fluroescent-antibody technique (24). Virus bodies resembling those of myxoviruses have been observed (2). The Negri bodies consist of a DNA matrix containing RNA granules (60). The virus is inactivated by ether.

Neutralizing and complement-fixing (CF) antigens are present in the virus particle. In gel-diffusion agar tests two lines of precipitate develop when fixed virus and specific sera are used. Chicken embryo cells infected with high egg passage (HEP) Flury strain adapted to tissue culture produced a hemadsorption phenomenon by using goose erthyrocytes (48). Two types of hemagglutinin were demonstrated in particles propagated in chick embryo cell cultures: (*a*) noninfectious hemagglutinating

Figure 51.2. Rabies, showing perivascular cuffing in Ammon's horn in a rabbit's brain. × 320. (Courtesy S. H. McNutt.)

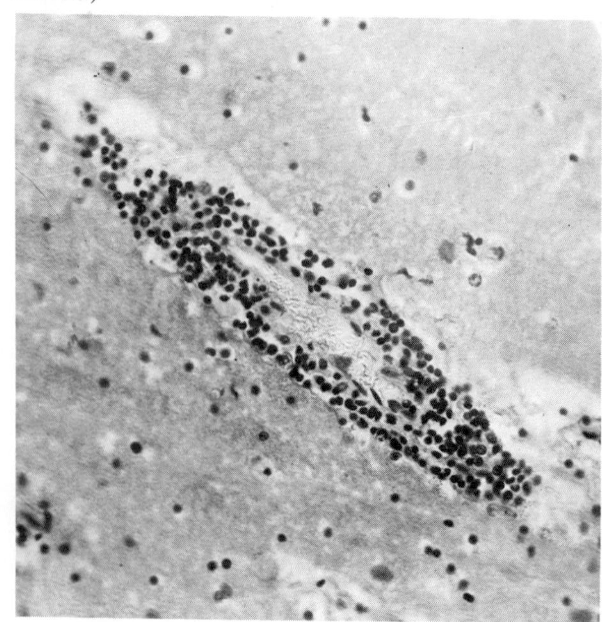

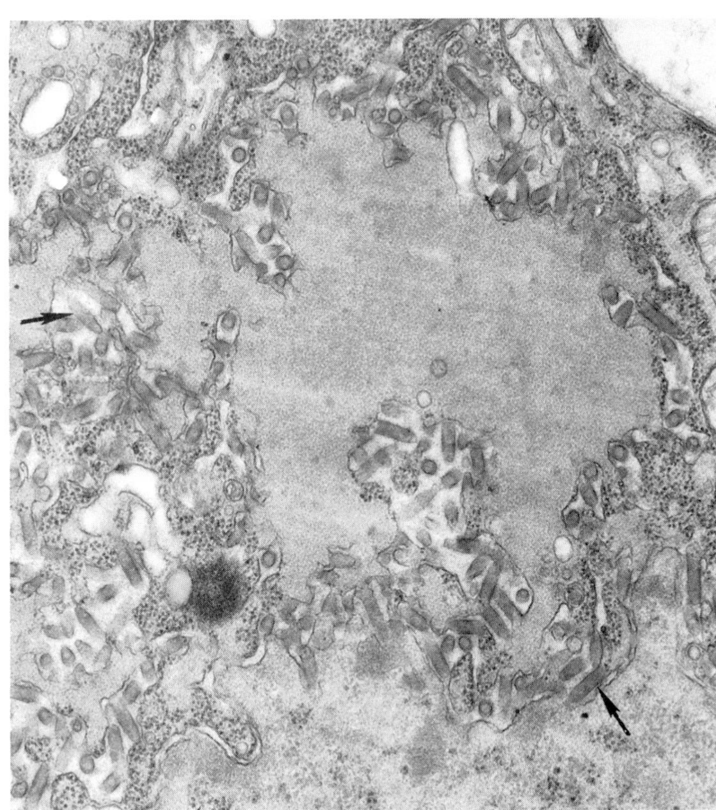

Figure 51.3. Rabies virus. Note fibrillar nature of cytoplasmic inclusion body in a mouse neuron with bullet-shaped virions, 75 × 180 nm (*arrows*), at its periphery. × 24,700. (Courtesy F. Murphy, Center for Disease Control.)

particles and (*b*) Hanin that was obtained after particle treatment with Nonidet P-40 followed by successive high speed and cesium chloride density gradient centrifugations (5). Hanin produces hemagglutination inhibition and virus-neutralizing antibodies in rabbits, and it also gives immunity to animals (5, 17).

On the basis of serological tests other rhabdoviruses have been placed into a subgroup with rabies virus (1, 51, 59). They include Lagos bat, Nigerian horse staggers, Mokola, Duvenhage, Obudhiang, and kotonkan viruses that were isolated in Africa. Except for Nigerian horse staggers virus, significant differences have been found between the other viruses in this subgroup and rabies virus. It is interesting that kotonkan virus may be related to bovine emphemeral fever virus.

Interference with poliomyelitis and also with western equine encephalitis virus has been observed in a tissue culture system, interferon being responsible in the latter instance. The virus in aqueous suspension is readily destroyed by acids, alkalies, phenol, formalin, chloroform, bichloride of mercury, and many other disinfectants. In very thin layers it is readily inactivated by ultraviolet light. It is destroyed by pasteurization. It deteriorates rather rapidly in suspensions, particularly dilute suspensions, at room temperature. Lyophilized virus may be kept for relatively long periods. Pieces of nerve tissue preserved in 50 percent glycerol solution will retain virulence for months at refrigerator temperatures. Virus in dried saliva loses virulence within a few hours at ordinary temperatures.

Cultivation. The virus of rabies can be cultivated in tissue cultures containing viable nerve cells. Webster and Clow (66) obtained multiplication in a medium consisting of embryonic mouse or chicken brain suspended in Tyrode's solution. Kligler and Bernkopf (33) and Dawson (20) showed that the virus could be propagated in chick embryos. Koprowski and Cox (39) were able to cultivate in chick embryos a virus strain which Harald N. Johnson had passed through a long series of day-old chicks by intracerebral passage. This strain is of special interest since it was passaged directly from the human patient into chicks, and it has proved useful in immunizing animals. It is known as the HEP Flury strain. Virus has also been grown in duck eggs and is now in use for immunization (54).

Kissling (32) cultivated rabies virus in hamster kidney cell cultures without a cytopathogenic effect. Fixed virus in cultures of human diploid and canine cell cultures produced a cytopathogenic effect. Subsequently, it was found that rabies virus could be grown in many cell types from various animal species including the baby hamster kidney (BHK 21) cells (1, 31, 69). Rabies virus grows to a significantly higher titer in BHK 21 cells than the WI 38 cells, a human diploid cell line. The latter line now is used to produce vaccine (7).

Immunity. The glycoprotein component of the virus will produce as much neutralizing antibody and be as protective as the intact virus particle. The attenuated virus vaccines and the glycoprotein each are capable of producing IgM and IgG. Rabies virus is sensitive to interferon, and this substance plays a role in the host response and protection. The role of cell-mediated immunity also may be important. Defective virus particles form in cell cultures, and it is possible that they play a role in the outcome of *in vivo* infection. Immunity to inactivated virus vaccine lasts for at least one year, and attenuated virus vaccines provide protection for at least 3 years.

Numerous serological tests have been developed for immunity studies and for the identification of rabies virus. Some tests have already been mentioned in the section on viral properties. Other tests include the soluble antigen fluorescent antibody (SAFA) (23), indirect radioimmunoassay, rapid fluorescent-focus inhibition, and indirect fluorescent antibody tests (44).

Although rabies virus does not propagate in the mammary gland of the goat, repeated instillation of the virus stimulates the production of neutralizing antibody in the milk serum IgG fraction (25). The active fraction has a sedimentation coefficient of 6.8 Svedberg units.

Transmission. Rabies is usually transmitted when the virus reaches and is eliminated by the salivary glands. Infections are set up in other individuals by the entrance of this infected saliva into their tissues through wounds or abrasions. Usually this is accomplished through bite wounds, but infections may also occur through contamination of existing wounds with salivary virus. Persons have been infected through scratch wounds or by contaminating existing abrasions on the hands while endeavoring to find the "bone in the throat" of dogs with rabic pharyngeal paralysis. It has been suggested that rabies transmission can occur by aerosol (15, 16).

Because of its unusual mode of transmission the disease is very seldom transmitted by herbivorous animals. Of the domestic animals only the dog and cat are of any importance in this respect. Insectivorous and fruit-eating bats also play important roles in rabies transmission. It should be kept in mind, however, that virus is eliminated through the saliva by all species of animals, and these animals should be handled by human attendants with due care.

It has been demonstrated by several workers that virus sometimes appears in the saliva before recognizable signs of the disease have appeared. Nicholas (50) demonstrated salivary virus in one dog on the 5th day prior to the appearance of signs; others have reported the 2nd and 3rd days. In dogs and most animals, virus has never been found in the salivary gland when it was absent from the brain. This finding has been reported, however, in vampire bats.

Virus does not appear in the saliva of all rabid animals. Whether it appears, and the frequency with which it appears, apparently depend upon the strain of virus and the animal species in which it develops. Fixed virus strains apparently never appear in the saliva of any animal. In the vampire bat, virus apparently has a strong predilection for the salivary glands, since in this species the saliva may be infectious for long periods while no nervous signs are exhibited. In studies reported by Johnson (29), 21 of 28 dogs in which virus had been demonstrated in the brain showed virus in their salivary glands (75 percent). In rabid foxes, salivary virus was demonstrated in 130 of 150 animals (87 percent); in rabid cattle, the ratio was 16:34 (53 percent).

The natural reservoir of rabies is in wild carnivora. In the United States wild foxes are reservoir hosts in many parts of the eastern portion of the country. In the north-central states skunks have been the main offenders. In the prairie states ground squirrels, ordinary squirrels, and coyotes harbor the disease. In South Africa (58) and many other areas the mongoose is the principal reservoir. Wolves (46) are the principal hosts in many undeveloped areas of the world. Rats may also be involved (65). In Trinidad and much of South and Central America, the vampire bat (*Desmodus rotundus*) is the principal host. Rabies virus behaves in the vampire bat population like other diverse infectious agents (45). Some die from the infection while others survive and ultimately the disease disappears until susceptible bats reenter the population. Virus usually is isolated just before or during the bovine disease outbreak. In areas where the vampire bat occurs, rabies has been recognized in fruit-eating and insectivorous bats, but it was supposed that these infections had been contracted from the vampire bat. In 1953 a case of rabies was diagnosed in an insectivorous bat in Florida (55). This area is far outside the range of the vampire. Shortly afterward incidents and surveys showed that rabies occurred in bats in a great many parts of the United States (13, 70). Cases have been recognized in about 40 states so situated as to suggest that the disease probably occurs in all. They have been found in three Canadian provinces (10) and in several countries of Europe (62).

It has been presumed that the nonhemophagous bats constituted a reservoir of infection for man and animals, but this has not yet been satisfactorily proved. These bats, when rabid, often attack man and animals. There have been no proved natural transmissions to animals, but there appear to be several well-documented cases in people. Certainly it seems that the disease is not very frequently transmitted to other species of animals by bats other than the vampires.

Domestic animals and man have often been infected by these wild animal hosts. In large cities and in densely populated areas where wild animals have been driven out, dogs constitute the host species. In many ways these animals are more dangerous for man than wild animals because of their intimate relationships with him.

It has long been recognized that not all bite wounds made by animals suffering from rabies result in the disease. As a matter of fact, it is estimated that before prophylactic treatment for rabies was developed, not more than one-fifth of all persons bitten actually developed the disease. We know that many rabid animals do not have virus in their saliva and thus are incapable of transmitting the disease, even though the disease causes them to attack and bite others. Also it is known that the dosage factor is important and that many minor bite wounds and scratches do not become contaminated with enough virus to establish infection. This is particularly true of bites through thick hair coats or, in the case of people, through clothing both of which undoubtedly soak up much of the saliva and prevent its entering the wound.

Rabies virus has been detected by a few workers in mammary tissue and in milk. Even if milk were regularly and heavily infected, and apparently this is not the case, there is practically no danger of the transmission of the disease by the ingestion of milk. In the past, various individuals failed to transmit rabies by ingestion. More recently, Fischman and Ward (22) reported that oral transmission was routinely observed in mother mice following cannibalism of their infant mice previously infected with virus. Transmission of virus to infant mice from an infected mother was demonstrated on rare occasions. This was not readily reproducible, so this mechanism of transmission from mother to offspring is unclear. Konradi (35) claimed to have demonstrated rabies virus in the fetuses of pregnant, rabid dogs. These findings indicate that the virus of rabies occurs in the blood at times. Generally, attempts to demonstrate virus in the blood fail.

Diagnosis. The signs of rabies are so characteristic in most instances that a diagnosis may be made from the clinical signs. This is not always true, however, especially in animals that are not commonly affected by the disease. In several instances, diseases that have been diagnosed as encephalitis, both in man and animals, were proved to be rabies. The nature of the disease, when the clinical diagnosis is not clear, can be confirmed only by laboratory examinations. Tissues from suspect cases for rabies diagnosis include salivary gland, brain stem, and cerebellum.

Some of the laboratory procedures are as follows.

1. *By mouse inoculation.* Swiss mice are regularly susceptible when inoculated intracerebrally with test suspensions. Leach (42) suggests that a 27-gauge needle one-fourth inch long be used and that this be forced directly into the brain at right angles with the external surface at a point a little off the median line and about halfway between the eyes and the ears. The mouse should be etherized before the injection is made. The material for injection is prepared by grinding a part of the Ammon's horn in a sterile mortar, suspending it in sterile broth in a proportion of one part of brain to nine of broth, and then centrifuging the mixture at 2,000 rpm for 5 minutes. The opalescent supernatant fluid is used for inoculation. For the mouse the standard dose is 0.03 ml injected with a 0.25-ml tuberculin syringe.

Paralysis of the hind legs of inoculated mice may occur as early as the 7th day or as late as the 25th day, and this is followed by death within 24 hours. Convulsions may be observed just before the paralytic signs occur. Although the incubation period is variable, the majority of inoculated mice show signs and die between the 8th and 14th days. When several mice are inoculated with the same material containing rabies virus, it is unusual for none of them to show within 10 days. It is not unusual, however, for one or two of them to exhibit longer incubation periods, and even for some of them to escape the infection entirely. Thus it is important that several animals should always be inoculated with suspected material.

Wilsnack and Parker (68) stated that the mouse-inoculation test is not accurate in detecting the presence of rabies antigen in the salivary glands and brains of infected animals because such tissues contain a material termed rabies-inhibiting substance (RIS), which renders the rabies virus nonlethal for mice by the intracerebral route. RIS does not impede detection of rabies antigen by immunofluorescent staining. Guinea pigs and rabbits usually exhibit longer incubation periods than mice, and some periods are much longer. Occasionally these species pass through a siege of convulsions before paralytic signs develop. Negri bodies can be found in the brains of animals inoculated with street virus by the time that signs are evident. Leach (42) states that they may sometimes be found in white mice as early as the 5th day after inoculation. When several animals have been inoculated and it is important that an early diagnosis be given, it is recommended that one or two of them be sacrificed as soon as signs are seen in order to hurry the search for Negri bodies.

If it has been demonstrated satisfactorily that an encephalitis-producing virus is concerned in a particular disease but it is not clear whether the virus is rabies, the specific identification can be made by conducting a virus-neutralization test. With an antiserum for rabies virus, tests may be conducted on Swiss mice to determine whether the questionable virus is neutralized by it *in vitro*. Inasmuch as there is no plurality of viruses in this disease, so far as has been demonstrated, neutralization with a known antirabies serum indicates that the unknown virus is rabies. This procedure has largely been supplemented by other tests for the diagnosis of rabies.

2. *By the demonstration of Negri bodies*. In 1903 Negri (49) described the inclusion bodies which now bear his name. These bodies are specific for rabies; thus their identification makes it possible to diagnose the disease very quickly (Figure 51.4). If they are not found, it is not permissible, however, to assume that the disease is not rabies, since a certain number of cases of the disease do not exhibit recognizable Negri bodies, and in others they are sparse and may be overlooked. Koch and Jahn (34) in Berlin reported that of 4,682 positive laboratory diagnoses, 4,125 (88.1 percent) disclosed Negri bodies and 557 (11.9 percent) failed to show them but were positive on animal inoculation. Damon and Sellers (18) in the United States found 189 (12.3 percent) of 1,531 cases positive by inoculation but negative microscopically. Hagan and Evans (27) in a fox-borne outbreak in New York found only 3.1 percent of rabid fox brains negative for Negri bodies but positive on inoculation, but the percentage amounted to 12.6 percent in cattle and 19.3 percent in dogs.

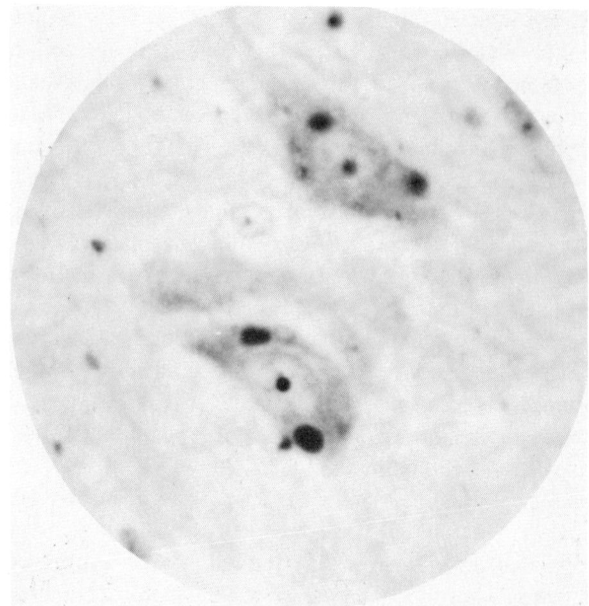

Figure 51.4. Negri bodies in motor cells of Ammon's horn in a dog. The clear vesicular nuclei with sharply stained nucleoli occupy the center of the cells. The Negri bodies are located outside the nuclei in the cytoplasm. × 1,200. (Courtesy S. H. McNutt.)

More recently Bahmanyar *et al.* (8) reported that a substantial portion of specimens found to be nonrabid by the fluorescent antibody test showed structures indistinguishable from Negri bodies in smear preparations stained with Seller's stain. Although smear preparations are still used, they have largely been supplemented by other tests.

3. *By fluorescent antibody technique (FAT)*. This method has supplanted the use of mice in the diagnosis of rabies. The correlation between this procedure and mouse inoculation is remarkably good, but the immunofluorescence staining test is more sensitive and accurate. Consequently it is the test of choice for the diagnosis of rabies. It is advisable to run the mouse inoculation test in conjunction with this method to detect the odd case that is positive by mouse inoculation and is negative by the immunofluorescence test.

The immunofluorescence test detects rabies antigen present in the tissues under inspection. Like the Negri body procedure a diagnosis can be made the same day the suspect brain is presented at the laboratory, but the fluorescent antibody diagnostic procedure is more accurate and sensitive. Residual virus may be found on slides after fixation unless the smear preparation is exposed to a fixative such as ethanol at 4 C for 4 hours. Ethanol fixation provides for excellent conjugate staining.

Recently the FAT test has been applied to corneal cell scrapings for the diagnosis of rabies. Comparative studies in foxes that were positive by FAT test on brain also were positive by the corneal test (67). The corneal test gave false-negative results only when the specimen was in a macerated state. Rabies antigen also was detected by FAT in frozen sections of facial tissue from three cases of human rabies (12).

4. *By tissue culture.* This method is more sensitive for the isolation of rabies virus than the suckling mouse (41). The BHK-21 tissue-cultured cells supplemented with diethylaminoethyl-dextran combined with the FAT provide an excellent method for isolation and identification of rabies virus in saliva samples from suspected cases.

Vaccination. There are two kinds of vaccines used to protect against rabies: (*a*) those that contain attenuated but active virus, and (*b*) those that contain inactivated virus. Many rabies vaccines have been made and used with variable success. No attempt will be made here to discuss or even name all of them. Those who wish further details should consult more comprehensive texts such as that of Van Rooyen and Rhodes (64). It should be emphasized that none of the present vaccines are successful in all cases with the possible exception of the newly developed vaccine produced in the human diploid cell line (7). In man, deaths from rabies have occurred in individuals who have received all types of vaccine, and the same is true in dogs. Mass immunization of dogs, however, has proved a very valuable means of controlling outbreaks in this species, which proves that the degree of immunity conferred is significant.

The vaccination of humans exposed to rabies has been practiced since Pasteur developed his vaccine (52). Recently preexposure immunization has been recommended for those individuals at risk. Postexposure treatment is seldom practiced in domestic animals since the danger to humans is considered too great if treatment were to fail. Preexposure vaccination has been used for many years to eradicate the disease in certain countries. Countries free of the disease, such as Great Britain, will use only inactivated virus vaccines in animals where warranted, but countries with endemic disease use either inactivated or attenuated virus vaccines or both for prophylaxis.

The original vaccines were used for treatment in humans, and until recently little improvement in vaccines or their use occurred. The early vaccines consisted of inactivated or partially inactivated infective nervous tissue which usually elicited a poor antigenic response. During the course of postexposure vaccination an individual received 14 to 21 daily doses, receiving up to 2.5 grams of brain tissue, sometimes resulting in permanent damage to the nervous system, and occasionally death. The effects were attributed to the high myelin content of the vaccine. During the 1950s two vaccines were introduced that are commonly used in humans for postexposure treatment. In South America the suckling mouse brain-tissue inactivated virus vaccine was introduced, but its use also has been associated with neurological complications. The duck embryo inactivated virus vaccine, although free from neurological side effects, gives frequent local reactions and occasionally produces allergic effects. Furthermore, the duck embryo vaccine virus is inferior in antigenicity to other inactivated virus vaccines currently in use. Recently, a safe and efficacious inactivated vaccine was developed that uses virus propagated in the human diploid cell line, WI-38 (7). This vaccine has been tested extensively in human volunteers, and it elicits a good antibody response with negligible side effects. In Iran 45 persons severely bitten by rabid dogs and wolves were treated after exposure with the WI-38 inactivated virus vaccine and one injection of rabies immune serum (7). The treatment resulted in complete protection, so it appears that effective biologics now exist for the postexposure treatment of rabies in man.

Rabies Biologics in Current Use. Rabies biologics in current use consist of attenuated virus vaccines, inactivated virus vaccines, antirabies serum biologics, and interferon.

1. *Attenuated virus vaccines.* Attenuated virus vaccines are as follows:

(*a*) Avianized (Flury) Vaccine. Although a number of strains of rabies virus have been cultivated in series in embryonated eggs, only one of these strains has been widely used as an immunizing agent. This strain was isolated by Leach and Johnson (43) from a child whose name was Flury. The strain was isolated by direct inoculation of the child's brain tissue into the brain of a day-old chick and was then carried by Johnson through 136 day-old chicks by serial intracerebral inoculation. By that time the pathogenicity for laboratory animals and dogs had been greatly reduced. The strain was then given to Koprowski and Cox (39), who carried it through another series of passages in chick embryos. After 40 to 50 passages the strain had lost its neutrotropic properties for the embryos; the virus now occurred in high concentration in all tissues, including the blood. This attenuated strain was then tested by Koprowski and Black (36) as a vaccine for dogs. It produced a solid immunity, and there were no undesirable reactions. Extensive field trials in several parts of the United States, Israel, and Malaya showed that the vaccine was a very good one. Not only is a high level of protection conferred on dogs by a single injection, but this immunity persists for at least 3 years in most dogs (63). Comparative experiments with inactivated vaccine (Semple, see below) by Koprowski and Black (37) showed that the immunity produced by the Flury vaccine was better at 1 year, and very much better at 2 years, than that produced by the other vaccine.

An additional advantage of the Flury vaccine over the brain-tissue vaccines is the absence of paralytic phenomena following its use. This will be discussed below.

Schroeder *et al.* (56) used this vaccine in Central America on more than 6,000 cattle living in an area where rabies (*derriengue*) transmitted by the vampire bat was prevalent. They reported no untoward results attributable to the vaccine itself and no reports of rabies in vaccinated animals, although the incidence in the unvaccinated controls was great. In the United States, however, a few cases of vaccine paralysis have occurred, indicating that this vaccine is probably a little too potent for cattle. Koprowski and Black (38) have produced what they call a high-egg passage (HEP) Flury vaccine by continuing chick embryo serial passage to the 178th generation. This strain has lost almost all pathogenicity for laboratory animals and seems to be innocuous for domesticated animals, although it appears to have retained much of its antigenicity. It is recommended for use on cattle. Some lots of commercially produced low-egg-passage (LEP) vaccines for dogs have deteriorated. The U.S. Department of Agriculture now requires that samples of all lots of vaccine on the market be collected from distributors and retested 5 months after the original potency test.

(*b*) Tissue-cultured attenuated vaccines. Two virus strains of rabies virus have been adapted to tissue culture systems for use as virus vaccines. Both the low-egg passage (LEP) and high-egg passage (HEP) of the Flury strain were cultivated in cell culture and are now used as articles of commerce. The tissue-cultured ERA strain also is given intramuscularly as an attenuated virus vaccine for cats, cattle, dogs, and other domestic animals. This strain was isolated from the brain of a rabid dog. Subsequently it was passaged in mice, hamster kidney tissue culture, chick embryo, and finally in porcine kidney cell culture.

The attenuated virus vaccines of chick embryo and tissue-culture origin are tested for efficacy by single vaccination of guinea pigs with a specified fraction of an animal dose. Both the vaccinated and control guinea pigs are given a challenge dose of fixed or street virus calculated to infect 80 percent of the control guinea pigs; 80 percent of the vaccinated guinea pigs must survive.

2. *Inactivated virus vaccines*. Several vaccines containing inactivated virus have been used in the past. A vaccine inactivated with chloroform (30) proved effective. Others were inactivated with phenol, ether, and formalin. In 1937, Hodes, Lavin, and Webster (28) described a vaccine inactivated with ultraviolet light. Habel (26) confirmed the finding that such vaccines were somewhat more potent than chemically altered vaccines made from the same materials. Irradiated vaccines have been used to some extent on people but not on animals. Semple (57), working with the British army in India as early as 1911, used fixed virus inactivated with phenol as a vaccine for rabies in man.

(*a*) Inactivated duck-embryo vaccine. A strain of rabies virus has been adapted to embryonated ducks' eggs. After beta-propiolactone inactivation it is then used as a vaccine which elicits a variable antibody response in humans (54). At present it is one vaccine approved for use in humans in the United States.

(*b*) Inactivated tissue-culture vaccine. The CVS strain is propagated in hamster kidney cell cultures. The phenolized vaccine contains virus that is propagated on primary hamster kidney cells. In the formalinized vaccine product virus is propagated in serum-free medium. Although the titer is lower due to the absence of serum, the use of an oil-in-water adjuvant reputedly enhances the immune response to the virus.

3. *Antirabies Serum Biologics*. The serum biologics available for treatment are as follows.

(*a*) Antirabies immune globulin (human origin). The production of this product originally was impeded by the difficulty in obtaining rabies immune plasma of the required antibody level (14). Production is now on a scale to satisfy clinical needs for use in humans. This product avoids adverse serum reactions.

(*b*) Antirabies serum (equine origin). Antirabies serum of equine origin, when used in conjunction with rabies vaccine, enhances the chance of survival in humans after a severe bite by a rabid animal (14). Unfortunately, one-third of the patients develop serum sickness or even anaphylaxis.

4. *Interferon*. There is evidence accumulating that interferon inducers produce interferon levels in laboratory animals such as the rabbit which protect them against challenge with lethal doses of rabies virus. To be protective the inducer must be given to the animals before virus challenge or within a few hours after injection of virus. These results suggest that interferon inducers may be used as a future means of treating individuals immediately after a bite by a rabid animal.

Recommended Animal Vaccination Procedures. Various agencies have been involved in the development of recommended vaccination procedures, notably the World Health Organization; Center for Disease Control, U.S. Public Health Service; and, to a lesser degree, the American Veterinary Medical Association (3, 4). As new improved biological products and increased knowledge become available about their use in animals and humans, new vaccination recommendations are provided to the health professions. The recommendations, in conjunction with local rabies statutes, constitute the guidelines to veterinary practitioners for their vaccination programs.

Rabies vaccines currently licensed in the United States by the U.S. Department of Agriculture are given in Table 51.2 and described in a compendium that is reviewed and revised yearly. This provides standardized recommendations for a viable rabies control program. The table provides the immunization schedules and the types of vaccines recommended for the various domestic animals. All vaccines are given intramuscularly in the rear leg of domestic animals. No vaccine is licensed for use in wildlife in the United States at present. If it became necessary to vaccinate wild animals, only inactivated virus vaccines should be used as some modified virus vaccines may cause rabies in wild animals. If vaccination is initiated, annual vaccination is suggested using the same dosage recommended for dogs.

Accidental inoculation or other exposure may occur to individuals administering animal rabies vaccines. Inactivated virus vaccines constitute no danger. The Flury LEP and HEP strains and the SAD strain vaccines apparently do not provide any hazard, but this is based largely on empirical observations. Available data on human exposures to other live virus vaccines for animal use are inadequate, so public health officials should be contacted for specific recommendations in these cases.

Control. Because rabies is transmitted almost exclusively by the bites of rabid animals, its control depends on the success achieved in controlling the activities of the species that is acting as the reservoir in a particular area. If the reservoir is in wild animals—in foxes, wildcats, bats, mongooses—the disease can be eliminated only by destroying these animals or by greatly reducing the population. This often is a very difficult and even an insoluble problem in some parts of the world. Because Baer (6) has shown that dogs and foxes can be immunized by oral feeding of sausage baits containing attenuated ERA vaccine, certain countries such as Switzerland and West Germany have used this technique in extensive field trials to immunize foxes in an effort to reduce sylvatic rabies.

When the dog is the principal reservoir host, the problem is simple in theory but often difficult in practice. England has eliminated rabies on several occasions by simple quarantine measures. Owners are required to keep their dogs under control at all times, and ownerless dogs are caught and impounded until owners are found for them, or they are destroyed. When the cooperation of the people can be obtained so that these measures can be made effective for 6 months, rabies will disappear. England and Australia have been successful in preventing the entrance of the disease over long periods by requiring a 6-month quarantine on all imported dogs. Hawaii has been equally successful with a 4-month period. Britain also requires a 6-month quarantine on all imported animals except race horses.

Muzzling of dogs has been employed as a means of rabies control. It is of limited value. Effective muzzles are hard to keep in place on certain dogs, some types are not effective, and many sympathetic people object to them and will not cooperate in their use.

In the United States vaccination of dogs has become an important factor in the control of rabies. If the reservoir of the infection is in dogs, the method is very effective. This has been demonstrated in many localities by the rapid subsidence of the disease after mass vaccination of dogs (11). When the reservoir is in animals other than dogs, vaccination of dogs is effective in preventing the establishment of a secondary reservoir in that species (40).

Most of the dog and other animal immunizations are carried out on individuals not known to have been exposed, and the recommended procedures outlined above are based on this assumption. If a dog or cat has been bitten by an animal known to have had rabies, it is generally best to urge the owner to consent to destroying the animal, since one cannot be sure that rabies will be prevented and one may risk human exposure if the animal becomes rabid. If the owner insists on keeping the ani-

Table 51.2. Compendium of animal rabies vaccines in the U.S., 1979

Generic name	Produced by	Marketed by (product name)	For use in	Dosage*	Age at primary vaccination	Booster recommended
Modified live virus						
Canine cell line origin, high egg passage, Flury strain	Norden	Norden (Endurall-R)	Dogs	1 ml	3 months and 1 year later**	Triennially
			Cats	1 ml	3 months	Annually
Canine tissue culture origin, High cell passage, SAD strain	Philips Roxane	Bio-Ceutic (Neurogenic-T-C)	Dogs	1 ml	3 months and 1 year later**	Triennially
			Cats	1 ml	3 months	Annually
Canine tissue culture origin, cell passage, SAD strain	Philips Roxane	Bio-Ceutic (Unirab)	Dogs	1 ml	3 months	Annually
Canine cell culture origin, high cell passage, SAD strain	Philips Roxane	Pitman-Moore (Rabvax)	Dogs	1 ml	3 months and 1 year later**	Triennially
			Cats	1 ml	3 months	Annually
Porcine tissue culture origin, high cell passage, SAD strain	Jensen-Salsbury	Jensen-Salsbury (ERA strain rabies vaccine)	Dogs	1 ml	3 months and 1 year later**	Triennially
			Cats	1 ml	3 months	Annually
			Cattle	1 ml	4 months	Annually
			Horses	1 ml	4 months	Annually
			Sheep	1 ml	4 months	Annually
			Goats	1 ml	4 months	Annually
Bovine kidney tissue culture origin, high cell passage, SAD strain	Pitman-Moore	Pitman-Moore (Rabies vaccine)	Dogs	1 ml	3 months	Annually
Hamster cell line origin, high cell passage, Kissling strain	Beecham	Beecham (Rabtect)	Dogs	1 ml	3 months	Annually
Inactivated vaccines						
Caprine origin	Bandy	Bandy (Rabies vaccine)	Dogs	2 ml	3 months	Annually
			Cats	2 ml	3 months	Annually
Murine origin	Rolynn	Ft. Dodge (Trimune)	Dogs	1 ml	3 months and 1 year later	Triennially
			Cats	1 ml	3 months	Annually
Murine origin	Rolynn	Ft. Dodge (Annumune)	Dogs	1 ml	3 months	Annually
Hamster cell line origin, high cell passage, Kissling strain	Beecham	Beecham (Rabcine)	Dogs	1 ml	3 months	Annually
			Cats	1 ml	3 months	Annually
Hamster cell line origin, high cell passage, Kissling strain	Beecham	Beecham	Cats	1 ml	3 months	Annually

*All vaccine must be administered intramuscularly at one site in the thigh.

**Three months is the earliest age recommended. Dogs vaccinated between 3 and 12 months should be revaccinated 1 year later.

This information was supplied by G. Baer, Center for Disease Control, U.S. Public Health Service, on behalf mal, it may be given multiple injections of vaccine and kept under secure control for at least 4 months. Other farm animals may be treated with multiple injections of vaccine in the same way, but there is no reliable data on whether animals will be saved to pay for the cost of the vaccine.

Compulsory vaccination of dogs has been found difficult to administer effectively in the United States because of lack of cooperation by many dog owners. New York State has found it better to carry out a well-organized educational program among dog owners, to provide free vaccination clinics in all involved areas, and to offer inducements to owners to have their dogs immunized. The inducement is that all dogs that carry special tags on their collars indicating that they have been vaccinated are allowed to be at large, whereas those who do not have such tags, when found at large, are retained by dog catchers and impounded. Owners may reclaim their pets only after paying a fine, and if the animal is not claimed within a reasonable time, it may be destroyed or a new owner found for it. In an infected district such freedom is not permitted until 30 days after attendance at the vaccination clinic in order that the dog may be fully protected before it is allowed to risk exposure.

The Disease in Man. Rabies in man presents essentially the same picture as that seen in animals. Both furious and paralytic forms of the disease occur, the latter being the most common. The incubation period varies within wide limits—from about 12 days to 6 or more months, but the average is between 30 and 60 days. Bites on the face generally have a short incubation period. The course of the disease is short—only a few days—and the mortality is practically 100 percent. There are no records of rabies being transmitted by a human case, but the saliva is often infective and attendants should be cautious in handling bed clothing and other materials contaminated with it. The number of cases of rabies diagnosed in man in the United States has averaged one to three per year within the last two decades. Hence it is not a very significant disease statistically. It has already been pointed out, however, that the mental anguish caused those who have been exposed to it and the discomfort of some thousands of persons who each year take prophylactic treatments for it make it a far more important public health hazard than statistics indicate. In many other countries it is a common disease in man that occupies considerable time and effort on the part of the health professions to control it.

Certain countries have preexposure immunization programs to prevent rabies in high-risk groups of people.

This is recommended because excellent biologics that are safe and efficacous are now available for use in humans. In all likelihood these products will be used more commonly in future years.

Postexposure treatment of humans is clearly indicated and should be initiated immediately after a bite by an animal suspected of having rabies. If the laboratory tests show that an animal does not have rabies, treatment can be discontinued. A complete series of vaccine injections must be administered if rabies antigen is detected in the laboratory tests.

Currently, the inactivated vaccines for human use are the human diploid cell line (WI-38) and the duck embryo vaccine with preference given to the diploid cell vaccine. The diploid cell vaccine recently became available in the United States. The rabies immune globulin, human, is preferable to the antirabies serum, equine, because it causes virtually no serum sickness or anaphylaxis.

Since yearly reviews of rabies vaccine procedures are made, it is advisable to contact your local health authorities for current rabies immunization recommendations.

REFERENCES

1. Abelseth. Can. Vet. Jour., 1964, *5,* 279.
2. Almeida. Virol., 1962, *18,* 147.
3. American Veterinary Medical Association. Panel Rpt., Canine Inf. Dis. Symposium, Jour. Am. Vet. Med. Assoc., 1970, *156,* 1664.
4. American Veterinary Medical Association. Panel Rpt., Canine Inf. Dis. Symposium, Jour. Am. Vet. Med. Assoc., 1971, *158,* 840.
5. Arai, Kondo, and Suzuki. Arch. Virol., 1976, *51,* 335.
6. Baer. Dev. Biol. Stand., 1976, *33,* 417.
7. Bahmanyar, Fayaz, Nour-salehi, Mohammadi, and Koprowski. Jour. Am. Med. Assoc., 1976, *236,* 2751.
8. Bahmanyar, Nour-salehi, Fayaz, and Mohammadi. Lancet, 1978, *1,* 302.
9. Bauer and Murphy. Inf. and Immun., 1975, *12,* 1157.
10. Beauregard. Can. Jour. Comp. Med., 1969, *33,* 220.
11. Brueckner. Proc. U.S. Livestock Sanit. Assoc., 1944, *48,* 78.
12. Bryceson, Greenwood, Warrell, Davidson, Pope, Lawrie, Barnes, Bailie, and Wilcox. Jour. Inf. Dis., 1975, *131,* 71.
13. Burns and Farinacci. Science, 1954, *120,* 548.
14. Cabasso. Am. Jour. Hosp. Pharm., 1976, *33,* 48.
15. Conomy, Leibovitz, McCombs, and Stinson. Neurology (Minneapolis), 1977, *27,* 67.

16. Constantine. Pub. Health Rpts. (U.S.), 1962, *77,* 287.
17. Cox, Dietzschold, and Schneider. Inf. and Immun., 1977, *16,* 754.
18. Damon and Sellers. Vet. Med., 1942, *37,* 253.
19. Darbyshire. Vet. Rec., 1953, *65,* 261.
20. Dawson. Am. Jour. Pub. Health, 1941, *17,* 177.
21. Dediaz, Fuenzalida, and Bell. Ann. Microbiol. (Paris), 1975, *126,* 503.
22. Fischman and Ward. Am. Jour. Epidemiol., 1968, *88,* 132.
23. Garnham, Wilkie, Nielsen, and Thorsen. Jour. Immunol. Methods, 1977, *14,* 147.
24. Goldwasser, Kissling, Carski, and Host. Bull. World Health Org., 1959, *20,* 579.
25. Guerin and Mitchell. Can. Jour. Microbiol., 1975, *21,* 655.
26. Habel. Pub. Health Rpts. (U.S.), 1947, *62,* 791.
27. Hagan and Evans. Proc. 14th Internat. Vet. Cong., London, 1949, *11,* 457.
28. Hodes, Lavin, and Webster. Science, 1937, *86,* 447.
29. Johnson, *In* Virus and rickettsial infections of man, 2nd ed., ed. Frank L. Horsfall, Jr. Lippincott, Philadelphia, 1952, p. 267.
30. Kelser. Jour. Am. Vet. Med. Assoc., 1930, *77,* 595.
31. King, Croghan, and Shaw. Can. Vet. Jour., 1965, *6,* 187.
32. Kissling. Proc. Soc. Exp. Biol. and Med., 1958, *98,* 223.
33. Kligler and Bernkopf. Proc. Soc. Exp. Biol. and Med., 1938, *39,* 212.
34. Koch and Jahn. *In* Kolle and Wassermann. Handbuch der pathogenen Mikroorganismen, 3rd ed., vol. III, G. Fischer, Jena, 1930.
35. Konradi. Zentrbl. f. Bakt., I Abt. Orig., 1908, *47,* 203.
36. Koprowski and Black. Jour. Immunol., 1950, *64,* 185.
37. Koprowski and Black. Proc. Soc. Exp. Biol. and Med., 1952, *80,* 410.
38. Koprowski and Black. Jour. Immunol., 1954, *72,* 503.
39. Koprowski and Cox. Jour. Immunol., 1948, *60,* 533.
40. Korns and Zeissig. Am. Jour. Pub. Health, 1948, *38,* 50.
41. Larghi, Nebel, Lazaro, and Savy. Jour. Clin. Microbiol., 1975, *1,* 243.
42. Leach. Vet. Med., 1938, *28,* 162.
43. Leach and Johnson. Am. Jour. Trop. Med., 1940, *20,* 335.
44. Lee, Hutchinson, and Ziegler. Jour. Clin. Microbiol., 1977, *5,* 320.
45. Lord, Fuenzalida, Delpietre, Larghi, Dediaz, and Lazaro. Bull. Pan Am. Health Org., 1975, *9,* 189.
46. McMahon. Vet. Rec., 1935, *15,* 1464.
47. Metevier. Jour. Comp. Path. and Therap., 1935, *48,* 245.
48. Minamoto, Kurata, Kaizuka, and Sazawa. Inf. and Immun., 1976, *13,* 1454.
49. Negri. Zeitschr. f. Hyg., 1903, *43,* 507.
50. Nicholas. Comp. rend. Soc. Biol. (Paris), 1906, *60,* 625.
51. Nozaki and Atanasiu. Ann. Microbiol. (Paris), 1976, *127,* 429.
52. Pasteur. Comp. rend. Acad. Sci., 1881–86. A series of papers.
53. Pawan. Ann. Trop. Med. and Parasitol., 1936, *30,* 401.
54. Peck, Powell, and Culbertson. Jour. Am. Med. Assoc., 1956, *162,* 1373.
55. Scatterday and Galton. Vet. Med., 1954, *49,* 133.
56. Schroeder, Black, Burkhart, and Koprowski. Vet. Med., 1952, *47,* 502.
57. Semple. Sci. Mem., Off. Med. and San. Depts., Govt. India, Calcutta, n.s. 44, 1911.
58. Snyman. Jour. S. Afr. Vet. Med. Assoc., 1937, *8,* 126.
59. Sokol and Koprowski. Proc. Natl. Acad. Sci. USA, 1975, *72,* 933.
60. Sokolov and Vanag. Acta Virol. (Eng. ed.), 1962, *6,* 452.
61. Starr, Sellers, and Sunkes. Jour. Am. Vet. Med. Assoc., 1952, *121,* 296.
62. Tierkel. *In* Advances in veterinary science, ed. C. A. Brandly and E. L. Jungherr. Academic Press, New York, 1959, vol. 5, p. 183.
63. Tierkel, Kissling, Eidson, and Habel. Proc. Am. Vet. Med. Assoc., 1953, p. 443.
64. Van Rooyen, C. E. and A. J. Rhodes. Virus diseases of man, 2nd ed. Thos. Nelson and Sons, New York, 1948.
65. Verlinde, Li-Fo-Sjoe, Versteeg, and Dekker. Trop. Geogr. Med., 1975, *27,* 137.
66. Webster and Clow. Jour. Exp. Med., 1937, *66,* 125.
67. Wiegand. Arch. Exp. Veterinaermed., 1975, *29,* 323.
68. Wilsnack and Parker. Am. Jour. Vet. Res., 1966, *27,* 39.
69. Witkor, Fernandes, and Koprowski. Jour. Immunol., 1964, *93,* 353.
70. Witte. Am. Jour. Pub. Health, 1954, *44,* 186.

Lagos Bat Virus and Shrew Virus

The Lagos bat virus and an isolate from shrews (Ib An 27377), both from Nigerian hosts, showed a relationship to rabies virus (3).

Both viruses were bullet-shaped, a characteristic of the family Rhabdoviridae, and they matured intracytoplasmically in association with a distinct matrix. By the use of reciprocal complement-fixation (CF) tests, rabies, Lagos bat, and the shrew viruses clearly were shown to share a common CF antigen. The same reagents employed in reciprocal CF tests with other members of the genus *Rhabdovirus* gave negative results. Reciprocal neutralization tests in mice further demonstrated the relationship among the three viruses as there was neutralization to all three viruses but the three agents were readily distinguishable by this test.

Minor antigenic differences among rabies strains have been reported (1, 2), but the magnitude of these differences was not comparable to those observed for the Lagos bat virus, shrew virus, and rabies virus. The authors suggest that the degree of cross-reactivity among the three viruses substantiates a distinct subgrouping within the genus *Rhabdovirus* (3).

REFERENCES

1. Crandell. Proc. Natl. Rabies Sympos. Natl. Commun. Dis. Center, Atlanta, Ga., 1966, p. 37.
2. Johnson. Am. Jour. Hyg., 1948, *47*, 189.
3. Shope, Murphy, Harrison, Causey, Kemp, Simpson, and Moore. Virol., 1970, *6*, 690.

Vesicular Stomatitis

SYNONYMS: Sore mouth of cattle and horses, possibly the same as mycotic stomatitis, *mal de yerbe* (Mexico); abbreviation, VS

The disease occurs naturally among horses, cattle, and swine. Formerly it was recognized most often among horses; in more recent years it has occurred chiefly in cattle. Until very recently the disease was rarely recognized in swine, but it is now known that the disease is enzootic in swine in some regions (32). Serological evidence that the disease occurs in feral swine, racoons, and deer in the southeastern part of the United States has been obtained, and the susceptibility of deer has been confirmed by inoculation tests (16).

VS occurs sporadically in the United States and Canada. Outbreaks are seen only during the months of July, August, September, and October; the highest incidence is in September. The disease disappears promptly after killing frosts in the fall.

During the foot-and-mouth outbreak in Mexico (1946–54) it was discovered that VS was prevalent in the more tropical parts. It occurred at all times of the year. Disease outbreaks have occurred in Argentina and Brazil (10). Hanson (15) suggests that the sporadic outbreaks in the United States and Canada may have their origin in this permanent reservoir.

Character of the Disease. As a rule this disease, *per se*, is not very serious. When it occurs in cattle or swine, its principal significance is that it may not be distinguished readily from foot-and-mouth disease (FMD). If naturally infected horses are found, or if horses are successfully infected by artificial inoculation, FMD can definitely be ruled out, because horses are not susceptible to that virus.

The signs of this disease have been described by Mohler (25). In horses and cattle the principal lesions are found in the mouth. Vesicles indistinguishable from those of FMD may be found on the tongue of the mucosa of the oral cavity. Apparently in many outbreaks in cattle vesiculation of the mouth cavity is not common, the lesions appearing only as papules. Vesicles, when present, appear early in the course of the disease and disappear quickly. Before these appear, the animals suffer from a febrile reaction, and there may be some inappetence. When the vesicles appear, the animals champ their jaws, drool a clear, ropy saliva from their lips, and generally refuse feed but eagerly accept water. Horses often rub their lips on the edges of the mangers, or other objects, manifesting itchiness. Unlike FMD, secondary lesions on other parts of the body are uncommon in horses and cattle in most outbreaks. Hanson (15) reports, however, that in one outbreak foot lesions occurred in cattle in about 50 percent of all cases. In swine, foot lesions apparently are quite common (31, 33). Teat lesions occur rather rarely in cattle in most outbreaks, yet Strozzi and Ramos-Saco (35) report an extensive outbreak in Peru in which the lesions were almost exclusively on the teats.

Inoculated animals usually show signs within 24 hours of the time of inoculation. In all species the course of the disease is short. After 3 or 4 days the animals usually resume normal eating habits and rapidly regain lost weight. The mouth lesions heal quickly without complications, and since these are the only lesions in most cases, the effects of the disease are much less severe than those of FMD. When foot lesions occur, bacterial complications may prolong the recovery time. In the uncomplicated cases, and most of them are of this type, the death loss is negligible.

In summary, the lesions consist of the vesicles that appear on the tongue and other parts of the oral mucosa, on the snouts of pigs, occasionally in the interdigital space of swine and cattle, rarely in the coronary band of horses, swine, and cattle, and sometimes on the surface of the udder and especially the teats of cattle.

The Disease in Experimental Animals. Horses, cattle, swine, and sheep are easily infected by inoculation with virus into the epithelium of the dorsum of the tongue (intradermal lingual injection). Lesions generally appear within 24 hours. Only in rare instances do secondary lesions appear in the feet or elsewhere. This virus differs from FMD virus in that it is not infective for cattle when inoculated intramuscularly (26).

Cotton (7) showed that the virus would cause infections in guinea pigs when it was injected into the footpads. The lesions cannot be distinguished from those of FMD. Kowalczyk and Brandly (19) showed that ferrets, chinchillas, and hamsters could be infected with the virus of VS, but dogs proved resistant by all routes tested. The susceptible species were infected by intranasal instillation and by intracerebral injection. Ferrets survived inoculation by the intranasal route and sometimes by intracerebral injection, but usually exhibited secondary lesions in the footpads. VSV causes abortion and neonatal death in pregnant ferrets (36). Hamsters and chinchillas succumbed to the inoculation by both routes and never showed evidence of secondary lesions.

Properties of the Virus. The virus particles are rods, 176 by 69 nm, with the suggestion of a coiled, headed filament capped by a spherical granule (3). Particles of a purified preparation display a precise cylindrical form (Figure 51.5). Defective T particles cause interference (Figure 51.6).

It is an RNA virus inactivated in 30 minutes at 58 C and also by visible light as well as ultraviolet light. The virus is stable between a pH 4 or 5 and 10. It survives in the soil for many days at 4 to 6 C and for long periods of time in exceedingly low temperatures. It is ether-sensitive because it contains considerable phospholipid. It is somewhat more resistant to chemicals than FMDV. It is quickly destroyed by 1 percent formalin and by a number of ordinary commercial disinfectants. VSV resists normal pasteurization temperature.

Cotton (7) showed that there are two immunogenic types of VSV—New Jersey and Indiana. They are separable by neutralization and CF tests. There is one antigen, and possibly a second, common to the two serotypes. The more virulent New Jersey type occurs more frequently than the Indiana type in United States outbreaks.

A third type called cocal virus was reported in 1964 (18). The agent is related to, but different from, type Indiana as determined by complement-fixation and neutralization tests. No relationship to the New Jersey type was detected. Its structure is similar to the Indiana and New Jersey types. Other variants have been isolated from birds in South Africa and Egypt and several genera of arthropods in the Caribbean and in Central and South

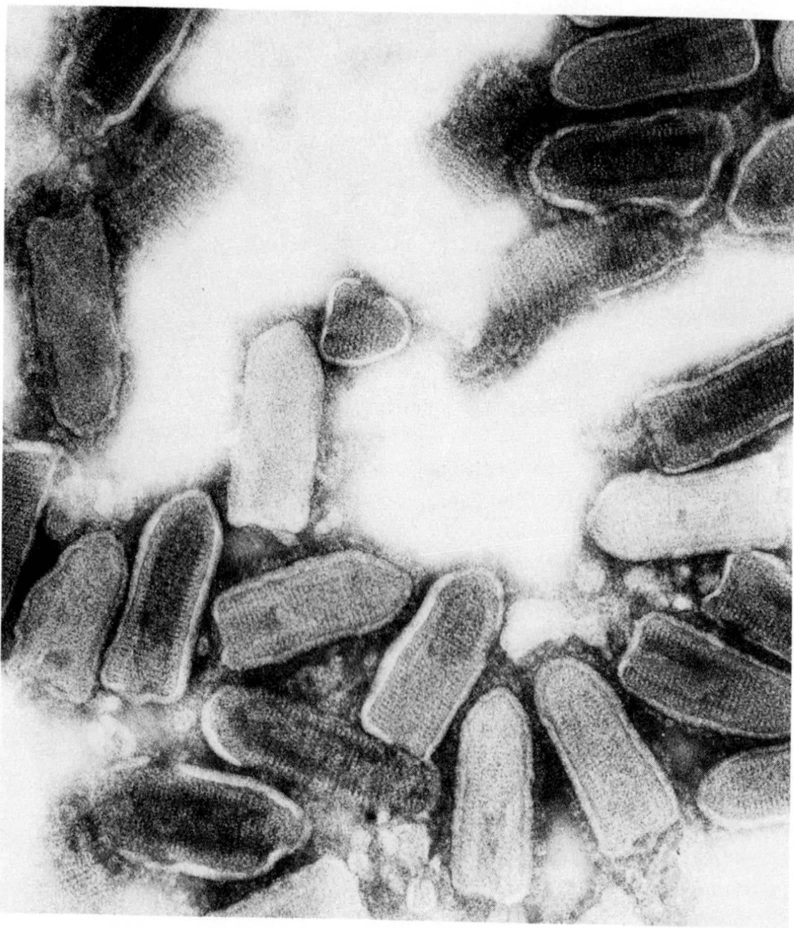

Figure 51.5. Purified preparation of vesicular stomatitis virus. Particles display a precisely cylindrical form. The envelope layer appears as a thickened line; the helically coiled nucleocapsid is seen as cross-striations having an interval of 4.5 nm. Negative stain. × 94,300. (Courtesy F. A. Murphy and J. Obljeski, Center for Disease Control.)

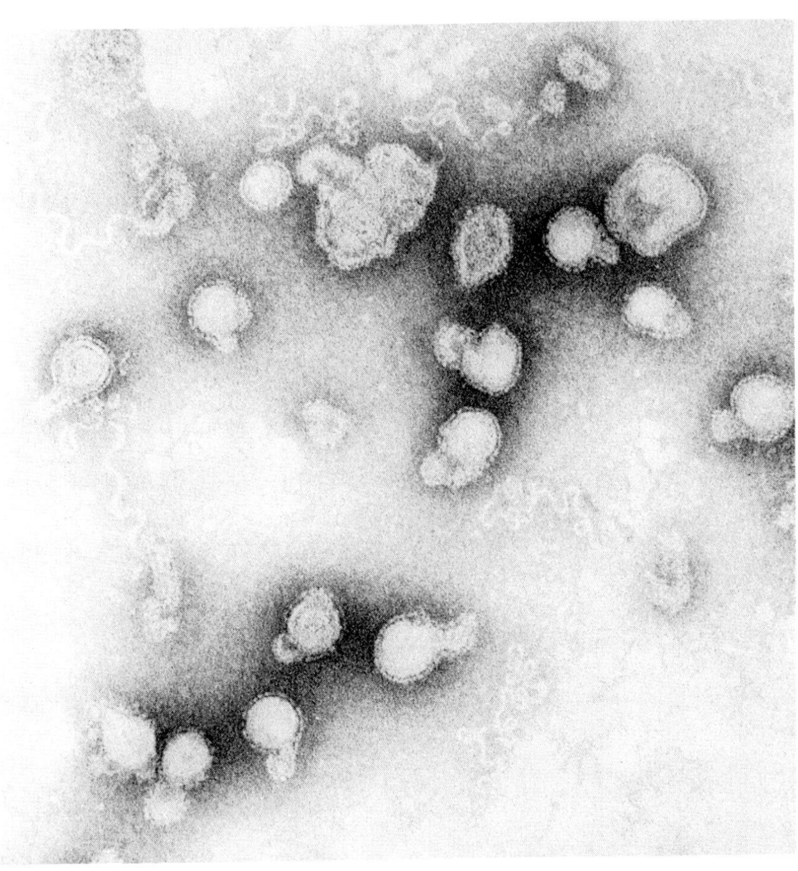

Figure 51.6. T (defective interfering) particles of vesicular stomatitis virus. Negative stain. × 105,621. (Courtesy F. A. Murphy and J. Obljeski, Center for Disease Control.)

America (1). In studies comparing strains of VSV isolated in South America with Indiana C serotype, Federer *et al.* (10) demonstrated that the Argentina and cocal strains were identical antigenically, but each differed considerably from Indiana C and the Brazil strain based on complement-fixation tests and cross-neutralization tests. It was proposed that the three antigenic groups represented by these strains be referred to as subtypes.

VSV replicates to high titers in various cell-culture systems and in the process also produces excellent interferon titers. As a consequence some investigators have studied the basic aspects of VSV replication (9, 30). Because excellent interferon levels are attainable with VSV, investigators have studied various aspects of its protective mechanism *in vitro* (12, 24, 29) and *in vivo* (8).

VSV titered with trypsin-modified mouse, goose, pigeon, and human erythrocytes shows hemagglutinating titers 2- to 32-fold higher than with aliquots of the same untreated erthyrocytes (28).

Cultivation. Burnet and Galloway (4) cultivated VSV on the chorioallantoic membrane of the embryonated hens' eggs. The embryos die within 1 or 2 days, or survive showing proliferative and necrotic changes on the membrane. There is also good growth in the allantoic cavity.

The virus has a rapid cytopathogenic effect in fluid cell cultures of chick embryo or chick kidney, and on epithelial cultures of cattle, pig, rhesus monkey, and guinea pig. In the agar overlay system plaques are produced in the monolayer of kidney cells.

VSV multiples in the leafhopper *Peregunus maidis,* a vector of a plant rhabdovirus, reaching titers of 10^6 plaque-forming units per insect in days 5 to 10 after inoculation (20). Thus a single host can be used to study the replication of both plant and animal rhabdoviruses.

The addition of concanavalin A to baby hamster kidney cell monolayers infected with VSV prevented the formation of mature virus particles (5). The removal of the lectin from the cells with alpha-methyl-d-glycoside 3 hours after infection was followed by the immediate release of mature virus particles.

Immunity. Antiserum can be prepared to neutralize this virus (37), but there are no practical uses for it. Horses and cattle that have recovered from natural infections maintain a serviceable immunity of at least 1 year's duration.

Complement (C) does have an effect on the neutralizing capacity of low titered human antisera. This requirement for complement fractions C_1 and C_3 can be overcome in the presence of higher antibody concentrations suggesting that contribution of the C system to viral neutralization *in vivo* may be chiefly in the early phase of infection when antibody is limited (21). Other serological procedures can be used for studying the humoral response to VSV.

In recent years there has been a great deal of research on cell-mediated response to VSV. This includes studies on delayed hypersensitivity using the macrophage migration inhibitory factor and interferon (2), measuring primary foot pad swelling in mice after local VSV infection and cytotoxic activity (38), and using *in vitro* phagocytosis of IgG-opsonized sheep erthyrocytes to measure the *in vivo* activation of mouse peritoneal macrophages (14).

Other exciting studies in VSV immunity deal with its potential role as a budding type virus that augments immunogenicity to tumor cells (13).

Transmission. It has long been recognized that VS does not spread nearly so readily as FMD. Because the virus is present in the saliva of affected animals, it has long been assumed that the disease was transmitted in a manner similar to FMD. This probably is correct for the New Jersey type, since there is no evidence to the contrary. On the other hand Ferris, Hanson, Dicke, and Roberts (11) have demonstrated the ability of a number of insects to transmit this virus. The stable fly (*Stomoxys calcitrans*), six species of tabanids, three species of *Chrysops*, and four species of mosquitoes were shown to be mechanical carriers of the virus. Indiana type virus has been isolated on four occasions from *Phlebotomus* sandflies collected in the tropical rain forest of Panama (34). While both types of spread probably occur, direct contact with infected animals appear to be more important than by arthropods.

Aedes aegypti tissues such as salivary gland, midgut, diverticulum, ovary, and Malpighian tubules are capable of supporting VSV growth (22, 23), but the salivary gland was the only organ capable of maintaining an appreciable amount of virus for periods longer than 9 days postinfection.

Diagnosis. The problem in diagnosis is distinguishing this disease from foot-and-mouth disease. In a country like the United States, where the latter does not occur, every outbreak has to be carefully examined for the possibility of its being FMD. A mistake in one direction might lead to disastrous conditions; in the opposite direction it might lead to serious and expensive restrictions that are unnecessary.

When the disease affects horses, there is no serious diagnostic problem because horses are not susceptible to FMD. The disease has some resemblance to contagious pustular stomatitis, but the mouth lesions are quite different.

Differentiation of the VS virus from that of FMD can be accomplished by animal inoculation tests (see Table 45.2 in Chapter 45) or by the complement-fixation test. In laboratories equipped for the test, the complement-fixation test is much more rapid and at least as accurate as the animal tests. The only laboratory in the United States now able to make this comparative test is the Plum Island Animal Disease Center of the U.S. Department of Agriculture.

Control. Drastic control methods are not justified in view of the mildness the disease usually exhibits. Infected premises should be quarantined and infected animals not moved until all signs have disappeared.

Cattle should not be vaccinated with FMD and VSV vaccines at the same time because an interference mechanism probably accounts for poor humoral antibody response to both vaccines (6).

The Disease in Man. Clinical reports have been published from time to time suggesting human infections with VS virus. Hanson *et al.* (17) furnished satisfactory proof that human infections occur, although they did not recover virus. During a period of 7 years while laboratory work and animal inoculation tests on this disease were going on at the Beltsville, Maryland, laboratories of the U.S. Department of Agriculture, 54 cases of human infections were recognized (27). These were observed in laboratory workers and animal handlers. The disease is comparatively mild and influenzalike. It is characterized by sudden onset, fever, chills, malaise, and muscle soreness in most instances; mild stomatitis and tonsillitis are seen in some cases. A few show a diphasic fever curve, the second peak appearing 4 to 5 days after the first. Except for some malaise and weakness most victims completely recover within 1 week. After recovery neutralizing antibodies develop. A survey of the Beltsville laboratories showed that 96 percent of all personnel who had been associated with the VS project during the 7-year period carried neutralizing antibodies for the virus, but only 57 percent of these recalled any clinical symptoms that could be related to their period of infection. It appears that VS is a much more common disease of man than has previously been suspected.

REFERENCES

1. Andrewes, Christopher. Viruses of vertebrates. Williams and Wilkins, Baltimore, 1964.
2. Bartfeld and Vilcek. Inf. and Immun., 1975, *12,* 1112.
3. Bradish, Brooksby, and Dillon. Jour. Gen. Microbiol., 1956, *14,* 290.
4. Burnet and Galloway. Brit. Jour. Exp. Path., 1934, *15,* 103.
5. Cartwright. Jour. Gen. Virol., 1977, *34,* 249.
6. Castaneda, Espinoza, Bernal, Jimenez, and Aguirre. Dev. Biol. Stand., 1976, *35,* 429.
7. Cotton. Jour. Am. Vet. Med. Assoc., 1926, *69,* 313.
8. Crick and Brown. Inf. and Immun., 1977, *15,* 354.
9. Doel and Brown. Jour. Gen. Virol., 1978, *38,* 351.
10. Federer, Burrows, and Brooksby. Res. Vet. Sci., 1967, *8,* 103.
11. Ferris, Hanson, Dicke, and Roberts. Jour. Inf. Dis., 1955, *96,* 184.
12. Friedman, Costa, Ramseur, Meyers, Jay, and Chang. Jour. Inf. Dis., 1976, *133,* 43.
13. Gillette and Boone. Int. Jour. Cancer, 1976, *18,* 216.
14. Hamburg, Manejias, and Rabinovitch. Jour. Exp. Med., 1978, *147,* 593.
15. Hanson. Bact. Rev., 1952, *16,* 179.
16. Hanson and Karstad. Proc. U.S. Livestock Sanit. Assoc., 1958, *62,* 309.
17. Hanson, Rasmussen, Brandly, and Brown. Jour. Lab. and Clin. Med., 1950, *36,* 754.
18. Jonkers, Shope, Aitken, and Spence. Am. Jour. Vet. Res., 1964, *25,* 236.
19. Kowalczyk and Brandly. Am. Jour. Vet. Res., 1954, *15,* 98.
20. Lastra and Esparza. Jour. Gen. Virol., 1976, *32,* 139.
21. Leddy, Simons, and Douglas. Jour. Immunol., 1977, *118,* 28.
22. Liu and Zee. Am. Jour. Trop. Med. and Hyg., 1976, *25,* 177.
23. Liu and Zee. Arch Virol., 1976, *52,* 259.
24. Marchenko, Pokidysheva, Malinovskaia, Aliav'eva, and Khesin. Vopr. Virusol., 1977, *3,* 344.
25. Mohler. USDA Bull. 662, 1918.
26. Olitsky, Traum, and Schoening. Jour. Am. Vet. Med. Assoc., 1926, *70,* 147.
27. Patterson, Mott, and Jenney. Jour. Am. Vet. Med. Assoc., 1958, *133,* 57.
28. Pugliese, Negro-Ponzi, Viano, and Santiano. Gen. Bact. Virol. Immunol., 1976, *69,* 78.
29. Rinaldo, Overall, and Glasgow. Inf. and Immun., 1975, *12,* 1070.
30. Rose. Proc. Natl. Acad. Sci. USA, 1977, *74,* 3672.
31. Sanders and Quin. North Am. Vet., 1944, *25,* 413.
32. Schoening. Proc. U.S. Livestock Sanit. Assoc., 1954, *58,* 390.
33. Schoening and Crawford. USDA Cir. 734, 1945.
34. Shelokov and Peralta. Am. Jour. Epidemiol., 1967, *86,* 149.
35. Strozzi and Ramos-Saco. Jour. Am. Vet. Med. Assoc., 1953, *123,* 415.
36. Suffin, Muck, and Porter. Jour. Clin. Microbiol., 1977, *6,* 437.
37. Wagner. Jour. Am. Vet. Med. Assoc., 1932, *81,* 160.
38. Zinkernagel, Adler, and Holland. Exp. Cell. Biol., 1978, *46,* 53.

Ephemeral Fever

SYNONYMS: Three-day sickness, stiff sickness, bovine epizootic fever, BEF

Ephemeral fever is an acute febrile disease of cattle characterized by high temperature, stiffness, and lameness. The mortality is low. The disease is widespread in Africa, and similar diseases have been reported in many tropical and subtropical regions of the Eastern Hemisphere (4, 14).

The epizootiology of ephemeral fever in Australia from its first recognition until 1968 was reviewed by George *et al.* (2). Major epizootics occurred during 1970–75, characterized by a rapid spread of disease in summer months.

Character of the Disease. The incubation period is about 2 to 3 days, and the disease begins suddenly with a high temperature accompanied by rigors, rough coat, running eyes and nose, swollen eyelids, and drooping ears. A characteristic feature of ephemeral fever is the presence of pain in the throat region. The animal shows it by refusing to swallow. Feeding and rumination are suppressed and milk production is reduced. Spontaneous recovery is usual and rapid. Prevalence of infection varies from 10 to 50 percent. Fatal cases in Africa are rare, but this was not true in an outbreak in Australia in 1936.

The usual postmortem lesion is "foreign-body" pneumonia. The mucous membranes of the respiratory and alimentary systems may be congested. The lymph glands may be swollen. Effusions into the pericardium and hemorrhages of the epicardium and myocardium are usually present. Secondary infections may mask the true lesions of the disease.

The pathogenesis of the disease in cattle was studied by Burgess and Spradbrow (1). The major clinical signs were fever lasting no more than 2 days, with increased respiratory rate, dyspnea and some degree of lameness. Hematological observations revealed a neutrophilia with a left shift and a lymphopenia at the time of peak clinical reaction. The net result is a slight leukopenia on the day after this reaction. The most prominent pathological changes involve the lungs and synovial tissues. Pulmonary emphysema and alveolar collapse with bronchiolitis, degenerative changes in synovial membranes, and increased synovial fluid were seen. Specific fluorescence indicating the presence of bovine emphemeral fever viral antigen could be detected at the time of peak clinical response in individual cells in the lungs, spleen, and lymph nodes as well as neutrophils. Before and after the peak fever some fluorescence was seen in cells that appeared to be reticular cells in the lymph nodes. Viral isolation in mice could be made from blood, lungs, spleen, and lymph nodes over a period of no more than 3 days. It is thought that viral growth takes place mainly in the reticuloendothelial cells in the lungs, spleen, and lymph nodes and not in vascular endothelium or lymphoid cells.

In a series of reports Tzipou studied the effects of BEF in experimental calves by various routes of inoculation and on the fetuses of pregnant cows. Both neonatal and young calves are susceptible to BEFV given intravenously unless they receive colostrum (10). Intracerebral inoculation produces fatal encephalitis (11). Heifers that were immune to BEF produced normal calves (12).

Hall *et al.* (3) produced experimental infection in Merino sheep without clinical signs of illness. BEF virus replicates in sheep inoculated intravenously, but the occurrence of natural infection is unknown.

Properties of the Virus. The blood of infected animals contains the virus. It appears to be host-specific and cell-specific. It is associated with the leukocytic-platelet fraction of the blood and probably with the platelets.

The virus is cone-shaped, 88 by 176 nm by electron microscopy (Figure 51.7) (7). It is readily inactivated by ether and deoxycholate (15). The virus is rapidly inactivated at high and low pH and within 10 minutes at 56 C. It retains its infectivity for long periods at −70 C, but declines readily at −20 C. One cycle of rapid freeze-thaw destroyed viral infectivity in Vero cells, but infectivity to baby mice by intracerebral inoculation was only reduced (9).

Cultivation. Mackerras *et al.* (8) propagated a strain of virus for 2.5 years by 81 serial passages in cattle, administering it by the intravenous route.

After passage in suckling mouse brains the virus readily propagates in monolayers of baby hamster kidney cell line (BHK 21) (15) and also in monkey kidney cell lines, MS, and Vero (5). Cytopathology usually becomes visible after three to four passages and develops 48 to 72 hours after inoculation. BEF virus strain 919 propagated in bovine kidney, testes, and synovial cell monolayers produces a cytopathic effect in 24 hours (9), but the effect was nonprogressive. Plaque formation occurs under agar overlay in Vero and MS cells (5).

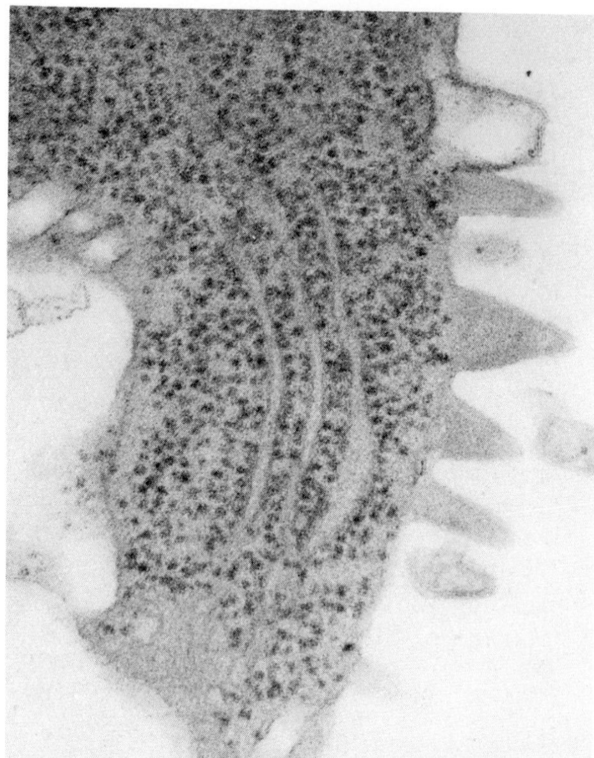

Figure 51.7. Bovine ephemeral fever virus–infected cell showing the characteristically broad-based cone shape of this virus. × 123,750. (From Frederick A. Murphy, William P. Taylor, Cedric A. Mims, and Sylvia G. Whitfield, *Arch. f. die gesam. Virusforsch.*, 1972, *38*, 243.)

Between the sixth and ninth intracerebral transfer in suckling mice the virus causes paralysis and death between 2 and 4 days after inoculation (15).

Immunity. It has been reported that an attack of the disease confers an immunity for about 2 years, but repeated attacks have been recorded in the field (8). The latter observation suggests that more than one serotype exists, but this has not been proved.

Cell-culture or mouse-adapted viruses in oil adjuvant given as multiple subcutaneous inoculations to cattle stimulate high neutralizing antibody titers. These cattle usually are resistant to challenge with virulent virus. In contrast Tzipori *et al.* (13) found that BEF vaccines prepared from suckling mouse brains infected with strain

525 elicited a short-lived immunity comparable to natural infection with apparently mild strains. The latter observation may explain the repeated attacks in the field.

Inaba *et al.* (6) observed that serial passage of bovine ephemeral fever virus in hamster lung cell, HmLu-1,

> deprived rapidly the virus of virulence for cattle with simultaneous loss of the ability to produce neutralizing antibody. The attenuated virus thus obtained, however, could prime cattle to produce neutralizing antibody rapidly to high titers following a subsequent inoculation of formalin-inactivated, $AlPO_4$ gel-adsorbed vaccine (K). Although one subcutaneous dose of live vaccine (L) prepared from the attenuated virus produces no detectable amounts of neutralizing antibody unless as heavy a dose as 10^7 $TCID_{50}$ was used, the priming effect of L vaccine was shown even with 10 $TCID_{50}$. Similar priming effect was also shown in mice by intracerebral inoculation of L vaccine. Maximal antibody response of cattle was obtained by one subcutaneous L vaccine dose of $\geqslant 10^5$ $TCID_{50}$ followed by 3 ml of K vaccine administered intramuscularly at intervals of 2 to 4 weeks. This LK method induced seroconversion in nearly all of initially seronegative cattle, and the neutralizing antibody thus produced persisted much longer than that following two doses of K vaccine given at one-month intervals. The LK method exerted little side effects in cattle. Cows vaccinated during pregnancy delivered healthy calves in term. No adverse effect on milk production was shown. The vaccine virus could not be passaged serially in calves by intravenous inoculation of the blood. Lyophilized L vaccine was stored at 4° C with little loss of infectivity for at least one year. Reconstituted vaccine could be used safely at least for 6 hours when kept at 4° C or even at room temperature.

All these findings by the Japanese investigators indicate the efficacy and safety of the LK vaccination method, although the final evaluation rests on large-scale field trials.

Transmission. The disease has not been transmitted in cattle by contact. Ceratopogonid gnats have been incriminated as important vectors of the disease.

The infection was not established in horses, sheep, goats, dogs, rabbits, guinea pigs, rats or mice by inoculation (8).

Diagnosis. The drooling and lameness associated with EF suggest vesicular disease, but there are no vesicular mouth or foot lesions. Inflammatory lesions of the joints and nasal and oral mucosa, and edematous lymph nodes are the usual lesions observed in fatal cases or sacrificed cattle during acute disease. The virus is associated with leukocyte-platelet fraction of the blood (8).

Neutralizing antibodies can be demonstrated in serum of cattle by virus neutralization in suckling mice or in cell culture. Other serological tests used in the diagnosis are the agar double-diffusion technique (5) and the complement-fixation test (8, 15).

Treatment. The benign nature of the disease obviates the necessity of medical treatment, and there is danger in administering drugs by mouth because paralysis of the pharyngeal muscles may allow the fluids to pass down the trachea into lungs and cause pneumonia.

The Disease in Man. It does not appear that this virus causes disease in man.

REFERENCES

1. Burgess and Spradbrow. Austral. Vet. Jour., 1977, *53*, 363.
2. George, Steadfast, Christie, Knott, and Morgan. Austral. Vet. Jour., 1977, *53*, 17.
3. Hall, Daddow, Dimmock, George, and Standfast. Austral. Vet. Jour., 1975, *51*, 344.
4. Henning. Animal diseases in South Africa, 2nd ed. Central News Agency, South Africa, 1949, p. 797.
5. Heuschele. Proc., 73rd Ann. Meet., U.S. Anim. Health Assoc., 1969, p. 6.
6. Inaba, Kurogi, Takahashi, Sato, Omori, Goto, Hanaki, Yamamoto, Kishi, Kodama, Harada, and Matumoto. Arch. f. die gesam. Virusforsch., 1974, *44*, 121.
7. Lecatsas, Theodoridis, and Erasmus. Arch. f. die gesam. Virusforsch., 1969, *28*, 390.
8. Mackerras, Mackerras, and Burnet. Austral. Council Sci. and Indus. Res. Bull., 136, 1940.
9. Tzipori. Austral. Jour. Exp. Biol. and Med. Sci., 1975, *53*, 273.
10. Tzipori. Austral. Vet. Jour., 1975, *51*, 251.
11. Tzipori. Austral. Vet. Jour., 1975, *51*, 254.
12. Tzipori and Spradbrow. Austral. Vet. Jour., 1975, *51*, 64.
13. Tzipori, Spradbrow, and Doyle. Austral. Vet. Jour., 1975, *51*, 244.
14. U.S. Livestock Sanitary Association. Foreign animal diseases. U.S. Livestock Sanit. Assoc., Trenton, N.J., 1954, p. 60.
15. Van der Westhuizen. Onderstepoort Jour. Vet. Res., 1967, *34*, 29.

Rhabdoviruses of Fish

There are presently three important rhabdovirus diseases of fish: (*a*) infectious hematopoietic necrosis (IHN), (*b*) viral hemorrhagic septicemia (VHS), and (*c*) spring viremia of carp (SVC). Other rhabdoviruses that have been described but will not be described here are pike fry rhabdovirus (PFR), serologically indistinguishable from grass carp rhabdovirus, and the American and European eel viruses.

Morphologically, these viruses are bullet-shaped and

similar to vesicular stomatitis virus, but VHSV has a less typical rhabdovirus morphology as the particles are pleomorphic with a preponderance of flexuous rods (3). SVC has a polypeptide composition similar to that of VSV, but IHN and VHS have a pattern similar to rabies virus. All viruses replicate to high titer in fathead minnow cells and the virus buds from the cell membrane. In serum-neutralization tests there is a low level of cross-reaction among PFR, IHN, and SVC viruses (3).

Yasutake has described the fish viral diseases from a clinical, pathology, histopathological, and comparative pathological viewpoint (4).

Viral Hemorrhagic Septicemia. This virus causes disease in brown trout, rainbow trout, and possibly other salmonids. It causes epizootics in 1- to 2-year-old trout, but on rare occasions in fry and brook trout. Some outbreaks have been reported in summer months, but most occur when the water temperature is lower than during the late winter or early spring. The disease was first reported in Egtved, Denmark, about 35 years ago and then spread to other European countries.

The disease usually occurs in 3 stages—acute, chronic, and nervous or latent. The acute stage occurs during the early part of the epizootic, and the mortality rate is high. The signs of illness are dark coloration, unilateral exophthalmos anemia, and hemorrhagic areas in the eyes and pectoral fins. During the chronic stage when the mortality is moderate the signs are more marked, and occasionally dropsy is seen, but some hemorrhagic conditions may be lacking in this stage. In the nervous stage mortality is usually low, and diseased fish will show rapid spiral, circular, and erratic swimming behavior.

Gross lesions during acute stage are many punctiform extravasations in the skeletal muscles and throughout the viscera. Hemorrhaging may occur in the chronic stage, but the kidney is often swollen, corrugated, and grayish. No lesions have been reported in the nervous stage (2).

The virus has been propagated in primary cell cultures of rainbow trout ovary and some continuous cell lines such as RTG-2 (trout gonad) and FHM (fathead minnow) cells. Optimal growth occurs at 12 to 14 C in or about 24 hours. The virus can be readily isolated in cell culture from infective liver, spleen, and kidney tissues. Histopathological and histopathogenesis studies are recorded by Yasutake (4).

Infectious Hematopoietic Necrosis. IHN virus causes disease primarily in juvenile trout and salmon. It has been established that IHN, sockeye salmon disease, and chinook salmon disease are caused by the same virus (1). IHN is enzootic in western Canadian and United States coastal areas. It has been reported in several midwestern states of the United States and more recently in New York State. These latter outbreaks usually were associated with transportation of infected eggs and fish from the western states.

IHN occurs in salmonids maintained at water temperatures lower than 15 C. There is a sudden increase in mortality of larger fish followed by other signs including pale gills, dark coloration, exophthalmos, ascites, petechiae in the buccal cavity, fecal casts, and hemorrhagic areas in the skeletal muscles of the dorsal fin area and bases of fins. Internal gross lesions include pale liver, kidney, and spleen and some petechiation of visceral areas. Survivors may show scoliosis. The histopathological and histopathogenesis studies are described by Yasutake (4).

Spring Viremia of Carp. It has been shown that this virus is also responsible for the condition known as *infectious swim bladder inflammation of carp*. SVC also was formerly known as *infectious abdominal dropsy* or *carp dropsy*.

SVCV grows best in cell culture at 22 C, but also replicates at 31 C, differentiating it from VHSV and IHNV. SVC virus does not replicate well in RTG-2 cells in contrast to the excellent growth of VHSV in this cell line.

REFERENCES

1. Amend, Yasutake, and Mead. Trans. Am. Fish Soc., 1969, *98,* 796.
2. Ghittino. *In* Symposium on the major communicable fish diseases in Europe and their control, No. C6896, Food and Agriculture Organization, Rome, 1972, p. 7.
3. Hill, Underwood, Smale, and Brown. Jour. Gen. Virol., 1975, *27,* 369.
4. Yasutake. *In* The pathology of fishes, ed. W. E. Ribelin and G. Migaki. Univ. of Wisconsin Press, ch. 8, p. 247.

52 The Retroviridae

The family Retroviridae consists of three subfamilies: Oncovirinae, Lentivirinae, and Spumavirinae. The subfamily Oncovirinae may eventually be divided into genera: *Oncovirus C* (type C RNA tumor viruses), *Oncovirus B* (type B RNA tumor viruses), and possibly *Oncovirus D* (type D RNA tumor viruses) and *Oncovirus R* (type R particles). The *Oncovirus C* genus may be further divided into mammalian, avian, and reptilian viruses. The taxonomy of the Retroviridae family is still being debated, and the structure of taxa is far from established. The important diseases of this family in domestic animals are given in Table 52.1.

THE SUBFAMILY ONCOVIRINAE

The animal RNA tumor viruses in the subfamily Oncovirinae have common biochemical, biophysical, structural, and growth properties. These viruses, isolated from eight or more different species, have been proved to have oncogenic properties in the natural host and some of them in other species under experimental conditions.

All of the oncoviruses have a chemical composition containing about 1 to 2 percent RNA, 60 to 70 percent protein, 30 to 40 percent lipid, and less than 1 percent carbohydrate. In a sucrose gradient they have a buoyant density of 1.16 to 1.18 g per cm^3.

Electron microphotographs show that in thin sections, particles of RNA tumor viruses budding from the cytoplasmic and vacuolar membranes are in an "immature" form and are "mature" when visualized in extracellular spaces. The size of these viruses is ± 100 nm in diameter.

Feline leukemia virus (FeLV) increases in diameter to 120 to 140 nm when the 14 to 30 nm of envelope spikes or knobs are included. The mature particles have an RNA electron dense nucleoid or core of 60 to 90 nm, either central (type C particles) or eccentric (type B particles) surrounded by an electron lucent space between the core and the envelope. There is a clear difference in maturation of B and C particles. The first indication of viral assembly of type C particles is the appearance of a crescent-shaped structure with concave orientation toward the cell center. The crescent closes at the time of budding to form a hollow sphere. The type B particle's core, in contrast, is complete before budding. Type A particles are seen in abundance in all replicating mammary mouse tumor viruses. Negative staining of the core of type C particles reveals coiled strands of 3 nm which represent the nucleoprotein.

The genome on RNA tumor viruses is generally thought to be an aggregate of 3 to 4 high molecular weight subunits (3.0 to 3.5 $\times$ 10^6 daltons) and several subclasses of low-molecular-weight RNAs. The genetic map of the RNA tumor viruses has been extensively studied in some strains of avian and murine viruses. Briefly, four genes are present in the Schmidt-Ruppin strain of Rous sarcoma virus, which is capable of replication and of fibroblast transformation. From the 5′ end of the RNA these genes are:

a. *gag*, which codes for a precursor polyprotein that is cleared to form the 4 virion core structural proteins

Table 52.1. Diseases in domestic animals caused by viruses in the Retroviridae family

Common name of virus	Natural hosts	Type of disease produced
Subfamily Oncovirinae		
Avian leukemia-sarcoma	Chickens	These strains of virus produce a variety of diseased conditions in birds—leukemia with or without solid tumors and solid tumor conditions such as visceral lymphomatosis, osteopetrotic lymphomatosis, and Rous sarcoma. Marek's virus, a herpesvirus, can also cause visceral lymphomatosis. It is a common entity causing considerable economic loss
Feline leukemia-sarcoma	Cats	This is a common disease of cats that manifests itself in a variety of ways—leukemias, lymphosarcomas, and nonspecific entities associated with the hematopoietic system
Malignant lymphoma	Cattle	The bovine leukemia-sarcoma strain of virus is responsible for producing many pathological forms comparable to those described for feline sarcoma virus strains
Canine leukemia-sarcoma	Dogs	Spontaneous lymphomas occur in the dog, but the disease incidence is lower than in the cat or chicken
Subfamily Lentivirinae		
Visna-maedi	Sheep, cattle	This virus can cause either the respiratory disease (maedi) or the nervous disease (visna) in sheep. The disease has a very long incubation period. In the respiratory form progressive lesions that lead to death occur in the lungs. In the nervous form lip trembling and abnormal head posture are followed by paraplegia, total paralysis, and death. Cattle have antibodies, but disease has not been observed
Equine infectious anemia	Horses; other species questionable	Diversity of signs and a variable course characterize the clinical disease. May appear in an acute, subacute, or chronic form. Anemia and hemorrhages are typical findings. Various insects such as stable flies and mosquitoes play significant roles in disease transmission

b. *pol,* which carries reverse transcriptase and RNase H activity on a single molecule

c. *env,* which forms a polyprotein which is cleaved to become the 2 envelope proteins

d. *src or onc,* which is by definition the transformation specific gene.

Transformation-defective viruses apparently lack *src,* and replication-defective viruses lack a functional *env* or another gene.

The growth properties of type C tumor viruses fall into two general categories: (*a*) endogenous xenotropic viruses, which are genetically inherited and will grow productively in cells of heterologous species and (*b*) the exogenous ecotropic viruses, which replicate in cells of the homologous species. The presently known xenotropic viruses isolated from baboons, cats, mice, and chickens are not oncogenic, while the ecotropic viruses isolated from the same animal species—woolly monkeys, cats, mice, and chickens are oncogenic. The exogenus ecotropic virus of cats that can be transmitted horizontally is only distantly related to the feline endogenous xenotropic virus as determined by antigenic and nucleic acid hybridization studies.

Recently, a third group of type C viruses, called the amphotropic agents, was recognized. They replicate well in cells from both homologous and heterologous animal species.

There are five principal groups based on the type of tumor and host range: (*a*) avian leukemia-sarcoma complex, (*b*) murine leukemia-sarcoma complex, (*c*) feline leukemia-sarcoma complex, (*d*) bovine leukemia, and (*e*) murine mammary tumors. The murine leukemia-sarcoma complex and murine mammary tumors are very interesting, but these groups are not discussed in this textbook.

Avian Leukemia-Sarcoma Complex

SYNONYMS: Big liver disease, hepatolymphomatosis, diffuse osteoperiostitis, osteopetrosis gallinarum, marble bone, thick-leg disease, leukosis complex

In 1908 Ellermann and Bang (5) produced evidence to indicate that a leukemic condition of fowls could be transmitted to other fowls by the inoculation of cell-free filtrates. In 1910 Rous transmitted a spindle-cell sarcoma by inoculation and in the following year showed that cell-free filtrates carried the tumor-inducing agent. Up to 1933, when their paper was written, Claude and Murphy (4) reported that no less than 27 different types of tumors of chickens had been proved transmissible. Not all of these had been transmitted by filtrates, but the authors listed 19 instances in which they felt that evidence of filtrate transmission was satisfactory.

Many of the transmissible tumors of chickens may be regarded as laboratory curiosities rather than important economic problems. There are some, especially those of the so-called leukosis complex, that are of great economic importance because they behave like highly infectious disease and thus involve large numbers of birds.

Earlier, most pathologists refused to believe that the virus-induced tumors were true neoplasms. It is generally admitted now, however, that they may not be distinguished morphologically from the majority of tumors that have not been associated with viral agents. Recently there has been a growing conviction by many workers that it may eventually be shown that many, or perhaps all, malignant tumors are virus-induced. There is no proof for such a belief now. Virus-induced tumors occur in a number of mammals, but none, except for some simple papillomas, have been identified in man.

The term *leukosis* is used to signify abnormal proliferation of primitive cells which are the precursors of leukocytes. The term is favored by some investigators over the older one, *leukemia,* which indicates that unusual numbers of such cells are found in the blood. There are many forms in which such cells are found in the tissues but not in the blood stream. The terms *pseudoleukemia* or *aleukemic leukemia* are sometimes used to differentiate these forms. There is good evidence that two types of viruses—Marek's virus (see Chapter 44 on herpesviruses) and the leukosis complex viruses included in this chapter—are responsible for the production of tumors listed under the heading of the avian leukosis complex.

An excellent review article on the avian leukemia-sarcoma group was written by Purchase and Burmester (15).

Character of the Disease. The avian leukosis (AL) viruses can be demonstrated in cell cultures of chick fibroblasts because they cause a cellular resistance, unrelated to interferon (8), to the Rous sarcoma virus which manifests itself as a cellular proliferation. This is termed the resistance-inducing factor (RIF). This method has made possible studies of the disease forms caused by the RIF virus. Vertical transmission of the virus from the dam through the egg to the progeny occurs. The RIF viruses are antigenic and produce neutralizing antibodies that can be measured by the tissue culture neutralization test. Morphologically, these viruses are similar. The leukosis viruses are less pathogenic than the Marek virus types with slower horizontal transmission (bird to bird) and also slower development of lesions in the infected birds.

Avian erythroblastosis virus (AEV) and avian myeloblastosis virus (AMV) are produced by the RIF group of viruses. The terms *erythroblastosis* and *myeloblastosis* are applied to diseases in which leukemia develops, that is, in which precursors of erythrocytes or of granulocytes occur in the blood stream. The disease is essentially one of the myeloid tissue of the bone marrow; the changes in the blood and other tissues are secondary. The air spaces and fatty tissue of the normal marrow are replaced with a grayish red tissue consisting of proliferating myeloid cells. Sometimes the proliferating cells are precursors of erythrocytes, in which case the disease is called *erythroblastosis* or *erythroleukosis;* in other cases they are precursors of the granulocytes, in which case the disease is called *myeloblastosis* or *myeloleukosis*. The filterable agent that acts as the stimulant may cause proliferation of either type; hence if a number of susceptible birds are inoculated with the blood, or filtrates of plasma, of a single bird suffering from either type, some of them are likely to develop one type and some of the other. Thus Stubbs and Furth (22) inoculated 25 birds with material from two chickens affected with leukosis, one of which was of the myeloid type and the other of the erythroid. Thirteen of these birds (52 percent) developed leukosis. Both types were represented in this series, distributed through both groups of birds irrespective of the type used for inoculation. Ellermann and Bang (5) earlier had found that a single virus might produce both types of the disease. After passage in the laboratory they invariably produce one type.

The affected bird becomes weak and anemic. The comb and wattles are pale, and the bird nearly always dies. The liver, spleen, and kidneys are found to be moderately enlarged and pale in color, the blood is thin and watery, and petechial hemorrhages are usually found in the loose areolar tissue and in the mucosa of the intestines. In practically every case, the immature myeloid cells, previously mentioned, are found in large numbers in the circulating blood, and the red cells are present in greatly reduced numbers.

Visceral lymphomatosis. This is a most frequently encountered type of tumor in chickens. Either the leukosis viruses or Marek's virus can cause this form. It consists of infiltrations of lymphocytic or mononuclear cells in the organs. Usually the liver presents the most conspicuous lesions. These are of two kinds, the nodular and the diffuse. The liver generally is greatly enlarged, and the body cavity may be filled with fluid (ascites). In the diffuse type the organ is grayish in color and granular in appearance. In the nodular form the areas of infiltration are in the form of discrete tumor masses of a grayish white color. In the one case the infiltrations are small and scattered throughout, whereas in the other they are more localized. The tumor tissue has about the same consistency as that of the liver.

The kidneys, ovaries, heart, lungs, and, in fact, almost all structures of the body may be infiltrated with such tumors. There is a tendency for the Marek's virus to produce tumors in these organs, such as the gonads, heart, and others, which are richly supplied with nerves. The blood picture usually is normal, but sometimes there may be a moderate increase in lymphocytic cells.

Osteopetrotic lymphomatosis. This condition has frequently been associated with other forms of lymphomatosis. Opinions differ as to whether it is etiologically associated, but recent evidence suggests the ALV may be involved (23). It is a comparatively uncommon condition. It is manifested by bone deformities, especially of the long bones, but it sometimes involves the pelvis and shoulder girdle. It is essentially a condensing osteitis in which the bones become greatly swollen and very dense, and often the marrow cavity may be largely or completely obliterated. When the lesions occur in the long bones of the legs, the deformities can be seen or felt by palpation. There is no osteoporosis.

Rous sarcoma virus. Rous (16) in 1910 described the first of a series of transplantable, malignant sarcomas of the chicken. In 1911 (17) he showed that the tumor could be induced with dried cells, with cells that had been destroyed with glycerol, and with cell-free filtrates. The tumor is now known as the Rous sarcoma I. It is a spindle-cell sarcoma which metastasizes freely and usually destroys its host within 1 month. This tumor has been extensively studied. In 1912 Rous, Murphy, and Tytler (18) described another chicken tumor transmissible with filtrates, an osteochrondosarcoma, and a third, a spindle-cell angiosarcoma. A considerable number of additions have been made to the list in later years.

The active principle of these tumors, particularly of tumor I, has been extensively studied by Murphy and coworkers (13, 14) and by Sittenfield, Johnson, and Jobling (21). In recent years Rubin and coworkers have dealt with the problems of assay of virus and host-virus relations *in vivo* and *in vitro* (19).

Properties of the Viruses. The avian leukosis viruses have been classified into 5 antigenic subgroups (types)—A, B, C, D, and E—each including different leukemia-inducing virus and different sarcoma viruses (Table 52.2). Subgroups A and B are the most important groups, and subgroup B shows serological evidence of heterogeneity within the subgroup and some cross-reaction with Group D. Viruses of ring-necked and golden pheasants belonging to subgroups F and G respectively have been described. There is a suggestion that the golden pheasant virus may belong to a new class of RNA viruses (7).

Table 52.2. Avian leukosis virus groups

Subgroups (types)	Rous Sarcoma Virus Strains: Nondefective	Pseudotypes	Leukosis viruses
A	SR-RSV-A	BH-RSV (RAV-1)	RAV-1
B	SR-RSV-B	BH-RSV (RAV-2)	RAV-2
C	PR-RSV-C	BH-RSV (RAV-49)	RAV-49
D	SR-RSV-D	BH-RSV (RAV-50)	RAV-50
E	RSV beta O	BH-RSV (RAV-60)	RAV-60

Abbreviations: RSV = Rous sarcoma virus; RAV = Rous associated virus. BH = Byran's high-titered virus; SR = Schmidt-Ruppin; PR = Prague C.

RNA avian tumor viruses produce antibody. There is cross-reactivity by neutralization and precipitation tests among virus strains that cause lymphomatosis, myeloblastosis, and erythroblastosis.

Rous sarcoma virus (RSV) was originally thought to be an entirely defective virus (9). This is true in a quantitative sense only, and a helper Rous-associated virus (RAV) is required to make some RSV particles an infective virus. More than 90 percent of different NP (cells that fail to produce infectious virus or protein coat antigen) cell lines studied contained virus particles as detected by electron microscopy. These mature particles, termed RSV-beta O, were infectious for certain types of avian cells not used in past studies. More recently a second particle, termed RSV-alpha O, has been isolated from NP cells, and it is unable to replicate in any known avian cells by itself. Thus, it remains to be seen if the latter type of particle represents the RSV genome in the protein coat of another uncharacterized helper RAV virus or whether it represents a true nondefective RSV population in the Bryan's high-titered RSV strain.

Furth's leukosis virus was probably a resistance-inducing factor (RIF) type of virus (6). It was preserved by desiccation, and infective blood mixed with 50 percent glycerol remained active for at least 104 days. The virus survived for 14 days at 4 C but not at 37 C. He also found that 10^{-7} per ml of infective plasma was sufficient to produce the disease by intravenous injection.

A number of arboviruses injected into a lymphoid tumor led to regression (20).

The Rous sarcoma virus is infectious for the rabbit and induces sarcomas in mice, rats, hamsters, primates, and chickens.

Cultivation. Most leukosis viruses multiply in cultures of chick embryo fibroblasts without causing a cytopathic effect or transformation. Virus replication can be detected by an immunofluorescence focal assay with type-specific chicken antisera or by failure of cells to transform when exposed to RSV, a phenomenon termed *interference* that can be used as an assay procedure in an RIF test.

Morphologic transformation of mesenchymal target cells into myeloblast cells occurs only with AMV. The transformed cells multiply exponentially and produce new virus. This test is used to assay virus. The virus also incorporates the enzyme ATPase during replication, and there is relationship between this activity and viral infectivity.

The RSV readily and quickly transforms cells in culture with formation of foci of transformed cells. Virus activity is measured as the number of focus-forming units (FFU) per unit volume.

Immunity. Chickens that are immunologically competent develop neutralizing antibody after exposure to leukosis virus. These birds usually are not viremic, but an occasional bird may harbor antibody and virus at the same time. Birds with antibody only do not develop tumors.

Transmission. Transmission experiments in the past were attended with great difficulties, not least of which is that the disease appears spontaneously in many birds and the control birds frequently show appreciable numbers of cases, which makes interpretation of the experiments subject to opinion. Careful culling of affected flocks generally has led to a reduction in the incidence of the disease. In areas where the incidence was previously high, usually it has decreased after a few years. Barber (1) found that when hatches of chicks were separated, some being reared where chickens had not previously been kept, the incidence of lymphomatosis varied according to the age at which such chicks were brought back to infected premises. Hutt and coworkers (11) found that divided lots of chicks brooded for the first 2 weeks at 40 and 200 feet away from infected pens showed a diminished incidence in those brooded at the greater distance.

Genetic factors undoubtedly influence susceptibility to lymphomatosis. The influence of these factors is summarized by Hutt (10) and Hutt and Cole (12), who point out that birds may be selected for resistance and that this process is occurring naturally in the field. Waters (24) and Waters and Prickett (25), working in experimental flocks kept under close quarantine, believe that they have shown that the disease is definitely infective and that the transmissible agent may be introduced into flocks in infected eggs used for hatching. Burmester (2) showed that adult hens could be immunized to the agent of lymphomatosis, that antibodies were produced, and that these were passed through the eggs to the newly hatched chicks.

The virus is transmitted horizontally through the feces and saliva. Vertical transmission occurs through the viremic hen but not the viremic rooster (19). Such hens and roosters usually fail to have antibody and are permanent shedders of the virus. The incidence of leukemia in vertical transmission is higher than in transmission by contact.

Ectoparasites could be involved in the transmission of leukosis viruses.

Diagnosis. At necropsy the various disease forms can be readily diagnosed. The isolation and classification of the leukosis viruses require a competence that is limited to a few laboratories engaged in leukosis research.

Control. It is now possible to establish a breeder flock that is free of leukosis viruses. The procedure that will be described does not eliminate leukosis caused by the Marek virus.

Basically three steps are involved in this program as suggested by Hughes *et al.* (9). A limited number of hens are tested for neutralizing antibody by the use of a color test devised by Calnek (3) which is accurate and simple. The eggs laid by the selected hens which have neutralizing antibody are tested for virus by the RIF assay method. Chicks reared in isolation and from hens selected for freedom from transovarian passage of virus are tested for RIF antibody at 16 to 20 weeks of age. The birds without RIF antibody are then used as the breeders for an RIF-free flock. With proper surveillance for RIF antibody and reasonable isolation it is possible to maintain an RIF-free flock.

The Disease in Man. It is not known to occur.

REFERENCES

1. Barber. Cornell Vet., 1943, *33,* 78.
2. Burmester. Proc. Soc. Exp. Biol. and Med., 1955, *88,* 153.
3. Calnek. Avian Dis., 1964, *8,* 163.
4. Claude and Murphy. Physiol. Rev., 1933, *13,* 246.
5. Ellermann and Bang. Zentrbl. f. Bakt., I Abt. Orig., 1908, *46,* 595.
6. Furth. Jour. Exp. Med., 1932, *55,* 465 and 495.
7. Hanafusa, Hanafusa, Metroka, Hayward, Rettenmier, Sawyer, Dougherty, and Stefano. Proc. Natl. Acad. Sci., 1976, *73,* 1333.
8. Hanafusa, Hanafusa, and Rubin. Virol., 1964, *22,* 591.
9. Hughes, Watanabe, and Rubin. Avian Dis., 1963, *7,* 154.
10. Hutt. Brit. Vet. Jour., 1951, *107,* 28.
11. Hutt, Ball, Bruckner, and Ball. Poultry Sci., 1944, *23,* 396.
12. Hutt and Cole. Science, 1947, *106,* 379.
13. Murphy, Helmer, Claude, and Sturm. Science, 1931, *73,* 266.
14. Murphy, Sturm, Claude, and Helmer. Jour. Exp. Med., 1932, *56,* 91.
15. Purchase and Burmester. *In* Diseases of poultry, 7th ed., ed. M. S. Hofstad and B. W. Calnek. Iowa State Univ. Press, Ames, Iowa, ch. 15, p. 418.
16. Rous. Jour. Exp. Med., 1910, *12,* 696.
17. Rous. Jour. Exp. Med., 1911, *13,* 397.
18. Rous, Murphy, and Tytler. Jour. Am. Med. Assoc., 1912, *59,* 1793 and 1912.
19. Rubin. Bact. Rev., 1962, *26,* 1.
20. Sharpless, Davies, and Cox. Proc. Soc. Exp. Biol. and Med., 1950, *73,* 270.
21. Sittenfield, Johnson, and Jobling. Am. Jour. Cancer, 1931, *15,* 2275.
22. Stubbs and Furth. Jour. Exp. Med., 1931, *53,* 269.
23. Walter, Burmester, and Fontes. Avian Dis., 1963, *7,* 79.
24. Waters. Science, 1947, *106,* 246.
25. Waters and Prickett. Poultry Sci., 1944, *23,* 321.

Feline Leukemia-Sarcoma Complex

In 1964 Jarrett and coinvestigators (43, 47) established that C-type viral particles were responsible for the incidence of feline lymphosarcoma in experimental cats. Later, Rickard *et al.* (62) observed C-type particles in a spontaneous case and transmitted the disease with cell-free filtrates (63). Several investigators subsequently observed C-type particles in feline lymphosarcoma and transmitted the disease with cell-free filtrates (31, 51, 64).

Leukemias and lymphosarcomas are undoubtedly the most frequently occurring malignancies in felids (24, 41, 76). Contrary to what happens in similar diseases of outbred mammalian species, cat leukemias, lymphomas, and fibrosarcomas are generally associated with viral particles that can be isolated in cell culture and identified with an electron microscope (43, 47, 49, 62, 78). These particles are infectious and generally oncogenic. Feline leukemia virus (FeLV) is a competent virus, whereas feline sarcoma virus (FeSV) is a defective virus requiring FeLV particles as helpers to replicate in cells. All the isolates of FeSV also have FeLV viral particles; the two viruses are indistinguishable serologically.

There are excellent reviews of the feline leukemia complex (1, 8, 26).

Character of the Disease. The true worldwide incidence of feline leukemia is difficult to assess as clinical diagnosis is difficult, but there is little doubt that the incidence and the mortality are high.

The disease that occurs most commonly in the cat is associated with the hematopoietic system (41). The signs of illness generally are nonspecific, such as depression, anorexia, and anemia. Without laboratory assistance this form of disease will likely be undiagnosed.

There are five distinct clinicopathological syndromes involving lymphoma, as follows.

1. *Alimentary lymphoma.* The majority of cells in these tumors have characteristics of B-cells. The tumors originate in the lymphoid tissue of the intestine and grow primarily in the wall of the gastrointestinal tract and/or in the mesenteric lymph nodes and Peyer's patches (distant from the primary tumor). The spleen and liver are sometimes involved, and the kidneys are frequently infiltrated (35, 36).

2. *Multicentric lymphoma.* The majority of the cells involved in these tumors appear to be T-cells. This form tends to involve lymph nodes bilaterally, which become enlarged and palpable. Splenomegaly is common, and the liver generally is enlarged. This syndrome also is characterized by depression and wasting (35, 36).

3. *Thymic or anterior mediastinal form.* The cells of these tumors have T-cell characteristics. The thymus is replaced by tumor tissue. The classical signs only become apparent in a terminal case when the tumors fill the entire thoracic cavity. The local lymph nodes are often involved. The animals generally collapse because compression of the thoracic fluid causes respiratory distress.

4. *Leukemia.* This disease has distinct characteristics. It originates in the bone marrow and causes an abnormally large cell population. Malignant cells spread and splenomegalia occurs due to the red pulp engorgement by leukemic cells. The liver is infiltrated, and the bone marrow is greatly enlarged. Lymph node enlargement is slight to moderate (5, 8, 12, 30–32, 35, 36, 61).

5. *Other forms.* Tumors induced by FeLV which are localized in single organs, such as the kidney, or in the nervous system are not very common and are difficult to classify.

Both FeLV and FeSV viruses are transmitted horizontally. In addition viremic mothers bear infected offspring, or more often, the fetuses are reabsorbed or stillborn. All felines are latently infected with vertically transmitted endogenous virus.

FeLV infections in cats can induce nonneoplastic diseases, such as anemia, glomeronephritis, or a syndrome like panleukopenia (48, 42). Fetal reabsorptions and abortions also can be associated with other viral diseases, and bacterial diseases that are motivated to FeLV-related immunosuppression lower the natural resistence of infected cats to common pathogens. It seems apparent that FeLV is involved in a wide spectrum of feline diseases and that only a percentage of these are related to neoplasia.

For details about lymphocytic leukemia and less common hematopoietic malignancies of cats in order of their frequency—reticuloendotheliosis, mast-cell leukemia, and granulocytic leukemia—the reader is referred to the articles by Gilmore and Holzworth (24) and Schalm (75) and also the textbook by Schalm (74). Rare leukemias of the cat such as eosinophilic, plasma-cell, and stem-cell leukemias as well as erythemic myelosis and erytholeukemia also are described in these sources.

The Disease in Experimental Animals. Various strains of feline leukemia virus (FeLV) are known to produce malignant lymphomas in newborn kittens (Figure 52.1). Older cats presumably are infected, but do not develop disease. At present very little is known about the replication of FeLV in experimental cats (40). It has been shown that the virus is present in tissues at 28 days after inoculation and persists throughout the disease process. Virus is detectable in the megakaryocytes of the spleen and bone marrow, which presumably leads to a viremia, since many viral particles are found in the blood platelets (51), and the viremia persists until death. Although

Figure 52.1. Experimental lymphoma in a neonatal kitten. The tumor mass principally involves the thymus gland. (Courtesy C. Rickard, J. Post, K. Lee, and J. Gillespie.)

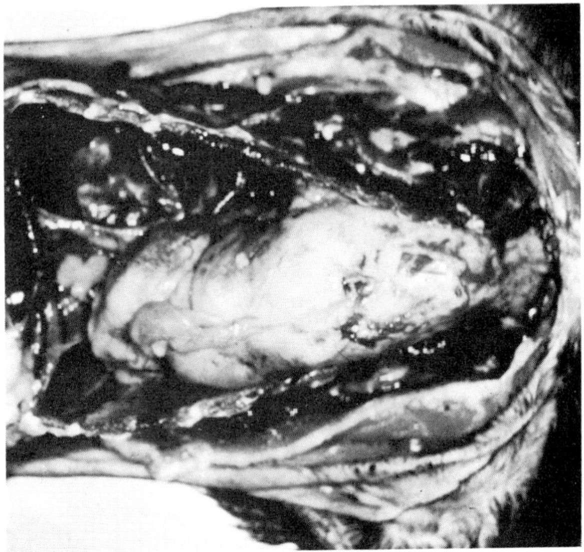

Kawakami *et al.* (49) found virus in the blood of some cats in the terminal stages of spontaneous and experimental disease, others did not show a viremia. FeLV produces leukemia in dogs.

The feline sarcoma virus (FeSV) has been isolated from spontaneous cases of cats with fibrosarcoma. It has a rather broad experimental host spectrum. This virus produces sarcomas in experimental fetal and day-old kittens, fetal and day-old puppies (20, 21, 63), newborn rabbits, fetal sheep (9, 81), and marmosets (6). This virus is defective and contains FeLV particles, with an excess of 100 to 1,000 times more FeLV particles than FeSV particles (4, 65, 66). FeLV particles facilitate the completion of viral replication and the release of the progeny virus from the infected cells.

Spontaneous fibrosarcomas are much less frequent than the leukemias.

FeSV inoculated into very young kittens causes their death within a few days. If the animals are 6 to 8 weeks old, they produce progressive tumors at the site of the inoculation within 3 to 10 weeks. Tumors also metastasize to many organs in the body, and these animals are viremic (11, 12, 16, 78). Sometimes they died within 3 to 5 weeks without the formation of tumors. Tumor regression can occur depending on the dose of inoculum and the age of the animal. The cats in which the tumors regressed generally had feline oncornavirus-associated cell membrane antigen (FOCMA) antibodies and remained viremic for at least 3 months because of the lack of an effective titer of neutralizing antibodies to eliminate the circulating virus (5, 12).

Properties of the Virus. The FeLV is similar in morphology and structure to other oncoviruses (69). Reverse transcriptase and ribonuclease H appear to be associated with the RNA as a protein of 10 daltons (p 10). The major core of protein p 30 is associated with protein p 15. Surrounding this core is an envelope from which glycoprotein spikes or knobs protrude (gp 71). Under the spikes is a layer of protein (p 15 E) that forms the envelope. The p 12 protein is supposedly associated with the inner coat, which is between the core and the envelope (7, 51, 64, 80). The virus is assembled by a process of budding from cell membranes. Type C particles have been observed in spontaneous and experimental cases (Figure 52.2). It is an RNA virus.

The antigens of oncoviruses are classified according to the degree of cross-reactivity exhibited. Thus, interspecies-specific determinants (30) cross-react among all mammalian C-type viruses (29, 30, 55, 57, 67, 68, 70–72). Species-specific determinants are shared by all oncovirus isolated from the same species (Figure 52.3). Type-specific determinants differentiate viral strains isolated within the species.

Feline endogenous virus, of which RD 114 is the prototype is an exception because the group or specific antigens are not related to the conventional feline oncovirus (23, 53, 60, 73). The endogenous p 30 has interspecies determinants shared with FeLV and/or FeSV, but the species-specific and type-specific antigens are different. These viruses are more closely related to baboon endogenous type C virus than to FeLV.

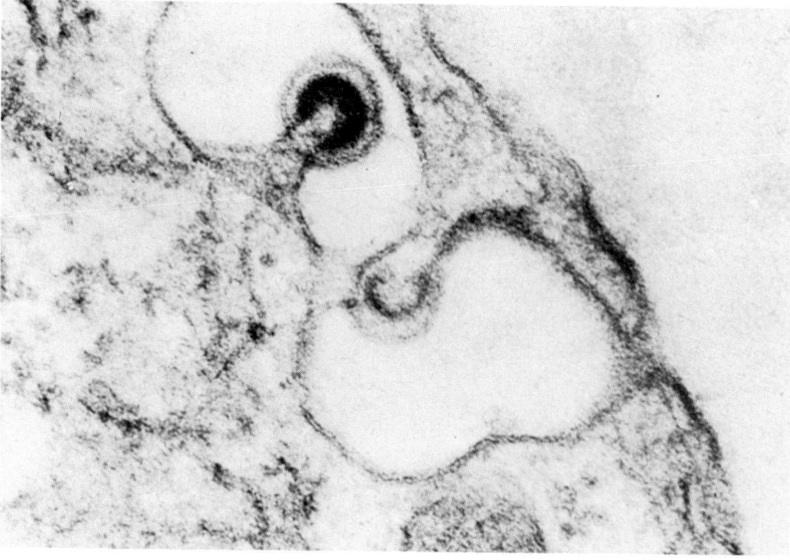

Figure 52.2. Budding C-type feline leukemia virus particle characteristic of C-type oncogenic RNA viruses. (Courtesy C. Rickard.)

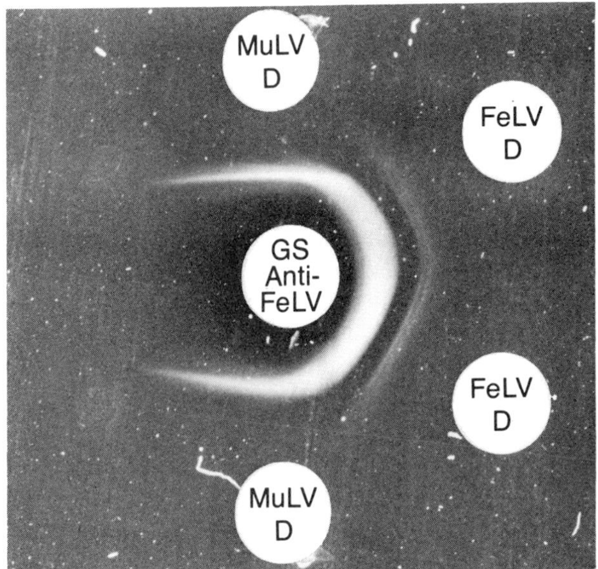

Figure 52.3. Demonstration of species and interspecies antigens by the immunodiffusion test. The broad interior line is the interspecies antigen/antibody complex showing its presence in the murine leukemia virus (MuLV) and feline leukemia virus (FeLV). The lighter exterior line demonstrates species-specific antigens. (Courtesy F. Noronha.)

Cultivation. FeLV strains replicate in cell cultures of human, canine, and porcine origin, but fail to replicate in selected cell-tissue cultures of murine, rat, or chicken origin. Sometimes virus grows as well in human cells as in feline cells, and virus recovered from both types of cultures was identical (40). Lee (52) found that murine sarcoma–feline leukemia hybrid virus of Fischinger and O'Connor (18) would replicate in many species of cells including dog, feline, cattle, and dolphin (Figure 52.4).

Feline embryonic cell cultures that were infected with a high multiplicity of FeLV (10^3 virus particles per tissue cell) yielded maximum titers of H-uridine-labeled particles at 24 hours (40). After this time there is a slight drop in virus titer to a level that is maintained indefinitely. Similar growth curves are reported for avian sarcoma viruses.

Immunity. Kittens of similar age and origin inoculated with FeLV become viremic at 4 to 6 weeks, but the tumors usually appear much later, usually 16 weeks to 2 years or more (37, 38, 82). Kittens naturally exposed to FeLV became viremic in 1 month to 6 months and developed tumors at 7 months or later.

Feline oncovirus-associated cell membrane antigen (FOCMA) is a transformation specific surface determinant expressed by both feline leukemia nonproducer and feline leukemia producer infected tumor cells (11). This antigen is not detected on cells from tumors of cats or on nontransformed FeLV replicating cells. FOCMA antibodies have been detected by membrane immunofluorescence in fixed cells as targets. The antibody was first detected in sera from cats inoculated with FeSV whose tumors had regressed. It is not present in inoculated cats in which the tumor progressed and caused death. Viremia frequently persisted in cats in which FeSV-induced tumors regressed completely. FOCMA antibodies were detected in these cats and in many inoculated and naturally infected viremic cats. It does not seem likely that these antibodies have virus-neutralization activities or are directed at virus components expressed by infected nontransformed FeLV replicating cells. The distinction between FOCMA antibodies and antibodies directed against FeLV-FeSV or other viral antigens has been confirmed by several other techniques (13). There is a correlation between the tumor-protective effects of FOCMA antibodies and a complement-dependent antibody (CDA) (8, 15, 25, 27). This strongly suggests that

Figure 52.4. A single focus (*F*) of transformed cells in the Crandell feline kidney cell line induced by the murine sarcoma–feline leukemia hybrid virus of Fischinger and O'Connor. May-Gruenwald-Giemsa. × 26. (Courtesy K. Lee.)

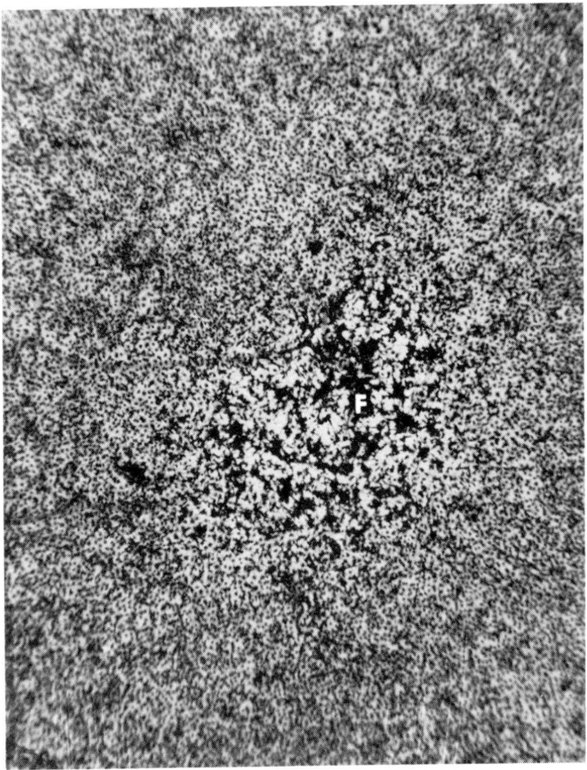

a major component of tumor immune surveillance is mediated by a lytic antibody and complement.

In an experimental trial approximately half of the kittens nursed by queens with high serum titers of neutralizing antibodies were subsequently protected the first week of life from progressive tumors induced by FeSV challenge. This protection disappeared by the 5th week of age. Vaccination of cats with live attenuated or gluteraldehyde killed FeLV tumor cells produced high titers of FOCMA antibody, and the immunized cats resisted the development of viremia from FeLV challenge.

Experimentally induced viremia has been prevented to some extent by immunization with FeLV-infected cells, or by passive administration of goat anti-FeLV and/or anti-MuLV (murine leukemia virus) anti-gp 70 and cat hyperimmune sera, but in all these cases the treatment was administered in a very early stage of infection (45, 46, 54, 58, 59).

Naturally exposed cats with preexisting low FOCMA antibody titers undergo a rapid secondary antibody response when immunized with allogenic tumor cells.

Heat-inactivated tumor cells also protect kittens from the fatal tumorogenic effects of FeSV. This vaccine induced FOCMA, but did not induce neutralizing antibodies. Tumor protection was evident in terms of progression rather than appearance, however, for the vaccinated kittens developed tumors that regressed, whereas the controls died with the tumors.

The antibodies directed to the *gag* gene products (p 30, p 15, p 12, p 10) do not have neutralizing properties, supposedly because these proteins are internal components of the virion (50). The major core protein, p 30, exists in the cytoplasm of cells actively producing virus and can be detected by immunofluorescence, immunodiffusion, complement-fixation, and radioimmunoprecipitation techniques. Antibodies against p 15, p 12, and p 10 have also been detected by the same procedures as p 30.

The *pol* gene product (reverse transcriptase) is also immunogenic and has been detected where other antigens are present.

The *env* gene products (gp 70 and p 15 E) are also present. The p 15 E is immunosuppressive. The presence of this antibody is correlated with a good prognosis, while its absence generally means that the animal is immunosuppressed. Gp 70 antibodies to gp 70 antigen are observed only in cats that overcome infection; conversely, cats persistently viremic do not have these antibodies. Animals with these antibodies in significant titer have neutralizing capabilities and are generally immune.

Transmission. The first report of horizontal transmission came from a household of 34 cats in which six cases of leukemia were reported within a 5-year period. Subsequently, many other multiple cat households with leukemia were discovered. Into one of these households ten FeLV-free kittens were introduced, and six became FeLV-positive within 5 months. The viremic contact cats died as a result of FeLV-related terminal diseases that included anemias or lymphomas. The nonviremic cats developed neutralizing viruses and FOCMA antibodies and remained healthy (3, 5, 10, 30, 41, 43, 47).

In laboratory experiments, normal kittens exposed by direct contact with naturally or experimentally infected viremic cats became viremic or developed virus-neutralizing antibodies. Control kittens of the same age and backgrounds (or even of the same litter) that were not exposed did not develop signs of disease or immunity.

Horizontal transmission seems to occur by the respiratory or gastrointestinal route. Replication of FeLV occurs in the tracheal, nasal, and oral epithelium, and in salivary gland tissue. Persistently viremic cats regularly shed between 10^4 and 10^5 infectious particles per ml of saliva, whereas urine and feces contained no virus. Viral transmission can be achieved by intranasal instillation or by aerosal (19). Evidence suggests that direct contact within cages is more effective in spreading FeLV than having cats in separate cages in the same room. It is believed that gastrointestinal transmission occurs more readily under natural conditions than via the respiratory route (12, 19, 37, 77, 82).

Common grooming and feeding utensils enhance the spread of virus. The virus also persists for several days in a moist room maintained at 22 C.

Diagnosis. It is difficult to make a diagnosis without laboratory assistance. Only a restricted number of cases of feline leukemia are true lymphoid leukemias characterized by absolute peripheral blood lymphocytosis and/or immature lymphoid cells in the blood. An analogous situation exists when the bone marrow is involved.

Tumors can be palpated when they are superficial, but involvement of internal organs only requires the use of x-ray equipment to provide a clinical diagnosis.

In the laboratory various techniques are used to make a diagnosis—hematologic, histopathological, serological, and virological procedures. A definite diagnosis involves serological and/or virological test procedures.

The most simple, rapid, and inexpensive test is the immunofluorescence method applied to blood smears, which detects interspecies antigens located in the infected blood cells (22, 34, 39). Another method, more precise but also more laborious, is the rescue of mouse sarcoma genome virus by FeLV for C 81 cat cell S + L − (17, 56). Positive results are manifested by transformation of cells that is manifested by the formation of foci. This latter procedure has the additional value of quantitatively assessing the extent of the infection.

There are other indirect methods as well. For instance, the virus can be isolated from infective tissues grown in feline embryonal cells and the presence of interspecies and/or other viral antigens can subsequently be determined by complement-fixation, diffusion, or radioimmunoassay techniques (79).

Electron microscopy has been used extensively in the past for identification of virus, but presently it is not used as frequently because of the cost and lack of sensitivity.

The FOCMA antibody is measured in target cells (cells actively producing virus and a high quantity of FOCMA antigens) that are not fixed, using a double immunofluorescence technique or cytotoxic dependent antibody (CDA) released from target cells tagged with chromium-51 as the indicator system (27, 28).

Prospective studies of Essex *et al.* (5, 9, 14) have shown that viremic cats with low or undetectable FOCMA titers develop leukemia. This is clear evidence of the importance of FOCMA antibody in immunosurveillance against feline leukemia and related diseases caused by these viruses.

The available test procedures provide the diagnostician with a vast knowledge of infection and the neutralizing and FOCMA antibody titers. On the basis of these tests a prognosis can be made regarding the patient.

Prevention and Control. It has been proved that the natural FeLV transmission usually occurs horizontally (44, 61) so that the establishment and isolation of FeLV-free colonies is the most important and effective prophylactic procedure. Cat colonies can be maintained FeLV-free for long periods if uninfected cats are not introduced. If new cats must be introduced in a cat colony free of oncovirus, the new animals must be surveyed for FeLV virus, at least by the immunofluorescence test. It is best to test the animal twice, at 1-month intervals, to insure that the animal does not have leukemia (31, 33). Young kittens are at the greatest risk from FeLV infection and subsequent disease. When an effective vaccine is developed, it will be particularly valuable in protecting these animals. Serotherapy and vaccination to cure and prevent FeLV/FeSV-induced cat tumors are feasible, but many problems remain to be solved in the near future to obtain an effective immunoprophylactic regimen.

The Disease in Man. According to a panel (2) there is no evidence at present to indicate the spread of feline tumor viruses to man. Whether cat tumor viruses contribute to the incidence of human lymphoma and sarcoma can only be determined by carefully designed epidemiological studies. Preliminary reports of such studies indicate clearly that cats, with or without leukemia or sarcoma, are not responsible for similar tumors in man.

REFERENCES

1. American Veterinary Medical Association Colloquium. Jour. Am. Vet. Med. Assoc., 1971, *158,* 1013.
2. American Veterinary Medical Association Panel. Jour. Am. Vet. Med. Assoc., 1971, *158,* 835.
3. Brody, McDonough, Frye, and Hardy. *In* Comparative Leukemia Research 1969, ed. R. M. Dutcher. S. Karger, Basel, 1970, p. 333.
4. Chan, Schiop-Stansly, and O'Connor. Jour. Natl. Cancer Inst., 1974, *52,* 473.
5. Cotter, Essex, and Hardy. Cancer Res., 1974, *34,* 1061.
6. Deinhardt, Wolfe, Theilen, and Snyder. Science, 1970, *167,* 881.
7. Dougherty and Rickard. Jour. Ultrastruct. Res., 1970, *32,* 472.
8. Essex. Adv. Cancer Res., 1975, *21,* 175.
9. Essex, Cotter, Sliski, Hardy, Stephenson, Aaronson, and Jarrett. Int. Jour. Cancer, 1977, *19,* 90.
10. Essex, Jakowski, Hardy, Cotter, Hess, and Sliski. Jour. Natl. Cancer Inst., 1975, *54,* 637.
11. Essex, Klein, Snyder, and Harrold. Int. Jour. Cancer, 1971, *8,* 384.
12. Essex, Klein, Snyder, and Harrold. Nature, 1971, *233,* 195.
13. Essex, Noronha, Oroszlan, and Hardy. *In* Prevention and detection of cancer, ed. H. E. Neiburgs. Marcel Dekker Inc., New York, 1978, p. 1401.
14. Essex, Sliski, Cotter, Jakowski, and Hardy. Science, 1975, *190,* 790.
15. Essex, Sliski, Hardy, and Cotter. Cancer Res., 1976, *36,* 640.
16. Essex and Snyder. Jour. Natl. Cancer Inst., 1973, *51,* 1007.
17. Fischinger, Blevins, and Nomura. Jour. Virol., 1974, *14,* 177.
18. Fischinger and O'Connor. Science, 1969, *165,* 714.
19. Francis, Essex, and Hardy. Nature, 1977, *269,* 252.
20. Gardner. Jour. Am. Vet. Med. Assoc., 1971, *158,* 1039.
21. Gardner, Arnstein, Johnson, Rongey, Charman, and Huebner. Jour. Am. Vet. Med. Assoc., 1971, *158,* 1046.
22. Gardner, Brown, Charman, Stephenson, Rongey, Hauser, Diegmann, Howard, Dworsky, Gilden, and Huebner. Int. Jour. Cancer, 1977, *19,* 581.
23. Gilden, Oroszlan, and Hatanaka. *In* Viruses, evolution and cancer, ed. Edouard Kurstack and Karl Maramorosch. Academic Press, New York, 1974, p. 235.

24. Gilmore and Holzworth. Jour. Am. Vet. Med. Assoc., 1971, *158,* 1013.
25. Grant, DeBoer, Essex, Worley, and Higgins. Jour. Immunol., 1977, *119,* 401.
26. Grant and Essex. *In* Cellular immunity to virus induced tumors, ed. J. W. Blasecki. Marcel Dekker, Inc., New York, in press.
27. Grant, Essex, Pedersen, Hardy, Stephenson, Cotter, and Theilen. Jour. Natl. Cancer Inst., 1978, *60,* 161.
28. Grant, Pickard, Ramaila, Madewell, and Essex. Cancer Res., 1979, *39,* 75.
29. Green, Bolognesi, Schaefer, Pister, Hunsmann, and Noronha. Virol., 1973, *56,* 565.
30. Hardy, Gerring, Old, deHarven, Brodey, and McDonough. Science, 1969, *166,* 1019.
31. Hardy, Hess, MacEwen, McClelland, Zuckerman, Essex, Cotter, and Jarrett. Cancer Res., 1976, *36,* 582.
32. Hardy, Hirshaut, and Hess. *In* Unifying concepts of leukemia, ed. R. M. Dutcher and L. Chiece-Bianche. S. Karger, Basel, 1973, p. 778.
33. Hardy, McClelland, Zuckerman, Hess, Essex, Cotter, MacEwen, and Hayes. Nature, 1976, *263,* 326.
34. Hardy, Old, Hess, Essex, and Cotter. Nature, 1973, *244,* 266.
35. Hardy, Zuckerman, MacEwen, Hayes, and Essex. Nature, 1977, *270,* 249.
36. Holmberg, Manning, and Osburn. Am. Jour. Vet. Res., 1976, *37,* 1455.
37. Hoover, Olsen, Hardy, Schaller, and Mathes. Jour. Natl. Cancer Inst., 1976, *57,* 365.
38. Hoover, Olsen, Hardy, and Schaller. Jour. Natl. Cancer Inst., 1977, *58,* 443.
39. Hoover, Olsen, Mathes, and Schaller. Cancer Res., 1977, *37,* 3707.
40. Jarrett. Jour. Am. Vet. Med. Assoc., 1971, *158,* 1032.
41. Jarrett. Int. Rev. Exp. Path., 1971, *10,* 243.
42. Jarrett, Anderson, Jarrett, Laird, and Stewart. Res. Vet. Sci., 1971, *12,* 385.
43. Jarrett, Crawford, Martin, and Davie. Nature, 1964, *202,* 567.
44. Jarrett, Jarrett, Mackey, Laird, Hardy, and Essex. Jour. Natl. Cancer Inst., 1973, *51,* 833.
45. Jarrett, Jarrett, and Mackey. Int. Jour. Cancer, 1975, *16,* 134.
46. Jarrett, Mackey, Jarrett, Laird, and Hood. Nature, 1974, *248,* 230.
47. Jarrett, Martin, Crighton, Dalton, and Stewart. Nature, 1964, *202,* 566.
48. Jarrett, Russel, and Hardy. *In* Advances in comparative leukemia research 1977, ed. P. Bentvelzen, J. Hilgers, and D. S. Yohn. North Holland Biomedical Press, Elsevier, 1978, p. 25.
49. Kawakami, Theilen, Dungworth, Munn, and Beale. Science, 1967, *158,* 1049.
50. Kahn and Stephenson. Jour. Virol., 1977, *23,* 578.
51. Laird, Jarrett, Crighton, and Jarrett. Jour. Natl. Cancer Inst., 1968, *41,* 867.
52. Lee. Jour. Am. Vet. Med. Assoc., 1971, *158,* 1037.
53. McAllister, Nicolson, Gardner, Rasheed, Rongey, Hardy, and Gilden. Nature, 1973, *242,* 75.
54. Noronha, Baggs, Schafer, Bolognesi. Nature, 1977, *267,* 54.
55. Noronha, Dougherty, Poco, Gries, Post, and Rickard. Arch. f. die gesam. Virusforsch., 1974, *45,* 235.
56. Noronha, Poco, Post, and Rickard. Jour. Natl. Cancer Inst., 1976, *57,* 129.
57. Noronha, Post, Norcross, and Rickard. Nature New Biol., 1972, *235,* 14.
58. Noronha, Schafer, Essex, and Bolognesi. Virol., 1978, *85,* 617.
59. Olsen, Hoover, Mathes, Heding, and Schaller. Cancer Res., 1976, *36,* 3642.
60. Oroszlan, Bova, White, Toni, Foreman, and Gilden. Proc. Natl. Acad. Sci., 1972, *69,* 1211.
61. Pedersen, Theilen, Keane, Fairbanks, Mason, Orser, Chen, and Allison. Am. Jour. Vet. Res., 1977, *38,* 1523.
62. Rickard, Barr, Noronha, Dougherty, and Post. Cornell Vet., 1967, *57,* 302.
63. Rickard, Gillespie, Lee, Noronha, Post, and Savage. Third Internatl. Sympos. Comp. Leukemia Res., ed. R. M. Dutcher. Paris. S. Karger, Basel, 1967.
64. Rickard, Post, Noronha, and Barr. Jour. Natl. Cancer Inst., 1969, *42,* 987.
65. Sarma, Basker, Gilden, Gardner, and Huebner. Proc. Soc. Exp. Biol. and Med., 1971, *137,* 1333.
66. Sarma, Log, and Theilen. Proc. Soc. Exp. Biol. and Med., 1971, *137,* 1444.
67. Schaefer, Claviez, Frank, Hunsmann, Moennig, Schwarz, Theilen, Bolognesi, Green, Langlois, Fischinger, and Noronha. Med. Microbiol. Immunol., 1977, *164,* 119.
68. Schaefer, Hunsmann, Moennig, Noronha, Bolognesi, Green, and Huper. Virol., 1975, *63,* 48.
69. Schafer and Bolognesi. In Contemporary topics in immunobiology, 6th ed., ed. F. Rapp and M. G. Hanna. Plenum, New York, 1977, p. 127.
70. Schafer, Lange, Bolognesi, Noronha, Post, and Rickard. Virol., 1971, *44,* 73.
71. Schafer, Lange, Pister, Seifert, Noronha, and Schmidt. Zbt. Naturforsch., 1970, *25b,* 1929.
72. Schafer and Noronha. Jour. Am. Vet. Med. Assoc., 1971, *158,* 1092.
73. Schafer, Pister, Hunsmann, and Moennig. Nature New Biol., 1973, *245,* 75.
74. Schalm, Oscar W. Veterinary hematology, 2nd ed. Lea & Febiger, Philadelphia, 1965.
75. Schalm. Jour. Am. Vet. Med. Assoc., 1971, *158,* 1025.
76. Schneider. *In* Advances in comparative leukemia research 1977, ed. P. Bentvelzen, J. Hilgers, and D. S. Yohn. North Holland Biomedical Press, Elsevier, 1978, p. 37.
77. Snyder and Dungworth. Jour. Natl. Cancer Inst., 1973, *51,* 781.
78. Snyder and Theilen. Nature, 1969, *221,* 1074.
79. Stephenson, Essex, Hino, Harauson, and Hardy. Proc. Natl. Acad. Sci., 1977, *74,* 1219.
80. Theilen, Dungworth, Kawakami, Munn, Ward, and Harrold. Cancer Res., 1970, *30,* 401.

81. Theilen, Snyder, Wolfe, and Landon. Fourth Internatl. Sympos. Comp. Leukemia Res., Cherry Hill, N.J., ed. R. M. Dutcher. S. Karger, Basel, 1970.
82. Yohn, Olsen, Schaller, Hoover, Mathes, Heding, and Davis. Cancer Res., 1976, *36,* 646.

Malignant Lymphoma of Cattle

SYNONYMS: Bovine lymphomatosis, bovine lymphocytomatosis, bovine leukosis, cattle leukemia

This is a progressive, fatal disease of cattle usually manifested by enlargement of some or all of the lymph nodes in clinically apparent cases. The glandular enlargements usually are preceded by blood changes. Many European workers believe that cattle may develop the blood changes without tumor formation.

The disease has been reported in the United States (18), Norway, Denmark, and Germany and probably exists elsewhere. In all the places mentioned it appears to be increasing rapidly in incidence. In the United States the records of the Meat Inspection Service of the Department of Agriculture suggest that the disease is becoming more prevalent. In all countries the disease appears to be distributed unevenly; that is, there are high and low incidence areas. In Denmark the incidence is reported to be as high as 40 cases per 100,000 cattle in some regions and as low as 1 in 100,000 in others. In the United States meat inspection statistics show a low of 5.3 and a high of 243.0 per 100,000 slaughtered cattle in different regions.

Character of the Disease. Evidence is emerging that bovine leukemia virus (BLV) is responsible for producing many pathological forms in natural disease similar to those described for avian and feline leukemia viruses. This concept is supported by the experimental studies in sheep with BLV (19).

Under field conditions the affected herd has cattle that show enlarged and firm superficial lymph nodes. Generally the disease progresses rapidly emaciation develops, and death ensues once the animal shows signs of illness. Sometimes an eyeball may protrude because of tumor formation in the orbit. Chronic bloating occurs in some because of enlargement of the thoracic nodes. Lameness and paralysis often occur because of pressures on parts of the spinal cord or peripheral nerves from the tumors. Lymphocytic infiltrations of some of the internal organs may result. Blood examinations may show as many as 50,000 large lymphocytes per mm^3. There is clear evidence that B-lymphocytes are the target cells for BLV infection (25, 27). A fall in the lymphocyte count at the time of tumor development is attributed to the loss of B-lymphocytes (10).

In experimental studies 69 sheep were infected with BLV from bovine lymphosarcoma tissues (19). Twenty-four animals developed lymphosarcoma and died 13 to 66 (average 29) months later. Circulating lymphocytes were increased to leukemia levels (70,000 to 403,000 per cu mm blood) in only eight sheep within 2 to 3 months of death. Various lymph nodes and visceral organs including heart, abomasum, uterus, kidneys, and urinary tract were commonly affected as in cattle with the adult form of lymphosarcoma. In one sheep the skin was involved. The liver was involved in only one case. This was in contrast to more frequent involvement reported in literature for naturally occurring lymphosarcoma. The neoplasms in experimental sheep are regarded as a mixture of reticulum or histiocytic cells and lymphoid cells with transitional forms supported by a usually sparse and diffuse fibroplasia and a web of silver-staining reticulin fibers.

Properties of the Virus. With the development of assay procedures for the study of BLV, marked advances have been made in studying the biochemical, biophysical, and biological characteristics of the virus. It clearly is a C-type virus and as such has the general features described for other C-type oncoviruses.

Earlier studies by various investigators (4, 11, 16, 24) presented evidence that a C-type particle may cause bovine leukemia.

Dutta and Sorensen (5) and Miller *et al.* (17) reported on the use of phytohemagglutinin (PHA) in cultured buffy-coat (BC) cells from cattle with persistent lymphocytosis or lymphosarcoma to enhance the appearance of C-type particles in these cell cultures. Ferrer *et al.* (6) enlarged on these observations and found that PHA also uncovered type C particles in BC cultures from clinically normal cows without lymphocytosis, as well. The use of PHA certainly has given investigators a new technique that will assist them in efforts to establish the etiological significance of these type C particles in bovine leukemia.

Gillette, Olson, and Tekeli (9) reported on the use of the immunoflourescence test for detection of bovine lymphosarcoma antigen in diseased cattle. Specific staining was limited to the cytoplasm of tumor cells and usually was weak. Specific flourescence was observed in tumor tissues from 40 to 66 percent of other cattle, but it was not seen in lymph nodes of healthy cows.

Other serological tests are used for the detection of

various antigenic components as well as the intact particle, including the complement-fixation, radioimmunoassay, immunodiffusion, and neutralization tests.

Most research activities are centered around studies of the various viral components (2, 8, 14, 15, 21, 23). These investigators are interested in determining which components are involved in infectivity and immunity. The approaches and findings are comparable to those described in this chapter on feline and avian leukemia-sarcoma complexes.

There is evidence that high-temperature, short-time pasteurization inactivates BLV in milk (1).

Immunity. At present there is little information on immunity in cattle. Based on our limited knowledge we can postulate that the mechanism is similar to that described for avian and feline leukemia.

It has been demonstrated that sera from three cows with natural cases of the adult form of lymphosarcoma inhibited the release of leukemia virus from a cell line of fetal lamb spleen infected with BLV (22). Sera from five of seven cattle experimentally infected with BLV also suppressed virus release. The phenomenon is reversible. On the other hand, sera from natural cases of cattle with the calf form and the thymic form of lymphosarcoma and normal bovine control sera failed to suppress viral release.

Cultivation. BLV replicates in a cell line from fetal lamb spleen (22). It also replicates in monolayers of bovine embryonic spleen cells or human diploid embryonic cells with the production of syncytia (7). Syncytial changes are observed in 4 to 6 days in the bovine cultures and in 6 to 8 days in the human diploid cultures. Pretreatment of the indicator cells with DEAE-dextran greatly increases the sensitivity of the system. As a consequence viral and antibody can be quantitated in a simple test system. These studies indicate cattle with the adult form of lymphosarcoma have neutralizing antibodies. With the development of a simple neutralization test in cell culture (7) studies of this type can be extended to include maternal and active humoral antibody studies and their correlation to protection.

Transmission. European investigators, particularly the Scandinavian and German scientists, for many years were convinced that the disease is transmissible. The evidence was based largely on epidemiological and hematological surveys. They noted its localized occurrence, multiple cases in single herds, and its apparent increased incidence in the last two or three decades.

Epidemiological evidence indicates that horizontal and vertical transmission can occur. Onuma *et al.* (20) have shown that BLV may be transmitted vertically from positive ewes to their progeny via the placenta and/or germinal cells but not from the sire to the lamb. Seroepidemiological evidence for the horizontal transmission of BLV showed that the disease can be transmitted from infected to noninfected cattle (26).

Diagnosis. Diagnosis often can be achieved by clinical, hematological, and/or necropsy examination. Virological or serological methods can be used to confirm a diagnosis.

It is conceivable that tissue culture can be used to isolate virus but the sensitivity of this assay procedure for this purpose has not been evaluated. The fluorescent-antibody test (FAT) affords another method for viral detection. Although the electron microscope can be used for particle visualization in suspected material, it lacks the sensitivity of the FAT.

Levy *et al.* (13) isolated and purified structural protein (BLV-24) of BLV. With this protein they developed a radioimmunoassay (RIA) test. This test was compared with the complement-fixation and immunodiffusion tests in a study of 363 cows and found to be more sensitive than the other two methods in detecting antibody in infected cattle. With this procedure all of the leukemic cattle, except those with juvenile lymphosarcoma, had high antibody titers greater than or equal to 10,000. Practically all cows with persistent leukemia were also positive but with lower titers. Approximately two-thirds of hematologically suspect animals and one-third of normal animals from BLV-exposed herds were positive, whereas all unexposed cows remained negative for antibodies to the BLV-24 antigen of BLV. This group (12) also showed that the complement-fixation test detected two times more positive animals than the hematological examination in the same group of cows. Another group (28) reported persistent levels of complement fixation (CF) antibodies to BLV in the leukosis herd.

Control. Slaughter of viremic and affected animals is recommended.

The Disease in Man. A seroepidemic study showed that high-risk humans, such as farmers, veterinarians, and farm families exposed to bovine leukosis herds did not develop precipitating antibodies to the BLV with the agar-gel immunodiffusion test (3). This is good evidence that BLV rarely, if ever, infects humans. Although 77 percent of the farm group consumed raw milk in the study, it is still advisable for people to drink pasteurized milk to eliminate any risk. It has been demonstrated that flash pasteurization inactivates the virus mixed with milk.

REFERENCES

1. Baumgartener, Olson, and Onuma. Jour. Am. Vet, Med. Assoc., 1976, *169,* 1189.
2. Deshayes, Levy, Parodi, and Levy. Jour. Virol., 1977, *21,* 1056.
3. Donham, Van der Maaten, Miller, Kruse, and Rubino. Jour. Natl. Cancer Inst., 1977, *59,* 851.
4. Dutcher, Szekely, Larkin, Coriell, and Marshak. Ann. N.Y. Acad. Sci., 1963, *108,* 1149.
5. Dutta and Sorensen. Fourth Internatl. Sympos. on Comp. Leukemia Res., Cherry Hill, N.J. ed. R. M. Dutcher. S. Karger, Basel, 1970.
6. Ferrer, Avila, Stock, Lin, and Guest. Fifth Internatl. Sympos. on Comp. Leukemia Res., Padova, Italy, ed. R. M. Dutcher and L. Chieco-Bianchi. S. Karger, Basel, 1972.
7. Ferrer and Diglo. Cancer Res., 1976, *36,* 1068.
8. Frenzel, Kaaden, and Mussgay. Zbt. Naturforsch., 1977, *32,* 301.
9. Gillette, Olsen, and Tekeli. Am. Jour. Vet. Res., 1969, *30,* 975.
10. Kenyon and Piper. Inf. and Immun., 1977, *16,* 898.
11. Lee, Takahashi, and Gillespie. Cornell Vet., 1970, *60,* 139.
12. Levy, Deshayes, Guillemain, and Parodi. Int. Jour. Cancer, 1977, *19,* 822.
13. Levy, Deshayes, Parodi, Levy, Stephenson, Devare, and Gilden. Int. Jour. Cancer, 1977, *20,* 543.
14. McDonald and Ferrer. Jour. Natl. Cancer Inst., 1976, *57,* 875.
15. McDonald, Graves, and Ferrer. Cancer Res., 1976, *36,* 1251.
16. McKercher, Wada, Staub, and Theilen. Ann. N.Y. Acad. Sci., 1963, *108,* 1163.
17. Miller. Jour. Natl. Cancer Inst., 1970, *43,* 1297.
18. Monlux, Anderson, and Davis. Am. Jour. Vet. Res., 1956, *17,* 646.
19. Olsen and Baumgartener. Cancer Res., 1976, *36,* 2365.
20. Onuma, Baumgartener, Olson, and Pearson. Cancer Res., 1977, *37,* 4075.
21. Onuma, Driscoll, and Olson. Arch Virol., 1977, *55,* 131.
22. Onuma, Olson, and Baumgartener. Jour. Natl. Cancer Inst., 1975, *54,* 1199.
23. Onuma, Olson, and Driscoll. Jour. Natl. Cancer Inst., 1976, *57,* 571.
24. Papparella, Cali, Rossi, and Lacobelli. Ann. N.Y. Acad. Sci., 1963, *108,* 1173.
25. Paul, Pomeroy, Castro, Johnson, Muscoplat, Sorensen. Jour. Natl. Cancer Inst., 1977, *59,* 1269.
26. Piper, Abt, Ferrer, and Marshak. Cancer Res., 1975, *35,* 2714.
27. Pomeroy, Paul, Weber, Sorensen, and Johnson. Jour. Natl. Cancer Inst., 1977, *59,* 281.
28. Tabel, Chander, Van der Maaten, and Miller. Can. Jour. Comp. Med., 1976, *40,* 350.

Canine Leukemia-Sarcoma Complex

Spontaneous lymphomas occur in the dog. Generally speaking there is little information about them, but the incidence of spontaneous lymphomas in dogs does not appear to be as high as the incidence in cats and chickens. Limited trials to determine the transmissibility and etiology with cell-free extracts of these tumors has met with failure. Within the last 10 years various investigators were successful in transplanting a canine lymphosarcoma (3), canine osteosarcoma (3), mixed-cell tumor (2), radiation-induced canine myelomonocytic leukemia (4), and radiation-induced canine granulocytic anemia (1) in perinatal puppies. Quite obviously, the problem is more difficult than that encountered with the domestic cat, mouse, and chicken; but the degree of technical difficulty is similar to that encountered with studies of leukemia in humans and cattle.

REFERENCES

1. Fritz and Norris. Fifth Internatl. Sympos. on Comp. Leukemia Res., Padova, Italy, ed. R. M. Dutcher and L. Chieco-Bianchi. S. Karger, Basel, 1972.
2. Jensen, Bowles, Kerber, Rangan, and Woods. Fifth Internatl. Sympos. on Comp. Leukemia Res., Padova, Italy, ed. R. M. Dutcher and L. Chieco-Bianchi. S. Karger, Basel, 1972.
3. Owen. Fifth Internatl. Sympos. on Comp. Leukemia Res., Padova, Italy, ed. R. M. Dutcher and L. Chieco-Bianchi. S. Karger, Basel, 1972.
4. Shifrine. Fifth Internatl. Sympos. on Comp. Leukemia Res., Padova, Italy, ed. R. M. Dutcher and L. Chieco-Bianchi. S. Karger, Basel, 1972.

THE SUBFAMILY LENTIVIRINAE

This is a new subfamily to which visna-maedi virus is assigned. Equine infectious anemia virus is provisionally placed in this subfamily. These viruses also contain reverse transcriptase and morphologically are similar to the oncogenic type C virus particles.

These viruses have characteristics that promote viral persistence such as viral genome integration selection of less virulent variants, selection of ts mutants, generation of defective interfering particles, and interferon production. Persistence may be influenced principally by the host's immune system, but the virus and the host together determine the outcome—persistence or no persistence of virus.

Visna-Maedi

The viruses known as *visna* and *maedi* are so similar that they are regarded as a single virus capable of producing nervous or respiratory manifestations.

Visna and maedi were present in Iceland and may also occur in Texel and in India. Maedi, progressive pneumonia of sheep in the United States, and lung disease (*zwolgerziekte*) in Holland (4) are the same disease or very closely related.

Ovine progressive pneumonia is prevalent in many major sheeping-producing areas in the United States, particularly in midwestern and northwestern states (3). Visna-maedi also has occurred in Canada (1, 10).

Character of the Disease. *Maedi (respiratory form).* Sheep that are 2 years of age or older are affected with emaciation and dyspnea. The disease is highly fatal. The incubation period is 2 years or longer, but sheep inoculated by various routes have lung lesions 1 month later. Infection also occurs after feeding or by contact.

At necropsy the lungs are much enlarged, weighing as much as double the normal. There is diffuse perivascular and peribronchiolar infiltration with mononuclear cells but little fibrosis.

The most common lesions in the lungs observed in natural cases of ovine progressive pneumonia from which virus was isolated were multiple lymphoid nodules and increased fibromuscular tissue (3).

Visna (nervous form). Early signs of illness in the disease are abnormal head posture and lip trembling. Other nervous manifestations lead to paraplegia and total paralysis. The incubation period is measured in months, and this slow, demyelinating disease persists for weeks or months, terminating in death. Pleocytosis in the cerebral spinal fluid may appear 1 month after injection with clinical signs appearing as long as 18 months later.

The lesions are typical of a diffuse encephalomyelitis with demyelination (9). In early reports visna was confused with *Rida,* a disease probably identical to scrapie in sheep (8).

The nervous disease is transmissible to sheep by intracerebral inoculation whereas the respiratory form (maedi) occurs after intranasal exposure. Present evidence suggests that visna is an encephalitic form of the lung disease (12).

Properties of the Virus. Visna and maedi viruses are antigenically related (13). Slight antigenic differences have been noted. In cross-neutralization tests in cell culture, maedi virus has a somewhat broader antigenic structure than visna virus (13).

The viruses are inhibited by the DNA inhibitors, 5-bromodeoxyuridine and actinomycin D. This doesn't necessarily imply that they are DNA viruses, only that cellular DNA is required for their synthesis (13). In fact it has been established that visna virus contains RNA (6). The analogy between visna virus and oncogenic RNA viruses has been extended by the demonstration of reverse transcriptase in purified visna virus (7). The morphology and maturation of the visna virus particle is somewhat comparable to the type C oncogenic virus particle observed in feline, murine, and avian leukemia. The visna virus particles vary in diameter from 60 to 90 nm, with a central core of 30 to 40 nm. Surface projections 10 nm in length have been observed (13). There is a suggestion of a concentric arrangement with the core, and a few helical rods 9 nm are seen. Particles appear to be released at the cell surface from two walled buds (11). Proviral DNA has been demonstrated by *in situ* hybridization in foci of cells of a lamb infected with visna virus (Figure 52.5) (5). Some of the cells also contain the major structural antigen p 30. This is an example of restriction in virus gene expression in the infected animal providing a mechanism for the persistence of virus in a chronic disease.

The virus particles are ether- and chloroform-sensitive, and inactivated readily by heat. Most are stable between pH 7.2 and 9.2 and survive storage for months at −70 C. Phenol (4 percent), formaldehyde (0.04 percent), and ethanol (50 percent) readily inactivate the virus. In the presence of toluidine blue, visna is sensitive to light.

Neutralizing antibodies are formed to visna and maedi virus strains with cross-neutralization generally resulting. Inhibitory substances have been found in the sera of cattle and other species. Most human sera of all ages inhibit these viruses; it is a heat-stable serum component believed to be a nonspecific inhibitor.

Cultivation. The virus strains are isolated from sheep tissues such as blood, spinal fluid, and saliva and propagated in cell cultures derived from ependyma or choroid plexus of sheep brain. Multinuclear giant cells are formed with subsequent cell destruction; cytopathic changes occur in 2 to 3 weeks. By serial transfer the time is shortened to 3 to 15 days depending on the viral dose. Virus can persist in cultures for at least 4 months.

Immunity. Sheep that show clinical signs die with the disease. There is no evidence that inapparent infections occur in sheep, but there is a suggestion of it in other species, such as cattle, that have a viral-neutralizing substance in their sera.

The agar-gel diffusion test detects antibody to ovine progressive pneumonia virus (2). The test antigen consists of concentrated nutrient medium removed every 2 weeks from a cell culture persistently infected with iso-

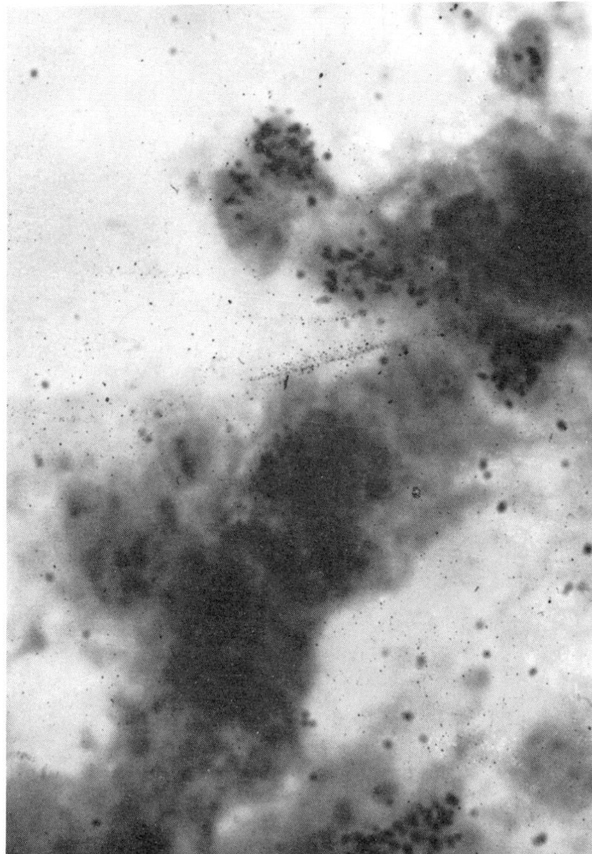

Figure 52.5. Demonstration of visna provirus by *in situ* hybridization. Section of choroid plexus from a sheep infected with visna virus, hybridized *in situ* with a radioactively labeled probe specific for the visna virus genome (9). Radioautograph developed after 16 weeks of exposure, stained with Giemsa. × 870. (Courtesy A. T. Haase, School of Medicine, University of California at San Francisco. From A. T. Haase, Opendra Narayan, Dianne Griffin, and Donald Price, *Science,* Vol. 195, Jan. 14, 1977, pp. 175–77. Copyright 1977 by the American Association for the Advancement of Science.)

late WLC-1 of ovine progressive pneumonia virus. Two lines of precipitate formed with some serums, but those taken early after viral exposure or 3 to 4 years after exposure often had 1 line of precipitate. All lambs inoculated with virus developed precipitating antibody one to six months later.

Diagnosis. Visna can be distinguished from Rida (scrapie) by clinical signs and pathological changes. Maedi can be differentiated from ovine adenomatosis by pathological changes (see "Character of the Disease" above for distinguishing features).

The immunodiffusion and neutralization tests can be used to detect antibody to virus. The isolation of virus can be made in cell cultures of sheep choroid plexus cells.

Control. A slaughter policy in 1951 in Iceland was apparently successful in eliminating both disease forms; however, the respiratory form reappeared in 1965.

The Disease in Man. The significance of a viral-neutralizing inhibitor in human sera is unknown.

REFERENCES

1. Bellavance, Turgeon, Phaneuf, and Sauvagean. Can. Vet. Jour., 1974, *15,* 293.
2. Cutlip, Jackson, and Laird. Am. Jour. Vet. Res., 1977, *38,* 1081.
3. Cutlip, Jackson, and Laird. Am. Jour. Vet. Res., 1977, *38,* 2091.
4. Deboer. Res. Vet. Sci., 1975, *18,* 15.
5. Haase, Stouring, Narayan, Griffin, and Price. Science, 1977, *195,* 175.
6. Harter, Rosenkranz, and Rose. Proc. Soc. Exp. Biol. and Med., 1969, *131,* 297.
7. Lin and Thomar. Bact. Proc., 1970, *6,* 702.
8. Sigurdsson. Brit. Vet. Jour., 1954, *110,* 255.
9. Sigurdsson, Palsson, and van Bogaert. Acta Neuropath., 1962, *1,* 343.
10. Stevenson. Can. Vet. Jour., 1978, *19,* 159.
11. Thomar. Virol., 1961, *14,* 463.
12. Thomar. Zeitschr f. Neurol., 1971, *199,* 155.
13. Thomar and Helgadottir. Res. Vet. Sci., 1965, *6,* 456.

Equine Infectious Anemia

SYNONYMS: Swamp fever, equine malarial fever; abbreviation, EIA

This is a disease of horses characterized by a diversity of signs and an exceedingly variable course. An excellent detailed account of the disease will be found in the monograph of Dreguss and Lombard (8) and the selected papers presented at the American Veterinary Medical Association Symposium on Equine Infectious Diseases (1) and at the Fourth International Conference on Equine Infectious Diseases (2).

Members of the horse family are the only known natural hosts. European workers have reported limited success in obtaining multiplication of the virus, sometimes accompanied by mild signs in sheep, goats, pigs, rabbits, and some other species, including man. Workers in the United States generally have not been able to confirm these findings. Infectious anemia of horses has been recognized in practically all parts of the world where horses are raised. It occurs mostly in rather small areas from which it shows little tendency to spread. The name *swamp fever* is derived from the fact that the disease is most frequent in animals pastured in low-lying areas. This is not always the case, however. Scott (23) saw the disease on lands in Wyoming that were 9,000 feet above sea level. Even at high altitudes, flat, swampy lands are found, and such lands apparently favor the disease. The disease has been seen in the United States for more than 70 years. It has been reported at one time or another from 42 of the 50 states. Formerly it was common in the Mississippi Delta region in mules that worked in the cotton fields, but tractors have now largely replaced work animals. Udall and Fitch (35) recognized a focus of the disease in northern New York in 1914. In 1947 an outbreak occurred in Thoroughbred horses at the Rockingham Race Track in Salem, New Hampshire. At least 47 cases were definitely diagnosed, and about 15 deaths occurred (29).

In 1970 Coggins and Norcross (5) reported on an immunodiffusion test which is remarkably accurate in its detection of virus carriers. It has become apparent that certain breeding establishments had the infection on the premises without being aware of its presence. Through the use of the test as a diagnostic procedure, it is evident that the disease is more prevalent in the United States than clinical reports would indicate.

The greater number of acute and subacute cases are seen during the late summer and early fall months, a circumstance which fits in well with the idea that most initial infections occur from the bites of bloodsucking flies and mosquitoes.

Character of the Disease. Infectious anemia may appear in an acute, subacute, or chronic form. The acutely ill animal develops signs suddenly. A temperature of 105 to 108 F commonly appears; the horse is very dejected, refuses feed, becomes anemic, and shows congested and even icteric mucous membranes. It often sweats profusely in warm weather and frequently develops a serous discharge from the nose. These attacks often last for 3 to 5 days, after which the animal appears to recover. It may be free of signs for many days, weeks, or months, but usually, sooner or later, other acute attacks occur. In any of these attacks, death may come.

The chronic form of the disease consists, essentially, of a series of short acute attacks, between which the normal intervals may be very long. Such animals may show no signs whatsoever, but most of them develop anemia and hypergammaglobulinemia, and the sedimentation rate of their corpuscles is greatly increased. The heart action becomes irregular, edematous swellings appear and disappear, and muscular weakness varies from slight to so much that the animal cannot stand or walk, or if it can walk, the gait may be very uncertain and wobbly. Such animals gradually become emaciated in spite of the fact that their appetite is often very great. Chronically infected animals have been kept under constant observation for periods in excess of 18 years (30), during which time their blood was constantly infective for other horses. With the availability of test procedures such as immunodiffusion and immunofluorescence tests, it is possible to determine whether some virus carriers are completely asymptomatic.

When horses are inoculated subcutaneously with infected blood, the incubation period generally is 12 to 15 days. Occasionally it is shorter, and frequently it is considerably longer—as long as 90 days in a few cases.

As has already been said, one of the striking features of this disease is the great variability in its duration. Acute episodes usually last from 3 to 5 days. Periods between episodes may be months or years. In all likelihood most infected animals eventually die of the disease unless their life span is terminated otherwise before the disease has run its full course. Experimentally it has been found that some animals, after carrying active virus for long periods, eventually become free of it. These recoveries apparently are the exceptions.

Animals dying of the acute form of the disease exhibit lesions of general septicemia. Hemorrhages occur in most of the parenchymatous organs; the spleen generally is enlarged and softened and its capsule is hemorrhagic. The lymph nodes of the abdominal cavity are swollen, and their peripheries generally are infiltrated with blood originating in hemorrhages in the organs from which their lymph sinuses drain. Splotchy hemorrhages occur on the serous membranes and in the mucous membrane of the intestines. The kidneys and liver show evidence of parenchymatous degeneration. Subcutaneous edema, emaciation, and evidences of anemia usually are apparent.

Animals that die after suffering from the chronic form of this disease show lesions similar to those described, but in addition there usually are characteristic changes in the liver and bone marrow. If the long bones are split lengthwise, the yellow marrow frequently is found to have disappeared more or less completely and to have been replaced with red marrow, an indication of tremendous stimulation of hematopoiesis in an effort on the part of the blood-forming tissues to compensate for the loss of red blood cells destroyed by the virus. The liver in such cases usually is reddish brown in color and enlarged because of great proliferation of the endothelial cells of the sinusoids, many of which are loaded with the brownish iron-containing pigment (hemosiderin) derived from destroyed blood cells. Other microscopic alterations include generalized lymphoproliferative changes with perivascular and hepatic lymphoid infiltrations, lymphoid hyperplasia in the lymph nodes and spleen; hepatic cell necrosis and glomerulitis (10). The mononuclear infiltration and necrosis in the liver are usually quite prominent in the disease. A proliferative glomerulitis with increased cellularity and thickening of glomerular tufts is prominent. The kidney lesion appears to be the result of immune complex deposition because the capillaries contain granular deposits of C′3 and IgG (10). A vasculitis has been described, but it is not a common finding. Inclusion bodies have not been demonstrated.

Information about the pathogenesis of the disease is known because assay procedures for viral assay and antibody detection are now available. At the end of 1 week after subcutaneous inoculation of the horse, the agent is detectable in the serum and leukocytes (10). During the first febrile period, the virus titer in the serum increases, probably reaching its peak. After the fever subsides, the titer decreases only to rise again during subsequent fever episodes. McGuire *et al.* (19) used the direct immunofluorescence test in a study of EIA viral antigen in tissues of 24 experimentally infected horses. Virus-infected cells were found in horses examined 6 to 40 days after inoculation. Horses examined for fluorescence before the 6th day after inoculation were negative, and those examined at 98, 218, and 915 days had no demonstrable fluorescence. Fluorescence was noted in the spleens of all 18 positive horses while fluorescence was seen in the splenic nodes of 14, livers of 12, and kidneys of 9. Fluorescence was observed occasionally in a number of other lymph nodes, various visceral organs, and the brain. Kupffer cells were infected with virus in the liver and macrophages in all other organs. EIA antigen also was observed in mononuclear cells in blood vessels of many organs. In all instances the antigen was located in the cytoplasm. The type of cell that was infected, and its distribution, are similar to those observed in certain other persistent virus infections (19).

The Disease in Experimental Animals. The only dependable animals for experimentation with this disease are members of the equine family.

Various European workers claim to have produced thermal reactions and even fatal terminations in swine with this virus. Virus multiplication has also been obtained in rabbits, chickens, and pigeons, and there are some records of finding virus in naturally infected birds on farms where the disease occurred in horses. Köbe (13) reports that small splenectomized pigs are especially suitable subjects for inoculation. Stein (26) reports that his attempts to infect calves, sheep, swine, dogs, cats, rabbits, guinea pigs, rats, mice, and pigeons were unsuccessful.

Properties of the Virus. The virus nature of the causative agent was determined by Carré and Vallée (3) in 1904 and has been amply confirmed by many others. The blood is infectious in all stages of the disease, and filtrates of Berkefeld or porcelain filters are about equally infectious. Virus is also found in washed blood cells, all parenchymatous organs, milk, urine, saliva, and feces.

The particle diameter of the virus is 100 to 120 nm with a nucleoid of about 50 nm (32) with maturation by budding from the plasma membrane. It is an RNA virus (21) that contains reverse transcriptase, an RNA-dependent DNA polymerase (7). The virus is inactivated by ether treatment; by heating at 58 to 60 C for 1 hour; and by phenol, formalin, and other chemicals (8, 31). It survives lyophilization and freezing for long periods of time. The virus contained in blood is quite resistant to heat, chemicals, and putrefaction. Dried blood retains virulence for some months if protected from sunlight. In thin layers the virus is quickly destroyed by sunlight, and thus it is believed that infected secretions, such as urine, will not long remain virulent on pastures. The infective agent can be separated from serum proteins and concentrated by DEAE cellulose chromatography (33). Chromatography and other methods were used in combination to purify and concentrate the virus.

The EIA agent can be detected in horse-leukocyte cell cultures by the indirect immunofluorescence test and in infected horse tissues by the direct immunofluorescence test (19).

Coggins and Norcross (5) described an immunodiffusion test for EIA which detects specific antibody in chronically infected horses for long periods of time. In an experiment to determine correlation between presence of antibody and infection with EIA virus, blood from 84 serologically test-positive horses representing acute, chronic, and inapparent EIA infection caused infection in 84 experimental ponies as determined by clinical signs of illness and production of EIA antibody (6). Blood from

77 serologically test-negative horses did not infect ponies and EIA antibody was not produced. Consequently the immunodiffusion test is accepted as being at least 95 percent accurate for the diagnosis of EIA infection.

A second antigen designated *C* was later described; it is a weaker antigen than the one described by Coggins and Norcross (5, 34). A polypeptide reacting in the immunodiffusion test has an approximate molecular weight of 28,000 daltons and also has group-specific activity. This is termed *antigen G*. Neither antigen is involved in EIA immunity.

The complement-fixation test described by Kono and Kobayashi (14) has been used to study various isolates of EIA virus. These isolates, made in Japan, the United States, and Germany, share common CF antigens. There is no evidence to suggest that EIA virus shares a common CF antigen with other equine viruses.

In horses infected with EIA, complement-fixing antibody disappears in the early stage of the disease while precipitating antibody persists. McGuire *et al.* (20) reported a complement-fixing inhibiting (CFI) antibody that was detected in the late stages of disease. This group also showed that IgG(T) immunoglobulin was responsible for the CFI antibody. It has been suggested that IgA-rich fraction also is related to CFI activity (37).

The EIA virus presumably is capable of producing neutralizing antibodies in horses as assayed by the cell culture technique (15). The antigens detected by neutralization tests are present on the virion surface which appear to be type-specific, and yet different isolates from the same horse vary in type (16). EIAV propagated on an equine dermal cell line agglutinated guinea pig erythrocytes (25). Viral fluids containing about $10^{7.5}$ mean tissue culture infective doses per ml showed hemagglutinating (HA) titers ranging from 16 to 32 units per 0.05 ml. Results of cesium chloride equilibrium density gradient centrifugation revealed that the hemagglutinin was inseparable from the virus particles. The hemagglutination reaction persisted over a wide range of temperature and pH, and the absence of divalent cations did not decrease it activity. The HA activity was stable at 4 C but not at 56 C. The activity was destroyed by virus-disrupting lipid solvents and moderately sensitive to a proteolytic enzyme. Neuraminidase enhanced HA activity slightly. Phospholipase C had no effect on HA titer, although it completely inactivated infectivity. It was relatively stable to ultraviolet irradiation. Thus, the hemagglutinin appears to be closely associated with virus particles, and its activity is dependent on the presence of its lipids and proteins. Hemagglutination was inhibited by sera from horses infected with EIA virus. Hemagglutinin receptors on the erythrocytes were inactivated by a proteolytic enzyme and formaldehyde, but were not influenced by neuraminidase or sodium deoxycholate.

Interferon is not produced in the serum of infected horses or in cell cultures infected with three different strains of EIA virus (17).

Cultivation. Primary peripheral horse leukocyte cultures are used for the propagation of the virus (12). A cytopathic effect may occur, but the changes are similar to spontaneous changes occurring in culture. To detect virus the CF test is applied using a standard antiserum (14) or the indirect immunofluorescence test is used (36). Exacting procedures and proper source of biological materials are essential to the success of a horse-leukocyte culture system.

Although reports in the literature might suggest otherwise, it is presently accepted that laboratory animals are insusceptible to EIA virus. Attempts to propagate the virus in the hen's embryonated egg have failed.

Immunity. Until recently all evidence suggested that only one immunological type of EIA virus existed. Kono *et al.* (15) reported that two strains used in their studies were immunologically heterologous by protection tests in horses and by reciprocal serum-neutralization tests performed in cell cultures. In the course of these experiments it also was shown that repeated inoculations of an attenuated horse leukocyte cell culture strain failed to produce disease or a viremia and withstood protection against its virulent parent strain. Furthermore, virus failed to replicate in these horses after challenge, but these same horses were not protected against a heterologous virulent horse virus. These experiments must be viewed with caution until confirmed because of the impact this newer knowledge may have on the control and prevention of EIA.

Obviously, there is still a great deal to be learned about the mechanism of immunity, or the lack thereof in the form of protection. It is clear that in natural infections the virus persists in most horses for long periods of time despite the presence of antibody in the form of precipitating, complement-fixing, and even neutralizing antibody. Chronically infected horses will not react to the injection of fresh virus. In a few animals that freed themselves from virus after a long course of infection, inoculation of virulent virus caused disease in some animals but not in others.

Many experiments have been directed toward prophylactic immunization (3), but these have usually been unsuccessful. The report of Kono *et al.* (15) is encouraging and undoubtedly calls for more study in this area.

There are no biological products now available in the United States for immunization against EIA.

Transmission. Infectious anemia is believed to be spread principally through the agency of insects, particularly of bloodsucking flies. *Stomoxys calcitrans,* the common stable fly, is capable of transmitting the disease and perhaps is the principal agent. Scott (24) believed that this fly was the principal agent concerned, and in this the Japanese Commission (11) concurred. Lührs (18) in Germany believes that mosquitoes, particularly *Anopheles maculipennis,* are the chief offenders. Other bloodsucking flies, particularly tabanids, probably are involved at times. Scott showed that infections in horses could be produced by a single prick with a hypodermic needle which had been infected by pricking an infected horse. This finding suggests that any type of insect that feeds first upon one animal and then another at short intervals could carry the disease. In the outbreaks at the New England race tracks in 1947 it was noted that there had been an influx of horseflies from nearby marshes shortly after sick horses had arrived.

There seems to be sufficient evidence to indicate that the disease may spread from one animal to another by simple contact without the intervention of insects. Fulton (9) believed that he had produced cases by injecting horses with water from swampy areas in pastures where infected horses were kept, and there are accounts of infections in horses kept within screened buildings with infected animals, all animals being watered out of common containers and all being fed from the floor, so there was ample opportunity for contamination of food and water with infectious excretions. Since infections can be produced, although somewhat irregularly, by feeding infectious material, it is reasonable to believe that natural infections can occur more or less directly.

Several authors have suggested that some of the roundworms parasitic in horses might play a part in the transmission of the disease. Stein, Lucker, Osteen, and Gouchenour (27) tested this hypothesis by injecting emulsions of washed parasites from animals suffering from infectious anemia. Out of a number of such experiments they succeeded only once in obtaining an infection. In this case the infecting material consisted of an extract prepared from strongyles.

Stein and Mott (28) state that it is difficult to transmit the disease by administering infective material *per os* or by direct contact. They were unable to obtain definite evidence that foals contracted the disease by suckling their infected dams or by associating with them. It was shown that the milk of infected mares sometimes contains virus, that the foals may be inapparent carriers, and that suckling foals may be infected artificially.

Rather conclusive evidence has been obtained that equine infectious anemia has been transmitted to susceptible horses by careless use of hypodermic syringes, tattooing needles, and other piercing instruments. Such instruments should be sterilized by boiling after they have been used on one animal and before they are used on another. Biological supply houses in the United States licensed by the U.S. Department of Agriculture to do interstate business are required to heat all antisera prepared from horses at 58 to 59 C for 1 hour to destroy any virus that may be present. This should eliminate the possibility of transmitting this disease by antitoxins or other antisera made in horses. As an added safeguard it is recommended that each horse be tested for antibody by the immunodiffusion test that detects viral carriers.

The persistence of the virus in the blood of chronically affected, apparently normal animals is astonishing. Schalk and Roderick (22) have published an account of one case which, after a number of acute attacks during a period of 3 months following inoculation with infected blood, lived in apparent health for 14 years, then suddenly developed acute signs and died. During this apparently normal period 18 other horses were inoculated with its blood at intervals of about 1 year, and all but one of these developed acute signs of infectious anemia. During the first 3 years after inoculation there were occasional febrile periods, but during the remainder of the time until the final illness there were only rare febrile periods, which may or may not have been due to the infection. The persistence of virus in the horse offers a mechanism which virtually assures its maintenance on premises unless carrier horses are eliminated by the immunodiffusion test procedure.

Diagnosis. Clinical pathological procedures and pathological alterations can be used to assist in the diagnosis of EIA. Clinical pathological alterations are related to the activity of the disease in a horse. Asymptomatic carriers have few detectable changes. The packed-cell volume and RBC counts decline during active disease. The hemolytic anemia probably is immunologically related. Sideroleukocytes are found in variable numbers in active disease. Hypergammaglobulinemia occurs. The WBC cell count varies, but associated with a decrease is a relative lymphocytosis as a result of a decrease in granulocytic type cells. There is a deranged coagulation hemostasis, so liver biopsies are ill-advised during active disease. Tests for liver changes are indicated. The principal distinctive alterations then are hepatic changes associated with periodic pyrexia, sideroleukocytosis, and anemia.

The only dependable animals for diagnostic inoculations are members of the equine family. Young animals are preferred to old, and individuals should be sought that lack precipitating antibody. Blood or tissue extracts may be injected parenterally. The test animals should be kept indoors and given good care; their temperatures should be taken twice daily. If the animals have not been previously exposed, they usually respond with a temperature reaction and other signs of the acute form of the disease. This reaction may be expected in most instances during the 2nd or 3rd week, but in a few cases the interval is much longer—sometimes as much as 3 months.

Various laboratory tests had been advocated from time to time by different workers, but none proved reliable. The immunodiffusion test described by Coggins and Norcross (5) is accepted in the United States and many other countries as a valid test for the diagnosis of EIA (Figure 52.6).

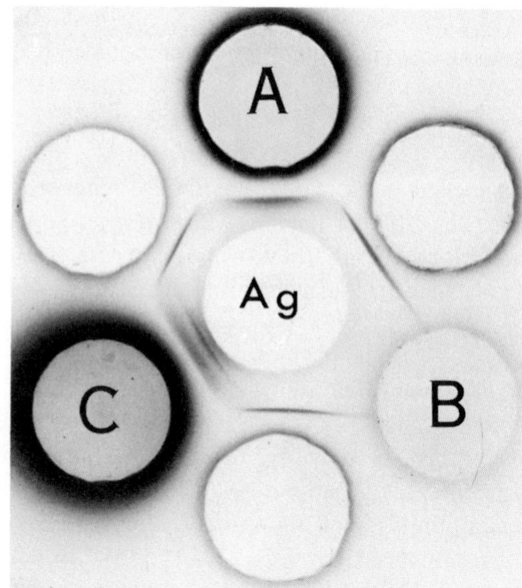

Figure 52.6. Agar-gel immunodiffusion test for the diagnosis of equine infectious anemia. Viral antigen is placed in the center well and a known positive control serum in the three outside unmarked wells. Serum from horses A and C indicate infection. The lack of a reaction at test serum B indicates no infection. (Courtesy L. Coggins, New York State College of Veterinary Medicine.)

The complement-fixation test has only limited value as CF antibodies do not persist beyond 2 months after an initial exposure to the virulent virus regardless of the existence of persisting virus or the recurrence of clinical disease (10). An occasional horse will have a second CF antibody response to an attenuated strain of EIA (15), but the titer persists only for a few days.

A radioimmunoassay procedure for the detection of EIA antigen and antibody has been described (4). Unfortunately, the sensitivity of the test procedure was less than anticipated, so at its present stage of development it is not recommended as a practical diagnostic test to detect low levels of antigen or antibody.

Control. Because the immunodiffusion test (5) detects viral carriers, officials have an accurate method for the control of the disease. Positive animals should be eliminated. In certain instances confirmation of the test may require the inoculation of a horse. This horse test necessitates a waiting period of 45 days combined with daily temperature readings on the animal. If there are no signs of illness or no rise in temperature, the test is considered negative.

The immunodiffusion test now is officially recognized as the diagnostic test acceptable to governments and the horse industry for control and elimination of the disease. Occasionally IgG(T) antibodies interfere with test results; however, the antibodies can be detected. These antibodies cause inhibition of adjacent positive control lines, but the problem is minimal because few horses have large amounts of EIAV P28 antigen-specific IgG(T) antibodies. As a matter of fact, total IgG(T) amounts are preferentially suppressed during EIAV infection.

Annual testing of horses for carriers is the principal feature of the control program. A 90- to 120-day retest on the premises is also recommended, especially on breeding farms where infection exists, until a complete negative testing is achieved.

In areas where the disease occurs, the use of common equipment—bridles, currycombs, and brushes—should be avoided. Surgical instruments, needles, and syringes should be thoroughly sterilized before use on each animal. Flies and insects should be controlled, and the horses should be kept from infected pastures.

REFERENCES

1. American Veterinary Medical Association Symposium. Jour. Am. Vet. Med. Assoc., 1969, *155,* 327.
2. Bryans, John T., and Heinz Gerber, eds. Equine Infectious Disease IV, *in* Proc. 4th Internatl. Conf. Equine Inf. Dis. Veterinary Publications, Inc., Princeton, N.J., 1978.

3. Carré and Vallée. Comp. rend. Acad. Sci., 1904, *139*, 26.
4. Coggins, Matheka, and Charman. *In* Proc. 4th Internatl. Conf. Equine Inf. Dis., ed. John T. Bryans and Heinz Gerber. Veterinary Publications, Inc., Princeton, N.J., 1978, p. 395.
5. Coggins and Norcross. Cornell Vet., 1970, *60*, 330.
6. Coggins, Norcross, and Nusbaum. Am. Jour. Vet. Res., 1972, *33*, 11.
7. Crawford and Archer. *In* Proc. 4th Internatl. Conf. Equine Inf. Dis., ed. John T. Bryans and Heinz Gerber. Veterinary Publications, Inc., Princeton, N.J., 1978, p. 395.
8. Dreguss and Lombard. Experimental studies in equine infectious anemia. Univ. of Penn. Press, Philadelphia, 1954.
9. Fulton. Jour. Am. Vet. Med. Assoc., 1930, *77*, 157.
10. Henson, McGuire, Kobayashi, Banks, Davis, and Gorham. *In* Proc. 2nd Internatl. Conf. Equine Inf. Dis., ed. John T. Bryans and Heinz Gerber. S. Karger, Basel, 1970, 178.
11. Japanese Commission. Review of report, Vet. Jour., 1914, *70*, 604.
12. Kobayashi. Virus, 1961, *11*, 249.
13. Köbe. Arch. f. Tierheilk., 1938, *73*, 399.
14. Kono and Kobayashi. Natl. Inst. An. Health Q., 1966, *6*, 194.
15. Kono, Kobayashi, and Fukunaga. Natl. Inst. An. Health, Q., 1970, *10*, 113.
16. Kono, Kobayashi, and Fukunaga. Arch. f. die gesam Virusforsch., 1971, *34*, 202.
17. Ley, Burger, McGuire, and Henson. Jour. Inf. Dis., 1970, *12*, 10.
18. Lührs. Zeitschr. f. Tierheilk., 1919, *31*, 369.
19. McGuire, Crawford, and Henson. Am. Jour. Path., 1971, *62*, 283.
20. McGuire, Van Hoosier, and Henson. Jour. Immunol., 1971, *107*, 1738.
21. Nakajima, Tanaka, and Ushimi. Arch. f. die gesam Virusforsch., 1970, *30*, 273.
22. Schalk and Roderick. N. Dak. Agr. Exp. Sta. Bull. 168, 1923.
23. Scott. Univ. Wyo. Bull. 121, 1919.
24. Scott. Jour. Am. Vet. Med. Assoc., 1920, *56*, 448.
25. Sentsui and Kono. Inf. and Immun., 1976, *14*, 325.
26. Stein. Infectious anemia. USDA, Farmers Bull. 2088, 1955.
27. Stein, Lucker, Osteen, and Gouchenour. Jour. Am. Vet. Med. Assoc., 1939, *95*, 536.
28. Stein and Mott. Vet. Med., 1946, *41*, 274.
29. Stein and Mott. Proc. U.S. Livestock Sanit. Assoc., 1947, *51*, 37.
30. Stein, Mott, and Gates. Jour. Am. Vet. Med. Assoc., 1955, *126*, 277.
31. Stein, Osteen, Mott, and Shahan. Am. Jour. Vet. Res., 1944, *5*, 291.
32. Tajima, Nakajima, and Ito. Arch. f. die gesam Virusforsch, 1970, *30*, 273.
33. Tanaka and Kirasawa. Natl. Inst. An. Health Q., 1962, *2*, 108.
34. Toma, Lauda, Iscaki, and Goret. *In* Proc. 4th Internatl. Conf. Equine Inf. Dis., ed. John T. Bryans and Heinz Gerber. Veterinary Publications, Inc., Princeton, N.J., 1978, p. 389.
35. Udall and Fitch. Cornell Vet., 1915, *5*, 69.
36. Ushimi, Nakajimi, and Tanaka. Natl. Inst. An. Health Q., 1970, *10*, 90.
37. Ushimi, Suguira, and Nakajima. *In* Proc. 4th Internatl. Conf. Equine Inf. Dis., ed. John T. Bryans and Heinz Gerber. Veterinary Publications, Inc., Princeton, N.J., 1978, p. 381.

THE SUBFAMILY SPUMAVIRINAE

The feline and bovine syncytium-forming viruses could be placed in this subfamily, particularly the feline syncytium-forming virus that contains reverse transcriptase. At present, it seems more reasonable to place them in the genus *Pneumovirus,* where the respiratory syncytial disease virus of man has been placed by the International Committee on Taxonomy of Viruses.

53 The Bunyaviridae

This family has one genus, *Bunyavirus,* and many other viruses forming two or more unnamed genera. Members of this family formerly were included under the general heading of arboviruses.

Viruses in this family contain single-stranded RNA in 3 or 4 linear segments. The molecular weight of the segments is 3.4 to 4.1, 2.1, and 0.5 × 10^6 daltons, and the total genome is 6 × 10^6 daltons. The particles are spherical, enveloped, and approximately 100 nm in diameter. Virions consist of a unit-membrane envelope with surface projections that may be randomly placed or clustered in arrays with icosahedral symmetry, containing helically wound symmetric ribonucleocapsids with circular configuration. The particles are formed by budding from intracytoplasmic (primarily Golgi) members (Figure 53.1). The buoyant density in potassium tartrate is 1.20 gm per cm^3. The particles are sensitive to ether, acid, and heat. The viruses hemagglutinate red blood cells.

Figure 53.1. A clearly defined budding viral particle. Chagres, a member of the phlebotomus fever group. × 122,500. (From F. A. Murphy, A. K. Harrison, and S. G. Whitfield, *Intervirology,* 1973, *1,* 309.)

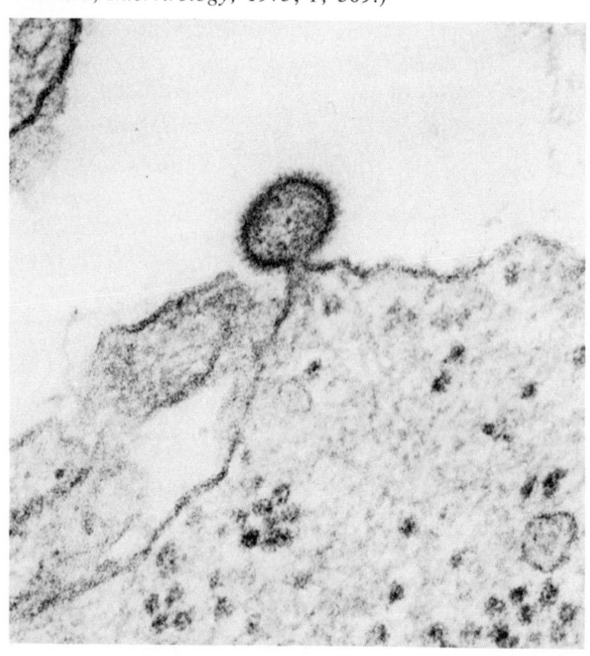

There are two important diseases of domestic animals—Nairobi disease of sheep and Rift Valley fever—that presently are limited to tropical climates. These virus diseases presently are included in the unnamed genera and will be the only two virus diseases described in this chapter.

Rift Valley Fever

SYNONYM: Infectious enzootic hepatitis of sheep and cattle

This disease takes its name from a geographic area in Kenya, Africa, where the disease was first described.

It occurs primarily in sheep and cattle. Outbreaks in goats have been described. It is highly contagious to man, and human cases invariably occur where the disease exists in animals.

So far as is known, this disease occurs only in Africa and the Middle East, except for human laboratory infections which have appeared in Europe, the United States, and Japan. It was first described by Daubney, Hudson, and Garnham (4) in 1931 in Kenya, but there is much evidence that the disease had occurred for many years in parts of equatorial Africa. In 1951 it suddenly appeared in South Africa (1). In 1978, this disease caused considerable mortality in humans and animals in Egypt. Outbreaks occur during warm, humid periods because mosquitoes are the principal transmitting agents.

Character of the Disease. The disease is most acute and causes the heaviest losses in sheep. Very young lambs often die in large numbers. The mortality rate in ewes is less but still serious. In the original outbreak described by Daubney, 3,500 lambs and 1,200 ewes died in a 2-week period.

In lambs, the disease is characterized by a high fever, prostration, and a rapid course which leads to death generally within 24 hours.

In ewes, abortions frequently are seen before lamb losses occur. Ewes are observed to be sick only a few hours before they die, or they are simply found dead in the corrals. Some vomit. Many have thick purulent nasal discharges. Some pass stools that consist of almost pure blood. Some show no signs other than abortion.

In cattle, the disease resembles that in sheep in every way, but the losses are not so high.

The incubation period of Rift Valley fever is very short. It may be no more than 24 hours in some cases and generally is not longer than 3 days.

In young lambs the course of the disease is rarely longer than 24 hours. In older animals it may be longer. After a short period of obvious illness pregnant ewes appear well, but often abort a few days later. In young lambs the mortality often is from 95 to 100 percent. In ewes it probably does not exceed 20 percent. In cattle of all ages the losses from death average about 10 percent, but many pregnant cows abort.

The most characteristic lesion in ruminants is focal necrosis of the liver. In many lambs the necrosis is so complete that sections are hardly recognizable. Findlay (5) and others have described inclusion bodies of an intensely acidophilic character in the nuclei of the liver cells. Other lesions consist principally of hemorrhages—in the lymph nodes, subendocardial and subepicardial, and in the gastric and intestinal mucosa. Blood examinations show severe leukopenia. In lambs especially it is sometimes difficult to find any mature leukocytes in blood films. Aborted fetuses show general hemorrhages and edema.

The Disease in Experimental Animals. The disease is readily produced in cattle and sheep by inoculation. White mice of the Swiss type are very easily infected. They die within 2 or 3 days after inoculation by any parenteral route. Infections can be produced by inoculation in monkeys, ferrets, hamsters, white rats, and possibly rabbits. Horses, swine, guinea pigs, and domestic and wild birds are not susceptible.

Properties of the Virus. This ungrouped member of the family is about 100 nm (Figure 53.2) (7). Infective virus persists for 3 months at room temperature and almost 3 years in serum kept at −4 C. It withstands lyophilization, but inactivation occurs in a 1 : 1,000 dilution of formalin and by pasteurization.

The virus has a hemagglutinin for red blood cells for day-old chicks at pH 6.5 and 25 C. The observation of interference between yellow fever and Rift Valley fever viruses was the first reported for serologically unrelated viruses.

Cultivation. The virus grows in cell cultures of the chick, rat, mouse, human, and lamb. Binn *et al.* (2) described its propagation and plaque formation in primary cell cultures of lamb kidney and of hamster kidney.

It produces a thickening of the chorioallantoic membrane of embryonated hens' eggs. Inoculation by the yolk-sac route is also successful.

Immunity. Animals and men that recover from a natural infection are solidly resistant thereafter. Sabin and Blumberg (8) have shown that neutralizing antibodies appear in the blood of man within a few days after recovery from infection and that these persisted, in one case, for as long as 12 years.

Smithburn (9) passed strains of Rift Valley fever virus serially in white mice by intracerebral injection and found that as they acquired neurotropic properties, they lost viscerotropism. He used these strains for immunizing ewes, finding that when injected subcutaneously, virus did not appear in the blood, and the animals suffered no damage from them. By this means the newborn lambs were protected during the period of greatest susceptibility.

Both neurotropic and field strains of Rift Valley fever virus have been adapted to embryonated eggs by Kaschula (6). The neurotropic strains are used successfully for field immunization. The immunity conferred is not as lasting or as solid as that conferred by actual infection.

Vaccines cannot be used on very young lambs or on pregnant ewes or cows. Safe protection of such animals can be conferred only by the use of convalescent serum.

Weiss (11) suggested that the 102nd intracerebral

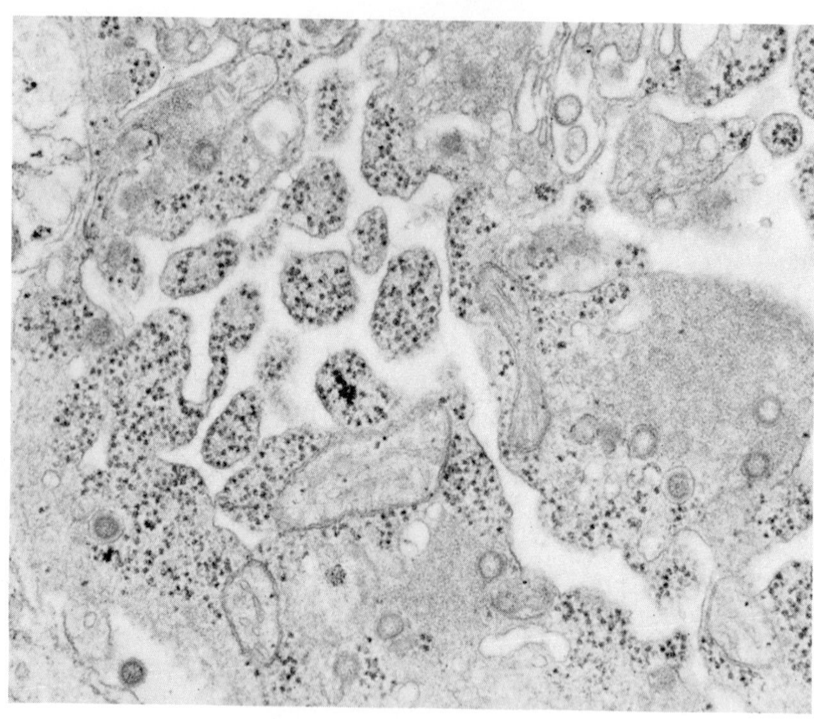

Figure 53.2. Rift Valley virus particles. × 49,600. (From F. A. Murphy, A. K. Harrison, and S. G. Whitfield, *Intervirology,* 1973, *1,* 307.)

mouse passage level virus is a safe vaccine for 1-day-old lambs. Formalin-inactivated virus vaccines are also available for animals (2).

Transmission. Daubney and Hudson, in their original investigations, found that Rift Valley fever could be easily transmitted by the inoculation of blood or tissue extracts. All investigators who have worked with this disease in the field or laboratory discovered that all persons who had intimate contact with infected animals developed the disease within 5 days after exposure. On the other hand, infected and susceptible sheep might be kept together and, in the absence of certain transmitting agents, the disease would not be transmitted. It was even shown that infected ewes did not infect their suckling lambs, and that infected lambs did not infect their mothers. In a recent communication (12) it was suggested that direct contact and aerosols may also play a role in animal infection under certain conditions (3).

Smithburn, Haddow, and Gillett (10) in 1948 succeeded in isolating the virus from 6 different lots of mosquitoes in the Semliki Forest in an uninhabited part of Uganda. These mosquitoes included several species of the genus *Eretmapodites,* and it was later shown that some of these could transmit the disease. The present evidence points strongly to these and perhaps other species of mosquitoes as the principal transmitting agents. Because there were no cattle or sheep in the Semliki Forest, the presence of infected mosquitoes strongly suggests the existence of a reservoir of virus in wild animals.

Diagnosis. The clinical behavior of the disease in sheep and cattle is at least highly suggestive. The presence of extensive liver necrosis should confirm the suspicion. Inoculation of white mice results in prompt fatal infections. Final confirmation must come from serological tests, using known antisera. These may be neutralization tests, using mice for the test species, or the complement-fixation, gel-diffusion, or hemagglutination-inhibition tests may be employed.

Control. The original outbreak described by Daubney *et al.* was controlled promptly when the flocks were driven into ranges at a higher altitude. Presumably this put the animals above the mosquito range. Immunization by means of the neurotropic vaccines is well tolerated by adult animals, and this offers a way to protect flocks and herds that must remain in regions inhabited by the vectors.

The Disease in Man. It has already been pointed out that veterinarians, laboratory workers, and herd and flock attendants almost invariably become infected when the disease appears. Butchers and housewives have also suffered from handling fresh meat that came from infected animals. The infections in these cases are obviously the result of direct contact with infected tissues. It is not clear whether human infections occur as a result of mosquito transmission.

The disease may be fatal. The attacks occur within a few days after exposure. The symptoms resemble those of influenza or dengue. The onset is sudden, with malaise, headache, and a feeling of chilliness. Fever develops quickly, and joint pains, often rather extreme, soon appear. Nausea and vomiting sometimes occur, and often there is some abdominal distress. The disease lasts only a few days, and recovery is complete. A formalin-inactivated virus vaccine is available for immunization of humans.

REFERENCES

1. Alexander. Jour. So. African Vet. Med. Assoc., 1951, *22,* 105.
2. Binn, Randall, Harrison, Gibbs, and Aulisis. Am. Jour. Hyg., 1963, *77,* 160.
3. Callis. Personal Communication, 1979.
4. Daubney, Hudson, and Garnham. Jour. Path. and Bact., 1931, *34,* 545.
5. Findlay. Brit. Jour. Exp. Path., 1933, *14,* 207.
6. Kaschula. Personal communication, 1957.
7. Murphy, Harrison, and Whitfield. Intervirol., 1973, *1,* 297.
8. Sabin and Blumberg. Proc. Soc. Exp. Biol. and Med., 1947, *64,* 385.
9. Smithburn. Brit. Jour. Exp. Path., 1949, *30,* 1.
10. Smithburn, Haddow, and Gillett. Brit. Jour. Exp. Path., 1949, *29,* 107.
11. Weiss. Onderstepoort Jour. Vet. Res., 1962, *29,* 3.
12. Yedloutschnig and Walker. Personal communication, 1979.

Nairobi Disease of Sheep

This arbovirus disease occurs in Kenya, Africa. It affects sheep which each year are brought down from the northern districts into Nairobi to be offered for sale. It has been described by Montgomery (2). It may cause disease in goats and, on occasion, mortality up to 10 percent. The disease is characterized by acute hemorrhagic gastroenteritis and respiratory signs in sheep. The mortality varies from 30 to 70 percent. Abortions may occur. The blood and tissues are always infective during the temperature reaction. The urine is said to be infective at this stage, but the feces ordinarily contain no virus.

The disease is transmitted by the adult forms of a tick, *Rhipicephalus appendiculatus,* which have fed as nymphs on infected sheep. Other species of *Rhipicephalus* and *Amblyomma* ticks may also act as vectors. Virus can be retained in the salivary glands of unfed nymphs and larvae for 1 year and may pass from one stage to another in the life cycle. Small rodents may act as a reservoir of the infection.

The virus was propagated in tissue-cultured cells of goat testes, goat kidney, and hamster kidney (1). A cytopathic effect of a consistent and uniform nature occurred only with hamster kidney cells. Intracerebral inoculation of suckling and adult mice with infective virus produces central nervous signs and death within 10 days. Either mice or baby hamster kidney cells (BHK-21 cell line) support replication of virus and provide systems for research and diagnosis.

Recovered animals possess a lasting immunity. Artificial immunization has been attempted only on a small scale. Control depends on eradication of the transmitting agent. *R. appendiculatus* also transmits East Coast fever of cattle; hence dipping of both sheep and cattle should be done, with benefit to both species.

REFERENCES

1. Howarth and Terptra. Jour. Comp. Path., 1965, *75,* 347.
2. Montgomery. Jour. Comp. Path. and Therap., 1917, *30,* 28.

54 The Arenaviridae

Member viruses are in a single genus, *Arenavirus*, and contain single-stranded RNA in linear segments. The molecular weight of four large RNA segments is 2.1, 1.7, 1.1, and 0.7 $\times$ 10^6 daltons; one to three small RNA segments are about 0.03 $\times$ 10^6 daltons. Virions are spherical or pleomorphic and 50 to 300 nm in diameter. Virions consist of unit-membrane envelope with surface projections containing varying numbers of ribosome particles (20 to 25 nm) either free in interior or, less commonly, connected by a linear structure. Virions are formed by budding from plasma membrane (Figure 54.1) Buoyant density in cesium chloride is 1.19 to 1.20 g per cm^3. Infectivity is sensitive to ether, acid, and heat. Most viruses have a limited rodent host range in nature in which maintenance is via persistent infection with viruria. There are a few important diseases of humans

Figure 54.1. Thin section of Lassa fever virus, an arenavirus. The virus is budding from plasma membrane and accumulating in extracellular spaces. $\times$ 55,500. (Courtesy F. A. Murphy, S. G. Whitfield, P. A. Webb, and K. M. Johnson, Center for Disease Control.)

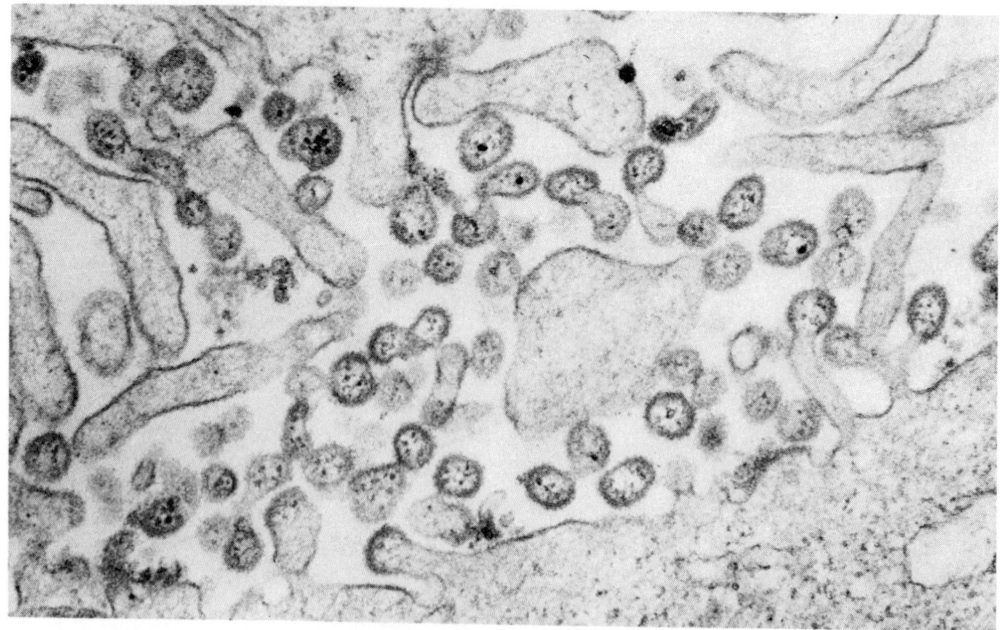

caused by arenaviruses, such as Lassa fever, but there is no evidence that any of these viruses causes disease in domestic animals.

Lymphocytic Choriomeningitis (LCM)

This disease of mice has great historical importance, as it was the first virus disease in which immunological tolerance was observed. Traub (4) showed that newborn mice or mice infected *in utero* with LCM developed such a state. Such tolerant mice continued to harbor the virus in high titers in the blood and organs, but no antibody was produced. In mouse colonies with this infection, birth and growth rates are lower and mortality is higher (3). Mice infected as newborns show no signs of illness, but develop a runting condition later in life (2). This chronic infection apparently leads to the production of an autoimmune disease (3). Depending on the disease form that the infection assumes in mice, the pathologic picture is one of a meningoplexal and perivascular infiltration by lymphoid cells, plasmacytes, macrophages, and other cells, with occasional areas of focal gliosis. There is often serous pleurisy and peritonitis, hepatitis, and also necrosis, hemorrhage, and serofibrinous exudate in lymphatic organs. Lymphoid cell infiltrations are present in the kidney, salivary gland, and pancreas. The renal lesions in this disease are comparable to those seen in Aleutian disease in mink, lupus glomerulitis in man, and a spontaneous glomerulonephritis found in sheep in the United States and England (1). There is a proliferation of the mesangial and endothelial cells with occasional thickening of the basement membrane.

REFERENCES

1. Abinanti. Ann. Rev. Microbiol., 1967, *21*, 467.
2. Hotchin. Cold Springs Harbor Sympos. Quant. Biol., 1962, *27*, 479.
3. Seamer. Arch. f. die gesam. Virusforsch., 1965, *15*, 169.
4. Traub. Science, 1935, *81*, 298.

55 The Coronaviridae

The coronaviruses contain single-stranded RNA. The enveloped particles vary in size from 70 to 120 nm in diameter. The nucleocapsid is probably helical and loosely wound, either 7 or 9 nm in diameter. The surface has characteristic pedunculated projections 20 nm in length (Figure 55.1). The buoyant density in cesium chloride is 1.15 to 1.16 g per cm^3. The particles are ether- and chloroform-sensitive with marked variation in sensitivity to acid conditions.

Replication occurs in the cytoplasm, and the virus is unaffected by DNA inhibitors. Maturation occurs by budding from membranes of the endoplasmic reticulum and cytoplasmic vesicles (Figure 55.2). The viruses in the genus are antigenically heterogenous, and there is some relationship between certain human and murine strains.

The type species for the single genus in this family is *Coronavirus* a-1 (avian infectious bronchitis virus).

Figure 55.1. Avian infectious bronchitis virus in negative stain preparation showing surface projections. × 298,900. (Courtesy J. C. Hierholzer, E. L. Palmer, S. G. Whitfield, H. S. Kaye, and W. R. Dowdle, Center for Disease Control.)

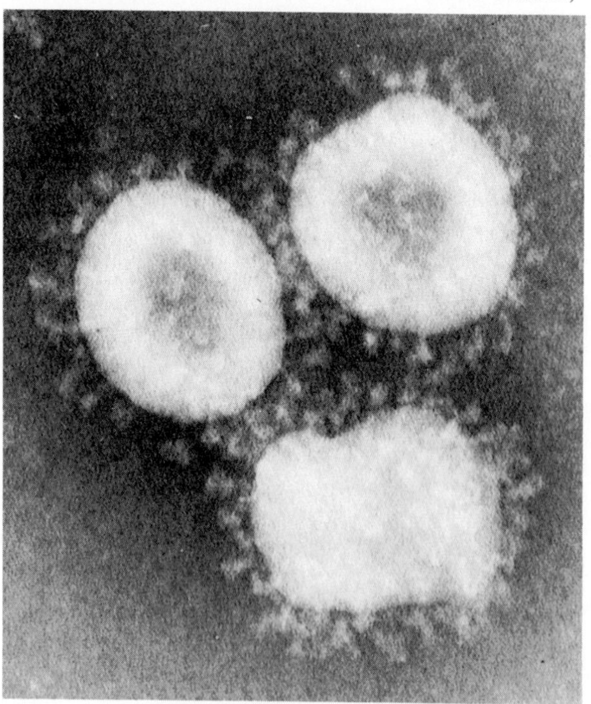

Figure 55.2. Maturation by budding of avian bronchitis virus into cytoplasmic vesicles of an embryonated hen's egg cell. (Courtesy B. Cowen.)

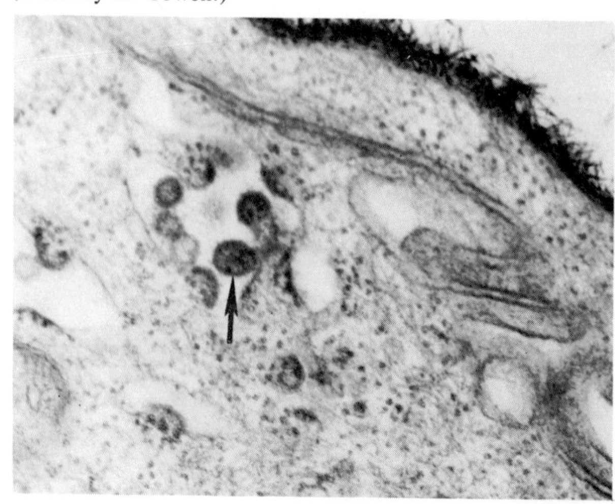

Other members of the group are mouse hepatitis virus, human respiratory virus, transmissible gastroenteritis virus of pigs, canine coronavirus, bovine coronavirus, hemagglutinating virus of pigs, feline infectious peritonitis, turkey bluecomb disease virus, and possibly an equine coronavirus as listed in Table 55.1. Four viruses in the family that form a distinctive antigenic cluster are transmissible gastroenteritis of pigs, feline infectious peritonitis, canine coronavirus, and human coronavirus strain 229 E. Calf diarrhea coronavirus, hemagglutinating encephalomyelitis virus of swine, mouse hepatitis virus type 3, and human coronavirus strain OC43 form another related antigenic group.

Avian Infectious Bronchitis

SYNONYMS: Chick bronchitis, gasping disease, *Coronavirus* a-1

This disease was first described by Schalk and Hawn (27) in 1931. These authors did not determine its cause. In 1933 Bushnell and Brandly (4) carried on some filtration studies and decided that a filterable agent was its cause. More extensive studies were reported by Beach and Schalm (2) in 1936 which showed that the causative agent was a virus that differed in several respects from that of infectious laryngotracheitis. This disease has been reported from North America, where it frequently causes serious losses, and also from many European countries and Japan.

Character of the Disease. This disease occurs in chicks from 2 days to 3 or 4 weeks of age. In some sections of the country it has become very important as a disease of partly grown and laying pullets and hens. The disease occurs often in hatcheries selling "started" chicks and from them is spread to flocks through the sale of the infected chicks. It causes large losses in establishments engaged in raising birds for the broiler trade, since

Table 55.1. Diseases in domestic animals caused by viruses in the Coronaviridae family, genus *Coronavirus*

Common name of virus	Natural hosts	Type of disease produced
Infectious bronchitis, multiple serotypes	Chickens	Acute, highly contagious respiratory disease with high mortality in young chicks. Kidney and oviduct damage may occur. Marked reduction in egg production and quality. Worldwide distribution.
Transmissible gastroenteritis, single serotype	Pigs	Acute, highly contagious enteric disease with vomiting, diarrhea, dehydration and high mortality rate in piglets under 2 weeks of age. Adult pigs also become infected and develop a milder or inapparent disease. Worldwide.
Hemagglutinating encephalomyelitis, single serotype	Pigs	Encephalomyelitis in piglets, also vomiting and wasting disease. High morbidity and mortality in piglets less than 2 weeks of age. Probably worldwide.
Neonatal calf diarrhea coronavirus, single serotype	Cattle	Diarrhea in neonatal calves with some mortality. Common in USA.
Canine coronavirus, one serotype	Dogs	Diarrheal disease in puppies with some mortality. Common in USA.
Transmissible gastroenteritis (bluecomb disease), one serotype	Turkeys	Enteritis in flocks, may have high mortality. Associated with cases of bluecomb disease.
Gastroenteritis	Horses	Diarrheal disease with mortality in neonatal foals. Single reference only of 40 cases in an endemic area.
Feline infectious peritonitis, one serotype described	Cats, domestic and wild	Cats with signs of illness usually terminate in death characterized by fever, anorexia, depression, and ascites. Probably worldwide, certainly widespread in USA and Europe.

in these plants large numbers of young birds are raised in very crowded conditions. Affected laying birds show a sharp decline in egg production, which may persist for several weeks. There is a marked loss of shell firmness and a deterioration in the internal quality of the egg. Virus may be present in the eggs from some hens during this period.

The disease is characterized by listlessness, depression, gasping, and râles, and by such rapid spread that nearly all exposed birds develop the disease at almost the same time. The outbreak runs a rapid course, and the mortality rate is from 25 to 90 percent in young chicks. The effect on birds from the age of 6 weeks up to shortly before the first egg is laid is not likely to be more than slight retardation in their development. In the laying flock the damage is due to depression of egg yield rather than to death losses. Exudate that may be mucoid or caseous is regularly found in the bronchi and sometimes in the nasal passages. In chicks that die, plugs of fibrinopurulent exudate often are found in the lower part of the trachea or in the larger bronchi. No inclusion bodies are found. Chicks that are inoculated into the trachea develop the disease after an incubation period of 24 to 48 hours as a rule, occasionally as long as 4 days, and death or recovery occurs in from 6 to 18 days.

From an outbreak of nephritis in previously vaccinated broilers an isolation of infectious bronchitis virus (IBV) was made which proved to be serologically distinct from other strains of IBV (6). Histopathological studies of the disease by the Cumming T strain showed that the virus had a strong affinity for the respiratory tract and kidney (24). The respiratory lesions were characterized by the desquamation of the ciliated end and glandular epithelium of the trachea followed by a rapid proliferation of residual basal cells with formation of a stratified, undifferentiated epithelial covering. Lymphocytic infiltration occurs in small areas of the trachial submucosa. Regeneration usually is complete on or about the 12th day. Lesions in the lungs usually are not severe. The air sacs are only slightly edematous. The lesions in the kidney originate in the tubules; initially there is a necrosis, followed by the formation of cystic tubules that contain epithelial debris and polymorphonuclear leukocytes in both cortex and medulla. Lymphocytes and plasma cells were present in the interstitium. Regeneration of tubular epithelial cells then occurred along with clearance of debris from lumina of the tubules. In the cortex the glomeruli and tubules were numerous but compressed at the 2nd week, but 3 weeks later the kidneys were normal.

Mixed infections sometimes occur when chicks harbor *Mycoplasma gallisepticum* and become infected with IBV. More severe disease ensues (5).

Properties of the Virus. Particles in cytoplasm are 200 nm in diameter and others in infected egg fluid 70 to 100 nm (11). Heat stability at 56 C varies with the strain, but none consistently survives more than 30 minutes at that temperature. A 1:10,000 dilution of $KMnO_4$ and 1 percent formalin inactivates the virus. It is ether-labile and labile to pH 3.

Low-passaged egg virus treated with trypsin will hemagglutinate chicken red blood cells at pH 7.2 in 45 to 60 minutes at room temperature. Egg-adapted strains were less active. No elution occurred (7).

By using the neutralization test in hens' eggs Hofstad (18) showed the presence of two antigenic types, Connecticut and Massachusetts, but with some cross-reaction. Iowa strains 97 and 609 represent additional serotypes. There are also additional field isolates that cannot be identified with existing recognized serotypes. The field strain most commonly isolated is the Massachusetts serotype.

Until there is agreement on the most suitable indicator system, on a standardized test procedure, and on the use of reference viruses and antiserum by various institutions, a satisfactory IBV classification scheme is not possible. As an example, 12 strains were evaluated in 2 different assay procedures, by chicken embryo assay eight serologic groups were identified. whereas there were four by plaque assay. Cross protection tests also are needed to determine the importance of IBV serotypes or variants on vaccine efficacy (8). By means of agar diffusion analysis antigen-antibody complexes of virus and antisera may be detected. None of the precipitating antigens can be specifically ascribed to IBV (12).

IBV has a density of 1.17 to 1.18 g/cm^3. In studies of various strains on polyacrylamide gels 7 polypeptides were observed with variations in the proportions of these polypeptides in particles of different densities and those from the different strains (22).

Suckling mice are susceptible by intracerebral inoculation to certain strains of IBV.

Cultivation. In 1937 Beaudette and Hudson (3) found that bronchitis virus can be propagated in chicken embryos. Characteristic dwarfing (15) and curling (17) of the embryo have been described.

Virus titration may be performed in chicken embryo-kidney cultures with chicken egg adapted strains by using cytopathic effects as revealed by the formation of

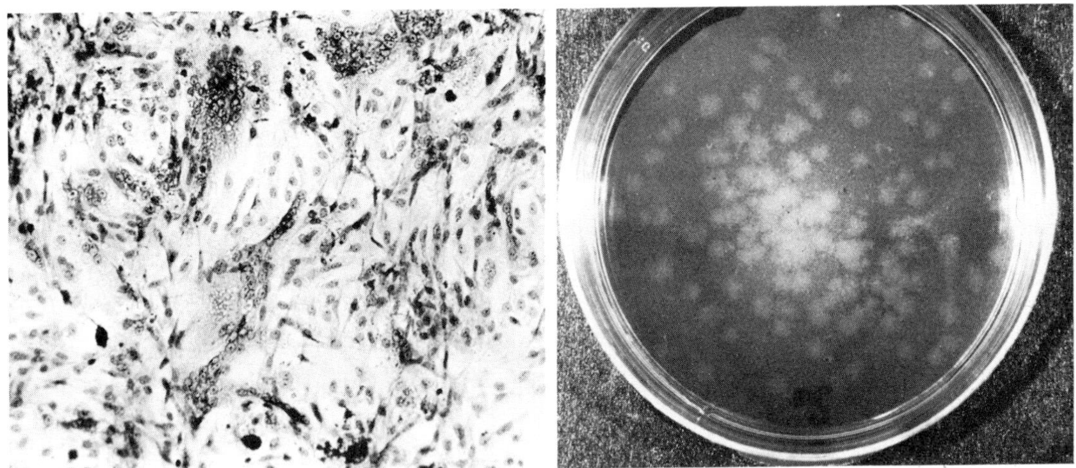

Figure 55.3 (*left*). Syncytia with necrosis induced by viral replication of avian bronchitis virus in chicken kidney cell culture. Giemsa stain. × 60. (Courtesy B. Cowen.)

Figure 55.4 (*right*). Necrosis of syncytia in Figure 55.3 manifested as plaques by the agar overlay method. (Courtesy B. Cowen.)

large syncytia followed by necrosis (Figure 55.3) and by the plaque technique (Figure 55.4) (12).

IBV produces marked pathological changes in tracheal organ cultures (16).

Immunity. Chickens that recover from natural infection are solidly immune for at least 6 to 8 months. Challenge of immunity is done by aerosol exposure, by intranasal inoculation, or by natural exposure. With adequate controls the natural exposure to virus is preferred. Challenge is evaluated by production of tracheal rales and by attempted isolation of virus from tracheal swabs.

Immunoglobulins induced by primary infection or by vaccination are IgG effective in the blood and presumably secretory IgA in the respiratory tract. The level of humoral neutralizing antibody does not necessarily correlate with immunity based on chicken protection tests. Maternal immunity is effective in providing passive protection for about 2 weeks after the chick is hatched (13). According to Winterfield, Fadly, and Hoerr (29), 1-day-old chicks possessing maternally derived immunity to Massachussetts-type IBV can be vaccinated against respiratory disease by the eye-drop route with the attenuated Holland strain of the Massachusetts type IBV. Inactivated virus vaccines have been unsuccessful.

For some years in the northeastern part of the United States a method of immunization recommended by Van Roekel *et al.* (28) was used with excellent success. This involved deliberately inoculating a small portion of flocks with virulent field virus when the birds were from 7 to 15 weeks of age. At this stage of their development birds are not seriously damaged by the disease. The mortality of younger birds and the disruption of production in laying flocks are not experienced in birds of this age. The method served very well, but had the disadvantage that active virus perpetuated the disease in the flock and in the community. This procedure has now been given up in favor of modified virus vaccines (10, 20). These vaccines are not avirulent, and trouble sometimes results from their use, but generally they are safer and apparently just as efficient as the virulent field virus. Vaccines are generally administered to flocks en masse by aerosol or sprays (9) or dusts (23), or they are given in the drinking water (21). Satisfactory immunity is not always attained by the use of these products (25). Successful vaccination has been further complicated by demonstration of multiple antigenic serotypes (14).

Transmission. Infections can readily be induced by inoculating minute amounts of virus into the respiratory apparatus. Natural infections, it seems certain, are contracted through inhalation of infective droplets. Levine and Hofstad (19) demonstrated experimentally that the infection can be airborne for a distance of at least 5 feet. Virus carriers have been demonstrated for periods longer than 20 weeks (1). Outbreaks have been traced to hatcheries which deal in "started chicks." Infection established in these chicks is carried to the farm of the purchaser. Egg-borne transmission is another possibility.

Diagnosis. In the absence of any nervous signs, coughing and gasping suggest infectious bronchitis in young chicks. Because nervous signs are not always apparent in Newcastle disease in chicks, a differential diagnosis is necessary. In older birds infectious bronchitis must be differentiated from laryngotracheitis, Newcastle disease, infectious coryza, and *Mycoplasma* infections.

Respiratory tissues are most useful for viral isolation. It is not usually possible to isolate virus after 10 to 14 days. Lung and trachea placed in 50 percent glycerol may be shipped to the laboratory without refrigeration. Inoculation of an infective-tissue suspension into the allantoic sac of a 9-to-11-day-old embryo causes stunting of the embryo. In initial passages stunting may not be prominent, but on continued passage all embryos will be stunted and some embryos die after 5 to 6 days of incubation.

IBV also can be identified in the hen's egg because it interferes with the production of hemagglutinin to the B-1 isolant of Newcastle disease virus (26). Many strains produce cytopathic effect and plaques in cell culture, providing still another means of diagnosis. A microneutralization using the cytopathic effect has been devised to test for neutralizing antibodies in serum and other body fluids as well as a plaque reduction test (30). The plaque reduction proved to be more sensitive. Its antigenic shifts do limit the usefulness of the neutralization test in diagnosis.

The fluorescent-antibody test has been used in detecting IBV in tracheal smears of acutely affected chickens with reasonable success.

Control. The disease is best controlled by disposing of entire flocks, cleaning and disinfecting the premises, and beginning over with clean stock. If infection occurs and depopulation is not possible, then vaccination can be used. Wherein possible, the prevalent serotype in a flock should be ascertained and the appropriate vaccine product selected for use.

The Disease in Man. The virus of avian infectious bronchitis is not infective for man or other mammals.

REFERENCES

1. Alexander and Gough. Res. Vet. Sci., 1977, *23*, 344
2. Beach and Schalm. Poultry Sci., 1936, *15*, 199.
3. Beaudette and Hudson. Jour. Am. Vet. Assoc., 1937, *90*, 51.
4. Bushnell and Brandly. Poultry Sci., 1933, *12*, 55.
5. Chu and Uppal. Dev. Biol. Stand., 1975, *28*, 101.
6. Chubb, Wells, and Cumming. Austral. Vet. Jour., 1976, *52*, 378.
7. Corbo and Cunningham. Am. Jour. Vet. Res., 1959, *20*, 876.
8. Cowen and Hitchner. Avian Dis., 1975, *19*, 583.
9. Crawley. Proc. Am. Vet. Med. Assoc., 1953, p. 342.
10. Crawley, Proc. Am. Vet. Med. Assoc., 1955, p. 343.
11. Cunningham. Am. Jour. Vet. Res., 1957, *18*, 648.
12. Cunningham. Am. Jour. Vet. Res., 1960, *21*, 498.
13. Cunningham, Dev. Biol. Stand., 1975, *28*, 546.
14. Cunningham, Dev. Biol. Stand., 1976, *33*, 311.
15. Delaplane. Proc. 19th Ann. Northeastern Pullorum Conf., 1947.
16. Dutta. Avian Dis., 1975, *19*, 429.
17. Fabricant. Cornell Vet., 1949, *39*, 414.
18. Hofstad. Am. Jour. Vet. Res., 1958, *19*, 740.
19. Levine and Hofstad. Cornell Vet., 1947, *37*, 204.
20. Luginbuhl and Jungherr. Poultry Sci., 1952, *31*, 924.
21. Luginbuhl, Jungherr, and Chomiak. Poultry Sci., 1955, *34*, 1399.
22. MacNaughton and Madge, Arch. Virol., 1977, *55*, 47.
23. Markham, Hammar, Gingher, and Cox. Poultry Sci., 1955, *34*, 442.
24. Purcell, Tham, and Surman. Austral. Vet. Jour., 1976, *52*, 85.
25. Raggi and Bankowski. Am. Jour. Vet. Res., 1956, *17*, 523.
26. Raggi and Pignattelli. Avian Dis., 1957, *19*, 334.
27. Schalk and Hawn. Jour. Am. Vet. Med. Assoc., 1931, *78*, 413.
28. Van Roekel, Bullis, Clarke, Olesiuk, and Sperling. Mass. Agr. Exp., Bull. 460, 1950.
29. Winterfield, Fadly, and Hoerr. Avian Dis., 1976, *20*, 369.
30. Wooley and Brown. Jour. Clin. Microbiol., 1977, *5*, 361.

Transmissible Gastroenteritis of Pigs

SYNONYM: Gastroenteritis in young pigs; abbreviation, TGE

This is a readily transmissible gastroenteritis of swine. The disease is highly fatal to pigs less than 10 days old. Older animals usually recover. In adult swine the disease is inapparent or mild. No animals other than swine are known to show signs of illness from this virus.

The disease was first reported in Indiana by Doyle and Hutchings (9) in 1946, although it is clear that it had existed much earlier. It occurs throughout the swine belt of the United States (north central states) and sporadically in other areas where swine are kept. TGE was described in England by Goodwin and Jennings (13) in 1959. It has since been reported in Canada, Taiwan, and many European countries and is now considered to be worldwide in distribution.

Character of the Disease: The disease generally spreads rapidly when it first enters a herd, involving animals of all ages. The older breeding animals generally show relatively mild signs varying from none at all to inappetence, vomiting, profuse scouring, severe weight loss, and even death in rare instances. They shed virus in various excretions, including milk of sows, during acute stages of illness. The older animals generally recover within a week, although the decrease in weight in feeder pigs may be a serious loss to the owner. Death losses in pigs under 2 weeks of age reach close to 100 percent. These suffer severe diarrhea, the bowel discharge being watery and whitish or whitish green in color. The animals suffer from severe thirst and frequently collect around the watering troughs, from which they drink excessively. Some die within 2 days, but most of the deaths are on the 4th or 5th day. Most piglets over 3 weeks of age survive, but often remain stunted afterward for a long period of time.

The period of incubation is relatively short—within 12 to 18 hours in many cases. The clinically sick animals in most instances are either well on the road to recovery or are dead within 1 week from the onset of signs. Some, especially very young pigs, may die within 2 or 3 days, and some survivors may show the effect of the disease for weeks afterward.

Besides gastroenteritis, there are few lesions in this disease. Emaciation and dehydration occur in animals that have lived long enough. Sometimes there are evidences of nephritis and hepatic degeneration. The stomach and intestines may exhibit severe inflammation. These lesions are nearly always found in older animals that die from the disease. In the young pigs, however, there may be little evidence of inflammation, but the intestines are distended with liquid ingesta (18). The wall of the intestinal tract is thin and almost transparent as a result of villi atrophy. The absence of chyle in the mesenteric lymphatics is a constant feature.

The Disease in Experimental Animals. The pathogenesis of TGE in newborn pigs has been studied to a certain degree by Lee (20), Young *et al.* (38), and Hooper and Haelterman (17). Ingestion and airborne infection constitute the means by which TGE virus enters the body to initiate the infection. The gastrointestinal route probably is the most important one, but virus also replicates to high titers in the nasal mucosa and lungs. When the virus reaches the highly susceptible epithelial cells of the small intestine, infection causes destruction of columnar epithelial cells with an accompanying marked shortening or contraction of the villi resulting in malabsorption. The shortened villi of the small intestine, particularly the jejunum, viewed through a dissecting microscope (×10) are quite characteristic of the disease (17). Other morphologic changes include vacuolation (13) and apical cytoplasm, and abundance of polyribosomes (35). There is a reduction in these cells of alkaline and acid phosphatase, adenosine triphophatase, succinic dehydrogenase, and nonspecific esterase (35). Lactose activity is not detected in the atrophic villi of the small intestine (8).

Dogs given TGE virus develop a serological response and virus is isolated from rectal swabs of dogs by inoculation of composite samples into susceptible piglets (24). There is evidence that a coronavirus antigenically related to TGE virus infects domestic cats (29).

Properties of the Virus. Various investigators (5, 7, 31) have studied certain biochemical and biophysical properties of the virus. This is an RNA virus which is ether-labile and trypsin-resistant. There are conflicting reports on its stability at pH 3, although the virus is entirely stable at pH 4 to 8. Amantadine-hydrochloride and puromycin reduce viral replication at least 98 percent as determined in a tissue-culture system (23). The virus is relatively heat-labile and also photosensitive. Phenol at 0.5 percent level destroys the virus held at 37 C for 30 minutes. The virus is quite stable when stored frozen, particularly in the tissue state. There is only a one-log drop in titer after storage at −18 C for 18 months. Virulent virus is stable to trypsin and proteolytic enzymes.

TGE virus has the morphological characteristics of a typical coronavirus, varying in size between 75 and 120 nm. Most particles are located in the cytoplasmic vacuoles with some budding from intracytoplasmic membranes. The polypeptides of purified preparations examined by polyacrylamide gel electrophoresis consist of 4 units as the major structural component of the surface projections (11). The phospholipid and glycolipid profiles of purified virus closely resemble those of the host cell (27). Using immunoelectrophoresis and counter-immunoelectrophoresis, 3 antigens were detected (1). Negatively stained viral preparations viewed by the electron microscope have spherical particles with clublike projections. Treating purified preparations with nonionic detergents removes virtually all of the viral lipid. Negatively stained preparations of this treated material revealed subunit spherical particles of between 50 and 60 nm, quite similar to those derived from members of oncovirnae (12).

A direct hemagglutination test has not been developed as the virus failed to cause hemagglutination of bovine porcine, guinea pig, or human erythrocytes (4, 31). A micro-indirect hemagglutination test was developed using viral-sensitized tanned sheep erythrocytes (32). This test is more sensitive than the serum neutralization test for detection of TGE antibody.

Present evidence suggests there is only 1 serotype of TGE virus. To substantiate this fact, Kemeny (19) compared 10 plaque purified isolates (8 American, 1 Japanese, and 1 English) and found they were indistinguishable by means of reciprocal plaque reduction neutralization tests.

Cultivation. Lee *et al.* (21) were able to grow the virus in porcine kidney cells, but did not note any cytopathogenic effects. More recently, Harada *et al.* (15) described strains that had the ability to destroy cells in pig kidney-cell cultures. Likewise, porcine thyroid and salivary gland cultures support viral replication. Virus also is propagated in canine kidney-cell cultures. The CPE produced by field strains usually is transient or slight in early passages; consequently, the piglet probably is a more sensitive experimental subject for detecting field virus. The plaque technique is more sensitive, achieving titers of 10^6 and 10^7 PFU (plaque forming unit) per ml of tissue-cultured virus, and reliable for the assay of TGE virus than the conventional fluid cell culture procedure (4, 23). Field strains of virus do not replicate as well as attenuated strains at 37 C and could not be passaged serially for more than 4 to 6 times at 33 C. Plaques produced in cell culture by attenuated strains were larger than those produced by field strains (16).

The interference phenomenon using bovine viral diarrhea-mucosal disease virus (22) or pseudorabies virus (26) has been used to demonstrate non-cytopathogenic strains of TGE virus in monolayer cultures.

Eto *et al.* (10) have propagated TGE through 20 transfers in the amniotic cavity of embryonated hens' eggs.

In piglets, the highest titers of virus are achieved in the jejunum and duodenum, usually 10^6 PID (pig infectious doses) per gram of infective material. Relatively high titers also are found in respiratory tissue and kidney early in the disease. The piglet is still commonly used for the cultivation of virus that is used for various purposes.

Immunity. There are some facts lacking about passive and active immunity to this disease. It is generally agreed that swine recovered from TGE usually are clinically protected when challenged with virulent test virus. However, immunity to reinfection or even to disease is probably not complete. It depends on the challenge dose, and swine infected as piglets have a lesser degree of immunity than older animals.

It has been observed that pigs born several weeks after the occurrence of an outbreak frequently escape the disease. When sows that have lost their litter of pigs from the disease are bred back immediately, the second litter escapes the disease. It appears that the immunity of such animals is passive, but the protection transmitted to piglets by immunized sows is not conferred by the absorption of globulin from the colostrum—rather it depends on the continuous supply of antibody in the milk from the dam (14). Unfortunately, sows vaccinated with attenuated virus vaccine do not afford the same degree of protection to their progeny regardless of the route of inoculation, including intramammary injection (3). This limited protection seemed to be the result of a low titer and the type of immunoglobulin class (IgG) in the sow's milk. Sows that recover from natural disease or inoculation with virulent virus have more neutralizing activity in the IgA fraction than the IgG fraction of the sow's milk. This suggests that the degree of invasiveness of a strain dictates the difference in the antibody class elicited in the colostrum (25). Inactivated TGE virus also fails to elicit an immunity in sows adequate to confer sufficient protection to their progeny through the colostrum and milk. Certainly, the mechanism of maternal immunity is unique and involves a new concept in the protection of neonates.

Some large swine farms that have suffered heavily from the disease follow the practice of feeding stored, frozen intestines from infected animals to their bred sows about a month before the farrowing date. The sows suffer from a mild diarrhea but recover, and their litters acquire enough immunity from their dams to protect them from the disease.

Neutralization tests can be done in piglets and in cell culture. The test in piglets was used for some time before cytopathic strains were described with limited and varying results by various investigators. The piglet test is seldom used now. In cell-culture systems, neutralization is determined in one of three ways: inhibition of CPE, plaque reduction, or stained monolayer test (36).

Transmission. The virus is present in all organs and fluids of the body as well as in the discharges. Because infection is readily produced by ingestion it seems certain that normal transmission is by contact, directly or indirectly, with the diarrheal discharges of the victims. Virus may persist in feces of recovered pigs at least for 10 weeks (21). The disease usually does not remain for long periods on farms unless there is a program of more or less continuous farrowing.

The disease usually occurs during the colder months of the years possibly because the virus is more stable in the frozen state and less subject to sunlight in the winter. In some instances the virus may be transferred by people from an infected premises to a clean area. Starlings may also be involved in its spread as starlings fed TGE virus have infective droppings for 32 hours after feeding (28). Furthermore, these birds are observed in large numbers among swine in the midwestern states of the USA.

Diagnosis. The diagnosis of this disease is easier than many others. The main features in differentiation from other swine enteric disorders are as follows: (*a*) rapidity of spread through all age groups, (*b*) lack of response to antibiotics, and (*c*) high mortality only in very young piglets and rapid recovery of older stock. Additional differences that separate it from swine enteric diseases include its lack of skin lesions, nervous signs, abortions, and stillbirths.

Laboratory confirmation is accomplished by virus isolation or by the demonstration of a rising titer of neutralizing antibodies. These procedures involve the use of tissue-culture and immunofluorescence tests in certain instances. Other tests that can be of use in diagnosis include microtiter complement-fixation and immunodiffusion tests (34) and a micro-indirect hemagglutination test for detecting antibody. For detection of antigen, immune electron microscopy (30) and the leukocyte aggregation assay are in current use (37).

Sibinovic *et al.* (33) developed a bentonite agglutination test based on the agglutination of TGE-treated bentonite particles by specific antibody. The test is complicated and of limited value in the diagnosis of TGE and does not correlate well with the neutralization test (2).

A ring-precipitation test has been described using concentrated TGE antigen and antiserum in small glass tubes (6).

Control. Apparently little can be done to stop outbreaks after they begin. Treatment of infected pigs has little or no value, especially in piglets under 10 days of age. Fortunately, on farms with an interval of several months between spring and fall farrowing periods, the disease seldom carries over into the next period. When farrowings are frequent on a farm where TGE is endemic, two procedures might be considered to reduce the losses of newborn pigs: (*a*) infect pregnant sows at least 2½ weeks prior to partuition so they will be immune at farrowing, and (*b*) isolate susceptible sows before and after farrowing in an area where they are least likely to be exposed to TGE virus. Vaccination of sows with attenuated or inactivated virus vaccine provides little or no maternal immunity protection to their progeny.

The Disease in Man. There is no evidence indicating that the virus of TGE is pathogenic for man.

REFERENCES

1. Bohac and Derbyshire. Can. Jour. Microbiol., 1975, *21,* 750.
2. Bohl. In Diseases of swine, 3rd ed., ed. Howard W. Dunne. Iowa State Univ. Press, Ames, Iowa, 1970, pp. 158–76.
3. Bohl, Fredrick, and Saif. Am. Jour. Vet. Res., 1975, *36,* 267.
4. Bohl and Kumagai. Proc. U.S. Livestock Sanit. Assoc., 1965, *69,* 343.
5. Bradfute, Bohl, and Harada. Quoted by Bohl in Diseases of Swine, 3rd ed., ed. Howard W. Dunne. Iowa State Univ. Press, Ames, Iowa, 1970.
6. Caletti and Ristic. Jour. Am. Vet. Med. Assoc., 1968, *29,* 1603.
7. Cartwright, Harris, Blandford, Fincham, and Gitter. Jour. Comp. Path., 1965, *75,* 386.
8. Cross and Bohl. Jour. Am. Vet. Med. Assoc., 1969, *154,* 266.
9. Doyle and Hutchings. Jour. Am. Vet. Med. Assoc., 1946, *108,* 257.
10. Eto, Ichihara, Tsunoda, and Watanabe. Jour. Jap. Vet. Med. Assoc., 1962, *15,* 16.
11. Garwes and Pocock. Jour. Gen. Virol., 1975, *29,* 25.
12. Garwes, Pocock, and Pike. Jour. Gen. Virol., 1976, *32,* 283.
13. Goodwin and Jennings. Jour. Comp. Path. and Therap., 1959, *69,* 87 and 313.
14. Haelterman. Proc. 17th Internatl. Vet. Cong. (Hannover), 1963, p. 615.
15. Harada, Kumagi, and Sasahara. Natl. Inst. Anim. Health, 1963, *3,* 166.
16. Hess and Bachmann. Inf. and Immun., 1976, *13,* 1642.
17. Hooper and Haelterman. Jour. Am. Vet. Med. Assoc., 1966, *194,* 1580.
18. Hutchings. Vet. Med., 1947, *42,* 297.
19. Kemeny. Can. Jour. Comp. Med., 1976, *40,* 209.
20. Lee. Ann. N.Y. Acad. Sci., 1956, *66,* 191.
21. Lee, Moro, and Baker. Am. Jour. Vet. Res., 1954, *15,* 364.
22. McClurkin. Can. Jour. Comp. Med. and Vet. Sci., 1965, *29,* 46.
23. McClurkin and Norman. Can. Jour. Comp. Med. and Vet. Sci., 1967, *31,* 299.
24. McClurkin, Stark, and Norman. Can. Jour. Comp. Med. and Vet. Sci., 1970, *34,* 347.
25. Morilla, Klemm, Sprino, and Ristic. Am. Jour. Vet. Res., 1976, *37,* 1011.
26. Phel. Arch. f. Exp. Vet.-Med., 1966, *20,* 909.
27. Pike and Garwes. Jour. Gen. Virol., 1977, *34,* 531.
28. Pilchard. Am. Jour. Vet. Res., 1965, *26,* 1177.
29. Reynolds, Garwes, and Goskill. Arch. Virol., 1977, *55,* 77.
30. Saif, Bohl, Hohler, and Hughes. Am. Jour. Vet. Res., 1977, *38,* 13.
31. Sheffy. Proc. U.S. Livestock Sanit. Assoc., 1965, *69,* 351.
32. Shimizu and Shimizu. Jour. Clin. Microbiol., 1977, *6,* 91.
33. Sibinovic, Ristic, Sibinovic, and Alberts. Am. Jour. Vet. Res., 1966, *27,* 1339.

34. Stone, Kemeny, and Jensen. Inf. and Immun., 1976, *13*, 521.
35. Thake. Am. Jour. Path., 1968, *53*, 149.
36. Witte and Easterday. Am. Jour. Vet. Res., 1968, *29*, 1409.
37. Woods. Am. Jour. Vet. Res., 1976, *37*, 1405.
38. Young, Ketchell, Luedke, and Sautter. Jour. Am. Vet. Med. Assoc., 1955, *126*, 165.

Hemagglutinating Encephalomyelitis Virus (HEV) of Pigs

In 1962 Greig *et al.* (3) described three natural outbreaks in Ontario, Canada, of encephalomyelitis in baby pigs. Since that time the disease has been described in England, the United States, Japan, and Denmark. In those countries where serological surveys have been conducted, the infection is very common in swine, particularly where there is a heavy swine population.

Character of the Disease. In the original Canadian outbreaks the affected animals were 4 to 7 days of age when signs of illness first appeared and death occurred usually within 3 days (8). The morbidity and mortality in infected litters approached 100 percent. The infection was characterized by depression, loss of condition, hyperesthesia, incoordination, and occasionally vomition. Concurrent illness in sows and older pigs characterized by inappetence, wasting, and vomition was seen in several instances, but its association with HEV infection was not proved. The disease was reproduced in baby pigs that received colostrum when administered infective material orally or by parenteral injection. In experimental studies unqualified success in the reproduction of clinical disease was only achieved with pigs 7 days of age or less. The signs of illness and histologic lesions of encephalomyelitis were closely similar to those observed in natural cases (2). Pigs from natural or experimental studies developed hemagglutinating antibodies. Pigs with hemagglutinating antibodies are immune.

In subsequent outbreaks described by other investigators (6) clinical disease was limited to piglets and similar to the signs described by Greig *et al.* Piglets that recover from acute disease may develop a chronic form characterized by loss of weight or failure to gain weight at a rate similar to nonaffected litter-mates.

Pathologic changes consist of a marked nonsuppurative encephalomyelitis characterized by perivascular mononuclear cuffing, gliosis, neural death, and satellitosis. Demyelinization has not been seen (9). Virus particles were seen in the cytoplasm of the neurons of an experimentally infected gnotobiotic piglet (7).

Properties of the Virus. Morphologically, virus particles are typical of coronaviruses. Six strains isolated by Greig and examined by electron microscope consist of spherical bodies ranging from 100 to 130 nm in diameter surrounded by a fringe of clublike surface projections 20 to 30 nm long (4). Consequently HEV is a coronavirus but with no apparent antigenic relationship to transmissible gastroenteritis virus of pigs. The HEV virus causes hemagglutination of chicken erythrocytes with a more permanent attachment to the red blood cells (4). There is no evidence of neuraminidase and thus no spontaneous elution. Red cells treated with neuraminidase are agglutinated equally well as nontreated cells. Concanavalin A, a phytoagglutinin, binds to the envelope causing a loss of hemagglutination and a transient interference with infectivity; it does not bind to particles stripped of their envelope (1).

The HEV virus is quite heat-labile but reasonably stable at refrigerator and freezer temperatures and in the lyophilized state (2). Ether and chloroform remove its infectivity and hemagglutinating activity.

Cultivation. HEV replicates in cell cultures of pig kidney cells. HEV virus has been adapted to growth in suckling mouse brain (5).

Immunity. Immunological studies suggest that this virus is not immunologically related to Teschen disease, but histologically it is impossible to distinguish between HEV and Teschen disease (2). It has been observed that following an epizootic in piglets on a farm, clinical disease did not recur for at least 18 months. This observation suggests that some factor(s), perhaps maternal immunity, is effective in protecting the piglets during a period of vulnerability. The high incidence of swine with antibody to HEV in the USA and other countries is another significant factor in the disease incidence.

Diagnosis. Clinical diagnosis may present some difficulty, particularly in distinguishing HEV from Teschen disease.

Virus can be isolated in cell culture and then identified by various means such as hemagglutination or electron microscopy. Serological tests used to demonstrate a rising titer in antibody by using acute and convalescent serum samples include hemagglutination inhibition (HI), agar gel diffusion, and serum-neutralization tests.

Control. There is no vaccine available at present. Knowledge of the immune status of a herd, particularly the sows, would provide a basis to the practitioner for devising means of controlling the disease by appropriate management procedures.

The Disease in Man. There may be an antigenic relationship between a human coronavirus (strain OC 43) and HEV of swine (5). Humans with sero-conversion to OC 43 antigen by various serological tests had diagnostic rises in antibody titer to HEV antigens. There is no evidence, however, that either virus causes disease in the heterologous host-humans and swine.

REFERENCES

1. Greig and Bouillant. Can. Jour. Comp. Med., 1977, *41*, 122.
2. Greig and Girard. Res. Vet. Sci., 1963, *4*, 511.
3. Greig, Mitchell, Corner, Bannister, Meads, and Julian. Can. Jour. Comp. Med. and Vet. Sci., 1962, *62*, 49.
4. Greig, Johnson, and Bouillant. Res. Vet. Sci., 1971, *12*, 305.
5. Kaye, Yarbough, Reed, and Harrison. Jour. Inf. Dis., 1977, *135*, 201.
6. Mengling and Cutlip. Jour. Am. Vet. Med. Assoc., 1976, *168*, 236.
7. Meyvisch and Hoorens. Vet. Path., 1978, *15*, 102.
8. Mitchell. Res. Vet. Sci., 1963, *4*, 506.
9. Werdin, Sorensen, and Stewart. Jour. Am. Vet. Med. Assoc., 1976, *168*, 240.

Neonatal Calf Diarrhea

SYNONYM: Bovine coronavirus

This disease was first described by Mebus and his coworkers. Coronaviruslike virions were isolated from the feces of experimental calves that were inoculated with feces from 7- to 10-day-old beef calves with natural disease (5, 6). The disease is a part of the acute diarrheal complex in neonatal calves that is a very common and serious economic disease in dairy and beef animals.

Character of the Disease. Most of our knowledge about the nature of this disease was developed by Mebus and his coworkers, who studied the disease in gnotobiotic and naturally born colostrum-fed and colostrum-deprived calves (2, 4).

After oral inoculation, the incubation period in gnotobiotic calves was about 20 hours. Initially, calves

Figure 55.5. Scanning electronmicrograph of lower ileum from a gnotobiotic calf infected with bovine diarrheal coronavirus. Villi are of irregular length, and numerous adjacent villi are fused. × 100. (Courtesy C. A. Mebus. From *Am. Jour. Vet. Res.*, 1975, *36*, 1723.)

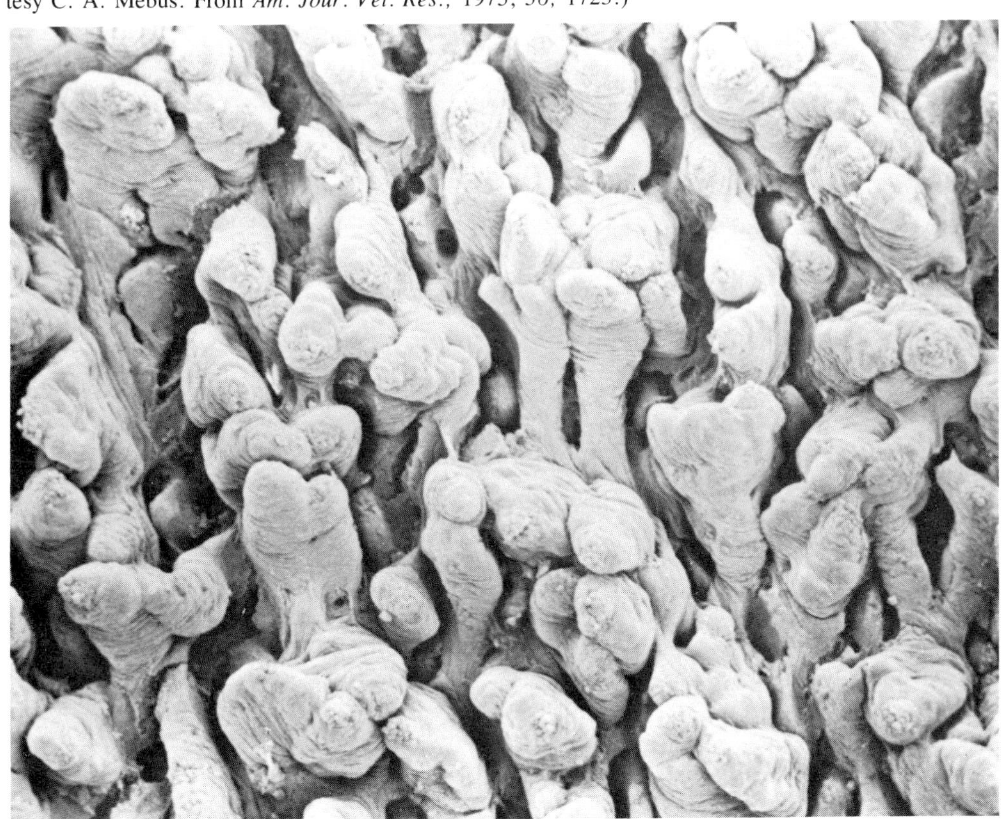

were moderately depressed, ate slowly, and passed liquid, yellowish feces. After the initial diarrhea, the liquid feces contained curds and mucus. This type of diarrhea continued, and the calves became depressed, weak, and gaunt 42 to 96 hours after onset of diarrhea. The packed blood cell volume for calves 42 to 96 hours after onset of diarrhea ranged from 49 to 61 percent, compared with 32 percent for a control calf. At necropsy, diarrheal gnotobiotic calves had liquid contents but no gross lesion in the small or large intestines. Histologically, by light microscopy, the small and large intestines were lined by normal epithelium at the onset of diarrhea. By immunofluorescent microscopy, the villous epithelial cell cytoplasm contained coronaviral antigen, and by transmission electron microscopy it contained virions. Lesions were not observed in the crypts of Lieberkühn. In the spiral colon, surface epithelial cells had a tall, columnar morphologic feature and were immunofluorescent positive for coronavirus.

The small intestine of calves 42 to 96 hours after the onset of diarrhea had, by light and scanning electron microscopy, severely shortened villi and fusion of adjacent villi occasionally (Figure 55.5). Villi were covered by cuboidal epithelial cells, some of which were immunofluorescent for coronavirus. However, as the interval between onset of diarrhea and necropsy increased, the number of immunofluorescent cells decreased. In the spiral colon, colonic ridges were atrophied, and the morphologic features of surface epithelial cells varied from cuboidal to low columnar. Scattered colonic crypts were dilated and lined by low cuboidal epithelial cells. Surface and crypt epithelial cells fluoresced for coronavirus.

Persistent diarrhea is believed to be caused by continued ingestion of milk and prolonged presence of immature villous epithelium, which results in a deficiency of enzymes required to complete the digestion of the milk, causing reduced absorptive capability. The volume of feces and curd in the feces are indications of the severity of intestinal alteration. Lesions and fluorescence are observed only in the mesenteric lymph nodes and not in other tissues.

Properties of the Virus. The virus has the biochemical and biophysical characteristics of a coronavirus.

Cultivation. The virus replicates in cell cultures of fetal bovine kidney cells with the formation of syncytia (3) (Figure 55.6). The virus also has been adapted to the suckling mouse brain (Figure 55.7).

Figure 55.6. Syncytium in fetal bovine kidney cells infected with bovine diarrheal coronavirus. (Courtesy C. A. Mebus, Plum Island Animal Disease Center, USDA.)

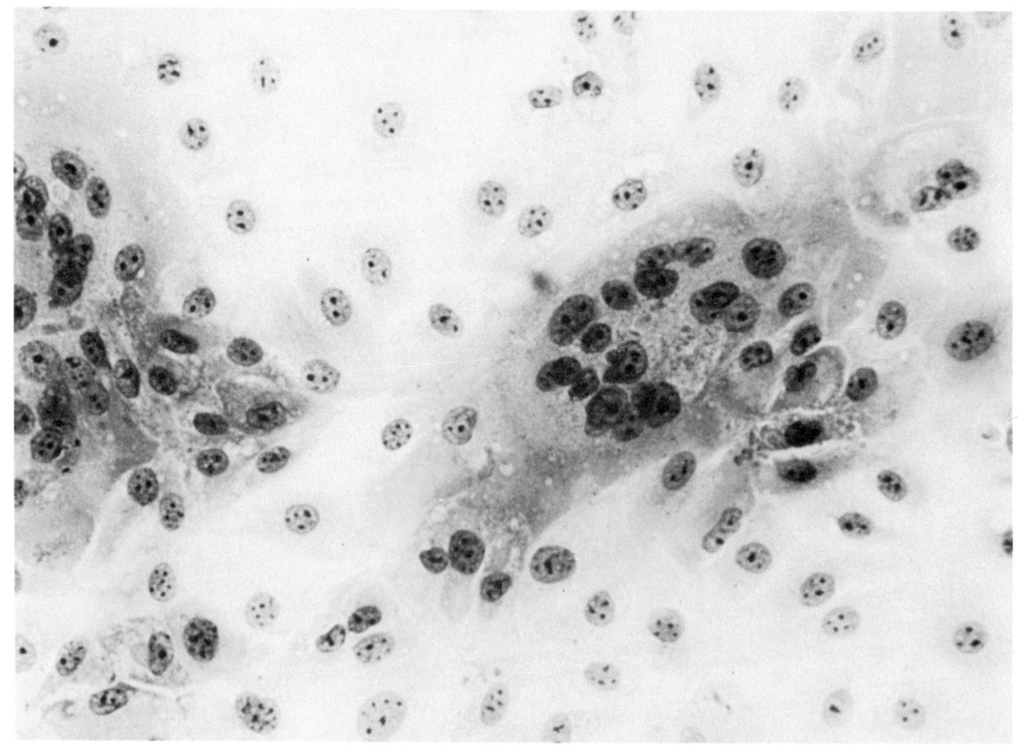

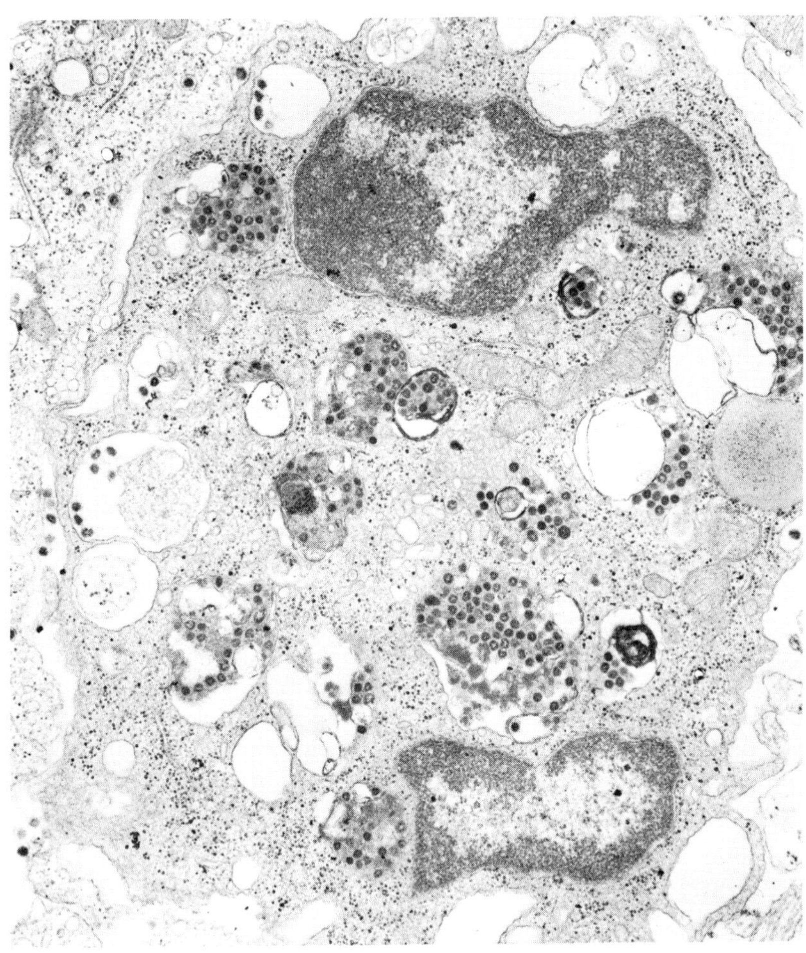

Figure 55.7. Calf diarrhea virus in suckling mouse brain. Virus particles have accumulated in vacuoles in a macrophage. × 25,000. (Courtesy A. K. Harrison, Center for Disease Control.)

Immunity. The mechanism for protection against this virus is located in the intestinal tract of the calf. The immunoglobulins principally responsible for immunity are IgA and IgM (1). Despite the presence of circulating IgG a calf is fully susceptible to the agent, which suggest this type of immunoglobulin in the blood does not provide protection. This is substantiated by limited but definite studies. Colostrum-fed calves were born normally, allowed to nurse, and thereafter fed autoclaved milk. Serum globulin values ranged from 1.7 to 2.6 g per dl, and coronaviral serum neutralization (SN) titers in the calves ranged from 324 to 537. When these inoculated calves were 4 and 5 days of age they developed diarrhea, but remained alert and in good condition. Sections from the cranial end of the small intestine had slight or no villous atrophy; sections from the caudal part of the small intestine had severe villous atrophy. A calf inoculated when 12 days old (SN titer of 537) developed severe diarrhea and villous atrophy in all levels of the small intestine.

Diagnosis. A precise etiological diagnosis is difficult to make on the basis of clinical signs. Other viruses (parvovirus or rotavirus) and certain bacteria cause an acute diarrheal disease in neonatal calves. Mixed infections may occur involving one or more of these other disease agents.

A precise diagnosis can be provided by the isolation of virus in cell culture and by demonstration of typical viral particles using electron microscopy with fecal material. At necropsy, the immunofluorescent procedure can be used to demonstrate viral antigen in epithelial cells of the villi. The demonstration of a rising antibody titer with acute and convalescent serums using the neutralization test in cell culture is another approach.

Control. This is an extremely difficult situation with no simple answer. Colostrum is extremely important to a neonate, and this is particularly true in diseases such as this one in which an infection involves a superficial tissue such as the intestinal tract and circulating antibody is not involved in protection. Management plays an important role in minimizing this disease—isolation and reasonably warm and clean quarters can reduce the losses. Symptomatic treatment provided early in the disease facilitates recovery.

The Disease in Man. There is no evidence that this virus causes disease in humans.

REFERENCES

1. Mebus. Jour. Am. Vet. Med. Assoc., 1978, *173,* 631.
2. Mebus, Newman, and Stair. Am. Jour. Vet. Res., 1975, *36,* 1719.
3. Mebus, Stair, Rhodes, and Twiehaus. Am. Jour. Vet. Res., 1973, *34,* 145.
4. Mebus, Stair, Rhodes, and Twiehaus. Vet. Pathol., 1973, *10,* 45.
5. Mebus, White, Stair, Rhodes, and Twiehaus. Vet. Med. Small An. Clin., 1972, *67,* 173.
6. Stair, Rhodes, White, and Mebus. Am. Jour. Vet. Res., 1972, *33,* 1147.

Canine Coronavirus

This disease was first described by Binn (2). The virus was isolated in 1971 from military dogs with suspected gastroenteritis and identified as a coronavirus.

Character of the Disease (3). Initial signs of illness in natural cases are loss of appetite, shortly followed or simultaneously followed by a loose stool. There may be mucus and/or variable amounts of blood in the feces. Stools often are orange in color and usually fetid. Vomiting sometimes occurs and occasionally is blood-tinged. Projectile diarrhea as a watery or bloody fluid has been observed. Dogs usually recover without treatment in 7 to 10 days. Relapses after 1 to 3 weeks are seen with death ensuing in some cases. Occasionally diarrhea will persist for 3 to 4 weeks even with symptomatic treatment. An occasional dog will die following a "convulsive-like" seizure. Young pups with severe diarrhea may die suddenly, especially under conditions of stress such as fatigue, mixed infection (parvovirus, for example), or sudden change in temperature. The disease is readily transmitted from infected to susceptible dogs that have direct contact with each other.

In experimental studies in neonatal beagle puppies the virus causes diarrhea that usually persists for 5 to 6 days (4). Contact animals developed the disease within 4 days. No mortality or complications in experimental puppies was reported. There was atrophy of the intestinal villi with healing within 7 to 10 days, and the pathological changes are similar to those observed in neonatal calf disease.

Properties of the Virus. Except for determining its typical morphological appearance under the electron microscope, studies of the canine coronavirus are rather limited. At present only one serotype has been recognized, but considerably more study on this important issue must be done in the future as it relates to prevention and control of the disease.

Some strains of virus can be cultivated in cell cultures derived from dog tissues, but they are fastidious and often difficult to propagate.

Diagnosis. A presumptive diagnosis is based on clinical signs, history of contagious diarrhea, and necropsy findings (1). Mixed infections must be considered. A rapid diagnosis may be obtained by observing characteristic viral particles in fresh fecal samples prepared by negative staining for electron microscopic examination. Caution must be exercised in interpreting results because artifacts can be misleading. When immunofluorescent reagents become available, this test also can be used.

Control. Treatment should be directed towards the control of diarrhea, vomiting, and dehydration in severely ill puppies.

REFERENCES

1. Appel, Cooper, Griesen, and Carmichael. Jour. Am. Vet. Med. Assoc., 1978, *173,* 1516.
2. Binn, Lazar, Keenan, Huxsoll, Marchwicki, and Strano. Proc. Annual Meeting of the U.S. Animal Health Assoc., 1974, *78,* 359.
3. Carmichael. James A. Baker Institute of Animal Health, Lab. Rep., Cornell Univ., 1978, 1.
4. Keenan, Jervis, Marchwicki, and Binn. Am. Jour. Vet. Res., 1976, *37,* 247.

Transmissible Gastroenteritis of Turkeys

SYNONYM: Bluecomb

This disease, often called bluecomb, has been recognized as a serious entity in turkeys for many years. It causes enteritis in turkeys and often results in high mortality.

The group at Minnesota under Pomeroy has studied the disease in some depth and initially established its etiology as a coronavirus. Various bluecomb isolates are closely related antigenically (2). Turkey flocks recovering from natural or laboratory-induced disease developed lifelong immunity.

To eliminate the disease in the turkey population in

Minnesota (USA), controlled depopulation and decontamination with a rest period before restocking achieved positive results (1). In some instances the indirect fluorescent antibody test can be used to detect serum antibody in birds that may be potential carriers.

REFERENCES

1. Patel, Gonder, and Pomeroy. Am. Jour. Vet. Res., 1977. *38,* 1407.
2. Pomeroy, Larsen, Deshmukh, and Patel. Am. Jour. Vet. Res., 1975, *36,* 553.

Gastroenteritis in Foals

There is only a single reference in literature about cases of acute diarrhea in horses caused by a coronavirus (1). Fecal specimens from 3 foals that died or were killed in the acute stage of the disease were examined by electron microscopy, and all 3 specimens contained typical coronavirus particles. These foals came from an endemic area in the United States where 40 or more cases of neonatal foal diarrhea were observed. The disease was characterized by profuse watery diarrhea fever, extensive lymphatic involvement, and a high rate of mortality despite treatment.

The investigators tested 65 equine sera for serum-neutralizing antibody against the calf diarrhea coronavirus. Some of the animals had titers to greater than 181. These serological results suggest the equine virus is antigenically related to the calf coronavirus. The serological and electron microscopy results suggest the existence of an equine coronavirus that causes diarrhea in neonatal foals.

REFERENCE

1. Bass and Sharper. Lancet, 1975, *7939,* 822.

Feline Infectious Peritonitis (FIP)

This disease was first described in 1963 by Holzworth (1). Sixteen naturally occurring cases, coupled with transmission studies, were described 3 years later (15). In recent years the disease has been diagnosed with increased frequency. The affected cats range in age from 3 months to 17 years. The proportion of males to females is significantly higher. The occurrence of the disease does not vary significantly with the season of the year. There is insufficient evidence to suggest that certain breeds of cats are more susceptible to the disease. The disease is widespread in domestic and large wild cats

located in the United States and Europe and probably throughout the world. The disease seems to be more serious in catteries where feline leukemia exists.

For detailed information about the disease the reader is referred to brief review articles by Jones (6), Pedersen (11), Horzinek and Osterhaus (3), and Ott (8).

Character of the Disease. FIP is a chronic, debilitating disease characterized by fibrinous peritonitis and often pleuritis (Figure 55.8) (2). Other clinical signs of illness include peritoneal and pleural effusion, depression, persistent or recurrent fever, inappetence, wasting, and anemia. Less common signs are thirst, constipation, neurological iritis, or hypopyon, harsh lung sounds, ventral edema, and bleeding gums. Masses occasionally are palpable in the abdomen, and these presumably are enlarged nodes or viscera with adhesions. Pain is noted in some cases. Most affected cats die within 5 weeks after diagnosis, and treatment is almost never effective. Often there is a relative or absolute hypergammaglobulinemia.

Most cats that are exposed to the virus become infected but show no signs of illness.

At necropsy FIP can be found earlier in the classical fibronecrotic (wet) form or in the granulomatous (dry) form, although a strict distinction cannot always be made (4, 11). In the fibronecrotic cases an inflammation of the

Figure 55.8. Elevated fibrinous plaques on the visceral and parietal peritoneum observed in a typical case of feline infectious peritonitis. (Courtesy J. Gaskin.)

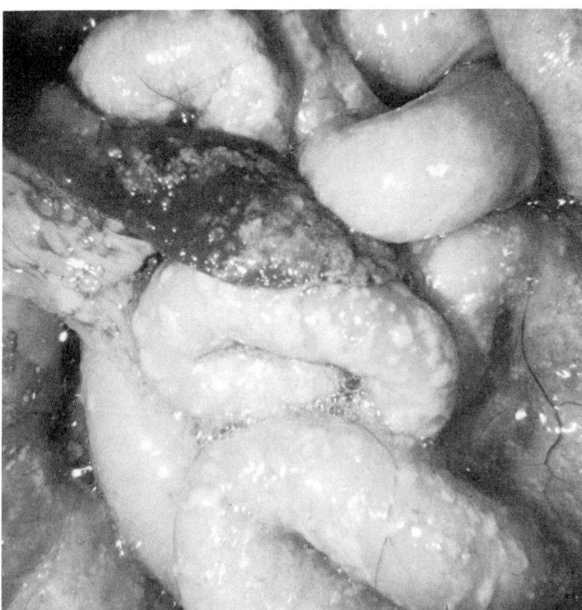

parietal and visceral surfaces of the peritoneum and/or pleura is most prominent. Small necrotic lesions are seen, and extensive accumulations of a yellowish viscid exudate containing fibrin flakes are found in the body cavities. The exudate adhering to the serosae is composed of fibrin, containing cells, mostly histiocytes, and necrotic masses. Focal necrotic lesions sometimes are observed in parenchymatous organs, usually the liver and kidneys, and granulomatous changes also may occur due to a histiocytic and lymphocytic reaction. In the dry form there are disseminated grey lesions, up to 2 mm, that are most abundant in the kidneys, central nervous system, mesenteric lymph nodes, and liver. The foci accumulate around the small blood vessels as a vasculitis. Ocular lesions are localized in the retina and meninges of the optical nerve and the nerve itself. Exudate may be in the ocular chambers. Lesions in the central nervous system are located in the meninges, ependyma, and plexus chorioideus and occasionally along the blood vessels in the parenchyma. The lesions in experimental cats, the only species known to be susceptible at present, vary in severity depending on the amount of infectious agent in the batch of infective material used for production of infection. When the dosage of the infective agent is high, the disease is more acute and the chronic type of disease observed in the field is not seen (13). Dilutions of the same inoculum produce the typical syndrome observed in practice.

Properties of the Virus. The viral properties of the FIP agent are characteristic, as anticipated of coronaviruses. The replication of the virus in cells of the cat and also in cell culture follow the pattern of other members of this family. The virus also is antigenically related to transmissible gastroenteritis of pigs. High titers to TGE were detected in sera and peritoneal fluids of FIP cases by the neutralization test (14). In their studies, Witte *et al.* found a one-way antigenic relationship between the 2 viruses, but Pederson *et al.* reported on cross-reactions in both directions (12).

In contrast, antibodies against TGE viral antigen could be detected by immunofluorescence in sera and ascites fluids from FIP-infected cats but not by the neutralization test. The possible existence of FIP serotypes may account for the difference in the neutralization test results (7).

Cultivation. Attempts to propagate the virus in primary feline cell cultures and continuous cell lines have failed, but *in vitro* growth of the virus has been demonstrated in cultures derived from peritoneal exudates of infected kittens (9).

Hoshina and Scott (5) have reported the replication of this virus in organ cultures derived from the small intestinal tract of 1-day-old to 9-week-old specific-pathogen-free kittens. Successful replication of the virus occurs in the brains of suckling mice, rats, and hamsters (4).

Immunity. Low antibody titers to FIP virus occur in healthy cats, but very high titers were found in diseased animals as determined by the homologous indirect immunofluorescence test (10). Virus-neutralizing antibodies have no protective value. It has been suggested that the persistence of virus in the presence of specific, high titering antibody gives rise to the immune pathology of FIP not unlike Aleutian disease in mink. Although immune complexes may contribute to the glomerular and vascular lesions such as fibrinoid necrosis of the media of small and medium-sized vessels, their existence in this disease are still to be proved.

Transmission. In limited serological studies it appears that the infection is common in cats, suggesting that only a small percentage develop clinical signs characteristic of FIP. Because the virus persists in chronically infected cats, they serve as the main reservoir of the agent, since the natural infection presumably only occurs in cats.

Diagnosis. The diagnosis of FIP is simple in terminal classical cases where extensive accumulations of exudate are present in either or both of the cavities. Because most clinical alterations now are presumed to be uncharacteristic, serological or virological methodology must be used to make a positive diagnosis of the disease.

Control. Presently, appropriate methods are difficult to recommend. In catteries where the disease is common, carrier cats should be eliminated by testing for neutralizing antibodies. Certainly, diseased cats should be isolated from healthy cats.

Administration of steroids in connection with supportive therapy has resulted in temporary remission and prolongation of the disease course of FIP (8).

The Disease in Man. It is not known to occur in man.

REFERENCES

1. Holzworth. Cornell Vet., 1963, *53,* 157.
2. Holzworth. Jour. Am. Vet. Med. Assoc., 1971, *158,* 981.
3. Horzinek and Osterhaus. Arch. Virol., 1979, *59,* 1.
4. Horzinek and Osterhaus. Jour. Small Anim. Prac., 1978, *19,* 623.
5. Hoshino and Scott. Cornell Vet., 1978, *68,* 411.
6. Jones. New Zeal. Vet. Jour., 1975, *23,* 221.
7. Osterhaus, Horzinek and Wirahadiredja. Zentrbl. Vet.-Med., 1978, *25B,* 301.

8. Ott. *In* Feline medicine and surgery, 2nd ed., ed. E. J. Catcott. American Veterinary Publications, Inc., Santa Barbara, Calif., 1975, p. 47.
9. Pedersen. Am. Jour. Vet. Res., 1976, *37,* 567.
10. Pedersen. Am. Jour. Vet. Res., 1976, *37,* 1449.
11. Pedersen. Fel. Pract., 1976, *6,* 42.
12. Pedersen, Ward, and Mengeling. Arch. Virol., 1978, *58,* 45.
13. Ward and Pedersen. Jour. Am. Vet. Med. Assoc., 1969, *154,* 26.
14. Witte, Tuch, Dubenkropp, and Walther. Berl. und Münch. tierärztl Wchnschr., 1977, *80,* 396.
15. Wolfe and Griesemer. Path. Vet., 1966, *3,* 255.

SECTION IV MISCELLANEOUS: DISEASES CAUSED BY UNCLASSIFIED VIRUSES OR OF UNCERTAIN VIRAL ETIOLOGY

56 Infectious Diseases of Domestic Animals Caused by Unclassified Viruses

There are a few diseases of the lower animals and man that are characterized by a long incubation period, insidious onset of clinical disease, protracted clinical course, high mortality, and pathologic changes different from acute viral disease (1). The conceptual approach of an infectious etiology, principally involving viruses, was developed by Sigurdsson (2) who coined the term *slow virus infections*. In recent years there has been great interest in the study of these animal viral diseases for two reasons: (*a*) the nature of the lesions, suggesting immunopathic disease, and their similarity to certain human diseases, and (*b*) the unusual characteristics of some of these agents which appear to have properties unlike other viruses. Some animal viral diseases such as visna-maedi, equine infectious anemia, ovine adenomatosis, murine lymphocytic choriomeningitis, and Aleutian disease viruses that fall into this category are discussed elsewhere in this book. Two rather unusual animal viruses—mink encephalopathy and scrapie—are described in the same section of this chapter. These agents and two human agents—kuru and Creutzfeldt-Jakob disease—comprise a group called the subacute spongiform virus encephalopathies, which have characteristics of slow viruses.

This chapter also describes some other animal virus diseases that are presently unclassified, such as Borna disease of horses, ulcerative stomatitis of calves, bovine papular stomatitis of calves, proliferative stomatitis of calves, and contagious pneumonia of calves. Three transmissible tumors of domestic animals—canine mastocytoma, canine venereal tumor, and ocular squamous cell carcinoma of cattle—may be caused by viruses; consequently, these diseases are also included in this chapter.

REFERENCES

1. Abinanti. Ann. Rev. Microbiol., 1967, *21*, 467.
2. Sigurdsson. Brit. Vet. Jour., 1954, *110*, 7.

Scrapie and Mink Encephalopathy

SYNONYMS: *Tremblant du Mouton,* Rida

Scrapie is a disease of sheep, occasionally of goats, characterized by a very long period of incubation, pruritus, nervous signs, and nearly always, death. The disease is obviously infectious and is generally considered to be of viral origin. If the causative agent is indeed a virus, it is a most unusual one. It has long been thought that the disease has hereditary features, and there is evidence to indicate that certain breeds of sheep are more susceptible than others.

Nussbaum *et al.* (20) established sheep flocks of predictable susceptibility to experimental scrapie by selection. They established that the type of scrapie caused by the SSBP-1 agent is largely under the genetic control of a single pair of autosomal genes, the dominant allele conferring susceptibility.

Scrapie has existed in Europe for 200 years or longer, particularly in England and Scotland, but it is also known on the continent. The first case in the United States was diagnosed in 1947 in Michigan in an animal that had been imported from Great Britain by way of Canada. In

1952 cases were recognized in California (19). Shortly afterward positive diagnoses of scrapie were made in Ohio, Illinois, New York, and Connecticut (30). Most of these cases occurred in the Suffolk breed, and most of them were traced to Canada, thence to importations from the British Isles. In 1952 isolated cases were reported in Australia and New Zealand in sheep imported from England.

Character of the Disease. The earliest sign frequently noticed is pruritus, although it is probable that more careful observation would detect certain nervous signs before the onset of pruritus. The itching is manifested by the animal's rubbing against objects and biting the itching areas, particularly the flanks. When rubbing, the animal draws back its lips, showing its teeth, and runs its tongue in and out. These signs can usually be elicited by rubbing or lightly pinching the skin over the lumbar region or in the flanks. Tremors of the muscles may be elicited in the same way. This sign has caused the French to call the malady *trembling disease*. Rubbing of the skin usually pulls out the wool, and the first impression is that the animal suffers from scabies. The skin is not encrusted, however, as it is in scabies; furthermore no mites can be found in scrapings. As the case advances, motor disturbances become more pronounced; the gait is affected, the animal weaves as it walks, the head is carried higher than normal, and the eyes assume a staring appearance. If the animal is frightened, it may fall down repeatedly because of its incoordination of locomotion, and sometimes the animal goes into convulsions. Paralysis, particularly of the hind quarters, then occurs in many cases, and finally the animal becomes recumbent and is unable to rise. Affected animals usually lose weight rapidly. Fever is not observed in any stage of the disease. It may possibly occur in an otherwise presymptomatic stage of the disease and escape attention.

Scrapie has an extraordinarily long incubation period. In the natural disease it is believed to be from 1 to 4 years. By inoculation it can be produced in 6 months or less, if the inoculum is given intracerebrally to day-old lambs. Older animals will generally have a longer incubation period, that is, up to 1 year or longer, but some will develop signs in less than 6 months. In goats the period of incubation is about the same as in sheep.

Most animals die 4 to 6 weeks after developing signs, but some survive considerably longer. The death rate in scrapie is essentially 100 percent.

There are no gross lesions in this disease. Most of our knowledge about the histological lesions of scrapie stems from the studies in laboratory animals. In mice infected with scrapie virus the spongiform changes can be seen in the cerebral cortex by electron microscopy (14). There was swelling and vacuolation of neurons, particularly the dendrites, with fusion of swollen cells. The changes are associated with plasma membranes. Curled fragments of membranes accumulated at points of cell fusion and at the margin of vacuoles within dendrites. The abnormal membranes are wider and more osmiophilic than normal plasma membranes. It is believed the alterations of neuronal membranes initiate the spongiform degeneration of neurons. Histologically, the retina and optic nerve are abnormal in hamsters infected with scrapie virus (3). There are varying degrees of thinning of the retina with the photoreceptor layer most severely affected. The optic nerve of infected hamsters appears more cellular than that of the controls.

Most who have worked with this disease believe that brain vacuoles are more numerous and more constant in scrapie than in normal animals. Zlotnik and Rennie (32), reviewing the matter, studied normal sheep from breeds that were known to be highly susceptible to scrapie and found vacuoles in all breeds and nearly all animals, but the numbers were always small, averaging about one to a microscopic field. In scrapie sheep they were identical in appearance but much more numerous. For more information about pathological changes see Abinanti (1).

The Disease in Experimental Animals. Scrapie has been transmitted by inoculation to mice, goats, mink, rats, hamsters, gerbils, and sheep. Wilson, Anderson, and Smith (31) passed the disease through nine generations of sheep by intracerebral inoculation. In some passages no more than 25 percent of the inoculated animals developed the disease. In some cases animals exhibited signs of pruritus, which was considered evidence of infection, and later became well. This raises the question of whether natural cases of scrapie may sometimes be nonfatal.

There is now good evidence that scrapie can be transmitted by intracerebral, subcutaneous, and intradermal inoculation of filtered brain material, although not all sheep will become infected (29). Pattison, Gordon, and Millson (24) succeeded in infecting all of 10 goats with brain material of a Welsh mountain sheep affected with scrapie, whereas no disease was produced in another lot of 10 goats injected in the same way with brain material from a normal animal of the same breed. The incubation period is reduced by serial goat passage of the agent. Virus has been segregated into itching and sleepy strains which breed true (25).

Chandler (4) transmitted an agent from a sleepy strain to Swiss mice by intracerebral injection, and after serial transfers, the incubation period was reduced to 3 to 4 months. The mice showed signs referable to the central nervous system. The agent withstood boiling and was similar to scrapie in this respect. Eklund *et al.* (6) extended these studies and showed that first passage mouse brain produced scrapie in goats injected intracerebrally.

Rennie and Zlotnick (28) reported the experimental transmission of mouse-passaged scrapie to goats, sheep, rats, and hamsters producing comparable brain lesions in all species. It is known that scrapie spreads from inoculated to uninoculated mice. The Compton strain can be transmitted from mice to hamsters and maintained in serial passage in hamsters with infective brain tissue suspension (9).

Eklund *et al.* (7) reported on a pathogenesis study in mice given the scrapie agent subcutaneously. The agent first appeared in the lymphatic tissues and over a period of many weeks spread slowly to the other tissues. It finally reached the spinal cord by the 12th week, and the brain by the 16th week. The highest concentrations of infective agent occurred in the CNS. Histological lesions were not detected until 8 weeks after the brain reached its maximum titer of the agent, and clinical signs appeared 9 weeks later. As the amount of the agent increased in the CNS, it decreased or disappeared entirely in the lymphoid tissues (2).

Hanson *et al.* (13) reported on the experimental transmission of the scrapie agent to mink producing a disease with clinical signs and pathological lesions indistinguishable from the naturally occurring transmissible encephalopathy of mink (TEM), a disease of undetermined origin. The most striking lesion observed in electron micrographs was a spongiform polioencephalopathy of the cerebral cortex and round-shaped lesion of electron lucent appearance surrounded by processes of nerve cells and glial cells. Mink that were given scrapie-infective brain from Suffolk sheep developed mink encephalopathy within 12 to 14 months. Mink given the Cheviot sheep infective brain remained normal for 20 months. Both inocula produced scrapie in mice after incubation periods between 15 and 16 months. The scrapie and TEM agents have a different host spectrum based on production of disease (13) but perhaps no differences in infection susceptibility. The TEM agent causes disease in three species of subhuman primates (23), in raccoons, and in striped skunks.

Marsh and Kimberlin studied the clinical signs, pathology, and pathogenesis of scrapie virus and transmissible mink encephalopathy virus in hamsters (16). The most noticeable clinical sign in scrapie-affected hamsters was a distinct cerebellar ataxia beginning 16 weeks after inoculation. Ataxia was not prominent in animals affected with transmissible mink encephalopathy. These animals gradually became more and more lethargic.

The pathology in the central nervous system in both diseases consisted of astrocytic hypertrophy, microvacuolation of the neuropile, and neuronal degeneration. The scrapie agent appeared to have a greater effect on nuclear masses, especially those present in brain stem and the central white matter of the cerebellum. The earliest lesions in both diseases were detected near pia-arachnoid surfaces and adjacent to the ventricular system. These initial sites of involvement suggest that the cerebrospinal fluid may be an important route by which inocula are disseminated to susceptible cells after intracerebral inoculation. Both agents multiplied rapidly in brain, reaching titers greater than $10^{8.0}$ LD_{50} per 0.05 ml before the onset of clinical signs. Viral titers in spleen were 4 to 6 logs lower than titers in brain at every stage measured during the symptomatic or clinical course of disease. It is believed that spongiform degeneration is a secondary change in TEM and vacuolation may be the result of lysosomal enzymes causing an increase in ganglioside catabolism (17).

Properties of the Virus. The infectious particle is apparently smaller than 50 nm. The agent withstands boiling for 30 minutes without losing infectivity (29). Previous reports that it withstands boiling were not confirmed by a test that employed a Seitz filtrate of 0.1 suspension of infected mouse brain (6). The suspension did withstand 80 C for 30 minutes, so it is unusually resistant to heating. It survived 0.35 percent formalin for 3 months (11) and also 10 to 12 percent formalin for periods ranging from 6 to 28 months at room temperature (23). Discrepancies exist regarding its ether-resistance. Scrapie infectivity present in a cell line is associated with the plasma membrane (5). Later studies suggested that the scrapie agent is a discrete infectious particle that should be separable from cellular membranes (27). These studies were substantiated by determinations of scrapie activity in subcellular fractions from infected hamster brains through the asymptomatic and symptomatic course of infection. Thus activity revealed the presence of substantial amounts of scrapie infectivity in the 100,000 × the force of gravity (G) supernatant fractions, indicating that association with physically discernible membrane structures is not necessary for the transmission of the scrapie agent (15). An increase of scrapie infectivity in the 100,000 × G supernatant fractions after vigorous homogenization of infected membrane-rich fractions suggests that the agent is identical in membrane-rich and 100,000 × G supernatant fractions.

Attempts to demonstrate the infective agent in the animal tissues by the fluorescent antibody technique have failed (18). No serological procedure is now available. The present attitude is to accept the idea that the infectious agent is viral, recognizing that it has features different from other conventional viruses, especially the experiments that suggest it is dialyzable (26). These experiments have not been confirmed, but the results are intriguing.

Cultivation. The 23rd cell subculture of midbrain from an infected sheep produced scrapie in mice. The 23 subcultures of the midbrain tissue required 14 months (12). No cytopathic effects were noted, but in comparison with normal cultures, the astrocytes had a wider range of cell and nuclear size and a greater order and intensity of multinucleation. The cells developed a tendency to proliferate and overlap as in cell cultures infected with certain oncogenic viruses.

Immunity. Little is known about immunity in scrapie. Attempts to demonstrate circulating antibody and/or specific antigen in scrapie disease in sheep have not met with success (7, 10).

Various reasons are given for the probable lack of protection against the scrapie agent (1). One theory suggests that the agent's initial affinity for lymphocytic tissue destroys its capacity to produce antibody and permits the agent to persist and eventually invade the CNS. The second concept embraces the idea that the slow production of the agent in the defense cells causes gradual disturbance of their function and hence the body does not recognize the agent as a foreign antigen and does not produce antibody. The third idea, and perhaps the one most readily accepted, suggests that the agent initiates subtle changes in the host tissues, particularly the CNS, making them unusually antigenic; and the ultimate damage is typical of an immunopathic disease in which the antigen-antibody complexes disrupt the normal physiological function of these cells. There is experimental evidence to support the latter concept (1).

Transmission. Epidemiological evidence suggests that the agent may enter the body through breaks in the skin and mucous membranes of susceptible sheep (2). Greig (11) alternated scrapie-infected and normal sheep on the same pasture, taking care that there were no direct contacts between the two groups. Ten of the 26 normal sheep eventually developed the disease, the first cases after about 3 years, the last after about 5 years. Greig concluded that the incubation period of the natural disease was very long and that the infective agent could persist for a time on grasslands. Reference has already been made to the possibility that genetic factors influence susceptibility. Stamp (29) states that the disease is found more often in some breeds of sheep than in others, and that purebred sheep appear to be more susceptible than crossbred.

Diagnosis. The diagnosis of scrapie at present rests largely on identification by the rather characteristic signs of illness. The vacuolization of the medullary neurons may be used as confirming evidence.

Control. In Europe, where the disease has long existed, no serious efforts to control it have been made. Some have suggested the slaughter of all animals in infected flocks and starting new flocks from uninfected sources. Greig (11) denies that this will succeed because he thinks that premises may remain infective for long periods.

Since the infection was introduced into the United States, attempts to control and eradicate it have been in progress. It remains to be seen whether these will succeed. The long incubation period of scrapie makes the task unusually difficult, since it is obvious that before clinical signs are apparent many animals will have been exposed and many of these will have been distributed to other flocks, carrying the disease with them. Infected flocks have been slaughtered and the owners indemnified from public funds, and attempts are made to trace all stock sold to other flocks, with particular emphasis on blood lines, and to keep these under surveillance by means of periodic inspections. It is hoped that by this means newly infected flocks can be detected early and eliminated before they spread the disease. Because it appears that all cases have been imported, directly or indirectly, from the British Isles, quarantine restrictions have been established to prevent importation of additional cases.

The Disease in Man. There is increasing concern that the scrapie agent may cause disease in man. A number of years ago 4 of 7 workers engaged in research on a neurological disease of sheep (swayback) developed a disease diagnosed as multiple sclerosis. Icelandic sheep inoculated with brain material from a patient that died with multiple sclerosis developed a disease clinically and histopathologically indistinguishable from scrapie (21).

Subsequent studies with similar human brain material yielded comparable results (22).

In 1957 Gajdusek and Zagas (8) described a degenerative disease of the CNS in human beings called *kuru*. The lesions of CNS are quite similar to those described for scrapie in sheep. There is increasing evidence that kuru, mink encephalopathy, scrapie, and Creutzfeldt-Jakob disease (spastic pseudosclerosis) agents have many similarities and may be closely related and also that their host spectrum may be broader than it was originally thought. Kuru is known to produce a lethal infection in chimpanzees, spider monkeys, and mice, and the Creutzfeldt-Jakob agent causes death in chimpanzees.

The public health significance of the two agents that naturally infect nonhuman animals is obscure at present and the problems of their importance to man are compounded by their long incubation period, genetic predisposition, and probable remission of clinical disease.

REFERENCES

1. Abinanti. Ann. Rev. Microbiol., 1967, *121*, 467.
2. Asher, Gibbs, and Gajdusek. Ann. Clin. Lab. Sci., 1976, *6*, 84.
3. Buyukmihci, Marsh, Albert, and Zelinski. Invest. Ophthalmol. Visual Sci., 1977, *16*, 319.
4. Chandler. Lancet, 1961, *1*, 1378.
5. Clarke and Millson. Jour. Gen. Virol., 1976, *31*, 441.
6. Eklund, Hadlow, and Kennedy. Proc. Soc. Exp. Biol. and Med., 1963, *112*, 974.
7. Eklund, Kennedy, and Hadlow. Jour. Inf. Dis., 1967, *117*, 15.
8. Gajdusek and Zagas. New Engl. Jour. Med., 1957, *257*, 974.
9. Gardash'ian. Biull. Eksp. Biol. Med., 1976, *81*, 199.
10. Gardiner. Res. Vet. Sci., 1966, *7*, 190.
11. Greig. Jour. Comp. Path. and Therap., 1950, *60*, 263.
12. Gustafson and Kanitz. Slow, latent, and temperate virus infections. NINDB Monograph 2, U.S. Pub. Health Service, Publ. 1378, 1965, p. 221.
13. Hanson, Eckroade, Marsh, Rhein, Kanitz, and Gustafson. Science, 1970, *172*, 859.
14. Lampert, Gajdusek, and Gibbs. Adv. Neurol., 1975, *12*, 465.
15. Malone, Marsh, Hanson, and Semancik. Jour. Virol. 1978, *25*, 933.
16. Marsh, and Kimberlin. Jour. Inf. Dis., 1975, *131*, 104.
17. Marsh, Sipe, Morse, and Hanson. Lab. Invest., 1976, *34*, 381.
18. Moulton and Palmer. Cornell Vet., 1959, *49*, 349.
19. News Item. Jour. Am. Vet. Med. Assoc., 1952, *121*, 263.
20. Nussbaum, Henderson, Pattison, Elcock, and Davies. Res. Vet. Sci., 1975, *18*, 49.
21. Palsson, Pattison, and Field. Slow, latent, and temperate virus infections. NINDB Monograph 2, U.S. Pub. Health Service, Publ. 1378, 1965, p. 49.
22. Palsson. Quoted by Abinanti in Ann. Rev. Microbiol., 1967, *121*, 467.
23. Pattison. Jour. Comp. Path., 1965, *75*, 159.
24. Pattison, Gordon, and Millson. Jour. Comp. Path. and Therap., 1959, *69*, 300.
25. Pattison and Millson. Jour. Comp. Path. and Therap., 1961, *70*, 182.
26. Pattison and Sansom. Res. Vet. Sci., 1964, *5*, 340.
27. Prusiner, Hadlow, Eklund, and Race. Proc. Natl. Acad. Sci. USA, 1977, *74*, 4656.
28. Rennie and Zlotnik. Vet. Rec., 1965, *77*, 984.
29. Stamp. Vet. Rec., 1958, *70*, 50.
30. Wagner, Goldstein, Doran, and Hay. Jour. Am. Vet. Med. Assoc., 1954, *124*, 136.
31. Wilson, Anderson, and Smith. Jour. Comp. Path. and Therap., 1950, *60*, 267.
32. Zlotnik and Rennie. Jour. Comp. Path. and Therap., 1958, *68*, 411.

Borna Disease

SYNONYMS: Enzootic encephalomyelitis, Near East equine encephalomyelitis

This disease is an encephalomyelitis of horses, and occasionally of sheep, which has occurred annually for a century or more in certain localities in Saxony.

Character of the Disease. The period of incubation of this disease is at least 4 weeks, in this respect differing from the other forms of virus encephalomyelitis in which it is very much shorter. The initial signs consist of a low fever, difficulty in swallowing, salivation, hyperesthesia, reflex irritability, spasms of the neck muscles, and other signs of cerebral irritation. These terminate in drowsiness and paralysis, either localized or general. The signs vary greatly. The course of the disease is also varied. Many cases die within 1 week after the appearance of the first signs; others may not die for 3 weeks. The mortality averages 90 percent.

There are no characteristic gross lesions, but microscopically the usual lesions virus encephalitis and myelitis are exhibited. These consist of perivascular infiltrations of lymphocytes (blood vessel "cuffing"), degeneration of ganglion cells, neuronophagia, and multiplication of neuroglia cells. The lesions are most marked in the brain stem. Lesions in the spinal cord are much less severe than those in the brain. A characteristic feature of Borna disease is the intranuclear bodies, commonly called *Joest bodies,* which were first described by Joest and Degen (1) in 1909. These inclusion bodies are seen in the ganglionic cells in the hippocampus and in the olfactory lobes, more rarely in other parts of the brain and cord. With the Giemsa stain they appear as reddish, round or oval bodies, varying in size, embedded in the nuclei, which are stained a light-blue color. Each of the bodies is surrounded by an unstained halo. They can be found in nearly all cases of Borna disease. In 1927 Zwick, Seifried, and Witte (3) isolated a virus from the brains of naturally infected horses and demonstrated its causal relationship to the disease.

Borna disease can be transmitted from horses to rabbits by intracerebral, intraocular, corneal, nasal, intravenous, intraperitoneal, or subcutaneous inoculation of brain material. Guinea pigs, rats, hens, and sheep can be infected by inoculation, but these species are not so susceptible as rabbits. The virus can be propagated indefinitely in rabbits by brain-to-brain inoculation. The incubation period in rabbits is 3 to 4 weeks, and the period of signs is 1 to 2 weeks. Death occurs in nearly all cases. A variety of nervous signs are exhibited by the animals, and general paralysis occurs before death ensues. Zwick and coworkers produced two cases of the disease in monkeys.

Properties of the Virus. Elford and Galloway estimate its size as between 85 and 125 nm. It is much more resistant than the other encephalitis viruses. In 50 percent glycerol, brain virus can be kept for at least 6 months. Zwick and Witte found that dried virus kept its virulence for more than 3 years. The brain of infected rabbits contains a complement-fixing antigen.

Cultivation. Successful propagation of the virus on the chorioallantoic membrane of the embryonated hen's egg maintained at 35 C is described. Ludwig and Thein (2) have developed persistently infected tissue cell cultures.

Immunity. Specific antibodies have been found in the central nervous system of horses infected with Borna disease virus (2). The antibodies are monospecific, recognizing identical antigens from infected brains of different animal species as well as from persistently infected tissue culture cells. Discrete immunoglobulin species (oligoclonal IgG) can be demonstrated in concentrated horse cerebrospinal fluid; the horses carry Borna virus antibody specificity. The higher antibody titers in the cerebrospinal fluid, compared with those in the serum, indicate that in these natural Borna virus infections local antibody production occurred in the central nervous system. Zwick, Seifried, and Witte (4) report the successful immunization of horses with lapinized virus. The method has been used successfully in the field.

Transmission. The mode of transmission of this disease is not known with certainty. Unlike the other forms of virus encephalitis of horses which occur almost

wholly during the warm periods of the year, Borna disease occurs throughout the year. Most of the cases are seen from February to July. About the time of year when the other forms of encephalitis appear, Borna disease cases become less frequent. The lack of seasonal occurrence suggests that insects play no part in its transmission. According to Joest and Degen, the virus is present in the salivary glands, in the saliva, and in the secretions of the nasopharynx. The fact that lesions may be demonstrated regularly in the olfactory tract is suggestive of an entry path by way of the nasopharynx. Successful feeding experiments have been reported; hence the digestive tract also may be a portal of entry.

The Disease in Man. It has not been reported in man.

REFERENCES

1. Joest and Degen. Zeitschr. f. Infektionskr. Haustiere, 1909, *6,* 348.
2. Ludwig and Thein. Med. Microbiol. Immunol. (Berlin), 1977, *163,* 215.
3. Zwick, Seifried, and Witte. Zeitschr. f. Infektionskr. Haustiere, 1927, *30,* 42.
4. Zwick, Seifried, and Witte. Arch. f. Tierheilk, 1929, *59,* 511.

Ulcerative Stomatitis

In 1947 Gibbons *et al.* (3) described an ulcerative stomatitis in calves. This could be reproduced in normal calves by blood transfer or scarification in some instances (1). The experimental animals showed a temperature, leukopenia, and diarrhea. Diarrhea was not a common sign in natural outbreaks, however. The investigators indicated that the disease was not like virus diarrhea-mucosal disease, but cross-immunity tests were not done.

In natural cases ulcerative stomatitis in calves is usually mild, but calves that are debilitated by parasitism, malnutrition, or hyperkeratosis may be severely affected with death ensuing. Ulceration and redness of the oral cavity characterize the disease.

In 1958 Pritchard *et al.* (8) reported on an infectious ulcerative stomatitis of cattle which they called *bovine infectious ulcerative stomatitis.* The disease does not cause mortality, but the morbidity may be 100 percent in some herds. It is characterized by erosions and ulcerations of the oral mucosa. The lesions are quite similar to those observed in ulcerative stomatitis of calves. The virus particle is spherical with a diameter between 125 and 150 nm. This agent has not been compared in cross-immunity tests with bovine virus diarrhea-mucosal disease virus or Gibbons's ulcerative stomatitis virus of calves, so its immunological relationship to these diseases is unknown.

Bovine Papular Stomatitis

Bovine papular stomatitis was first described in the United States by Griesemer and Cole in 1960 (4). It had been described earlier in various countries in Europe and also in eastern Africa and Australia, which suggests that it is worldwide in distribution. The disease is caused by a virus that usually produces a mild infection in calves characterized by proliferative papular lesions in and around the mouth. The course is prolonged but afebrile, and recovery ensues without treatment. In experimental calves the lesions persisted as long as 98 days.

Virus grows in bovine kidney cells without the production of a cytopathic effect (5).

In natural and experimental cases lesions were limited to the oral cavity, esophagus, and the forestomachs. The principal microscopic changes were focal hydropic degeneration, hyperplasia of the mucosa or epidermis, and the formation of intracytoplasmic inclusion bodies (6).

The gross lesions may be confused with the early changes of foot-and-mouth disease, vesicular stomatitis, bovine virus diarrhea-mucosal disease, the oral form of infectious bovine rhinotracheitis in young calves, and other types of stomatitis occurring in cattle.

Proliferative Stomatitis

According to Olson and Palionis (7) this condition is caused by a filterable agent. It is rarely seen as a primary disease, but usually accompanies conditions such as hyperkeratosis (chlorinated naphthalene poisoning) and avitaminosis A. It has been named as a primary condition in one large herd of Hereford calves that had a severe ulcerative and proliferative stomatitis. A few of the cows had proliferative lesions on the tests (2). Very young calves that are healthy are susceptible to injection with infective material. Immunity follows an active infection. The virus appears to be different from that of vesicular stomatitis, cutaneous papilloma of cattle, and oral papilloma of the dog.

The virus produced localized papular lesions on the hands of two attendants who were working with the experimental calves (7).

REFERENCES

1. Gibbons. *In* Diseases of cattle, 2nd ed., ed. Walter J. Gibbons. Am. Vet. Publications, Inc., Santa Barbara, Calif., 1963.
2. Gibbons. *In* Diseases of cattle, 2nd ed., ed. Walter J. Gibbons, Am. Vet. Publications, Inc. Santa Barbara, Calif., 1963.
3. Gibbons, Lee, Johnson, and Robinson. Quoted by Gibbons *in* Diseases of cattle, 2nd ed., ed. Walter J. Gibbons, Am. Vet. Publications, Inc., Santa Barbara, Calif., 1963.
4. Griesemer and Cole. Jour. Am. Vet. Med. Assoc., 1960, *137*, 404.
5. Griesemer and Cole. Am. Jour. Vet. Res., 1961, *22*, 473.
6. Griesemer and Cole. Am. Jour. Vet. Res., 1961, *22*, 482.
7. Olson and Palionis. Jour. Am. Vet. Med. Assoc., 1953, *123*, 419.
8. Pritchard, Claflin, Gustafson, and Ristic. Jour. Am. Vet. Med. Assoc., 1958, *132*, 273.

Contagious Pneumonia of Young Calves

SYNONYM: Calf pneumonia

Calf pneumonia in many large breeding herds is one of the most serious of the disease problems. The disease occurs in animals as old as 6 months and perhaps even older, but generally is seen in calves from 10 days to 4 months old. It is not usually a serious problem in small herds where the annual calf crop is small and where many young calves are not kept in close association. Larger establishments frequently maintain special calf barns, or nursery units, where the young calves are kept together for the first several months of their lives. Often these are models of construction, but it is in such units that the infection usually takes its greatest toll. The disease is highly contagious, and the fresh calves that are brought in from time to time serve as the means for continuing the disease in the herd.

It is generally believed that there is a direct connection between a common diarrheal disease of young calves, known as *white scours* or *calf scours*, and this highly contagious pneumonia. The diarrheal disease usually precedes the pneumonia, since it ordinarily occurs when the calf is from 1 day to perhaps 10 days old. Scours, however, occurs in calves that do not later have pneumonia, and pneumonia occurs in animals that have not previously scoured.

An etiological connection between scours and pneumonia has not been certainly established. For many years strains of *Escherichia coli* have been isolated from the intestinal discharges and tissues of calves dying of scours, and this organism was regarded as the causative agent by the earlier workers even though it was not usually possible to reproduce the disease by feeding large quantities of such cultures. From the lungs of calves dying from pneumonia a miscellaneous collection of bacteria have been isolated; streptococci, *Corynebacterium pyogenes,* and *Pasteurella multocida* and *hemolyticum* are the most frequent. Since it has never been possible to reproduce the characteristic pneumonia in calves with such cultures, it has been assumed that they were secondary invaders. The fact that the pneumonia spread so readily among groups of animals has suggested to many that a viral agent might be the initial pathogen which paved the way for the bacteria which are so prominent in the lesions. In 1942 Baker (1, 2) described a virus that he regarded as the primary agent in this disease. Moll (3) in 1952 was able to reproduce and extend Baker's work. It is presumed that the virus with which he worked was the same as the one which Baker described, although no comparisons of them were made. In all likelihood other bovine viruses that cause diarrhea and/or pneumonia are involved in the syndrome characterized as contagious pneumonia of calves.

Character of the Disease. The disease is seen at all times of the year, but is most prevalent during the winter months when animals are kept closely crowded in weatherproof buildings in which the ventilation often is very faulty. The disease is manifested by loss of appetite, high fever, unthriftiness, prostration, a scanty nasal discharge, and rapid breathing. The older and stronger the animal is originally, the better it will withstand the disease, and the more likely it is to recover. The younger, weaker calves may die after a course of only a few days; the larger, stronger animals may run a course of several weeks. If recovery from the acute phase of the disease occurs, permanent unthriftiness often remains because of the damage to the lung tissue from the bacterial agents that invariably accompany the virus.

The lesions are found most commonly in the anterior and ventral lobes. Usually the lesions occur bilaterally. The pneumonia tissue is dark red, or dark red mottled with gray. The affected tissue is firmer than normal and is not dry like hepatized tissue but is rather moist. Fibrinous exudate is sometimes found on the pleura, but this is exceptional. Usually the pleura over the pneumonic areas is smooth, moist, and glistening. The nonpneumonic areas frequently show emphysema. If the disease has been protracted, small abscesses commonly are found in the pneumonic areas, and the bronchi are filled with thick mucopurulent exudate. The pneumonic tissue in these cases is practically always mottled with grayish areas made up of large collections of neutrophilic leukocytes. When diarrhea accompanies the disease, the small intestine, especially the mucosa of the ileum, is covered with a sticky mucus.

The Disease in Experimental Animals. Baker found that a transmissible pneumonia of white mice could be produced by introducing calf lung filtrates into their air passages. Filtrates of mouse lung virus readily produced disease in calves when it was introduced into their air passages, and the disease was transmitted by pen contact from artificially inoculated calves to normal ones.

The disease was typical in every way of natural infection. Artificially inoculated calves developed fever in 2 to 4 days, and this lasted for 3 to 5 days, the peak usually being from 104 to 106 F. Diarrhea usually appeared the day after fever began and signs of pneumonia about the 5th day after inoculation. The pneumonic signs usually were mild, and the calves ordinarily recovered. Destroyed animals exhibited evidence of catarrhal enteritis, and pneumonic foci occurred in the ventral lobes of the lung. Calves that recovered from the disease were resistant to reinfection, and their serum contained neutralizing antibodies. Neutralizing antibodies for the mouse virus also developed in calves that suffered from the naturally occurring disease.

Properties of the Virus. Early in the course of the disease the virus is found only in the lungs and intestines, but 3 to 4 days from the onset of fever the virus is generally distributed throughout the body. It readily passes a Berkefeld N filter and can be recovered from infected tissues by introducing filtrates into the air passages of etherized white mice in the manner used to recover influenza viruses of man and swine.

Frozen and dried virus specimens were active after storage for 4 months. Specimens frozen at −4 C remained active for longer than 1, but less than 4 weeks, and storage in 50 percent glycerol for a week resulted in complete loss of virulence (2).

Cultivation. No attempts to cultivate this virus on artificial media have been reported.

Immunity. Clinical experience and Baker's work indicate that one attack of this disease confers immunity to reinfection.

Transmission. It is quite clear that natural transmission of this disease commonly occurs through inhalation of infective droplets projected into the air of the calf quarters through the coughing of affected animals.

REFERENCES

1. Baker. Cornell Vet., 1942, *32,* 202.
2. Baker. Jour. Exp. Med., 1943, *78,* 435.
3. Moll. Univ. of Wis. thesis, 1952.

Transmissible Canine Mastocytoma

In 1959 and 1963 Lombard *et al.* (2, 3) reported the transmission of a canine mastocytoma with either cellular or cell-free inocula of tumor material in puppies from 1 to 30 days of age. The donor, an 11-year-old female Doberman pinscher, had a mast-cell leukemia and also neoplastic mast-cell infiltrations of spleen, liver, lymph nodes, kidney, and skin. Rickard and Post (4) also transmitted the disease with cellular and cell-free inocula from a spontaneous case in a 9-year-old beagle that had leukemia and visceral mast-cell neoplasms but was conspicuously lacking in skin tumors. Both groups were able to maintain the infectious agent by serial passage in infant puppies, but not all experimental puppies developed the neoplastic growths.

As a rule, newborn puppies were injected either by the intravenous or intraperitoneal routes (2, 4). Mast-cell tumors developed at the subcutaneous inoculation sites and in the omentum following intraperitoneal injections. Marked mast-cell infiltrations occurred in most visceral organs and resulted in death. Practically all diseased puppies developed a mast-cell leukemia unless they died or were killed early in the course of the disease. Some developed gastric or duodenal ulcers, presumably from the pharmacological action of the histamine or serotonin in the mast-cell granules (4). The experimental dogs of Lombard *et al.* had dermal nodules like the dog from which the original material was derived. In contrast the isolate of Rickard and Post failed to produce dermal lesions except at inoculation site, but then the spontaneous case from which the isolate was derived also was lacking in skin tumors. Both groups prepared their cell-free inocula by ultracentrifugation. In addition, Lombard and Maloney (2) filtered some material through a Millipore HA or no. 12 Mandler filter. These treatments strongly support the idea that the infectious agent is a virus.

Mast cells obtained from a canine mastocytoma were maintained in cell culture for 11 weeks. Some cultures were examined after 9 weeks (1). Although the overall morphologic appearance was sufficient to allow their identification as mast cells, the tumor cells differed in several respects from descriptions of normal tissue mast cells. In contrast to normal tissue mast cells, the tumor cells exhibited peripheral accumulations of microfilaments, randomly dispersed microtubules, and small clusters of smooth endoplasmic reticulum. The tumor mast cells also presented three granule types: (*a*) spherical granules with an amorphous and electron dense matrix; (*b*) irregularly shaped granules possessing a limiting external membrane and an internal matrix containing laminated and/or coiled structures; and (*c*) granules containing loosely coiled, unorganized membrane structures similar in appearance to myelin whorls. The canine mastocytoma is an excellent source of mast cells as they can be obtained in large numbers without contamination by extraneous cell types. The cells can be maintained *in vitro* for extended periods of time.

REFERENCES

1. Cobb, Birkedal-Hanson, and Denys. Jour. Oral Pathol., 1975, *4,* 244.
2. Lombard and Maloney. Fed. Proc., 1959, *18,* 490.
3. Lombard, Maloney, and Rickard. Ann. N.Y. Acad. Sci., 1963, *108,* 1086.
4. Rickard and Post. Third Internatl. Sympos. Comp. Leukemia Res., Paris. S. Karger, Basel, 1967.

Canine Venereal Tumor

The canine venereal tumor was the first tumor transmitted by tissue transplantation (6).

Character of the Disease. The tumor affects both sexes and it has a worldwide distribution, occurring as an endemic disease in some parts of the world.

In female dogs the tumor usually is found beneath the mucosa in any part of the vagina often extending to the adjoining vestibule and labia. In males, the tumors vary in appearance with small reddish nodules appearing on the affected part of the penis in the early stage of infection. They may become quite large with infiltration of tumor cells into the scrotum. The tumors usually persist for a long period of time, and dogs rarely die as a result of these localized tumors. Histologically it has been characterized as a round-cell sarcoma while a few pathologists have termed it an endothelioma, contagious granuloma, or lymphosarcoma (2). A large number of tumor cells are found together with leukocytes and erythrocytes in the serous fluid exuding from the tumor surface. Tumor cells undergoing mitotic division probably are spontaneously transferred into the mucosa of the external genitalia of another dog during copulation. Metastasis rarely occurs.

Chromosome studies are often used in tumor investigations. Makino (4) studied 17 spontaneous cases of canine venereal tumors that were obtained from geographically separate localities at different times. These tumors were uniformly characterized by tumor stem cells having a lower number of chromosomes (usually 59) than the normal dog tissue (78). In cells with well-delineated chromosomes there usually were 17 metacentric (J-shaped) chromosomes and 42 acrocentric (rod-shaped) chromosomes.

Cultivation. An *in vitro* method for growing colonies of canine transplantable venereal tumor cells in a semisolid agar media was described and used to monitor serological responses to this tumor (1). It also is possible to produce tumor cells in monolayer or tumor tissue fragments *in vitro* for about 56 days in medium-199 (5).

Immunity. Dogs that recover from the disease appear to be immune to some degree, so the tumors seldom reoccur. Passive and active immunity studies to canine transmissible venereal sarcoma were reported by Powers (7). Passive immunity was substantiated by treatment of dogs with tumors and also by the inhibition of tumors in dogs that were given immune dog serum and inoculum at the same time. Dogs that recovered from neoplasma withstood challenge with infectious material demonstrating an active immunity. Tumor-specific antibody was demonstrated by the passive cutaneous anaphylaxis technique in newborn littermate puppies. Tumor-blocking and inhibitory serum factors are present in the clinical course of canine venereal tumor as demonstrated by their *in vitro* method for growing tumor cells in semisolid agar (1).

Transmission. The disease has not been reproduced with cell-free extracts in the dog, but transplantation attempts have succeeded. Sticker (9) produced tumors in foxes by the subcutaneous or intraperitoneal inoculation of tumor material. Shirasu (8) transplanted the tumor in the cheek pouch of the hamster. Forty successive transfers in dogs have been reported by Karlson and Mann (3).

The Disease in Man. There is no evidence that the disease is transmissible to man.

REFERENCES

1. Bennett, Debelak-Fehir, and Epstein. Cancer Res., 1975, *35*, 2942.
2. Feldman. Neoplasms of domesticated animals. W. B. Saunders & Co., Philadelphia, 1932.
3. Karlson and Mann. Ann. N.Y. Acad. Sci., 1952, *54*, 1197.
4. Makino. Ann. N.Y. Acad. Sci., 1963, *108*, 1106.
5. Mohanty and Rajya. Vet. Pathol., 1977, *14*, 420.
6. Novinsky. Zentbl. f. die Med. Wiss., 1876, *14*, 790.
7. Powers. Am. Jour. Vet. Res., 1968, *29*, 1637.
8. Shirasu. Jap. Jour. Vet. Sci., 1958, *11*, 245.
9. Sticker. Ztschr. f. Krebsforsch., 1904, *1*, 413.

Ocular Squamous Carcinoma of Cattle

SYNONYM: Cancer eye of cattle

Squamous cell carcinomas involving the conjunctival mucous membranes and skin around the eyes of cattle are not uncommon, particularly in those breeds or individuals in which the skin around the eyes is unpigmented. They occur most frequently in the Hereford breed but are seen also in others. In two studies made on large numbers of cattle presented for slaughter in the midwestern part of the United States, about 0.5 percent in one case and 1.25 percent in the other were afflicted with this disease. In 40 percent of all these cases there were metastatic lesions in other organs. The disease seems to be most frequent in range cattle raised in hot, dry regions. The hot sun and the dust have long been suspected of being contributing causes. The tumor is seen in older animals, mostly in ones that are at least 4 years of age.

It has been suspected that an infectious agent may be involved in the causation of this tumor, but there is very little evidence to support such a hypothesis. Sykes, Dmochowski, and Russel (2) studied certain plaques occurring in the eyes of cattle which Russell, Wynne, and Loquavam (1) considered to be precursors of the malignant growths. Growing cells from these plaques in tissue cultures, they found inclusion bodies and other changes which they believe indicate the presence of a virus.

REFERENCES

1. Russell, Wynne, and Loquavam. Cancer, 1956, *9*, 1.
2. Sykes, Dmochowski, and Russell. Proc. Soc. Exp. Biol. and Med., 1959, *100*, 527.

57 Infectious Diseases of Domestic Animals of Uncertain Viral Etiology

Since Pasteur and Koch laid the groundwork for determining the causative agents of infectious diseases, research workers have identified these agents in most of our better-known diseases of man and animals. In the beginning workers generally tried to incriminate bacteria, but gradually it was learned that other kinds of agents were responsible for many diseases; hence we now recognize pathogenic protozoa, fungi, rickettsiae, mycoplasmas, and viruses. We also know that many clinical entities are caused by the action of two or more of these types operating in conjunction. The causative factor or factors of a few of the well-known infectious diseases still remain to be elucidated, and new entities appear from time to time, the causes of which are not always determined immediately. Thus we always have a certain number that cannot be accurately assigned to any etiological group. This chapter is devoted to brief descriptions of two important diseases of domestic animals that at present are in this category.

Infectious or Epizootic Infertility of Cattle

SYNONYMS: Epivaginitis (epivag), specific bovine venereal epididymitis and vaginitis, catarrhal vaginitis of cattle

Epivaginitis is a chronic disease of cattle transmitted by coitus. It occurs in east, south, and central Africa (1, 2, 3). A clinically similar disease has been described by Kendrick *et al.* (4) in California.

It is generally believed that epivaginitis is viral in etiology, although this has not been established. McIntosh *et al.* (5) have cultivated in mice and embryonated hens' eggs a virus associated with vaginitis of cattle. Cows and heifers infected with material from both the mouse- and egg-propagated lines of this strain showed definite, though mild, signs of vaginitis. Daubney *et al.* (2) have suggested that there may be two types of infectious vaginitis and that the virus of McIntosh *et al.* may be the cause of the milder form. The agent isolated by Kendrick and coworkers in California was more pathogenic for chick embryos than the McIntosh strain; it also differed from the latter in being more difficult to adapt to mice. Serum-neutralization tests were not done to establish the identity of the two agents.

The incubation period in cattle is about 2 to 8 days. The vagina is affected and there is a vaginal exudate. Examination reveals diffusely reddened areas in the anterior part of the vaginal mucosa and cervix but no ulcers, vesicles, or granular lesions. The acute infective stage may last for 2 weeks to 9 months. Most cows and heifers recover eventually, but 15 to 25 percent may become permanently sterile. In bulls the characteristic lesion is an enlargement and hardening of the epididymis. Occasionally an orchitis may develop and result in degeneration and atrophy of the testes.

Transmission is by coitus, and the disease can be controlled by artificial insemination.

REFERENCES

1. Anderson, Plowright, and Purchase. Jour. Comp. Path. and Therap., 1951, *61*, 219.

2. Daubney, Hudson, and Anderson. East African Agr. Jour., 1938, *4,* 31.
3. Henning. Animal diseases in South Africa, 2nd ed. Central News Agency, South Africa, 1949, p. 863.
4. Kendrick, McKercher, and Saito. Jour. Am. Vet. Med. Assoc., 1956, *128,* 357.
5. McIntosh. Onderstepoort Jour. Vet. Res., 1954, *26,* 479.

Sweating Sickness of Cattle

This is an acute disease of unknown etiology, possibly viral in origin, known to occur only in certain parts of the southern part of the continent of Africa. It is manifested by characteristic signs among which is a moist eczema that sometimes involves the entire body. The name *sweating sickness* is a misnomer; the victims do not sweat. The disease is tick-transmitted. A good general account of this disease may be found in Henning's textbook (2).

The disease is important only in cattle, particularly calves. It also occurs in sheep and swine. The disease is occasionally seen in older cattle, but most cases are in animals less than 1 year old, and the most severe cases are usually in young calves. Following an incubation period of 4 to 7 days, anorexia and fever suddenly appear. The temperature may reach 108 F, but later in the disease the fever disappears. The affected animal is depressed and listless. A moist eczema soon appears, sometimes in restricted areas but often involving the skin of the entire body. The skin feels cold and the hair becomes matted with the moist secretions. The hair in the eczematous areas may easily be pulled out leaving raw places, and often the victim loses a great deal of its hair. The skin is very sensitive to touch and to hot sunlight. The body develops an unpleasant sourish odor. The ear tips and the end of the tail may become necrotic and slough off. Screwworms often invade the exposed tissues and greatly complicate the condition. The mucous membranes of the mouth develop necrotic areas from which the epithelium easily peels off. The mouth becomes so sore that the animal may refuse to eat, and there may be a copious flow of saliva, which causes frothing of the mouth. There may be severe conjunctivitis and keratitis with the development of corneal opacities. The nasal and vaginal mucosae develop lesions like those of the mouth. Nervous signs sometimes are evident.

Sweating sickness generally leads to death in 2 to 4 days when the animal is severely affected. Less severe cases may recover after a course of 1 to 2 weeks.

The mortality varies greatly in different areas and in different age groups. It is greater in the younger victims. The mortality rate according to different observers varies from 10 to 50 percent and higher. The pathological changes are confined to the skin and mucous membranes, as already described.

The cause of this disease is unknown, but it may be caused by a virus. Some have doubted its infectiousness but most workers long ago agreed that its epizootiology strongly indicated an infectious disease (1). Inoculations of blood and tissues into experimental cattle have failed to produce the disease in the hands of all who have tried them. In 1954 Neitz (3) supplied evidence that the disease was transmissible and that at least one vector is the tick *Hyalomma transiens*. The disease agent apparently undergoes biological changes in this arthropod, and it is transmitted transovarially through at least five generations without loss of virulence for cattle.

No effective method of treating affected animals has been developed other than supportive measures and force-feeding of victims that will not eat voluntarily. Because the tick is the only known transmitter, preventive measures lie in eradicating the vector or adopting other measures of protecting cattle from its bites.

REFERENCES

1. Du Toit. 9th and 10th Rpt., Director Vet. Educ. and Res., Union of So. Africa, 1924, p. 233.
2. Henning. Animal diseases in South Africa, 3rd ed. Central News Agency, South Africa, 1956.
3. Neitz. Jour. So. African Vet. Med. Assoc., 1954, *25,* 1.

Index

HAGAN AND BRUNER'S INFECTIOUS DISEASES OF DOMESTIC ANIMALS

Designed by G. T. Whipple, Jr.
Composed by The Composing Room of Michigan, Inc.
in 10 point VIP Times Roman, 2 points leaded,
with display lines in Times Roman Bold.
Printed offset by the Murray Printing Company
on Allied Laural Text, 50 pound basis.
Bound by the Murray Printing Company
in Holliston book cloth
and stamped in All Purpose foil.

Library of Congress Cataloging in Publication Data

HAGAN, WILLIAM ARTHUR, 1893–1963.
Hagan and Bruner's Infectious diseases of domestic animals.

Includes index.
1. Communicable diseases in animals. I. Bruner, Dorsey William, 1906– joint author. II. Gillespie, James Howard. III. Timoney, John Francis. IV. Title. V. Title: Infectious diseases of domestic animals.
SF781.H3 1981 636.089'69 80-15937
ISBN 0-8014-1333-8

Library of Congress Cataloging in Publication Data

HAGAN, WILLIAM ARTHUR, 1893–1963.
Hagan and Bruner's Infectious diseases of domestic animals.

Includes index.
1. Communicable diseases in animals. I. Bruner, Dorsey William, 1906– joint author. II. Gillespie, James Howard. III. Timoney, John Francis. IV. Title. V. Title: Infectious diseases of domestic animals.
SF781.H3 1981 636.089′69 80-15937
ISBN 0-8014-1333-8

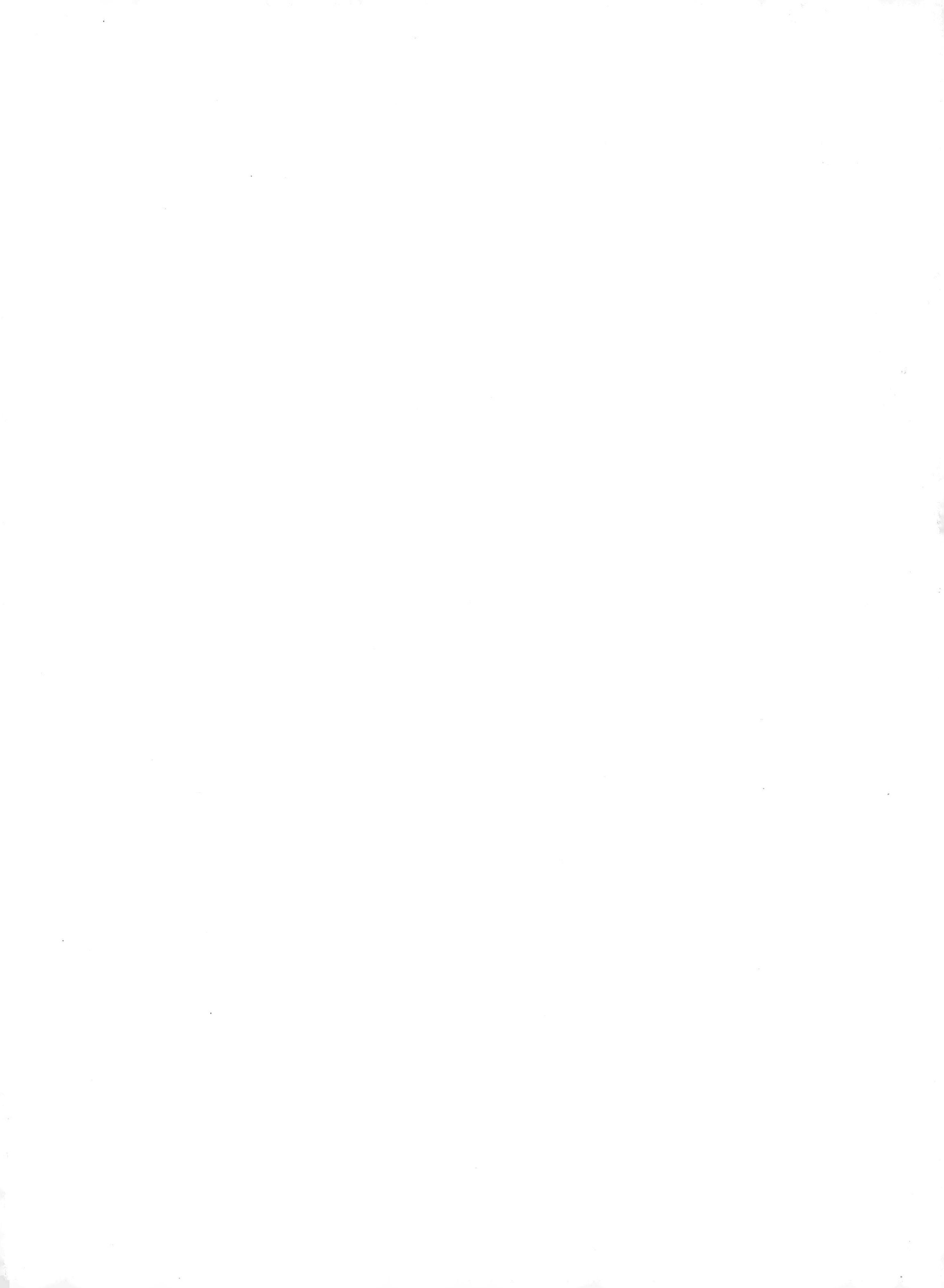